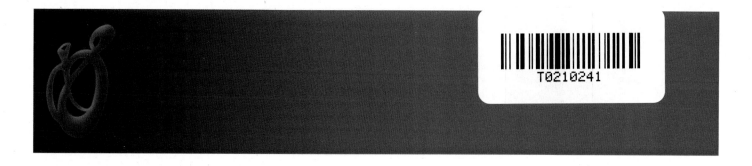

ESSENTIAL
ECHOCARDIOGRAPHY

A Companion to Braunwald's Heart Disease

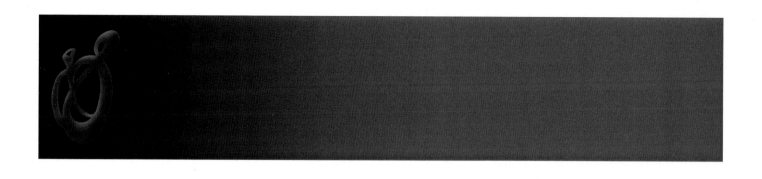

ESSENTIAL ECHOCARDIOGRAPHY
A Companion to Braunwald's Heart Disease

Scott D. Solomon, MD
The Edward D. Frohlich Distinguished Chair
Professor of Medicine, Harvard Medical School Director
Director, Noninvasive Cardiology
Brigham and Women's Hospital
Boston, Massachusetts

Justina C. Wu, MD, PhD
Assistant Professor of Medicine
Co-Director, Noninvasive Cardiology
Brigham and Women's Hospital
Boston, Massachusetts

Linda D. Gillam, MD, MPH, FACC, FASE, FESC
Dorothy and Lloyd Huck Chair
Department of Cardiovascular Medicine
Medical Director, Cardiovascular Service Line
Morristown Medical Center/Atlantic Health System
Morristown, New Jersey
Professor of Medicine
Sidney Kimmel Medical College
Thomas Jefferson University
Philadelphia, Pennsylvania

Illustration Editor

Bernard E. Bulwer, MD, FASE
Noninvasive Cardiovascular Research
Cardiovascular Division
Brigham and Women's Hospital
Boston, Massachusetts

ELSEVIER

ELSEVIER

1600 John F. Kennedy Blvd.
Ste 1800
Philadelphia, PA 19103-2899

Essential Echocardiography

ISBN: 978-0-323-39226-6

Notices

Knowledge and best practice in this field are constantly changing. As new research and experience broaden our understanding, changes in research methods, professional practices, or medical treatment may become necessary.

Practitioners and researchers must always rely on their own experience and knowledge in evaluating and using any information, methods, compounds, or experiments described herein. In using such information or methods they should be mindful of their own safety and the safety of others, including parties for whom they have a professional responsibility.

With respect to any drug or pharmaceutical products identified, readers are advised to check the most current information provided (i) on procedures featured or (ii) by the manufacturer of each product to be administered, to verify the recommended dose or formula, the method and duration of administration, and contraindications. It is the responsibility of practitioners, relying on their own experience and knowledge of their patients, to make diagnoses, to determine dosages and the best treatment for each individual patient, and to take all appropriate safety precautions.

To the fullest extent of the law, neither the Publisher nor the authors, contributors, or editors, assume any liability for any injury and/or damage to persons or property as a matter of products liability, negligence or otherwise, or from any use or operation of any methods, products, instructions, or ideas contained in the material herein.

Library of Congress Cataloging-in-Publication Data
Names: Solomon, Scott D., editor. | Wu, Justina C., editor. | Gillam, Linda
   D., editor.
Title: Essential echocardiography : a companion to Braunwald's Heart disease
   / [edited by] Scott D. Solomon, Justina C. Wu, Linda D. Gillam ;
   illustration editor, Bernard E. Bulwer.
Other titles: Essential echocardiography (2019) | Complemented by
   (expression): Braunwald's heart disease. 10th edition.
Description: Philadelphia, PA : Elsevier, [2019] | Complemented by:
   Braunwald's heart disease / edited by Douglas L. Mann, Douglas P. Zipes,
   Peter Libby, Robert O. Bonow, Eugene Braunwald. 10th edition. 2015. |
   Includes bibliographical references and index.
Identifiers: LCCN 2017045233 | ISBN 9780323392266 (pbk. : alk. paper)
Subjects: | MESH: Echocardiography
Classification: LCC RC683.5.E5 | NLM WG 141.5.E2 | DDC 616.1/207543--dc23 LC record
   available at https://lccn.loc.gov/2017045233

Executive Content Strategist: Dolores Meloni
Senior Content Development Specialist: Rae Robertson
Publishing Services Manager: Catherine Jackson
Project Manager: Tara Delaney
Design Direction: Renee Duenow

Printed in India

Last digit is the print number: 9 8 7 6 5 4 3 2

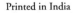

Contributors

Theodore Abraham, MD
Meyer Friedman Distinguished Professor of Medicine
Director, Echocardiography
University of California at San Francisco
San Francisco, California

Vikram Agarwal, MD, MPH
Noninvasive Cardiovascular Imaging Program
Department of Medicine (Cardiology) and Radiology
Brigham and Women's Hospital
Boston, Massachusetts

Lillian Aldaia, MD
Department of Cardiovascular Medicine
Morristown Medical Center, Gagnon
Cardiovascular Institute
Morristown, New Jersey

M. Elizabeth Brickner, MD
Professor
Department of Internal Medicine
Division of Cardiology
UT Southwestern Medical Center
Dallas, Texas

Bernard E. Bulwer, MD, FASE
Noninvasive Cardiovascular Research
Cardiovascular Division
Brigham and Women's Hospital
Boston, Massachusetts

Romain Capoulade, PhD
Echocardiography
Massachusetts General Hospital
Boston, Massachusetts

Maja Cikes, MD, PhD
Assistant Professor
Department for Cardiovascular Diseases
University of Zagreb School of Medicine
University Hospital Centre Zagreb
Zagreb, Croatia

Sarah Cuddy, MBBCh
Brigham and Women's Hospital Heart and
    Vascular Center
Boston, Massachusetts

Jan D'hooge, PhD
Professor
Department of Cardiovascular Sciences
University of Leuven
Leuven, Belgium

Rodney H. Falk, MD
Division of Cardiovascular Medicine
Brigham and Women's Hospital
Boston, Massachusetts

Patrycja Z. Galazka, MD
Division of Cardiovascular Medicine
Brigham and Women's Hospital
Boston, Massachusetts

Linda D. Gillam, MD, MPH, FACC, FASE, FESC
Dorothy and Lloyd Huck Chair
Department of Cardiovascular Medicine
Medical Director, Cardiovascular Service Line
Morristown Medical Center/Atlantic Health System
Morristown, New Jersey
Professor of Medicine
Sidney Kimmel Medical College
Thomas Jefferson University
Philadelphia, Pennsylvania

Alexandra Goncalves, MD, MMSc, PhD
Cardiovascular Division
Brigham and Women's Hospital
Boston, Massachusetts
Department of Physiology and Cardiothoracic Surgery
University of Porto Medical School
Porto, Portugal

John Gorcsan III, MD
Professor of Medicine
Director of Clinical Research
Washington University in St. Louis
St. Louis, Missouri

John D. Groarke, MBBCh, MSc, MPH
Brigham and Women's Hospital Heart and Vascular Center;
Cardio-Oncology Program
Dana-Farber Cancer Institute/Brigham and Women's Hospital
Boston, Massachusetts

Deepak K. Gupta, MD
Assistant Professor of Medicine
Division of Cardiovascular Medicine
Vanderbilt Translational and Clinical Cardiovascular Research Center
Vanderbilt University Medical Center
Nashville, Tennessee

Rebecca T. Hahn, MD, FACC, FASE
Director of Interventional Echocardiography
Center for Interventional and Vascular Therapy
Columbia University Medical Center
New York, New York

Sheila M. Hegde, MD
Cardiovascular Division
Brigham and Women's Hospital
Boston, Massachusetts

Carolyn Y. Ho, MD
Cardiovascular Division
Brigham and Women's Hospital
Boston, Massachusetts

CONTRIBUTORS

Stephen J. Horgan, MB, BCh, PhD
Cardiology Fellow
Morristown Medical Center
Morristown, New Jersey

Judy Hung, MD
Associate Director
Echocardiography
Division of Cardiology
Massachusetts General Hospital
Boston, Massachusetts

Eric M. Isselbacher, MD, MSc
Director, Healthcare Transformation Lab
Co-Director, Thoracic Aortic Center
Massachusetts General Hospital
Associate Professor of Medicine
Harvard Medical School
Boston, Massachusetts

Kurt Jacobsen, RDCS
Lead Sonographer
Echocardiography Lab
Brigham & Women's Hospital
Boston, Massachusetts

Konstantinos Koulogiannis, MD
Associate Director
Cardiovascular Core Lab
Department of Cardiovascular Medicine
Morristown Medical Center
Morristown, New Jersey

André La Gerche, MBBS, PhD
Laboratory Head
Department of Sports Cardiology
Baker Heart and Diabetes Institute
Cardiologist
St. Vincent's Hospital
Melbourne, Victoria, Australia
Visiting Professor
Department of Cardiovascular Medicine
KU Leuven
Leuven, Brabant, Belgium

Jonathan R. Lindner, MD
M. Lowell Edwards Professor of Cardiology
Knight Cardiovascular Institute and Oregon National
Prime Research Center
Oregon Health & Science University
Portland, Oregon

Dai-Yin Lu, MD
Instructor
National Yang-Ming University School of Medicine
Taipei, Taiwan
Visiting Scientist
Department of Cardiology
The Johns Hopkins University School of Medicine
Baltimore, Maryland

Judy R. Mangion, MD, FACC, FAHA, FASE
Associate Director of Echocardiography
Department of Cardiovascular Medicine
Brigham and Women's Hospital
Boston, Massachusetts

Warren J. Manning, MD
Section Chief, Non-invasive Cardiac Imaging & Testing
Cardiovascular Division
Beth Israel Deaconess Medical Center
Professor of Medicine and Radiology
Harvard Medical School
Boston, Massachusetts

Leo Marcoff, MD
Director of Interventional Echocardiography
Department of Cardiovascular Medicine
Morristown Medical Center
Morristown, New Jersey
Assistant Professor of Medicine
Sidney Kimmel Medical College
Thomas Jefferson University
Philadelphia, Pennsylvania

Thomas H. Marwick, MBBS, PhD, MPH
Director and Chief Executive, Professor
Baker Heart and Diabetes Institute
Melbourne, Victoria, Australia

Federico Moccetti, MD
Oregon Health & Science University
Portland, Oregon
Cardiovascular Division
University Hospital Basel
Basel, Switzerland

Monica Mukherjee, MD, MPH
Assistant Professor of Medicine
Department of Cardiology
Johns Hopkins University
Baltimore, Maryland

Denisa Muraru, MD, PhD
Department of Cardiac, Thoracic, and Vascular Sciences
University of Padua
Padua, Italy

Jagat Narula, MD, DM, PhD
Associate Dean for Global Affairs and Professor
Departments of Medicine and Cardiology
Icahn School of Medicine at Mount Sinai
New York, New York

Faraz Pathan, MBBS
Imaging Cardiovascular Fellow
Menzies Institute for Medical Research
Hobart, Tasmania, Australia

Elke Platz, MD, MS
Assistant Professor
Department of Emergency Medicine
Brigham and Women's Hospital
Harvard Medical School
Boston, Massachusetts

Jose Rivero, MD, RDCS
Cardiovascular Department
Brigham and Women's Hospital
Boston, Massachusetts

Mário Santos, MD, PhD
Faculty of Medicine
Department of Physiology and
Cardiothoracic Surgery
Cardiovascular R&D Unit
University of Porto
Department of Cardiology
Porto Hospital Center
Porto, Portugal

Sara B. Seidelmann, MD, PhD
Cardiovascular Division
Brigham and Women's Hospital
Boston, Massachusetts

Keri Shafer, MD
Adult Congenital Heart Disease Cardiologist
Brigham and Women's Hospital
Instructor
Boston Children's Hospital
Harvard Medical School
Boston, Massachusetts

Amil M. Shah, MD, MPH
Assistant Professor of Medicine
Harvard Medical School
Associate Physician
Division of Cardiovascular Medicine
Brigham and Women's Hospital
Boston, Massachusetts

Douglas C. Shook, MD, FASE
Chief, Division of Cardiac Anesthesia
Department of Anesthesiology, Perioperative and Pain Medicine
Brigham and Women's Hospital, Harvard Medical School
Boston, Massachusetts

Scott D. Solomon, MD
The Edward D. Frohlich Distinguished Chair
Professor of Medicine, Harvard Medical School
Director, Noninvasive Cardiology
Brigham and Women's Hospital
Boston, Massachusetts

Jordan B. Strom, MD
Division of Cardiovascular Disease
Beth Israel Deaconess Medical Center
Instructor in Medicine
Harvard Medical School
Boston, Massachusetts

Timothy C. Tan, MBBS, PhD
Clinical Associate Professor
Department of Cardiology
Westmead Hospital
University of Sydney
Westmead, Australia
Conjoint Associate Professor
Department of Cardiology
Blacktown Hospital, Western Sydney University
Blacktown, Australia

Eliza P. Teo, MBBS
The Department of Cardiology
Royal Melbourne Hospital
Melbourne, Australia

Seth Uretsky, MD, FACC
Medical Director of Cardiovascular Imaging
Department of Cardiovascular Medicine
Morristown Medical Center
Morristown, New Jersey
Professor of Medicine
Sidney Kimmel School of Medicine
Thomas Jefferson University
Philadelphia, Pennsylvania

Rory B. Weiner, MD
Inpatient Medical Doctor
Cardiology Division
Massachusetts General Hospital;
Assistant Professor of Medicine
Harvard Medical School
Boston, Massachusetts

Leah Wright, BAppSc
Baker Heart and Diabetes Institute
Melbourne, Victoria, Australia

Justina C. Wu, MD, PhD
Assistant Professor of Medicine
Co-Director, Noninvasive Cardiology
Brigham and Women's Hospital
Boston, Massachusetts

Preface

Echocardiography, or cardiac ultrasound, is the most commonly used imaging technique to visualize the heart and great vessels. It remains an essential tool for cardiovascular evaluation and management despite the emergence of other imaging techniques such as cardiac magnetic resonance, computed tomography, and nuclear imaging (SPECT and PET). Echocardiography has proven diagnostic and prognostic value in the vast majority of cardiovascular diseases. Compared to other techniques, it is relatively noninvasive, inexpensive, and has none of the harmful effects of ionizing radiation. Because it is increasingly portable and available in virtually any clinical setting, it may be used by a wide variety of practitioners, including cardiologists, intensivists, emergency physicians, anesthesiologists, and others.

The practice of echocardiography requires a strong knowledge of the physical principles underlying ultrasound, an understanding of cardiac anatomy and physiology, and an appreciation of the ultrasonic appearance of both normal variants and different cardiovascular diseases. Moreover, echocardiography, at its core, is a hands-on technique in which obtaining high-quality images is dependent on the skill and training of the operator.

Essential Echocardiography: A Companion to Braunwald's Heart Disease, is designed as a textbook in echocardiography for anyone interested in learning the technique, including practicing cardiologists, cardiology fellows, sonographers, anesthesiologists, critical care physicians, emergency physicians, radiologists, residents, and medical students. The text is designed to be simple enough to serve as an introduction to the field, yet comprehensive enough to serve as a reference for experienced practitioners. Written by expert echocardiographers and sonographers with an emphasis on the practical rather than the esoteric, the book focuses on the basic principles of anatomy, physiology, and the hands-on approaches necessary to acquire and interpret echocardiographic images with a rigorous focus on clinical care. The abundant illustrations, most of which are also available on Expert Consult, underscore the importance of visual learning in echocardiography. The images selected comprise an extensive collection of classic and clear examples, representing decades of experience over multiple institutions and also recent advances in the field.

Echocardiography remains a vital and evolving technology. As a part of the *Heart Disease* family, *Essential Echocardiography* will ensure that students and practitioners of cardiology will have the tools and skills necessary to apply ultrasonic imaging to the care of cardiac patients.

Scott D. Solomon, MD
Justina C. Wu, MD, PhD
Linda D. Gillam, MD, MPH, FACC, FASE, FESC
Eugene Braunwald, MD

Contents

CONTENTS

Video Contents ▶

Braunwald's Heart Disease
Family of Books

BRAUNWALD'S HEART DISEASE COMPANIONS

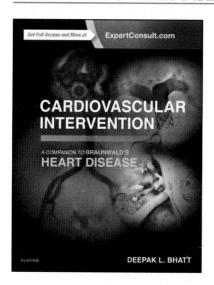

BHATT
*Cardiovascular
Intervention*

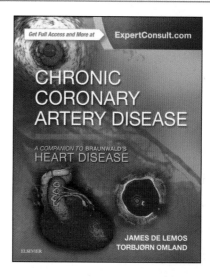

DE LEMOS AND
OMLAND
*Chronic Coronary
Artery Disease*

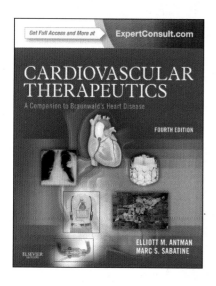

ANTMAN AND
SABATINE
*Cardiovascular
Therapeutics*

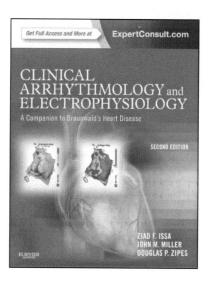

ISSA, MILLER,
AND ZIPES
*Clinical Arrhythmology
and Electrophysiology*

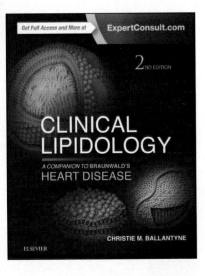

BALLANTYNE
Clinical Lipidology

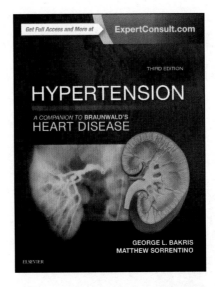

BAKRIS AND
SORRENTINO
Hypertension

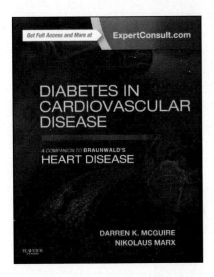

MCGUIRE AND
MARX
Diabetes in Cardiovascular Disease

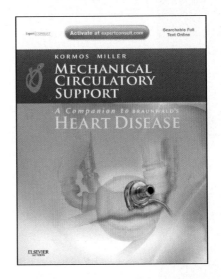

KORMOS AND
MILLER
Mechanical Circulatory Support

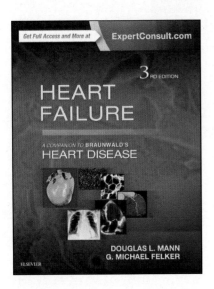

MANN AND
FELKER
Heart Failure

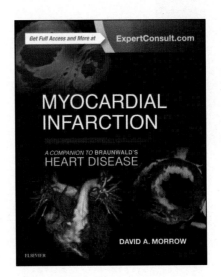

MORROW
Myocardial Infarction

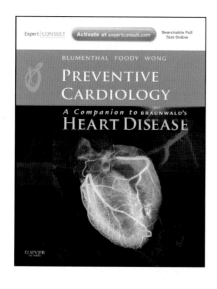

BLUMENTHAL, FOODY,
AND WONG
Preventative Cardiology

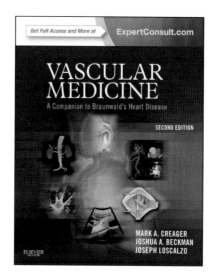

CREAGER, BECKMAN,
AND LOSCALZO
Vascular Medicine

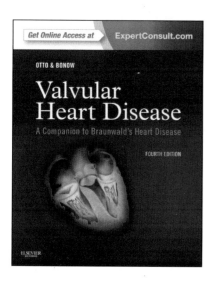

OTTO AND
BONOW
Valvular Heart Disease

BRAUNWALD'S HEART DISEASE REVIEW AND ASSESSMENT

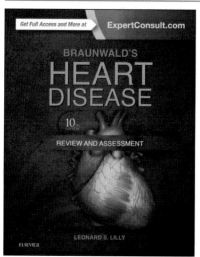

LILLY
Braunwald's Heart Disease

BRAUNWALD'S HEART DISEASE IMAGING COMPANIONS

BRAUNWALD'S HEART DISEASE FAMILY OF BOOKS

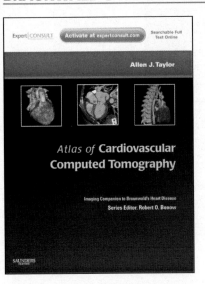

TAYLOR
Atlas of Cardiovascular Computer Tomography

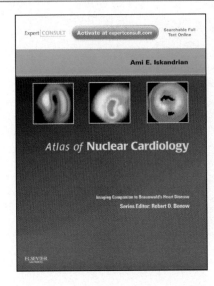

ISKANDRIAN AND GARCIA
Atlas of Nuclear Cardiology

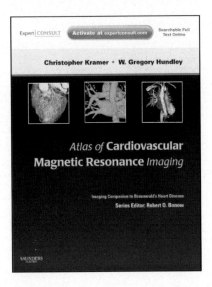

KRAMER AND HUNDLEY
Atlas of Cardiovascular Magnetic Resonance Imaging

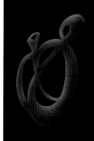

1

Physical Principles of Ultrasound and Generation of Images

Maja Cikes, Jan D'hooge, Scott D. Solomon

INTRODUCTION

Ultrasound imaging is ubiquitous in medical practice and is used to image all regions of the body, including soft tissues, blood vessels, and muscles. The machines used for ultrasound imaging range from small hand-held ultrasound devices no bigger than a smartphone to more elaborate and complex systems capable of advanced imaging techniques such as three-dimensional (3D) imaging. Although imaging of the heart and great vessels has traditionally been referred to as "echocardiography," the fundamental physical principles of image generation are common to all ultrasound devices. These principles should be familiar to the end-user because they are essential to understanding the utility and limitations of ultrasound and to the interpretation of ultrasound images and can help optimize the use of ultrasound systems to obtain the highest-quality images.

GENERATION OF IMAGES BY ULTRASOUND

The generation of images by ultrasound is based on the *pulse-echo principle*.[1-3] It is initiated by an electric pulse that leads to the deformation of a piezoelectric crystal housed in a transducer. This deformation results in a high-frequency (>1,000,000 Hz) sound wave (ultrasound), which can propagate through a tissue when the transducer is applied, resulting in an *acoustic compression wave* that will propagate away from the crystal through the soft tissue at a speed of approximately 1530 m/s. As with all sound waves, each compression is succeeded by decompression: the rate of these events defines the *frequency* of the wave. In diagnostic ultrasound imaging, this applied frequency is generally between 2.5 and 10 MHz, which is far beyond the level audible by humans, and is thus termed *ultrasound*.

The principal determinants of the ultrasound wave are: (1) *wavelength* (λ), which represents the spatial distance between two compressions (and is the primary determinant of axial resolution, as defined later), (2) *frequency* (f), which is inversely related to wavelength, and (3) *velocity of sound* (c), which is a constant for any given medium (Fig. 1.1A and B). These three wave characteristics have a set relationship as $c = \lambda f$. An increase in the frequency (i.e., shortening of the wavelength) implies less deep penetration due to greater viscous effects leading to more attenuation. As the acoustic wave travels through tissue, changes in tissue properties, such as tissue density, will induce disruption of the propagating wave, leading to partial reflection *(specular reflections)* and scatter *(backscatter)* of its energy (Fig. 1.2, Box 1.1).[4] Typically, specular reflections originate from interfaces of different types of tissue (such as blood pool and myocardium or myocardium and pericardium), whereas backscatter originates from within a tissue, such as myocardial walls. In both cases, reflections propagate backwards to a piezoelectric crystal, again leading to its deformation, which generates an electric signal. The amplitude of this signal (termed the *radiofrequency [RF] signal*) is proportional to the amount of deformation of the crystal (i.e., the amplitude of the reflected

wave). This signal is then amplified electronically, which can be modified by the "gain" settings of the system that will amplify both signal and noise. In addition to defining the amplitude of the returning signal, the depth of the reflecting structure can be defined according to the time interval from emitting to receiving a pulse, which equals the time required for the ultrasound to travel from the transducer to the tissue and back. The data on amplitude and depth of reflection are used to form *scan lines*, and the overall image construction is based on repetitive operations of the previously mentioned procedures of image (scan line) acquisition and (post-) processing. During image acquisition, transducers emit ultrasound waves in pulses of a certain duration *(pulse length)*, at a certain rate, termed the *pulse repetition frequency* (PRF), which is one of the determinants of the temporal resolution of an echo image (obviously limited by the duration of the pulse-echo measurement [i.e., its determinants]), as elucidated further (see Fig. 1.1C).

The data obtained from scan lines can be visually represented as A- or B-mode images (Fig. 1.3). The most fundamental modality of imaging RF signals is A-mode, where A = amplitude, in which such signals are imaged as amplitude spikes at a certain distance from the transducer; however, because visualization of the A-mode signals is relatively unattractive, A-mode is not used as an image display option; further processing is used to create a B-mode (B = brightness) image in which the amplitudes are displayed by a gray scale (see Fig. 1.3). To achieve such gray scale encoding, multiple points of the signal (i.e., pixels) are, based on the local amplitude of the signal, designated with a number that further represents a color on the gray scale. The B-mode dataset can then be displayed as an M-mode (M = motion) image, which displays the imaged structures in one dimension over time (distance of the imaged structures from the transducer is shown on the y-axis, and time is recorded on the x-axis; optimal for assessments requiring high temporal resolution and for linear measurements) or as a 2D image. By convention, strong, high-amplitude reflections are given a bright color and weak, low-amplitude reflections are dark (Box 1.2).

Another point in processing the RF signal overcomes a potential technical limitation of echocardiography; namely, reflections from tissues more distant from the transducer are inherently smaller in amplitude, due to attenuation (see Box 1.1). In practice, this implies that the segments of the ultrasound image depicting, for example, the atria in the apical views would be less bright than the myocardium. However, *attenuation correction* can compensate for this effect, automatically amplifying the signals from deeper segments, defined as *automatic time-gain compensation* (TGC) (Fig. 1.4). In addition to the automatic TGC, most systems are equipped with TGC sliders that enable modification of the automated TGC by the operator during image acquisition. Because the attenuation effect can be variable among patients, the acquisition of echocardiographic images should commence with a neutral setting of the sliders, which are then individually modified according to the patient and the current echocardiographic view. Of note, attenuation cannot be corrected for after

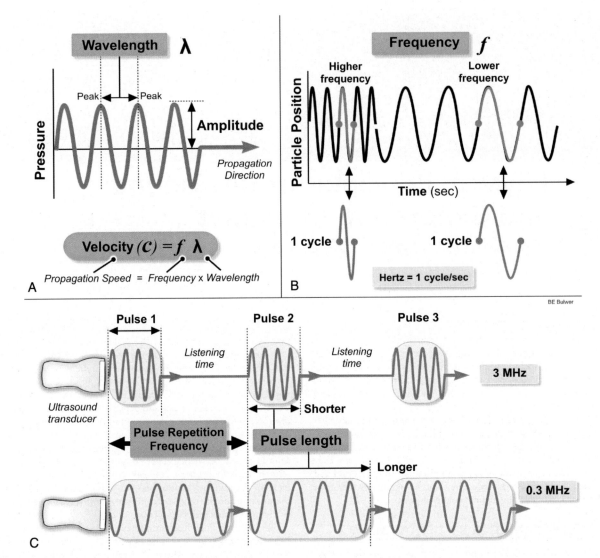

FIG. 1.1 (A and B) Depiction of an (ultra)sound wave as a sine wave. The wave propagates through tissue at a given wavelength that is determined by frequency (to which it is inversely related) and at a given amplitude that quantifies the amount of energy (i.e., the pressure change) transported by the wave. For sound waves, frequency is observed as pitch, whereas amplitude is observed as loudness of the tone. (C) Pulse length (duration) is primarily determined by the transducer frequency, to which it is inversely related (e.g., higher-frequency transducers can emit pulses of shorter pulse length). These pulses are emitted at a certain rate, termed the *pulse repetition frequency*. *(Courtesy of Bernard E. Bulwer, MD, FASE.)*

image acquisition. The final step in image optimization, which can be performed during post-processing, is *log-compression*—most often applied in diagnostic imaging as the "dynamic range." This method enables the increase of image contrast by modifying the number of gray values, thus leading to nearly black-and-white images (low dynamic range) or more gray images (high dynamic range).[2]

Typically, the duration of the pulse-echo event is approximately 200 μs, taking into consideration the usual wave propagation distance during a cardiac examination (~30-cm distance from the chest wall to the roofs of the atria and back) and the speed of ultrasound propagation through soft tissue. This implies that approximately 5000 pulse-echo measurements can be undertaken every second, while approximately 180 of these measurements are performed in the construction of a typical 2D image of the heart, by emitting pulses in 180 different directions within a 90-degree scanning plane, reconstructing one scan line for each transmitted pulse. In summary, a construction of one echocardiographic image requires approximately 36 ms (180 measurements × 200 μs), which translates to approximately 28 frames created per second. However, the number of frames (i.e., the *frame rate*) can be multiplied by various techniques, some of which are implemented in most current systems, such as the multiline acquisition that constructs two or four lines in parallel, leading to a fourfold increase in the 2D image frame rate.[2] For more information on high frame rate imaging, see Box 1.3.

Resolution of Echocardiographic Images

Resolution is defined as the shortest distance between two objects required to discern them as separate. However, resolution in echocardiography, being a dynamic technique, consists of two major components: spatial and temporal resolution. Furthermore, spatial resolution mainly comprises axial and lateral resolution, depending on the position of the objects relative to the image line, and various determinants will influence each component of image resolution (Figs. 1.5 to 1.7).[1–3,5,6] Temporal resolution (i.e., frame rate) represents the time between two subsequent measurements (i.e., the ability of the system to discern temporal events as separate).

Axial resolution refers to resolution along the image line (i.e., two objects located one behind another, relative to the image line) (see Fig. 1.6). Its principal determinant is pulse length (which is, similarly to wavelength, inversely related to frequency), such that a shorter ultrasound pulse will allow for better axial resolution (typically 1.5 to 2 times the wavelength).[2,6] Pulse length is predominantly defined by the characteristics of the transducer: a higher-frequency transducer provides shorter pulses, yielding better axial resolution. In practical terms, a typical scanning frequency of 2.5 MHz implies a wavelength of approximately 0.6 mm, at which an axial resolution of approximately 1 mm is obtained. However, higher frequencies have reduced penetration due to more attenuation by soft tissue, implying that a compromise between axial resolution and image depth needs to be

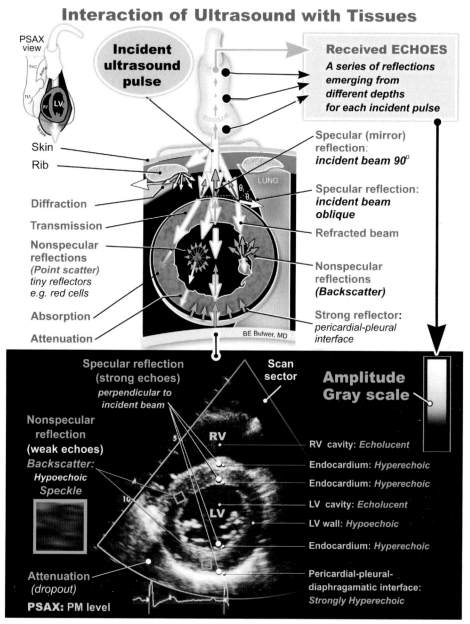

FIG. 1.2 **The interaction of the transmitted wave with an acoustic interface (i.e., cardiac structures).** A segment of the transmitted wave is reflected at the interface, while another part is transmitted through the tissue. Such a wave can be refracted, while the transmitted wave may also reflect and return to the transducer (thus carrying information on signal amplitudes) as a specular reflection (mainly occurring at the interfaces of different types of tissue, such as myocardium and pericardium), or as backscatter reflection (mainly originating from within the myocardial walls). *LV*, Left ventricle; *PM*, papillary muscle; *PSAX*, parasternal short-axis view; *RV*, right ventricle. *(Modified from Bulwer BE, Shernan SK, Thomas J. Physics of echocardiography. In: Savage RM, Aronson S, Shernan SK, eds.* Comprehensive textbook of perioperative transesophageal echocardiography. *Philadelphia: Lippincott, Williams & Wilkins; 2009:15.)*

made. Therefore high-resolution imaging is predominantly limited to pediatric echocardiography, where transducers up to 10 to 12 MHz can be used for infants, as opposed to 2.5- to 3-MHz transducers typically used in adult echocardiography.

Lateral resolution refers to the spatial resolution perpendicular to the beam (i.e., two objects located next to each other, relative to the image line) (see Fig. 1.7). It is predominantly determined by beam width, which depends on depth and the size of the transducer footprint (Box 1.4). Lateral resolution will thus be increased with a narrower beam (i.e., larger transducer footprint and/or shallower scanning depths).

Elevation resolution—resolution perpendicular to the image line—is somewhat similar to lateral resolution. In this case the determinant is the dimension of the beam in the elevation direction (i.e., orthogonal to the 2D scan plane). Elevation resolution is more similar to lateral in newer systems with 2D array transducer technology (compared with 1D transducers).

Temporal resolution, as mentioned previously, is predominantly determined by PRF, which is limited by the determinants of the duration of the pulse-echo event—the wave propagation distance (the distance from the chest wall to the end of the scanning plane) and the speed of ultrasound propagation through soft tissue (which is considered constant). Frame rate can be increased either by reducing the field of view (a smaller sector requires the formation of fewer image lines, allowing for a faster acquisition of a single frame) or by reducing the number of lines per frame (line density), controlled by a "frame rate" knob on the system. Reduced line density jeopardizes spatial resolution because it sets the image lines further apart. There is an intrinsic trade-off between the image field of view, spatial resolution, and temporal resolution and should be kept in mind as a potential shortcoming of the technique (Box 1.5). For advice on image optimization, see Box 1.6.

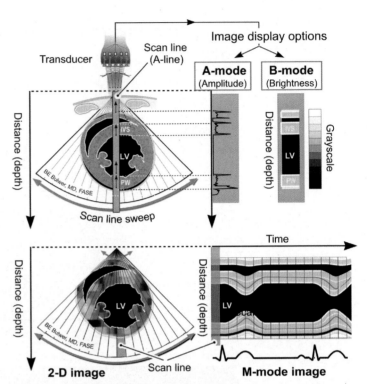

FIG. 1.3 Generation of images by ultrasound. After an ultrasound pulse is emitted by the piezoelectric crystals located in the transducer *(upper left)*, it travels through tissue, reflects from structures, and propagates backwards to the transducer. The received signals undergo processing and are displayed according to their amplitudes and depth of reflection *(upper right)*. The fundamental A-mode display images the signals as amplitude spikes *(upper right)*. On B-mode, these amplitude spikes are translated to a gray scale, such that the least reflective tissues (e.g., blood pool) are visualized as black *(upper right)*. B-mode images can further be displayed as a two-dimensional cross-sectional image *(bottom left)* or in M-mode, which visualizes the imaged structures in one dimension over time *(bottom right)*. Note that reflections with the highest amplitudes originate from tissue interfaces such as the myocardium and pericardium or blood pool and myocardium *(upper and lower panels)*. *IVS,* Interventricular septum; *LV,* left ventricle; *PW,* posterior wall. *(Courtesy of Bernard E. Bulwer, MD, FASE; Modified from Solomon SD, Wu J, Gillam L, Bulwer B. Echocardiography. In: Mann DL, Zipes DP, Libby P, Bonow RO, Braunwald E, eds.* Braunwald's heart disease: a textbook of cardiovascular medicine. *10th ed. Philadelphia: Elsevier; 2015:180.)*

Phased Array and Matrix Array Transducers

As opposed to mechanically rotating transducers used in earlier echocardiography systems, contemporary 2D imaging is based on electronic beam steering. This is achieved by an array of piezoelectric crystals (typically up to 128 elements), while the time delay between their excitation enables emission of the ultrasound wave in various directions across the scan plane and the generation of multiple scan lines (Fig. 1.8). The sum of signals received by individual elements translates to the RF signal for a certain transmission, a process referred to as *beam forming* (Box 1.7), which is crucial for acquiring high-quality images. Three-dimensional imaging relies on matrix array transducers, which are based on a 2D matrix of elements, thus enabling the steering of the ultrasound beam in three dimensions. This allows for both simultaneous multiplanar 2D imaging, as well as for volumetric 3D imaging.[2]

Second Harmonic Imaging

Current ultrasound systems are based on fundamental and harmonic imaging. In fundamental imaging the transducer listens for the ultrasound of equal frequency to the emitted wave. However, at higher amplitudes of the transmitted wave, wave distortion may occur during propagation, causing harmonic frequencies (multiples of the transmitted frequency), which can be received by the transducer when properly implemented (Fig. 1.9). Such second harmonic images have significantly improved signal-to-noise ratio and in particular improved endocardial border definition. However, this comes at the cost of poorer axial resolution (due to longer transmitted pulses), which may cause some structures, such as heart valves, to appear thicker on harmonic imaging. The transition between fundamental and harmonic imaging is achieved by the selection of transmit frequency: lower frequencies automatically enable

harmonic imaging, which is discernible by both the transmit and receive frequency displayed on the screen (e.g., 1.7/3.4 MHz), whereas a single displayed frequency implies fundamental imaging.[1,2,5]

PRINCIPLES OF DOPPLER IMAGING

Although imaging of the morphology of cardiac structures is increasingly complemented by other modalities such as magnetic resonance imaging (MRI) or computed tomography (CT) imaging, the diagnostic role of echocardiographic imaging in the evaluation of valvular function and noninvasive assessment of hemodynamics remains fairly unique. Such assessments are based on the *Doppler principle*, which allows for the

Time (Depth) Gain Compensation (TGC)

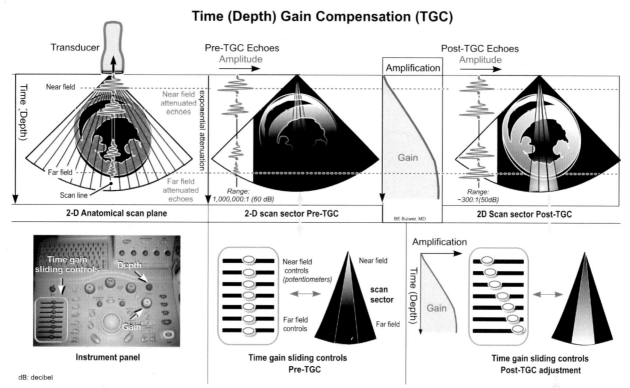

FIG. 1.4 Attenuation correction settings. Optimal settings of time-gain compensation (TGC) can provide a uniform display of signal intensity for echoes from similarly reflecting structures, across various depths of the scan sector. *(From Bulwer BE, Shernan SK. Optimizing two-dimensional echocardiographic imaging. In: Savage RM, Aronson S, Shernan SK, eds.* Comprehensive textbook of perioperative transesophageal echocardiography. *Philadelphia: Lippincott, Williams & Wilkins; 2009:59.)*

BOX 1.3 High Frame Rate Imaging

Multiple approaches have been proposed to increase frame rate (i.e., time resolution) of the echocardiographic recordings. Most high-end commercially available systems reconstruct 2 to 4 image lines from each transmitted pulse, but 3D imaging systems reconstructing up to 64 lines for each transmit are commercially available. Although this "parallel beam forming" results in better time resolution of the images, it typically comes at the cost of reduced spatial resolution and/or signal-to-noise ratio of the images. Finding the optimal compromise between these parameters is a major challenge for all vendors of ultrasound equipment. Alternative imaging techniques to speed up the acquisition process but with potentially less effects on spatial resolution and signal-to-noise ratio (e.g., multiline transmit and diverging wave imaging) are being developed. Two popular approaches that are currently being explored are "multiline transmit" imaging and "diverging wave" imaging. For the former a number of pulse-echo measurements are done in multiple directions in parallel, a challenge being to avoid crosstalk between the simultaneously transmitted pulses. In the latter technique the whole field of view (or a large part of it) is insonified by a very wide (i.e., defocused) ultrasound beam, allowing to reconstruct the whole image with a very small number of transmits (i.e., 1 to 5). In this way, frame rate is increased tremendously (up to 1 to 5 kHz), the challenge being to preserve spatial resolution and contrast of the images (i.e., image quality). Despite these remaining challenges, fast imaging approaches will undoubtedly enter clinical diagnostics in the years to come.

compared with it moving away. The Doppler effect can be applied to measuring blood (and tissue) velocities, by measuring the difference between the frequency of emitted and received ultrasound, which will be reflected off moving red blood cells. Should the blood cells be moving in the direction of the transducer, the reflected waves will be compressed and the frequency of the received ultrasound will be higher compared with the emitted ultrasound. Conversely, the frequency of the received ultrasound will be lower with blood cells moving away from the transducer. This difference between the emitted and received frequency is termed the *Doppler shift* or *Doppler frequency*, which is directly proportional to the velocity of the reflecting structures (red blood cells, i.e., blood flow):

$$f_d = 2f_t v \, (\cos \theta) \, / c$$

where f_d is the Doppler frequency, f_t is the original transmitted ultrasound frequency, v is the magnitude of the velocity of blood flow, θ stands for the angle between the ultrasound beam and the blood flow (i.e., the angle of incidence/the angle of insonation), and c is the velocity of ultrasound through soft tissue (1530 m/s). The main limitation of the Doppler equation is the angle of incidence, such that its increase decreases the calculated velocity: cos 0 degrees = 1, which implies that data acquisition with the ultrasound beam parallel to the direction of blood flow would be ideal; conversely, cos 90 degrees = 0, implying that motion orthogonal to the ultrasound beam cannot be detected regardless of the velocity magnitude. Practically, an angle lower than 20 degrees is considered adequate for acceptable measurements (of note, there is no possibility of velocity overestimation due to this phenomenon). To optimize alignment, Doppler imaging can be used in conjunction with 2D imaging, which allows for optimal placement of the Doppler cursor prior to Doppler data acquisition. Furthermore, should the angle of incidence be known, it can be corrected for in the Doppler equation of the velocity estimate by means of a feature available on many ultrasound systems, usually termed *angle correction*. However, this is acceptable for laminar flow conditions (typically in vascular ultrasound, in particular of nonstenosed vessels), whereas the exact direction of flow within the heart is, in fact, unknown. For this reason, it is not recommended to use angle correction in cardiac ultrasound (or if applied, use with caution and awareness of the issue).

calculations of blood velocities within the heart or in blood vessels.[1–3,5,6] The Doppler effect states that the frequencies of transmitted and received waves differ when the acoustic source moves towards or away from the observer (due to wave compression or expansion, depending on the direction of motion) (Fig. 1.10). For example, this is noticed as a higher-pitched sound of the siren as the ambulance approaches the observer,

Spatial Resolution Parameters

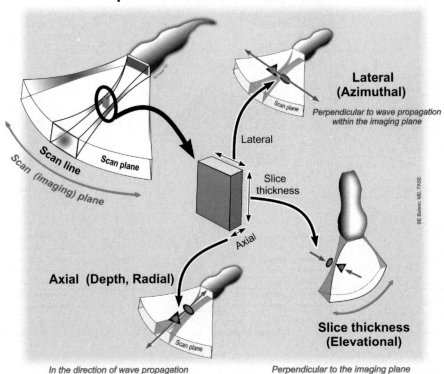

FIG. 1.5 Components of spatial resolution. Lateral resolution refers to the spatial resolution perpendicular to the beam, **axial resolution** refers to resolution along the image line, and **elevation resolution** is also perpendicular to the image line; however, its determinant is the dimension of the beam in the elevation direction. *(Modified from Bulwer BE, Shernan SK. Optimizing two-dimensional echocardiographic imaging. In: Savage RM, Aronson S, Shernan SK, eds.* Comprehensive textbook of perioperative transesophageal echocardiography. *Philadelphia: Lippincott, Williams & Wilkins; 2009:54.)*

Continuous Wave Doppler

The Doppler modalities used in echocardiography are pulsed wave (PW) and continuous wave (CW) Doppler (Fig. 1.11), as well as color flow mapping (color flow Doppler). In CW, separate piezoelectric crystals continuously emit and receive ultrasound waves, and the difference between the frequencies of these waves (the Doppler shift) is calculated continuously. In PW Doppler, ultrasound is emitted in pulses, as is the case with standard image acquisition. According to the Doppler equation, the Doppler shift is translated to velocity, which is then displayed over a certain time frame (determined by the *sweep speed* of the image), and is termed the *spectrogram*. As red blood cells travel at different velocities within the ultrasound beam, various receive frequencies will be detected, implying that a spectrum of Doppler shifts will be calculated and displayed on the spectrogram—thus termed *spectral Doppler* (Fig. 1.12). In CW the spectrum is rather broad due to the large sample volume, which accounts for a wide range of detected velocities, as opposed to PW. Although ultrasound is well beyond the limits of human hearing, the frequencies of the Doppler shift for typical blood velocities are actually within the audible range and can be heard during an examination: a higher-pitched sound corresponds to higher velocities (larger Doppler shift), whereas lower velocities generate a lower-pitched sound (smaller Doppler shift). Furthermore, because the ultrasound waves are emitted (and received) continuously in CW (i.e., the ultrasound system is not "waiting" for the reflection and return of the emitted pulse), the location of the reflected sound cannot be determined and therefore no spatial information is available by CW. However, all frequency shifts (i.e., velocities) along the beam are measured, which allows for high-velocity measurements by CW, typically used in the assessment of high velocities (turbulence) across the aortic valve in patients with aortic stenosis or in the approximation of pulmonary artery pressure from the velocity of the tricuspid regurgitation jet. As is the case in 2D imaging the attenuation effect also takes place in CW, as a consequence of which velocities from deeper tissue contribute less to the displayed signal (Fig. 1.13). For advice on CW Doppler optimization, see Box 1.8.

Pulsed Wave Doppler

As opposed to CW, in PW Doppler ultrasound is emitted and received in a similar manner to 2D imaging: individual pulses are emitted as brief, intermittent bursts. After emitting such a pulse, the transducer "listens" to returning signals only during a short, defined time interval following pulse emission. This time interval corresponds to the time required for the pulse to reach a certain depth and travel back to the transducer. The depth is defined by the *sample volume*—in practical terms, a cursor that the operator places at a certain depth along the transmitted beam, on the superimposed 2D image; technically, this implies adjusting the timing between signal emission and reception.[7] Furthermore, the previously mentioned pulse-echo measurement is repeated along a specific line, at a specific repetition rate, termed the *PRF* (i.e., the number of pulses transmitted from transducer per second). Such pulses require time to reflect and travel back to the transducer; thus the interval at which they are transmitted has to be long enough for the ultrasound system to be able to discern whether the reflected signal originates from the given pulse or a later one. Based on this concept the velocity of blood can be measured at a specific location in the heart by PW, thereby providing spatial information on flows. Therefore PRF represents the sampling rate of the ultrasound machine: higher blood velocities imply higher Doppler shift frequencies, requiring a higher sampling rate to detect the shift (Box 1.9). Notably, PRF should not be mistaken for the frequency of the ultrasound wave: in analogy to music, the PRF denotes the rate at which a certain note is repeated, whereas the ultrasound wave frequency corresponds to the pitch of a certain note.[5] The PRF is a principal determinant of the maximal Doppler shift (i.e., the maximal velocity within the sample volume that the ultrasound system can accurately quantify). This maximal velocity is also referred to as the *Nyquist frequency* (or the *Nyquist limit*) and is the maximal velocity that can be accurately interrogated within a certain sample volume. It is directly related to PRF, which is inversely related to the distance between the transducer and sample volume. The Nyquist limit equals one-half of the PRF. When imaging flows with velocities higher than double the PRF value, sampling of the waveform is inaccurate, disabling the accurate assessment of velocities, which can be detected by the appearance of *aliasing*

Transducer Frequency, Spatial Pulse Length, and Axial Resolution

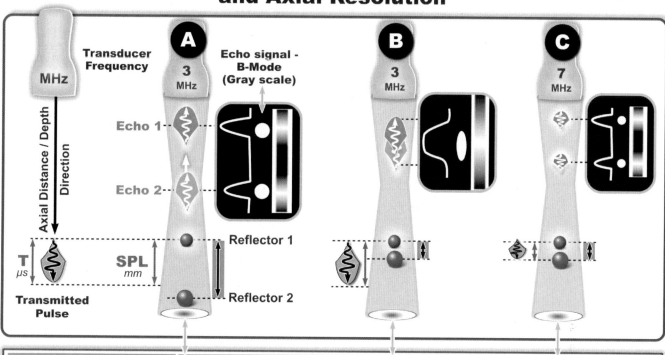

Transducer Frequency (f)	3 MHz As f↓, SPL↑, T↑	3 MHz As f↓, SPL↑, T↑	7 MHz As f↑, SPL↓, T↓
Echo Signal - B-Mode (gray scale)	**2 distinct signals**	**1 merged signal**	**2 distinct signals**
Axial Resolution (AR) (Image quality / detail)	Resolved (Good detail) ✓	Unresolved (Less detail) ✗	Resolved (Better detail) ✓✓
RATIO- Reflectors: ½ SPL	> ½ SPL	< ½ SPL	> ½ SPL

BE Bulwer, MD, FASE

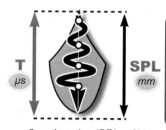

3 cycle pulse (SPL = 3λ)

The Longer the Pulse Duration (T)
or Spatial Pulse Length (SPL),
The Lower the Axial Resolution
↓Image detail - ↓Accuracy ✗
2 adjacent Reflectors appear as 1 Signal

The Shorter the pulse duration (T)
or Spatial pulse length (SPL),
The Better the Axial Resolution
↑Image detail - ↑Accuracy ✓
2 adjacent Reflectors appear as 2 Signals

Period = time or duration of 1 cycle, i.e., time for 1λ = 1/F

Pulse Duration (T) = no. of cycles (n) x Period

Spatial Pulse Length (SPL) = no. of cycles (n) x Wavelength

$$SPL = n\lambda = \frac{n\,c}{f}$$

Velocity $(C) = f\,\lambda$

Propagation Speed (m/s)   Frequency x Wavelength (m/s) (mm)

$$\lambda\,(mm) = \frac{C\,(mm/\mu s)}{f\,(MHz)}$$

$$\text{Axial Resolution (AR)} = \frac{SPL\,(mm)}{2}\,(mm)$$

Maximal AR = 0.5 SPL: The *smallest distance between 2 reflectors* (structures) that can be resolved as two distinct structures on the ultrasound image.
Transducer *f* and SPL are the major determinants of axial resolution (AR)

FIG. 1.6 Features of axial resolution are based on pulse duration (spatial pulse, length), which is predominantly defined by the characteristics of the transducer (i.e., its frequency). (A) The two reflectors (echo 1 and echo 2) are located apart enough to be resolved by the separately returning echo pulses. (B) The two reflectors (echo 1 and echo 2) are located too close, and the returning echo pulses will merge. (C) An increase in the transducer frequency from 3 to 7 MHz will shorten the spatial pulse length (and pulse duration), thus permitting the returning echoes from these reflectors to be resolved. *(Courtesy of Bernard E. Bulwer, MD, FASE.)*

Lateral Resolution (LR)

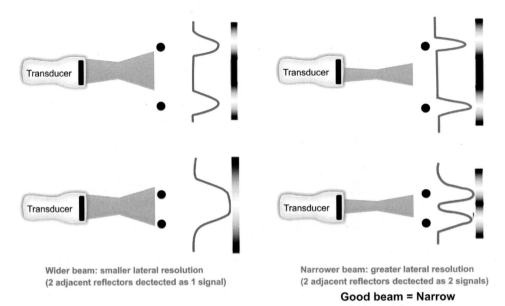

Wider beam: smaller lateral resolution
(2 adjacent reflectors detected as 1 signal)

Narrower beam: greater lateral resolution
(2 adjacent reflectors detected as 2 signals)

Good beam = Narrow

FIG. 1.7 Lateral resolution is predominantly determined by beam width, such that a narrower beam will allow for greater lateral resolution.

BOX 1.4 Beam Width

As a first approximation the beam width can be calculated as: 1.22.λ. d/D with "λ" the wavelength, "d" the focal depth, and "D" the dimension of the transducer footprint. The ratio of d/D is called the f-number of the transducer. From the previous equation, it is clear that transducer size directly impacts the spatial resolution for a given depth. Unfortunately, for cardiac applications, transducer footprint needs to remain limited (and hence the spatial resolution) due to the limited size of the acoustic window towards the heart (i.e., the intercostal space). Although, for example, fetal cardiac imaging is possible with a cardiac ultrasound probe, image resolution will intrinsically be much better when using a large, curved array as used in obstetrics.

BOX 1.5 The Trade-off Between Temporal and Spatial Resolution

The trade-off between spatial resolution, temporal resolution, signal-to-noise ratio and field of view of the echocardiographic data is intrinsic and application dependent. Indeed, when measuring, for example, the dimensions of a given cardiac structure, time resolution may be less critical and system settings could be adjusted to get the best possible spatial resolution and signal-to-noise ratio at the cost of time resolution. On the other hand, when making a functional analysis of the heart (e.g., when applying speckle tracking), improved time resolution may be important and justify reducing the overall image quality. It is thus important to realize that optimal acquisition settings are application dependent.

BOX 1.6 Image Optimization General Points

- For optimal spatial resolution, use highest possible transducer frequency
- For optimal temporal resolution, use narrowest possible sector and highest frame rate setting (i.e., lowest line density)
- Optimize depth and focus according to imaged structure; use minimal depth settings
- Optimize gain and dynamic range settings to obtain optimal image contrast: start with a black blood pool, increasing gain to a minimal amount that allows for definition of the heart structures
- Time gain compensation should be used to homogenize the image at various depths; start at a neutral position of the sliders

transducer and downwards in case of flow towards the transducer, allowing for higher velocities to be measured. Finally, a lower or higher PRF needs to be applied depending on the depth of the measured flow: to "reach" flows at greater depths (further from the transducer) and carry the information back to the receiver, a lower PRF needs to be used, compared with flows closer to the transducer. In practice, this is particularly obvious when measuring pulmonary vein flow in the apical views: a dedicated "low PRF" button on the ultrasound system can be helpful to obtain an instantaneous shift in PRF and improve signal quality. In analogy, higher velocities can be sampled without aliasing at sample volume positions closer to the transducer. For advice on PW Doppler optimization, see Box 1.10 and Fig. 1.15.

Color Flow Doppler

Color Doppler processing is based on PW Doppler imaging technology; however, in color flow Doppler the time shift between subsequent measurements is determined at multiple sample volumes along multiple scan lines. The calculated velocities are linked to a preset color scheme by means of a specific color map (displayed on the ultrasound image, Fig. 1.16), according to which the direction of flow and its velocity amplitudes can be determined. By convention, flow away from the transducer is colored in blue, whereas flow towards the transducer is coded in red. The color flow Doppler data are displayed superimposed on a 2D or M-mode image, allowing for visualization of flow patterns with

in the generated image. Aliasing occurs due to the inability of the system to accurately determine the velocity or direction of flow at velocities exceeding the Nyquist limit (Fig. 1.14). To avoid aliasing, a higher PRF should be used, although a lower PRF will enable a better estimation of the blood flow velocity—thus the lowest PRF possible without introducing aliasing should be used. Depending on the machine, the PRF adjustment is referred to as "scale," "velocity range," or "Nyquist velocity."[1–3,5,6] In addition, the baseline of the spectrogram should be shifted upwards in case of flow away from the

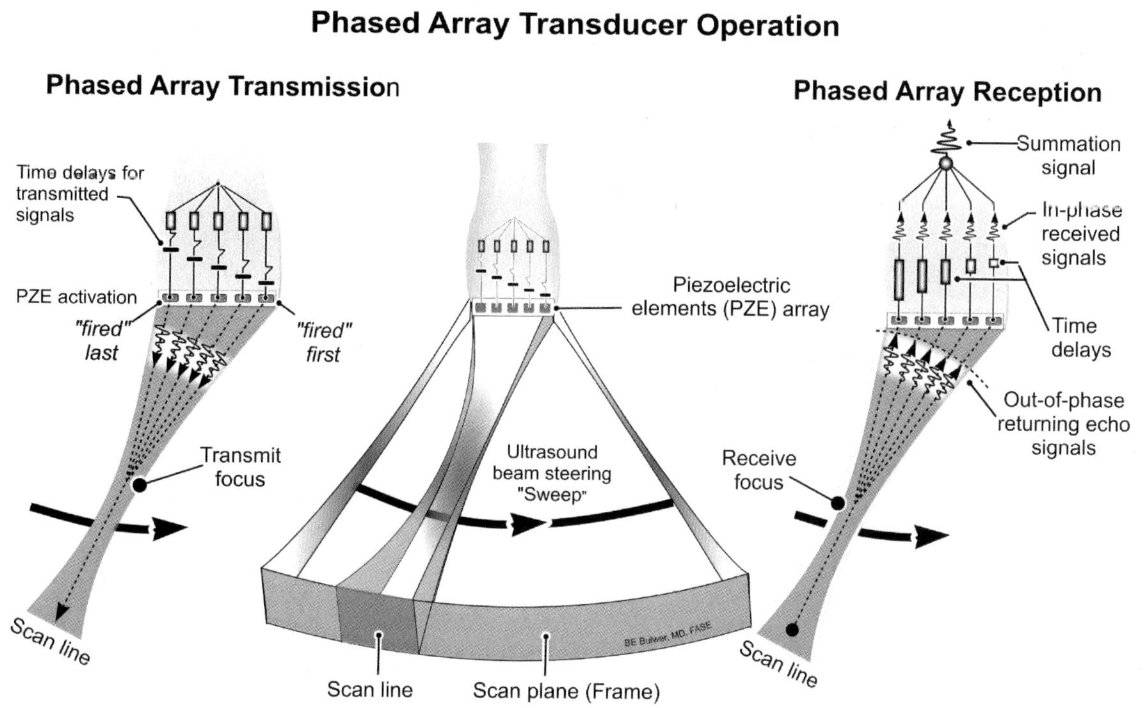

Phased Array Transducer Operation

Phased Array Transmission

Phased Array Reception

FIG. 1.8 **The phased array transducer technology.** Current echocardiography transducers steer the ultrasound beam (also termed *sweep*) across the scan plane, thus creating a fairly wide scan sector *(center)*. During ultrasound transmission the time delays in activating the piezoelectric crystals induce the sweep of the scan line over the scan plane *(left)*. During reception, the reflected echo signals are out of phase when received by each crystal and need to be shifted in time (i.e., phased) prior to summation and further processing *(right)*. *(Courtesy of Bernard E. Bulwer, MD, FASE; Modified from Solomon SD, Wu J, Gillam L, Bulwer B. Echocardiography. In: Mann DL, Zipes DP, Libby P, Bonow RO, Braunwald E, eds.* Braunwald's heart disease: a textbook of cardiovascular medicine. *10th ed. Philadelphia: Elsevier; 2015:180.)*

BOX 1.7 Beam Forming

Phased array transducers enable steering and focusing of the ultrasound beam simply by adjusting the electrical excitations of the individual transducer elements (see Fig. 1.7, *left panel*). Similarly, during reception, the received signals coming from individual transducer elements will be delayed in time to correct for the differing time of flight of a given echo to the individual transducer elements as a result of the differences in path length to each of these elements (see Fig. 1.7, *right panel*). The former is referred to as "transmit focusing," whereas the latter is "receive focusing." Interestingly, during receive focusing, one can dynamically adjust the focus point as one knows a priori from which depth echo signals are arriving at a given time point after transmission given the sound velocity is known. As such, the time delays applied to the signals coming from the different elements is adjusted dynamically in time to optimally focus the ultrasound beam at all depths. Similarly, given that focusing works better close the probe (see Box 1.4), some elements near the edge of the probe can be switched off when (receive) focusing close to the probe to reduce the effective transducer size, thereby making its ability to focus worse. The advantage of this approach is that the beam width becomes more uniform as a function of depth and thus so does the lateral image resolution. These beam-forming modalities are referred to as "dynamic receive focusing" and "dynamic apodization," respectively, and are implemented on all cardiac ultrasound systems.

---

additional information on the spatial location of the flow, nature of the flow (turbulence, direction of flow), geometry of potential connections between the heart chambers or great vessels, etc. Due to the same basic principles of PW Doppler, color flow Doppler is also subject to aliasing, whereas a high variance of velocity in a particular pixel is mostly displayed as shades of green, which is indicative of turbulent flow. Similar to PW Doppler, the appearance of aliasing can be reduced by increasing the PRF (however, PRF is coupled to velocity resolution) or by reducing the transmission frequency (rarely performed). The generation of a color

flow Doppler image requires more "computing" time, and, to retain an acceptable temporal resolution, it is suggested that the region of color flow imaging (i.e., the color box) is kept to the minimal size required.[1,2,5] For advice on color flow Doppler optimization, see Box 1.11.

Doppler Echocardiography in the Assessment of Hemodynamics

Doppler echocardiography is predominantly used for the assessment of velocities of blood flow within the heart and great vessels, which are determined by the driving pressure gradients between these structures (i.e., across heart valves). Analogously, the measured velocities of blood flow across a certain valve can be used in the assessment of pressure gradients between the relevant chambers: based on conservation of energy, the *Bernoulli equation* defines the relation between pressures and velocities for fluids in chambers separated by an orifice:

$$P_1 - P_2 = \frac{1}{2}\rho\left(V_2^2 - V_1^2\right) \quad + \quad \rho\int_1^2 \frac{dv}{dt} d\vec{s} \quad + \quad R(\vec{v})$$

Connective Acceleration   Flow Acceleration   Viscous Friction

where P_1 and P_2 represent the pressures, and V_1 and V_2 represent the velocities proximal and distal to the orifice.[1]

In daily practice a simplified form of the Bernoulli equation may be used, not taking into account flow acceleration and viscous friction:

$$P_1 - P_2 = 1/2\rho\left(V_2^2 - V_1^2\right)$$

Velocities proximal to the stenosis (i.e., orifice) are usually rather low (when comparing with those distal to the stenosis) and may thus generally be ignored, which further simplifies the equation:

$$P_1 - P_2 = 4V^2$$

Some of the most frequent applications of the Bernoulli equation in the assessment of hemodynamics include the evaluation of the peak systolic gradient across the aortic valve in aortic stenosis: Doppler echocardiography can assess the peak velocity of antegrade blood flow across the stenosed aortic valve, whereas applying the modified Bernoulli equation

PRINCIPLES OF ULTRASOUND AND INSTRUMENTATION

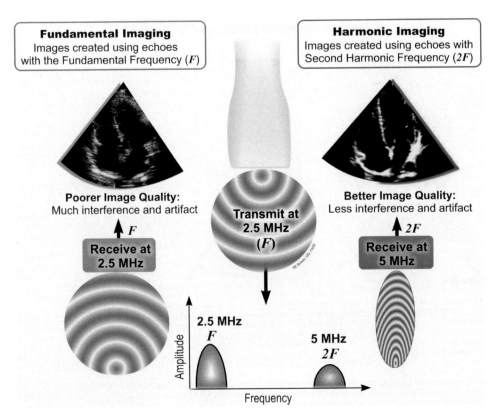

FIG. 1.9 Tissue harmonic imaging. Tissue harmonic imaging allows for improved image quality by using second-order harmonics in which specific frequencies of ultrasound induce tissue vibrations at twice the frequency. Listening for such higher frequencies of returning ultrasound allows for dramatic improvement of the signal-to-noise ratio. Second-harmonic imaging provides images with clearly ameliorated tissue definition and less affected by acoustic noise and artifacts *(right). (Courtesy of Bernard E. Bulwer, MD, FASE; From Solomon SD, Wu J, Gillam L, Bulwer B. Echocardiography. In: Mann DL, Zipes DP, Libby P, Bonow RO, Braunwald E, eds.* Braunwald's heart disease: a textbook of cardiovascular medicine. *10th ed. Philadelphia: Elsevier; 2015:181.)*

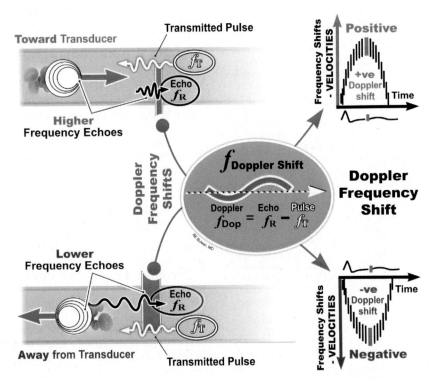

FIG. 1.10 The Doppler principle and Doppler frequency shift. Ultrasound emitted from the transducer reflects off moving red blood cells and returns to the transducer: if reflected from red blood cells moving in the direction of the transducer, the echo returns at a higher frequency (shorter wavelength) than the emitted ultrasound pulse *(upper left)*; conversely, if blood cells are moving away from the transducer, a lower-frequency echo will be reflected back to the transducer *(lower left)*. The difference between the transmitted and the returning frequency equals the Doppler shift, which is used by Doppler echocardiography systems to calculate velocities of blood flow. These velocities are graphically displayed by spectral Doppler as a time velocity spectrum (spectrogram), where a positive Doppler shift (implying flow toward the transducer) is depicted above the baseline, and a negative Doppler shift (flow away from the transducer) is drawn below the baseline *(right)*. In color flow Doppler the direction of flow can be detected according to the color-coded velocities. *(Courtesy of Bernard E. Bulwer, MD, FASE; Modified from Solomon SD, Wu J, Gillam L, Bulwer B: Echocardiography. In Mann DL, Zipes DP, Libby P, Bonow RO, Braunwald E, eds.* Braunwald's Heart Disease: A Textbook of Cardiovascular Medicine. *10th ed. Philadelphia: Elsevier; 2015:182.)*

Continuous-Wave Doppler (CW) Principle

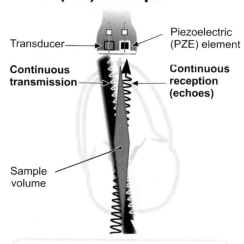

Transducer — Piezoelectric (PZE) element

Continuous transmission → ← **Continuous reception (echoes)**

Sample volume

1. Two PZE crystals:
   - *one transmitting (100%)*
   - *one receiving (100%)*
2. Continuous operation *(duty factor = 1)*
3. Large sample volume
4. No range/depth specificity: *cannot distinguish the exact anatomical location of the velocities measured*
5. Detects wider range of velocities
6. No aliasing at high velocities

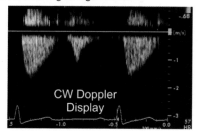

CW Doppler Display

Pulsed-Wave Doppler (PW) Principle

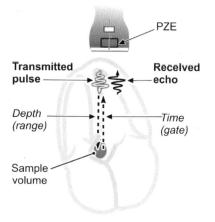

PZE

Transmitted pulse → ← Received echo

Depth (range) ← → *Time (gate)*

Sample volume

1. One PZE crystal:
   - *same crystal transmitting (~1%)*
   - *same crystal receiving (~99%)*
2. Pulse-Echo operation
3. Small sample volume
4. Range/depth specificity: *can distinguish the exact anatomical location of the velocities measured*
5. Detects narrower range of velocities
6. Aliasing at higher velocities

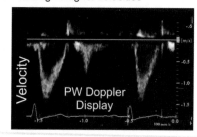

Velocity

PW Doppler Display

FIG. 1.11 **Comparison of continuous wave (CW) Doppler and pulsed wave (PW) Doppler.** *(Courtesy of Bernard E. Bulwer, MD, FASE; Modified from Solomon SD, Wu J, Gillam L, Bulwer B. Echocardiography. In: Mann DL, Zipes DP, Libby P, Bonow RO, Braunwald E, eds.* Braunwald's heart disease: a textbook of cardiovascular medicine. *10th ed. Philadelphia: Elsevier; 2015:182.)*

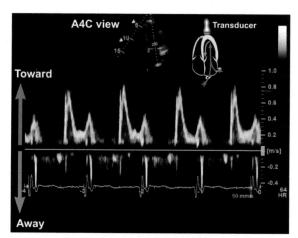

A4C view   Transducer

Toward

Away

FIG. 1.12 **The properties of spectral Doppler.** The velocity of blood flow is graphically displayed on the y-axis, and time is on the x-axis. Flow direction can also be determined, depending on the relation of the spectrogram to the baseline: flow toward the transducer is imaged above and flow away from the transducer is imaged below the baseline. The signal intensity reflects the quantity of red blood cells that are moving at a specific velocity range. In continuous wave the spectrum is rather broad due to the wide range of velocities detected by the beam, as opposed to pulsed wave (which is imaged here). *A4C,* Apical four-chamber.

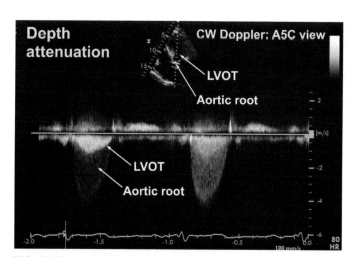

Depth attenuation   CW Doppler: A5C view

LVOT
Aortic root

LVOT
Aortic root

FIG. 1.13 **The depth attenuation effect seen on continuous wave (CW) Doppler in aortic stenosis.** With minimal gain settings, it can be appreciated that the velocities from deeper tissues contribute less to the spectrogram: the Doppler signal from the aortic root is attenuated and much weaker than that from the left ventricular outflow tract (LVOT). With higher Doppler gain (second heart cycle), the effect is less obvious. *A5C,* Apical five-chamber.

BOX 1.8 Continuous Wave Doppler Optimization Points

- Optimize beam alignment with the direction of measured velocity (direction of flow)
- Optimize gain to create a uniform Doppler profile free of "blooming": to prevent loss of data due to insufficient gain, start with an overemphasized image, decreasing the gain to a minimal required amount
- Optimize the "compress" control (assigns a certain shade of color to varying amplitudes): extreme values can affect the quality of the spectral analysis
- The "low velocities reject" button discards the signals of lower amplitude, providing a cleaner image and more precise measurements
- The "filter" reduces noise occurring from reflectors originating from the myocardium and other heart structures

BOX 1.9 High Pulse Repetition Frequency Pulsed Wave Doppler

High PRF PW Doppler is also optional on some systems and can be recognized by the occurrence of several sample volumes along the Doppler beam. The measurement concept is based on the fact that the PW Doppler system knows exactly when to sample the echo signal (i.e., at the sample volume). As such, a new pulse can already be transmitted (to a more proximal/distal sample volume) before the echoes of the original transmit have received without inducing artifacts. Thus the PRF (and Nyquist limit) can be increased by emitting one (or more) new pulses prior to receiving the signal of the first pulse from the expected depth. However, such construction of the spectrogram implies that the exact location of the origin of the signal along the Doppler beam cannot be known.

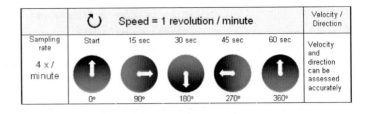

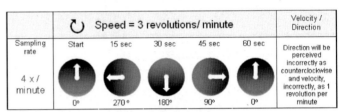

FIG. 1.14 The explanation of aliasing based the "wagon wheel" example, stemming from the wagon wheel illusion seen in old western motion pictures (an example from sampling theory): envision a rotating clock hand—in the *top panel*, it rotates at one revolution per minute. If one would "sample" the clock 4 times per minute (every 15 seconds) by shooting a picture, one could easily "capture" the motion of the clock, could comprehend that the direction of rotation is clockwise, and could perceive the rate of rotation. However, if the rotational speed were to be increased to two revolutions per minute, maintaining the sampling rate, one would "capture" only the hand at 12 o'clock and 6 o'clock, still being able to discern the rate of rotation, but not the direction *(middle panel)*. Ultimately, if the revolution velocity increased to three revolutions per minute (in the same direction), retaining the same sampling rate, the perceived rate of rotation would be one revolution per minute while the perceived direction would be counterclockwise *(bottom panel)*. In analogy to pulsed wave Doppler, at a certain sampling rate of the system, increasing velocities of blood flow cannot be assessed adequately, neither for their velocity, nor direction of blood flow. *(From Solomon SD. Echocardiographic instrumentation and principles of Doppler echocardiography. In: Solomon SD, ed. Essential echocardiography—a practical handbook with DVD. Totowa, NJ, Humana Press; 2007:12.)*

allows for the estimation of the peak instantaneous transvalvular gradient, relevant for the assessment of aortic stenosis severity. Another frequently used example refers to the assessment of peak systolic right ventricular and pulmonary artery pressure: it is derived by adding the peak velocity of the tricuspid regurgitation jet, which indicates the pressure gradient between the right ventricle and right atrium in systole, to the right atrial pressure estimate (which can also be determined by echocardiography, according to the diameter and respiratory collapse of the inferior vena cava). However, the Bernoulli equation can be used in all cases in which a velocity gradient is present: valvular stenosis or regurgitation, as well as abnormal connections (ventricular septal defect, etc.). Importantly, it should be kept in mind that Doppler echocardiography enables the measurement of velocity, from which pressures and flows are inferred—the absolute pressures in cardiac chambers can only be measured invasively.[1]

Another physical principle that is frequently used in the assessment of hemodynamics is the *continuity of flow equation*, which states that the same volume/flow passes through different cross sections of a tube (i.e., the heart), assuming no loss of fluid (i.e., no shunt). This equation is typically applied in the assessment of volumes/flows and valve areas: by multiplying the cross-sectional area (CSA) of the interrogated orifice by the time velocity integral (TVI, i.e., the integration of blood velocity across an orifice during one cardiac cycle) at the corresponding level, the magnitude of flow can be assessed (Fig. 1.17).

Furthermore, because a CSA of a diseased valve may be difficult to measure, valve area can be calculated by estimating the flow proximal to the valve and the TVI at the level of the valve. A frequently used example includes the assessment of aortic valve CSA in aortic stenosis: according to the continuity equation, the flow through the left ventricular outflow tract (LVOT) equals that through the aortic valve, that is:

$$TVI_{LVOT} \times Area_{LVOT} = TVI_{AV} \times Area_{AV} \rightarrow Area_{LVOT} = (TVI_{AV} \times Area_{AV}) / TVI_{LVOT}$$

BOX 1.10 Pulsed Wave Doppler Optimization Points

- Optimize beam alignment and gain, use the compress, reject and filter settings as for CW Doppler
- Position the sample volume with particular caution: even slight changes can affect the measurements significantly (Fig. 1.15)
- Shift the baseline upwards or downwards to use the entire display for either forward or backward flow (useful in unidirectional flows)
- Optimize the PRF: use as high as possible to detect high velocities, avoiding aliasing
- Use low PRF for flows distant from the transducer
- Use high PRF with caution if the origin of flow is relevant

CW, Continuous wave, *PRF,* pulse repetition frequency.

Obviously, such a calculation is prone to pitfalls that are mainly due to erroneous measurement of the LVOT diameter, suboptimal positioning of the PW Doppler sample volume in the LVOT, or malacquisition of the peak velocities by CW Doppler across the aortic valve.

An overview of hemodynamic data that can be derived from Doppler echocardiography is given in Fig. 1.18. More detailed explanations of specific measurements and entities will be given in further chapters of the book.

Effect of Sample Volume Position

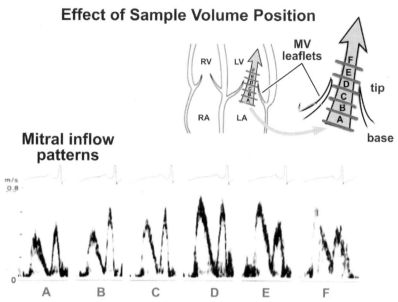

FIG. 1.15 The effect of sample volume position on the mitral inflow pattern. For the assessment of left ventricular diastolic function, the pulsed wave Doppler sample volume should be positioned at the tips of the mitral valve leaflets, which would correspond to the mitral inflow pattern shown under the letter "E." As can be observed, even small deviations from this position can dramatically impact the pattern as well as the obtained measurements, thus rendering an inaccurate assessment of diastolic function. *LA,* Left atrium; *LV,* left ventricle; *MV,* mitral valve; *RA,* right atrium; *RV,* right ventricle. *(Modified from Appleton CP, Jensen JL, Hatle LK, Oh JK. Doppler evaluation of left and right ventricular diastolic function: a technical guide for obtaining optimal flow velocity recordings. J Am Soc Echocardiogr. 1997;10(3):271-292, with permission.)*

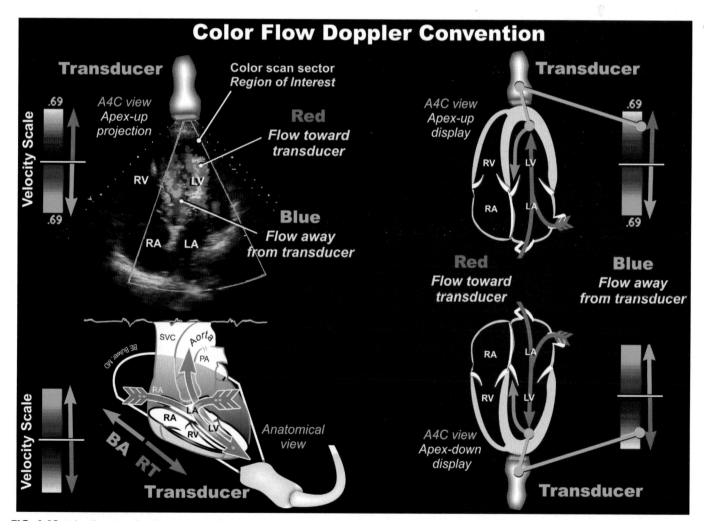

FIG. 1.16 Color flow Doppler imaging. Color flow Doppler is superimposed on the two-dimensional image. By convention, blood flow with mean velocities traveling toward the transducer is encoded in red, and mean velocities moving away from the transducer are color-coded in blue. Similar to other forms of PW Doppler, high velocities and turbulent flow are subject to aliasing, which is in color flow Doppler depicted as a multicolored mosaic pattern (typically green and yellow). The color-velocity scale illustrates incremental velocities in both directions from the baseline, such that higher velocities appear in increasingly lighter hues. *A4C,* Apical four-chamber; *BA RT,* blue away - red toward; *LA,* left atrium; *LV,* left ventricle; *RA,* right atrium; *RV,* right ventricle. *(Courtesy of Bernard E. Bulwer, MD, FASE; Modified from Solomon SD, Wu J, Gillam L, Bulwer B. Echocardiography. In: Mann DL, Zipes DP, Libby P, Bonow RO, Braunwald E, eds. Braunwald's heart disease: a textbook of cardiovascular medicine. 10th ed. Philadelphia: Elsevier; 2015:183.)*

Doppler Tissue Imaging

The principles of Doppler imaging are also applied to Doppler tissue imaging (DTI)—a modality in which the measured velocities are those of myocardial motion, rather than blood flow. This is obtained by the use of contrasting filters: when imaging blood flow, low velocities of strongly reflecting structures (such as the myocardium) should be filtered out; conversely, the filters omit high velocities of low scattering structures (such as red blood cells) while performing DTI.[8,9]

The basic quantification performed by DTI is that of velocities of myocardial motion (with regard to the transducer) at all points

within the cardiac cycle, at any segment of the myocardium, thus also providing insight to regional myocardial function. The typical DTI waveforms reveal systolic contraction (S′), early diastolic relaxation (E′), and late diastolic relaxation velocities (A′). DTI data can be obtained by both pulsed wave (spectral) Doppler and color Doppler. Accordingly, the inherent limitations of Doppler imaging, such as angle dependence, apply to DTI as well, reinforcing the necessity of optimal beam alignment with the direction of myocardial motion. Furthermore, it should be noted that the absolute recorded velocities are not equal for the PW and color DTI technique: PW DTI velocities represent peak velocities and are thus higher than those obtained by color DTI.[8,9]

One of the principal advantages of DTI is its high temporal resolution (usually between 150 and 200 Hz), which is typically obtained by imaging myocardial walls within narrow sectors. Conversely, one of the shortcomings of DTI-based velocity measurements is their dependency on the overall motion of the heart. Thus additional modalities have been developed to better assess the deformation (as opposed to motion) of specific myocardial segments. In the DTI approach the calculation of spatial gradients of the obtained velocities of neighboring myocardial segments allows for the quantification of local myocardial deformation (i.e., strain-rate). However, strain-rate curves may be rather "noisy," and a temporal integration of such curves is often performed to extract strain values. In more practical terms, strain-rate represents the speed of myocardial deformation (s⁻¹) and can be expressed for both systolic

---

BOX 1.11 Color Flow Doppler Optimization Points

- Optimize the size of the color box to the smallest necessary size
- Optimize gain settings: start with overemphasized gain such that background noise is detectable, reduce until disappearance of background noise
- Optimize the Nyquist scale according to the measured velocities: with high velocities, chose a high Nyquist limit (e.g., mitral regurgitation), and a low Nyquist limit when measuring low velocities (e.g., pulmonary vein flow)

Hemodynamic Doppler Assessment of
LV Stroke Volume

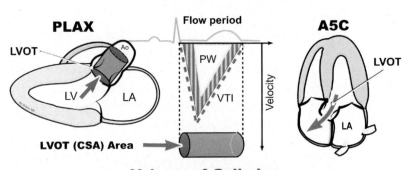

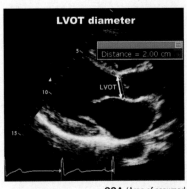
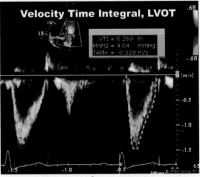

FIG. 1.17 Stroke volume calculation from Doppler measurements, which can be applied on all four heart valves. *A5C,* Apical five-chamber view; *CSA,* cross-sectional area; *HR,* heart rate; *LA,* left atrium; *LV,* left ventricle; *LVOT,* left ventricular outflow tract; *PLAX,* parasternal long-axis view; *PW,* pulsed wave Doppler; *SV,* stroke volume; *VTI,* velocity time integral.

- Volumetric measurements
  - Stroke volume (SV) & cardiac output (CO)
  - Regurgitant volume (RV) and fraction (RF)
  - Pulmonary-systemic flow ratio (Qp/Qs) ⎫
                                          ⎬ Continuity equation
- Valve area
  - Stenotic valve area
  - Regurgitant orifice area ⎭

- Pressure gradients
  - Maximal instantaneous gradient
  - Mean gradient ⎫
                  ⎬ Bernoulli equation
- Intracardiac pressures
  - Pulmonary artery pressures (PAP)
  - Left atrial pressure (LAP)
  - LV end-diastolic pressure (LVEDP) ⎭

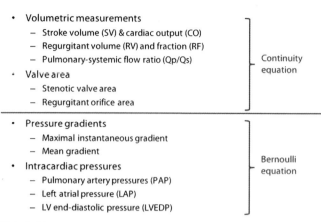

FIG. 1.18 Hemodynamic data obtainable by Doppler echocardiography.

and diastolic events, whereas strain corresponds to the amount of deformation (%), typically referring to systolic deformation. The mentioned quantification can be performed for all three major components of myocardial deformation: longitudinal, radial, and circumferential deformation (Fig. 1.19).[8,9]

2D Speckle Tracking Echocardiography

For information on this topic, refer to Chapter 6.

Suggested Readings

Armstrong, W. F., & Ryan, T. (Eds.). (2010). *Feigenbaum's Echocardiography* (7th ed.). Philadelphia: Lippincott Williams & Wilkins.

Bijnens, B. H., Cikes, M., Claus, P., & Sutherland, G. R. (2009). Velocity and deformation imaging for the assessment of myocardial dysfunction. *European Journal of Echocardiography, 10,* 216–226.

D'hooge, J., & Mertens, L. L. (2016). Ultrasound physics. In W. W. Lai, L. L. Mertens, M. S. Cohen, & T. Geva (Eds.), *Echocardiography in Pediatric and Congenital Heart Disease: From Fetus to Adult* (2nd ed.) (pp. 2–18). Chichester: John Wiley and Sons.

Solomon, S. D. (Ed.). (2007). *Essential Echocardiography—A Practical Handbook with DVD.* Totowa, New Jersey: Humana Press.

Szabo, T. L. (Ed.). (2014). *Diagnostic Ultrasound Imaging: Inside Out* (2nd ed.). Amsterdam: Elsevier.

A complete reference list can be found online at ExpertConsult.com.

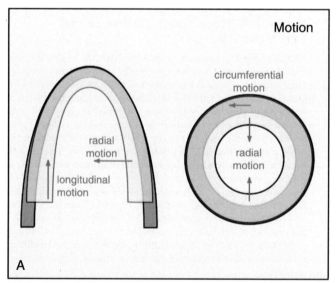

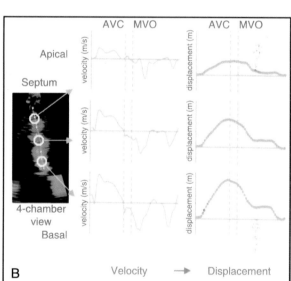

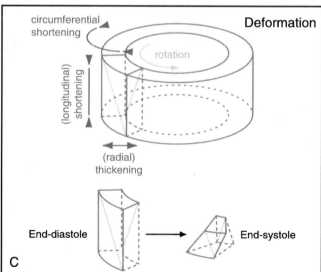

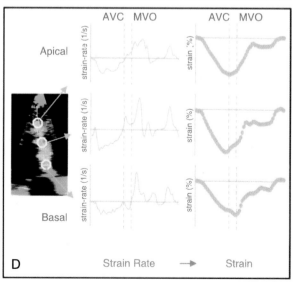

FIG. 1.19 Three major components of myocardial motion and deformation: longitudinal, radial, and circumferential (A and B). The total deformation of a myocardial segment from end-diastole to end-systole includes shortening, thickening, and shearing (B). Typical waveforms of myocardial velocity and displacement (C), as well as strain-rate, strain (D) over a cardiac cycle of a normal individual. *AVC,* Aortic valve closure; *MVO,* mitral valve opening. *(From Bijnens BH, Cikes M, Claus P, Sutherland GR: Velocity and deformation imaging for the assessment of myocardial dysfunction. Eur J Echocardiogr. 2009;10(2):216-226. Reprinted with permission.)*

M-Mode Imaging

Judy R. Mangion

INTRODUCTION

M-mode echocardiography provides superior temporal resolution, and therefore subtle changes are more readily appreciated with m-mode than with two-dimensional or three-dimensional methods. M-mode methods may include more precise measurement of cardiac chambers (provided they are obtained on-axis), independent motion of valvular vegetations, early closure or early opening of valve structures with respect to timing in the cardiac cycle (Fig. 2.1), identification of prosthetic valves and their function, assessment of paradoxical interventricular septal motion and dyssynchrony of the left ventricle, as well as fluttering of valve leaflets seen in association with valvular regurgitation (Fig. 2.2). The exaggerated motion, as well as restricted motion, of various cardiac structures is readily appreciated with m-mode.

An m-mode echocardiogram provides one-dimensional information regarding a particular cardiac structure as it relates to time and distance, with time displayed on the horizontal axis and depth or distance displayed on the vertical axis. The strength of the reflected echo is represented as the brightness of structures appearing on the image display (Fig. 2.3). The limitations of m-mode echocardiography relate to having to draw conclusions in one dimension about a three-dimensional structure. Furthermore, measurements are dependent on the identification of clearly defined borders, which may not be obtainable in technically challenging patients. With respect to m-mode's derived ejection fractions, calculations may not be accurate when regional wall motion abnormalities are present.

Although m-mode echocardiography was described more than 50 years ago by Edler and Hertz, new concepts and technologies that take advantage of m-mode techniques continue to expand. For example, color m-mode echocardiography evolved in the 1990s to provide rapid evaluation of time-related events, such as diastolic mitral regurgitation, and has also been used to provide less load-dependent information regarding diastolic function. Color m-mode techniques have also been applied to the assessment of myocardial deformation or strain, in which a curved m-mode is traced along an area of interest of the myocardium and information is displayed in both parametric and graphic format, allowing sensitive evaluation of normal and abnormal patterns of ventricular contractility. M-mode images of the left ventricle are often displayed simultaneously during left ventricular strain analysis to improve interpretation of the curves with respect to the cardiac cycle. Although m-mode echocardiography has been around for a long time and the field of echocardiography has dramatically changed with numerous technological advances, m-mode recordings can still oftentimes provide additional and complementary information, resulting in a more accurate and complete echocardiographic assessment of the heart.

This chapter provides case examples of normal m-mode exams, as well as a diverse spectrum of abnormal m-mode exams illustrating classic cardiac anomalies. Each figure legend provides a "clinical pearl" highlighting important concepts involved in either technically obtaining or interpreting each m-mode image.

NORMAL M-MODE MEASUREMENTS

Normal M-Mode Examination of the Aortic Root, Aortic Cusp Separation, and Left Atrial Dimension

Traditionally, m-mode measurements have been used to quantify aortic root size, aortic valve cusp separation, and left atrial dimensions. These measurements are obtained from the parasternal long-axis imaging plane. By convention, m-mode measurements are made leading edge to leading edge, which differs from two-dimensional measurements, which are made inner edge to inner edge. The m-mode cursor is placed perpendicular to the structure being measured. Fig. 2.4 illustrates the proper m-mode technique for measuring the aortic root, aortic valve cusps, and left atrium. The aortic root is measured in end-diastole, just before the onset of the QRS complex. The aortic valve cusp separation is measured in midsystole. The normal appearance of the aortic cusps during systole is that of an "open box," which reflects holosystolic opening of the valve leaflets. By convention, the left atrium is measured during ventricular systole or atrial diastole, when the left atrium is maximally filled with blood.

Normal M-Mode Examination of the Left Ventricle

The m-mode examination of the left ventricle is also obtained from the parasternal long-axis imaging plane. By convention, left ventricular dimensions are made at end-diastole and end-systole, whereas measurements of left ventricular wall thicknesses, including the interventricular septum and posterior wall of the left ventricle, are usually measured only at end diastole. By convention, the m-mode cursor is placed perpendicular to the long axis of the left ventricle at the level of the mitral valve chordae. Fig. 2.5 illustrates the proper m-mode technique for measuring left ventricular internal dimensions at end systole and end diastole, as well as septal and posterior wall thicknesses in end diastole. In the absence of left ventricular regional wall motion abnormalities, m-mode recordings of the left ventricle have been shown to be an accurate method for calculating left ventricular ejection fraction via the method of Teicholtz. According to this method, the left ventricular dimension in diastole squared minus the left ventricular dimension in systole squared is divided by the left ventricular dimension in diastole squared.

Normal M-Mode Examination of the Mitral Valve

The normal m-mode recording of the mitral valve—like that of the aortic root, left atrium, and left ventricle—is also obtained from the parasternal long-axis imaging plane. The m-mode cursor is placed perpendicular to the long axis of the left ventricle at the level of the tips of the mitral leaflets. The anterior leaflet and posterior leaflet are noted to open fully in diastole and close completely during systole (Fig. 2.6).

Normal M-Mode Examination of the Pulmonic Valve

The normal m-mode recording of the pulmonic valve is usually obtained from the parasternal short-axis view, but it can also be obtained from the right ventricular outflow tract view and main pulmonary artery and bifurcation view (Fig. 2.7). Like the normal aortic valve, the normal pulmonic valve opens throughout systole and has the appearance of "an open box." Normal m-mode letter designations for the pulmonic valve are as follows: a = atrial contraction, b = onset of ventricular systole, c = ventricular ejection, d = during ventricular ejection, and e = end of ventricular ejection.

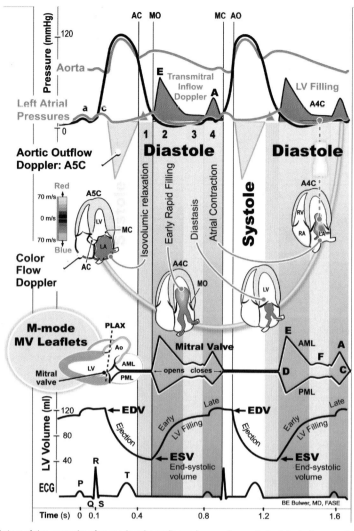

FIG. 2.1 This figure provides an overall view of the strengths of m-mode echocardiography as a diagnostic tool, including superior temporal resolution, which allows for more precise measurements, and timing of motion of cardiac structures with respect to the cardiac cycle. *AC,* Aortic valve closure; *AML,* anterior mitral leaflet; *EDV,* end diastolic volume; *ESV,* end systolic volume; *LV,* left ventricle; *MO,* mitral valve opening; *PLAX,* parasternal long axis; *PML,* posterior mitral leaflet. *(Courtesy of Bernard E. Bulwer, MD, FASE.)*

Normal M-Mode Examination of the Tricuspid Valve

The normal m-mode recording of the tricuspid valve is obtained from the right ventricular inflow view (Fig. 2.8). Usually, only the anterior leaflet of the tricuspid valve is transected by the m-mode cursor. M-mode letter designations for the tricuspid valve are as follows: D = onset of diastole, E = maximal opening of the leaflet, F = most posterior position of the leaflet, E–F slope = closing motion of the leaflet, A = leaflet reopening with atrial contraction, and C = leaflet closure following ventricular systole.

M-MODE ECHOCARDIOGRAPHY IN THE IDENTIFICATION OF ABNORMAL CARDIAC STRUCTURE AND FUNCTION

Bicuspid Aortic Valve

M-mode echocardiography can often be useful in helping establish the diagnosis of a bicuspid aortic valve (Fig. 2.9). The classic appearance of a bicuspid aortic valve on m-mode echocardiography is eccentric closing of the valve leaflets. If present, this is strongly suggestive of a bicuspid aortic valve, although in some cases, bicuspid aortic valves may open symmetrically.

Subaortic Membrane

M-mode echocardiography can also be helpful in confirming the diagnosis of a fixed subaortic membrane (Fig. 2.10). In this case, an m-mode

cursor placed through the aortic valve leaflets will demonstrate early closure of the leaflets in systole. In this case, the subaortic membrane decreases the pressure differential between the systemic circulation and left ventricle, causing the aortic valve to close early.

Mitral Valve Prolapse

M-mode echocardiography has also been used to diagnose mitral valve prolapse (Fig. 2.11). An m-mode cursor placed at the tip of the mitral leaflets in the parasternal long-axis view can demonstrate late systolic prolapse of the mitral leaflets into the left atrium. Because of the dependence of the ultrasound beam, however, mitral valve prolapse can be missed or overdiagnosed with m-mode echocardiography alone. For this reason, the diagnosis of mitral valve prolapse be confirmed by two-dimensional methods, which should demonstrate systolic prolapse of greater than 2 mm beyond the plane of the mitral annulus and into the left atrium.

Systolic Anterior Motion of the Mitral Valve

M-mode echocardiography is especially useful for establishing the presence of systolic anterior motion (SAM) of the mitral valve, causing dynamic left ventricular outflow tract obstruction (Fig. 2.12). This is often seen in the setting of hypertrophic obstructive cardiomyopathy; however, it can also occur in the absence of hypertrophic cardiomyopathy. In the parasternal long-axis view, as the left ventricular chamber decreases in systole, the anterior cusp of the mitral valve comes into forceful contact

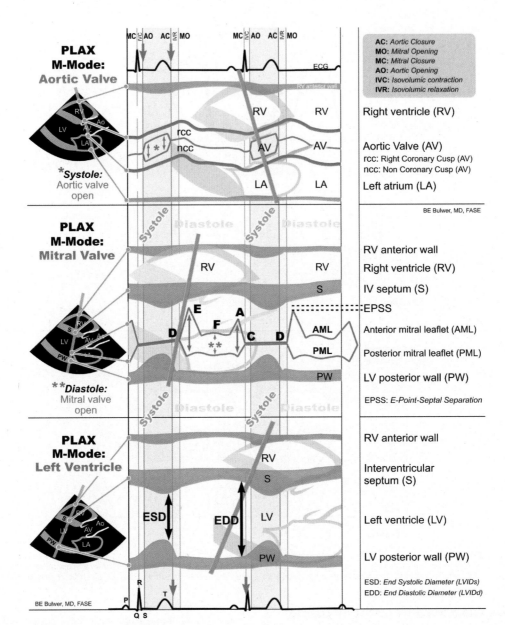

FIG. 2.2 This figure illustrates the most common m-mode measurements obtained from the parasternal long-axis view, including measurements of the aortic root, cusp separation of the aortic valve leaflets, mitral valve opening and closure, and left ventricular measurements including internal dimensions in diastole and systole and septal and posterior wall thickness in end-diastole. *(Courtesy of Bernard E. Bulwer, MD, FASE.)*

with the protruding interventricular septum. The m-mode recording is especially useful in providing information pertaining to the timing of the SAM of the mitral valve (i.e., early systolic, holosystolic, or late systolic).

Severe Aortic Insufficiency (Austin Flint Murmur)

M-mode echocardiography can also provide clues with respect to quantifying the severity of aortic insufficiency. In cases of severe aortic insufficiency, the aortic regurgitant jet can impinge on the anterior leaflet of the mitral valve, causing diastolic fluttering as well as early closure of the anterior leaflet of the mitral valve (Figs. 2.13–2.15), or the so-called Austin Flint murmur heard on clinical exam, which can be mistaken for the murmur of mitral stenosis. In cases of severe acute aortic insufficiency, a sudden increase in diastolic volume overload causes increased resistance by the ventricle to diastolic filling, resulting in early diastolic closure of the mitral valve.

Valvular Vegetations

Because of its higher frame rates (i.e., number of times per second the image is updated on ultrasound), m-mode echocardiography can sometimes identify vegetations that may be missed with two-dimensional

echocardiography. M-mode echocardiography may demonstrate the presence of a mobile mass on one of the valves with independent motion (Fig. 2.16), which is highly suspicious for vegetation in patients with a strong clinical suspicion of endocarditis.

Rheumatic Mitral Valve Deformity

M-mode imaging can also be helpful in establishing the diagnosis of rheumatic mitral stenosis (Fig. 2.17). In this case there is reduced opening of the mitral leaflets during diastole due to fusion of the commissures. When used in combination with spectral Doppler of the mitral valve to measure gradients, pressure half-time–derived mitral valve areas, and direct planimetry of the mitral valve area, the added information provided by m-mode can often assist in making a more accurate judgment as to the severity of mitral stenosis, particularly when there are discrepant data.

Cardiomyopathy and Elevated Left Ventricular Filling Pressures

The m-mode examination of the mitral valve can also provide insight into hemodynamics in patients with cardiomyopathy. A classic m-mode

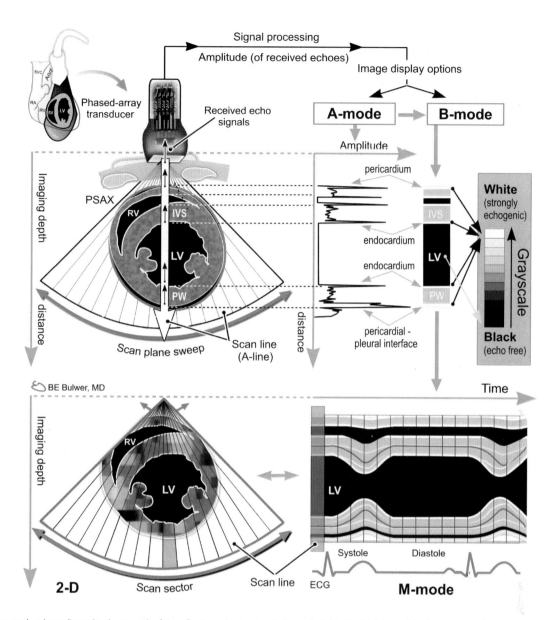

FIG. 2.3 With m-mode echocardiography, the strength of the reflecting echo structure is demonstrated by the brightness of the image on the ultrasound screen. Time is represented in milliseconds; with respect to the cardiac cycle (systole and diastole), it is displayed on the horizontal axis. Distance of the reflecting cardiac structure is displayed on the vertical axis. *EDV,* End diastolic volume; *IVS,* interventricular septum; *LV,* left ventricle; *PSAX,* parasternal short axis; *PW,* posterior wall; *RV,* right ventricle. (*Courtesy of Bernard E. Bulwer, MD, FASE.*)

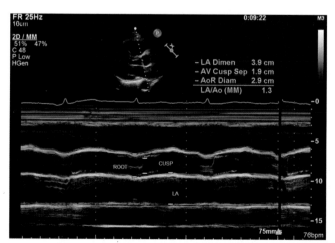

FIG. 2.4 Normal m-mode examination of the aortic root, aortic valve cusps, and left atrium. Measurements are obtained in the parasternal long-axis imaging plane. Note the holosystolic opening of the aortic valve cusps. By convention, m-mode measurements are made leading edge to leading edge, which differs from two-dimensional measurements. The m-mode cursor is placed perpendicular to the aortic valve leaflets. *Ao,* Aorta; *AoR,* aortic root; *AV,* aortic valve; *Cusp,* aortic leaflet separation; *LA,* left atrium; *Root,* aortic root.

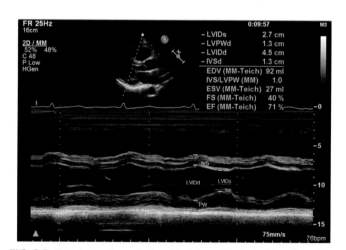

FIG. 2.5 Normal m-mode examination of the left ventricle obtained from the parasternal long-axis imaging plane. Left ventricular dimensions are made at end diastole and end systole, whereas septal and posterior wall thicknesses are usually measured only at end diastole. The m-mode cursor is placed perpendicular to the long axis of the left ventricle at the level of the mitral valve chordae. *Ao,* Aorta; *AV,* aortic valve; *EDV,* end diastolic volume; *EF,* ejection fraction; *ESV,* end systolic volume; *FS,* fractional shortening; *IVS,* interventricular septum; *LVIDd,* left ventricular internal dimension in diastole; *LVIDs,* left ventricular internal dimension in systole; *LVPWD,* left ventricle posterior wall diastole; *PW,* posterior wall.

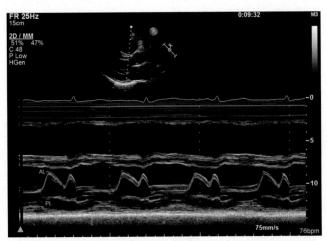

FIG. 2.6 Normal m-mode examination of the mitral valve leaflets from the parasternal long-axis imaging plane. The m-mode cursor is placed perpendicular to the long axis of the left ventricle at the level of the tips of the mitral leaflets. *AL,* Anterior leaflet; *PL,* posterior leaflet.

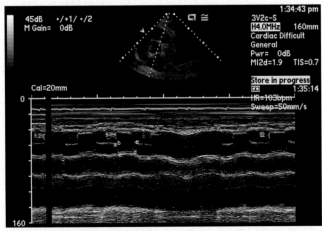

FIG. 2.7 Normal m-mode examination of the pulmonic valve obtained from the parasternal short-axis view. This recording may also be obtained from the parasternal right ventricular outflow view and the main pulmonary artery and bifurcation view. Note the holosystolic opening of the cusps, similar to the aortic valve. Often, m-mode of the pulmonic valve only transects the right posterior leaflet. In this example, both the anterior and right posterior leaflets are transected. The m-mode letter designations for the pulmonic valve are as follows: *(a),* atrial contraction; *(b),* onset of ventricular systole; *(c),* ventricular ejection; *(d),* during ventricular ejection; *(e),* end of ventricular ejection.

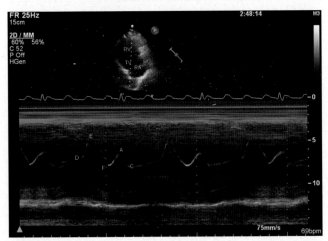

FIG. 2.8 Normal m-mode examination of the tricuspid valve obtained from the right ventricular inflow view. Usually only the anterior leaflet of the tricuspid valve is transected. *RA,* Right atrium; *RV,* right ventricle; *TV,* tricuspid valve. The m-mode letter designations for the tricuspid valve are as follows: *(D),* onset of diastole; *(E),* maximal opening of the leaflet; *(F),* most posterior position of the leaflet; *(E–F slope),* closing motion of the leaflet; *(A),* leaflet reopening with atrial contraction; *(C),* leaflet closure following ventricular systole.

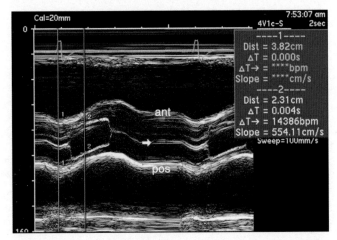

FIG. 2.9 M-mode examination of a bicuspid aortic valve obtained from the parasternal long-axis view. Note that in this case the closing of the valve is asymmetric *(arrow)*. If present, this may be an important clue in establishing the diagnosis of bicuspid aortic valve. In some situations, bicuspid aortic valves may open symmetrically. *ant,* Anterior; *pos,* posterior.

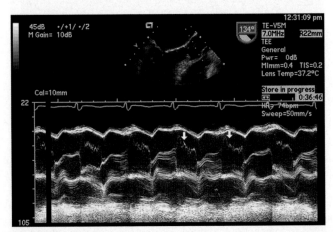

FIG. 2.10 M-mode examination of the aortic valve demonstrating early systolic closure of the leaflets *(arrows)* due to a fixed subaortic membrane. The membrane decreases the pressure differential between the systemic circulation and left ventricle, causing the aortic valve to close early. This image was obtained with a transesophageal probe from a longitudinal view of the aortic valve.

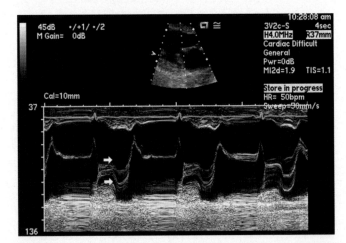

FIG. 2.11 M-mode examination of the mitral valve demonstrating classic late systolic bileaflet mitral valve prolapse *(arrows)*; the image was obtained from the parasternal long-axis view. Because of dependence on the ultrasound beam, prolapse can be missed or overdiagnosed with m-mode echocardiography alone; therefore the diagnosis needs to be confirmed by two-dimensional methods, demonstrating systolic prolapse of greater than 2 mm beyond the plane of the mitral annulus and into the left atrium.

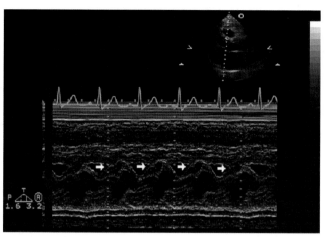

FIG. 2.12 M-mode examination of the mitral valve, parasternal long-axis view, demonstrating systolic anterior motion of the mitral valve *(arrows)*, which is causing dynamic obstruction of the left ventricular outflow tract. This is often observed in the setting of hypertrophic obstructive cardiomyopathy. However, it can also occur in the absence of hypertrophic cardiomyopathy. In the setting of hypertrophic obstructive cardiomyopathy, the anterior cusp of the mitral valve comes into forceful contact with the protruding interventricular septum as the left ventricular chamber decreases in systole. The m-mode recording provides information pertaining to the timing of systolic anterior motion of the mitral valve.

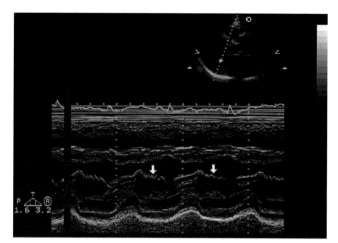

FIG. 2.13 M-mode examination of the mitral valve, parasternal long-axis view, demonstrating high-frequency diastolic fluttering of the anterior mitral leaflet *(arrows)* due to severe aortic insufficiency. This is the equivalent of the Austin Flint murmur.

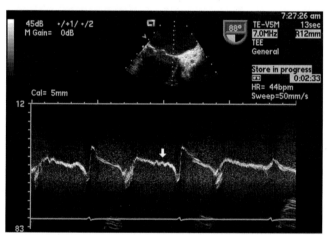

FIG. 2.14 M-mode examination of the mitral valve, midesophageal two-chamber view, also demonstrating high-frequency diastolic fluttering of the anterior mitral valve leaflet *(arrow)* due to severe aortic insufficiency, impinging on the leaflet.

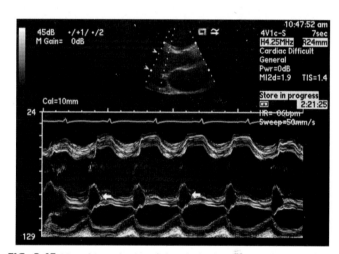

FIG. 2.15 M-mode examination of the mitral valve, parasternal long-axis view, demonstrating early diastolic closure of the mitral valve *(arrows)* due to severe acute aortic insufficiency. The sudden increase in diastolic volume overload causes increased resistance by the ventricle to diastolic filling, causing early diastolic closure of the mitral valve.

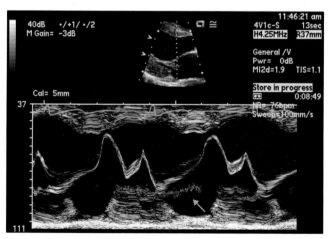

FIG. 2.16 M-mode examination of the mitral valve demonstrating a large mobile mass with independent motion on the atrial surface of the posterior leaflet in a patient with suspected endocarditis *(arrow)*. Because of its higher frame rates, m-mode echocardiography can sometimes identify vegetations that may be missed with two-dimensional echocardiography.

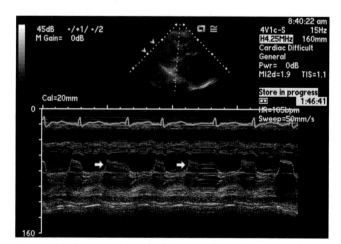

FIG. 2.17 M-mode examination of the mitral valve affected by rheumatic valvular heart disease. There is reduced opening of the mitral valve leaflets during diastole *(arrows)* due to fusion of the commissures.

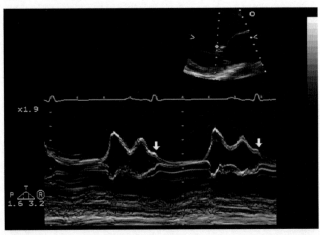

FIG. 2.18 M-mode examination of the mitral valve demonstrating a "b-notch" on the anterior mitral valve leaflet *(arrows)* in a patient with a dilated cardiomyopathy. Although not always present, the b-notch, when identified, is indicative of markedly elevated left ventricular end-diastolic pressure.

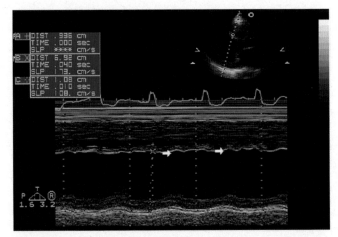

FIG. 2.20 M-mode examination of the left ventricle, parasternal long-axis view, in a patient with left bundle branch block. Note the paradoxical septal motion, or delayed contraction of the interventricular septum in systole *(arrows)*.

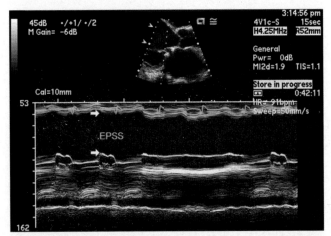

FIG. 2.19 M-mode examination of the mitral valve demonstrating enlarged E-point septal separation (EPSS) *(arrows)* in a patient with dilated cardiomyopathy due to a reduced stroke volume with poor systolic function. In general, a normal EPSS should be less than 1 cm. EPSS on m-mode can provide a useful marker of overall left ventricular systolic function.

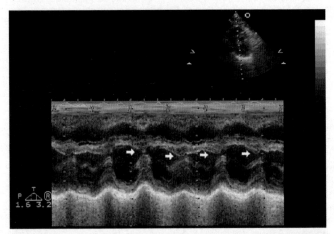

FIG. 2.21 M-mode examination of the left ventricle, parasternal long-axis view, demonstrating exaggerated respiratory variation of the position of the interventricular septum ("septal bounce") *(arrows)*. This is a nonspecific finding in suspected constrictive pericarditis. If clinical suspicion of cardiac constriction is high, it should warrant additional directed comprehensive two-dimensional and Doppler evaluation.

finding in patients with dilated cardiomyopathy is the "b-notch" on the anterior mitral valve leaflet (Fig. 2.18). Although not always present, the b-notch, when identified, is indicative of a markedly elevated left ventricular end-diastolic pressure.

Cardiomyopathy and Reduced Left Ventricular Ejection Fraction

M-mode interrogation of the mitral valve has also been commonly used to estimate left ventricular ejection fraction in patients with global left ventricular systolic dysfunction. The m-mode examination in this case will demonstrate an enlarged E point septal separation (EPSS) (Fig. 2.19). This is due to a reduced stroke volume with poor left ventricular systolic function. In general, a normal EPSS should be less than 1 cm. The greater the EPSS distance on m-mode, the worse the overall left ventricular systolic function.

Left Ventricular Dyssynchrony

M-mode interrogation of the left ventricle has also been used to establish the presence of left ventricular dyssynchrony in patients with heart failure being considered for cardiac resynchronization therapy (CRT). Fig. 2.20 illustrates an m-mode recording of the left ventricle in a patient with left bundle branch block (LBBB). In this patient, there is marked paradoxical septal motion or delayed contraction of the interventricular septum in systole. Measurement of the septal-to-posterior wall motion

delay (SPWMD), which is defined as the distance between the timing of septal and posterior wall contraction, has been used to predict a positive response to CRT therapy, with greater than 130 ms being used as the cutoff to predict a positive response to CRT.

Constrictive Pericarditis

M-mode interrogation of the left ventricle can also be helpful in detecting an exaggerated respiratory variation of the position of the interventricular septum ("septal bounce") (Fig. 2.21). Although this is a nonspecific finding in suspected constrictive pericarditis, its identification, along with a strong clinical suspicion of cardiac constriction, should warrant additional directed comprehensive two-dimensional and Doppler evaluation for other markers of cardiac constriction.

Cor Pulmonale

M-mode examination of the left ventricle can also be helpful in identifying echocardiographic evidence of right heart failure or cor pulmonale complicated by evidence of both pressure and volume overload of the right ventricle (Fig. 2.22). M-mode interrogation can readily identify both systolic and diastolic flattening of the interventricular septum (the "D-shaped septum"). Systolic flattening of the septum represents pressure overload of the right ventricle from pulmonary hypertension, whereas diastolic flattening of the septum represents volume overload of the right ventricle, which is often secondary to severe wide-open tricuspid insufficiency.

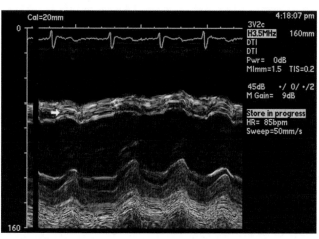

FIG. 2.22 M-mode examination of the left ventricle, parasternal long-axis view, in a patient with severe cor pulmonale, demonstrating both systolic and diastolic flattening of the interventricular septum ("D-shaped septum") *(arrow)*. Systolic flattening of the septum represents pressure overload of the right ventricle from pulmonary hypertension, while diastolic flattening of the septum represents volume overload of the right ventricle. Here, this was secondary to severe wide-open tricuspid insufficiency.

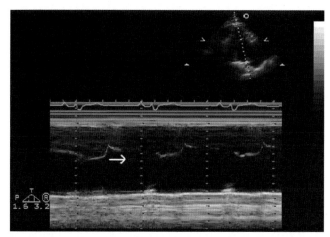

FIG. 2.24 M-mode examination of the tricuspid valve, right ventricular inflow view, in Ebstein anomaly. Note the decreased diastolic opening of the anterior leaflet due to deformation *(arrow)*; compare with Fig. 2.8, showing a normal m-mode view of the tricuspid valve. The Ebstein anomaly is a congenital deformity characterized by downward displacement of part or all of the tricuspid valve into the right ventricular cavity.

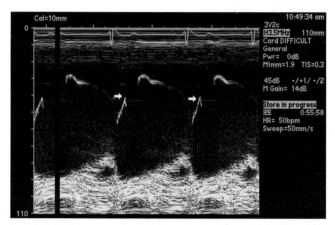

FIG. 2.23 M-mode examination of the pulmonic valve, main pulmonary artery view, demonstrating early systolic closure of the pulmonic valve ("flying w") *(arrows)* associated with severe pulmonary hypertension and due to the elevated filling pressure of the right ventricle. Often there may also be an absent a wave (atrial wave) of the m-mode tracing.

Severe Pulmonary Hypertension

M-mode examination of the pulmonic valve from the parasternal short-axis or main pulmonary artery view can also assist in identifying the presence of severe pulmonary hypertension (Fig. 2.23). This can be readily identified by demonstrating early systolic closure of the pulmonic valve ("flying w") associated with severe pulmonary hypertension and due to the elevated filling pressure of the right ventricle. Often there may also be an absent a wave (atrial wave) of the m-mode tracing as well.

Ebstein Anomaly

Ebstein anomaly is a congenital deformity characterized by downward displacement of part or all of the tricuspid valve into the right ventricular cavity. M-mode examination of the tricuspid valve from the right ventricular inflow view can be helpful in establishing the diagnosis of Ebstein anomaly (Fig. 2.24). Typically there is decreased diastolic opening of the anterior leaflet due to deformation (compare with Fig. 2.8, a normal m-mode view of the tricuspid valve).

Increased Right Atrial Pressure

An elevation in right atrial pressure—seen in different cardiac pathologies including cardiac tamponade, cardiac constriction, and both left- and right-sided heart failure—can be confirmed by an m-mode tracing of the inferior vena cava near its communication with the right atrium. Fig. 2.25 illustrates an m-mode examination of the inferior vena cava obtained in

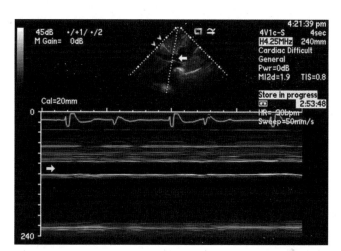

FIG. 2.25 M-mode examination of the inferior vena cava, subcostal view, in the presence of markedly elevated right atrial pressure (such as tamponade, constriction, or cor pulmonale). Note the markedly dilated (greater than 2 cm) and plethoric (no inspiratory collapse) inferior vena cava *(arrows)*. The m-mode cursor is placed at the junction of the inferior vena cava and right atrium. The estimated right atrial pressure in this scenario is at least 20 mm Hg.

the subcostal view in the presence of markedly elevated right atrial pressure. Note the markedly dilated (greater than 2 cm) and plethoric (no inspiratory collapse) inferior vena cava (IVC) *(arrows)*. The m-mode cursor is placed at the junction of the inferior vena cava and right atrium. The estimated right atrial pressure in this scenario is at least 20 mm Hg. In situations of low filling pressures, m-mode recordings of the IVC can confirm greater than 50% inspiratory collapse of the IVC.

M-Mode Examination of Prosthetic Valves

M-mode recordings can also be useful in differentiating various types of prosthetic valves, particularly when patients are unaware of the type of valve they may have. M-mode can differentiate single-disk, bileaflet, and ball-in-cage mechanical valves and bioprosthetic valves. It can also confirm normally functioning prosthetic valves from those with evidence of valve dysfunction. Fig. 2.26 illustrates an m-mode examination of a normally functioning St. Jude bileaflet mechanical aortic valve prosthesis; it was obtained with transesophageal echocardiography from a midesophageal longitudinal view demonstrating opening of both prosthetic valve leaflets in systole *(arrows)*. Fig. 2.27 illustrates a transthoracic m-mode examination of a normally functioning St. Jude bileaflet mechanical mitral valve prosthesis; it was obtained from the parasternal long-axis view, demonstrating opening of both prosthetic valve leaflets in diastole *(arrows)*.

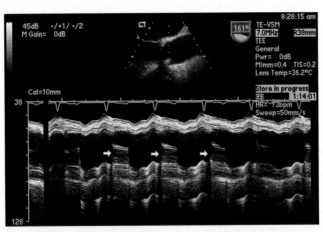

FIG. 2.26 M-mode examination of a normally functioning St. Jude bileaflet mechanical aortic valve prosthesis, longitudinal view, obtained with transesophageal echocardiography. To demonstrate correct motion of both prosthetic valve leaflets in systole (arrows), m-mode echocardiography continues to be an important part of the evaluation of prosthetic valve function.

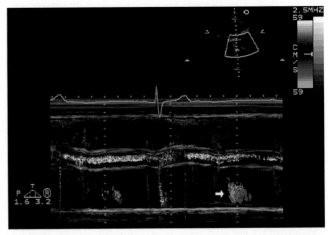

FIG. 2.28 Color m-mode examination of the aortic root and left atrium, parasternal long-axis view, in a patient with mild diastolic mitral regurgitation (arrow) attributable to heart block. This demonstrates that m-mode echocardiography is an ideal modality for confirming the timing of events with respect to the cardiac cycle.

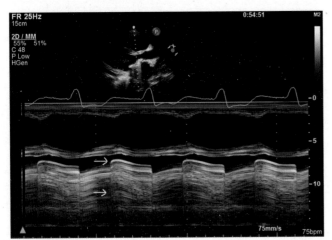

FIG. 2.27 M-mode examination of a normally functioning St. Jude bileaflet mechanical mitral valve prosthesis, parasternal long-axis view. To demonstrate correct motion of both prosthetic valve leaflets in diastole (arrows), m-mode echocardiography continues to be an important part of the evaluation of prosthetic valve function.

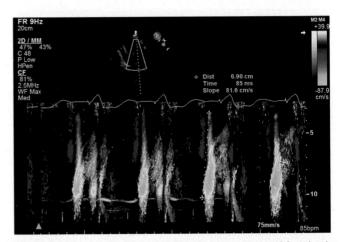

FIG. 2.29 Color m-mode examination of the left ventricle, apical four-chamber view, demonstrating normal propagation velocity of blood flow in the left ventricle of 81.6 cm/s during diastole, which is indicative of a normal diastolic filling pattern. Normal propagation velocities are measured by the initial slope of the E wave on color m-mode and are always greater than 45 cm/s. Note that the Nyquist color scale is moved up to 39.4 cm/s (arrow), allowing color Doppler flow to be visualized all the way from the base of the mitral annulus to the left ventricular apex.

Color M-Mode Echocardiography

Color m-mode echocardiography is an ideal modality for confirming the timing of events with respect to the cardiac cycle, which can be especially useful in valvular regurgitant lesions. Color m-mode has also been used in the assessment of left ventricular diastolic function and is thought to be less pre- and afterload-dependent than spectral Doppler. In this situation, the initial propagation velocity (Vp) of blood flow in the left ventricle is measured. Fig. 2.28 illustrates a color m-mode examination of the aortic root and left atrium from the parasternal long-axis view in a patient with mild diastolic mitral regurgitation (arrow) attributable to heart block. Fig. 2.29 illustrates a color m-mode examination of the left ventricle, from the apical four-chamber view, demonstrating a normal Vp of blood flow in the left ventricle of 81.6 cm/s during diastole, which indicates a normal diastolic filling pattern. Normal propagation velocities are measured by the initial slope of the E wave on color m-mode and are always greater than 45 cm/s. To make these color m-mode recordings, the Nyquist color scale is moved up to 39.4 cm/s (arrow), allowing color Doppler flow to be visualized all the way from the base of the mitral annulus to the left ventricular apex. Fig. 2.30 illustrates a color m-mode examination of the left ventricle from the apical four-chamber view, demonstrating a diastolic filling pattern consistent with impaired left ventricular relaxation. In this case, the Vp measures 40.2 cm/s and is mildly reduced. Fig. 2.31 demonstrates a color m-mode examination of the left ventricle from the apical four-chamber view, showing a diastolic filling pattern consistent with markedly delayed

propagation or restrictive physiology. In this example, the Vp measured significantly less than 45 cm/s (blue arrow). Note that the accuracy of the measurement of the Vp of early diastolic filling on color m-mode is improved by increasing the sweep speed to 100 mm/s (yellow arrow).

Strain Imaging of the Myocardium (Parametric M-Mode Echocardiography)

Strain imaging represents a load-independent technology, now well validated, for measuring regional myocardial deformation of the ventricular myocardium; this is measured in terms of percent to reflect the relative shortening of the myocyte during systole. Fig. 2.32 illustrates a parametric curved m-mode examination of the left ventricle from the apical four-chamber view demonstrating a normal strain pattern of the left ventricle. In this example, a curved m-mode line is traced along the interventricular septum from apex to base. The wide orange band in systole represents shortening, whereas the wide yellow band in diastole represents lengthening. The four red curves below the parametric image represent four separate strain measurements from apex to base, with the apex (top curve) showing the least amount of strain or deformation during systole (arrow). Different strain patterns have been shown to differentiate various cardiomyopathies, including cardiac amyloidosis as well as hypertrophic

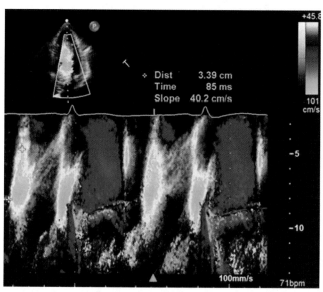

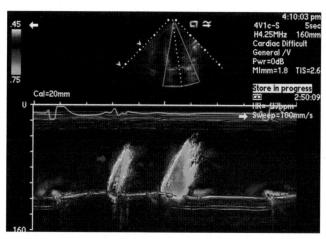

FIG. 2.31 Color m-mode examination of the left ventricle, apical four-chamber view, demonstrating a diastolic filling pattern consistent with markedly delayed propagation or restrictive physiology. In this example the propagation velocity measured significantly less than 45 cm/s (*blue arrow*). Note that the accuracy of the measurement of the propagation velocity of early diastolic filling on color m-mode is improved by increasing the sweep speed to 100 mm/s (*yellow arrow*).

FIG. 2.30 Color m-mode examination of the left ventricle, apical four-chamber view, demonstrating a diastolic filling pattern consistent with impaired left ventricular relaxation. In this case, the propagation velocity measures 40.2 cm/s and is mildly reduced. Color m-mode in a useful tool in the assessment of diastolic function of the left ventricle and is thought to be less flow-dependent than pulsed-wave Doppler.

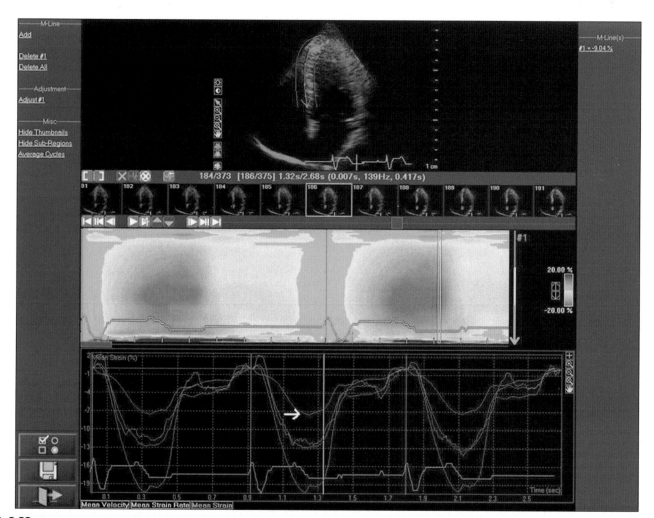

FIG. 2.32 Parametric curved m-mode examination of the left ventricle, apical four-chamber view, demonstrating normal strain pattern of the left ventricle. Strain imaging represents load-independent, cutting-edge technology for measuring regional myocardial deformation of the ventricular myocardium and is measured in terms of percent so as to reflect the relative shortening of the myocyte during systole. In this example, a curved m-mode line is traced along the interventricular septum from apex to base. The wide *orange* band in systole represents shortening, whereas the wide *yellow* band in diastole represents lengthening. The four *red* curves below the parametric image represent four separate strain measurements from apex to base, with the apex (*top curve*) showing the least amount of strain or deformation during systole (*arrow*).

and hypertensive cardiomyopathies. This is an exciting and active area of investigation in the field of echocardiography that is likely to significantly improve the diagnostic capabilities of cardiac ultrasound in the future.

SUMMARY

M-mode echocardiography, because of its superior temporal resolution, remains important in today's echo lab because of its ability to time rapidly moving structures within the heart, such as the valves, in relation to the cardiac cycle. It is capable of providing additional clues to answering complex clinical questions, and represents an inexpensive tool, in the vast and widely expanding echocardiography tool box.

Suggested Readings

Feigenbaum, H. (2010). Role of m-mode echocardiography in today's echo lab. *Journal of the American Society of Echocardiography, 23,* 240–257.

Sahn, D. J., DeMaria, A., Kisslo, J., & Weyman, A. (1978). The committee on M-mode standardization of the American Society of Echocardiography: recommendations regarding quantitation in M-mode echocardiography: results of a survey of echocardiographic measurements. *Circulation, 58,* 1072–1083.

Weyman, A. E. (1994). M-Mode echocardiography: principles and examination techniques. In *Principles and Practice of Echocardiography* (2nd ed.) (pp. 282–301). Philadelphia: Lea & Febiger.

3 Principles of Contrast Echocardiography

Jonathan R. Lindner

INTRODUCTION

Contrast echocardiography is a broad term used to describe an array of approaches that can be used to improve and expand diagnostic capabilities by acoustic enhancement of the blood pool during cardiac ultrasound imaging.[1,2] Ultrasound contrast agents are generally composed of gas-filled encapsulated microparticles, usually microbubbles that are 1–5 μm in diameter, or nanoparticles.[1] The most common clinical application of contrast echocardiography has been to better delineate the endocardial contours of the left ventricular (LV) cavity, termed *left ventricular opacification* (LVO; Fig. 3.1).[3,4] Although there are many reasons clinicians opt for performing LVO in a given patient, the most frequent indication is to better evaluate global or regional LV systolic function (Videos 3.1 and 3.2). Justification for this application of LVO is based on (1) the inability to fully examine LV myocardial thickening in 10%–20% of unselected patients; (2) the frequent use of echo to guide management in critically ill patients who have difficult acoustic windows due to positive pressure ventilation or inability to cooperate with the ultrasound examination; and (3) frequent use of echo to make critical decisions based on the presence of segmental wall motion, where every myocardial segment needs to be well seen with a high degree of reader confidence (e.g., stress echocardiography, point-of-care echo for detection of myocardial ischemia or evaluation of heart failure). There are many other clinical situations where LVO has had a positive impact in clinical echocardiography (Box 3.1).

Refinements in contrast ultrasound technology that improve the detection of microbubble signal in the coronary circulation relative to myocardial tissue signal have permitted the imaging of the myocardial microcirculation. These techniques are broadly referred to as myocardial contrast echocardiography (MCE). The most basic approach to MCE is to spatially evaluate the presence of an intact microcirculation. The presence of a functional microvascular bed can be used to assess myocardial viability, to characterize a cardiac mass as a tumor rather than thrombus based on the presence of functional microvessels, and to detect therapeutic or spontaneous reperfusion in acute myocardial infarction (Fig. 3.2; Videos 3.3–3.5).[5–10] Quantitative or semiquantitative assessment of perfusion requires not only quantification of the intact microvasculature but also temporal information of microbubble transit through the microcirculation. This measurement generally requires destruction of microbubbles within the acoustic sector and evaluation of signal reappearance.[11] This approach can be used to detect resting ischemia, flow heterogeneity during stress echocardiography, or microvascular dysfunction, or to assess the presence/adequacy of collateral blood flow.

In this chapter, the basic principles of contrast echocardiography will be described, including an overview of contrast agents and the specific imaging modalities that have been developed to improve microbubble signal-to-noise ratio during clinical imaging. Clinical applications of contrast echocardiography are detailed in Chapter 12.

MICROBUBBLE CONTRAST AGENTS

Signal enhancement during contrast echocardiography relies on the dynamic interaction of ultrasound pressure waves, with a highly compressible and expandable particle that is smaller in scale than the wavelength of ultrasound applied. As will be described later, particle expansion and compression during ultrasound pressure peaks and nadirs, respectively, produces volumetric oscillations of these particles, which is the primary source of ultrasound signal generation.[12–14] The rationale for using microbubbles, as ultrasound contrast agents is based on their compressibility/expandability, and on their in vivo stability. Air and high-molecular-weight gases that have been used in microbubble contrast agent preparations are several orders of magnitude more compressible than water or tissue. During most forms of clinical contrast echocardiography, contrast oscillation and the subsequent acoustic energy response occurs for particles that are resident within the vascular compartment of interest (e.g., the LV cavity or myocardial microcirculation).

The initial description of contrast enhancement by microbubbles was made by Gramiak and Shah, when a cloud of echo signals was detected in the right heart, coming from the formation of microbubbles formed by fluid dynamic forces during rapid, high-pressure intravenous injection of a water-soluble fluorophore used at the time for measurement of cardiac output during heart catheterization.[15] Over the ensuing years, several different forms of nonencapsulated microbubbles generated by hand agitation or low-frequency sonication were investigated, including for myocardial enhancement by MCE after intracoronary injection.[16–19] These techniques were limited by the wide range of microbubble sizes produced, the inability of most of these microbubbles to pass to the left heart after intravenous injection, and the potential for large bubbles to become entrapped within the microcirculation when given as an intra-arterial injection.

The safety, reproducibility, and widespread clinical feasibility of producing LV cavity and myocardial opacification with intravenous contrast administration microbubble contrast agents relied on the advent of small but stable and acoustically active microbubbles that are able to pass freely through pulmonary and systemic capillaries.[1] Many of these microbubble agents also have a relatively narrow size distribution (relatively monodisperse).[20] Those that do not, termed *polydisperse agents*, still contain relatively few microbubbles that are greater than the average functional capillary diameter of 5–7 μm when taking into account intraluminal projection of the glycocalyx.[21,22] The creation of these stable size-controlled microbubbles that produce a strong acoustic signal relied on two major modifications: (1) a change in the gases used for the microbubble core material, and (2) microbubble encapsulation.

A partial list of some of the microbubble contrast agents that are currently commercially produced, marketed, and used in patients are shown in Fig. 3.3. One of the common features of these agents is that the gas core is not composed of ambient atmospheric air components, which are for the most part nitrogen and oxygen. The reason for this compositional modification is based on mathematical models that have been used to predict the stability of a gas bubble. The rate of disappearance for a gas bubble in any given medium is dependent on the bubble size, the surface tension, and constants that describe the solubility and diffusion capacity of the gas in the bubble.[23] Accordingly, the stability of microbubble contrast agents used in humans is improved when they contain gases with low diffusion coefficients and low solubility in water or blood, which is described by the ratio of the amount of gas dissolved in the surrounding liquid to that in the gas phase, or the Ostwald coefficient.[24] These gases also must be inert, safe to use in humans, and cleared readily through respiration. These requirements are met in contemporary agents by using high-molecular-weight gases such as perfluorocarbons that remain in gas form at room and body temperature—for example, octafluoropropane (C_3F_8), decafluorobutane (C_4F_{10}), or sulfur hexafluoride (SF_6).

The encapsulation of the microbubbles represents a second common feature of contemporary contrast agents. On the most basic level, encapsulation with a "shell" composed of biocompatible materials such as protein (albumin) or lipid surfactants enhances in vivo stability by providing a barrier function that reduces outward diffusion of the gas core. Encapsulation also has an important role reducing surface tension of microbubbles, which allows tight control of microbubble size distribution, and both "on the shelf" and in vivo stability of small gas-filled particles. The use of air (mostly nitrogen) as the primary gas core component in microbubble contrast agents is still possible, provided encapsulation is performed with a relative thick and impermeable shell. However, first-generation contrast agents such as Albunex, which contained air and an

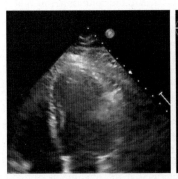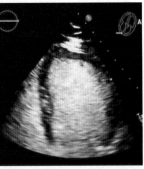

FIG. 3.1 Transthoracic echocardiography images in the apical four-chamber imaging plane in a patient illustrating poor endocardial definition in the non-contrast-enhanced study *(left)*, which improves with the intravenous administration of a stable encapsulated microbubble contrast agent *(right)*.

BOX 3.1 Clinical Scenarios or Conditions Where Left Ventricular Opacification Improves Diagnostic Yield

Detection of segmental wall motion abnormalities (rest or stress)
Quantification of LV ejection fraction
Quantification of LV volumes
Detection of LV or atrial thrombus
Detection and characterization of LV masses
Confirmation of the presence of apical hypertrophic cardiomyopathy
Evaluation of eosinophilic cardiomyopathy
Detection of ventricular pseudoaneurysms
Evaluation of ventricular noncompaction cardiomyopathy
Augmentation in Doppler signals
Detection of aortic thrombus or dissection

LV, Left ventricular.

albumin shell, still did not prove to be stable enough for reproducible LVO or for myocardial opacification, particularly in those with reduced cardiac output that result in long transit times from intravenous injection to systemic circulation, or in those receiving supplemental oxygen.[25,26] The problem of air diffusion can be solved by the use of even more impermeable "air-tight" shells composed of thick layers of biopolymers. However, this compositional modification results in relatively inflexible microbubbles that can only be imaged well with very high acoustic powers.[27]

The chemical nature and self-assembly of the components of the microbubble outer shell are heavily influenced by the gas composition and the process used to entrain gas into an encapsulated particle. For example, much of the albumin in the shell of microbubble agents is predicted to exist in a denatured form, owing to the temperature and pressure environment during manufacture. Because of the somewhat hydrophobic nature of perfluorocarbons, lipids in the microbubble shell arrange not as a bilayer configuration, as found in cell membranes, but rather as a monolayer configuration with inner orientation of the hydrocarbon residues.[20,28] In research studies, nanoparticle ultrasound contrast agents with lipid bilayer configuration or multilamellar membranes based on a core that is mostly aqueous have also been produced.[29–31] However, signal on conventional imaging has been low for these agents, due to the small amount of entrained gas.

Investigational Ultrasound Contrast Agents

There have been many investigational contrast agents that are not currently in routine clinical use that have been specially formulated for a unique diagnostic or therapeutic purpose (Box 3.2). One general direction has been to create nanoparticle contrast agents that are approximately an order of magnitude smaller than most conventionally produced microbubbles. There are several reasons for wanting to use submicron acoustically active nanoagents. Based on experience with liposomes, smaller lipid-based agents could have longer intravascular circulation times before removal by the reticulo-endothelial phagocytic organs.[31,32] Because of the inverse relationship between bubble size and its ideal resonant frequency (discussed later),[12,33] smaller microbubbles may also be advantageous with high-frequency ultrasound applications, such as intracardiac ultrasound, intravascular ultrasound, or small animal imaging. With regard to using microbubbles as therapeutic delivery vehicles, very small contrast agents may also potentially extravasate, especially in inflamed or ischemic tissues where endothelial permeability is increased. The major limitation of nanobubbles is their instability. Accordingly, most of the experience with these agents has been with agents such as the multilamellar nanoparticles or perfluorocarbon emulsion (mostly liquid phase) nanodroplets, discussed previously, that do not produce strong acoustic signals with conventional contrast imaging protocols and frequencies.

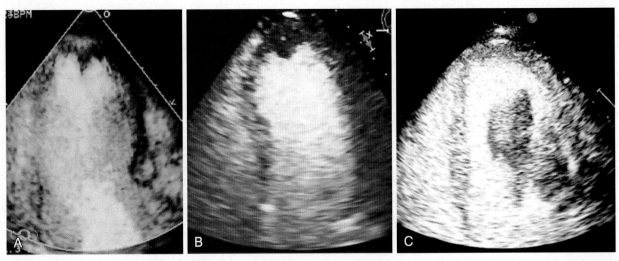

FIG. 3.2 Transthoracic contrast echocardiography images in the apical imaging planes from separate patients illustrating (A) a perfusion defect reflecting microvascular no-reflow in the anteroseptal territory after reperfused LAD infarction, (B) an apical thrombus, and (C) a large cardiac mass due to metastatic melanoma, which can be differentiated from thrombus by the presence of contrast reflecting a functional microcirculation.

Shell	Gas	Size	Proprietary Name
Lipid	C_3F_8	1-3 μm	Definity
	C_4F_{10}	2 μm	Sonazoid
	SF_6	2-3 μm	Sonovue/Lumason
	Air	2-3 μm	Levovist
Albumin	C_3F_8	2-4 μm	Optison
Polymer (PLGA)	PFC	2-3 μm	AI-700
Polymer/Albumin	Air	2-3 μm	Cardiosphere

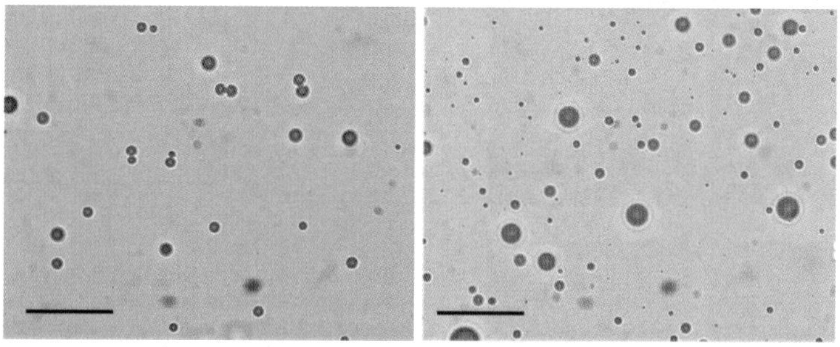

FIG. 3.3 Partial list of commercially produced microbubble contrast agents *(top)*, and light microscopy images of lipid-shelled perfluorocarbon contrast agents *(bottom)*, illustrating relatively monodisperse *(left)* and polydisperse *(right)* size distribution.

BOX 3.2 Potential Future Applications of Contrast Ultrasound in Cardiovascular Medicine

Molecular imaging (e.g., atherosclerosis, ischemic memory)
Acceleration of clot lysis (sonothrombolysis)
Acoustically targeted gene or drug delivery
Augmentation of tissue ablation with HIFU
Augmentation of tissue perfusion through shear pathways

HIFU, High-intensity focused ultrasound.

Some of the limitations of nanoparticle ultrasound contrast agents could potentially be solved by the creation of phase-shifting nanodroplets.[34] These encapsulated particles are an order of magnitude smaller in diameter than microbubbles, possess a condensed liquid-phase perfluorocarbon core, and require activation, whereby the diameter increases upon vaporization of the core to gas phase during the negative pressure phase of an acoustic field.[35] These agents have recently been shown to produce myocardial microvascular opacification. Their use could potentially create novel ways of performing quantitative flow imaging or for reducing far-field attenuation caused by high gas-phase concentration within the LV cavity.[36] Barriers to their use include the need to reproducibly convert from liquid to gas phase and to avoid large particles that lodge in the microcirculation.

There has been extensive investigation into the use of targeted microbubble contrast agents that can be employed for ultrasound-based molecular imaging.[37,38] The most common approach has been to conjugate binding ligands to the surface of lipid-shelled perfluorocarbon microbubbles using a molecular spacer that projects the ligand away from the bubble surface and that theoretically produces a lever arm that reduces the force necessary to achieve bubble ligation. Tens of thousands of ligands can be conjugated to the surface of each microbubble.[39] The most common approach to imaging these agents has been to perform ultrasound imaging 5–10 minutes after intravenous injection to detect retained microbubbles with minimal background signal from freely circulating microbubbles.[40] Since microbubble-based ultrasound contrast agents are confined within the vascular space, the biologic processes that have been targeted have generally involved events that occur at the blood pool-endothelial interface. Clinical areas of greatest interest in cardiovascular medicine include molecular imaging of tissue ischemia, vascular inflammation or atherosclerosis, thrombus formation, and angiogenesis.[38,41] Active research is also investigating how to improve microbubble adhesion through ligand, spacer arm, or microbubble shape modification, and novel ultrasound algorithms to detect the signal from retained microbubbles.

Novel microbubble agents have also been formulated for therapeutic purposes. Although a discussion of the full range of these agents is beyond the purview of this chapter, it is worth noting the ultrasound-facilitated delivery of genes has been augmented using cationic microbubbles to which cDNA can be charge-coupled, and by targeting these agents to the vascular endothelium.[42-44] Similarly, ultrasound-facilitated drug delivery has been augmented by microbubbles that are specifically designed to carry either lipophilic drugs that can be loaded into an oil rim in the microbubbles or in the lipid shell, or hydrophilic drugs placed directly or indirectly on the microbubble surface.[45]

MICROVASCULAR BEHAVIOR OF MICROBUBBLES

The rheology or vascular kinetics of conventional microbubble contrast agents in the microcirculation has been of great interest for safety consideration, understanding tissue-specific differences in the temporal changes in video intensity, and tracer kinetic modeling for perfusion imaging. There are several approaches that can be used to assess rheology. One approach to microbubble rheology has been to compare the transfer functions of microbubbles to that of technetium-labeled red blood cells (RBCs) through the myocardial microcirculation. To avoid confounding effects of recirculation and differential clearance from the blood pool, these studies were performed with intraarterial injections. These studies demonstrated similar first pass tracer kinetics for albumin microbubbles and RBCs through the myocardial circulation.[46] A different approach is to use intravital microscopy to directly visualize microbubbles within an intact microvascular network. This technique has demonstrated that microbubbles transit the microcirculation of normal muscle beds unimpeded, do not coalesce or aggregate, and have a similar velocity profile as RBCs in arterioles, venules, and capillaries.[47,48]

The safety issues related to rheology are based on the need to ensure that microbubbles do not lodge in the systemic microcirculation. After intravenous injection, the pulmonary circulation, which possesses capillaries

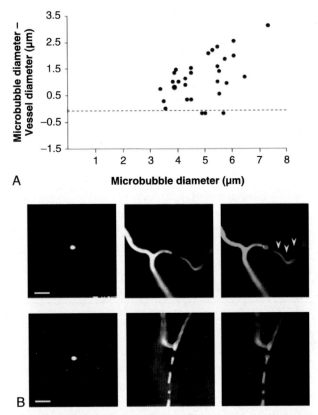

FIG. 3.4 Microbubble lodging in the microcirculation. (A) Example of the relationship between the diameter of microbubbles retained in a microvascular bed and the difference between the microbubble and vessel size illustrating size-dependent lodging. (B) Fluorescent microscopy illustrating lodged microbubbles (*left panels*), capillaries defined by fluorescent dextran (*middle panels*), and a merged image (*right panels*) with lower plasma volume (*arrows*) beyond the lodged bubble. (*From Kaufmann BA, Lankford M, Behm CZ, et al. High-resolution myocardial perfusion imaging in mice with high-frequency echocardiographic detection of a depot contrast agent. J Am Soc Echocardiogr. 2007;20(2):136–143.*)

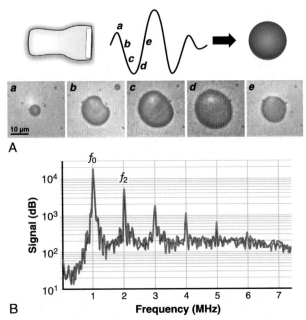

FIG. 3.5 Acoustic emission from volumetric oscillation of microbubbles during ultrasound imaging. (A) The microscopy images at the bottom obtained 330 ns apart illustrate microbubble volumetric compression and expansion that occurs during high- and low-pressure phases, respectively, represented schematically by the location of frames *a–e* on the acoustic pulse. (B) Frequency-amplitude histograms measured by passive cavitation detection with a broad-band hydrophone. Peaks at the fundamental (f_0) and second harmonic (f_2) are denoted. (*A, Microbubble images courtesy of M. Postema, A. Bouakaz, and N. de Jong, Erasmus University.*)

of a similar diameter as the heart, acts as a filter for microbubbles that are larger than average capillary diameter (~5 μm), thereby preventing systemic transit (Fig. 3.4).[49] There are potential exceptions to this process. One possibility is that the presence of any occult right-to-left shunting could result in systemic lodging. The extent of lodging is expected to be proportional to the number of larger microbubbles, and, accordingly, is of greater concern for agents with more polydisperse size ranges. Even for these agents, <1%–2% of microbubbles are of sufficient size to lodge, and microscopy has indicated that retention is often a transient event due to gradual deflation.[47] Nonetheless, the presence of a "significant" right-to-left shunt remains a contraindication to microbubble contrast agents, despite the recognition that approximately 20% of nonselected subjects referred for echocardiography have the presence of a patent foramen ovale, which has not resulted in any major events on large safety studies. In small animal models where pulmonary arteriovenous shunting is proportionally high (3%–8% of transpulmonary flow), passage of microbubbles sufficiently large to be trapped by the systemic circulation can occur and can be used to assess regional blood flow after clearance of microbubbles from the blood pool.[49]

Systemic lodging can also occur if microbubbles were to coalesce, aggregate, or enlarge after injection. The latter is possible from thermal increase in gas volume when bubbles are introduced to body temperature. This process has been noted for some experimental non-encapsulated microbubble contrast agents composed of mostly liquid emulsions with a low boiling point that can undergo uncontrolled increase in dimension after intravenous injection. For agents that are approved for use in humans, this problem has been resolved through the use of smaller molecular weight perfluorocarbon gases and bubble encapsulation. Another theoretical issue is rectified diffusion, where dissolved air in blood enters into a relatively nitrogen- or oxygen-free

microbubble according concentration gradient, particularly during the negative pressure phase of ultrasound, which produces bubble expansion. This phenomenon has not been detected to any degree during in vivo imaging. Fortunately, aggregation and coalescence in vivo also do not occur, due to the relatively low concentration of microbubbles diluted in blood.[47]

Although microbubbles that reach the systemic circulation have a similar rheology as RBCs in the normal coronary microcirculation, there are some exceptions that occur after microvascular injury. Microbubble clearance from the blood pool generally relies on the functions of the monocytic/phagocytic cells of reticuloendothelial organs. For many of the contrast agents, this process relies on opsonization, whereby serum complement mediates receptor-mediated uptake in cells, such as Kupffer cells of the liver.[50,51] In areas of vascular inflammation or postischemic injury, lipid microbubbles can adhere directly to the endothelium or to adherent leukocytes, which results in a microvascular retention.[52–56] Opsonization is amplified by the use of lipids in the microbubbles' shell that possess a strong negative charge which tends to amplify opsonization, and also with the absence of shell components such as polyethylene glycol, which provide steric hindrance to bubble-cell interaction.[54] With strong enough negative charge or with certain lipid components in the shell, microbubbles can even be retained within the normal microcirculation.[57] This phenomenon has not resulted in any safety concerns, but rather has been leveraged as a technique for detecting recent but resolved myocardial ischemia, which results in an increase in microbubble retention.[55]

Detection of Microbubble Ultrasound Signal

Microbubbles and other ultrasound contrast agents are effective because their size and deformability allow them to compress and expand in the sinusoidal pressure environment of an ultrasound field (Fig. 3.5). The degree of signal enhancement is related to the magnitude and type of microbubble oscillation about its equilibrium radius. There have been many different models that have been used to describe the determinants of bubble volumetric resonance.[33] The parent equation is the Rayleigh-Plesset equation, which describes the bubble dynamics according to pressures applied, surface tension, and boundary conditions.[23]

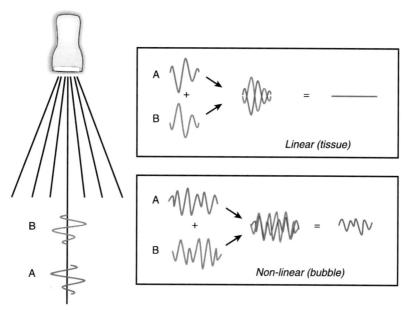

FIG. 3.6 Schematic depicting pulse-inversion contrast ultrasound imaging. Two or more sequential pulses (denoted as A and B) are transmitted for each line that are phase-inverted. The summation of the returning signals for tissue (a linear scatterer at low power) is eliminated, whereas a nonlinear microbubble signal is not.

One of the earliest applications of this model was to understand how bubble collapse contributes to the physical degradation of ship propellers. Ensuing descriptions of bubble oscillation in an acoustic field based on the parent equation were used to describe energy losses that occur from thermal damping (heat loss into the medium), viscous damping (work to produce resonance in a viscous medium), and radiation damping, part of which is manifest as sound emission.[12,33,58] These models were useful for defining how the magnitude of sound-producing oscillation is dependent on the compressibility and density of the gas core, the viscosity and density of the surrounding medium, the frequency and power of ultrasound applied, and microbubble radius. For encapsulated microbubbles, which are traditionally used as ultrasound contrast agents, viscoelastic damping from the shell is another important factor that influences bubble oscillation.[12,58,59] In practical terms, for any given ultrasound power and frequency, less oscillation and acoustic signal is generated from microbubbles that have thick, stiff shells. This concept has been confirmed by comparing the acoustic signal from microbubbles with different shell thickness in vitro and in vivo.[27,60] However, even microbubbles with extremely rigid shells can produce strong enhancement when imaging at sufficiently high power to release free gas bubbles through defects produced in the shell.

Resonant frequency is another important determinant of acoustic emission from ultrasound contrast agents. The ideal resonant frequency for a microbubble is inversely related to the square of its radius, and is influenced by the viscoelastic and compressive properties of the shell and gas.[12,33] When acoustic pressures at or near the resonant frequency are sufficiently high, nonlinear oscillation of microbubbles occurs, whereby microbubble size is not linearly related to the acoustic pressure and alternate compression and expansion are asymmetric.[13] It is this nonlinear behavior that produces unique acoustic signatures that can be used to selectively detect microbubble signals.

The first nonlinear acoustic response that is seen as ultrasound pressure is increased is the production of harmonics, where particularly strong signals are emitted not only at the frequency of ultrasound transmission (the fundamental frequency) but also at multiples (harmonics) of the fundamental frequency (see Fig. 3.5).[32] Despite the lower receive amplitude for harmonic peaks compared with fundamental signal, filtering all but harmonic signals can enhance the signal-to-noise ratio and relative microbubble signal during contrast imaging, since tissue produces relatively less harmonics.[61,62] With higher acoustic pressures, there is exaggerated microbubble oscillations, which leads to microbubble destruction by several mechanisms and transient release of free gas bubbles.[14,63] The degree of destruction depends on both the shell composition and the ultrasound power. "Power" on ultrasound systems is commonly displayed on

diagnostic imaging systems in relative pressure scale (dB) or the mechanical index (MI), which is directly proportional to the acoustic pressure (peak negative pressure in MPa) and is inversely proportional to the square root of the frequency. For most agents, nondestructive low-power MCE imaging is performed at an MI of 0.1–0.2, whereas purposeful destruction of microbubbles employed during MCE perfusion imaging is performed at an MI of >0.8.

Contrast-Specific Imaging Methods

Commercial ultrasound imaging systems have been modified to incorporate imaging protocols that are designed to specifically detect the nonlinear signals from microbubbles and to null fundamental and even harmonic signal from tissue.[1,64] Although now rarely performed, high-MI MCE perfusion methods produces the highest microbubble signal through inertial cavitation (microbubble destruction). When this occurs, filtering for signals at the harmonic frequency range can give strong microbubble signals. High-MI MCE perfusion, however, produces the greatest undesirable tissue signal. The high tissue signal has been addressed by filtering for signals between the harmonic peaks, which represents the broadband signal produced by microbubble destruction, or by offline digital subtraction of images void of microbubbles. Another approach has been to perform multipulse decorrelation algorithms (e.g., power Doppler imaging) that display rely on the "disappearance" of microbubbles from their destruction between subsequent pulses. Nonetheless, the technical difficulty of performing high-power MCE, which requires image acquisition with long interframe delays, has resulted in the adoption of low-MI "real-time" imaging techniques for imaging tissue perfusion.

When imaging at a low acoustic power (MI 0.1–0.3), harmonic signals are produced from nonlinear microbubble behavior with only a small amount of tissue signal. However, the microbubble signal is low so that it is necessary to use signal processing techniques that completely eliminate tissue to optimize contrast signal-to-noise ratio.[1,64] One approach is termed *pulse-inversion* or *phase-inversion* (Fig. 3.6). For each transmitted line, successive pulses are sent that are phase-inverted (phase-shifted by 180 degrees). At low MI, the mostly linear backscatter will return at the fundamental frequency and can be eliminated by summing the two phase-shifted signals. The nonlinear signal that comes from stable cavitation of microbubbles does not cancel by summation, and a signal is displayed according to the amplitude of this signal. Another approach is to use amplitude modulation (Fig. 3.7). With this technique, alternating pulses with either low or very low (termed *half-amplitude*) acoustic power are applied. Linear signals that return from tissue are similar in

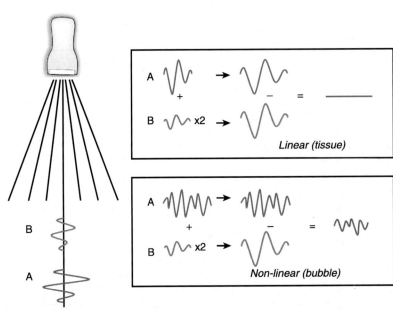

A

B

B

A

FIG. 3.7 Schematic depicting power-modulation imaging. Two or more sequential pulses (denoted as A and B) are transmitted for each line, which include a full-amplitude pulse at low power and a half-amplitude pulse (very low power). By doubling the returning signals from half-amplitude pulse and subtracting from those from the full amplitude pulse, tissue signal is eliminated, whereas microbubble signal is not.

phase and frequency for each pulse, and can be eliminated by doubling the half-amplitude signal and subtracting it from the low-power signal. Microbubbles stop producing nonlinear signals during the very low power (half-amplitude) pulse. Hence doubling the low-power linear signal will not result in complete cancellation of the signal. Some ultrasound systems have maximized microbubble signal to noise by combining both phase-inversion and amplitude modulation.

SAFETY OF MICROBUBBLE CONTRAST AGENTS

Microbubbles that are commercially produced and have been approved by regulatory authorities are among the safest contrast agents that are used for all forms of cardiovascular noninvasive imaging. The safety issues that are unique to microbubbles relate to three primary factors: (1) their microvascular behavior and likelihood for microvascular obstruction; (2) the physical and biochemical bioeffects from acoustic cavitation; and (3) interaction of microbubbles with components of the innate and adaptive immune processes of the body.

The issue of microvascular behavior has been described previously. Microbubble contrast agents that have been approved for human use lack the physical properties that lead to entrapment. Through encapsulation, microbubble size distribution is controlled so that capillary or precapillary lodging is minimized. Microbubbles do not aggregate in vivo, coalesce, or expand.[47] These properties are important for the use of microbubbles as flow tracers, but also to ensure there are no ischemic complications or increases in pulmonary artery systolic pressure from microvascular obstruction.[65-67] Even in patients with at least moderate preexisting pulmonary hypertension, full-dose administration of a polydisperse-sized microbubble agent does not increase pulmonary pressure or reduce pulmonary vascular resistance.[65] Because of concern with pulmonary vascular lodging concern, the experimental nonencapsulated microbubble agents with low boiling point gases (e.g., dodecafluoropentane) that can undergo uncontrolled increase in dimension have not been approved for use in humans. Similarly, phase-transition nanoparticles composed with large perfluorocarbons that undergo vaporization and intentional growth when insonified will need to be closely scrutinized for size control during any regulatory approval process.

Microbubble agents, or more precisely their shell components, interact with components of the immune system. Immune clearance by the reticuloendothelial organs, such as Kupffer cells of the liver or splenic monocytic cells, is one of the primary methods of clearance of microbubbles from the blood pool.[50,68] This process is recapitulated by circulating or peripherally activated/adherent leukocytes as well.[52,54] There

are several mechanisms that underlie microbubble interactions with phagocytic cells. Lipid-shelled microbubbles are opsonized through local activation of serum complement, which mediates microbubble attachment to leukocyte or sometimes activated endothelial cell complement receptors.[52] Lipid binding scavenger receptors (e.g., CD36, SR-A, Lox-1) could also potentially bind lipid microbubbles nonspecifically.[69] While albumin-shelled microbubbles can also be opsonized, the primary mechanism for interaction with immune cells appears to be mediated by specific integrins that are capable of binding denatured albumin.[52]

Because complement can be activated by microbubble shell components,[57] there is risk of non-IgE-mediated immune reactions, termed *pseudoanaphylaxis*. Experience with liposomal drugs provides knowledge that these reactions are lipid dose dependent.[70,71] Hence they are more likely to occur with microbubbles that have a large volume of incipient lipid, not in the form of microbubbles (e.g., micelles), that is coinjected. Fortunately, serious pseudoanaphylactic reactions are rare and have only been described with lipid not albumin-shelled microbubbles.[66,72,73] Approximately 1 of every 10,000 patients (0.01%) receiving ultrasound contrast materials will have a serious cardiopulmonary reaction. In a retrospective propensity-match population, hospital inpatients receiving ultrasound contrast agents during echocardiography were found to have a lower not higher mortality rate.[67] Postmarketing registries also further confirmed that there is no significant increase in death or serious adverse events in patients receiving these agents. Similar to what has been found with liposomes, administration of some lipid-shelled microbubbles can produce back or flank pain. This reaction is thought to be attributable to a mild form of complement-mediated microbubble attachment to glomerular endothelial cells, which does not produce renal ischemia but may activate pain receptors downstream from complement activation.[74]

The process of stable cavitation has not been associated with any biologic processes that would raise safety concerns. On the other hand, inertial cavitation, or abrupt microbubble disruption, can produce a variety of effects, including transient endothelial microporation, vascular permeability, cell activation manifest by increased intracellular calcium and endocytosis, and even petechial hemorrhage.[75,76] Several of these bioeffects have been leveraged for applying microbubbles as vehicles for targeted tissue delivery of therapeutic genes or drugs, or for the acceleration of clot lysis in acute thrombotic events.[42,45,77,78] Bioeffects are strongly dependent on the ultrasound amplitude (pressure), ultrasound frequency, and dose of microbubbles. Extensive safety studies performed in the course of regulatory approval and postmarketing studies in humans have not detected any evidence of tissue injury, troponin release, microvascular disruption, or inflammation produced during MCE, even when high MI imaging is performed. However, because there have been case reports of premature ventricular contractions during very high-power imaging,[79] the package inserts for some agents warn that safety has not been established at the highest MI range for clinical scanners.

Despite the established safety record of the approved microbubble contrast agents, in 2007 the US Food and Drug Administration mandated labeling revision, including a "black box" warning for serious cardiopulmonary adverse events in those receiving ultrasound contrast agents. This action was based on several life-threatening events out of >1 million doses administered that occurred in critically ill patients and that were not necessarily directly attributed to microbubble administration. Many of the safety studies mentioned previously were performed subsequent to this action and resulted in the easing of restrictions for ultrasound contrast use and for the need for hemodynamic monitoring. Currently, the only major contraindications to the use of ultrasound contrast agents are large intracardiac right-to-left shunts or previous hypersensitivity to the contrast agent or to blood products in the case of albumin-shelled agents. There are also warnings for the use of ultrasound contrast agents in subjects who are pregnant (Category C), lactating, or in the pediatric age range, based primarily on the lack of information rather than any specific safety concern. Small preliminary studies have suggested that microbubbles are safe to use in the general pediatric population.[80] There are also warnings against the use of commercially produced ultrasound contrast agents for intraarterial injection, although some agents have been used off-label for defining the perfusion territory of coronary arteries in the course of planning for alcohol septal ablation in patients with hypertrophic cardiomyopathy.[81]

Suggested Readings

Kaufmann, B. A., Wei, K., & Lindner, J. R. (2007). Contrast echocardiography. *Current Problems in Cardiology, 32*, 51–96.

Bhatia, V. K., & Senior, R. (2008). Contrast echocardiography: evidence for clinical use. *Journal of the American Society of Echocardiography, 21*, 409–416.

de Jong, N., Hoff, L., Skotland, T., & Bom, N. (1992). Absorption and scatter of encapsulated gas filled microspheres: theoretical considerations and some measurements. *Ultrasonics, 30*, 95–103.

Lindner, J. R. (2009). Molecular imaging of cardiovascular disease with contrast-enhanced ultrasonography. *Nat Rev Cardiol, 6*, 475–481.

A complete reference list can be found online at ExpertConsult.com.

4 Principles of Transesophageal Echocardiography

Douglas C. Shook

INTRODUCTION

Transesophageal echocardiography (TEE) is an additional and complementary method of obtaining ultrasound images of the heart and surrounding structures. A flexible TEE probe is introduced, via the mouth, into the esophagus of the patient. The tip of the TEE probe contains a miniaturized phased array transducer capable of producing imaging planes in a full 180-degree spectrum (multiplane imaging; Fig. 4.1A). TEE has all the imaging capabilities of transthoracic echocardiography (TTE), including two-dimensional (2D) and three-dimensional (3D) imaging, and color, spectral, and tissue Doppler. Most TEE images are obtained with the tip of the probe in the esophagus, with additional images obtained from the stomach (see Fig. 4.1B). Given the proximity of the esophagus to the heart, TEE can use much higher transmission frequencies, resulting in better image quality and spatial resolution compared to standard TTE imaging. This is especially true for posterior structures adjacent to the esophagus such as the left atrium, left atrial appendage, pulmonary veins, atrial septum, and left-sided valves. TEE is generally used as an adjunct or follow-up test to an initial TTE exam if additional information is sought or the TTE images are inconclusive. Table 4.1 summarizes the advantages and disadvantages of TTE versus TEE.

In 1999, the American Society of Echocardiography and the Society of Cardiovascular Anesthesiologists published guidelines for a comprehensive intraoperative TEE examination that consisted of 20 2D views.[1] In 2013, the TEE guidelines were updated to include 28 2D views.[2] The initial 20 views from the 1999 paper focused primarily on intraoperative imaging and decision making. The updated 2013 guidelines included additional views, such as imaging the left atrial appendage, that are obtained regularly in the nonoperative application of TEE. In addition, the guidelines also added 3D imaging and use of biplane imaging. 3D echocardiography is a valuable imaging modality that is particularly suited for TEE.[3–5]

INDICATIONS

Indications for TEE fall into two basic categories: diagnostic and procedural (Table 4.2). Diagnostic indications for TEE include the evaluation of cardiac and surrounding structures, where TTE is either nondiagnostic or will likely be nondiagnostic. Commonly this includes the evaluation of far field TTE structures that are in the near field for TEE imaging, given the probe location in the esophagus. Examples of this include imaging the left atrial appendage to rule out thrombus or plan suitability for percutaneous left atrial occlusion device placement.[6,7] In addition, TEE is used to evaluate cardiac valvular pathophysiology because its superior image quality often facilitates medical and surgical planning and decision making. Examples of this include planning of surgical or percutaneous valve interventions, evaluation of valve masses including infectious complications such as endocarditis, and evaluation of prosthetic valve dysfunction. It is not possible to review all the diagnostic indications for TEE, but given the invasive nature of the procedure, it is important that the findings sought should alter the medical or surgical management of the patient.

Procedural indications for TEE include both surgical and interventional evaluation and guidance. The utility of TEE for the evaluation and guidance of cardiac surgical procedures is recognized by cardiologists, anesthesiologists, and surgeons.[8–10] Recent practice guidelines describing the indications for perioperative imaging have been published by the American Society of Anesthesiologists and the Society of Cardiovascular Anesthesiologists.[11] TEE should be used in all open heart and thoracic aortic surgical procedures and should be considered in coronary artery bypass procedures. The objectives of the TEE exam include confirmation and/or refinement of the preoperative diagnosis, detecting new or unsuspected pathology, and assessing the results of the surgical intervention. TEE should also be used for transcatheter intracardiac procedures. TEE is especially useful for structural heart interventions such as atrial septal defect or patent foramen ovale closure, atrial appendage occlusion, and catheter-based valve repair or replacement. The utilization of TEE is equivocal for dysrhythmia treatment. In noncardiac surgery, TEE may be indicated when the surgery or the patient's condition might result in severe hemodynamic, pulmonary, or neurologic compromise. TEE is indicated during unexplained life-threatening circulatory instability that persists despite corrective therapy.

Appropriate use criteria for the ordering of echocardiographic examinations have been established to assist clinicians in determining when echocardiography is indicated for specific clinical scenarios.[12] The writing taskforce developed 202 indications for echocardiographic imaging. The proposed list of indications was not meant to be exhaustive. Specifically they evaluated 15 clinical indications for TEE for appropriateness. The criteria did not include intraoperative indications for TEE. Table 4.3 lists the 15 clinical indications and their appropriateness for TEE as an initial or supplemental test.

COMPLICATIONS

TEE is a semiinvasive procedure that carries potential risks to the patient. Because of the invasive nature of the exam, indications for TEE should be followed and best practice guidelines adhered to for every patient. Overall, TEE is a low-risk procedure, but complications have been reported for both diagnostic and interventional/intraoperative TEE. A review of the literature by Hiberath et al.[13] reported major TEE complications in 0.2%–0.5% of patients having nonoperative, diagnostic TEEs, with an estimated mortality less than 0.01%. TEE in patients under general anesthesia may carry some additional risk. Probe placement is not facilitated by the patient swallowing the probe; rather, the probe must be gently pushed into the esophagus. In addition, the patient cannot respond to painful stimuli, which may indicate possible injury during the exam. Despite these challenges, reported morbidity rates in the operative setting are similar to diagnostic TEEs ranging from 0.2% to 1.2%. The largest single-center intraoperative study to date was reported by Kallmeyer et al., with associated morbidity and mortality at 0.2% and 0%, respectively.[14] The sites of potential injury during a TEE exam include the oral cavity (dental/lip trauma), oropharyngeal (laceration, perforation), esophageal (laceration, perforation, false passage), and gastric locations (laceration, perforation, bleeding; Fig. 4.2).

Additional more rarely reported complications include cardiac arrhythmias such as atrial fibrillation or nonsustained ventricular tachycardia, which may be related to the comorbidities of the patient population, TEE procedure, or sedation-related complications during the case.[15,16] Complications in patients receiving sedation include hypoxia, unplanned need for endotracheal intubation, bronchospasm,

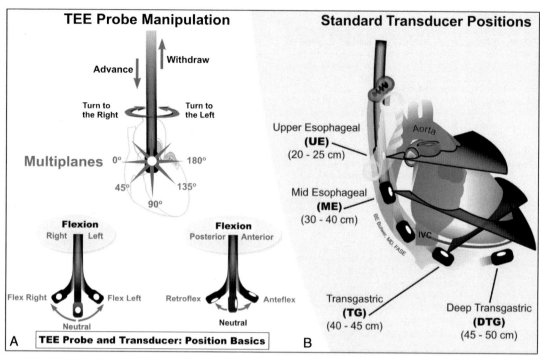

FIG. 4.1 (A) TEE probe manipulation, and (B) imaging levels during a standard exam. *TEE,* Transesophageal echocardiography. *(Courtesy of Bernard E. Bulwer, MD, FASE.)*

TABLE 4.1 Advantages and Disadvantages of Transesophageal Echocardiography Versus Transthoracic Echocardiography

ADVANTAGES	DISADVANTAGES
Useful in percutaneous and surgical procedures, as well as at the bedside	Semiinvasive—usually requires sedation, hence associated risks with probe intubation (gastrointestinal and pulmonary implications) and sedation effects (hypotension). Long procedures may necessitate general anesthesia. Generally a minimum of two staff members required: one operator and one person to monitor the sedation needed.
Higher resolution: better to definitively diagnose or characterize vegetations, thrombi, masses, intracardiac shunts. Superior imaging of valves, especially the mitral and aortic, left atrium, left ventricle, aorta and arch, and interatrial septum, as well as the pulmonary veins.	May not view the LV apex or right-sided structures well (structures that are further from probe, particularly in large patients).
"Continuous" acoustic window when compared with TTE (no ribs to cause shadowing).	"Blind spot" of acoustic shadowing where the trachea is interposed between the esophagus and heart. Much of the abdominal aorta is out of range.
Superior imaging of the mitral valve and mitral prostheses in general, with the ability to precisely localize valvular and paravalvular defects.	Mechanical aortic prostheses can cause excessive shadowing. May be technically difficult to achieve the best angle of insonation for interrogating aortic gradients (i.e., less reproducible for assessing aortic stenosis gradients). Maneuvers to increase or decrease preload may be more difficult (e.g., Valsalva maneuver), although most patients can cooperate. Real-time three-dimensional imaging and reconstruction dependent on a slow regular heart rate and "stable" window (i.e., still patient).

From Solomon SD, Wu J, Gillam L. Echocardiography. In: Mann DL, Zipes DP, Libby P, et al. eds. Braunwald's Heart Disease: A Textbook of Cardiovascular Medicine. *10th ed. Philadelphia: Elsevier; 2015:179–260.*

laryngospasm, or intolerance of the exam. Malposition of the endotracheal tube during intraoperative TEE was noted in 0.03% of the cases reported by Kallmeyer et al.[14] The absorption of ultrasound energy or heating of the TEE transducer during an exam could lead to thermal injury to the surrounding tissue.[17] This is particularly noticeable when using ultrasound intense imaging, such as live 3D imaging, from a singular window over a prolonged period of time. Most probes have a safety sensor designed to automatically shut off the transmission of ultrasound waves when the surrounding tissue is heated to a preset temperature threshold.

To reduce the risk of injury, each patient should be evaluated for relative or absolute contraindications to TEE on a case-by-case basis (Table 4.4).[11,13] Depending on the specific contraindication, a risk-benefit analysis should be discussed with the patient and involved clinicians to determine

the appropriateness of the procedure for the patient. Patients may require additional preprocedural workup, such as a referral to a gastroenterologist to better assess the risk of the procedure (e.g., history of dysphagia or upper gastrointestinal [GI] bleed). Potential procedural modifications in patients with relative contraindications include limiting either the length of the exam or confining the level of the exam to the midesophagus in patients with distal esophageal or gastric contraindications. The experienced echocardiographer can minimize the amount of probe manipulation during the procedure or choose a smaller probe such as a pediatric probe. If a patient has an absolute contraindication or a relative contraindication where the risks outweigh the benefits, an alternative imaging or diagnostic modality should be sought. Alternatives include cardiac computed tomography (CT) or magnetic resonance imaging (MRI) for diagnostic exams, and intracardiac ultrasound (ICE) or epiaortic ultrasound in the interventional

TABLE 4.2 Indications for TEE

INDICATION	EXAMPLES
1. Diagnostic TEE when TTE is nondiagnostic or likely will be nondiagnostic, and the findings will alter patient care management	• Evaluation of structures and abnormalities in the in the TTE far field such as the left atrial appendage • Prosthetic valves • Poor TEE windows • Valve endocarditis and paravalvular abscesses • Patients on ventilators
2. Perioperative TEE (cardiac and noncardiac surgery and critical care)	• All open heart procedures • All thoracic aortic procedures • Some coronary artery bypass graft surgeries • Some noncardiac operations when the surgery or suspected cardiac pathophysiology might result in hemodynamic, pulmonary, or neurologic compromise • All unexplained life-threatening circulatory instability that persists despite corrective therapy • Critical care patients when TEE information is expected to alter management
3. Interventional TEE	• Guiding percutaneous transcatheter procedures

Modified from Hahn RT, Abraham T, Adams MS, et al. Guidelines for performing a comprehensive transesophageal echocardiographic examination: recommendations from the American Society of Echocardiography and the Society of Cardiovascular Anesthesiologists. Anesth Analg. 2014;118(1):21–68.

suite or operating room, respectively.[18,19] Whenever a patient has suffered a potential complication related to a TEE procedure, such as blood noted on the probe after removal, a full workup is indicated to evaluate the possibility of injury anywhere from the mouth to the abdomen.

PATIENT MANAGEMENT

TEE probe placement is performed with either sedation for most diagnostic procedures or with general anesthesia for patients who are not candidates for sedation or are in the operating room or interventional suite. In either case, the patient must be consented for the procedure, fully reviewing the risks and benefits of the procedure and anesthetic technique. Patients receiving sedation should have their oropharynx topicalized with a local anesthetic prior to beginning the procedure. This facilitates introduction of the TEE probe and reduces the amount of sedation needed to keep the patient comfortable during the exam. Each institution must follow their local guidelines for the care of patients receiving sedation by either nonanesthesia personnel or involving an anesthesiologist during the procedure. Practice guidelines for sedation by nonanesthesia providers have been established by the American Society of Anesthesiologists.[20] Most patients are sedated with a short-acting benzodiazepine and/or opiate because of their synergistic effect for amnesia and comfort. Nonanesthesia providers should be trained to manage mild to moderate sedation (Table 4.5).[21] Patients at a moderate level of sedation have a purposeful response to verbal or tactile stimulation. Spontaneous respiration is typically adequate, without need for intervention, and hemodynamic support is rarely needed. Deep sedation must be immediately recognized and avoided by nonanesthesia providers. If a patient has multiple comorbidities and is deemed a poor candidate for mild to moderate sedation by a nonanesthesia provider, then an anesthesiologist needs to be consulted for administering sedation, including possible airway and/or hemodynamic management. Most procedures in the operating room and

TABLE 4.3 Suggested Appropriate Use Criteria for TEE

TEE AS INITIAL OR SUPPLEMENTAL TEST	INDICATION FOR EXAM	APPROPRIATE USE
General use	Use of TEE when there is a high likelihood of a nondiagnostic TTE due to patient characteristics or inadequate visualization of relevant structures	Yes
General use	Routine use of TEE when a diagnostic TTE is reasonably anticipated to resolve all diagnostic and management concerns	No
General use	Reevaluation of prior TEE finding for interval change (e.g., resolution of thrombus after anticoagulation, resolution of vegetation after antibiotic therapy) when a change in therapy is anticipated	Yes
General use	Surveillance of prior TEE finding for interval change (e.g., resolution of thrombus after anticoagulation, resolution of vegetation after antibiotic therapy) when no change in therapy is anticipated	No
General use	Guidance during percutaneous noncoronary cardiac interventions including but not limited to closure device placement, radiofrequency ablation, and percutaneous valve procedures	Yes
General use	Suspected acute aortic pathology including but not limited to dissection/transsection	Yes
General use	Routine assessment of pulmonary veins in an asymptomatic patient status post pulmonary vein isolation	No
Valvular disease	Evaluation of valvular structure and function to assess suitability for, and assist in planning of, an intervention	Yes
Valvular disease	To diagnose infective endocarditis with a low pretest probability (e.g., transient fever, known alternative source of infection, or negative blood cultures/atypical pathogen for endocarditis)	No
Valvular disease	To diagnose infective endocarditis with a moderate or high pretest probability (e.g., staph bacteremia, fungemia, prosthetic heart valve, or intracardiac device)	Yes
Embolic event	Evaluation for cardiovascular source of embolus with no identified noncardiac source	Yes
Embolic event	Evaluation for cardiovascular source of embolus with a previously identified noncardiac source	Uncertain
Embolic event	Evaluation for cardiovascular source of embolus with a known cardiac source in which a TEE would not change management	No
Atrial fibrillation/flutter	Evaluation to facilitate clinical decision making regarding anticoagulation, cardioversion, and/or radiofrequency ablation	Yes
Atrial fibrillation/flutter	Evaluation when a decision has been made to anticoagulate and not to perform cardioversion	No

Modified from American College of Cardiology Foundation Appropriate Use Criteria Task Force, American Society of Echocardiography, American Heart Association, et al: ACCF/ASE/AHA/ASNC/HFSA/HRS/SCAI/SCCM/SCCT/SCMR 2011 appropriate use criteria for echocardiography. A report of the American College of Cardiology Foundation Appropriate Use Criteria Task Force, American Society of Echocardiography, American Heart Association, American Society of Nuclear Cardiology, Heart Failure Society of America, Heart Rhythm Society, Society for Cardiovascular Angiography and Interventions, Society of Critical Care Medicine, Society of Cardiovascular Computed Tomography, Society for Cardiovascular Magnetic Resonance, American College of Chest Physicians. J Am Soc Echocardiogr 24(3):229–267, 2011.

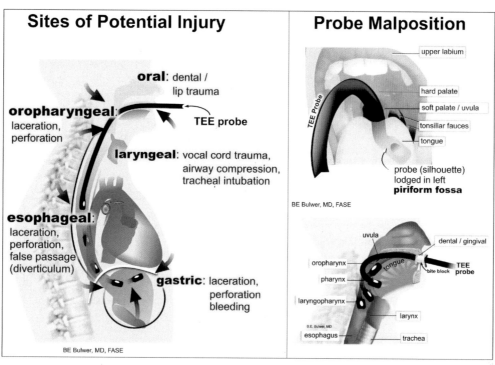

FIG. 4.2 Sites of potential injury from TEE probe insertion and manipulation during an exam. *TEE*, Transesophageal echocardiography. *(Courtesy of Bernard E. Bulwer, MD, FASE.)*

TABLE 4.4 Suggested Contraindications to TEE

ABSOLUTE	RELATIVE
Perforated viscous	Restricted cervical mobility (atlantoaxial joint disease, severe arthritis)
Esophageal stricture	Radiation to the chest
Esophageal trauma	Hiatal hernia
Esophageal tumor	GI surgery
Esophageal scleroderma	Recent upper GI bleed
Esophageal diverticulum	Esophagitis
Mallory-Weiss tear	Peptic ulcer disease
Active upper GI bleeding	Thoracoabdominal aneurysm
Recent upper GI surgery	Barrett's esophagus
Esophagectomy	Dysphagia
Esophagogastrectomy	Coagulopathy

TEE may be used in patients with absolute or relative contraindications if the benefits outweigh the risks provided appropriate precautions are applied and discussed with the patient and clinical providers.
Modified from Hilberath JN, Oakes DA, Shernan SK, et al. Safety of transesophageal echocardiography. J Am Soc Echocardiogr. 2010;23(11):1115–1127 quiz 1220–1221.

interventional suite that need TEE guidance require general anesthesia and the involvement of an anesthesiologist.

In a sedated patient, insertion of the TEE probe is usually performed with the patient in a left lateral decubitus position. The probe must be checked to ensure there are no physical defects noticeable and confirm it is not locked in a particular position, as this could induce injury. After placement of an oral bite block, the well-lubricated probe is gently advanced in the midline of oropharynx until it reaches the back of the hypopharynx. The patient should be awake enough to swallow upon command as the probe is gently advanced into the esophagus. Slight anteflexion of the probe and/or guidance with one or two fingers may be necessary to ensure proper probe placement. The probe should never be advanced if resistance is felt. Some patients may not be amenable to probe

placement with moderate sedation or have other risk factors, such as an increased oxygen requirement or hemodynamic instability, that precludes TEE with standard sedation. In these cases, an anesthesiologist should be consulted to assist with the procedure.

In the operating room or interventional suite, the patient is usually intubated and supine. The TEE probe is typically introduced from the head of the bed. It is important to confirm the patient is deeply anesthetized or has been paralyzed prior to probe placement, since a bite block is not used during placement of the probe. The bite block can push the tongue posteriorly, making placement much more difficult. The mouth is flexed open and the lubricated probe is gently advanced into patient's posterior pharynx, which can be facilitated by using one to two fingers of the opposite hand to guide the probe. Once the probe is in the posterior pharynx, the mandible is lifted anteriorly to help open the entrance to the upper esophagus. The probe should pass into the esophagus with very little resistance. If resistance is felt, the assistance of a laryngoscope or a video laryngoscope can help guide placement. A bite block is still used after the probe has been placed, to protect both the probe and the patient's mouth and teeth.

THE COMPREHENSIVE TEE EXAM

A comprehensive 28-view exam with a suggested image acquisition pathway is outlined in the most recent American Society of Echocardiography and Society of Cardiovascular Anesthesiologists guidelines from 2013.[2] The suggested 28 views form the basis for a comprehensive evaluation of cardiac structure and function (Figs. 4.3–4.6). The normal TEE exam is outlined in Videos 4.1–4.28. All the suggested views are not needed in every patient, so the exam should be tailored and prioritized per the pathophysiology of the patient. This is especially important in patients receiving sedation, as they may not be able to tolerate a prolonged examination. Additional nontraditional views, not included in the 28 standard, may also be necessary to fully characterize the patient's anatomy and pathophysiology. Multiple views of each cardiac structure, taken at different esophageal and gastric levels, should be obtained as part of the comprehensive examination (see Fig. 4.1). It is relatively common that undiagnosed anatomy or pathophysiology is learned during the examination that needs to be incorporated into the patient's medical or surgical/interventional decision-making process.[22,23]

38

PRINCIPLES OF ULTRASOUND AND INSTRUMENTATION

TABLE 4.5 Continuum of Depth of Sedation: Definition of General Anesthesia and Levels of Sedation/Analgesia[21]

	MINIMAL (ANXIOLYSIS)	MODERATE (CONSCIOUS SEDATION)	DEEP	GENERAL ANESTHESIA
Responsiveness	Normal response to verbal stimulation	Purposeful response to verbal or tactile stimulation	Purposeful response after repeated or painful stimulation	Unarousable, even with painful stimulation
Airway	Unaffected	No intervention required	Intervention may be required	Intervention often required
Spontaneous ventilation	Unaffected	Adequate	May be inadequate	Frequently inadequate
CV function	Unaffected	Usually maintained	Usually maintained	May be impaired

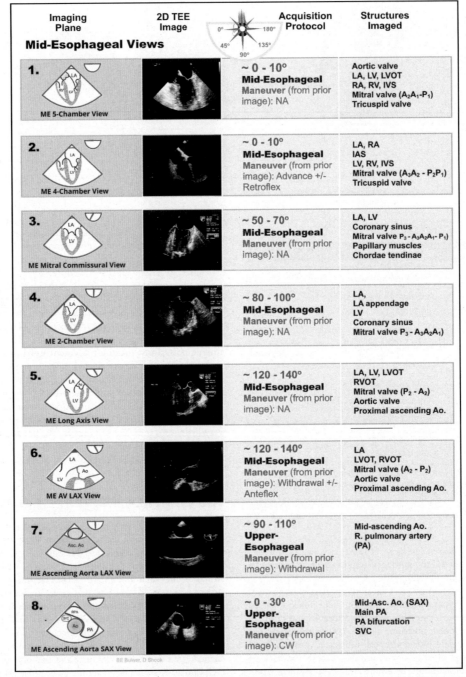

FIG. 4.3 The initial eight midesophageal views. Each view has an imaging plane, 2D TEE image, method of acquisition, which has a progression from the previous image using terminology from Fig. 4.1A, and the primary structures imaged. *Ao,* Aorta; *CW,* clockwise turning of the TEE probe; *IVS,* interventricular septum; *LA,* left atrium; *LAX,* long-axis; *LV,* left ventricle; *LVOT,* left ventricular outflow tract; *ME,* midesophageal; *PA,* pulmonary artery; *RA,* right atrium; *RV,* right ventricle; *RVOT,* right ventricular outflow tract; *SAX,* short-axis; *SVC,* superior vena cava. (*Courtesy of Bernard E. Bulwer, MD, FASE; Modified from Hahn RT, Abraham T, Adams MS, et al. Guidelines for performing a comprehensive transesophageal echocardiographic examination recommendations from the American Society of Echocardiography and the Society of Cardiovascular Anesthesiologists. Anesth Analg. 2014;118(1):21–68.*)

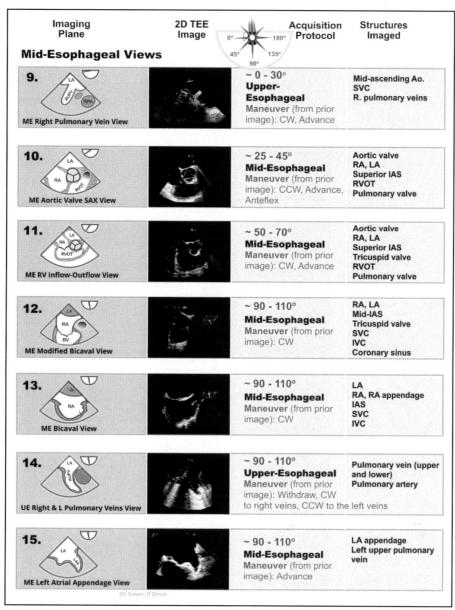

FIG. 4.4 Midesophageal views 9–15. Each view has an imaging plane, 2D TEE image, method of acquisition, which has a progression from the previous image using terminology from Fig. 4.1A, and the primary structures imaged. *Ao,* Aorta; *CCW,* counterclockwise turning of the TEE probe; *CW,* clockwise turning of the TEE probe; *IAS,* interatrial septum; *IVC,* inferior vena cava; *LA,* left atrium; *ME,* mid-esophageal; *RA,* right atrium; *RVOT,* right ventricular outflow tract; *SVC,* superior vena cava; *UE,* upper-esophageal. *(Courtesy of Bernard E. Bulwer, MD, FASE; Modified from Hahn RT, Abraham T, Adams MS, et al: Guidelines for performing a comprehensive transesophageal echocardiographic examination: recommendations from the American Society of Echocardiography and the Society of Cardiovascular Anesthesiologists. Anesth Analg. 2014;118(1):21–68.)*

The named 28 views typically describe anatomy that is present in the center of the image. For example, the midesophageal (ME) aortic valve short-axis (SAX) view has the aortic valve in the center of the screen in a SAX orientation. The simplest way to create this view is to start from the ME four-chamber view and withdraw the probe up the esophagus until the aortic valve is seen in the center of the screen. Then advance the angle of the ultrasound beam until the aortic valve is seen in short axis. This typically occurs between 25 and 45 degrees, but it is important to understand the relationship of the heart to the esophagus is different in every patient. The degree of ultrasound beam rotation needed to create the view is determined by the anatomy seen in the image and not the degree range noted in published literature. In some patients, the ME aortic valve SAX view may be obtained at 10 degrees, and in another patient, the same view is obtained at 90 degrees. The echocardiographer should have an advanced understanding of cardiac anatomy and apply this knowledge to the acquisition of TEE images. It is the anatomy of the heart that defines each image and not the suggested degrees of ultrasound beam rotation or suggested position of the probe.

MID- AND UPPER-ESOPHAGEAL IMAGING

Most echocardiographers begin at the ME level, as these views make up most of the images in the comprehensive exam (see Figs. 4.3 and 4.4). At the ME level, the esophagus is immediately posterior to the dome of left atrium. Therefore the left atrium is seen at the apex of the TEE image in all the ME views except for two, the ME ascending aorta long-axis (LAX) view and the ME ascending aorta SAX view. These two views are described at the ME level, but to obtain them, the probe needs to be withdrawn above the level of the left atrium. Each view is created by manipulating the TEE probe to center the structure of interest by either advancing or withdrawing the probe in the esophagus, anteflexing or retroflexing the tip of the probe, and flexing the tip of the probe to the left or right. Once the cardiac structure is centered in the screen, changing the angle of the ultrasound beam will create the additional views needed to complete the examination of that structure (Video 4.29). Each view should assess the 2D image and incorporate color-flow, spectral, and tissue Doppler as needed to give a comprehensive understanding of the

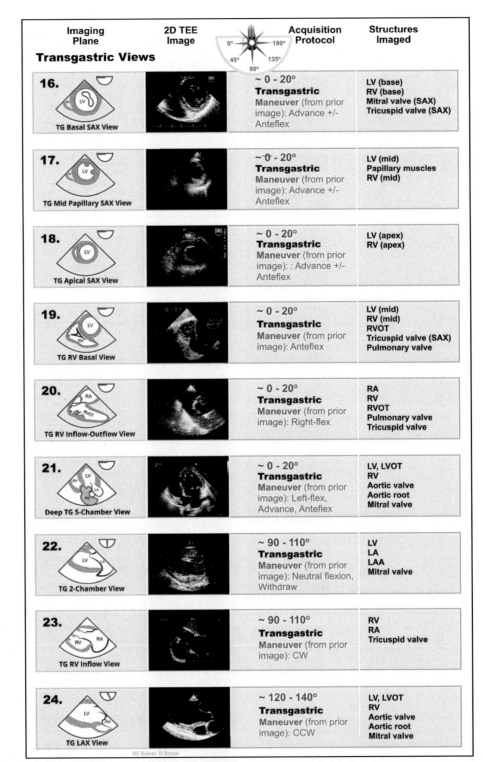

FIG. 4.5 Transgastric views 16–24. Each view has an imaging plane, 2D TEE image, method of acquisition, which has a progression from the previous image using terminology from Fig. 4.1A, and the primary structures imaged. *Ao*, Aorta; *CCW*, counterclockwise turning of the TEE probe; *CW*, clockwise turning of the TEE probe; *LA*, left atrium; *LAA*, left atrial appendage; *LAX*, long-axis; *LV*, left ventricle; *RA*, right atrium; *RV*, right ventricle; *RVOT*, right ventricular outflow tract; *SAX*, short-axis; *TG*, transgastric. *(Courtesy of Bernard E. Bulwer, MD, FASE; Modified from Hahn RT, Abraham T, Adams MS, et al: Guidelines for performing a comprehensive transesophageal echocardiographic examination: recommendations from the American Society of Echocardiography and the Society of Cardiovascular Anesthesiologists. Anesth Analg. 2014;118(1):21–68.)*

patient's pathophysiology. In addition, live and/or gated 3D imaging should also be incorporated as needed to round out the comprehensive examination (Fig. 4.7).

TRANSGASTRIC IMAGING

The probe is then advanced into the stomach to obtain the transgastric (TG) views (see Fig. 4.6). Most of these views complement the ME views

and provide additional information that cannot be obtained from the ME probe position. For example, parallel alignment of the Doppler beam for evaluation of flows across the left ventricular outflow tract and aortic valve can only be obtained from the TG probe level (deep TG 5-chamber and TG LAX views). The TG SAX views of the left ventricle complement the ME views of the left ventricle, because all the walls of the ventricle at a particular level can be viewed at the same time (basal septal, anterior, lateral, and inferior walls). In contrast, the ME views show all the levels of

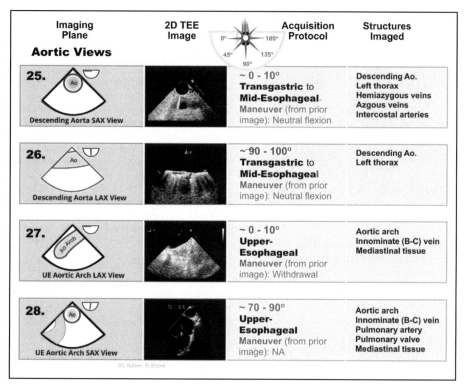

Imaging Plane	2D TEE Image	Acquisition Protocol	Structures Imaged
Aortic Views	0° — 180° / 45° — 135° / 90°		
25. Descending Aorta SAX View		~ 0 - 10° **Transgastric** to **Mid-Esophageal** Maneuver (from prior image): Neutral flexion	Descending Ao. Left thorax Hemiazygous veins Azgous veins Intercostal arteries
26. Descending Aorta LAX View		~ 90 - 100° **Transgastric** to **Mid-Esophageal** Maneuver (from prior image): Neutral flexion	Descending Ao. Left thorax
27. UE Aortic Arch LAX View		~ 0 - 10° **Upper-Esophageal** Maneuver (from prior image): Withdrawal	Aortic arch Innominate (B-C) vein Mediastinal tissue
28. UE Aortic Arch SAX View		~ 70 - 90° **Upper-Esophageal** Maneuver (from prior image): NA	Aortic arch Innominate (B-C) vein Pulmonary artery Pulmonary valve Mediastinal tissue

BE Bulwer, D Shook

FIG. 4.6 Aortic views 25–28. Each view has an imaging plane, 2D TEE image, method of acquisition, which has a progression from the previous image using terminology from Fig. 4.1A, and the primary structures imaged. *Ao,* Aorta; *LAX,* long-axis; *SAX,* short-axis; *UE,* upper-esophageal. *(Courtesy of Bernard E. Bulwer, MD, FASE; Modified from Hahn RT, Abraham T, Adams MS, et al: Guidelines for performing a comprehensive transesophageal echocardiographic examination: recommendations from the American Society of Echocardiography and the Society of Cardiovascular Anesthesiologists. Anesth Analg. 2014;118(1):21–68.)*

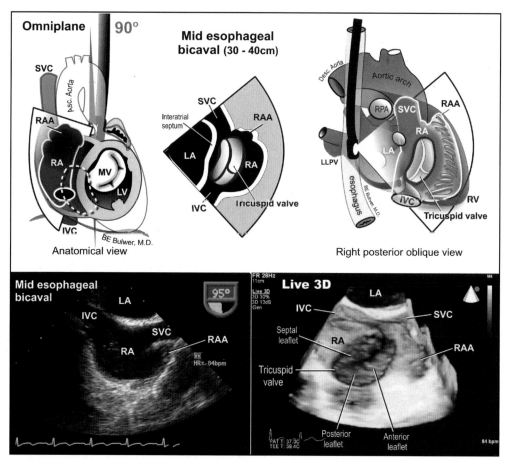

FIG. 4.7 Integrating transesophageal echocardiography probe position with anatomy and 2D and 3D imaging to form a complete exam. *IVC,* Inferior vena cava; *LA,* left atrium; *LV,* left ventricle; *RA,* right atrium; *SVC,* superior vena cava. *(Courtesy of Bernard E. Bulwer, MD, FASE.)*

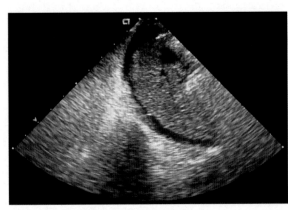

FIG. 4.8 Right pleural effusion.

a left ventricular wall (basal, mid, and apical) at the same time. In sedated patients, the TG views can be more uncomfortable, especially when significant probe flexion is needed to obtain the view, such as the deep TG five-chamber view.

THORACIC AORTA

As the probe is withdrawn from the stomach, the probe is turned to the patient's left to image the remaining aortic views to complete the comprehensive exam (see Fig. 4.7; Video 4.30). These views include the descending aorta SAX and LAX view. The left thorax is also imaged during probe withdrawal to evaluate for left pleural effusion. Once the probe reaches the arch, the upper esophageal aortic arch LAX and SAX views can be obtained. One additional view not included in this progression is imaging the right thorax for effusion or other pathology (Fig. 4.8). To accomplish this, the TEE probe is turned to the patient's right, past the right ventricle from the ME four-chamber view.

INTERVENTIONAL ECHOCARDIOGRAPHY

The scope and complexity of structural heart intervention continue to broaden. Just as intraoperative TEE guidance and decision making has become a standard indication for optimal operative outcomes, TEE imaging for structural heart disease has become a standard for successful intervention.[24,25] Percutaneous interventions in the cardiac catheterization lab that used to primarily include atrial and ventricular septal defect closure are now being performed on all chambers and valves of the heart. The need for precise, real-time adjunctive imaging is now paramount to the success of these procedures. The term *interventional echocardiography* represents the acknowledgment that the echocardiographer is now a coproceduralist in structural heart intervention.[26] Interventional TEE is used to guide and assess the progress and outcome of interventions in a real-time, continuous, and stepwise fashion. There is constant communication between the echocardiographer and interventionalist regarding anatomic structure and function, as well as to provide feedback regarding the progress of the procedure. All the modalities of TEE are integrated as part of the exam, including both 2D and 3D imaging. This evolving indication for TEE in patient care represents the ever-changing indications for advanced imaging that all echocardiographers need to remain prepared for as new technological advances are incorporated into daily practice.

CONCLUSION

TEE provides complementary and additional information regarding the anatomy and pathophysiology of the heart, great vessels, and thorax. It is a semiinvasive procedure that carries some risk to the patient due to the invasive nature of the exam and associated need for sedation or general anesthesia to perform the exam. When the indications for a TEE exam are met and a risk/benefit analysis discussed, TEE adds vital information for patient diagnosis, planning, and guidance of surgical/interventional procedures and outcomes.

Suggested Reading

American Society of Anesthesiologists and Society of Cardiovascular Anesthesiologists. (2010). Task Force on Transesophageal Echocardiography: practice guidelines for perioperative transesophageal echocardiography. An updated report by the American Society of Anesthesiologists and the Society of Cardiovascular Anesthesiologists Task Force on Transesophageal Echocardiography. *Anesthesiology, 112,* 1084–1096.

Hahn, R. T., Abraham, T., Adams, M. S., et al. (2014). Guidelines for performing a comprehensive transesophageal echocardiographic examination: recommendations from the American Society of Echocardiography and the Society of Cardiovascular Anesthesiologists. *Anesthesia and Analgesia, 118,* 21–68.

Hilberath, J. N., Oakes, D. A., Shernan, S. K., et al. (2010). Safety of transesophageal echocardiography. *Journal of the American Society of Echocardiography, 23,* 1115–1127; quiz 1220–1221.

Savage, R. M., Aronson, S., & Shernan, S. K. (Eds.). (2011). *Comprehensive Textbook of Perioperative Transesophageal Echocardiography* (2nd ed.). (pp. 487–565). Philadelphia: Lippincott Williams & Wilkins.

A complete reference list can be found online at ExpertConsult.com.

5 Principles of Three-Dimensional Ultrasound

Alexandra Goncalves, Denisa Muraru

INTRODUCTION

Since 1974, when the first three-dimensional echocardiography (3DE) images of the heart were obtained by Dekker and colleagues,[1] 3DE technology has greatly evolved. The development of the real-time volumetric acquisition technique, along with significant technological advances in computer and transducer technologies, have significantly improved the image quality and the practical feasibility of 3DE, allowing its implementation in clinical practice. 3DE data sets can be acquired from either transthoracic (TTE) or transesophageal (TEE) approach, allowing real-time visualization of the cardiac structures from any spatial point of view. 3DE has been demonstrated to be superior to two-dimensional echocardiography (2DE) in various clinical scenarios, such as (1) quantification of cardiac chamber volumes and function,(2) assessment of the mechanisms and severity of heart valve diseases, (3) evaluation of cardiac complex anatomy and defects in congenital valve diseases, and (4) patient selection and monitoring during cardiac interventional procedures (Boxes 5.1 and 5.2).[2] However, to take the best use of this technique, a full understanding of its technical principles, as well as of its strengths and limitations, is essential.

Fully Sampled Matrix Array Transducers

Considerable advancements in hardware and software, involving microelectronic techniques, image formation algorithms, and digital processing, have led to the development of fully sampled matrix array transducers, which enabled the volumetric 3DE acquisition with good imaging quality within a short acquisition time (Fig. 5.1). At present, matrix array transducers are composed of nearly 3000 piezoelectric elements (as opposed to only 128 elements in a conventional 2DE phased-array transducer), with operating frequencies ranging from 2 to 4 MHz for TTE and from 5 to 7 MHz and TEE imaging. The piezoelectric elements are arranged in rows and columns to form of a rectangular grid (i.e., matrix configuration), individually connected and simultaneously active (fully sampled). The electronically controlled phased firing of the piezoelectric elements enable to generate a scan line that propagates radially (y, axial direction) and can be steered both laterally (x, azimuthal direction) and in elevation (z, vertical direction) to acquire a pyramidal volumetric data set (see Fig. 5.1 A and B).

Currently matrix-array probes are available for both TTE and TEE imaging and, in addition to the conventional 2D-Doppler imaging, they enable three different acquisition modalities: multiplane 2DE imaging, real-time (or live) 3DE imaging, and multibeat ECG-gated 3DE imaging, all three with/without color flow information (Chapter 10, "3D Image Acquisition").

Previous 3DE equipment could only acquire and display in real-time volumetric data sets of a relatively small size (about 30° × 50°). These pyramids were sufficiently large to allow a partial display of the ventricles or of the valvular structures; the larger volumes needed to encompass the whole structure required at least four smaller component volumes acquired over a series of consecutive cardiac cycles to yield a 90° × 90° image (see Fig. 5.1C). However, the technology evolved and the current 3DE systems have the capability of acquiring and displaying single-beat volumes as 90° × 90° pyramids in real time (see Fig 5.1A), with improved temporal and spatial resolution (even though significantly lower than by multi-beat acquisition).

A major technological breakthrough that allowed manufacturers to develop fully sampled matrix array transducers was the electronics miniaturization and microbeamforming. Several miniaturized circuit boards have been incorporated into the matrix-array transducer, allowing partial beamforming to be performed in the transducer itself, reducing both power consumption and the size of the connecting cable. In addition, more advanced crystal manufacturing processes (such as the PureWave crystal technology), by increasing the efficiency of transduction and of conversion process between electrical power and ultrasound energy, helped reduce heat production.[3]

PHYSICS OF THREE-DIMENSIONAL ULTRASOUND

3DE is an ultrasound technique; consequently it is limited by the speed of ultrasound in human body tissues (~1540 m/s in myocardial tissue and blood).[4] The image depth determines the distance a single pulse has to travel backward and forward, resulting in the maximum number of pulses per second. The acquisition is performed by a pyramidal volume with the desired beam spacing in each dimension (spatial resolution), which is related to the volumes per second that can be imaged (temporal resolution). As a consequence, similarly to 2DE, there is an inverse relationship between temporal resolution, acquisition volume size, and spatial resolution, as represented in the equation:

$$\text{Volume rate (temporal resolution)} = \frac{1{,}540 \times \text{Number of parallel received beams (volume size)}}{2 \times \left(\dfrac{\text{volume width/}}{\text{lateral resolution}} \right)^{2} \times \text{Volume depth (spatial resolution)}}$$

According to the structure of interest and specific requirements, the volume rate can be augmented by decreasing the volume width or depth, or by increasing the number of parallel receiving beams (line density). However, decreasing the volume width or depth can limit the capability to acquire the whole structure of interest, and increasing the number of parallel receiving beams may adversely affect the signal-to-noise ratio and the image quality. Manufacturers have developed several approaches to overcome this issue, such as the development of multibeat ECG-gated acquisition, real-time zoom acquisition, and parallel receive beamforming.

Multibeat ECG-Gated Acquisition

This technique uses a number of ECG-gated subvolumes acquired from consecutive cardiac cycles (see Fig. 5.1C), stitched together in position and size, to increase the size of the pyramidal volume maintaining the volume rate (>30 Hz). Nevertheless, the pyramidal volume should be optimized to the smaller volume capable to encompass the cardiac structure of interest, for the highest spatial resolution. The main limitation of gated imaging is the occurrence of stitching artifacts, shown as subvolume malalignments in the pyramidal imaging, which may impede proper image interpretation or quantification. Those can occur by transducer movement, cardiac translation motion due to respiration, or change in cardiac cycle length (arrhythmias; Fig. 5.2 and Video 5.1).[5]

Real-Time Zoom Acquisition

Real-time zoom mode is ideal for the study of a restricted structure of interest, with high spatial and temporal resolution. The operator can adjust the area of acquisition with the minimum lateral and elevation width, and the ultrasound system automatically crops the adjacent structures to provide a real-time display of the structure of interest. If the structure of interest is large, the temporal resolution can be further increased by using a multibeat zoom acquisition. The main disadvantage of real-time zoom is the limited ability to show the anatomic relationships between the structure of interest and surrounding structures. However, it is of great use to study the mitral valve, particularly by TEE, and whenever a large ECG-gated acquisition is not feasible (arrhythmias, patient unable to breath hold, etc.; Fig. 5.3 and Videos 5.2 and 5.3).[6,7]

Parallel Receive Beamforming

Beamforming is a technique used to process signals so that directionally or spatially selected signals can be sent or received from sensor arrays. Parallel receive beamforming uses a high-end imaging engine, wherein the system

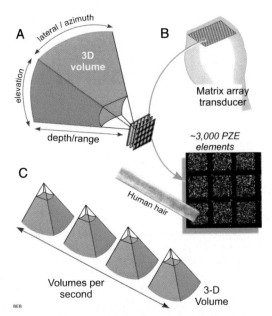

FIG. 5.1 The electronically controlled phased firing of the piezoelectric elements enable to generate a scan line that propagates radially (*y*, axial direction) and can be steered both laterally (*x*, azimuthal direction) and in elevation (*z*, vertical direction) to acquire a pyramidal volumetric data set (A), by fully sampled matrix array transducers (B). Volume pyramids can be acquired over a series of consecutive cardiac cycles, using a number of electrocardiogram-gated subvolumes (C). *(Courtesy of Bernard E. Bulwer, MD, FASE.)*

transmits one wide beam and receives multiple narrow beams in parallel, and requires a platform with higher volume/information rate. The transmit beamformer transmits timed pulses thousands of times per second, and the receive beamformer generates multiple beams through parallel and real-time processing of echo. The number of receive beams generated in parallel by the receive beamformer determines the maximum information rate the imaging system can achieve. In this way, the volume rate/temporal resolution ratio is increased by a factor equal to the number of received beams. Nevertheless, the finite speed of sound through tissue imposes a physical limit on the maximum number of pulses that can be fired per second, as it takes hundreds of microseconds for a round trip pulse to reach the deepest depth, and then to propagate back to the acoustic array. Conversely, the size of the volume, target volume rate, and lateral resolution determines the total number of beams needed per second. For example, to obtain a full volume (90° × 90°), 16-cm depth pyramidal volume at 25 volumes/s, the system needs to receive 100,000–200,000 beams/s, depending on the lateral resolution. Since the emission rate is around 5000 transmitted pulses, the system needs to form 20 to 40 beams in parallel for each transmit pulse, and even higher for real-time imaging of motion. However, there are limits to the increase in the number of parallel beams, since it leads to an increase in size, cost, and power consumption of the beamforming electronics, as well as deterioration of the signal-to-noise ratio and contrast resolution.[8] To overcome this problem, manufactures have been developing innovative technologies for beamforming, image forming, and processing (nSIGHT imaging, Philips Healthcare; XDclear and cSound, GE Healthcare; coherent volume formation, Siemens Healthcare; etc.), which allow us to increase the spatial resolution, clarity, and overall quality of the 3DE images, and to reduce noise.

Similar to what occurs with conventional 2DE imaging, the use of 3D color Doppler further impacts the spatial and temporal resolution of the 3DE images. The use of 3D color Doppler in real time is limited by lower frame rates and by the smaller volume size. Conversely, the multibeat 3D color full-volume can be affected by stitching artifacts. The TEE approach for 3D color acquisition provides higher spatial resolution and superior image quality than TTE. The limited spatial and temporal resolution of 3D color Doppler used to be a major limitation, but it has greatly improved with the advancing technology, and color Doppler volumes can be currently obtained with up to 40 voxels/s (Fig. 5.4 and Video 5.4).

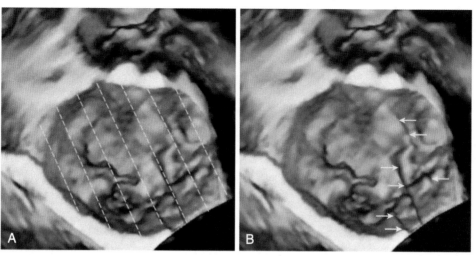

FIG. 5.2 Multibeat acquisition of the mitral valve by 3D TEE in a patient with P1 flail while breathing normally. Several stitching artifacts (B, *yellow arrows*) between the subvolumes (delimited by the white dashed lines in A) are shown.

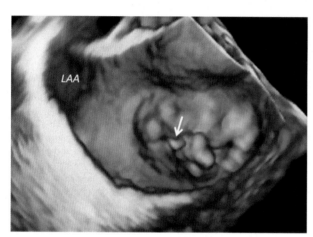

FIG. 5.3 Real-time 3D zoom acquisition of the mitral valve by 3D TEE in a patient with Barlow disease and P2 flail with ruptured chord *(arrow)*, in atrial fibrillation. *LAA*, Left atrial appendage.

Finally, the image quality of the 3DE data sets is also affected by the point spread function. The point spread function describes the imaging system response to a point input, which is represented as a single pixel. The degree of spreading (blurring) of any point object varies according to the dimension employed. In current 3DE systems, the degree of spreading (blurring) is around 0.5 mm in the axial (y) dimension, 2.5 mm in the lateral (x) dimension, and 3 mm in the elevation (z) dimension. As a result, higher resolution images should be expected when acquired using the axial dimension (i.e., parasternal views), rather than the elevation dimension (i.e., apical views), and when acquiring the structure of interest in the center of the pyramidal volume sector, rather than in an eccentric position.

As a consequence, to obtain effective 3DE images, it is pivotal that the appropriate acquisition window and modality are selected, and that acquisition settings are optimized according to the desired structure of interest.

DISPLAY OF THREE-DIMENSIONAL ECHOCARDIOGRAPHIC IMAGES

The 3DE graphic reproduction of cardiac structures on flat 2D monitors has been made possible using computer graphics techniques. Since the different structures (blood, pericardial fluid, air) within the heart have distinct physical properties and different abilities to reflect ultrasound, segmentation is performed by setting a threshold of echo intensity. Once segmented, the 3DE data set can be displayed using a series of rendering options: 2D tomographic slices, volume rendering, surface rendering, and wireframe rendering.

Two-Dimensional Echocardiography Tomographic Slices

The volumetric data set can be sliced or cropped to obtain multiple simultaneous 2D views of the same 3D structure. This method allows the observation of any cutting plan from any acoustic window, overcoming the limitations of conventional 2DE. The optimized cross-sectional planes of the heart provide accurate measurements of chamber dimensions and valve areas, as well as improved evaluation of the morphology and function.[9,10] This functionality can also be used at the time of image acquisition, because it allows the evaluation of several 2DE views simultaneously during the study; thus it can increase the quality of the data acquired. The current software tools for 3DE volume segmentation along the three axes (x, y, z) can be used in real time or during postprocessing for qualitative assessment, as well as for linear and area measurements.

Volume Rendering

This technique uses different types of algorithms to preserve all 3DE information and to project it onto 2D planes for manipulation and viewing.[11] These algorithms cast a light beam through the collected voxels; then the voxels are weighted to obtain a voxel gradient intensity that, integrated with different levels of opacification and shadowing, allow the structures to appear solid (i.e., tissue) or transparent (i.e., blood pool). In addition, a variety of shading techniques (distance shading, gray-level gradient coding, and texture shading) are used to generate a 3D display of the different depths of cardiac structures.[4] As opposed to 2D tomographic images, the tissue characterization is lost when displaying structures in the volume-rendered mode, in which various color shades depend exclusively on the depth of the structure relative to the cropping plane and of the total depth of the volume data set in which the structure is contained (i.e., higher color gradient for smaller volume depths). Volume rendering is commonly used to visualize cardiac anatomy—in particular the structures with complex morphology like heart valves, which require greater anatomical detail for clinically meaningful imaging (Fig. 5.5 and Video 5.5).

Since all the 3DE acquisitions are virtually pyramidal in shape, the display of inside structures requires cropping, which represents a process of virtual electronic "cutting" of one or more parts of the data set to remove the irrelevant cardiac tissues from the field of view. To reach the cardiac structure of interest, the cropping can be performed either during or after 3DE data set acquisition. The use of zoom acquisition practically eliminates the need for cropping. Specific tools for cropping have been

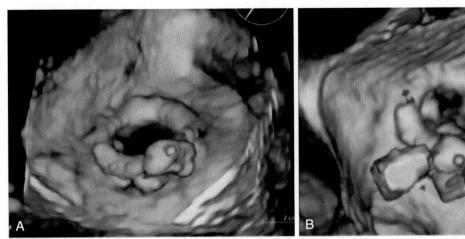

FIG. 5.4 3D TEE imaging of a mitral bioprosthesis after percutaneous periprosthetic leak closure using two vascular plugs (A) and 3DTEE color Doppler imaging showing multiple residual leaks between the devices (B).

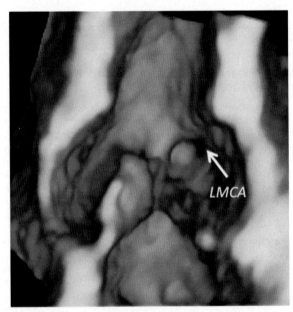

FIG. 5.5 3D TEE volume rendering of the aortic root, showing the crown-like insertion of the aortic cusps and the interleaflet triangle between the left and the non-coronary cusps, as well as the ostium of the left main coronary artery (LMCA, *arrow*).

implemented on the latest 3DE scanners, allowing an easier and faster 3DE image processing for clinical use. When the cropping is performed during the acquisition process, it provides data sets with better temporal and spatial resolution, but these will not be amenable to "uncropping" at a later stage. Uncropped images displaying the relationship between multiple anatomic structures may be also important for the data set orientation in the 3D space and for the identification of individual structures. The cropping can be performed in any plane, and the respective "cropping plane" can be rotated to visualize the structure of interest from any desired perspective, irrespective of its orientation and position within the heart. This provides exclusive images of cardiac anatomy, which may be difficult or impossible to obtain using conventional 2DE.

Surface Rendering

This type of display shows the surfaces of structures or organs in a solid appearance. It can be obtained by manual tracing and now also using semiautomatic border detection algorithms to trace the endocardium in cross-sectional images generated from the 3D data set segmentation.

These contours can be combined together to generate a 3D shape that can be visualized in detail as a solid or a wireframe object used to create a 3D perspective.[12] The combination of solid and wireframe

surface-rendering techniques can be useful to appreciate cardiac structure geometry and motion, such as right or left ventricular (LV) volume changes during the cardiac cycle.

Wireframe Rendering

This is the simplest of the available display techniques for 3DE. It identifies equidistant points on the surface of a 3D object obtained from manual tracing, or using semiautomatic border detection algorithms, to trace the endocardial contour in cross-sectional images. Finally, it connects these points using lines (wires) to create a mesh of small polygonal tiles. Smoothing algorithms are used to smooth angles and provide realistic appearances to the structures of interest. This rendering technique processes a relatively low amount of data, and it is used predominantly in relatively flat endocardial boundaries such as the cardiac chamber walls (Fig. 5.6 and Videos 5.6 and 5.7).

CLINICAL APPLICATIONS OF THREE-DIMENSIONAL ECHOCARDIOGRAPHY

Quantification of Cardiac Chambers

Conventional 2DE assessment of cardiac chamber size requires manual measurements of areas and linear dimensions to be performed in one or two tomographic planes of the respective chamber. Using various formulas (area-length, discs' summation, etc.) and geometric assumptions about the shape of the chamber (ellipsoid) and the relative position of the tomographic planes (orthogonal to each other and displaying the largest cavity dimension), these simple measures can be used to calculate the chamber volumes. However, all these geometric assumptions are rarely verified in practice. Cardiac chambers may assume different shapes in various pathologic conditions, and the recommended tomographic views on which the measurement should be obtained may be foreshortened and/or not representative of the overall chamber size/function. Small differences in probe position and rotation may lead to different measurements, especially in the case of complex-shaped chambers (i.e., right ventricle) or regional abnormalities. By conventional echocardiography, when the standard apical four-chamber and/or two-chamber views are not possible to obtain, the quantification of cardiac chambers is inherently limited and less accurate. Finally, manual measurements on still frames are affected by errors and by the operator's subjectivity in image selection and/or interpretation.

By virtue of its unique volumetric acquisition, the assessment of cardiac chamber volumes and function by 3DE requires no calculations or geometric assumptions, offering superior accuracy and reproducibility in comparison with conventional measures.[12] Provided that the cardiac chamber can be included completely within a pyramidal 3DE data set with an adequate image quality of the endocardium, there is virtually no constraint related to the use of a specific acoustic window with 3DE.

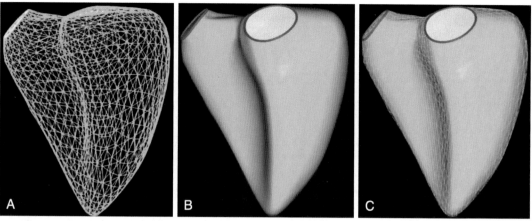

FIG. 5.6 Right ventricular 3D model ("beutel," cast) by 3D TTE, shown using wire-frame display (A); surface rendering (B); and combined wire-frame and surface-rendering display (C).

In addition, the multislice display of a 3DE data set (i.e., simultaneous 2DE tomographic views of several long and short axes of the cardiac chamber, which can be repositioned and reoriented after acquisition) enables a comprehensive analysis of the morphology and function of all myocardial segments, with no more oblique views or need of interpolation from few slices, covering a very limited portion of the myocardium. Finally, the possibility to acquire large volumes of the heart, including more than one chamber, opens new opportunities for the 3DE quantification of the functional interdependence among various cardiac structures, which would be impossible to evaluate from multiple tomographic planes dedicated for each structure.

On the other hand, the benefits of 3DE for cardiac chamber quantification come at the expense of few common limitations, such as (1) reliance on a good quality of the acoustic window; (2) patient cooperation for breath hold and regular rhythm; (3) lower spatial and temporal resolution than 2DE; (4) intervendor differences in software tools, algorithms, and measurements; and (5) reliance on operators' specific expertise in using various software tools and validating their measurements.

CLINICAL APPLICATIONS OF THREE-DIMENSIONAL ECHOCARDIOGRAPHY

Left Ventricular Structure and Function

The noninvasive calculation of global LV ejection fraction (EF) is one of the mainstays for echocardiography use. It has a vast impact on medical decisions, particularly when considering patients with heart failure or valvular heart disease. Using 3DE, LV volumes and EF have been generally assessed from multibeat full volume LV data sets obtained from several (4–7) consecutive heartbeats. This type of acquisition, however, can be affected by stitching artifacts in arrhythmic or uncooperative patients, thus limiting the wide clinical use of 3DE for LV quantification. Nowadays, large LV data sets can be obtained with acceptable temporal resolution from a single beat, and automated models based on segmentation algorithms and a priori knowledge have been developed. However, these models are not able to account for major structural changes, such as large LV aneurysms, mitral valve flail, or congenital defects. Systematic verification of the accuracy of the automated LV endocardial contour identification by software is mandatory, and manual corrections ("editing") should be applied whenever necessary.[13] From a single LV data set, in a few minutes, the LV geometry and function parameters (depending on the specific 3DE platform) that can be obtained simultaneously include global and segmental LV volumes, stroke volume, EF, shape (i.e., sphericity index), mass, regional and global systolic function analysis (longitudinal, circumferential, radial, and area strain, rotation, twist, torsion by 3D speckle tracking, 3DSTE), and synchronicity (systolic dyssynchrony index, SDI).[14] Besides the panel presenting the final results of LV measurements, the 3DE LV analysis also yields time–volume curves and various parametric

17-segment "bull's eye" displays of segmental and global LV function indices (Fig. 5.7 and Videos 5.8–5.10).

3DE imaging has clearly improved the accuracy in the evaluation of LV volumes, ejection fraction (EF), and wall motion analysis.[15] Multiple studies have demonstrated better accuracy and higher levels of agreement and reproducibility between the 3DE and other imaging techniques, such as radionuclide ventriculography and cardiac magnetic resonance (CMR), when compared with conventional 2DE methodology.[16,17] Several studies reported a significant underestimation of 3DE LV volumes, when compared with CMR,[17–19] which has been explained by the lower spatial resolution of 3DE in comparison with CMR,[15,18] adversely affecting its ability to differentiate between the myocardium and the trabeculae. Improved recognition of the trabeculae and papillary muscles (which should be included within the LV cavity for the measurement of LV volumes) and better agreement with CMR are likely to be obtained with 3DE software improvements, systematic methodology of assessment, and with the increasing use of high-performing automatic border detection algorithms.

LV mass calculations by M-mode and 2DE are subject to the same limitations in accuracy and reproducibility affecting the LV volume quantification.[12] 3DE may obviate the inaccurate geometric assumptions inherent to 2DE, which become exaggerated in remodeled ventricles.[20] Several comparative studies against CMR have demonstrated that 3DE is more reproducible and accurate than conventional echocardiographic methods in measuring LV mass,[21,22] despite some difficulties in the LV epicardial border tracing, particularly if incompletely visualized within the pyramidal data set in dilated ventricles. The LV mass measurement is now recommended to be performed by 3DE, especially in abnormally shaped ventricles or in individuals with asymmetric/localized LV hypertrophy.[20] Of note, the interpretation of LV hypertrophy from 3DE mass measurements should take into account dedicated normative values, specifically identified for 3DE.[23]

The LV sphericity index is a parameter reflecting LV shape, and it is obtained by dividing the 3DE LV end-diastolic volume to the volume of a sphere, the diameter of which equals the LV major end-diastolic long axis. As the LV becomes more globular (i.e., dilated cardiomyopathy), the LV sphericity index increases, approaching the value of 1. LV sphericity by 3DE was able to predict LV remodeling in patients with acute myocardial infarction, better than clinical, electrocardiographic, and echocardiographic parameters.[24]

The SDI[25] is defined as the standard deviation of time to minimal regional volume, expressed as a percentage of cardiac cycle duration and might be used as an additional tool for patients' selection for cardiac resynchronization therapy (CRT). Observational studies on SDI value in CRT patients showed its ability to predict response to CRT,[26] but notably different thresholds of abnormality, and measurement variability due to different technical factors and observers, have been reported.[27]

When compared with the 2D speckle tracking echocardiography (STE) method, 3DSTE saves time and is potentially more accurate and reproducible.[28,29] Since the speckles are tracked within a volumetric

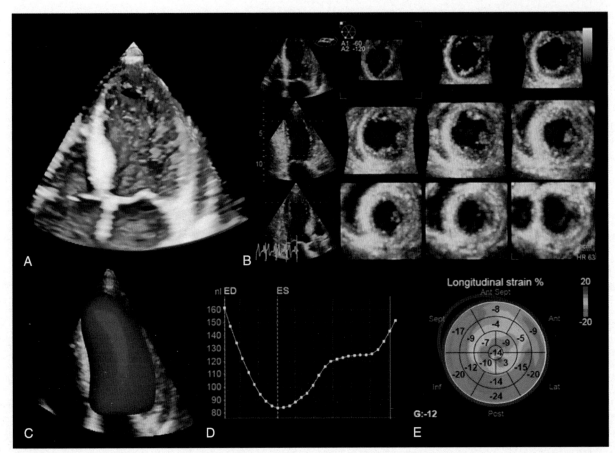

FIG. 5.7 Example of comprehensive left ventricular analysis by 3D TTE from a single multibeat acquisition in a patient with anterior myocardial infarction: anatomic 3D rendering for morphology analysis (A); multislice display for regional wall motion score analysis (B); surface-rendered left ventricular 3D model from which left ventricular volumes, ejection fraction, and shape (sphericity) are computed (C); curve displaying the left ventricular volume changes during the cardiac cycle (D); bull's-eye display of the 3D longitudinal strain values, showing impaired deformation in the apical and anterior segments of the left ventricle (E).

region of interest, 3DSTE is not affected by the through-plane motion of speckles, requires a lower temporal resolution of the data set than the 2DSTE method, and provides all LV strain parameters from the same apical LV data set. Area strain, integrating both longitudinal and circumferential deformation, represents a promising 3DSTE parameter of global and regional LV systolic function.[30–32] At the current stage of development, the use of 3DSTE is mainly limited for research purposes, due to insufficient evidence regarding its clinical added value, the intervendor differences of 3DSTE-derived LV strain measurements,[33] and the need for specific normative ranges.[9,34]

During stress echocardiography, 3DE is able to overcome some limitations of 2DE. Using the matrix array transducer, there is no need to change the transducer rotation during scanning, as two (for parasternal window) or three (for apical window) image planes can be visualized simultaneously and acquired at peak stress. Moreover, 3DE full volume acquisition provides shorter acquisition times, reduces operator dependence in image acquisition,[35] avoids foreshortening, and allows a higher detection rate of LV ischemia at the apex when compared with 2DE.[36–38] However, its lower temporal resolution may become insufficient at peak stress with dobutamine, yet not with dipyridamole infusion (which does not affect significantly the heart rate).[38] Along with further improvements in image quality and display, frame rate, and automated algorithms for LV regional function quantification, 3DE may assist in a more precise and objective approach for the evaluation of LV ischemia during stress echo in the near future.

Right Ventricular Structure and Function

Right ventricular (RV) function is an independent determinant of patient clinical status and prognosis in various disease states. Due to its complex anatomic shape, the accurate quantification of RV size and function by conventional echocardiography remains challenging. According to

current guidelines,[39] 3DE is recommended for assessing and monitoring RV size and function, due to its superior accuracy and reproducibility compared with 2DE. 3DE-derived EF is the only true global echocardiographic measure of RV systolic function, since all the other parameters (TAPSE, TDI S wave, fractional area change, longitudinal strain) are obtained from the RV inflow view only. Dedicated 3DE software for RV quantification enables RV volumes and ejection fraction measurement. It is based on volumetric semiautomatic endocardial border detection at end diastole and end systole.[40] The mainstream studies were performed using software that required manual tracing of RV endocardium in the different cut planes (i.e., sagittal, four-chamber, and coronal), obtained from the full-volume 3DE data set (Fig. 5.8 and Video 5.11). Recently, a more user-friendly, automated, and less time-consuming analysis tool has been commercially released to facilitate its clinical use.[41] The accuracy of 3DE for RV function measurement has been documented in patients with different pathologies (pulmonary hypertension, pulmonary regurgitation, secundum atrial septal defects, corrected tetralogy of Fallot, Ebstein anomaly, RV cardiomyopathy, etc.),[42] and normal reference range values for RV volumes and function have been described.[43] Despite optimal correlation with CMR and radionuclide ventriculography,[44] it has been reported that RV volumes by 3DE are underestimated in comparison with CMR RV volumes.[40,42,43] This is mainly due to the lower image spatial resolution of 3DE and the need for manual interpolation of difficult-to-see endocardial borders of RV outflow. The underestimation of volumes decreases when manual correction of automatically identified endocardial contours is performed, yet at the cost of an increase in the time required for analysis. The recent ASE/EACVI guidelines advocate for the use of 3DE for assessing the RV size and EF in clinical laboratories with appropriate equipment and expertise.[12] Seeing the recent improvements in imaging quality and in software algorithms, it is likely that 3DE will become the standard method for RV volume and EF quantification in clinical practice, similarly as for the LV.

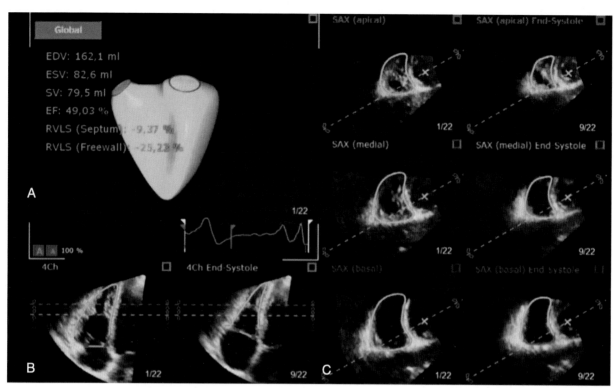

FIG. 5.8 Example of right ventricular quantitative analysis from a 3D TTE data set. A dedicated software enables to derive a 3D model of the right ventricle (A), based on automatic endocardial border detection, shown in different cut planes (short-axes at three different levels, B; four-chamber view, C), and tracking of these contours throughout the cardiac cycle. A shows the derived quantitative measurements from the 3D model. *EDV,* End-diastolic volume; *EF,* ejection fraction; *ESV,* end-systolic volume; *RVLS,* right ventricular longitudinal strain; *SV,* stroke-volume.

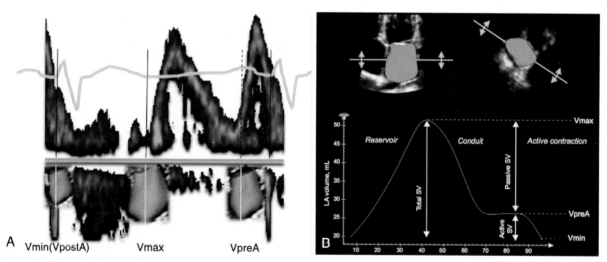

FIG. 5.9 Example of left atrial volumes and phasic function analysis from a 3D TTE data set. The timing of minimal, maximal, and pre-A volume measurements is shown superimposed on the ECG and Doppler mitral inflow trace (A). Semiautomated analysis of the left atrial volume changes throughout the cardiac cycle enables to evaluate the reservoir, the conduit, and the booster pump function (B).

Left and Right Atria

A growing interest has been recently dedicated to atrial cavities, due to their prognostic value in various cardiovascular conditions and the rapid development of cardiac electrophysiology interventional procedures. Current guidelines for cardiac chamber quantification using echocardiography recommend the calculation of atrial volumes using either the biplane discs' summation (by Simpson's rule) or the area-length algorithms.[2,12,46] However, both algorithms are heavily dependent on correct positioning and angulation of imaging planes, and on unverified geometric assumptions about atrial shape. As a result, 2DE significantly underestimates atrial size in comparison with volume measurements by cardiac computed tomography[47] and CMR.[48,49]

Since it does not imply any geometric assumption, 3DE provides a more accurate[50–54] and reproducible[55] measurement of atrial volumes than 2DE.[2] With 3DE, atrial volumes at multiple time points during the cardiac cycle are automatically calculated, and several atrial function parameters are provided in a time interval that is comparable with the time needed to obtain the maximal atrial volume with conventional 2DE (Fig. 5.9 and Video 5.12). Since 3DE atrial volumes are significantly larger than 2DE volumes, dedicated reference limits for each technique should be used when assessing LA/RA size and function.

LA volume assessment by 3DE offers an incremental capability to predict cardiovascular events[56,57] with respect to 2DE. There are recent data showing that both minimal LA volume[58–61] and total LA emptying

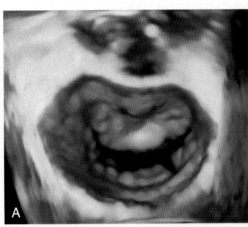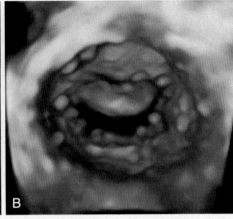

FIG. 5.10 Mitral valve rendering by 3D TEE displayed from the left atrial perspective ("surgical view," A) and from the left ventricular perspective (B). Note the presence of a small indentation ("cleft") between the P2 and P3 scallops, which is best appreciated from the surgical view.

fraction by 3DE[59,62–64] have incremental prognostic power over LA maximal volume. In patients with rheumatic mitral stenosis, a more spherical LA shape, as assessed by 3DE, was independently associated with an increased risk for embolic cerebrovascular events, adding incremental value in predicting events beyond that provided by age and LA function.[64]

RA size is a predictor of outcome in pulmonary hypertension, in Eisenmenger syndrome, and in chronic systolic heart failure.[65] RA volumes obtained with 3DE were demonstrated to be larger compared with 2DE-derived volumes,[66] similar to RA volumes obtained with CMR[53] and smaller than those obtained by CT.[67] The poor correlation between 2DE and 3DE RA volumes underlies the limitations of 2DE related to geometric assumptions and foreshortening,[68] as demonstrated for the other cardiac chambers. RA volume index by 3DE allows for the identification of high RA pressure in patients with acutely decompensated heart failure.[69] Thus 3DE has the potential to become the primary technique to assess the atrial size and function in clinical practice.

Valvular Heart Disease

3DE is an important clinical tool in the assessment of valvular heart disease, and it has been demonstrated to be superior to 2DE in a variety of scenarios. The ability to orientate a structure from the axial direction of the beam allows new perspectives of the valvular structures, on its face view ("surgeon's view") and on its ventricular view, and provides a better understanding of the morphology and spatial relation among the intracardiac structures. This was shown to improve the diagnostic confidence and the communication between the heart team, during clinical decision making for mitral valve repair, for selecting patients for percutaneous interventions, and during the effective performance of these procedures.[70,71] 3DE main limitations in the assessment of valvular heart disease result from the limited temporal resolution (10–20 volumes/s). A higher frame rate can be achieved when the image is acquired with several heartbeats, but relying on assumptions of periodicity of heart motion from beat to beat limits its applicability in patients with variable R-R intervals. Future advances in 3DE may allow wider angle acquisition and color flow imaging to be completed in a single cardiac cycle, and potentially the measurement of flow dynamics in an automated fashion.

Mitral Valve

The mitral apparatus is a complex dynamic structure formed by the mitral annulus, leaflets, commissures, and subvalvular apparatus, composed of the chordae tendineae, papillary muscles, and LV wall attachments. 3DE has the ability to represent in detail those structures, enabling both LV perspective and the generation of the "surgeon's views," facilitating the progress of anatomic and functional interpretation, with high accuracy for precise location of abnormal MV segments and recognition of prolapse, flail leaflet, or chordae rupture (Fig. 5.10 and Videos 5.13 and

5.14).[71] 3D TEE is superior to 2D TEE for diagnosing the location and the extent of complex MV disease, either of degenerative or ischemic aetiology.[72] Moreover, it improves the diagnostic confidence for selecting patients for percutaneous interventions, such as the MitraClip, and improves the communication between the heart team during the performance of invasive procedures. Particularly, during MitraClip deployment, 3D TEE facilitates the best alignment for septum puncturing, for A2P2 mitral leaflets gasping,[73] and for the immediate assessment of complications.[70,74] Similarly, during balloon mitral valvotomy, 3DE improves the visualization of mitral valvular and subvalvular apparatus from the ventricular perspective, providing a detailed anatomic evaluation of the leaflets motion, chordae and mitral commissures shortening and fusion, and papillary muscles fibrosis or rupture.[75]

Furthermore, 3DE provides tools for the evaluation of mitral stenosis and mitral regurgitation that overcome some 2DE limitations.[76] The evaluation of mitral stenosis traditionally depended on mitral transvalvular gradient and mitral valve area, estimated by pressure half-time, proximal isovelocity surface area (PISA), or 2DE direct valve planimetry. However, 3DE is currently suggested as the new standard for mitral valve area quantification.[77,78] When using 3DE, any orientation of the cardiac structures can be achieved, and independently of the stenotic valve opening angle, the optimal plane of the smallest mitral valve orifice can be obtained. When compared with 2DE, this methodology showed better agreement with the mitral orifice area calculations derived from the Gorlin formula.

Considering mitral regurgitation, 3DE has shown that the true proximal flow convergence region (vena contracta) is generally more hemielliptical than hemispheric, and that erroneous assumption of spherical PISA, obtained from 2DE, underestimates mitral regurgitation severity.[79,80] These data result from the ability to manipulate the cut planes (x, y, and z) through the data set, creating four-chamber and two-chamber views and cropping the image plane perpendicularly, orientated to the narrowest cross-sectional area of the jet in en face view.[2] At this point, the regurgitant orifice can be measured by manual planimetry of the color Doppler signal, even if the jet has an eccentric position. This method has demonstrated special usefulness in functional mitral regurgitation and complex mitral regurgitant flows, for which severity is usually underestimated by 2DE,[81] and an excellent correlation between 3D anatomic EROA-derived regurgitant volume and mitral regurgitant volume calculated by CMR was found.[82] In addition, dedicated automatic software for visualization and effective regurgitant orifice area (EROA) calculation has been developed (Siemens Medical Solutions).[83,84] The operator initializes the analysis by setting the location of the jet and valve coaptation point and after specifying the desired isovelocity value and the direction of interest, which is followed by fully automatic segmentation of the valve annulus and isovelocity surface area computation (Fig. 5.11). In vitro and in vivo experiments established the accuracy of this method in measuring surface area, EROA, and regurgitant flow.[84,85] A subsequent study highlighted that 3D PISA analysis reclassifies the severity of the MR, and specific cutoffs should be further established for the 3D assessment of MR severity.[86] 3D TTE and TEE are now recommended

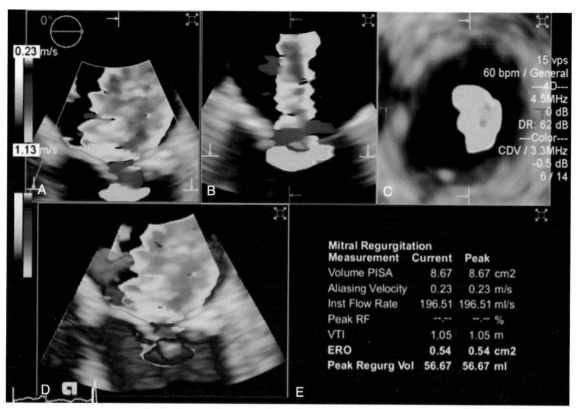

FIG. 5.11 3D TEE semiautomatic recognition and measurement of three-dimensional proximal isovelocity surface area in mitral regurgitation. (A) 4—chambers/sagittal view; (B) 2—chambers/coronal view; (C) short-axis/axial view; (D) three-dimensional view of the mitral regurgitation flow; (E) effective regurgitant orifice area and regurgitant flow quantification.

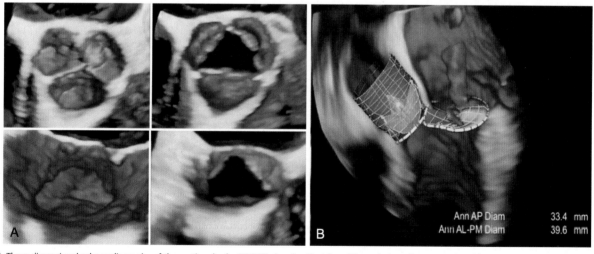

FIG. 5.12 Three-dimensional echocardiography of the aortic valve by 3D TEE, showing the tricuspid morphology (best appreciated from the aortic root perspective, A, *upper images*) with irregular thickening of the cusps due to calcifications, as well as the ellipsoidal shape of the aortic annulus (best appreciated from the ventricular perspective, A, *lower images*). Using dedicated software, automated quantification of both aortic and mitral valve annulus and leaflet geometry can be obtained (B).

for the interpretation of mitral valve disease in routine clinical practice, and 3D TEE is recommended for guidance of interventional mitral valve procedures.

The 3DE valve models, developed from TEE acquisitions, provide detailed data of the mitral valve anatomy, including measurements of size, shape, degree of nonplanarity of the MV annulus, mitral leaflet surface area, and prolapse height. However, the first models were time-consuming and required significant expertise.[70] Recently, dedicated software for quantification has been developed, providing automated measurements for the aortic and mitral valve in seconds, along with modeling and measuring of the valves over time (i.e., the diameter of the mitral valve annulus variation throughout the cardiac cycle; Fig. 5.12 and Videos 5.15 and 5.16). Thus far its clinical use is still being explored.

Aortic Valve

The analysis of the aortic valve using echocardiography can be challenging, as it usually presents thin leaflets and the imaging is obtained with an oblique angle of incidence of the ultrasound. However, 3DE provides incremental value over 2DE in the assessment of aortic valve morphology,[87] in providing data on the spatial relationship with the surrounding structures, and it allows en face alignment of the cut plane of the aortic annulus orifice, irrespective of the spatial orientation of the aortic root in the body. This alignment might be impossible to obtain in 2DE short-axis view, particularly in the presence of aortic root pathology or in horizontally positioned hearts.

After image acquisition, the use of the MPR provides tools for the perfect orthogonal alignment of the LV outflow tract and the aortic

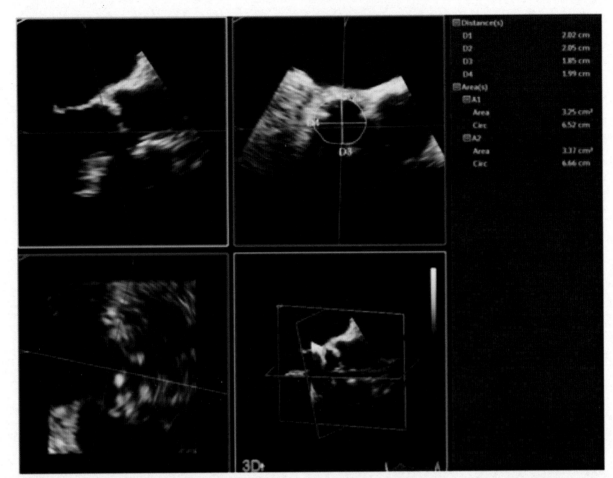

FIG. 5.13 3D TEE measurement of the diameter, area, and perimeter of aortic annulus, using the multiplanar tools for perfect orthogonal alignment.

annulus; as a consequence, its diameter and area can be precisely measured (Fig. 5.13). Images obtained in this way have shown that the LV outflow tract is mostly elliptical and not circular, and that estimation of the LV outflow tract area from the 2DE parasternal long-axis view often underestimates the true area.[88] As a result, by avoiding assumptions in the continuity equation, 3DE aortic valve areas have a better correlation to invasively measured aortic valve area and improved accuracy and reproducibility, compared with 2D TEE values.[89] Other alternative to avoid errors in the calculation of aortic valve area by the continuity equation is to use stroke volume data from 3DE semiautomated LV endocardial border detection.[89] Likewise, the aortic annulus is mostly elliptical, and its precise measurement is crucial for prosthesis size selection in patients referred to transcatheter aortic valve implantation (TAVR).[70] 3DE with the use of multiplanar (MPR) tools presents the real short-axis view of the annulus, allowing the measurement of its area by planimetry and its larger and shorter diameters, reducing the potential error occurring from 2DE circularity assumption.[90] During TAVR, 3DTEE can assist in guiding the procedure and in the assessment of complications (see "Echocardiography in Context of Percutaneous Valve Repair/Replacement" for details).

Aortic regurgitation evaluation can be performed by 3DE vena contracta planimetry, using the MPR tools previously described for mitral regurgitation evaluation. This method does not make assumptions of geometry, improves precision, and had a good correlation with aortic regurgitation severity measurement by aortography and with CMR.[91,92] However, up to now, in absence of more substantial clinical data, the aortic regurgitation assessment should follow the principle of comprehensive evaluation and integrated approach.[93]

Tricuspid Valve

3DE allows the visualization of tricuspid valve (TV) leaflets and apparatus, chordae tendineae, papillary muscles, and moderator band, from any perspective, improving its morphologic evaluation.[94] The TV can be

visualized either from the right atrial or RV perspective. These views may be especially helpful in localizing leaflet disease such as leaflet prolapse, perforation, or vegetation, as well as localizing the origin of regurgitation jets, or planimetering the tricuspid orifice area in case of tricuspid stenosis.[94,95]

3DE has shown that the tricuspid annulus is less nonplanar compared with the mitral annulus, and presents a round or oval shape.[96] It has a saddle shape with higher points toward the right atrium, along the anterior and posterior sectors of the annulus, and inferior points, in the direction of the RV, at the medial and lateral sectors of the annulus. The unique possibility of evaluating the distinct shape of the TV annulus may have implications for the innovative design of tricuspid annuloplasty rings, which are mostly planar at this point.

Moreover, 3DE measurements of the tricuspid annulus are accurate compared with CMR imaging and may have important implications in the surgical decision-making processes.[97] Using dedicated software for TV analysis from 3DE data sets allows the semiautomated quantitative analysis of TV annulus area and diameters, annular nonplanarity, and leaflet tenting. Software-generated reconstruction of TV annulus and leaflets can be used to obtain a 3D printed model of the TV with highly conserved fidelity.[98] The prospects for applications of 3D printing in transcatheter interventional TV procedures and presurgical planning for challenging cases are particularly attractive.[99] The automated tracking of TV geometry parameters throughout the cardiac cycle provides novel insights into the normal tricuspid annulus dynamics and the pathophysiology of functional tricuspid regurgitation (Fig. 5.14 and Videos 5.17 and 5.18).

In addition, the concepts of 3DE color flow might be applied to tricuspid regurgitation assessment. The feasibility for obtaining the area of vena contracta from the tricuspid regurgitant jet has already been established,[100] the area of the vena contracta obtained by 3DE and its width measured by 2DE correlate poorly.[101] These data support the concept that the vena contracta of the regurgitant tricuspid jet has a complex geometry and deserves future studies within the technical advances of 3DE capabilities.

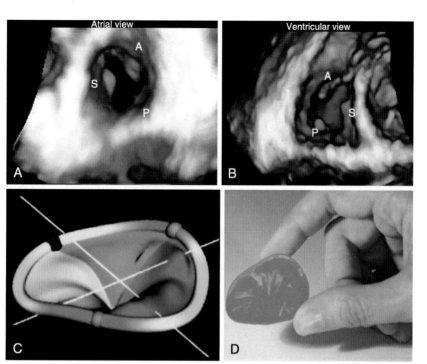

FIG. 5.14 Qualitative and quantitative analysis of a normal tricuspid valve from a 3D TTE data set. (A and B) show the anatomy of the tricuspid valve leaflets from 3D rendered images (A, Anterior leaflet; P, posterior leaflet; S, septal leaflet). (C) Shows a surface-rendered 3D model of the tricuspid valve annulus and leaflets, showing its elliptical and saddle-shape. In (D), the 3D printed model of the tricuspid valve is shown.

TABLE 5.1 Summary of the Main Advantages and Limitations of 3D Echocardiography in Comparison With Conventional 2D and Doppler Echocardiography

ADVANTAGES	LIMITATIONS
The third dimension (i.e., depth) of complex, nonplanar cardiac structures is displayed (no through-plane motion) and is taken into account for quantitative analyses	Clinical utility highly depending on the quality of the acoustic window and of baseline 2D images of the patient
Comprehensive assessment of the entire structure of interest in a unique image, frequently obviating the need of performing several acquisitions from different perspectives of the same structure	Optimal data set quality and analysis require a stable R-R interval and patient's cooperation for breath hold, to ensure multibeat acquisitions without stitching artifacts
No geometric assumptions regarding a specific shape or orientation of cardiac structures	Quantitative measurements require the use of various vendor-specific analysis tools (at times available only offline) and a sufficient amount of training and experience with each software
Full control of the position and the orientation in space of any tomographic planes	Data set postprocessing (cropping, slicing, navigation) and/or quantitative analysis adds additional time to the routine echo examination
Unique anatomically sound perspectives (en face views, surgical views, etc.)	Loss of tissue characterization in 3D rendered images
Possibility to analyze the spatial relationship and the functional interplay among cardiac structures contained in a large 3D volume of the heart	Trade-off between volume size and spatial and temporal resolution (i.e., large fields of view are affected by lower temporal resolution; 3D color Doppler imaging has low temporal resolution when performed in real time etc.)
Measurements from 3D data sets are more accurate and reproducible than those obtained from 2D images	The accuracy of the measurements depends on data set image quality, 3D image settings (gain, temporal resolution, etc.) and the accuracy of border tracing/tracking.
Facilitates the understanding of true cardiac anatomy and the communication with surgeons or clinicians less familiar with tomographic ultrasound image interpretation	Since it is only a complementary technique, it cannot substitute a complete 2D Doppler examination; unexpected or unusual findings from 3D rendered images often require confirmation by a focused reevaluation using conventional 2D Doppler or multiplanar scanning to reliably rule out artifacts

Prosthetic Valves

3D TEE has improved the visualization and the assessment of complications, such as prosthetic valve endocarditis or paravalvular regurgitation. The aortic prosthetic ring can be well visualized from the LV outflow tract and from aortic perspective in unique views.[102] However, the bioprosthetic leaflets or mechanical prosthetic occluders in the aortic position are visualized poorly, and frame rate constraints can limit the 3DE capability for identification of small mobile vegetations, compared with 2DE. Conversely, the mitral mechanical and bioprosthetic valve ring, leaflets, and struts can be visualized clearly from different perspectives, and 3D TEE allows the precise description of number of sites of dehiscence and its configuration. Using MPR 3D color flow imaging, it is possible to quantify the area of dehiscence and to assist in the decision of surgical or percutaneous intervention.[70]

CONCLUSION

At the present time, 3DE is complementary to 2DE in clinical practice (Table 5.1). However, this is a rapidly evolving field, and further improvements in image quality, higher temporal and spatial resolution, and software are foreseen in the near future. Moreover, reference parameters and specific cutoff values are needed to provide proper interpretation and global use of 3DE measurements. As a result, while 3DE is used in a limited way by most echocardiography laboratories currently, we anticipate widespread use of 3DE as the technology improves and expect that its contribution to the assessment of cardiac structure and function, especially to support interventional procedures, will grow rapidly.

Suggested Reading

Badano, L. P., Boccalini, F., Muraru, D., et al. (2012). Current clinical applications of transthoracic three-dimensional echocardiography. *Journal of Cardiovascular Ultrasound, 20,* 1–22.

Lang, R. M., Badano, L. P., Mor-Avi, V., et al. (2015). Recommendations for cardiac chamber quantification by echocardiography in adults: an update from the American Society of Echocardiography and the European Association of Cardiovascular Imaging. *European Heart Journal of Cardiovascular Imaging, 16,* 233–270.

Lang, R. M., Badano, L. P., Tsang, W., et al. (2012). EAE/ASE recommendations for image acquisition and display using three-dimensional echocardiography. *European Heart Journal of Cardiovascular Imaging, 13,* 1–46.

Muraru, D., Badano, L. P., Sarais, C., et al. (2011). Evaluation of tricuspid valve morphology and function by transthoracic three-dimensional echocardiography. *Current Cardiology Reports, 13,* 242–249.

Zamorano, J. L., & Goncalves, A. (2013). Three dimensional echocardiography for quantification of valvular heart disease. *Heart, 99,* 811–818.

A complete reference list can be found online at ExpertConsult.com

6 Principles and Practical Aspects of Strain Echocardiography

Dai-Yin Lu, Monica Mukherjee, Theodore Abraham

INTRODUCTION

Assessment of regional and global ventricular function has long relied on visual assessment. However, this approach is subjective and variable leading to significant interobserver variability in interpretation. The heart is a mechanical organ and undergoes cyclic deformation in systole and diastole. This cyclic deformation can be measured and for decades was restricted to those undergoing open-heart surgery when metal beads were sown onto particular locations on the left ventricle (LV); deformation was then assessed via fluoroscopy. Approximately 20 years ago, magnetic resonance methods were introduced that allowed noninvasive assessment of deformation. Later, tissue Doppler-based methodology was used to track tissue motion by echocardiography. Further refinement of these techniques enabled echo-based assessment of regional deformation via determination of strain.

PRINCIPLES OF STRAIN IMAGING

Strain is a measure of tissue deformation. Strain is defined as a change in length of an object relative to its original length (i.e., reduction to half its original length is 50% strain; Fig. 6.1). Strain rate (SR) is the rate at which this deformation (length change) occurs. Although myocardial deformation is a three-dimensional phenomenon, echo-based interrogation techniques have generally been limited to interrogating one or more of three imaging planes—longitudinal, circumferential, and radial (Fig. 6.2). More recently, 3D strain has been introduced.

Strain and SR allow a clinician to determine regional and global myocardial function at the same level as a muscle physiologist by providing parameters similar to shortening fraction and shortening velocity, respectively.[1]

Echo-based techniques measure deformation by two primary methods—tissue Doppler and speckle-based. In tissue Doppler imaging (TDI), SR is the difference in velocity between two points along the myocardial wall (velocity gradient) normalized to the distance between the two points (Fig. 6.3). A similar velocity gradient exists between the endocardium and the epicardium, because the endocardium moves faster. This concept is used to derive myocardial velocity gradient (radial SR). This velocity gradient depicts the rate of change of myocardial wall thickness during systole and diastole. Thus SR measures the rate at which the two points of interest move toward or away from each other. Integration of SR yields strain, the normalized change in length between these two points (Fig. 6.4).

In speckle-tracking methodology, the system tracks unique acoustic patterns within the myocardium termed *speckles*. These speckles can be tracked over time, and speckle displacement can be used to calculate tissue velocity and strain (Fig. 6.5). This method is relatively angle-independent, because it is not based on the Doppler principle. Because speckle tracking can be automated, this technique lends itself to semiautomated measurements of strain. One such method allows the generation of bull's-eye plots of longitudinal segmental strain (Fig. 6.6 and Video 6.1). Another similar technique uses arrows to display the direction and amplitude of motion at various points in the heart (velocity vector imaging). Speckle tracking imaging can use preexisting B-mode images; however, it is performed at much lower frame rates (40–90 frames per second) and may not be as accurate in timing mechanical events as Doppler-based imaging (100–250 frames per second).

Commonly measured strain parameters include systolic and diastolic SRs, and systolic strain (Fig. 6.7). Peak systolic SR is the parameter that comes closest to measuring local contractile function in clinical cardiology. It is relatively volume independent and is less pressure independent than strain. In contrast, peak systolic strain is volume dependent and does not reflect contractile function as well as SR.

TWIST AND TORSION

Myocardium are three-dimensional continuous fibers that change direction from subendocardial right-handed helix to a subepicardial left-handed helix.[2] The fibers arranged in counter-direction generate sliding or shear deformation during contraction.[3] When viewed from apex to base, the apex rotates counterclockwise during systole, while base rotates in clockwise (Fig. 6.8). Twist is the apex-to-base difference in rotation, which is expressed in degrees. Torsion refers to the normalized twist, where the twist angle is divided by the distance between LV base and apex, which is expressed in degrees per centimeter. The systolic twist and diastolic untwist can be influenced by age, change of preload or afterload, diastolic dysfunction, cardiomyopathy, and valvular heart disease.[4]

REGIONAL AND GLOBAL FUNCTION

Left Ventricle

Circumferential and radial strain values are obtained in standard parasternal short axis view at mitral valve, papillary muscle, and apex level. Longitudinal strain is calculated from apical two-, three-, and four-chamber views, with basal, mid, and apical segments in each of the six walls. Timing of aortic valve closure (AVC) is used to define end-systole in a cardiac cycle. To avoid underestimation, it is important to get a circular LV images when performing circumferential and radial strain analyses, and avoid foreshortened apical chamber views in longitudinal strain

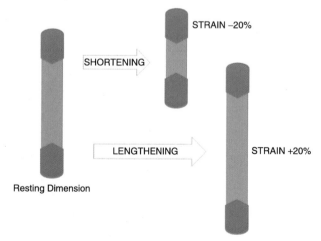

FIG. 6.1 Strain is a dimensionless index defined as change in length normalized to the original length. This reduction in length of the myocardial segment by 20% would indicate a strain of −20%. Conversely, a lengthening of a myocardial segment by 20% would yield a strain of +20%. Strain rate is the rate at which these length changes occur.

55

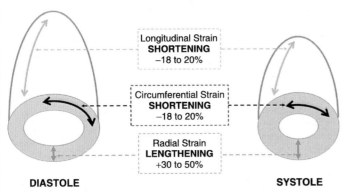

Longitudinal Strain
SHORTENING
–18 to 20%

Circumferential Strain
SHORTENING
–18 to 20%

Radial Strain
LENGTHENING
+30 to 50%

DIASTOLE

SYSTOLE

FIG. 6.2 Myocardial deformation is a three-dimensional phenomenon. However, echocardiographic interrogation of strain occurs along three primary directions—longitudinal (apex to base), circumferential (along the short axis curvature), and radial (endocardial to epicardial). There is systolic shortening and diastolic lengthening in the longitudinal and circumferential directions. There is systolic thickening and diastolic thinning in the radial direction.

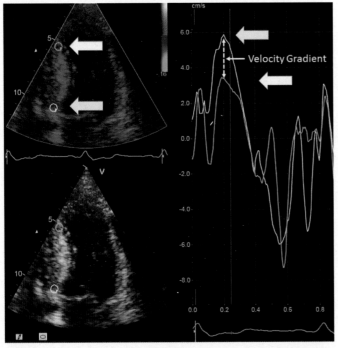

FIG. 6.3 Tissue velocity–based strain imaging measures tissue velocities along to locations in the long axis direction. The difference in peak velocities normalized to the distance between them yields myocardial velocity gradient or strain rate.

analysis. Global longitudinal strain (GLS), calculated as the average from all segments, is commonly used as a measure of global LV function. Fig. 6.9 shows typical segmental speckle-tracking strain in a healthy normal heart. Timing of end systole needs to be defined clearly to identify postsystolic shortening from systolic shortening. Normal GLS value is reported between 18% and 25% in healthy participants.[5] However, there is intervendor variability.

Right Ventricle

The RV wall is thinner than the LV myocardium, and these two ventricles have different shapes. DTI has been validated in quantification of RV myocardial deformation in healthy individuals. RV longitudinal velocities demonstrate a typical base-to-apex gradient with higher velocities at the base (Fig. 6.10A). The deformation properties within the LV are more homogeneous. Conversely, the SR and strain values are less homogeneously distributed in the right ventricle and show a reverse base-to-apex gradient, with the highest values in the apical segments and outflow tract (see Fig. 6.10B).[6] This reverse pattern can be explained by the complex geometry of the thin-walled, crescent-shaped right ventricle, and the less homogeneous distribution of regional wall stress. DTI-derived and speckle tracking-derived strain and SR can be used to evaluate RV dynamics, and both were found to be feasible and generally comparable.[7] Strain and SR correlate well with radionuclide RV EF. Systolic velocity and strain best correlated with invasively determined right ventricular stroke volume and change in right ventricular function after vasodilator infusion (Fig. 6.11).[8] SRs and strain quantitate regional right ventricular systolic function in children and adults with various conditions.[9,10]

Left Atrium

Under normal conditions, the left atrium (LA) is a low-pressure, highly expandable chamber, but in the presence of acute and chronic injury, the left atrial wall stretches and stiffens.[11,12] LA volume is not a specific marker for LA function, as it reflects the chronic effect of LV filling pressure but may also be increased in patients with atrial arrhythmias or in athletes whose LV filling pressure is actually normal.

Assessment of LA strain with two-dimensional (2D) speckle tracking and Doppler-based strain provide additional information on LA mechanics. Components of atrial function include reservoir, conduit, and active booster contraction. The LA strain and SR demonstrate atrial physiology and closely follow LV dynamics during the cardiac cycle. LA reservoir function is displayed by "total" strain, and contractile function is presented by the negative strain following the beginning of the "P" wave. There are two different ways to define the reference (zero) point: One is to define the onset of P wave as baseline, and then the first negative peak strain corresponds to atrial contractile function, peak positive strain as conduit function, and the total sum represents reservoir function. The other is to set the peak of QRS complex as baseline, and then

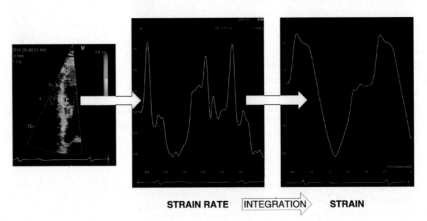

STRAIN RATE | INTEGRATION | **STRAIN**

FIG. 6.4 In tissue velocity-based strain imaging, a region of interest is placed in a particular location on the myocardium. This measures strain rate at that location. Integration of strain rate deals strain.

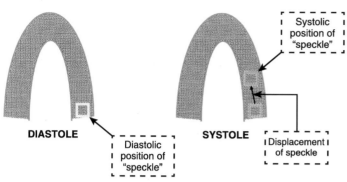

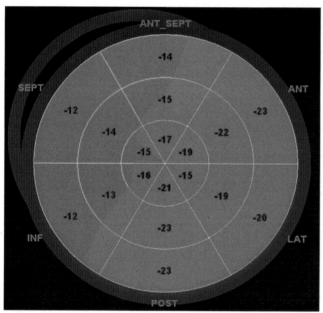

FIG. 6.5 Two-dimensional strain imaging uses speckle tracking methodology. A speckle is a particular acoustic pattern that can be computationally identified within the myocardium. For strain estimation, a speckle is identified at end diastole (*yellow box*) and tracked until end systole (*blue box*). The distance traveled by the speckle is displacement, which is used to calculate strain, the temporal derivative of which in turn yields strain rate.

FIG. 6.6 A representative example of two-dimensional strain output. Segmental strain rate tracings are provided for each apical view: four-chamber (*upper left*), two-chamber (*upper right*), and apical long (*lower left*). Peak strain values are converted into a color code depicted as a bull's-eye plot (*lower right*).

peak positive longitudinal strain represents atrial reservoir function, and strains during early and late ventricular diastole equal to conduit and atrial contractile function (Fig. 6.12).[13,14] Global strain and SR are calculated by averaging values observed in all LA segments,[15,16] either with a 15-segment model (six segments in the apical four-chamber view, six in the two-chamber view, and three in the three-chambers views)[17] or a 12-segment (six segments in the four-chamber view and six more in the two-chamber views) model.[18] LA deformation assessment has an established role in assessing LA performance and LV diastolic function. For patients with atrial fibrillation, those who have higher atrial strain and SR appear to have a greater likelihood of staying in sinus rhythm after cardioversion (Fig. 6.13).[19]

CORONARY ARTERY DISEASE AND ISCHEMIC CARDIOMYOPATHY

Strain and SR appear to be sensitive indicators for subclinical diseases, including diabetic or nonischemic cardiomyopathy, myocardial ischemia, arterial hypertension, and valvular heart disease. They are also useful in evaluation of myocardial damage after infarction, as well as outcome after revascularization.[20–28] Myocardial ischemia is associated with reduction in peak systolic strain and often accompanied by postsystolic shortening. Infarct or severe ischemia is associated with systolic lengthening. These changes in strain and SR are dynamic (i.e., rapid reduction in ischemia and immediate return to normal upon restoration of blood flow; Fig. 6.14). Bull's-eye plots of 2D strain (speckle-tracking method) are not time-consuming, semiautomated, and easy to generate and interpret. Some examples of regional ischemia are shown in Fig. 6.15 and Video 6.2 . Another important application of strain imaging is to combine with low-dose dobutamine stress echocardiography to assess myocardial viability. Augmentation of strain and SR after dobutamine infusion helps identify viable muscle. Postsystolic shortening occurs in the presence of active myocardial contraction and hence reflects viable myocardium. However, it should not be used as the only parameter indicating viability, since postsystolic shortening may be also present in myocardium with transmural necrosis or scar.

NONISCHEMIC CARDIOMYOPATHY

In the presence of overt cardiomyopathy demonstrated by conventional echocardiography, strain imaging is generally not needed. Nevertheless, it can be of great help when diseases are in early stages or to predict prognosis. GLS appears to have superior prognostic value to left ventricular ejection fraction (LVEF) for predicting major adverse cardiac events.[29] Strain mapping depicts a global reduction in GLS, with the typical preservation of function noted in the basal inferior and inferolateral segments (Fig. 6.16)

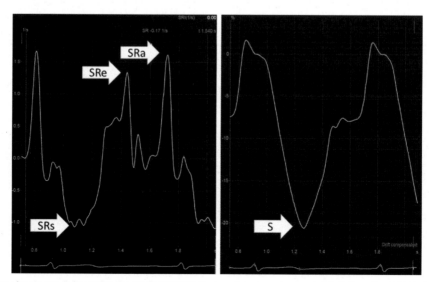

FIG. 6.7 Representative tracings of strain rate (*left panel*) and strain (*right panel*). Commonly measured parameters include peak systolic strain rate (SRs), early and late diastolic strain rates (SRe and SRa, respectively), and peak systolic strain (S).

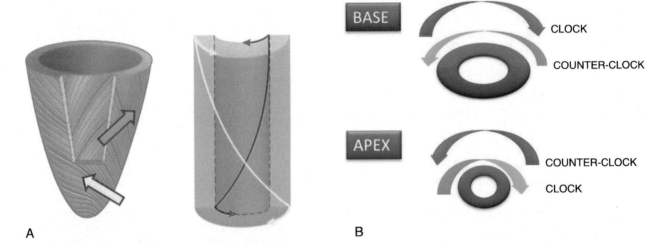

FIG. 6.8 A, Subepicardial fibers wrap around the left ventricle (LV) in a left-handed helix *(yellow arrows),* and subendocardial fibers wrap around the LV in a right-handed helix *(green arrows).* **B,** The outer epicardial layer *(red arrows)* in LV base rotates in a clockwise direction, whereas the inner endocardium *(blue arrows)* rotates in an opposite direction. For the apex, the epicardial layer rotates in a counterclockwise direction, and the endocardium rotates in clockwise rotation. The overall LV rotational direction is dominated by the epicardial rotation because the epicardial layer has a larger radius. *(A adapted from Partho P, Sengupta A, Tajik J, et al: Twist mechanics of the left ventricle: principles and application.* JACC Cardiovasc Imaging. *2008;1(3):366–367.)*

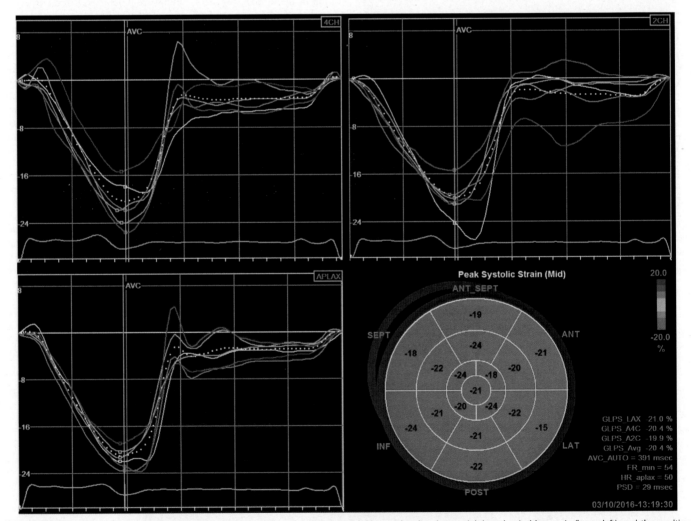

FIG. 6.9 Representative strain tracings from three apical views—four-chamber *(upper left),* two-chamber *(upper right),* and apical long-axis *(lower left),* and the resulting "bull's-eye" plot *(lower right).* In this example, segmental strain values are all normal and represented by shades of red in the bull's-eye plot. Global longitudinal strain was −20% (normal range).

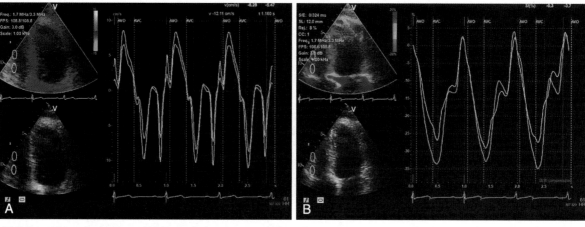

FIG. 6.10 (A) RV lateral free wall velocities and (B) longitudinal strain assessed using color DTI in a normal subject. Note the base-to-apex gradient in velocities and apex-to-base gradient in longitudinal strain. Yellow tracing = basal; green tracing = apical.

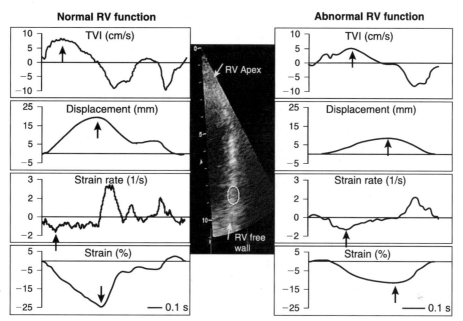

FIG. 6.11 Strain appears superior to other Doppler-based indices such as the index of myocardial performance and tissue Doppler-based isovolumic acceleration. Representative traces from the basal RV free wall illustrating tissue velocity (TVI), tissue displacement, strain rate, and strain from a normal subject *(left)*, and a subject with abnormal RV function *(right)*. *(From Urheim S, Cauduro S, Frantz R, et al: Relation of tissue displacement and strain to invasively determined right ventricular stroke volume. Am J Cardiol. 2005;96(8):1173–1178.)*

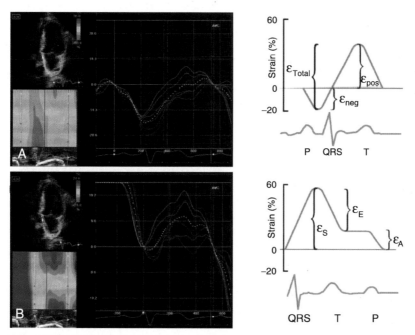

FIG. 6.12 Speckle tracking-derived left atrial (LA) global longitudinal strain can be demonstrated with triggering on the (A) starting of the P wave or (B) peak of the QRS wave. ε_S = peak positive strain, ε_E = strain during early diastole, and ε_A = strain during late diastole. *(Right panel from Hoit BD: Left atrial size and function: role in prognosis. J Am Coll Cardiol. 2014;63(6):493–505.)*

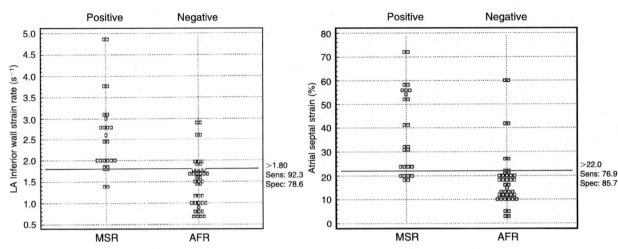

FIG. 6.13 A cutoff value of 1.8 s⁻¹ for atrial inferior wall peak systolic strain rate was associated with sinus rhythm maintenance, with a sensitivity of 92% and specificity of 79% *(left panel)*. For atrial septal peak systolic strain, a cutoff value of 22% was associated with a sensitivity of 77%, specificity of 86% *(right panel)*. MSR, Maintenance of sinus rhythm; AFR, recurrence of atrial fibrillation. *(From Di Salvo G, Caso P, Lo Piccolo R, et al: Atrial myocardial deformation properties predict maintenance of sinus rhythm after external cardioversion of recent-onset lone atrial fibrillation: a color Doppler myocardial imaging and transthoracic and transesophageal echocardiographic study. Circulation. 2005;112(3):387–395.)*

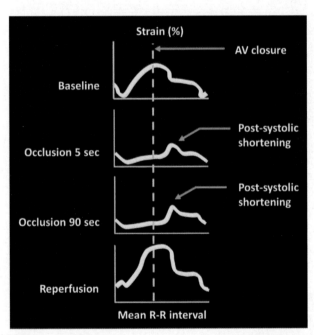

FIG. 6.14 A 78-year-old woman undergoing coronary angioplasty with serial posterior wall regional strain (%) averaged for mean heart cycle. During the ischemia period, peak strain value was clearly decreased in systole, with the appearance of postsystolic thickening phenomenon. After reperfusion there was an increase in myocardial systolic thickening caused by reactive hyperkinesia. *(Modified from Jamal F, Kukulski T, D'hooge J, et al: Abnormal postsystolic thickening in acutely ischemic myocardium during coronary angioplasty: a velocity, strain, and strain rate Doppler myocardial imaging study. J Am Soc Echocardiogr. 1999;12(11):994–996.)*

Hypertrophic Cardiomyopathy

Hypertrophic cardiomyopathy (HCM) is characterized by scattered regions of fiber disarray within the hypertrophic areas.[30,31] Regional analysis differentiates abnormal hypertrophic regions of cardiac muscle in which there was no systolic shortening from adjacent normal regions.[32–34] The thickest segments of myocardium are usually associated with greatest reduction or even absence of deformation (Fig. 6.17). In a study with patients having familial nonobstructive HCM, average longitudinal strain was reduced in affected individuals compared with healthy controls, despite apparently normal systolic function. In addition, there was no significant difference in the values obtained by TDI versus 2D strain echocardiography.[32] An early diastolic SR ≤7 s⁻¹ differentiated

accurately (0.96 positive and 0.94 negative predictive value, respectively) between patients with HCM and physiologic hypertrophy in athletes (Fig 6.18).[35] Furthermore, strain analysis may offer prognostic stratification. A GLS cutoff value of 15% measured at rest is an independent indicator of cardiac events and symptomatic exacerbation in patients with HCM.[36]

Chemotherapy-Related Cardiotoxicity

Chemotherapy-related cardiotoxicity is usually defined as a reduction of LVEF greater than 5% in symptomatic or 10% in asymptomatic patients from baseline to an LVEF <55%.[37] However, reduction in LVEF is not a sensitive parameter, since it appears late in the disease process, after significant cardiotoxicity has already developed. Myocardial deformation indexes have been applied to detect early-stage myocardial injury in patients receiving chemotherapy. The myocardial deformation parameters decreased rapidly, as early as 2 hours after the first dose of anthracyclines.[38] In a recent systemic review, 13 publications with 384 patients demonstrated consistently that reduction in myocardial deformation occurred earlier than reduction in LVEF, despite the heterogeneity of patient age, cancer type, strain methodology, and timing of follow-up, and GLS being the most consistent parameter. Furthermore, a 10% to 15% early reduction in GLS by speckle tracking during chemotherapy appears to be the most useful parameter for the prediction of cardiotoxicity, with a drop in LVEF or heart failure.[39] The Expert Consensus Statement from the American Society of Echocardiography and the European Association of Cardiovascular Imaging suggested that a relative percentage reduction of GLS <8% from baseline might not be meaningful, whereas a >15% reduction from baseline is likely to be abnormal.[40] Because of intervendor variability, it is important that similar equipment and protocol for calculating strain should be used when patients undergo serial evaluations.

Other Cardiomyopathies

Duchenne muscular dystrophy (DMD) is one of the most common X-linked recessive neuromuscular disorders. Boys with DMD lose independent ambulation by the age of 12 and die of respiratory failure or cardiomyopathy in their late teens or early 20s. A report in 2006 showed that radial strain was significantly lower in asymptomatic boys with DMD, when conventional echocardiography failed to show any abnormality.[41]

Friedreich ataxia (FRDA) is an inherited neurodegenerative disorder associated with cardiomyopathy and impaired glucose tolerance. SR offers a means of further characterizing the myocardial abnormalities in patients with FRDA. Early diastolic myocardial velocity gradient appear to relate most closely to the genetic abnormality and the consequential reduction in frataxin protein (Fig. 6.19).[42]

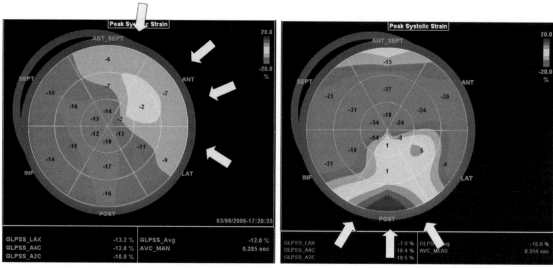

FIG. 6.15 Representative two-dimensional strain polar color plots demonstrating ischemia in the left anterior descending territory *(left panel)* evidenced by low strain in the anterior septal, anterior and anterolateral walls *(arrows)*, and in the circumflex territory *(right panel)*, demonstrating reduced strain and dyskinesis in the inferolateral region *(arrows)*.

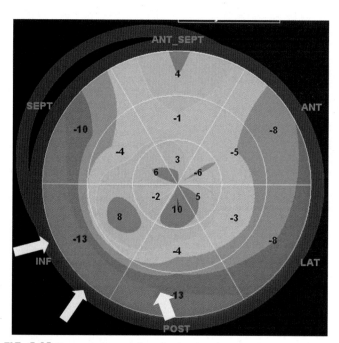

FIG. 6.16 Representative two-dimensional strain polar color plot in a patient with nonischemic cardiomyopathy demonstrating reduced strain globally with preserved systolic function, normal strain, in the basal infer-septum, inferior and infero-lateral walls.

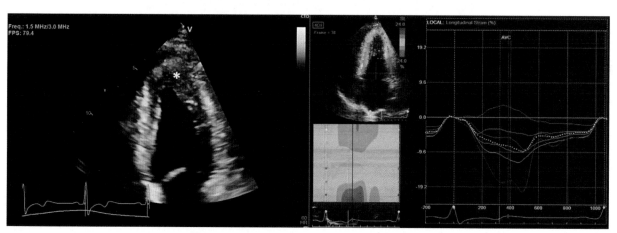

FIG. 6.17 In apical hypertrophic cardiomyopathy, the thickest segments in the apex *(asterisk)* are usually associated with greatest reduction or even absence of deformation.

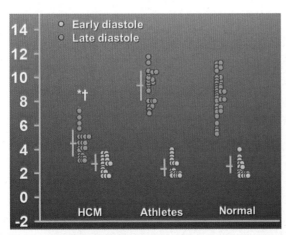

FIG. 6.18 An early diastolic *(yellow dots)* strain rate ≤7 s^{-1} differentiated between patients with HCM and physiologic hypertrophy in athletes. *(Modified from Palka P, Lange A, Fleming AD, et al: Differences in myocardial velocity gradient measured throughout the cardiac cycle in patients with hypertrophic cardiomyopathy, athletes and patients with left ventricular hypertrophy due to hypertension. J Am Coll Cardiol. 1997;30[3]:760–768.)*

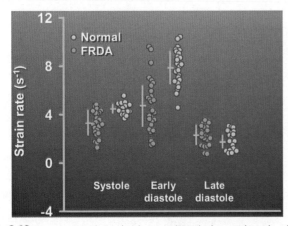

FIG. 6.19 In patients with Friedreich ataxia (FRDA), the systole and early diastolic strain rate were reduced compared with control subjects. In contrast, the late diastolic strain rate is higher in patients with FRDA than in control subjects. *(Modified from Dutka DP, Donnelly E, Przemyslaw P, et al: Echocardiographic characterization of cardiomyopathy in Friedreich's ataxia with tissue Doppler echocardiographically derived myocardial velocity gradients. Circulation. , 2000;102(11):1276–1282.)*

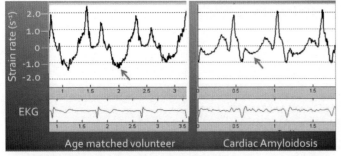

FIG. 6.20 The systolic strain rate in a patient with cardiac amyloidosis *(right panel, arrow)* is −0.4 s^{-1}, which is marked smaller in the absolute value compared with an age-matched control *(left panel, arrow).*

DILATED CARDIOMYOPATHY AND DYSSYNCHRONY ANALYSIS

Mechanical dyssynchrony is discoordinate ventricular contraction resulting from either an electrical condition delay or abnormal ventricular contraction. It has been reported as a more sensitive marker

of myocardial dysfunction than LVEF.[43,44] Cardiac resynchronization therapy (CRT) is a catheter-based therapy for patients with heart failure and left ventricular dyssynchrony. Several large clinical trials have established the benefits of CRT on hospitalization or survival in patients with severe LV dysfunction and a QRS duration wider than 120 ms.[45–47] However, about one-third of patients selected based on electrocardiogram criteria do not respond to CRT. Measurement of regional electromechanical activities with TDI information helps identify mechanical dyssynchrony and is useful in selecting patients who might get more benefit from CRT.[48,49] Strain analyses by speckle tracking or TDI were used to detect and define intraventricular dyssynchrony, and they were demonstrated as reliable markers in predicting responders to CRT.[50–52] Use of the strain delay index with longitudinal strain by speckle tracking has a strong value for predicting response to cardiac resynchronization therapy in both ischemic and nonischemic patients.[48] Another important issue for CRT efficacy is to find optimal lead position in the left ventricular free wall. Several series have demonstrated that an LV lead position, coinciding with the regions of latest mechanical activation, yields superior outcomes compared with discordant positions.[53]

VALVULAR HEART DISEASE

The timing for surgical intervention in asymptomatic or mild symptomatic moderate to severe valvular heart disease is largely based on symptoms, lesion severity, and negative LV volumetric remodeling or functional decline. Reduction in LVEF indicates impairment of contractility. However, it is often a late consequence of myocardial injury and sometimes not fully reversible after surgery. Subclinical myocardial dysfunction may be a potential guide for the timing of surgical intervention.[54] Recent studies have suggested that strain imaging provides additional clinical value in aortic and mitral valve diseases.[55–57] In patients with severe aortic stenosis, impaired LV strain and SR were noted, although LVEF was preserved. After aortic valve replacement, a significant improvement in these parameters was observed. These subtle changes in LV contractility can be detected by 2D speckle tracking imaging.[58] Another report on percutaneous aortic valve replacement showed improvements of strain and SR in TDI.[59] In patients with mitral stenosis who underwent percutaneous mitral balloon valvotomy (PMBV), GLS is a powerful predictor of long-term outcome after successful PMBV and provides incremental prognostic value over traditional parameters.[60] In patients with asymptomatic mitral regurgitation, strain and SR help identify subclinical LV dysfunction and correlate with contractile reserve with exercise; strain and SR are significantly greater in patients with adequate contractile reserve.[26] However, these results were largely based on observational studies, and prospective randomized control trials are needed before routine use of strain imaging can be recommended regarding to timing of surgery.

INFILTRATIVE DISEASE

Amyloidosis

Cardiac amyloidosis (CA) (see Chapter 24) is a manifestation of amyloidosis. As extracellular misfolding fibrillar proteins deposit in heart muscle, LV wall becomes thickened with the presentation of restrictive cardiomyopathy, followed by overt heart failure or sudden death.[61] Patients with amyloidosis had severe diastolic dysfunction, and myocardial deformation was significantly decreased (Fig. 6.20).[62] When compared with conventional mitral inflow spectral Doppler velocities (E wave and A wave), strain imaging of the right and LVs are more insightful and sensitive for the early identification of cardiac amyloidosis.[63,64] A specific pattern of longitudinal strain characterized by worse longitudinal strain in the mid- and basal ventricle with relative sparing of the apex[63] is typical for amyloid cardiomyopathy, which may help distinguish from hypertensive cardiomyopathy or hypertrophic cardiomyopathy (Fig. 6.21).[65,66]

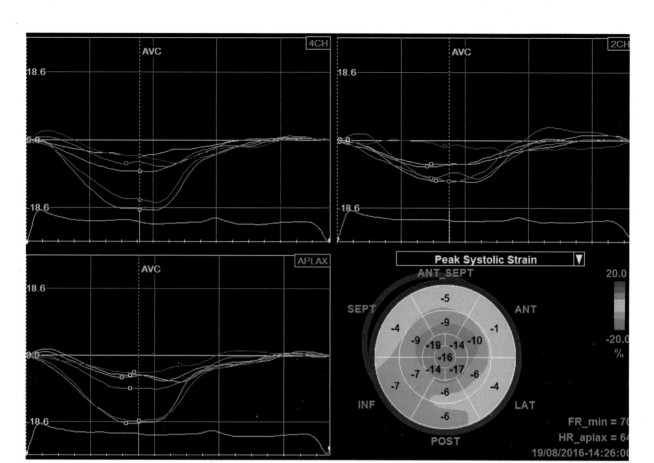

FIG. 6.21 Two-dimensional speckle-tracking longitudinal strain ("bull's-eye plot") demonstrates reduced strain at the base and mid-levels, with apical sparing in patients with cardiac amyloidosis (cherry on sundae pattern).

Suggested Readings

Mirea, O., Duchenne, J., & Voigt, J. U. (2016). Recent advances in echocardiography: strain and strain rate imaging. *F1000Res, 5*. pii: F1000 Faculty Rev-787.

Opdahl, A., Helle-Valle, T., Skulstad, H., & Smiseth, O. A. (2015). Strain, strain rate, torsion, and twist: echocardiographic evaluation. *Current Cardiology Reports, 17*(3), 568.

Smiseth, O. A., Torp, H., Opdahl, A., et al. (2016). Myocardial strain imaging: how useful is it in clinical decision making? *European Heart Journal, 37*(15), 1196–1207.

Voigt, J. U., & Flachskampf, F. A. (2004). Strain and strain rate. New and clinically relevant echo parameters of regional myocardial function. *Z Kardiol, 93*(4), 249–258.

A complete reference list can be found online at ExpertConsult.com.

7

Understanding Imaging Artifacts

Maja Cikes, Jan D'hooge

INTRODUCTION

Imaging artifacts encompass patterns in the image that seem to suggest the presence of structures that are in reality not present. They may in fact relate to both the appearance of nonexistent structures, as well as the concealing of existing structures. Artifacts are mostly caused by physical interactions between the imaged tissue and ultrasound itself that are more complex than assumed by the ultrasound system; however, they can also result from malfunctioning ultrasound equipment or their inadequate settings, as well as from interference caused by other electronic equipment. Imaging artifacts can occasionally encumber an echocardiographic examination (particularly for novices), and the knowledge of these occurrences should thus be used to minimize their effect. In this chapter, the most common artifacts have been categorized according to the authors' discretion, although they recognize that alternative ways of classifying these artifacts are possible, as no standard nomenclature exists and reference to certain artifacts in the literature is limited (Table 7.1).

B-MODE ARTIFACTS

Shadowing (Attenuation) and Dropout Artifacts

Shadowing (i.e., attenuation) artifacts obscure certain (segments of) underlying structures. When imaging structures with mechanical properties (i.e., mass density and/or compressibility) substantially differ from soft tissue (e.g., metals such as used in prosthetic valves or air/contrast bubbles), very strong reflections will occur, resulting in little or no transfer of ultrasound energy to more distal regions, as (almost) all energy will have been reflected. This will manifest as a strong reflection in the area of the reflector, followed by an "acoustic shadow" that represents a signal void (Fig. 7.1, yellow dashed arrows, Video 7.1).

This shadowing will affect not only the two-dimensional (2D) image but also the color Doppler signal, which could be, for example, highly relevant in the assessment of regurgitant jets in the setting of prosthetic heart valves. Heavily calcified tissue is a similarly strong reflector; resorting to alternative scanning windows can mostly circumvent such artifacts. For more information on negative shadows, refer to Box 7.1 and Fig. 7.2.

Similarly, superficial structures leading to notable attenuation of ultrasound may significantly impair its penetration. As a result, the ribs or lung tissue can diminish the ability to image underlying structures, giving rise to **"dropout" artifacts** that typically occur at some phases of the respiratory cycle. Such artifacts can be reduced or avoided by scanning at different intervals of the respiratory cycle (i.e., breath hold), and occasionally only by choosing another transducer position (Fig. 7.3, Videos 7.2 and 7.3). A dropout artifact is thus similar to a shadowing artifact that occurs very near the transducer, thereby causing part of the image to become invisible.

Reverberation Artifacts

During image generation, the signal of the reflected wave arriving at the transducer is transformed to electrical energy (i.e., the radiofrequency signal) to be used in the image reconstruction process (for more details, see Chapter 1). However, a certain portion of the reflected wave is not converted to electrical energy and is merely reflected on the transducer surface to start repropagating through the tissue as if it were another ultrasound transmission. This secondary "transmission" is yet again reflected by the tissue and ultimately detected by the transducer (Fig. 7.4, *upper panel*). Since the ultrasound system assumes all echo signals are resulting from the original transmission, these secondary reflections that arrive late (as they have to travel back and

TABLE 7.1 Types of Artifacts Encountered in Echocardiography and Potential Approaches to Their Resolution

TYPES OF ARTIFACTS	RESOLUTION APPROACH
B-mode Artifacts	

• Shadowing (attenuation) and dropout artifacts
  • Excess/deficit attenuation
  • Excess reflection of energy (see Figs. 7.1, 7.6; Video 7.1)
  • Dropout artifact—shadowing of superficial structures during parts of the cardiac cycle (see Fig. 7.3, Videos 7.2 and 7.3)
	• Alternative imaging planes
	• Increase transmit power
	• Adjust time gain compensation

• Reverberation artifacts
  • Transducer-related reverberation (see Fig. 7.4)
  • Internal reverberation (see Fig. 7.5, Video 7.4)
    • Step ladder (reverberating structure large compared to pulse length; see Figs. 7.1, 7.6, 7.7; Videos 7.1 and 7.7)
    • Comet tail (reverberating structure small compared to pulse length; see Fig. 7.8, Video 7.8)
	• Alternative imaging planes
	• Decrease transmit power

• Multiple reflection artifacts (see Fig. 7.9)
  • Near-field clutter (see Fig. 7.10, Videos 7.5 and 7.6)
  • Ghost or mirror image (see Figs. 7.7, 7.11; Videos 7.7, 7.9, and 7.10)
	• Alternative imaging planes
	• Decrease transmit power

• Side-lobe artifacts (see Figs. 7.7, 7.12, 7.13, 7.14; Videos 7.7, 7.11, 7.12, 7.13)	• Respiratory maneuvers (if caused by lungs/ribs) • Decrease gain • Apply color Doppler • Change position of imaged structure towards center of field of view • Change transmit focus position and/or transmit frequency
• Refraction (lens) artifacts (see Fig. 7.15, Video 7.14)	• Alternative imaging planes • Decrease gain
• Beam width artifacts/partial volume artifacts (see Fig. 7.16)	• Use a 2D array for 2D imaging (improved elevation beam width)
Doppler Artifacts	
• (Color) Doppler mirror image artifacts (see Fig. 7.17)	• Alternative imaging planes
4D Echocardiography Artifacts	
• Stitch artifacts (see Fig. 7.18)	• Patient breath hold

4D, Four-dimensional; 2D, two-dimensional.

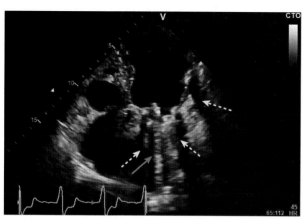

FIG. 7.1 Apical four-chamber view of a patient with a prosthetic mitral valve, which is the origin of multiple acoustic shadows—that is, signal voids (*yellow dashed arrows*)—due to proximal strong reflecting structures. Furthermore, the cusps of the mitral prosthesis give rise to step ladder artifacts (as explained further in the text; *blue arrows*), seen throughout the central portion of the left atrium and beyond the roof of the left atrium. These artifacts can also be appreciated on the cine loop of this figure (Video 7.1).

BOX 7.1 Negative Shadows

Although shadowing is typically seen as a darker zone (i.e., signal void) distal to a highly reflecting (most common) or absorbing (less common) structure, the opposite can also occur in that a structure is attenuating less than what is assumed by the scanner's automatic time gain compensation (refer to Chapter 1). As a result, the distal echo signals are overamplified by the scanner, resulting in a brighter zone distal to the low-attenuating structure, which is referred to as a "negative" shadow. A typical example is that of a cyst, as the liquid in the cyst is attenuating the ultrasound wave less than soft tissue, while the scanner automatically corrects for attenuation, assuming it is imaging soft tissue only. An example of such a negative shadow following a cyst in the liver is given in Fig. 7.2. In cardiac imaging, negative shadows do not normally occur.

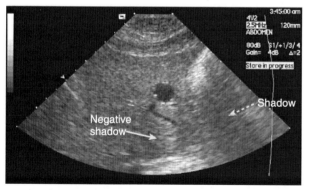

FIG. 7.2 Example of a shadow (*yellow dashed arrow*) and negative shadow following a cyst (*yellow arrow*) in the liver.

---

forth twice) will thus be depicted at a greater depth, mimicking a reflecting structure at a greater distance (see Fig. 7.4, *lower panel*).[1]

In fact, the secondary reflections will also be partially reflected at the transducer surface, resulting in an apparent third transmit; this process can be repeated multiple times. Although these second- and/or higher-order reflections always occur, they are normally negligible in amplitude with respect to the primary echo amplitudes and can therefore simply be ignored. However, when strong reflections of the primary wave occur, the reverberated signal (i.e., the signal caused by two or more round-trips) can be substantial and give rise to image artifacts (i.e., **reverberation artifacts**). This type of artifact can typically be recognized as the repetition of a strongly reflecting structure at

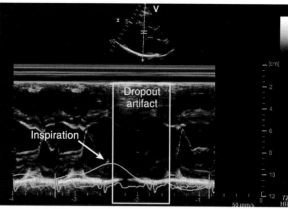

FIG. 7.3 Dropout artifact imaged on an M-mode trace of the parasternal long-axis. In this case, during inspiration (as appreciated from the respirometer trace—*white arrow*) the tissue close to the transducer (e.g., ribs or lung tissue) causes attenuation of the echo signal, thus obscuring the underlying image. The cine loop of the corresponding B-mode image can be found under Videos 7.2 and 7.3, where it can be appreciated that the visibility of the underlying structures clearly depends on the phase of the respiratory cycle. Video 7.2 is taken during normal respiration, while Video 7.3 shows a corresponding cine loop taken during breath hold at end-expiration, demonstrating the relevance of scanning at various intervals of the respiratory cycle for the optimization of image acquisition.

integer multiple distances from the transducer. When the reflecting structure causing the reverberation is moving, so will the induced reverberation (with an amplified motion amplitude; Video 7.4). If, on the other hand, this structure is not moving (e.g., a rib), the induced artifact will be stationary as well (i.e., a **stationary reverberation artifact**; Videos 7.5 and 7.6).

Similarly, reverberations can occur within structures that are being visualized. Indeed, on their way back to the transducer, reflections from the primary wave can meet strong reflectors that cause these reflections to start propagating in the direction away from the transducer again (Fig. 7.5). As such, these waves are propagating with some time lag with respect to the primary wave and create secondary reflections. Obviously, similar as for the transducer-related reverberations described previously, higher-order reflections can arise by multiple round-trips between both boundaries of the object. Structures with well-aligned, flat, strong reflecting boundaries (due to a strong mismatch in mechanical properties), such as catheters or the metallic leaflets of a prosthetic valve, are most likely to give rise to this acoustic "ping-pong." When the reverberating structure is substantially larger than the length of the ultrasonic pulse, individual "ping-pong" reflections can be detected (Fig. 7.6, blue arrows; Fig. 7.7, yellow arrows; and corresponding Video 7.7), in which case the name "**step ladder**" artifact is used. On the other hand, if this structure is small compared with the pulse length, all "ping-pong" reflections start to interfere, giving a more hazy appearance in the image referred to as a "**comet tail**" artifact (Fig. 7.8). Depending on the attenuation the reverberating wave experiences, the "step ladder" or "comet tail" fades out faster (i.e., higher attenuation; see Fig. 7.6) or slower (i.e., lower attenuation; see Fig. 7.1, blue arrow; see Video 7.1 and Fig. 7.8).

Various reverberation artifacts can often be seen behind valvular ring calcifications, pericardial calcifications, mechanical valve prostheses, and left ventricular assist device cannulas (see Figs. 7.1, 7.6–7.8). Of note, change of probe frequency will typically not eliminate these artifacts. For additional information on "ring down" artifacts and the diagnostic utility of reverberation artifacts, refer to Boxes 7.2 and 7.3 as well as Video 7.8.

Multiple Reflection Artifacts

Although the ultrasound system assumes that the transmitted wave travels to the target of interest and back in a direct manner, this is not necessarily the case. Indeed, similar to reverberations—where the acoustic wave propagates back-and-fourth between structures along the image line—more complex propagation paths of the acoustic wave can occur. For example, the wave can bounce off on some structure in order to continue to propagate away from the transducer but in another direction, to then be reflected and reach the transducer (Fig. 7.9). The detected echo signal is thus not

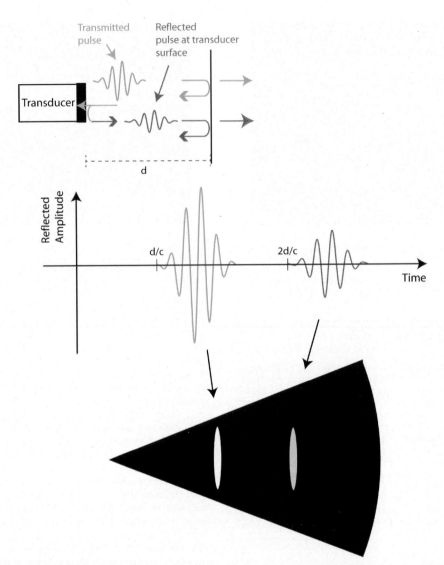

FIG. 7.4 The generation of a reverberation artifact. A transmitted pulse *(green)* reflects form a structure and results in an echo signal *(green)*. The reflected pulse will partially reflect at the surface of the transducer *(red)* and be the source of secondary echo signals *(red; upper panel)*. The additional time required for the "back-and-forth" travel of the signal causes the ultrasound system to depict the artifact distal to the true image, positioned at a distance that is an integer multiple of the true distance (d) between the transducer and the reflective structure *(lower panel)*. *(Modified from D'hooge J, Mertens LL. Ultrasound physics. In: Lai WW, Mertens LL, Cohen MS, Geva T, eds. Echocardiography in pediatric and congenital heart disease: from fetus to adult, Second Edition. Chichester: John Wiley and Sons; 2016:8.)*

related to structures along the image line at the calculated distance, thereby giving rise to a **multiple reflection artifact**. Given that the path followed by the acoustic wave can go outside of the field-of-view of the image and can involve more than two reflecting surfaces, it can become very challenging to understand the origin of some of these artifacts.

A typical example of a multiple reflection artifact is **near-field clutter**, which is caused by acoustic waves bouncing around between structures close to the probe (e.g., skin, muscle/fat layers, and ribs). It can be cumbersome to discern this clutter artifact from, for example, thrombi in the LV apex (Fig. 7.10; see Videos 7.5 and 7.6). Several features notable in the case of clutter (and not in apical thrombi) include the possibility of imaging the presence of blood flow within the apex by color Doppler imaging (particularly with lower velocity settings), a higher likelihood of clutter in a well-contracting apex, no obvious dependency of clutter "motion" in relation to myocardial motion, as well as a "shading" of the apex, which extends across the LV walls. Should these features not be sufficient for the discrimination between near-field clutter and apical thrombi/cardiac structures, other imaging views and/or contrast echocardiography should be used.

When multiple reflections occur in a very systematic manner, they can give rise to a **ghost or mirror image**. For example, when the pericardium is very reflective (i.e., bright), the reflected pericardial echo signal is very strong. On its way back to the transducer, this pericardial reflection will also generate echo signals from the structures it encounters. Obviously, these echo signals will propagate back in the direction of the pericardium. Given the pericardium is very reflective, the echo signals arriving at the pericardium are yet again reflected and now start propagating toward the transducer where they are detected. As such, it would appear that an acoustic wave was transmitted for imaging from the pericardium toward the transducer (i.e., the strong pericardial echo) and an apparent image is created distal to the pericardium. This image thus resembles the original echo image and is mirrored around the pericardium (i.e., a **mirror image**; Fig. 7.11, corresponding Video 7.9 and 7.10). Interestingly, the mirror image is not necessarily exactly the same as the original image, as the pericardium is curved. As such, the reflections will typically not be parallel to the original lines, resulting in the acoustic analogue of looking in a curved mirror. As a result, the mirrored structures can be distorted. Moreover, as the pericardial reflection occurs in three-dimensional (3D), out-of-plane curvature of the pericardium can result in the mirrored image plane being different from the original image plane (see Fig. 7.11; see also Videos 7.9 and 7.10). Similar to the pericardial example given, a mirror image of the aorta can sometimes be seen in transesophageal imaging (see Fig. 7.7 and corresponding Video 7.7).[1,3] Note that mirroring does not only apply to the pericardium (where it most often found), but can occur at any strong reflector.

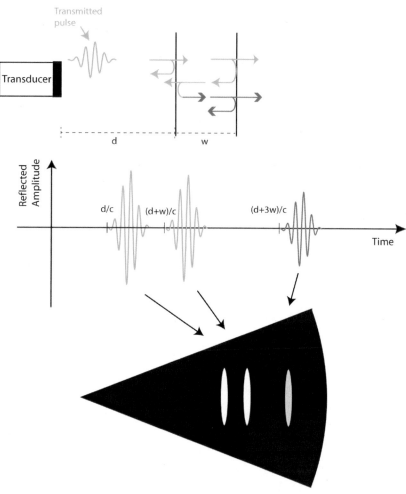

FIG. 7.5 The generation of an internal reverberation artifact. A transmitted pulse *(green)* partially reflects form two parallel structures resulting in the expected echo signals at a time corresponding to a distance "d" and "d+w" *(green)*. However, the reflection from the distal boundary reflects at the proximal one *(red)* resulting in a late echo signal *(red)*. The additional time required for the "back-and-forth" travel within the layer causes the ultrasound system to depict the artifact distal to the true boundaries, positioned at a distance equal to twice the thickness (w) of the layer. Most often, this process is repeated resulting in a series of additional (artefactual) echo signals. *d*, distance; *w*, thickness of the layer; *c*, ultrasound propagation speed.

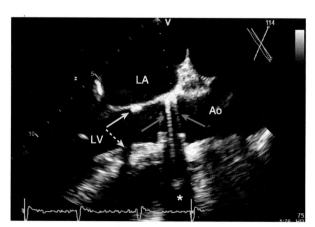

FIG. 7.6 Transesophageal echocardiographic long-axis view of the left ventricle (midesophageal view at 114 degrees) of a patient with an aortic valve prosthesis and mitral valve calcifications. The aortic valve prosthesis creates step ladder artifacts *(blue arrows)* as well as a shadow *(star)*. A larger calcification seen at the ventricular side of the anterior mitral leaflet *(yellow arrow)* also creates a shadow, which obscures the full thickness of the interventricular septum posterior to the artifact *(yellow dashed arrow)*. *Ao,* Aorta; *LA,* left atrium; *LV,* left ventricle.

Side Lobe Artifacts

Image reconstruction is based on the assumption that all echo signals are coming from structures located on the line along which the ultrasound wave was transmitted. As shown previously, this assumption does not always hold due to multiple reflections taking place (i.e., along the image line leading to reverberation artifacts; due to more complex acoustic paths resulting in multiple reflection artifacts). Intrinsically, a phased array transducer will not only transmit acoustic energy along the direction of the image line to be reconstructed (i.e., the main lobe) but will also transmit energy in other directions (i.e., the side lobes), as illustrated schematically in Fig. 7.12.

Similar to higher-order reflections observed as reverberations, the echo amplitudes of the side lobes are typically negligible to the ones coming from the main lobe and can likewise be ignored. However, should the main lobe be imaging an anechogenic region (such as one of the heart's cavities), the relative contribution of the side lobes can become significant and incorrectly shown in the image. As such, structures imaged by side lobes will "spill over" in the anechogenic region, causing a **"side lobe" artifact**. Some sources of side lobe artifacts include lung (Fig. 7.13; Video 7.11), the fibrous skeleton of the heart, aortic valve cusps (Fig. 7.14, Videos 7.12 and 7.13), aortic plaque (see Fig. 7.7, *left panel, blue arrowhead,* and corresponding Video 7.7), as well as the atrioventricular groove.

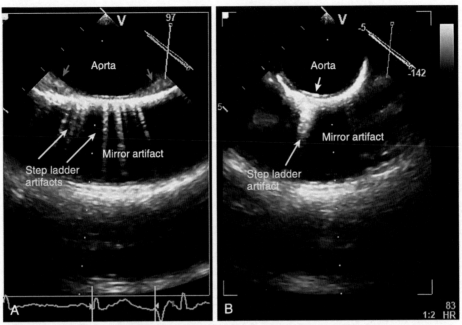

FIG. 7.7 The descending thoracic aorta imaged by biplane transesophageal echocardiography in the long axis (A) and short-axis (B): the aortic wall (in particular the endothelial calcification—*white arrowhead*, B) generates reverberations seen in the form of step ladder artifacts (*yellow arrows*). Furthermore, this calcification is the origin of a side lobe artifact (*blue arrowheads*, A, see further text for more detail). Finally, a mirror artifact resembling an additional aortic lumen can also be seen posterior to the aorta in both planes. This figure is one of many examples of various artifacts seen in one echocardiographic image. For a cine loop of this figure, refer to Video 7.7.

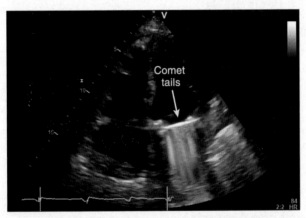

FIG. 7.8 Comet tail artifact caused by a mechanical mitral valve covering the entire left atrium. Note a hazier appearance of the comet tail artifact, compared with step ladder artifacts (Fig. 7.1 [*blue arrow*], Fig. 7.6 [*blue arrow*], Fig. 7.7 [*yellow arrow*]).

BOX 7.3 Reverberations as a Source of Information

The step ladder artifact can also be used to extract information. Indeed, the distance at which the step ladder is repeated is directly linked to the thickness of the reverberating structure (e.g., the prosthetic valve leaflet). As such, the reverberation artifacts allow for a very precise measurement of the thickness of the structure (using the so-called cepstrum method that automatically measures the distance at which the echo signal is repeated). This measurement is much more precise than a caliper-based B-mode measurement of the thickness of the structure causing the reverberation.

Similarly, comet tail artifacts are commonly used as a noninvasive, easy to perform semiquantitative tool for the assessment of extravascular lung water in the evaluation of B-lines by lung ultrasound (Video 7.8).[2]

Refraction Artifacts

Although ultrasound imaging assumes that the ultrasonic beam travels along a straight path to the structures of interest, this assumption can be violated when imaging through an object with different acoustic properties leading to refraction (i.e., redirection) of the propagating wave (for further explanation, see Chapter 1) at the surface of this object. As such, morphologic distortions can occur (as the true echo signals arrive from another direction than anticipated), which may not be trivial to detect. This artifact due to redirection of the ultrasound wave is referred to as a **"refraction" or "lens" artifact**. The thoracic or abdominal wall (structures such as costal cartilage, fasciae, and adipose tissue) as well as the pleura, pericardium, or even diaphragm may act as such a refraction-inducing medium (i.e., lens). This artifact can also present itself as doubling of structures in the image (Fig. 7.15, Video 7.14). Refraction artifacts are mainly recognized, as they form anatomically rather improbable structures (see Fig. 7.15, Video 7.14). In most cases, it is necessary to resort to an alternative echocardiographic window in order to avoid the lens effect of the refracting structure.[4]

BOX 7.2 The Changing Meaning of Ring-Down Artifacts

The "comet tail" and "step ladder" artifacts are sometimes referred to as "ring down" artifacts, as the reverberated echo signal gradually drops amplitude as if it were a bell ringing down after being hit. Although this ring-down artifact was originally related to near-field artifacts caused by ringing down of the transducer after it was "hit" with an electrical impulse, state-of-the-art transducers make use of very good damping (i.e., backing) materials, thereby essentially eliminating this ring down. Older literature may thus refer to the "ring down" artifact as transducer-related near-field artifacts, while more recently the same terminology was used to refer to reverberation artifacts associated with attenuation (i.e., the "comet tail" artifact).

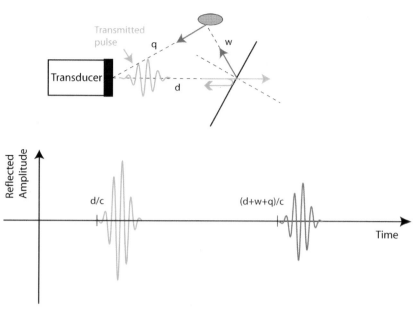

FIG. 7.9 The generation of multiple reflection artifacts. The transmitted wave *(green)* reflects at a tissue boundary at a distance "d" from the transducer. Part of the energy is reflected (due to scattering), causing an echo at the appropriate time. However, part of the energy bounces off *(red)* and meets other structures that cause a late arriving echo signal *(red)*. *d,* distance from transducer to imaged tissue; *w,* thickness of the layer; *q,* distance from other reflector to transducer; *c,* ultrasound propagation speed.

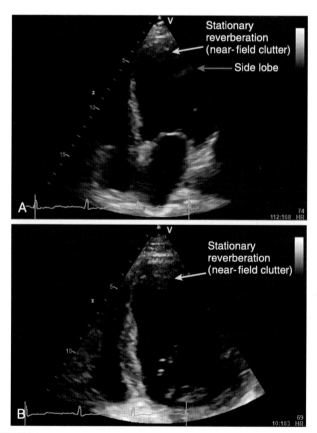

FIG. 7.10 Apical four-chamber view (A) and the same view focused on the left ventricle (B): stationary reverberation artifacts caused by the ribs, creating a ghost echo that may mimic a left ventricular apical thrombus *(yellow arrow)*; this specific type of artifact is also referred to as near-field clutter. A side-lobe artifact (explained in the text) can also be seen on panel A *(blue arrow)* as well as on the corresponding video (for cine-loop images, see Videos 7.5 and 7.6).

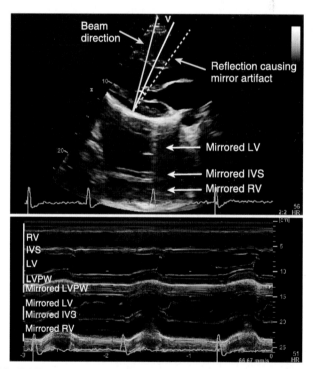

FIG. 7.11 *Upper panel:* Parasternal long axis view showing a strongly reflecting pericardium resulting in the generation of a mirror image posterior to the true left ventricle: mirrored left ventricle (LV), interventricular septum (IVS), and right ventricle (RV), white arrows. The upper panel also demonstrates the direction of ultrasound originating from and reflecting back to the transducer *(yellow line)*, as well as the direction of the reflection created at the pericardial surface *(yellow dashed line)*, responsible for the mirror artifact seen distal ("below") to the true parasternal long axis image. Note that the angle between the beam direction *(yellow line)* and the plane perpendicular to the pericardium *(white line)* equals that between the perpendicular plane and reflection *(dashed line)*. Namely, the concave surface of the pericardium distorts the direction of the reflected beam, such that the reflections in fact mirror the image in a distorted way. This can be better appreciated on the M-mode image *(lower panel)*—for example, from visible motion of the mitral leaflets within the mirrored LV cavity (not seen in the "true" cavity), a somewhat different motion of the myocardial walls as well as a greater RV cavity in the mirrored image. For a cine-loop image of this parasternal long axis, see Video 7.9. Video 7.10 demonstrates the left ventricular short axis plane of the same patient, imaged at the level of the papillary muscles. However, the mirrored image clearly depicts the mitral valve leaflets, due to the distortion of the reflected beam. *LVPW,* Left ventricular posterior wall.

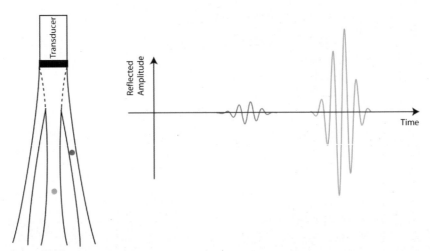

FIG. 7.12 Reflections originating from side lobes *(red)* are typically smaller in amplitude than those from the main lobe *(green)*. Should the main lobe be covering an anechogenic region, the amplitude of the side lobe reflections will supersede that of the reflections from the main lobe, and the side lobe reflections will erroneously be mapped on the image. *(From D'hooge J, Mertens LL. Ultrasound physics. In: Lai WW, Mertens LL, Cohen MS, Geva T, eds.* Echocardiography in pediatric and congenital heart disease: from fetus to adult, *2nd ed. Chichester: John Wiley and Sons; 2016:7).*

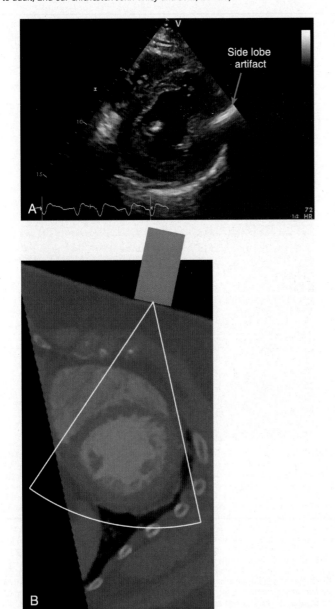

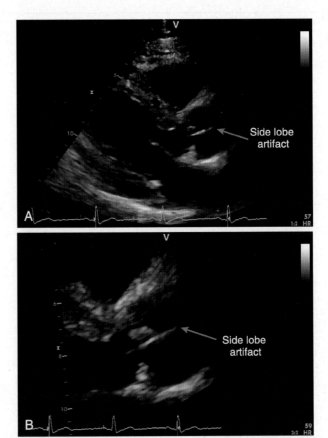

FIG. 7.14 Parasternal long axis view (A) and the same view zoomed on the aortic valve and left ventricular outflow tract (LVOT) (B) displaying a side lobe artifact visible as a bright, sharp line at the level of the aortic cusps, from which it originates *(arrow)*. The corresponding cine loops can be found under Videos 7.12 and 7.13.

FIG. 7.13 Parasternal short-axis view of the left ventricle exhibiting a side lobe artifact originating from the neighboring lung tissue (A) (clearly appreciated on computed tomography, B) that is filled with air and is thus very reflective, thereby creating a ghost echo across the left ventricular lateral wall *(blue arrow)*. A cine loop of part A of this figure can be seen on Video 7.11.

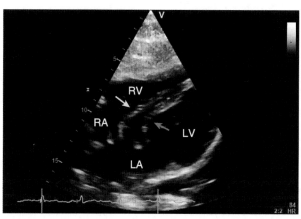

FIG. 7.15 A refraction artifact causing a double image of the interventricular septum *(yellow arrow)* in the subcostal view (the true interventricular septum is marked with a *blue arrow*). The cause of the artifact in this case is most likely the surface of the diaphragm. A cine loop of this figure can be seen under Video 7.14. *LA,* Left atrium; *LV,* left ventricle; *RA,* right atrium; *RV,* right ventricle.

Beam-Width Artifacts/Partial Volume Artifacts

Although 2D echocardiography displays a 2D cross-section of the heart, acoustic waves are intrinsically 3D, implying that all echo signals arising from the out-of-plane direction will be interpreted by the system as coming from the imaging plane itself. As such, structures that are located out-of-plane can be projected into the imaging plane due to extending of the acoustic wave in the elevation direction (i.e., the direction orthogonal to the scan plane). These artifacts are referred to as **"beam-width"** or **"partial volume" artifacts**. Similarly, Doppler recordings can suffer from picking up velocities out-of-plane and displaying them within the imaging plane (Fig. 7.16).

(COLOR) DOPPLER MIRROR IMAGE ARTIFACTS

B-mode mirror image artifact is created by a strong reflector that acts as a secondary acoustic source and images from the reflector toward the transducer (discussed previously); (color) Doppler imaging inherits this property and can give rise to (color) Doppler mirror image artifacts. From the perspective of the reflector, the blood flow velocities are of opposite sign

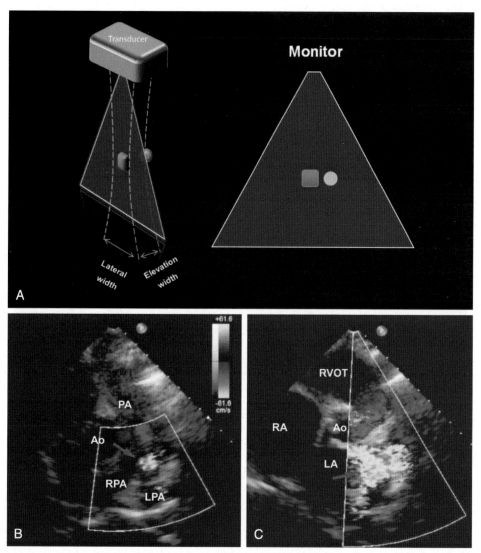

FIG. 7.16 **The generation of beam-width artifacts.** (A) The features of the ultrasound beam, such as its lateral width and elevation, impair lateral resolution and induce the occurrence of beam-width artifacts, respectively. The blue square (which is within the imaging plane) is adequately positioned in the center of the beam; yet the green circular object (which is outside the imaging plane) is inadequately recognized within the scanning plane, due to the elevation width of the beam. (B) Parasternal short-axis image focused on the pulmonary arteries shows unexplained turbulent flow into the left pulmonary artery (LPA; *arrow*), without clear shunting or stenosis. (C) By tilting the probe out of the scanning plane, massive mitral regurgitation *(arrow)* towards the left atrium (LA) is picked up by the beam as if occurring in the pulmonary artery (PA). *Ao,* Aorta; *RA,* right atrium; *RPA,* right pulmonary artery; *RVOT,* right ventricular outflow tract. *(From Bertrand PB, Levine RA, Isselbacher EM, Vandervoort PM. Fact or artifact in two-dimensional echocardiography: avoiding misdiagnosis and missed diagnosis. J Am Soc Echocardiogr. 2016;29(5):381–391).*

(opposite direction) when compared with those seen by the transducer. Thus the colors depicted by color Doppler imaging in the mirror image are equally reversed. An example of a pericardial color Doppler mirror image is given in Fig. 7.17.

Another example of a color Doppler mirror image artifact described in the literature is the occurrence of color Doppler flow visible in the left atrium in patients with prosthetic mitral valves, suggestive of mitral regurgitation.[5] Obviously, it is clinically highly relevant not to mistake such artifactual flow for valvular regurgitation, which may even lead to inappropriate surgical revision procedures. The described flow can most easily be recognized by assessing the flow pattern and duration determined by PW Doppler, which in this case equals that of left ventricular outflow tract (LVOT) flow, rather than that of mitral regurgitation.

FOUR-DIMENSIONAL ECHOCARDIOGRAPHY STITCH ARTIFACTS

In order to keep space-time resolution of four-dimensional (4D) imaging systems adequate, a full volume image of the heart is formed by acquiring multiple smaller volumes acquired over multiple heartbeats and subsequently fuse (i.e., stitch) these smaller volumes to a single recording. However, the stitching procedure can fail due to motion between the acquisitions of the different subvolumes (i.e., spatial misalignment) and/or due to changes in heart rate (i.e., temporal misalignment; Fig. 7.18), generally referred to as **"stitching" artifacts**. If caused by respiratory motion, stitch artifacts may be prevented by the patient's breath hold, while they otherwise limit the diagnostic utility of the images, particularly in arrhythmias. Newer systems that employ single-beat acquisition of full volume data circumvent this technical limitation of 4D echocardiography at the cost of reduced spatiotemporal or contrast-to-noise ratio of the data set.

Suggested Readings

Bertrand, P. B., Levine, R. A., Isselbacher, E. M., & Vandervoort, P. M. (2016). Fact or artifact in two-dimensional echocardiography: avoiding misdiagnosis and missed diagnosis. *Journal of the American Society of Echocardiography, 29*, 381–391.

D'hooge, J., & Mertens, L. L. (2016). Ultrasound physics. In W. W. Lai, L. L. Mertens, M. S. Cohen, & T. Geva (Eds.), *Echocardiography in Pediatric and Congenital Heart Disease: From Fetus to Adult* (2nd ed.) (pp. 2–18). Chichester: John Wiley and Sons.

Linka, A. Z., Barton, M., Attenhofer Jost, C., & Jenni, R. (2000). Doppler mirror image artifacts mimicking mitral regurgitation in patients with mechanical bileaflet mitral valve prostheses. *European Journal of Echocardiography, 1*(2), 138–143.

Miglioranza, M. H., Gargani, L., Sant'Anna, R. T., et al. (2013). Lung ultrasound for the evaluation of pulmonary congestion in outpatients: a comparison with clinical assessment, natriuretic peptides, and echocardiography. *JACC Cardiovascular Imaging, 6*(11), 1141–1151.

Solomon, S. D. (2007). Echocardiographic instrumentation and principles of Doppler echocardiography. In S. D. Solomon (Ed.), *Essential Echocardiography - A Practical Handbook with DVD* (pp. 3–17). Totowa, NJ: Humana Press.

A complete reference list can be found online at ExpertConsult.com.

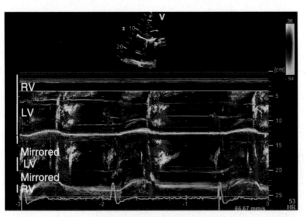

FIG. 7.17 Color M-mode image showing the true (proximal, *full yellow line*) and mirrored (distal, *dashed yellow line*) structures of the heart. In the mirrored part of the image the velocities measured are of opposite sign and the color encoding is thus inversed. Note that the mirrored color flow velocities are taken along the mirrored image line which is typically not along the original image line as explained above (see Fig. 7.11). *LV*, Left ventricle; *RV*, right ventricle.

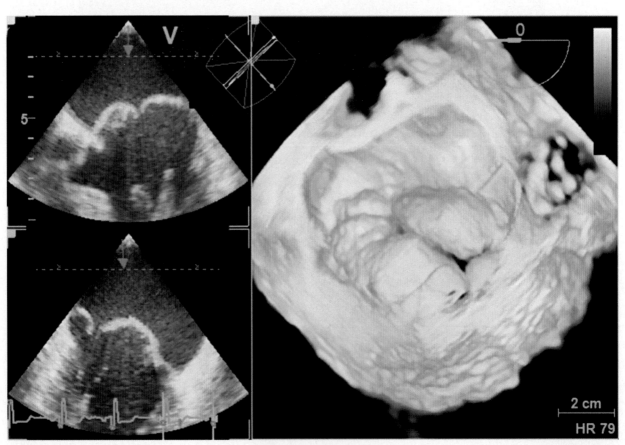

FIG. 7.18 Example of incorrect fusion (i.e., stitching) of four subvolumes acquired in four subsequent heart beats by 4D echocardiography.

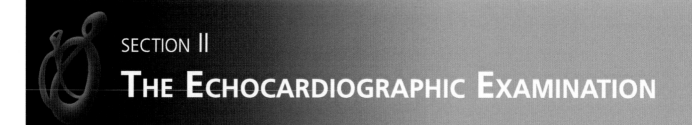

8 Principles of Transthoracic Imaging Acquisition: The Standard Adult Transthoracic Echocardiographic Examination

Bernard E. Bulwer

INTRODUCTION

In the adult two-dimensional (2D) transthoracic echocardiographic (TTE) examination, a standard series of cross-sectional anatomical views are recommended by the American Society of Echocardiography (ASE).[1-6] Each echocardiographic view is described using three aspects of the examination, namely (1) the transducer positioned at a specified anatomical "window" on or near the thorax, (2) the cardiac scan plane transected by the transducer beam, and (3) the anatomical structure or region of interest (Fig. 8.1).[1-12] The 2D TTE examination is the basis for the comprehensive assessment of cardiac structure and function (Figs. 8.2–8.21; see also Fig. 8.1).

The 2D TTE examination supplanted the M-Mode examination—a one-dimensional "motion-mode" examination, which remains a useful adjunct to the 2D TTE protocol. The 2D TTE examination is also complemented by additional echocardiography protocols. These include Doppler echocardiography (color flow, spectral, and tissue Doppler) and three-dimensional (3D) echocardiography (Figs. 8.22–8.24).[13-18] Myocardial segmentation nomenclature and assessment is integral to the 2D TTE examination (Fig. 8.25).[19]

Transducer Positions

The bony chest wall and the air-filled lungs are major obstacles to transmission of the ultrasound beam. Consequently, optimal examination of the adult heart requires placing the ultrasound transducer at specified positions or "windows" on or near the chest wall. Four primary transducer positions or "windows" are recommended. For patients with normal levocardia, the examination begins at (1) the left parasternal window—P, followed by (2) the apical window—A, (3) the subcostal or subxiphoid window—SC, and (4) the suprasternal notch window—SSN (Fig. 8.2).[1-6]

Cardiac Imaging Plane

By convention, tomographic imaging of most human organs and structures are described according to the anatomical position and the standard anatomical planes—median (sagittal), transverse (horizontal or axial), and frontal (coronal). Thanks to its embryology, the heart is unique in its disregard for this cardinal principle.[5-7] Three orthogonal imaging planes are used as reference for each standard echocardiographic view: (1) long-axis—LAX, (2) short-axis—SAX, and (3) four-chamber—4C planes (Figs. 8.3 and 8.4).[1,4,5]

The cardiac LAX plane lies parallel to the left ventricular (LV) long-axis, transects the LV apex, the center of the aortic valve (AV), and anteroposterior diameter of the mitral valve (MV). The LAX planes of the LV can be acquired from both the left parasternal and apical windows (Fig. 8.5; see also Figs. 8.1 and 8.4).[1-6]

The cardiac SAX plane transects the heart orthogonal to the LV long axis, starting from the cardiac base—at the aortic valve level (AVL), then slicing toward the LV apex. SAX planes of the LV can be acquired from both the left parasternal and subcostal windows (see Figs. 8.1, 8.4, and 8.5).[1-6]

The cardiac 4C plane transects both atria, both ventricles, and their intervening septae. This 4C plane is oriented orthogonal to both the cardiac LAX and SAX planes. The 4C planes of the heart can be acquired from both the apical and subcostal windows (see Figs. 8.1, 8.4, and 8.5).[1-6]

Region or Structure of Interest

The third component used to describe each standard echocardiographic view is the structure or region of interest (see Figs. 8.1 and 8.8).[1-6] Using this nomenclature, the echocardiographic view obtained with (1) the transducer positioned at the left parasternal window—P, oriented along (2) the cardiac long-axis plane—LAX, with (3) focus on the *left ventricular (LV) inflow and outflow* (i.e., with the mitral and aortic valves in focus) is called the *parasternal long-axis view—LV inflow-outflow*, or *PLAX* for short

Likewise, the echocardiographic view of obtained with (1) the transducer positioned at the left parasternal window—P, oriented along (2) the cardiac short-axis plane—SAX, with (3) focus on the *mitral valve* is called the *parasternal short-axis view—mitral valve level*, or *PSAX-MVL*, for short. The echocardiographic views obtained at the apical window, A, or subcostal window, SC, that transect the *cardiac four-chamber plane* are hence referred to as the *apical four-chamber view, A4C view*, or the *subcostal four-chamber view, SC-4C view*, and so on (Fig. 8.6; see also Fig. 8.1).

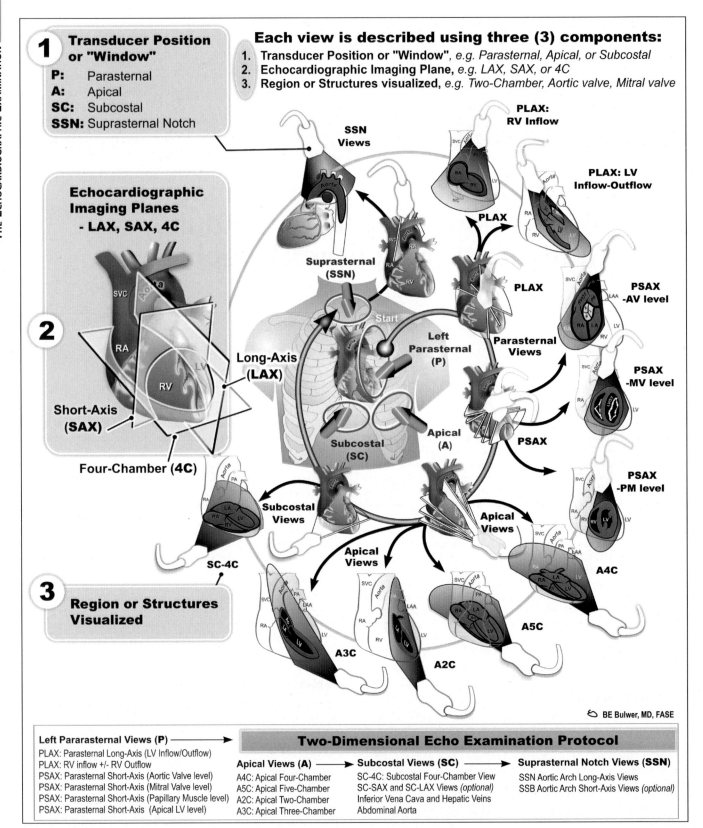

1 **Transducer Position or "Window"**

- **P:** Parasternal
- **A:** Apical
- **SC:** Subcostal
- **SSN:** Suprasternal Notch

Each view is described using three (3) components:

1. Transducer Position or "Window", *e.g. Parasternal, Apical, or Subcostal*
2. Echocardiographic Imaging Plane, *e.g. LAX, SAX, or 4C*
3. Region or Structures visualized, *e.g. Two-Chamber, Aortic valve, Mitral valve*

Echocardiographic Imaging Planes - LAX, SAX, 4C

2

Long-Axis (LAX)

Short-Axis (SAX)

Four-Chamber (4C)

3 **Region or Structures Visualized**

SSN Views — Suprasternal (SSN)

Start — Left Parasternal (P)

Subcostal (SC) — Apical (A)

PLAX: RV Inflow

PLAX: LV Inflow-Outflow

PLAX — Parasternal Views

PSAX -AV level

PSAX -MV level

PSAX -PM level

A4C

A5C

A3C — A2C

SC-4C — Subcostal Views

Apical Views

↳ BE Bulwer, MD, FASE

Left Parasternal Views (P) ⟶

PLAX: Parasternal Long-Axis (LV Inflow/Outflow)
PLAX: RV inflow +/- RV Outflow
PSAX: Parasternal Short-Axis (Aortic Valve level)
PSAX: Parasternal Short-Axis (Mitral Valve level)
PSAX: Parasternal Short-Axis (Papillary Muscle level)
PSAX: Parasternal Short-Axis (Apical LV level)

Two-Dimensional Echo Examination Protocol

Apical Views (A) ⟶

A4C: Apical Four-Chamber
A5C: Apical Five-Chamber
A2C: Apical Two-Chamber
A3C: Apical Three-Chamber

Subcostal Views (SC) ⟶

SC-4C: Subcostal Four-Chamber View
SC-SAX and SC-LAX Views *(optional)*
Inferior Vena Cava and Hepatic Veins
Abdominal Aorta

Suprasternal Notch Views (SSN)

SSN Aortic Arch Long-Axis Views
SSB Aortic Arch Short-Axis Views *(optional)*

FIG. 8.1 Graphical summary of the standard examination protocol and nomenclature of the two-dimensional (2D) transthoracic echocardiographic views (American Society of Echocardiography [1980]). Note the transducer scan planes and cross-sectional anatomical planes. *(Modified from Bulwer BE, Shernan SK, Thomas JD. Physics of echocardiography. In: Savage RM, Aronson S, Shernan SK, eds. Comprehensive textbook of perioperative transesophageal echocardiography. Philadelphia: Lippincott, Williams & Wilkins; 2009:1–41.)*

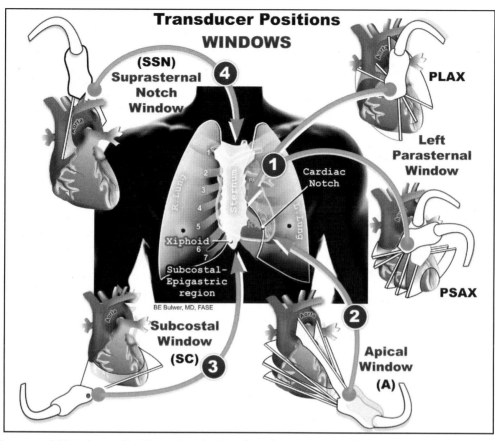

FIG. 8.2 The standard recommended transducer positions in transthoracic echocardiography. *PLAX,* Parasternal long-axis; *PSAX,* Parasternal short-axis. *(Courtesy of Bernard E. Bulwer, MD, FASE.)*

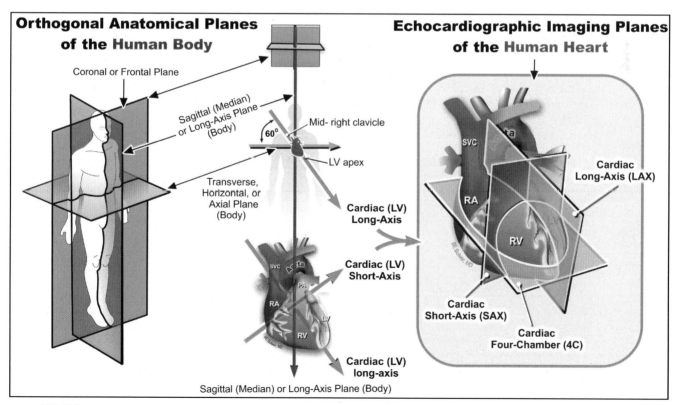

FIG. 8.3 The orthogonal anatomical imaging planes and the echocardiographic imaging planes compared. *(Courtesy of Bernard E. Bulwer, MD, FASE.)*

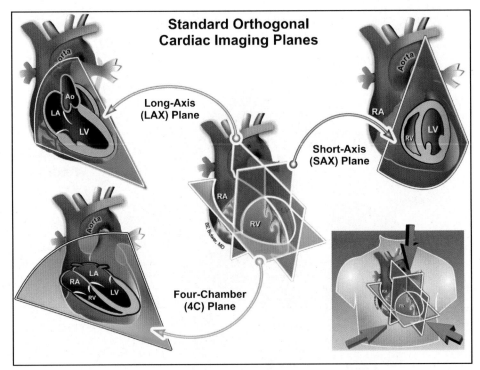

FIG. 8.4 The standard orthogonal cardiac imaging planes and cross-sectional projections. *(Courtesy of Bernard E. Bulwer, MD, FASE.)*

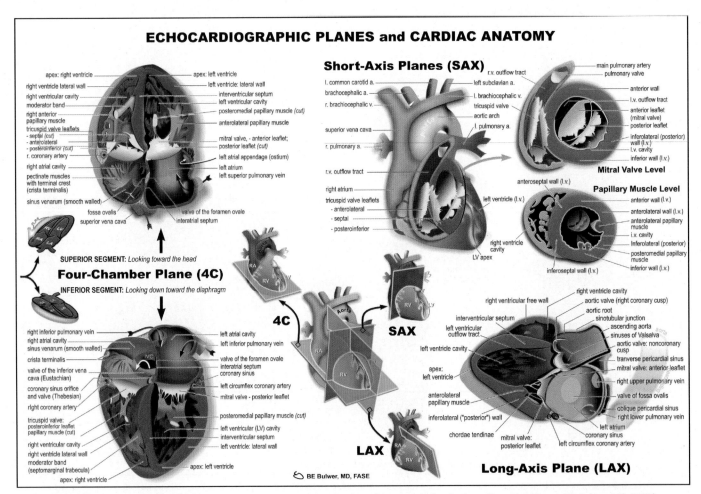

FIG. 8.5 The orthogonal echocardiographic imaging planes and their corresponding anatomical projections. *(Courtesy of Bernard E. Bulwer, MD, FASE.)*

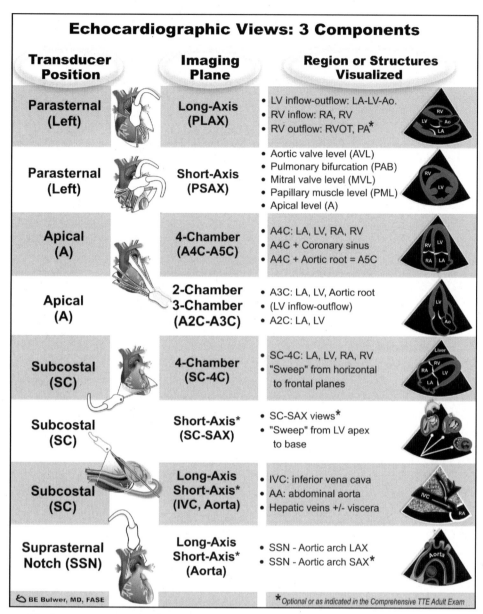

FIG. 8.6 Graphical summary of the three components used to describe the standard transthoracic echocardiographic (TTE) views in the adult: (1) transducer position or "window," (2) cardiac imaging plane, and (3) the cardiac region or structure of interest. *(Courtesy of Bernard E. Bulwer, MD, FASE.)*

An overview of the standard adult TTE views used to examine the major cardiac chambers and valves are summarized in Fig. 8.7.[1-6]

IMAGE ORIENTATION STANDARDS

Phased array transducers used in echocardiography are designed with a transducer index mark. This serves as a guide to the transducer scan plane orientation, the recommended transducer maneuvers, and the resultant image display. By the ASE convention, the index mark indicates the part of the image plane that appears on the right side of the image display (see Figs. 8.8 and 8.9).[3-5,7,8]

TWO-DIMENSIONAL ECHOCARDIOGRAPHY: TOMOGRAPHIC SCAN PLANE ORIENTATION AND DISPLAY PROTOCOL

A graphical exposé of the following transducer scan planes, orientation, and views in adult 2D TTE) examination are presented[1-6,9-12]:

1. Left parasternal views (see Figs. 8.9–8.11)
2. Apical views (see Figs. 8.12–8.15)
3. Subcostal views (see Figs. 8.16 and 8.17)
4. Suprasternal notch views (see Figs. 8.18–8.20)

COMPLEMENTARY PROTOCOLS: DOPPLER, THREE-DIMENSIONAL ECHOCARDIOGRAPHY, AND MYOCARDIAL SEGMENTATION

Color flow Doppler and spectral Doppler echocardiography are essential in the comprehensive assessment of intracardiac flows and transvalvular hemodynamics.[13-15] These protocols are integrated into the 2D TTE examination (see Figs. 8.22 and 8.23).[13-17]

Newer tissue Doppler and 3D echocardiography techniques are also increasingly integrated within the workflow of the 2D TTE examination (see Figs. 8.23 and 8.24).[16-18] They have added utility in the assessment of myocardial systolic and diastolic performance, hemodynamic function, and cardiac chamber quantification.

The contractile behavior of the myocardial walls is an essential part of the echocardiographic assessment of patients with coronary artery disease. The 2D TTE examination serves as the basis for correlating the ventricular myocardial segments with their corresponding coronary artery supply (Fig. 8.25).[19]

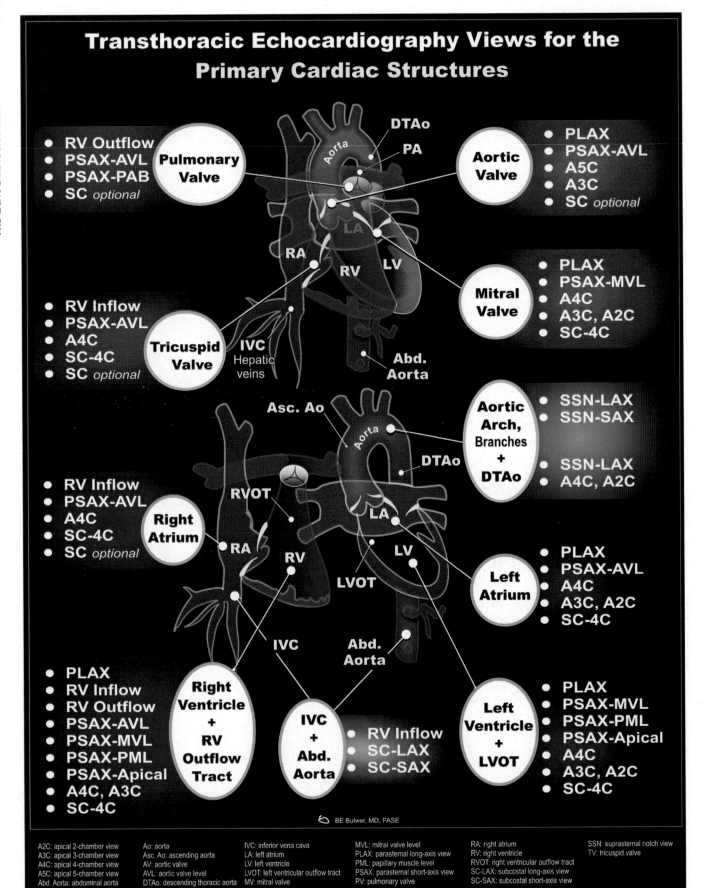

Transthoracic Echocardiography Views for the Primary Cardiac Structures

Pulmonary Valve
- RV Outflow
- PSAX-AVL
- PSAX-PAB
- SC *optional*

Aortic Valve
- PLAX
- PSAX-AVL
- A5C
- A3C
- SC *optional*

Mitral Valve
- PLAX
- PSAX-MVL
- A4C
- A3C, A2C
- SC-4C

Tricuspid Valve
- RV Inflow
- PSAX-AVL
- A4C
- SC-4C
- SC *optional*

Aortic Arch, Branches + DTAo
- SSN-LAX
- SSN-SAX
- SSN-LAX
- A4C, A2C

Right Atrium
- RV Inflow
- PSAX-AVL
- A4C
- SC-4C
- SC *optional*

Left Atrium
- PLAX
- PSAX-AVL
- A4C
- A3C, A2C
- SC-4C

Right Ventricle + RV Outflow Tract
- PLAX
- RV Inflow
- RV Outflow
- PSAX-AVL
- PSAX-MVL
- PSAX-PML
- PSAX-Apical
- A4C, A3C
- SC-4C

IVC + Abd. Aorta
- RV Inflow
- SC-LAX
- SC-SAX

Left Ventricle + LVOT
- PLAX
- PSAX-MVL
- PSAX-PML
- PSAX-Apical
- A4C
- A3C, A2C
- SC-4C

BE Bulwer, MD, FASE

A2C: apical 2-chamber view
A3C: apical 3-chamber view
A4C: apical 4-chamber view
A5C: apical 5-chamber view
Abd. Aorta: abdominal aorta

Ao: aorta
Asc. Ao: ascending aorta
AV: aortic valve
AVL: aortic valve level
DTAo: descending thoracic aorta

IVC: inferior vena cava
LA: left atrium
LV: left ventricle
LVOT: left ventricular outflow tract
MV: mitral valve

MVL: mitral valve level
PLAX: parasternal long-axis view
PML: papillary muscle level
PSAX: parasternal short-axis view
PV: pulmonary valve

RA: right atrium
RV: right ventricle
RVOT: right ventricular outflow tract
SC-LAX: subcostal long-axis view
SC-SAX: subcostal short-axis view

SSN: suprasternal notch view
TV: tricuspid valve

FIG. 8.7 Primary cardiac structures and the standard transthoracic echocardiographic views used in their assessment. *(Courtesy of Bernard E. Bulwer, MD, FASE.)*

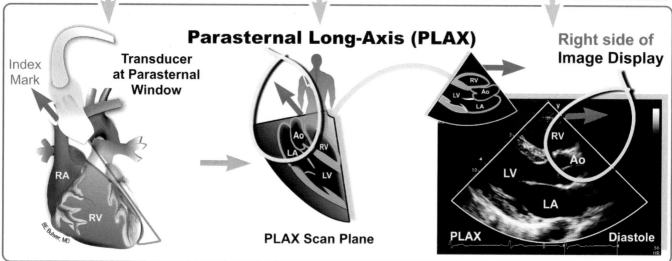

Parasternal Long-Axis (PLAX)

Parasternal Short-Axis (PSAX)

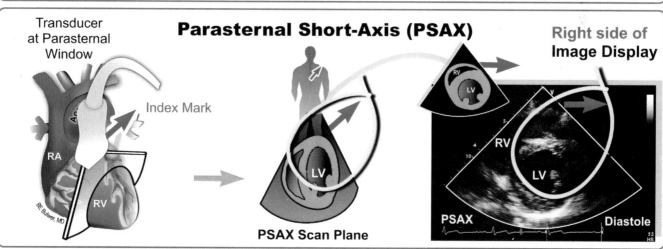

Apical 4-Chamber (A4C)

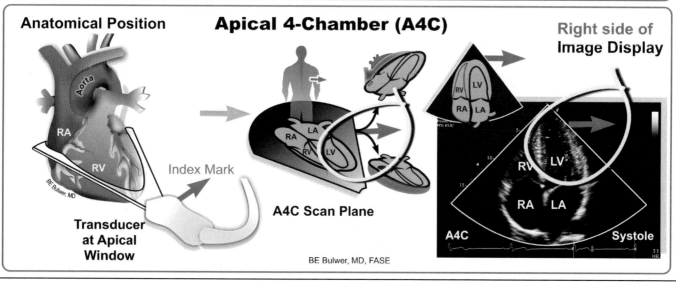

FIG. 8.8 Image display convention recommended by the American Society of Echocardiography (1980). The index mark located on the transducer indicates the part of the echocardiographic imaging plane that appears on the right-hand side of the image display. *(Courtesy of Bernard E. Bulwer, MD, FASE.)*

Parasternal Long-Axis Scan Planes and Views

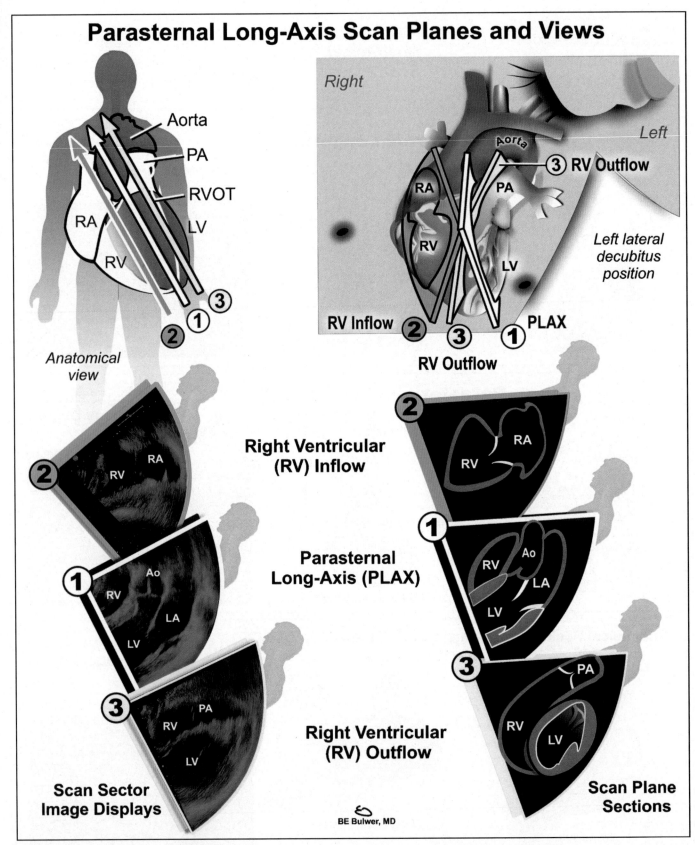

FIG. 8.9 Panorama of the standard left parasternal long-axis (PLAX) views showing their anatomical orientation *(above)*, their corresponding cross-sectional anatomy *(below right)*, and image displays *(below left)*. The PLAX view (scan plane 1)—typically the first to be obtained in the two-dimensional transthoracic echocardiography examination (see Fig. 8.1)—is aligned along the long-axis of the left ventricular (LV), aortic root (Ao), and left atrium (LA), and transects both the mitral and aortic valves. The RV inflow view (scan plane 2) transects the right atrium (RA), right ventricle (RV), and the tricuspid valve. The RV outflow view (scan plane 3) transects the RV outflow tract and pulmonary valve. Note that when the transducer is positioned at the left parasternal window, the first cardiac chamber transected is the RV—which appears in the near field of the image display. *(Courtesy of Bernard E. Bulwer, MD, FASE.)*

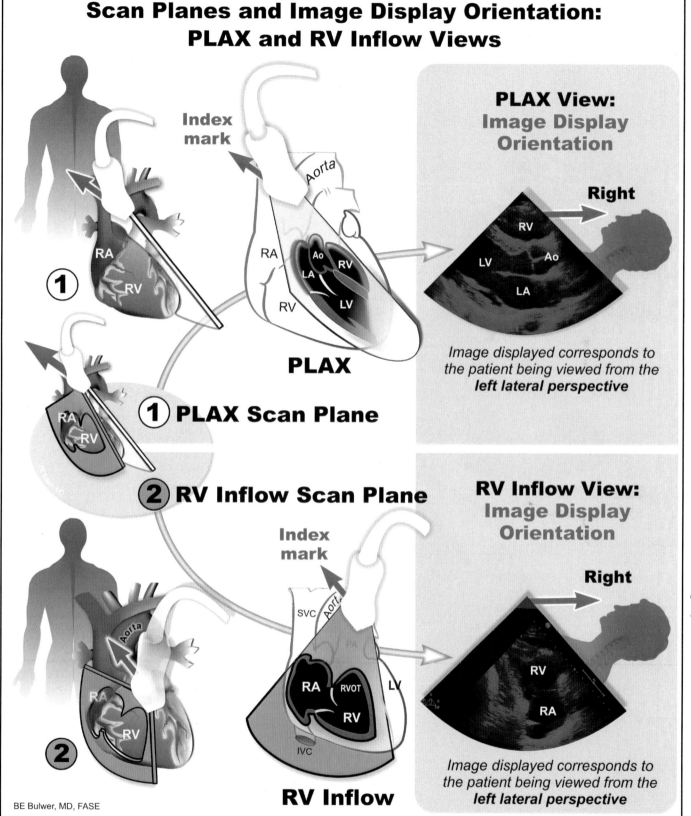

Scan Planes and Image Display Orientation: PLAX and RV Inflow Views

Index mark

Aorta

RA

Ao

RV

LA

RV

LV

PLAX

① **PLAX Scan Plane**

② **RV Inflow Scan Plane**

Index mark

SVC

Aorta

RA

RVOT

LV

RV

IVC

RV Inflow

PLAX View: Image Display Orientation

Right

RV

LV

Ao

LA

Image displayed corresponds to the patient being viewed from the **left lateral perspective**

RV Inflow View: Image Display Orientation

Right

RV

RA

Image displayed corresponds to the patient being viewed from the **left lateral perspective**

BE Bulwer, MD, FASE

FIG. 8.10 Orientation of the parasternal long-axis views of the left ventricular inflow-outflow (PLAX) and the right ventricular (RV) inflow, showing their anatomical orientation *(left-hand column)*, cross-sectional anatomy (central column), and corresponding image displays *(right-hand column)*. Note the orientation of the index mark in the anatomical position—directed toward the right shoulder (~10 o'clock position), compared with the corresponding image display. *(Courtesy of Bernard E. Bulwer, MD, FASE.)*

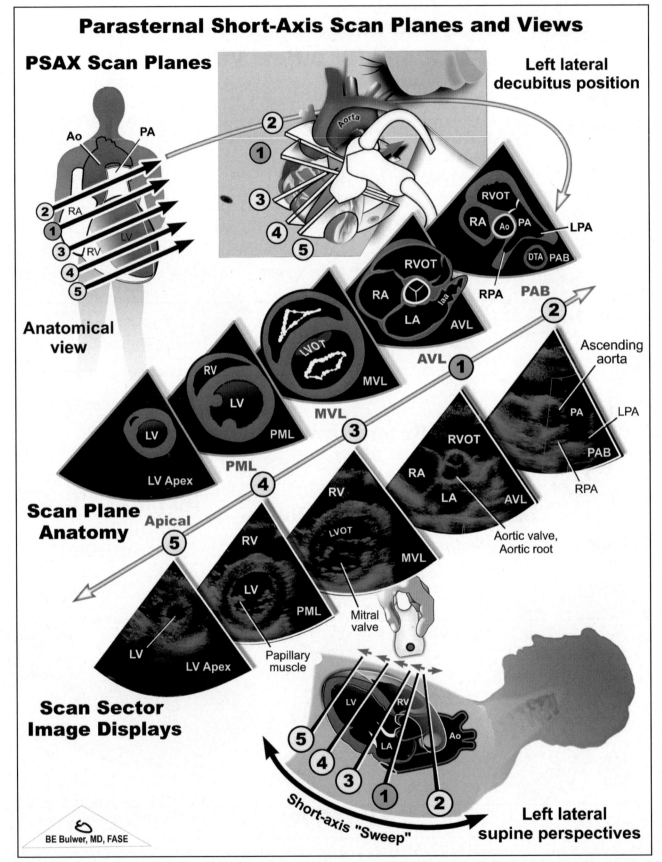

Parasternal Short-Axis Scan Planes and Views

PSAX Scan Planes

Left lateral decubitus position

Anatomical view

Scan Plane Anatomy

Scan Sector Image Displays

Short-axis "Sweep"

Left lateral supine perspectives

BE Bulwer, MD, FASE

FIG. 8.11 Panorama of the standard left parasternal short-axis (PSAX) views showing their anatomical orientation *(top panel)*, the corresponding cross-sectional anatomy (mid-panel), and image displays *(below)*. Note that the PSAX views are oriented orthogonal to the long-axis (LAX) views (see Figs. 8.1 and 8.9). The PSAX family of views are acquired following the examination of the parasternal long-axis family of views (see Fig. 8.1). The PSAX view at the aortic valve level (AVL, scan plane 1) is typically the first PSAX view to acquire (since it is reliably obtained by rotating the transducer scan plane 90 degrees clockwise, starting from the PLAX view). The PSAX-AVL serves as the reference plane for the scan planes labeled 2–5. *(Courtesy of Bernard E. Bulwer, MD, FASE.)*

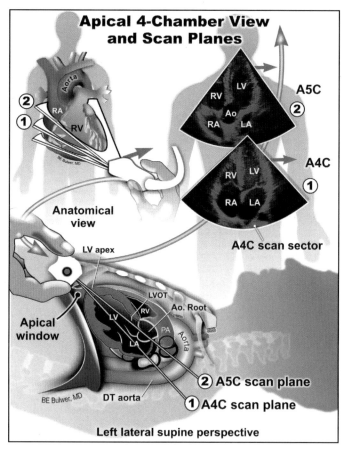

FIG. 8.12 Panorama of the standard apical views with the transducer positioned at the apical (A) window, transecting the left ventricular (LV) apex and the four-chamber (4C) plane. Note their anatomical orientation *(top left)*, corresponding cross-sectional anatomy viewed from the left lateral supine perspective *(bottom panel)*, and the corresponding image displays *(top right)*. The A4C view transects the LV apex and all four cardiac chambers (LA, LV, RA, and RV) and septae, with their junction (internal cardiac crux) clearly visible. When the A4C scan plane is superiorly directed, it transects the LV outflow tract and the aortic root (Ao) or "fifth" chamber; hence the term *apical five-chamber* or *A5C view*. Optimally acquired apical views should transect the true anatomical apex of the LV. The apical views are acquired following examination of the left parasternal views (see Fig. 8.1). *(Courtesy of Bernard E. Bulwer, MD, FASE.)*

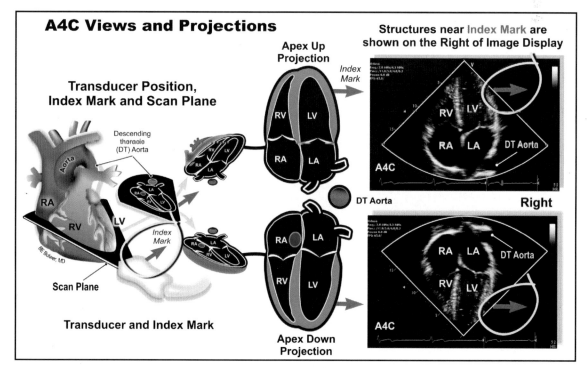

FIG. 8.13 Anatomical orientation and scan plane projections of the apical four-chamber (A4C) view. Two image display options are recommended. Most laboratories use the apex-up projection to display the A4C view, as this is consistent with other imaging protocols such as cardiac computed tomography and cardiac magnetic resonance imaging. The apex-down projection is preferred in pediatric echocardiography. *(Courtesy of Bernard E. Bulwer, MD, FASE.)*

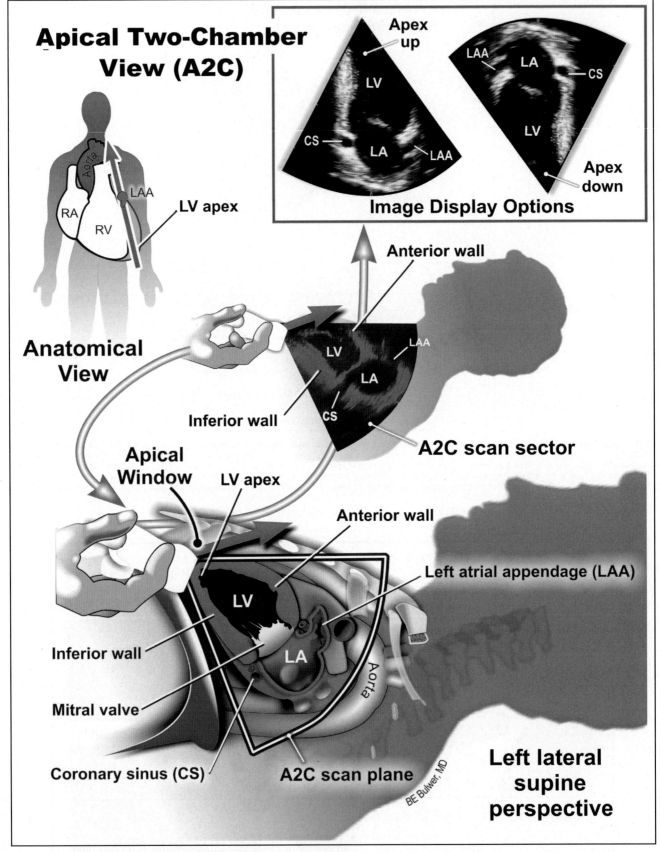

Apical Two-Chamber View (A2C)

Aorta

RA

RV

LAA

LV apex

Anatomical View

Apical Window

LV apex

Inferior wall

LV

LA

CS

Anterior wall

LAA

A2C scan sector

Apex up

LV

CS

LA

LAA

LAA

LA

CS

LV

Apex down

Image Display Options

Anterior wall

Left atrial appendage (LAA)

LV

LA

Aorta

Inferior wall

Mitral valve

Coronary sinus (CS)

A2C scan plane

Left lateral supine perspective

BE Bulwer, MD

FIG. 8.14 The apical two-chamber (A2C) view depicting its anatomical orientation *(top left)*, corresponding cross-sectional anatomy viewed from the left lateral supine perspective *(bottom panel)*, and the corresponding image display options *(top right)*. Note the transducer positioned at the apical window, with the scan plane transecting the left ventricular (LV) apex, the LV chamber, and the left atrium (LA), and the intervening mitral valve (MV). The A2C view is examined following acquisition of the A4C and A5C views (see Fig. 8.1). *(Courtesy of Bernard E. Bulwer, MD, FASE.)*

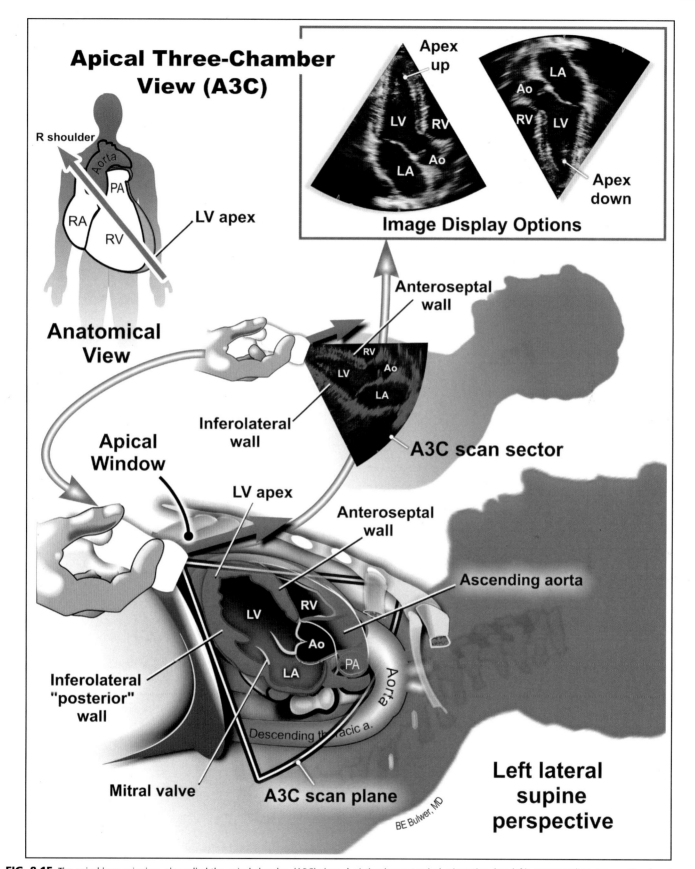

FIG. 8.15 The apical long-axis view, also called the apical-chamber (A3C) view, depicting its anatomical orientation *(top left)*, corresponding cross-sectional anatomy viewed from the left lateral supine perspective *(bottom panel)*, and the corresponding image display options *(top right)*. Note the transducer positioned at the apical window, with the scan plane aligned along the long-axis of the left ventricular (LV), aortic root (Ao), and left atrium (LA), and transects both the mitral and aortic valves. Note The A3C view, unlike the parasternal long-axis view, transects the LV apex and apical segments. It is examined following acquisition of the A4C and A5C views (see Fig. 8.1). *(Courtesy of Bernard E. Bulwer, MD, FASE.)*

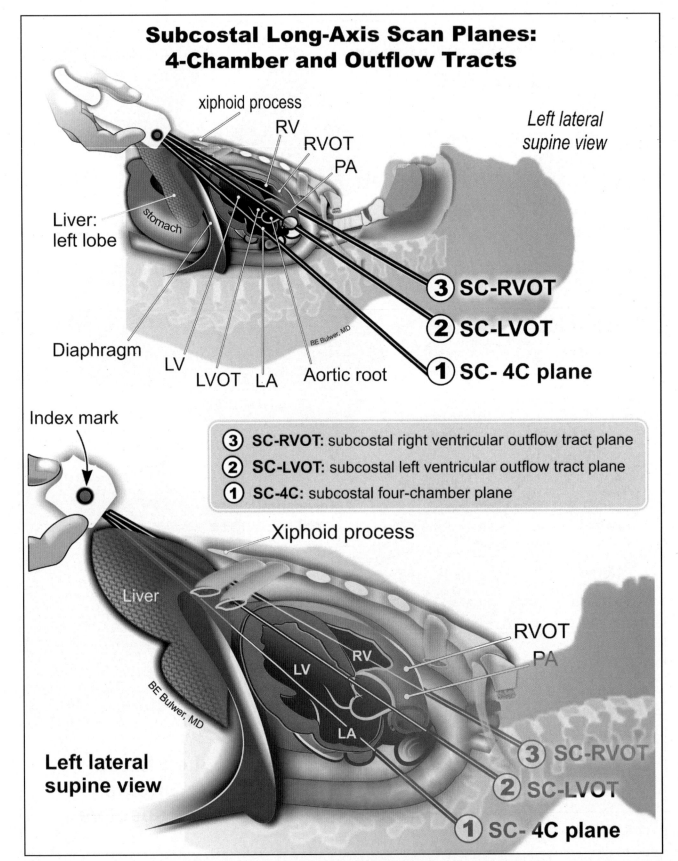

Subcostal Long-Axis Scan Planes:
4-Chamber and Outflow Tracts

xiphoid process

Left lateral supine view

RV
RVOT
PA

Liver: left lobe
stomach

③ SC-RVOT
② SC-LVOT
① SC- 4C plane

Diaphragm
LV
LVOT   LA   Aortic root

BE Bulwer, MD

Index mark

> ③ **SC-RVOT:** subcostal right ventricular outflow tract plane
> ② **SC-LVOT:** subcostal left ventricular outflow tract plane
> ① **SC-4C:** subcostal four-chamber plane

Xiphoid process

Liver

RVOT
PA

RV
LV

LA

③ SC-RVOT
② SC-LVOT

Left lateral supine view

① SC- 4C plane

BE Bulwer, MD

FIG. 8.16 Subcostal scan planes and corresponding image displays illustrating (1) the subcostal four-chamber view, (2) long-axis view of the inferior vena cava (IVC), and (3) long-axis view of the abdominal aorta (AA). In the adult two-dimensional (2D) transthoracic echocardiographic (TTE) examination, cardiac views obtained from the parasternal and apical windows are generally sufficient to comprehensively assess cardiac structure and function. The subcostal window is therefore used primarily to assess the interatrial and interventricular septae (on the subcostal four-chamber view), and to assess the proximal inferior vena cava, hepatic veins, and the proximal abdominal aorta. In the pediatric examination, subcostal short-axis views of the IVC and AA are typically the first step in the pediatric 2D TTE protocol *(bottom panels)*. They are used to establish situs or position of the heart and organs, as part of the sequential segmental analysis of the cardiac chambers. *(Courtesy of Bernard E. Bulwer, MD, FASE.)*

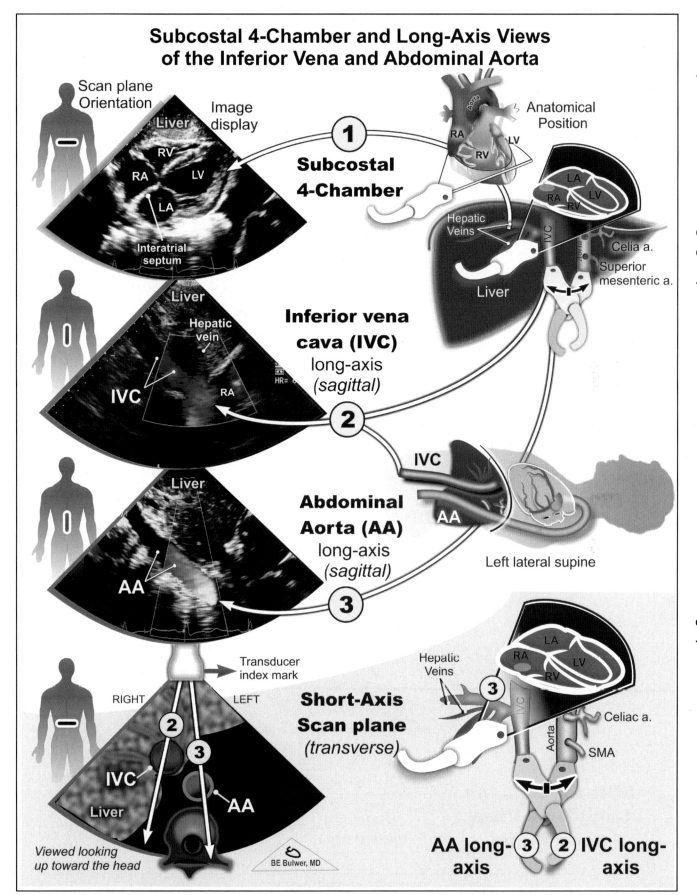

Subcostal 4-Chamber and Long-Axis Views of the Inferior Vena and Abdominal Aorta

FIG. 8.17 Left lateral supine anatomical perspectives of the subcostal scan plane swept along (1) the subcostal four-chamber (SC-4C) plane, (2) the plane swept superiorly through the left ventricular outflow tract, and (3) through the right ventricular outflow tract. If the parasternal and apical windows are obliterated or inaccessible, or as in pediatric echocardiography, the subcostal window can be used to obtain a family of views that approximate short-axis, long-axis, and four-chamber views. *(Courtesy of Bernard E. Bulwer, MD, FASE.)*

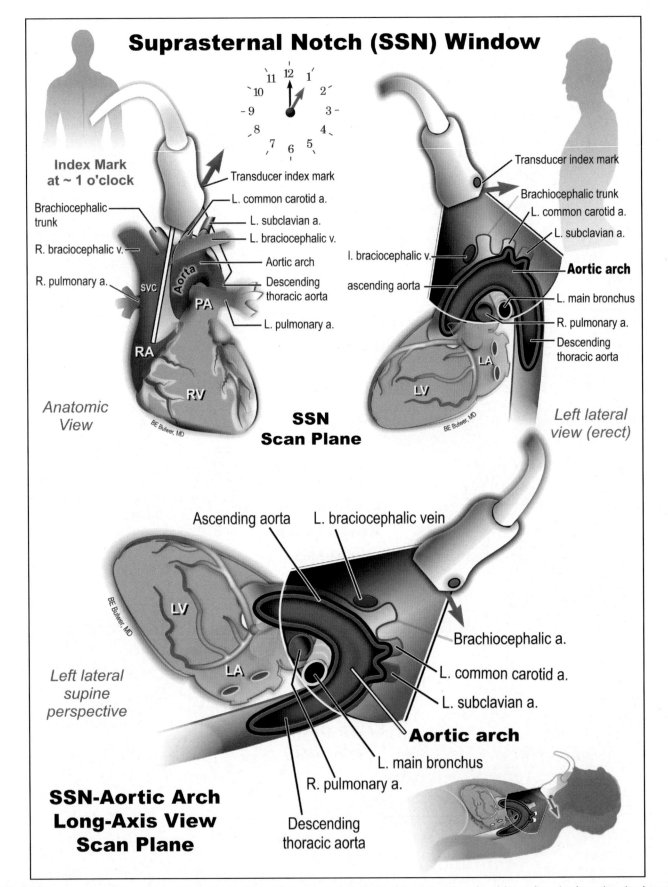

Suprasternal Notch (SSN) Window

Index Mark at ~ 1 o'clock

Transducer index mark

Brachiocephalic trunk

R. braciocephalic v.

R. pulmonary a.

SVC

Aorta

PA

RA

RV

L. common carotid a.

L. subclavian a.

L. braciocephalic v.

Aortic arch

Descending thoracic aorta

L. pulmonary a.

Anatomic View

SSN Scan Plane

BE Bulwer, MD

Transducer index mark

Brachiocephalic trunk

L. common carotid a.

L. subclavian a.

l. braciocephalic v.

ascending aorta

Aortic arch

L. main bronchus

R. pulmonary a.

Descending thoracic aorta

LA

LV

Left lateral view (erect)

BE Bulwer, MD

Ascending aorta

L. braciocephalic vein

LV

LA

BE Bulwer, MD

Brachiocephalic a.

L. common carotid a.

L. subclavian a.

Aortic arch

L. main bronchus

R. pulmonary a.

Descending thoracic aorta

Left lateral supine perspective

SSN-Aortic Arch Long-Axis View Scan Plane

FIG. 8.18 Panoramic perspectives of the suprasternal notch (SSN) scan plane across the long-axis of the aortic arch. In the adult two-dimensional transthoracic echocardiographic examination, the SSN window is used primarily to assess the aortic arch, the distal ascending aorta, and the proximal descending thoracic aorta. The proximal portions of the branches of the aortic arch—the brachiocephalic artery (innominate trunk), the left common carotid artery, and the left subclavian artery—can also be examined using the SSN view. In the pediatric examination, the SSN window is also used to assess the ascending aorta, the main pulmonary artery and branches, as well as the left atrium with its four tributary pulmonary veins (Figs. 8.19 and 8.20). *(Courtesy of Bernard E. Bulwer, MD, FASE.)*

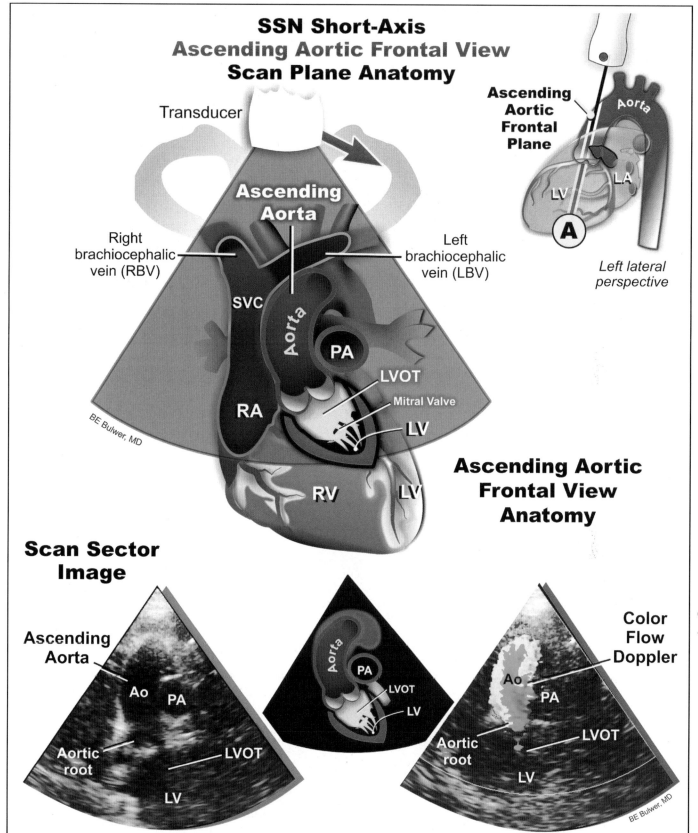

FIG. 8.19 The suprasternal notch (SSN) window, transducer orientation, and anatomical scan plane used to obtain the SSN-ascending aortic frontal view *(upper panels)*, with the corresponding scan sector image displays *(lower panels)*. (Courtesy of Bernard E. Bulwer, MD, FASE.)

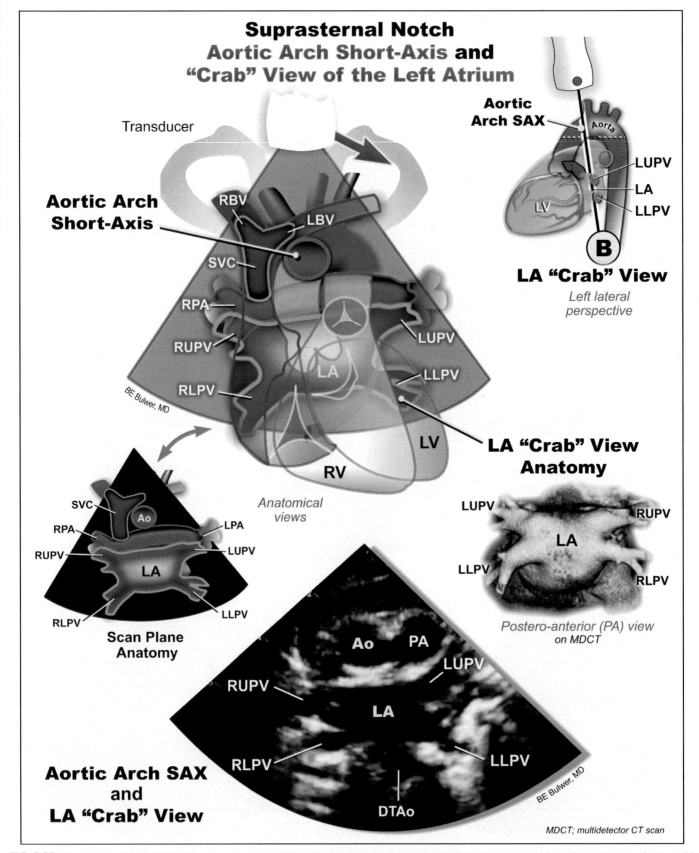

FIG. 8.20 The suprasternal notch (SSN) window, transducer orientation, and anatomical scan plane used to obtain the SSN aortic arch short-axis view *(upper and mid panels)*, with the corresponding scan sector image displays *(lower panel)*. In the pediatric examination, this view is important for visualization of the pair of upper (RUPV, LUPV) and lower (RLPV, LLPV) pulmonary veins as the empty into the left atrium—hence the commonly used term *crab* view of the left atrium (LA). *(Courtesy of Bernard E. Bulwer, MD, FASE.)*

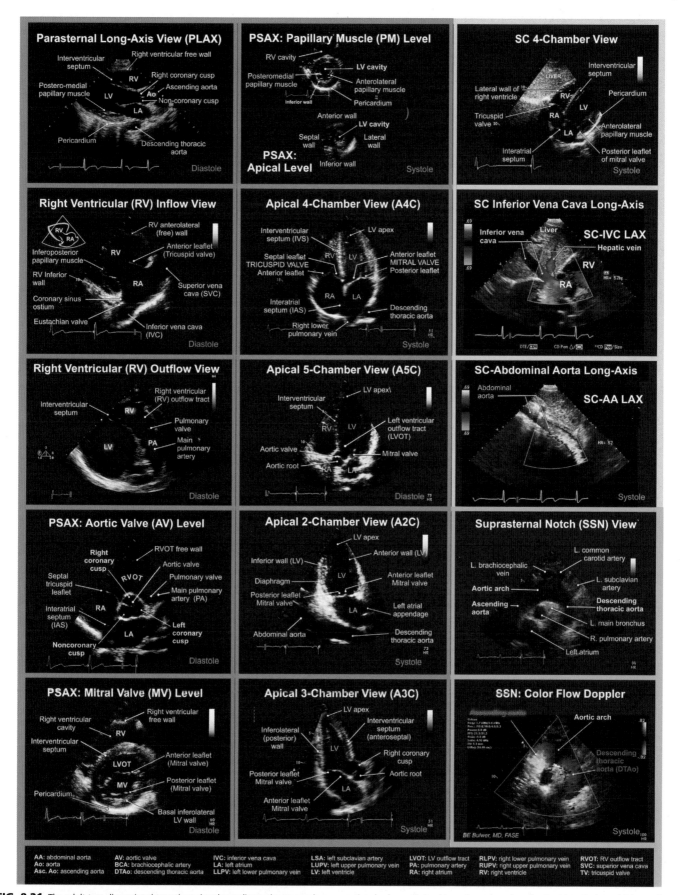

FIG. 8.21 The adult two-dimensional transthoracic echocardiography protocol: cross-sectional echocardiographic anatomy based on the American Society of Echocardiography nomenclature and standards. *(Courtesy of Bernard E. Bulwer, MD, FASE; Modified from Solomon SD, Wu J, Gillam L. Echocardiography. In: Mann DL, Zipes DP, Libby P, et al., eds.* Braunwald's heart disease: a textbook of cardiovascular medicine. *10th ed. Philadelphia: Elsevier; 2015:186.)*

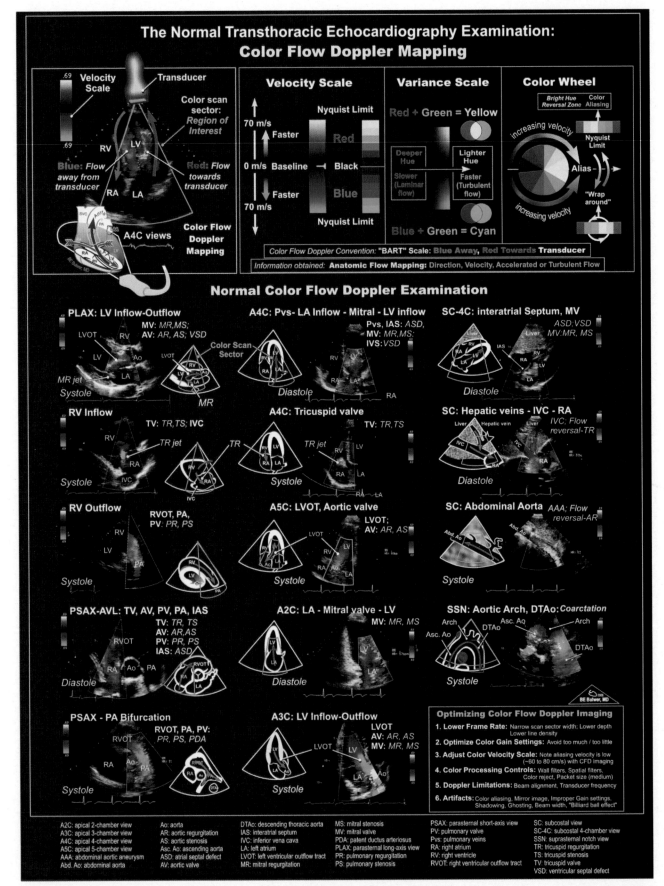

FIG. 8.22 Chart summary of the color flow Doppler echocardiography protocol, a major addition to the standard two-dimensional (2D) transthoracic echocardiography examination. Here, mean color-coded velocities are mapped onto the 2D images in real-time. This major addition to the 2D examination facilitates the rapid intuitive assessment of normal and abnormal intracardiac flow patterns. Color-coded, Doppler-derived blood velocities are displayed using conventional color scales, with velocities moving toward the transducer color-coded red, and velocities moving away from the transducer color-coded blue *(top panels)*. *(Courtesy of Bernard E. Bulwer, MD, FASE.)*

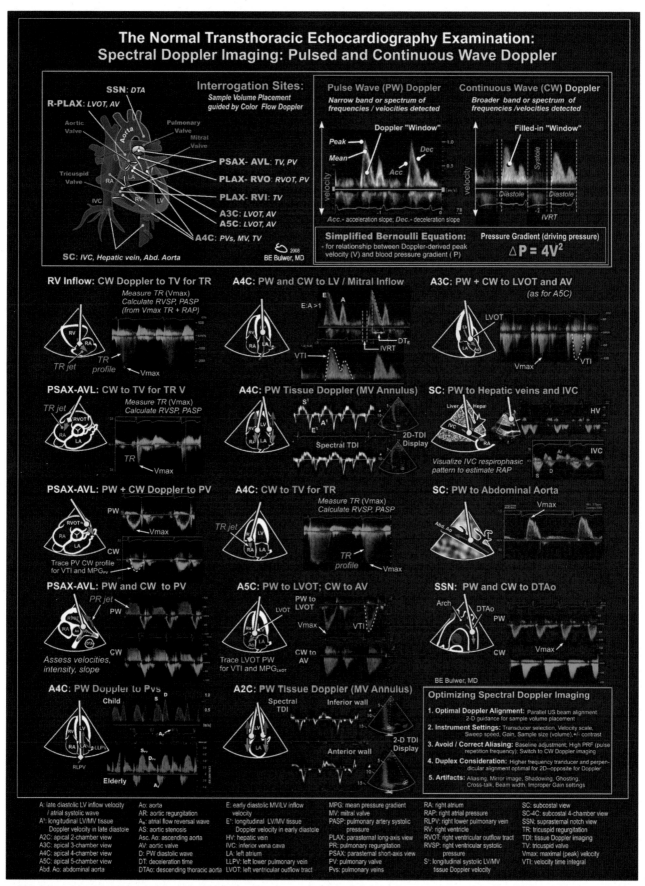

FIG. 8.23 Chart summary of the spectral Doppler echocardiography protocols—pulsed-wave (PW) and continuous-wave (CW) Doppler. Within the cardiovascular system, a wide spectrum of blood flow velocities exists—minimum, maximum, and mean. Spectral Doppler echocardiography is used to quantify this wide spectrum of velocities, hence the term *spectral*. These modalities are central to the quantitative assessment of intracardiac and transvalvular velocities and pressure gradients, the latter derived by employing the Bernoulli equation. Spectral Doppler-derived blood velocities are graphically displayed by convention, with velocities moving toward the transducer displayed above the baseline, and velocities moving away from the transducer displayed below the baseline. *(Courtesy of Bernard E. Bulwer, MD, FASE.)*

THE ECHOCARDIOGRAPHIC EXAMINATION

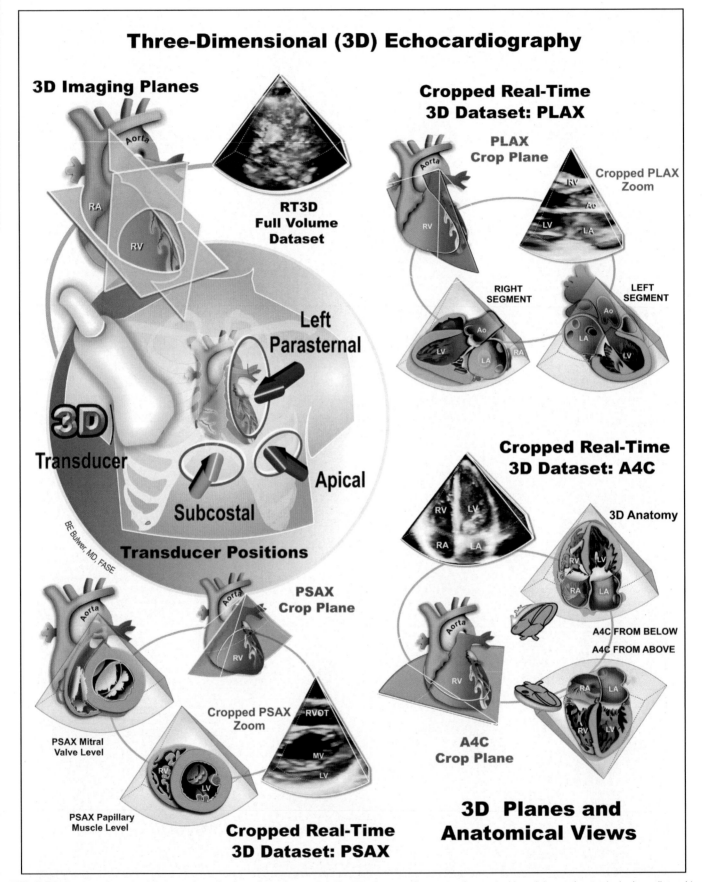

Three-Dimensional (3D) Echocardiography

3D Imaging Planes

RT3D Full Volume Dataset

Cropped Real-Time 3D Dataset: PLAX

PLAX Crop Plane

Cropped PLAX Zoom

RIGHT SEGMENT

LEFT SEGMENT

Left Parasternal

3D Transducer

Apical

Subcostal

Transducer Positions

BE Bulwer, MD, FASE

Cropped Real-Time 3D Dataset: A4C

3D Anatomy

A4C FROM BELOW
A4C FROM ABOVE

A4C Crop Plane

PSAX Crop Plane

Cropped PSAX Zoom

PSAX Mitral Valve Level

PSAX Papillary Muscle Level

Cropped Real-Time 3D Dataset: PSAX

3D Planes and Anatomical Views

FIG. 8.24 The three-dimensional (3D) transthoracic echocardiography protocol. The 3D volumes or datasets can be acquired in real time at the standard echocardiographic windows, and then cropped along the orthogonal cardiac imaging planes: the long-axis plane (LAX), short-axis (SAX), and four-chamber (4C) planes. *(Courtesy of Bernard E. Bulwer, MD, FASE.)*

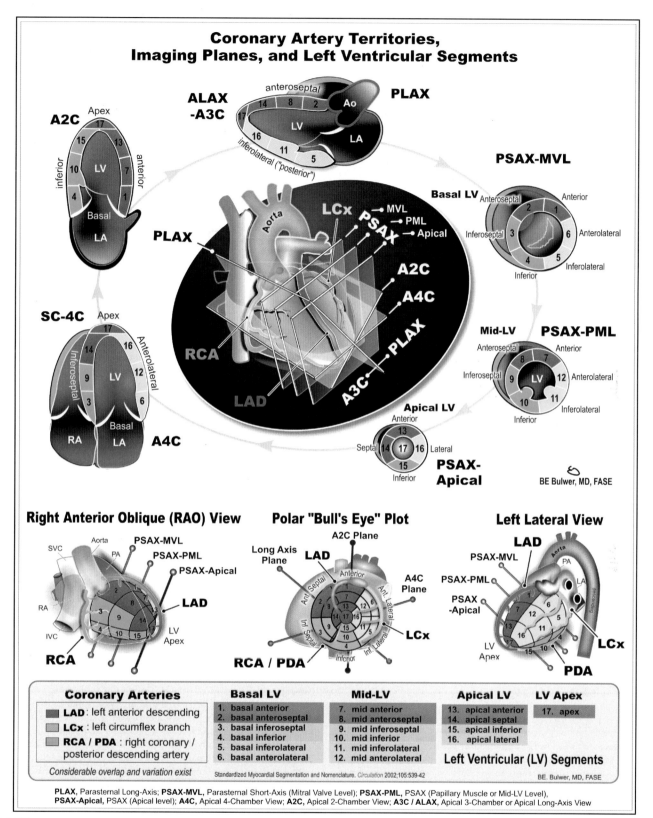

FIG. 8.25 The two-dimensional transthoracic echocardiographic views showing the superimposed 17-segment model of the left ventricular segments, and their corresponding coronary artery territories. Correlation of regional wall motion abnormalities with their corresponding coronary blood supply is the basis for the echocardiographic assessment of coronary artery disease. *(Courtesy of Bernard E. Bulwer, MD, FASE.)*

Suggested Reading

Bulwer, B. E., & Rivero, J. M. (2013). *Echocardiography Pocket Guide—The Transthoracic Examination.* Sudbury, MA: Jones and Bartlett Learning.

Cerqueira, M. D., Weissman, N. J., Dilsizian, V., et al. (2002). Standardized myocardial segmentation and nomenclature. *Circulation, 105,* 539–542.

Henry, W. L., DeMaria, A., Gramiak, R., et al. (1980). Report of the American Society of Echocardiography report on nomenclature and standards in two-dimensional echocardiography. *Circulation, 62,* 212–217.

Seward, J. B., Jamil Tajik, A., et al. (1990). Nomenclature, image orientation, and anatomic-echocardiographic correlation with tomographic views. In J. N. Schapira, & J. G. Harold (Eds.), *Two-Dimensional Echocardiography and Cardiac Doppler* (2nd ed.) (pp. 68–120). Baltimore: Williams & Wilkins.

Weyman, A. (1994). Cross-sectional echocardiographi examination. In A. Weyman (Ed.), *Principles and practice of Echocardiography* (2nd ed.) (pp. 75–97). Philadelphia: Lea & Febiger.

A complete reference list can be found online at ExpertConsult.com

9 The Transthoracic Examination, View by View

Bernard E. Bulwer

INTRODUCTION

This chapter presents the views acquired during the normal two-dimensional (2D) adult comprehensive transthoracic echocardiography (TTE) examination. These views are based on the standards recommended by the American Society of Echocardiography (see Chapter 8).[1] Optimal image acquisition is a prerequisite for optimal interpretation and reporting of the adult transthoracic echocardiogram by the echocardiographer/cardiologist expert. This involves competency in cardiac sonographer skills and training,[2] as well as optimizing patient and instrument settings (see Chapter 11).

The comprehensive adult 2D TTE examination (TTE) begins at the left parasternal window, followed by the apical, subcostal, and suprasternal notch windows (Tables 9.1–9.6). Each standard echocardiographic view is described using three components (see Table 9.1; see also Chapter 8): (1) transducer position or window, namely the parasternal (P), apical (A), subcostal (SC), and suprasternal notch (SSN) windows; (2) echocardiographic imaging plane, namely long-axis (LAX), short-axis (SAX), or four-chamber (4C) planes; and (3) cardiac structures or regions of interest.

At each window, each echocardiographic view must be optimized and recorded. This includes video loops, still frames, and recommended pertinent measurement (Figs. 9.1–9.10 and corresponding Videos 9.1 – 9.28).[1-10] The typical sequence of the modalities employed are as follows:

1. 2D examination for cross-sectional anatomy of the cardiac structures
2. M-mode examination for timing of cardiac events and linear measurements
3. Color flow Doppler examination for the initial visual assessment of normal and abnormal flows, and a guide to quantitative assessment of velocities using spectral Doppler
4. Spectral Doppler examination—namely continuous-wave (CW) Doppler to measure maximum transvalvular velocities and gradients, followed by pulsed-wave (PW) Doppler to detect flows at specific anatomical sites when indicated
5. Tissue Doppler imaging (TDI) to assess myocardial velocities
6. Three-dimensional (3D) echocardiography incorporated when available and as indicated (see Chapter 10)

LEFT PARASTERNAL VIEWS

The left parasternal window (P) or transducer position is where the adult TTE examination begins. Here a family of left parasternal long-axis (PLAX) and left parasternal short-axis (PSAX) views are acquired and assessed (see Tables 9.1 and 9.2; see also Figs. 9.1–9.4). All four cardiac chambers, the four cardiac valves, and the juxtacardiac portions of the great vessels are examined. Complementary views from the A, SC, and SSN windows are necessary for the comprehensive assessment of cardiac structure and function (see Figs. 9.5–9.10).

The PLAX view of the left ventricle (LV) inflow-outflow tract, or simply PLAX, is the starting point for the adult TTE echo exam (see Tables 9.1 and 9.2; see also Fig. 9.1). The PLAX view sets the stage for the assessment of several important parameters of global and regional cardiac structure and function. Important L-sided structures are optimally aligned and measured: LV walls and cavity, mitral and aortic valves (MV, AV).

The initial assessment of right ventricle (RV) function and the pericardium also begins with the PLAX view.

The RV Inflow view is used to evaluate right ventricular inflow, from right atrium (RA) to RV via the tricuspid valve (TV; see Tables 9.1 and 9.2; see also Fig. 9.2). It can be used to assess the inferior two-thirds of RV, TV, RA, and the inferior vena cava (IVC) and coronary sinus as they empty into the RA. This view is useful for the evaluation of right heart pressures, specifically the RV systolic (RVSP) and pulmonary artery systolic (PASP) pressures. The RV outflow view is often used to examine the RV outflow tract (RVOT), pulmonary valve (PV), and proximal pulmonary artery (PA; see Table 9.1; see also Fig. 9.2).

The PSAX views are aligned orthogonal to the long-axis of the LV or aorta (see Tables 9.1 and 9.3; see also Figs. 9.3 and 9.4). The PSAX views are important for examination of all four cardiac valves: AV, MV, PV, and TV; both ventricles, LV, RV; both atria (LA, RA); and both septae, interatrial septum (IAS) and the interventricular septum (IVS). The PSAX views are acquired at multiple levels (see Figs. 9.3 and 9.4; see also Table 9.3)—namely at levels of (1) the aortic valve (AVL); (2) pulmonary artery bifurcation (PAB); (3) the MV; (4) papillary muscle (PML) or mid-LV; and (5) LV apical level and apical cap (apex).

APICAL VIEWS

The apical views (see Figs. 9.5–9.8; see also Tables 9.1 and 9.4) are the most important views in the TTE exam (along with the parasternal views). They play a central role in the assessment of ventricular systolic and diastolic function, as well as atrioventricular valve structure and function. The apical views transect the true cardiac apex and are aligned parallel to the cardiac long-axis. The typical order of examination of the apical views are (1) the apical four-chamber (A4C) view, (2) the apical five-chamber (A5C) view, (3) the apical two-chamber (A2C) view, and (4) the apical three-chamber (A3C) or apical long-axis (ALAX) view.

SUBCOSTAL VIEWS

In adult echocardiography, the SC views complement the examination of the parasternal and apical views—specifically, both atria, LA, RA; both ventricles, LV, RV; the interatrial and interventricular septae; the mitral and tricuspid valves; the IVC and hepatic veins; and the proximal abdominal aorta (AA; see Fig. 9.9; see also Tables 9.1 and 9.5).

In patients with advanced chronic obstructive pulmonary disease (COPD) and chest trauma/postchest surgery patients, in whom the parasternal and apical windows are often obliterated or unavailable, the SC window can be used as a substitute. Here, a family of short-axis and long-axis views can be acquired that correspond to those normally obtained from the left parasternal and apical windows.

SUPRASTERNAL NOTCH VIEWS

In the comprehensive 2D TTE adult examination, the suprasternal notch views are typically the final views acquired in the adult TTE examination. Here, the aortic arch and branches, the vena cave (SVC, IVC) en route to the RA, and proximal branches of the main pulmonary artery are examined (see Fig. 9.10; see also Tables 9.1 and 9.6).

TABLE 9.1 Standard Two-Dimensional Adult Transthoracic Echocardiography Views

WINDOW	CARDIAC IMAGING PLANE	REGION-STRUCTURES OF INTEREST
Parasternal Views (see Figs. 9.1–9.4)		
Parasternal (P)	Long-axis (LAX)	LV inflow-outflow, LA, MV, LV, LVOT, RVOT, IVS, Aortic root, descending thoracic aorta
P	LAX	RV inflow, TV, RV, coronary sinus, IVC
P	LAX	RV outflow: RVOT, PV, PA
P	Short-axis (SAX)	Aortic valve level: AV, TV, PV, IAS, LA, IAS, coronary arteries; IVC
P	SAX	PA bifurcation: main PA, PV, RPA, LPA, coronary arteries
P	SAX	Mitral valve level: MV, basal LV walls, LVOT, IAS
P	SAX	Papillary muscle level: LV walls, papillary muscles; IAS
P	SAX	Apical level: apical LV walls; LV apex (apical tip)
Apical Views (see Figs. 9.5–9.8)		
Apical (A)	Four-chamber (4C)	LV, RV, LA, RA, MV, TV, pulmonary veins
A	Five-chamber (5C)	AV, LV, LVOT
A	Two-chamber (2C)	LV walls, LV, LA, LAA, MV
A	Three-chamber (3C); or long-axis (LAX)	LV walls, LV inflow-outflow, LA, MV, LV, LVOT, RVOT, IVS
Subcostal Views (see Fig. 9.9)		
Subcostal (SC)	Four-chamber	IAS, LV, RV, LA, RA, MV, TV
SC	Long-axis (LAX)	Inferior vena cava (IVC), hepatic veins
SC	LAX	Abdominal aorta (AA)
SC	Optional views	Family of SAX and LAX views of the heart when transthoracic windows unavailable, or in the pediatric examination. SAX views of IVC and AA
Suprasternal Notch Views (see Fig. 9.10)		
Suprasternal notch	Long-axis	Aortic arch and branches, distal ascending aorta, proximal descending thoracic aorta
Suprasternal notch	Optional views	Short-axis views of the aortic arch with "crab" view of the LA and pulmonary veins, frontal view of the ascending aorta

AA, Abdominal aorta; *AV*, aortic valve; *IAS*, interatrial septum; *IVS*, interventricular septum; *IVC*, inferior vena cava; *LA*, left atrium; *LV*, left ventricle; *LVOT*, left ventricular outflow tract; *MV*, mitral valve; *PA*, pulmonary artery; *PV*, pulmonary valve; *RA*, right atrium; *RV*, right ventricle; *RVOT*, right ventricular outflow tract; *TV*, tricuspid valve

TABLE 9.2 Parasternal Long-Axis Views: Normal Examination (see Figs. 9.1 and 9.2)

TRANSDUCER POSITION (WINDOW)	2D ± M-MODE ± 3D	CFD	SPECTRAL DOPPLER (PW, CW)
Parasternal long-axis (PLAX): LV inflow-outflow	PLAX 2D • Use increased depth to rule out effusions, and then decrease depth. • 2D zoom of the MV and AV • Measure the aortic root leading edge to leading edge on 2D. • Measure the LA at the largest dimension during the end of ventricular systole on PLAX view or on the PSAX/AV level view. • Measure the LVIDd, IVSd, LVPwd at the end of diastole just when the MV closes and measure at the level of the mitral chordae level (MM or 2D). • Measure the LVIDs at the end of systole at the same level that the diastolic measurements were made (MM or 2D). • M-mode MV/AV, Aortic root/LA, LV • 3D full-volume (optional)	CD to AV/MV, Zoom (on/off)	CW if VSD
RV inflow	2D depth 20 cm, then 15–16 cm Zoom on the TV	Color Doppler TV for TR	CW Doppler for Max; TR velocity
RV outflow (optional)	2D Zoom on the PV	Color Doppler PV for PR	—

2D, Two-dimensional echocardiography; *3D*, three-dimensional echocardiography; *AV*, aortic valve; *CFD*, color flow Doppler echocardiography; *CW*, continuous-wave Doppler echocardiography; *IVS*, interventricular septum; *LA*, left atrium; *LV*, left ventricle; *LVIDd*, LV internal diameter at end diastole; *LVIDs*, LV internal diameter at end systole; *LVPwd*, LV posterior wall thickness at end diastole; *MM*, M-mode/motion-mode; *MV*, mitral valve; *PR*, pulmonary regurgitation; *PV*, pulmonary valve; *PW*, pulsed-wave Doppler echocardiography; *RV*, right ventricle; *TR*, tricuspid regurgitation; *TV*, tricuspid valve; *VSD*, ventricular septal defect.

TABLE 9.3 Parasternal Short-Axis Views: Normal Examination (see Figs. 9.3 and 9.4)

TRANSDUCER POSITION (WINDOW)	2D ± M-MODE ± 3D	CFD	SPECTRAL DOPPLER PW, CW
Parasternal short-axis (PSAX): aortic valve level (AVL)	2D to AV • Zoom AV 2D 2D to TV 2D to PV M-mode (optional) 3D full-volume (optional)	CFD to AV CFD to TV for TR CFD to PV for PR	CW to TR max velocity
PSAX: pulmonary artery bifurcation (PAB)	2D image of PAB	CFD for PR and PDA	PW-CW of PV
PSAX: Mitral valve level (MVL)	2D image at the MV and basal LV walls	CFD to MV	—
PSAX: papillary muscle level (PML)	2D image at PML, mild LV walls	—	—
PSAX: apical level	2D image at LV apical walls and LV apical segment	—	—

2D, Two-dimensional echocardiography; *3D*, three-dimensional echocardiography; *AV*, aortic valve; *CFD*, color flow Doppler echocardiography; *CW*, continuous-wave Doppler echocardiography; *LV*, left ventricle; *MV*, mitral valve; *PDA*, patent ductus arteriosus; *PR*, pulmonary regurgitation; *PV*, pulmonary valve; *PW*, pulsed-wave Doppler echocardiography; *TR*, tricuspid regurgitation; *TV*, tricuspid valve.

TABLE 9.4 Apical Views (see Figs. 9.5–9.8)

TRANSDUCER POSITION (WINDOW)	2D ± M-MODE ± 3D	CFD	SPECTRAL DOPPLER PW, CW	TISSUE DOPPLER IMAGING (TDI)
Apical four-chamber (A4C)	2D image; depth 15–16 cm. LV and LV walls • Optimize endocardial borders for LV volumetric EF assessment MV assessment 2D Measurement of LA volume- measure LA volume at the end of systole and the shorter length of the LA 3D full-volume (optional) Evaluate RV function on 2D focus RV image. TAPSE (tricuspid annular plane systolic excursion)	CFD to MV for MR, MS CFD the Pulmonary veins, PW of right upper or lower pulmonary vein Color M-Mode flow propagation velocity CFD to TV and CW for TR max velocity.	PW Doppler at the tips of the mitral leaflets for MV inflow CW Doppler of the MV	TDI (PW) of MV annulus (lateral and septal) Color TDI to LV walls TDI of TV annulus
Apical five-chamber view (A5C)	2D visualization of the AV-Zoom on the valve	CFD to the AV	PW Doppler of the LVOT (1–2 cm) from the valve leaflets, closing AV click CW for transaortic velocities	
Apical two-chamber view (A2C)	2D image LV and LV walls • Optimize endocardial borders for LV volumetric EF assessment Volumetric measurement of the LA	CFD to MV		TDI (PW) of MV annulus (anterior and inferior) Color TDI to LV walls
Apical three-chamber view (A3C) or apical long-axis (ALAX) view	2D image for wall motion evaluation	CFD to AV and MV	—	—

2D, Two-dimensional echocardiography; *3D*, three-dimensional echocardiography; *AV*, aortic valve; *CFD*, color flow Doppler echocardiography; *CW*, continuous-wave Doppler echocardiography; *EF*, ejection fraction; *LA*, left atrium; *LV*, left ventricle; *LVOT*, left ventricular outflow tract; *MR*, mitral regurgitation; *MS*, mitral stenosis; *MV*, mitral valve; *PW*, pulsed-wave Doppler echocardiography; *RV*, right ventricle; *TR*, tricuspid regurgitation; *TV*, tricuspid valve

TABLE 9.5 Subcostal Views (see Fig. 9.9)

TRANSDUCER POSITION (WINDOW)	2D ± M-MODE ± 3D	CFD	SPECTRAL DOPPLER PW, CW	TISSUE DOPPLER	3D
Subcostal views	Subcostal four-chamber (SC-4C) • On-off zoom	CFD to interventricular and interatrial septum CFD to TV, CW if TR velocity (optional)	Optional	Optional	Optional
	Subcostal view short-axis view at the AV level 2D	Color Doppler	Optional	Optional	Optional
	Subcostal view • IVC-Long-axis 2D image Respiratory Changes of the IVC; Use M-mode or 2D (sniff) IVC/Hepatic vein • LV short axis	Color Doppler	PW Doppler	—	—
	Subcostal view • Abdominal aorta-long-axis	2D color Doppler	PW Doppler	—	—

2D, Two-dimensional echocardiography; *3D*, three-dimensional echocardiography; *AV*, aortic valve *CFD*, color flow Doppler echocardiography; *CW*, continuous-wave Doppler echocardiography; *IVC*, inferior vena cava; *LV*, left ventricle; *PW*, pulsed-wave Doppler echocardiography; *SC*, subcostal; *SSN*, suprasternal notch view; *SVC*, superior vena cava; *TR*, tricuspid regurgitation; *TV*, tricuspid valve

TABLE 9.6 Suprasternal Notch Views (see Fig. 9.9)

TRANSDUCER POSITION (WINDOW)	2D	COLOR FLOW DOPPLER	SPECTRAL DOPPLER PW, CW	TISSUE DOPPLER	3D
SSN	2D image Aortic arch, distal ascending aorta, proximal descending aorta	CFD	PW/CW	—	—

2D, Two-dimensional echocardiography; *3D,* three-dimensional echocardiography; *CFD,* color flow Doppler echocardiography; *CW,* continuous-wave Doppler echocardiography; *PW,* pulsed-wave Doppler echocardiography; *SSN,* suprasternal notch view.

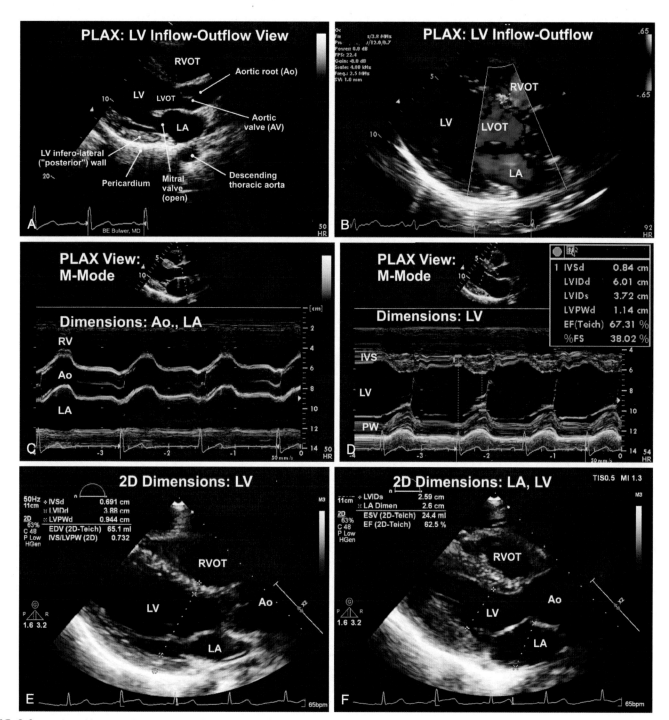

FIG. 9.1 Parasternal long-axis (PLAX) view—left ventricular (LV) inflow-outflow. (A) PLAX of the heart showing the LV inflow, and outflow (LVOT), the outflow portion of the right ventricle (RV), and related structures. This view is usually the first view obtained in the transthoracic examination, and can provide a quick overview of several aspects of cardiac structure and function. Significant findings should be sought using subsequent echocardiographic windows and views. Quantitative measures of cardiac chamber size and dimensions should also obtained on this view. (B) PLAX showing color flow Doppler (CFD) interrogation of the mitral and aortic valves. The examination may reveal flow patterns indicative of valvular stenosis or regurgitation. Ventricular septal defects involving the interventricular septum may also be detected on CFD. (C) M (motion) of the PLAX at the level of the aortic valve (AV). These measurements are useful when LV geometry is normal. (D) M-mode along the PLAX at the level of the LV. These measurements are useful when LV geometry is normal. (E) Linear LV dimensions measured using the parasternal long-axis (PLAX) view. These are preferred over M-mode linear measures which are prone to off-axis measurements, made worse in the presence of remodeled LV geometry. (F) End-systolic frame showing measurement of the LV internal diameter during systole (LVIDs) and the left atrial.

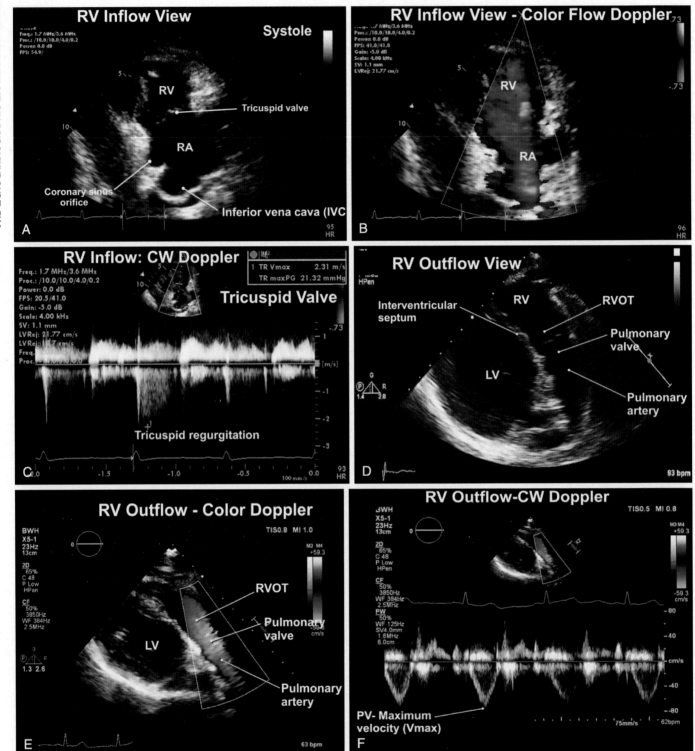

FIG. 9.2 **Right ventricular inflow and outflow views.** Right ventricular (RV) inflow view. This view is useful for Doppler interrogation of the tricuspid valve. (A) RV Doppler interrogation of the tricuspid valve on the RV inflow view. Diastolic flow from the right atrium (RA) into the RV moves in a direction toward the transducer—hence appearing red (by convention). Flow away from the transducer (e.g., tricuspid regurgitation) would appear blue. (B) Continuous-wave (CW) Doppler to the tricuspid valve showing spectral profile predominantly below the baseline. This finding represents mild tricuspid regurgitant flow away from the transducer. (C) The long-axis view of the RV outflow track and main pulmonary artery (MPA) is often performed in the initial assessment of flow across the RV outflow tract (RVOT), the pulmonary valve, and the MPA. (D) Color flow Doppler showing the normal systolic flow velocities across the pulmonary valve. Blue flow is indicative of flow away from the transducer. (E) Pulsed-wave (PW) Doppler assessment of flow at the level of the pulmonary valve. Velocities below the baseline are indicative of forward flow away from the transducer.

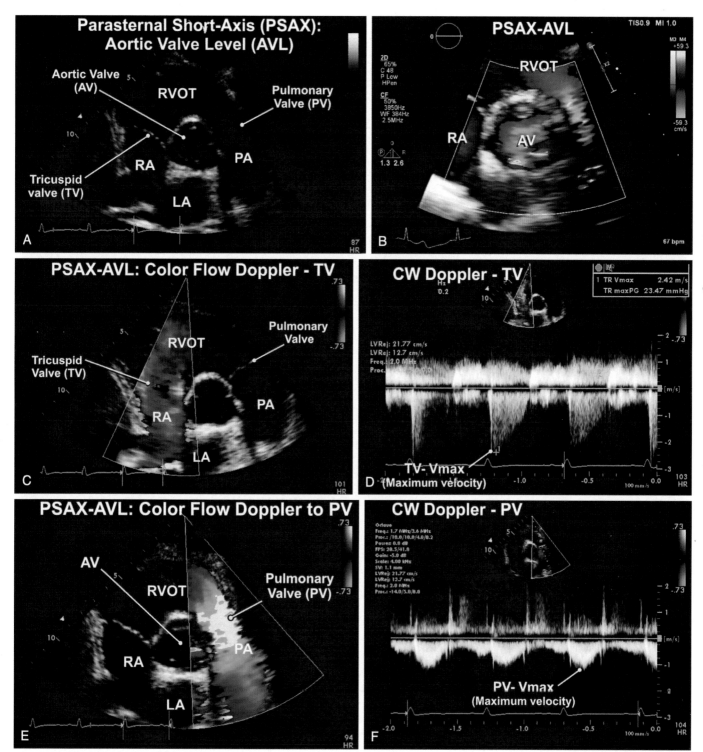

FIG. 9.3 **Parasternal short-axis (PSAX) view—aortic valve level (AVL).** (A) The PSAX-AVL view at the base of the heart is important in the assessment of the three cardiac valves: the aortic, tricuspid, and pulmonary valves. (B) Zoomed view of the aortic valve showing flow across the aortic valve on color flow Doppler. (C) The routine assessment of flows across the tricuspid valve, including tricuspid regurgitant (TR) flows is performed on the PSAX-AVL view on color flow Doppler. (D) Maximum velocities (Vmax) of TR flows is routinely measured using continuous-wave (CW) Doppler. This is used to estimate RV systolic pressures/pulmonary artery systolic pressures (PASP) using the Bernoulli equation. (E) Color flow Doppler assessment is the important first step in the evaluation of flows across the pulmonary valve. (F) The Vmax across the pulmonary valve is routinely measured using the CW Doppler.

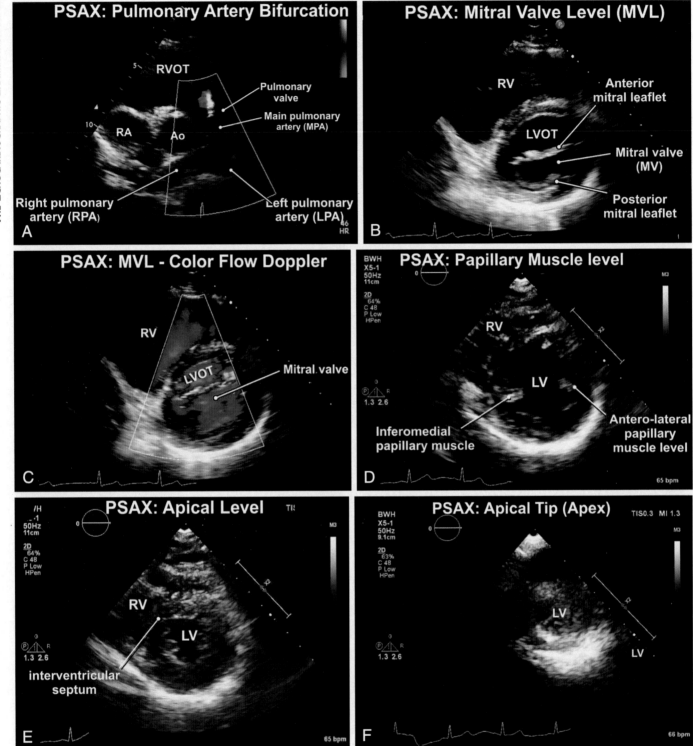

FIG. 9.4 Parasternal short-axis (PSAX) views—at the levels of the pulmonary artery bifurcation (PSAX-PAB), mitral valve (PSAX-MVL), papillary muscle (PSAX-PML), and left ventricular apex. (A) Diastolic frame of the PSAX-PAB is shown, along with a small pulmonary regurgitant jet. The ostia of the coronary arteries can be examined using this view. (B) A diastolic frame on the PSAX-MVL view is shown, with the mitral leaflets in their open position. Polarimetry of the mitral valve orifice on both two-dimensional and three-dimensional echocardiography is measured on this view. (C) Color flow Doppler is useful to assess abnormal flow patterns across the MV on the PSAX-MVL view. Localization of the affected MV scallops can be identified on color flow Doppler. (D) Assessment of ventricles, the LV walls, and the interventricular septum is routinely performed using the PSAX-PML view. This complements the regional wall motion assessment of the LV segments performed. (E) More distally, assessment of the regional walls of the LV is also routinely performed on the PSAX view at the level of the LV apical segments. (F) LV torsion can be routinely observed by PSAX views at the apical tip of the LV. This can be quantified on speckle-tracking echocardiography.

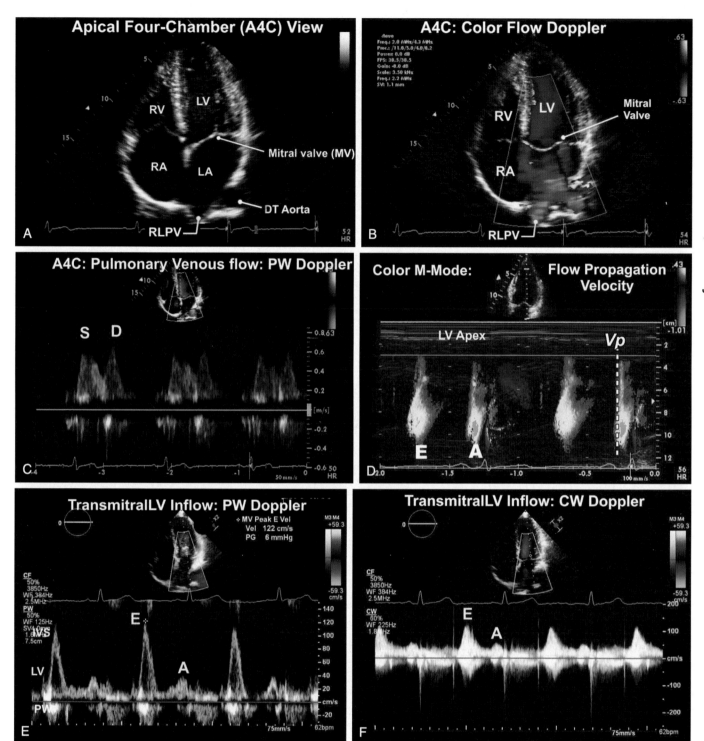

FIG. 9.5 Apical four-chamber (A4C) view—left atrial and left ventricular filling. (A) The A4C showing the four cardiac chambers and the atrioventricular valves. This view plays a critical role in the assessment of ventricular systolic and diastolic function, and is optimally aligned to assess left atrial and left ventricular filling. (B) Color flow Doppler assessment is initially used to assess flows within the cardiac chambers and across the mitral and tricuspid valves. (C) Left atrial filling is assessed using PW Doppler interrogation of pulmonary venous flow. This is used as a composite measure of LV diastolic function assessment. (D) Color Doppler M-mode of flow propagation of velocities within the LV is routinely measured. The slope (Vp) of the early rapid diastolic flow of LV filling is also used as a composite measure in the assessment of LV diastolic function. (E) Left ventricular transmitral filling is routinely assessed as a composite measure of LV diastolic function. Flow at the tip of the mitral leaflets is measured using PW Doppler. (F) Peak flows and gradients across the mitral valve is assessed using CW Doppler.

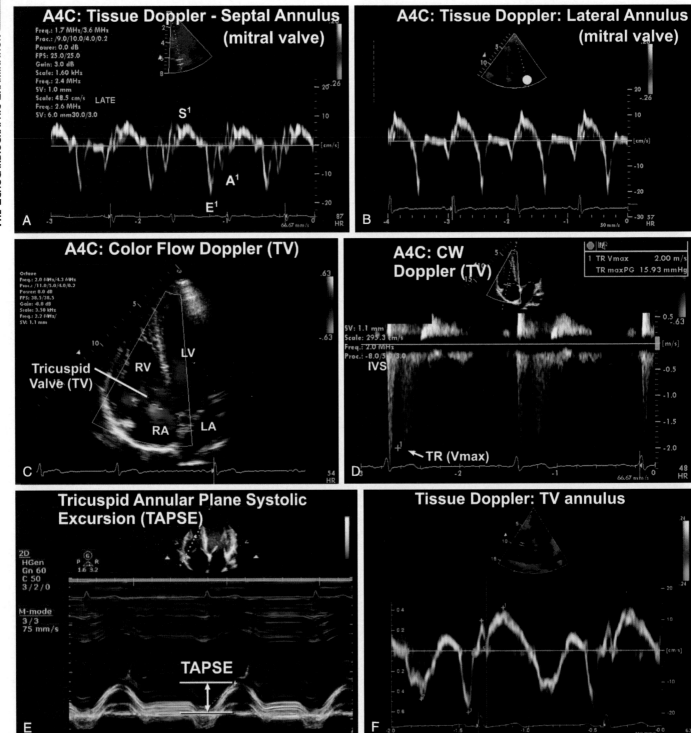

FIG. 9.6 Apical four-chamber (A4C) view—tissue Doppler imaging at the mitral annulus and right ventricular function assessment. (A) Tissue Doppler imaging (TDI) of the mitral valve annulus on the A4C views. TDI is useful in the assessment of longitudinal diastolic and systolic myocardial mechanics. (B) Both the septal and mitral annulus are routinely assessed during the comprehensive adult transthoracic echocardiography examination. (C) Assessment of flow across the tricuspid valve (TV) on the A4C view. This complements the assessment of tricuspid regurgitation that initially begins on the PSAX view at the level of the aortic valve. (D) Continuous-wave (CW) Doppler assessment of tricuspid regurgitation (TR) across the TV. From this, right atrial systolic pressure and pulmonary artery systolic pressure can be assessed using the maximum velocity (Vmax) of the TR jet. (E) Complementary measures of right ventricular systolic function includes the measurement of the tricuspid annular plane systolic excursion (TAPSE) on M-mode and RV fractional area change. (F) Tissue Doppler imaging (TDI) of the RV myocardial velocities is now routinely performed on the A4C view.

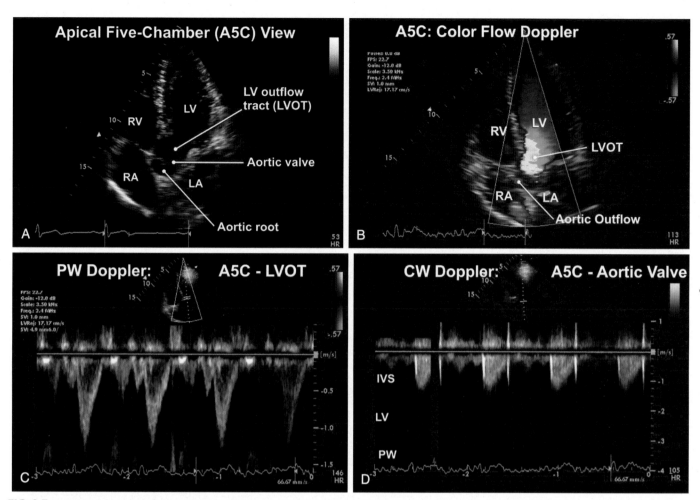

FIG. 9.7 Apical five-chamber (A5C) view. (A) Apical five-chamber (A5C) view showing the aortic root and LV outflow tract. The A5C view also complements the evaluation of the four cardiac chambers, intervening, and atrioventricular valves. (B) Color flow Doppler interrogation of flow velocities across left ventricular outflow tract (LVOT) and the aortic valve on the A5C view. This view is important for evaluating pathology of the aortic valve and LVOT. (C) The A5C view is ideal for evaluation of flows across the LV outflow tract and the aortic valve. Frame showing PW Doppler assessment of velocities and gradients across the left ventricular outflow tract. This is useful for evaluation of LVOT obstruction in hypertrophic cardiomyopathy and subvalvular aortic stenosis. (D) Continuous-wave (CW) Doppler is useful for evaluation of the transaortic velocities and pressure gradient. This measurement is used for calculation of peak velocities and gradients across the aortic valve in aortic stenosis.

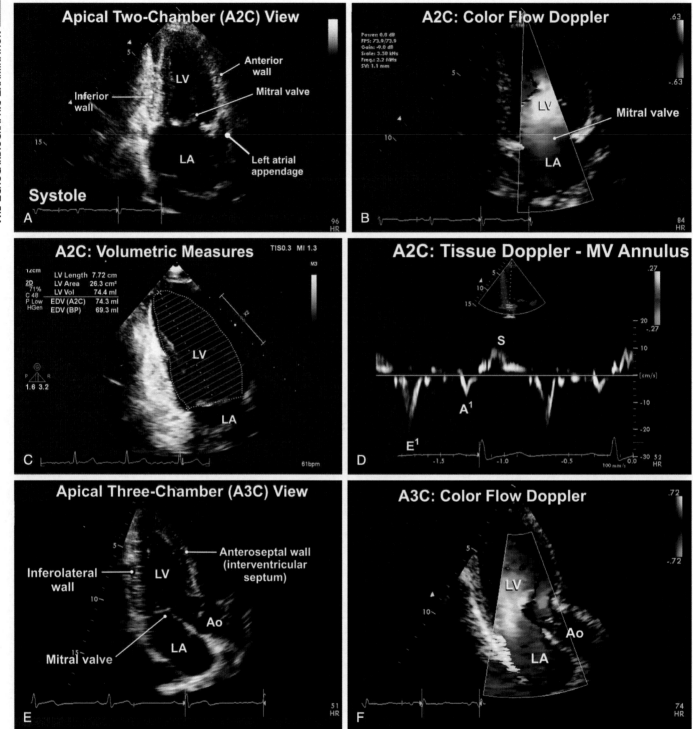

FIG. 9.8 Apical two-chamber (A2C) and apical three-chamber (A3C) views. (A) The A2C view showing the left-sided cardiac chambers and the intervening mitral valve. Measures of cardiac chamber size and dimensions should also obtained on this view. (B) Color flow Doppler evaluation of the mitral valve on the A2C) view. (C) Diastolic frame showing the measurement of left ventricular area, as part of the assessment of LV volumes using the biplane method of disks (Simpson's rule). This method is used to measure left atrial areas and volumes on the A2C view. (D) Tissue Doppler assessment of the left ventricular annulus is also performed on the A2C view. Here, measurement of the inferior mitral annulus is shown. (E) The A3C or the apical long-axis (ALAX) view is aligned along the LV long-axis like the PLAX view. However, it enables visualization of the LV apex. Measures and assessments conducted on the PLAX and A5C views can be performed and corroborated using the A3C view. (F) Color flow Doppler assessment of LV inflow and outflow across the mitral and aortic valves on the A3C view.

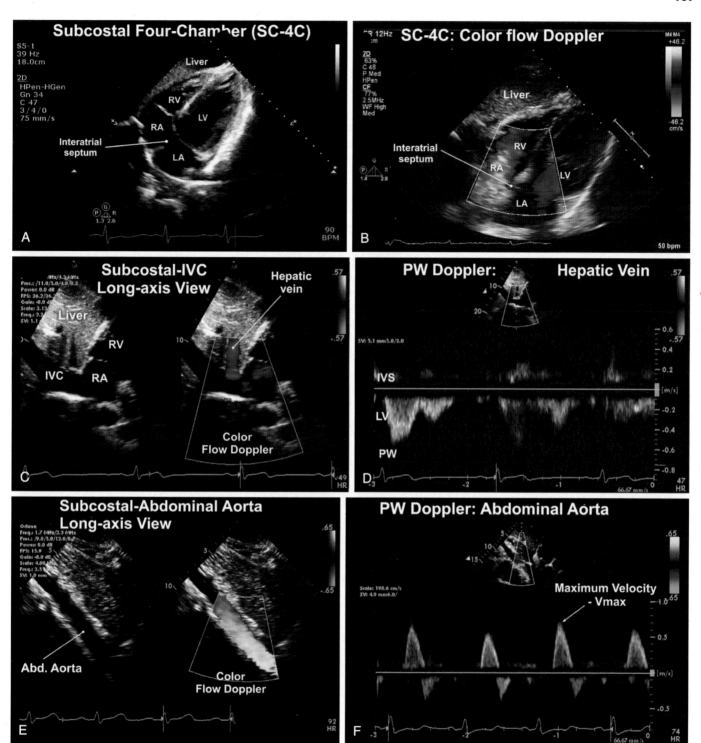

FIG. 9.9 Subcostal views. (A) The subcostal four-chamber (SC-4C) view permits optimal viewing of the interatrial septum and atrial septal defects. It complements the assessment of the parasternal and apical views of the four-cardiac chambers and atrioventricular valves. (B) Color flow Doppler interrogation of the interatrial septum on the subcostal four-chamber (SC-4C) view shows an intact interatrial septum. (C) The subcostal-IVC view permits evaluation of inferior vena cava (IVC) dimensions, respirophasic behavior, and Doppler evaluation of IVC and hepatic vein flow. (D) On the subcostal-IVC view, pulsed (PW) Doppler evaluation of the hepatic veins normally shows a spectral velocity profile of flow (below baseline), mostly during systole. This pattern is reversed in severe tricuspid regurgitation due to flow reversal. (E) Subcostal long-axis views of the proximal abdominal aorta (left). Color flow Doppler examination of the abdominal aorta shows laminar red flow velocities toward the transducer. (F) PW Doppler examination of the aortic valve shows the characteristic biphasic velocity profiles, with forward flow above the baseline and peak velocities below 1 m/s.

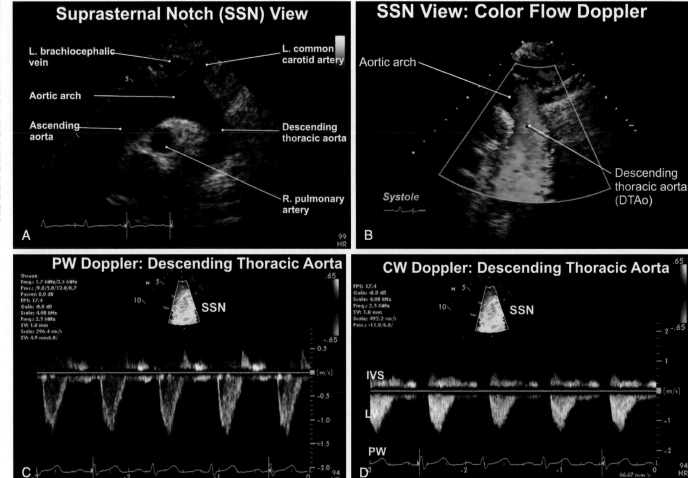

FIG. 9.10 Apical two-chamber (A2C) and apical three-chamber (A3C) views. (A) The suprasternal notch (SSN) view is best for visualization of the aortic arch and branches and for evaluation of coarctation of the aorta. (B) Color flow Doppler evaluation of the proximal descending thoracic aorta shows normal (blue) flow away from the transducer. (C) Evaluation of flow in the descending thoracic aorta is best visualized and assessed on the suprasternal notch (SSN) view. Coarctation of the aorta, which classically affects the postductal portion distal to the left subclavian artery origin, requires pulsed (PW) and continuous-wave Doppler assessment. (D) Continuous-wave (CW) Doppler assessment of flow in the descending thoracic aorta. This is used to evaluate peak flows across the descending thoracic aorta.

Suggested Reading

Quinones, M. A., Otto, C. M., Stoddard, M., et al. (2002). Recommendations for quantification of Doppler echocardiography: a report from the Doppler quantification task force of the nomenclature and standards committee of the American Society of Echocardiography. *Journal of the American Society of Echocardiography, 15,* 167–184.

Seward, J. B., Jamil Tajik, A., Hagler, D., & Edwards, W. D. (1990). Nomenclature, image orientation, and anatomic-echocardiographic correlation with tomographic views. In J. N. Schapira, & J. G. Harold (Eds.), *Two-Dimensional Echocardiography and Cardiac Doppler* (2nd ed.) (pp. 68–120). Baltimore: Williams & Wilkins.

Solomon, S. D., Wu, J., Gillam, L., & Bulwer, B. E. (2015). Echocardiography. In D. L. Mann, D. P. Zipes, P. Libby, et al. (Eds.), *Braunwald's Heart Disease—A Textbook of Cardiovascular Medicine* (pp. 340–560). Philadelphia: Elsevier.

Weyman, A. (1994a). Cross-sectional echocardiographic examination. In A. Weyman (Ed.), *Principles and Practice of Echocardiography* (2nd ed.) (pp. 75–97). Philadelphia: Lea & Febiger.

Weyman, A. (1994b). Standard plane positions—standard imaging planes. In A. Weyman (Ed.), *Principles and Practice of Echocardiography* (2nd ed.) (pp. 98–123). Philadelphia: Lea & Febiger.

A complete reference list can be found online at ExpertConsult.com.

10 Three-Dimensional Echocardiography: Image Acquisition

Jose Rivero, Alexandra Goncalves, Bernard E. Bulwer

INTRODUCTION

In the modern echocardiography laboratory, three-dimensional transthoracic echocardiography (3D-TTE) complements the standard two-dimensional transthoracic echocardiographic (2D-TTE) examination. 3D-TTE adds value, improves workflow, and substantially improves accuracy in the quantification of cardiac chambers by avoiding errors inherent in the geometric assumptions made in 2D-TTE (Figs. 10.1 and 10.2, and Video 10.1). 3D TTE provides a more accurate assessment of cardiac morphology and pathology, native and prosthetic valve structure and function, and guidance in interventional intracardiac procedures.

This chapter presents an overview of the basic 3D-TTE image acquisition and optimization techniques used in the echo lab. Optimal utilization of 3D-TTE requires an understanding of the clinical or research application (Box 10.1 and Table 10.1). A comprehensive understanding of the clinical application helps determine the optimal 3D-TTE technique employed in image optimization, acquisition, rendering, display, and analysis (Fig. 10.3 and Videos 10.2–10.6). The specific clinical applications of 3D-TTE employed in the assessment of cardiac structure and function are covered elsewhere in this book (see Chapter 5).

THE THREE-DIMENSIONAL TRANSTHORACIC ECHOCARDIOGRAPHY DATA ACQUISITION PROTOCOL

The optimization of both patient and machine preparation for 3D-TTE, consistent with the 2D-TTE examination, is important (see Chapter 11). Electrocardiography (ECG) gating is critical for 3D trigger-mode imaging. Therefore it is important to obtain a good ECG signal with clearly visible R-waves. Until recently, the 3D-TTE exam required switching from the standard 2D phased array transducer to a 3D matrix array transducer. Today, the most recent 3D "all-in-one" transducer designs facilitate simultaneous 2D and 3D image acquisition using a single probe. This improves workflow efficiency (see Fig. 10.2). The following steps are generally required during 3D-TTE image acquisition (Box 10.2; see also Fig. 10.3 and Videos 10.2–10.6).

1. 2D image optimization
2. Acquisition modes
   - Narrow volume vs. wide (full) volume
   - Single-beat vs. multibeat
   - 3D zoom
   - 3D color
3. Rendering
4. Final image display and analysis

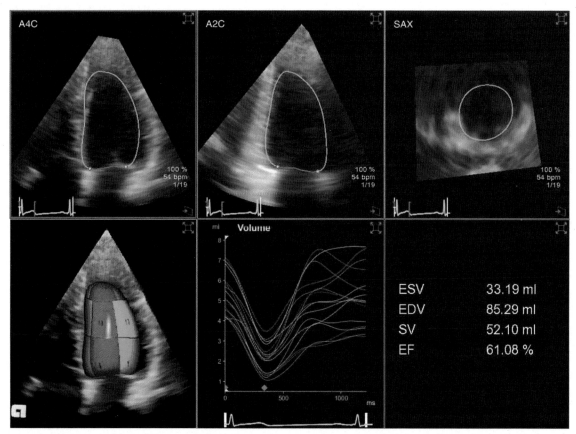

FIG. 10.1 Three-dimensional transthoracic echocardiography (3D-TTE) 3D-TTE employed in the assessment of LV volumes and ejection fraction (EF). 3D-TTE substantially improves the workflow and accuracy in the quantification of cardiac volumetric measures, and avoiding errors inherent in the geometric assumptions made in 2D-TTE, such as LV foreshortening. See also Video 10.1 . (See text and Box 10.1.) *EDV,* End-diastolic volume; *EF,* ejection fraction (LV); *ESV,* end-systolic volume; *SV,* stroke volume.

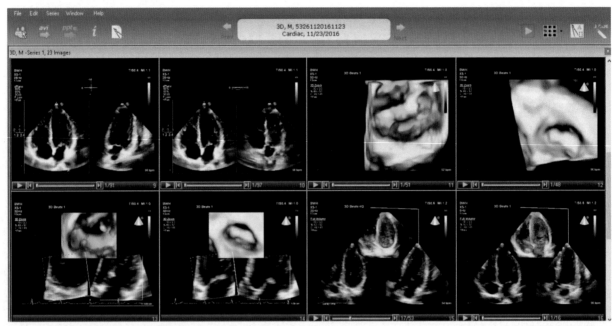

FIG. 10.2 Three-dimensional transthoracic echocardiography (3D-TTE) delivers improved workflow in the modern echocardiography laboratory. Until recently, the 3D exam involved switching from the two-dimensional (2D) phased array transducer to a separate 3D matrix array transducer. However, newer 3D transducer designs facilitate simultaneous 2D and 3D image acquisition using a single probe. (See text and Boxes 10.2 and 10.3.)

BOX 10.1 Clinical and Research Applications of Three-Dimensional Echocardiography

Clinical and Research Applications
Ventricular structure and function: LV, R:
- Ventricular volumes
- LV mass
- LV Geometry/shape
- LV dyssynchrony
- Stress echocardiography
Atria volumes
Intracardiac shunts
Valvular structure and function:
Native valve anatomy
Native valve pathology
- Mitral stenosis, regurgitation
- Aortic stenosis, regurgitation
Prosthetic valves
Invasive procedures:
- Transcatheter guidance procedures
- Intracardiac biopsies
- Ablation procedures in electrophysiology

TABLE 10.1 Examples of Choice of Three-Dimensional Transthoracic Echocardiography Acquisition Mode in the Echo Lab

CLINICAL APPLICATION	MODE
Ventricular volumes (LV, RV) Atrial volumes Ejection fraction Whole heart	Full volume (wide-angle, multibeat)
Valve anatomy Valvular pathology Shunt lesions Small structures visualized within narrow sector	Live 3D zoom (color)
Guidance for transcatheter procedures	Live 3D zoom (color)
Native heart biopsies Electrophysiology ablations	Live 3D

LV, Left ventricle; *RV*, right ventricle; *3D*, Three-dimensional.

TWO-DIMENSIONAL IMAGE OPTIMIZATION

Optimal 3D image acquisition is contingent on acquiring an optimal 2D image, as the same physical principles of B-mode imaging apply (Box 10.3; see Chapter 11). If the 2D images are poor, so will be the resultant 3D images. Appropriate transducer frequency selection is necessary for acquisition of the 3D data set. Using a lower-frequency transducer improves image penetration, and is important at greater depths. Harmonic imaging modality is also recommended, as this improves the blood-tissue definition. In order to obtain the best possible images, the operator should (1) optimize the region of interest by reducing the angle, depth, and density of the 3D scan sector volume; (2) maximize the number of subvolumes and increase system gain; (3) avoid or minimize imaging artifacts, including image drop-out or attenuation artifact; and (4) optimize time-gain compensation (TGC). Most times, it is better to overgain on the 2D image, as the 3D data set can be optimized postacquisition if there is too much gain, to a lower optimal gain setting.

ACQUISITION MODES

Two major image acquisition modes are used in 3D-TTE: (1) real-time (live) 3D imaging and (2) electrocardiographically triggered multibeat 3D imaging (see Fig. 10.3 and Table 10.2). In real-time (live) 3D-TTE, multiple 3D pyramidal data sets per second are acquired during a single heartbeat (Fig. 10.4; see also Fig. 10.3 and Videos 10.2–10.6). In contrast, in ECG-triggered multibeat 3D image acquisition, multiple narrow volumes (subvolumes) are acquired over several heartbeats, typically 2–7, and stitched to generate a single 3D volume (Fig. 10.5 and Video 10.7; see also Fig. 10.3 and Videos 10.2–10.6). The subvolumes are acquired with each beat, displayed, and updated with acquisitions obtained during the subsequent beats. This mode is clinically useful for 3D left ventricular function assessment and LV mass.

With both real-time (live) 3D and ECG-triggered multibeat 3D acquisition modes, the acquired 3D-TTE data sets may be narrow volume or wide volume, and with options for 3D zoom and 3D color flow Doppler (Figs. 10.6–10.8; see also Fig. 10.3 and Videos 10.2–10.7). Full volume 3D image acquisition produces a larger 3D dataset or full volume of the entire heart (see Fig. 10.7). The advantage of single beat acquisition is that that it can minimize stitch artifacts due to arrhythmias and respiratory cardiac translation. Its main disadvantage, however, can be the limited temporal resolution. Multibeat 3D acquisition has higher temporal resolution compared with single-beat acquisition, but its main disadvantage is its susceptibility to motion or stitch artifacts.

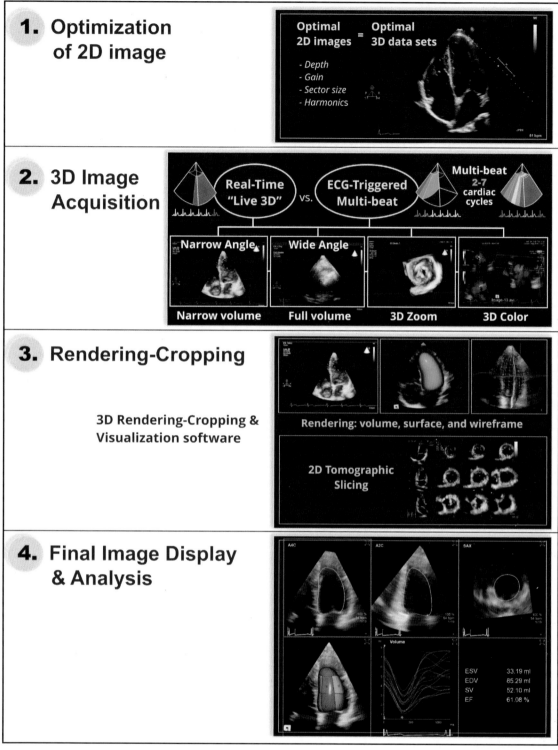

1. Optimization of 2D image

Optimal 2D images = Optimal 3D data sets
- Depth
- Gain
- Sector size
- Harmonics

2. 3D Image Acquisition

Real-Time "Live 3D" vs. ECG-Triggered Multi-beat — Multi-beat 2-7 cardiac cycles

Narrow Angle | Wide Angle

Narrow volume | Full volume | 3D Zoom | 3D Color

3. Rendering-Cropping

3D Rendering-Cropping & Visualization software

Rendering: volume, surface, and wireframe

2D Tomographic Slicing

4. Final Image Display & Analysis

A4C | A2C | SAX

Volume

ESV	33.19 ml
EDV	85.29 ml
SV	52.10 ml
EF	61.08 %

FIG. 10.3 Optimizing the three-dimensional (3D) transthoracic echocardiography imaging involves a series of techniques, including optimization of the two-dimensional image, acquisition of the 3D image based on the clinical question, rendering the image, finalizing the image display, and postprocessing analysis. See also Videos 10.2–10.6. (See text and Box 10.2.)

3D zoom facilitates focusing on a desired region of interest (see Figs. 10.3 and 10.8). The narrower the sector, the higher the temporal resolution. Adjust box size accordingly, based on the region of interest.
- Optimize the 2D image; change to a lower-frequency transducer (good 2D image equals good 3D data set).
- Change focus, beam size, and location if necessary.
- Preview image, and ensure the region of interest is within the sector; adjust lateral and elevation width, and focus on the region of interest. This improves the frame rate.

- Adjust 3D gain settings.
- Adjust the image using the trackball to ensure optimal visualization.
- Rotating the knob (on most instruments) enables image manipulation with reference to a central axis.

There are useful additional 3D acquisition and display protocols, using proprietary software. Simultaneous multiplane 3D imaging is a useful protocol that significantly improves workflow by providing simultaneous display of orthogonal images (Figs. 10.9 and 10.10, and Videos 10.8 –10.10).

BOX 10.2 Typical Workflow in Three-Dimensional Transthoracic Echocardiography

1. Optimize the two-dimensional (2D) images, including imaging depth, sector size
2. Use lower-frequency transducer to improve penetration
3. Apply tissue harmonic imaging
4. Apply automated gain optimization
5. Increase overall gain compensation, usually by more than 50% (55–60 units)
6. Ensure that the region of interest is fully within the scan sector by using multiplane scanning
7. Apply three-dimensional (3D) zoom
8. Optimize box size and position; make sure the region of interest is within the box size range
9. Activate 3D zoom
10. For 3D color zoom, add the color over the selected anatomic area of interest
11. Ensure that the color box occupies the entire selected area
12. Remember the trade-off between image acquisition and frame rate: the larger the area, the larger the volume, the lower the frame rate.
13. If necessary, acquire six-beat electrocardiography data set for higher color frame rates.

BOX 10.3 Steps to Optimization of the Two-Dimensional Image in Three-Dimensional Transthoracic Echocardiography

1. Optimize your two-dimensional images, including imaging depth, sector size.
2. Change transducer frequency to penetration harmonics.
3. Make sure your region of interest is encompassed within the sector by using multiplane scanning.
4. Use an automated gain optimization tool on your machine.
5. Turn the overall gain compensation to a little more than half (55–60 units).
6. Optimize the electrocardiography.
7. Set the number of beats for acquisition (2-4-6 beats) six beats for added color Doppler.
8. Once you are ready, ask your patient to take a breath in, and then slowly exhale.
9. See the image is optimal and ask patient to hold breath.
10. Press Full Volume, review, check for stitches artifacts, and approve.

CROPPING AND RENDERING

Following optimal acquisition of the 3D data set, proprietary software are used to render and display the 3D images using three general formats: (1) volume rendering, (2) surface rendering, and (3) 2D tomographic slicing (see Fig. 10.3). With volume rendering, the acquired 3D data set is subjected to various algorithms (e.g., ray casting or share warp) to project the 3D data set unto the 2D image display for viewing. The resultant image can then be manipulated, rotated, and cropped to display the desired region of interest, and is useful in the assessment of complex relationships such as the intracardiac valves and related anatomy. 3D volumes can be cropped to transect the cardiac short-axis to visualize the aortic and mitral valves, as viewed from the apex or to visualize the cardiac chambers consistent with the standard 2D imaging planes from a 3D perspective (see Fig. 10.10 and Video 10.10).

The 3D data set can also be surface-rendered. Surface rendering facilitates visualization of the region of interest by using manual tracing or proprietary algorithms. These can display contours of cardiac structures using contours that can be visualized as solid shapes or wireframes of the 2D images (Fig. 10.11 and Videos 10.11 and 10.12). Surface rendering is

TABLE 10.2 Comparison of Real-Time (Live) and ECG-Triggered Three-Dimensional Echocardiography

Real-time (live) 3D-TTE	ECG-triggered multibeat 3D-TTE
• Images acquired in a single heartbeat	• Multiple volumes acquired over several heartbeats, typically 2–7, and stitched single 3D data set
Narrow volume	Wide (full) volume
3D zoom	3D zoom
Live 3D color	3D color
Advantages: • Less affected by cardiac dysrhythmias • Less affected by respiratory movements (translation)	Advantages: • Better temporal resolution • Better spatial resolution
Disadvantages: • Poor temporal resolution • Poor spatial resolution	Disadvantages: • Prone to stitch artifacts due to cardiac dysrhythmias, respiratory and patient motion

ECG, Electrocardiography; *3D-TTE,* three-dimensional transthoracic echocardiography.

useful in the basement of cardiac chambers and dynamic volumes during the cardiac cycle (compare with Fig. 10.1).

Following both real-time (live) 3D and multigate 3D image acquisition, the acquired 3D data set can be cropped to display the desired anatomical or cut plane. Multiple cropping options are available, depending on the vendor software. The American Society of Echocardiography (ASE) and the European Association of Echocardiography (EAE) have posited protocols for orientation and display of 3D-TTE images (Table 10.3), but in current clinical practice, 3D-TTE is used to complement, not substitute, the comprehensive 2D-TEE examination.

IMAGE DISPLAY AND ANALYSIS

Simultaneous multiplane 3D imaging facilitates the simultaneous display of 2D image planes that can be adjusted, rotated, tilted, or elevated using predefined or operator-determined settings. Multiplane 3D imaging facilitates higher-frame rates. This modality uses a dual screen that simultaneously displays 2D images in real-time images (Figs. 10.12 and 10.13, and Video 10.13). The first image is typically displayed on the left a reference plane, and the second or additional images can be viewed using predefined or operator-determined lateral rotation or elevated plane. By default, images are displayed orthogonal or 90 degrees to each other, with each image adjustable using its own reference plane.

In addition, simultaneous multiplane 3D imaging also facilitates simultaneous color flow Doppler mapping, where such data is superimposed on the 2D image. This is useful in quantitation and valvular assessment (see Fig. 10.13). Such simultaneous displays and standard measurements based thereon lead to a greatly reduced need for transducer manipulation, thereby improving workflow, increasing productivity, and improving diagnosis and quantification.

CHALLENGES AND OPTIMIZATION IN THREE-DIMENSIONAL DATA ACQUISITION

The key trade-off in 3D imaging is between volume rate and spatial resolution (Fig. 10.14). By adjusting the imaging volume sizes, volume rates are improved while maintaining spatial resolution. The larger beat sample volume obtained, the better the temporal resolution.

ELECTROCARDIOGRAPHY GATING AND BREATH HOLD

Gated sets are more challenging in patients with arrhythmias or in respiratory distress. In both of these situations, the likelihood of stitching artifacts is higher (Fig. 10.15 and Videos 10.14 and 10.15). If the clinical question to be answered requires a larger 3D data set

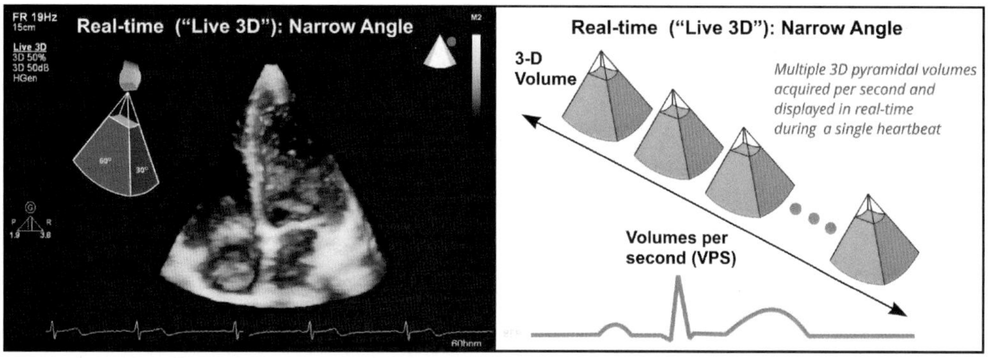

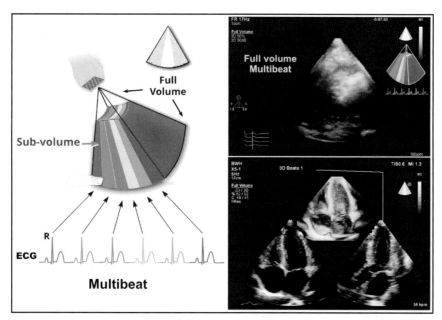

FIG. 10.4 Real-time (live) or narrow angle three-dimensional (3D) transthoracic image acquisition (see text). *(Courtesy of Bernard E. Bulwer, MD, FASE.)*

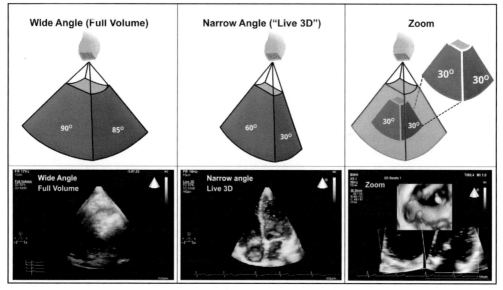

FIG. 10.5 Multibeat image acquisition in three-dimensional (3D) transthoracic echocardiography. Electrocardiograph (ECG)–triggered multiple-beat 3D data acquisition. Note that with each consecutive beat, a narrow pyramidal volume is obtained. Each narrow volume of data is then stitched together for form a single 3D full volume (90 degrees × 90 degrees). Wide or full volume mode 3D acquisition sector delivers the largest data set, delivers the better spatial resolution, and therefore facilitates improved assessment complex pathologies. In addition, full volume 3D data sets can be cropped and postprocessed, thereby facilitating improved analyses. See also Video 10.7 and Fig. 10.3. *(Courtesy of Bernard E. Bulwer, MD, FASE.)*

FIG. 10.6 Narrow volumes and wide volume three-dimensional (3D) image acquisition compared (see text). *(Courtesy of Bernard E. Bulwer, MD, FASE.)*

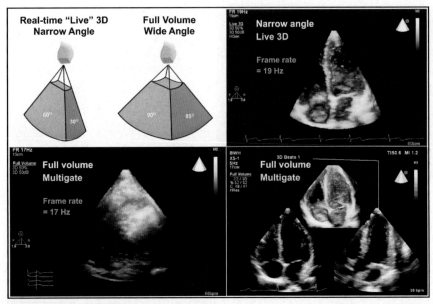

FIG. 10.7 Narrow volume versus full volume image acquisition (see text). *(Courtesy of Bernard E. Bulwer, MD, FASE.)*

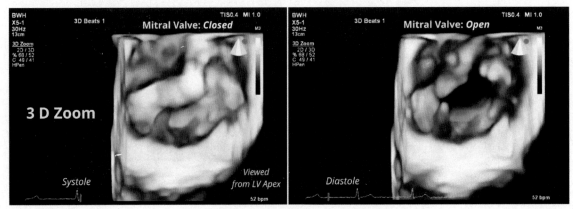

FIG. 10.8 Three-dimensional zoom (see text).

volume, the ECG tracing will need to be optimized with a clear R wave and by using the patient breath hold technique to prevent stitching artifacts. This in turn avoids cardiac translation. Stitching artifacts are clearly demonstrated on acquired perpendicular images (series of short axis cuts). Larger volumes require more beat acquisition, which can affect the spatial resolution. If the objective is to obtain an anatomic data set (e.g., with a dilated left ventricle), the sector size can be reduced to only include the region of interest. In this case, the left ventricle increases the volume rate and temporal resolution, and preserves spatial resolution. The same can be done for the right ventricle and other cardiac structures or chambers. It is similar to having a focused gated 3D image acquisition; volume rate higher or equal to 15 volumes per second is considered optimal for LV and RV acquisition.

THREE-DIMENSIONAL GAIN OPTIMIZATION

Gain settings are also another important factor in the data set optimization (Fig. 10.16). The same principles need to be taken into consideration with 3D data sets as well as 2D imaging. Low gain setting will result in echo dropout on 2D as well as in the 3D data set. Optimization of the 2D images using the overall gain settings, TGC setting, changing frequencies, using vendors' automated gain setting system, will improve final data set

optimization. There is not a simple formula or setting—if the 2D image is poor, the resulting 3D images will be suboptimal.

- Optimize 2D images, depth, and image sector.
- Change transducer frequency to penetration harmonics.
- Make sure your region of interest is encompassed within the sector by using multiplane scanning.
- Use automated gain optimization tool on your machine.
- Turn your overall gain compensation to a little more than half (55–60 units).
- Turn on Live 3D and look for dropout areas in the data set and appreciate the depth of your 3D image.

LIVE THREE-DIMENSIONAL OPTIMIZATION

Live 3D is a single pyramidal volumetric data over time that requires adequate frame rates. Most of its limitation derives from limited display of entire anatomic structures. It is useful clinically as a complement of 2D images to provide additional information not otherwise seen by conventional 2D imaging. It allows for quick access display from the control panel and no gating (it can be obtained without ECG). Live 3D is clinically relevant in prepost, during catheterization lab procedures (i.e., TAVR, closure devices, native heart biopsies). Optimization of live 3D echocardiography is summarized in Box 10.4.

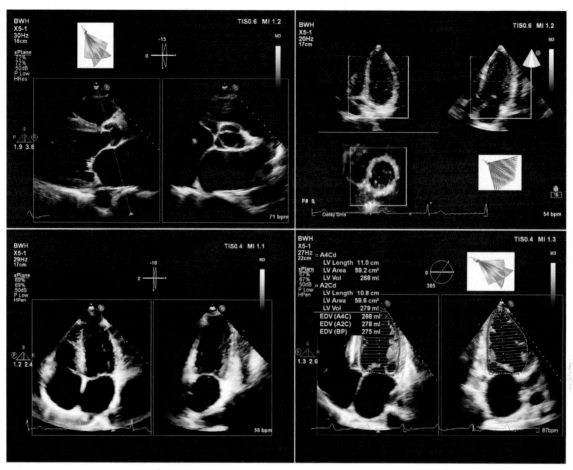

FIG. 10.9 Two-dimensional orthogonal views obtained with matrix probe.

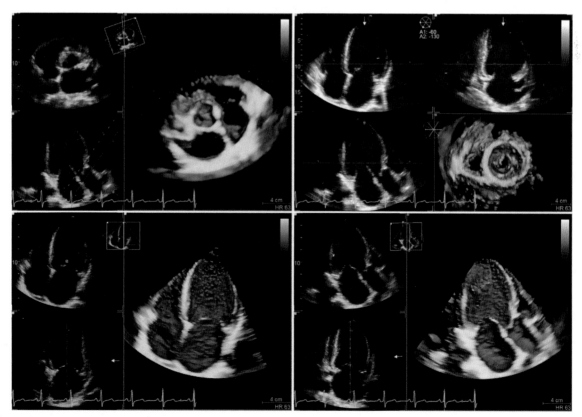

FIG. 10.10 Cropping of selected views, consistent with current protocols advanced by the American Society of Echocardiography and the European Association of Echocardiography. See also Videos 10.10.

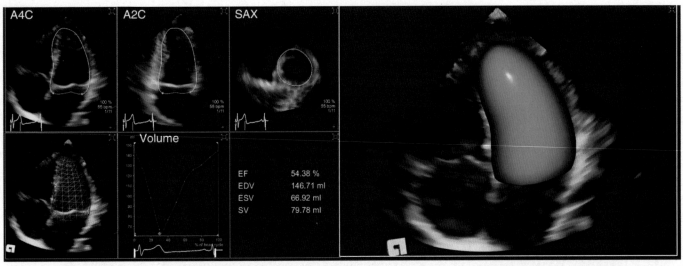

FIG. 10.11 Volume rendering *(above)* and surface rendering *(below)* in three-dimensional transthoracic echocardiography (see text). See also Videos 10.11 and 10.12.

TABLE 10.3 **ASE/EAE Recommended Protocol for Three-Dimensional Transthoracic Echocardiography Protocol**

Aortic valve	PLAX—No color flow Doppler; PLAX—Color flow Doppler Narrow angle Zoom
Mitral valve	PLAX—No color flow Doppler; PLAX—Color flow Doppler Narrow angle Zoom A4C—No color flow Doppler; A4C—Color flow Doppler Narrow angle Zoom
Tricuspid valve	RV inflow view—No color flow Doppler RV inflow view—Color flow Doppler Narrow angle Zoom A4C—No color flow Doppler; A4C—Color flow Doppler Narrow angle Zoom
Pulmonary valve	RV outflow view—No color flow Doppler RV outflow view—Color flow Doppler Narrow angle Zoom
Left ventricle	A4C Narrow angle Wide angle
Right ventricle	A4C with RV tilt to center RV Narrow angle Wide angle

A4C, Apical four-chamber; *ASE,* American Society of Echocardiography; *EAE,* European Association of Echocardiography; *PLAX,* parasternal long-axis.

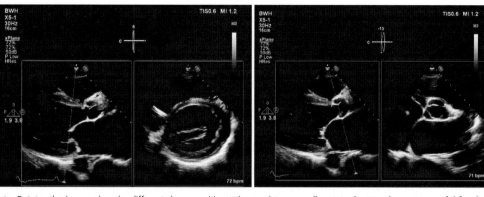

FIG. 10.12 Multi iRotate. Rotates the image plane by different degrees without the need to manually rotate the transducer; very useful for those difficult cases that the operator has limited access to rib spaces and for rapid image acquisition in stress echocardiograms.

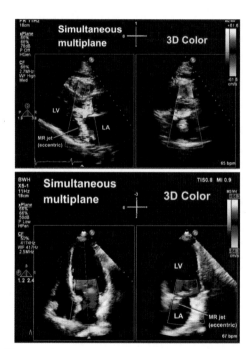

FIG. 10.13 Simultaneous multiplane three-dimensional image acquisition using matrix array transducer, showing simultaneous biplane image acquisition (top left) and triplane image acquisition (top right). This image display mode also facilitates the use of two-dimensional (2D) color (bottom left), as well as quantification of standard 2D measures, including LV ejection fraction (bottom right). See also Video 10.13.

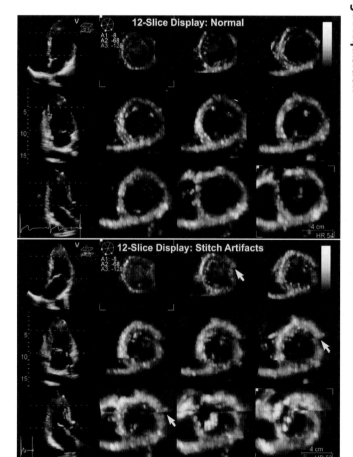

FIG. 10.15 Three-dimensional imaging pitfalls: stitch artifact (12 slice). When looking for stitch artifacts, it is important to examine the image plane perpendicular or orthogonal to the sweep plane. For example, when looking at images acquired using the apical four-chamber plane, stitch artifacts should be sought on the short-axis views (see text). See also Videos 10.14 and 10.15.

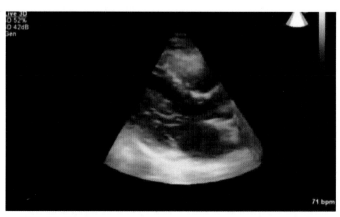

FIG. 10.14 Three-dimensional imaging pitfalls: poor resolution (see text).

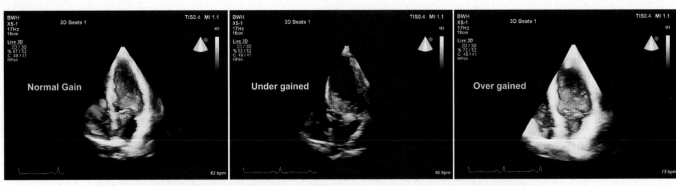

FIG. 10.16 Three-dimensional imaging pitfalls: over gaining and under gaining (see text).

BOX 10.4 Steps to Optimization of Live Three-Dimensional

1. Optimize your two-dimensional images, depth, and image sector.
2. Change transducer frequency to penetration harmonics.
3. Make sure your region of interest is encompassed within the sector by using multiplane scanning.
4. Use automated gain optimization tool on your machine.
5. Turn your overall gain compensation to a little more than half (55–60 units).
6. Turn on the three-dimensional (3D) bottom.
7. In most devices, a multiplane reconstruction display is offered; this helps discern if the anatomic area you want to acquire is encompassed in the 3D image for display.
8. Rotate your 3D data set with the trackball; use the multiplane reconstruction for elevation back, front or width.

Suggested Reading

Badano, L. P., Boccalini, F., Muraru, D., et al. (2012). Current clinical applications of transthoracic three-dimensional echocardiography. *Journal of Cardiovascular Ultrasound, 20*, 1–22.

Badano, L. P., Lang, R. M., & Goncalves, A. (2015). Three-dimensional echocardiography. In P. Lancellotti, J. Zamorano, G. Habib, & L. Badano (Eds.), *EACVI Textbook of Echocardiography* (2nd ed.) (pp. 59–69). Oxford: Oxford University Press.

Badano, L. P., & Muraru, D. (2016). Three-dimensional echocardiography. In R. M. Lang, S. A. Goldstein, I. Kronzon, et al. (Eds.), *ASE's Comprehensive Echocardiography* (2nd ed.) (pp. 3–10). Philadelphia: Elsevier.

Badano, L. P., Muraru, D., Dal Lin, C., & Iliceto, S. (2013). Instrumentation and data acquisition. In R. Lang, S. K. Shernan, G. Shirali, & V. Mor-Avi (Eds.), *Comprehensive Atlas of 3D Echocardiography. Philadelphia* (pp. 13–28). Lippincott Williams & Wilkins.

Lang, R. M., Badano, L. P., Mor-Avi, V., et al. (2015). Recommendations for cardiac chamber quantification by echocardiography in adults: an update from the American Society of Echocardiography and the European Association of Cardiovascular Imaging. *European heart journal Cardiovasc Imaging, 16*, 233–270.

Lang, R. M., Badano, L. P., Tsang, W., et al. (2012). EAE/ASE recommendations for image acquisition and display using three-dimensional echocardiography. *Journal of the American Society of Echocardiography, 25*, 3–46.

Thavendiranathan, P., Liu, S., Datta, S., et al. (2012). Automated quantification of mitral inflow and aortic outflow stroke volumes by three-dimensional real-time volume color-flow Doppler transthoracic echocardiography: comparison with pulsed-wave Doppler and cardiac magnetic resonance imaging. *Journal of the American Society of Echocardiography, 25*, 56–65.

Optimization of the Patient and Equipment

Jose Rivero, Kurt Jacobson, Bernard E. Bulwer, Linda D. Gillam

INTRODUCTION

Optimal performance of the comprehensive two-dimensional (2D) transthoracic echocardiography (TTE) examination depends on the interaction between the operator (sonographer and/or physician), instrument (ultrasound system), and patient (Fig. 11.1). This chapter will focus on techniques for optimizing acquisition that relate to the patient and ultrasound system, including optimizing the patient and transducer positions as well as using maneuvers and machine settings to optimize the 2D imaging, spectral, and color Doppler display.

OPTIMIZING PATIENT AND TRANSDUCER POSITIONS

The TTE examination is built on the framework of standard views (e.g., parasternal long axis, apical four chamber), as discussed in Chapter 9. Optimal acquisition of TTE images/Doppler for these views is dependent on appropriate patient and transducer positioning (Fig. 11.2). While some patients have easily accessible echocardiographic windows, others are far more challenging, resulting in studies that are often described as "technically difficult." The sonographer has a variety of tools available to assist in obtaining the best possible echocardiographic images/Doppler signals for each patient. They include positioning the patient, manipulating the transducer, and the effective utilization of ultrasound machine settings. The standard echocardiographic windows therefore are primarily a guide, as nonstandard windows and maneuvers may be necessary, based on individual patient characteristics (Table 11.1). Additionally, nonstandard views may be required to delineate pathology and answer the clinical question posed. The goal therefore is to use whatever patient and transducer positions, maneuvers, and machine settings are needed to deliver the optimal image and/or Doppler display. The use of contrast is discussed in detail in Chapters 3 and 12, but it should be noted here that appropriate use of echocardiographic contrast agents is a critical component of image optimization.

The ultrasound transducer is separated from its target organ, the heart, by the bony chest wall and the air-filled lungs. These can greatly impede ultrasound beam transmission and have a negative impact on image quality. The rationale for the various TTE transducer positions or "windows," including patient maneuvers during the examination, is the desire to minimize obstacles to beam transmission, thereby optimizing image quality.

The comprehensive TTE examination generally begins at the left parasternal window, with the patient in the left lateral decubitus position, his/her left arm up and away from the chest, and the transducer positioned at the left sternal border at or near the third intercostal space (see Fig. 11.2). Sometimes the patient's medical condition, prior surgery, or congenital abnormalities may necessitate a more exploratory approach, but this is generally the best starting point. The left lateral decubitus position pulls the heart closer to the chest wall, displacing the air-filled lungs, thereby expanding the window. Breath holding at end-expiration or acquiring images during shallow breathing often helps. Parasternal long and short axis views can be acquired here. It is essential that parasternal views be recorded on axis—that is, with the long axis of the heart pointed due left or horizontally in parasternal long axis views. Frequently, the image recorded is one in which the long axis of the ventricle points up toward the upper left corner of the image, typically reflecting a lower than ideal window. With such off-axis views, it will be impossible to obtain accurate measurements of the left ventricular (LV) cavity and walls, and the short

axis views obtained from the same window will be ovoid rather than circular, making it difficult to assess septal contour and regional wall motion. Off-axis views can be avoided by trying higher windows and repositioning the patient, often further over in the left lateral decubitus position (Figs. 11.3 and 11.4, and Videos 11.1 and 11.2). That said, while basal and mid-ventricular short axis views can and should be obtained from the optimized parasternal view, it will typically be necessary to move the transducer down and away from the sternum to capture a short axis image of the true apex. With the transducer rotated 90 degrees from this new window, typically midway between the parasternal long axis and apical four-chamber views, a long axis of the apex can be achieved that can minimize the risk of missing true apical wall motion abnormalities and thrombi. Note that the standard parasternal views do not show the true apex. In the case of the ascending aorta, moving up an intercostal space and tilting slightly downward can often yield an effective window, as can right parasternal views (discussed later).

The apical views are best obtained with the patient in the steep left lateral decubitus position that brings the LV apex closer to the chest wall, with the transducer positioned at or near the palpable apex beat (see Fig. 11.2). Positioning the patient near the edge of the examination bed or using a cutout window facilitates transducer maneuvers at the apex. For apical views, care should be taken to move sufficiently lateral and down far enough to see the true apex of the heart, avoiding foreshortened images. Images acquired at end expiration or with the patient holding a small breath can assist with many apical images, particularly the apical two-chamber and apical three-chamber views. Especially in patients with known regional wall motion abnormalities, it may be helpful to also move

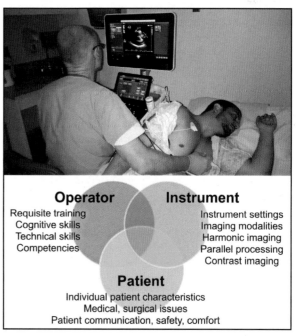

FIG. 11.1 Schematic representing the interaction between the operator, instrument, and patient (model shown here) in optimizing echocardiography image acquisition. (*Courtesy of Bernard E. Bulwer, MD, FASE.*)

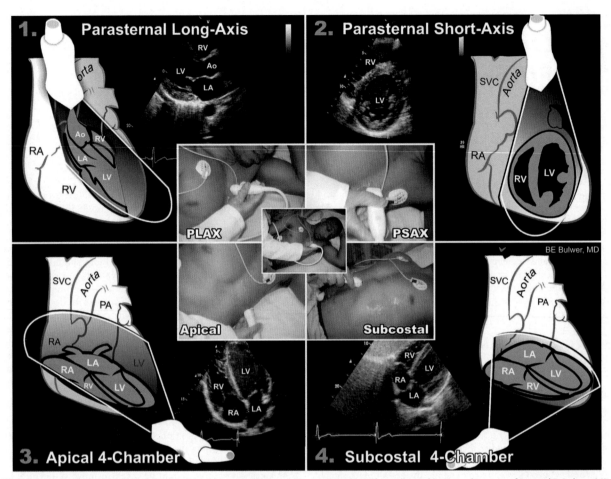

FIG. 11.2 Composite displaying patient positioning, transducer windows, and the corresponding echocardiographic views. *(Courtesy of Bernard E. Bulwer, MD, FASE.)*

TABLE 11.1 Patient Characteristics and Examination Considerations

PATIENT CHARACTERISTICS	EXAMINATION CONSIDERATIONS
Normal individual variation	The recommended transducer positions or "windows" are a good guide. However, acquire views using the best windows that optimize the desired images.
Normal patient with "difficult windows"	Consider repositioning patient, inspiratory maneuvers, transducer options, and instrument settings.
Body habitus, including obesity	Consider using lower-frequency transducers (less than 2.5 MHz) as necessary ± ultrasound contrast agents.
Lung disease (e.g., emphysema, pneumothorax)	Hyperinflated lungs lower or eliminate the parasternal windows. Subcostal windows may be the best windows in patients with emphysema. Consider use of ultrasound contrast agents.
Chest wall pathology (e.g., scoliosis, pectus excavatum)	Nonstandard views and/or patient position may provide the best views.
Patients in critical care units or emergency room	Targeted or focused examination may be all that is possible. Transesophageal echocardiography (TEE) as indicated. Consider use of ultrasound contrast agents.
Post chest surgery	The subcostal examination may be the only "free" window. Other imaging options (e.g., TEE or contrast agents) may be necessary.

the transducer down an interspace from what appears to the optimal apical view and then have the patient take a breath in. This may reveal segments apical to those seen on the earlier view and unmask aneurysms ± thrombi.

The subcostal (subxiphoid) views are optimally acquired with the patient lying supine with knees flexed, which relaxes the abdominal muscles (see Fig. 11.2). Elevating the head of the bed often helps, as gravity pulls the heart closer to the transducer. Acquiring images at end-inspiration facilitates this further. Respiratory variation in the size of the inferior vena cava (IVC), which is used to estimate the right atrial pressure, can be assessed with M-mode or 2D imaging while the patient takes a vigorous sniff. However, care must be taken to ensure that the appearance of a diminution in the size of the IVC is not artifactually created by simply losing the correct imaging plane with the sniff. Biplane 2D imaging derived from 3D images can be helpful in this regard.

For the suprasternal notch (SSN) views, the patient remains in the supine position, but with the neck extended or hyperextended and the head rotated to facilitate transducer positioning. Placing a pillow under the shoulders promotes neck hyperextension. Right parasternal views that are essential for assessing patients with aortic stenosis are best acquired just to the right of the sternum, with the transducer oriented as it was in the parasternal long axis. The patient should be lying on her or his right side, with the right arm up and away from the torso. The smaller imprint of the nonimaging Pedoff transducer facilitates suprasternal and right parasternal Doppler interrogation (Table 11.2).

OPTIMIZING TWO-DIMENSIONAL IMAGING: MACHINE SETTINGS

To create the brightness-mode (B-mode) anatomical image, which is based on the relative strengths (amplitudes) and depths (timing) of the returning echoes, the echoes received by the transducer must undergo a

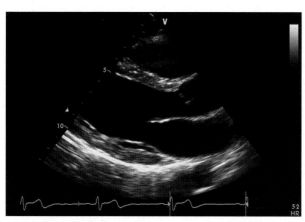

FIG. 11.3 Proper parasternal long axis view. Note that the long axis of the left ventricle is aligned horizontally on the image. The apex is typically not seen in this view. See also Video 11.1.

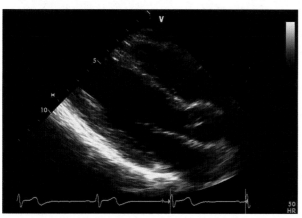

FIG. 11.4 Off-axis parasternal long axis view. Note that the long axis of the left ventricle is aligned diagonally. This can be converted to a proper parasternal view by moving the transducer up and/or repositioning the patient. See also Video 11.2.

TABLE 11.2 Examination Tips for Optimal Image Acquisition

AIM	METHODS AND TECHNIQUES
Minimize translational motion of the heart	• Quiet or suspended respiration (at end-expiration)
Optimize image resolution	• Image at minimum depth necessary • Highest possible transducer frequency • Adjust gains, dynamic range, transmit, and lateral gain controls appropriately • Frame rate ≥30/s • Harmonic imaging
Avoid apical foreshortening	• Steep lateral decubitus position • Cutout mattress • Do not rely exclusively on the palpable apical impulse • Move the transducer down an interspace from the initial apical window and check to see if deep inspiration reveals more apical segments (± aneurysm) than initially suspected
Maximize endocardial border delineation	• Tissue harmonic imaging • Use contrast agents to enhance delineation of endocardial borders
Identify end diastole and end systole	• Use ventricular cavity size and mitral valve motion rather than reliance on electrocardiogram (end diastole = maximal dimension, and end-systole = minimal dimension)
Optimize parasternal windows	• Apex should be directed horizontally. If not, try a higher parasternal window and/or reposition the patient.

according to the agent and transducer used, and the reader is encouraged to work with contrast and system applications specialists to ensure that settings are optimized.

OPTIMIZING THE SPECTRAL DOPPLER EXAMINATION

Doppler echocardiography is integral to the comprehensive TTE examination. It makes possible the noninvasive assessment of blood flow velocities, direction, and flow patterns, based on the Doppler principle. In contrast to B-mode echocardiography, which uses the amplitudes of the received echoes to create the anatomical image, Doppler echocardiography harnesses the change or shift in frequency of the returned echoes to detect and quantify blood flow velocities (Figs. 11.9 and 11.10). By convention, signals from blood cells moving toward the transducer are displayed above the baseline, with signals from blood moving away from the transducer being displayed below the baseline.

Blood flow velocities change during the cardiac cycle. These velocities can be assessed and displayed as a histogram of red cell velocity plotted over time—hence the term *spectral Doppler*. The two spectral Doppler modalities routinely employed in the comprehensive echocardiographic exam are pulsed-waved (PW) and continuous-wave (CW) Doppler. PW Doppler (see Fig. 11.10) assesses blood flow velocities at specific anatomical sites and within small sample volumes. Hence PW Doppler has the advantage of being "range specific," with the ability to localize the site at which flow is recorded. This translates to an ability to detect regurgitant lesions and shunts. A major disadvantage of PW Doppler is that it cannot accurately record velocities above the Nyquist limit, which is inversely related to the distance of the sample volume from the transducer. Therefore the imaging window chosen for PW Doppler interrogation should be as close as possible to the region of interest. CW Doppler overcomes this aliasing limitation, but cannot distinguish the site at which flow is recorded beyond identifying it as originating from along the line of insonation, so-called range ambiguity.

sophisticated series of processing steps prior to being displayed as a one-dimensional (M-mode), 2D, or three-dimensional (3D) image over time formats. The returning weak echo signals must be amplified with the overall "strength" of the image influenced by overall gain control, time-gain compensation controls (based on imaging depth) (Fig. 11.5), and lateral gain compensation controls (based on medial to lateral position in the imaging field). Additional adjustments involve log-compression (dynamic range control) to optimize the grayscale image.

There are several controls that influence the contrast of the ultrasound image and that can be used to achieve a balance between too black and white versus too gray. The dynamic range (compression; Fig. 11.6) sets the range between the strongest and weakest echoes that can be displayed by compressing or decompressing them into fewer or greater shades of gray. With full compression, the image will have high contrast and appear to be largely black and white. Another control is reject, which is used to filter out weaker (gray) echoes and may be used to eliminate weak echoes that obscure the image. The expert sonographer can optimize image quality through adjustment of several of these and other instrument settings ("knobology") that are available in modern full-featured instrument platforms (Figs. 11.7 and 11.8; Table 11.3).

USE OF CONTRAST

The use of contrast is discussed in detail in Chapters 3 and 12, but it is important to note here that contrast can be very helpful in optimizing images. In this discussion, which is focused on optimizing the patient and equipment, the use of contrast-specific presets, which use harmonic imaging and lower power settings (mechanical index) than used for non-contrast-enhanced imaging, is emphasized. The optimal settings vary

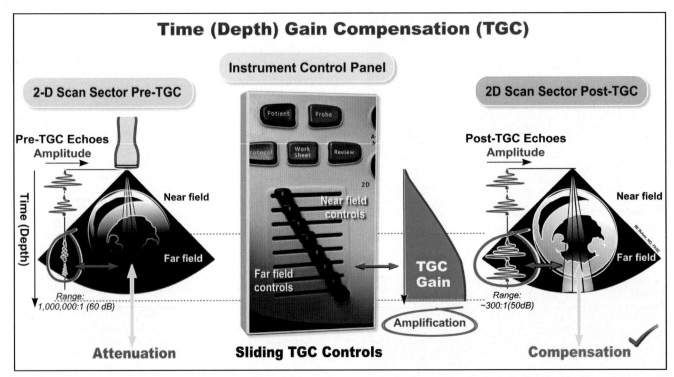

FIG. 11.5 Time-gain (or depth-gain) compensation principle. As ultrasound travels from the transducer to the imaged target, progressive attenuation or loss of strength/amplitude occurs. Echoes arising from greater depths take longer times to return and suffer from greater attenuation, thus demanding greater compensation for optimal display. *(Courtesy of Bernard E. Bulwer, MD, FASE.)*

Therefore these two spectral Doppler modalities are complementary and routinely employed together.

Blood flow velocity measurements are subject to variables controlled by the sonographer. Chief among them is the beam-blood flow angle, the Doppler angle of insonation. This relationship described by the Doppler equation emphasizes that the ability to accurately record blood velocity is optimized when the angle of insonation is 180 degrees (i.e., parallel to flow). It also follows that it is not possible to accurately measure Doppler-derived blood velocities when the transducer is aligned perpendicular to the direction of flow. Closer inspection of the cosine function incorporated into the Doppler equation reveals that the accuracy is most significantly affected when the angle of insonation is more than 30 degrees away from parallel to flow (see Fig. 11.9).

Because of the phenomenon of angle dependency, Doppler signals are typically recorded from prespecified TTE windows (Fig. 11.11). However, it must be emphasized that these are starting points, and the signal must be optimized to yield the highest possible velocities that are exclusively toward or away from the transducer. Situations in which there are strong positive and negative flow signals, which is a display that can be created when the angle of insonation is 90 degrees, are to be avoided. While angle correction has been proposed as a means of correcting for suboptimal angles of insonation, its use has been discouraged, as it is limited to only planar rather than 3D correction. Instead, the sonographer should try to adjust the angle of insonation, listening to the pitch of the signal on the audio and looking for the highest velocity in the spectral display.

Color-flow Doppler (discussed later) may help guide spectral Doppler evaluation, particularly when CW is being used—for example, to capture the highest velocity of the tricuspid regurgitant jet. Color will direct placement of the Doppler cursor ± sample volume. Therefore color flow mapping and spectral Doppler interrogation are typically performed in a complementary fashion. In addition, the adjustment of various instrument settings is required for optimization of spectral Doppler velocity measurements, avoidance of erroneous (aliased) velocities, and artifacts (Box 11.1).

For PW, an important consideration is the need to capture modal, the most commonly occurring velocities in any scenario in which blood flow is being quantitated. For these applications, the gain of a PW spectrum should be turned down to the minimum that allows a complete spectral display. While adjusting the brightness and contrast of the display of already acquired spectra can compensate for suboptimally recorded signals, this is not the preferred approach.

OPTIMIZING THE COLOR FLOW DOPPLER EXAMINATION

Color flow is, in essence, a parametric display of pulsed Doppler signals; it displays color-coded blood flow velocities, by convention, mapped onto the B-mode (2D, M-mode, or 3D) image (Figs. 11.12 and 11.13). Typically flow away from the transducer is mapped in shades of blue, while flow toward the transducer is mapped in shades of red, i.e., blue away, red toward (BART). As with spectral PW Doppler, the maximum velocities that can be unambiguously displayed are defined by the Nyquist limit. The primary color assigned to a pixel is the mean velocity, but the variation around that mean can be captured by superimposing a color-coded (typically green) measure of variance (see Fig. 11.12; Box 11.2).

As with other forms of Doppler, color Doppler is angle-dependent. A consideration that is relatively unique to color flow is the frame rate. Frame rate can be optimized by minimizing the size of the color area of interest (color box), reducing the depth and narrowing the overall width of the imaging sector (see Box 11.2).

SUMMARY

Echocardiography is inherently an operator- and patient-dependent imaging modality. The measure of a good sonographer is being able to optimize the examination through a combination of patient and transducer positioning, with appropriate adjustment of machine settings as outlined in this chapter.

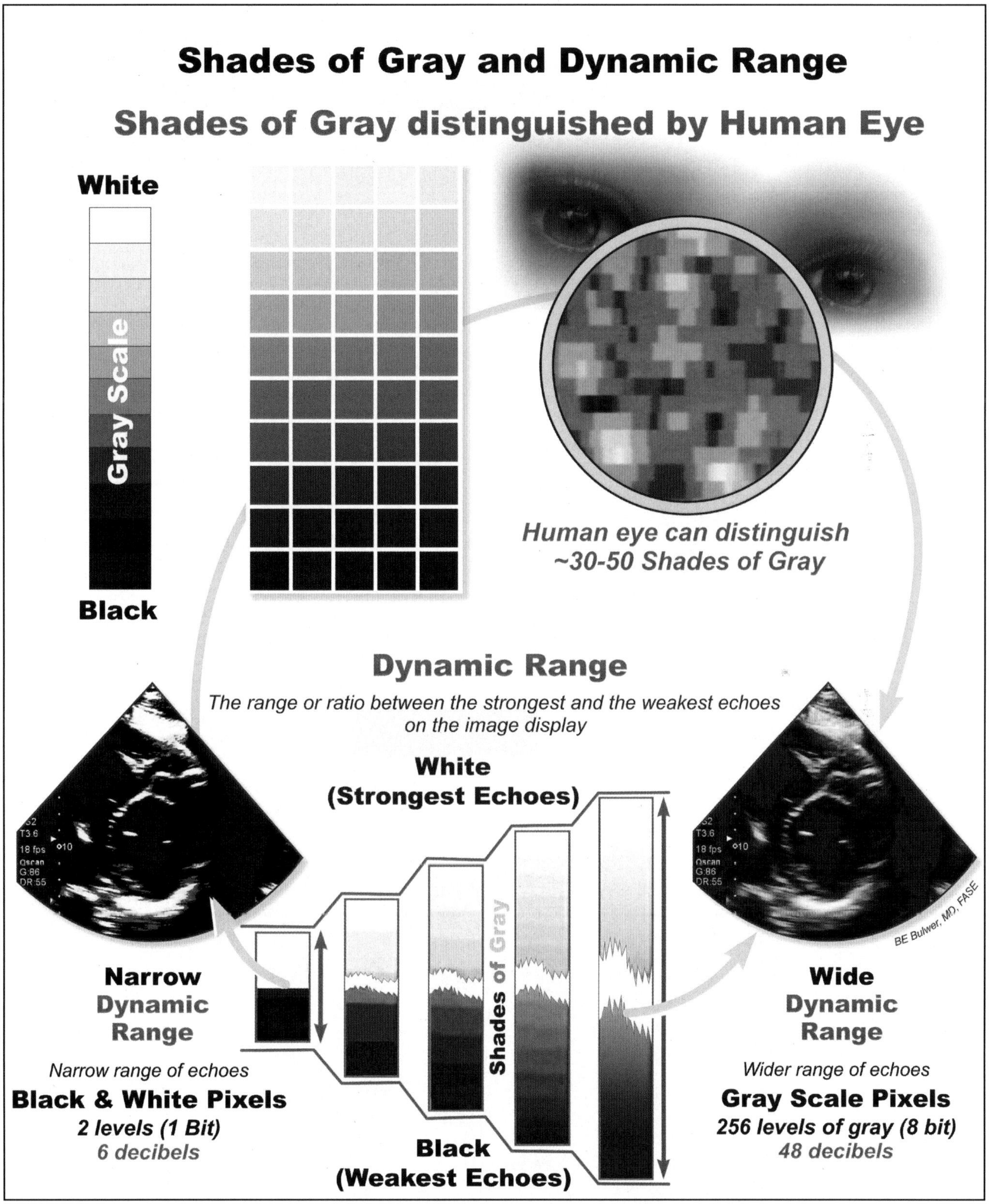

FIG. 11.6 Shades of gray and dynamic range. The ability of the normal human eye to distinguish shades of gray is influenced by overall brightness of the environs and the intensity of ambient and background lighting. Dynamic range adjustments are used to optimize the image by increasing (decompress) or decreasing (compress) the shades of gray. *(Courtesy of Bernard E. Bulwer, MD, FASE.)*

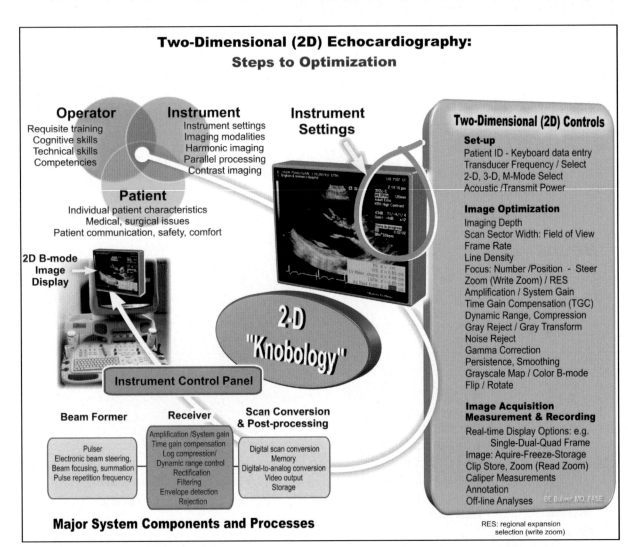

FIG. 11.7 Steps to optimization of the two-dimensional image. Note the annotated instrument knobs. *(Courtesy of Bernard E. Bulwer, MD, FASE.)*

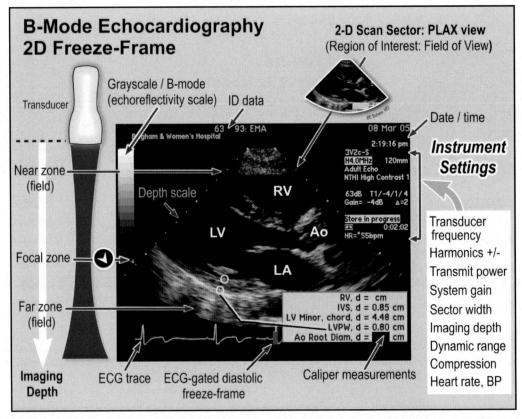

FIG. 11.8 B-mode freeze frame two-dimensional image display. Note the various elements of the display, as well as the instrument settings that require optimization during image acquisition. *(Courtesy of Bernard E. Bulwer, MD, FASE.)*

TABLE 11.3 Echocardiography Instrumentation

2D	Two-dimensional echocardiography; commonly referred to as "B-mode"
3D	Three-dimensional echocardiography
Acoustic power	Transmit power; acoustic energy output of the ultrasound beam per unit time (in watts [W]); control feature that adjusts the amount of energy delivered to the patient; use high-power default setting to optimize image quality (better signal-to-noise ratio); acoustic output indices: mechanical index (MI) and thermal index (TI) typically displayed on image frame.
Annotation keys	Function keys to enter labels or measurements on the B-mode image display
Archiving	Transferring echo images to storage media (e.g., CDs, DVDs, USB drives, online/network upload)
B-mode	Brightness modulation of amplitudes of the received echo signals using gray scale; display formats include M-mode, 2D, and 3D options
Calipers	Function tools for measurements, typically activated by pointing device
Cine loop/ Playback	For review of recently acquired images within system memory before applying freeze or save functions
Color B-mode	B-mode contrast-enhancing technique using various color options
Colorize	*See* color B-mode
Depth	Distance from the transducer; adjust as needed to visualize specified region of interest; depth scale visible on scan sector; frame rate decreased with greater imaging depth due to finite speed of ultrasound
Depth gain	Depth-gain compensation (DGC); *see* time-gain compensation (TGC)
Dynamic range/log compression	Range of echo intensities ranging from threshold (smallest) to saturation (largest) that can be displayed on the B-mode ultrasound image; increasing the dynamic range increases the number of gray shades. Decreasing the dynamic range decreases number of gray shades (image appears more black and white).
Edge enhancement	Selective enhancement of the gray scale pixel differences to improve tissue definition
Field of view	FOV; region of interest (ROI) or scan sector width; pie-shaped image with scan sector swivel or sweep angle ± 45° (typical range 15°–90°); *see* scan sector; sector width
Focus	Narrowest region of the ultrasound beam that exhibits the best spatial resolution; also called focal zone, focal spot, focal point
Focus, dynamic	Technique for adjusting the focus of an ultrasound beam
Focus number and position	For increasing the number of transmit focal zones or moving the position of the focal zone
Frame	Digital memory of cardiac ultrasound display (typical display is composed of 512 × 512 pixels). Still-frame or freeze-frame of B-mode display; display scan sector
Frame average	Temporal filter for averaging frames to display an aesthetically smoother image
Frame rate	The rate or frequency at which the ultrasound equipment can process and display image frames in real-time (frames/sec); ~30 frame/s processing power needed to display flicker-free images in real-time. To increase frame rate: narrow scan sector, decrease imaging depth, and decrease line density.
Freeze	Freeze-frame; still-frame of video image display
Frequency	*See* transducer frequency, pulse repetition frequency (PRF); multifrequency
Gain	System gain; used to amplify weak echoes and improve image contrast; avoid excessive gain (especially in the operating theatre setting)
Grayscale map	Scale displayed with B-mode (brightness-mode or grayscale) images that indicates echo strength or intensity; structures that produce echoes with the highest intensities appear white (echoreflective, "echobright"); structures that produce few no echoes appear black (echolucent or "echo free"); the human eye can discern 16–32 intermediate shades of gray out of a potentially displayable 256 shades of gray.
Harmonic imaging	A technique to improve image quality; improved signal-noise ratio, reduced side lobe artifacts, and improved lateral resolution compared with fundamental frequency imaging. Physical principles are discussed in Chapter 1.
Image Optimization	Includes: Presets, transducer frequency, imaging depth, focal points, gain/TGC, auto-optimize functions
Line density	Scan line density; adjust to optimize B-mode frame rates or spatial resolution; the number of scan lines within scan sector; frame rate and temporal resolution decreased with increased line density due to finite speed of ultrasound
Mechanical index	Acoustic output measure to describe the nonthermal and biosafety effects of ultrasound (e.g., cavitation, microbubble rupture); compares two parameters: peak rarefaction pressure and center frequency of the transmitted ultrasound
M-mode	Time-motion-mode (T-M-mode); one-dimensional echocardiography over time, with time on the *x*-axis and depth on the *y*-axis
Probe	Transducer housing, but loosely called the transducer
PRF (Pulse Repetition) Frequency	Pulse rate or PRF; the number or separate pulses that are sent out every second by the transducer; the pulse-echo operation requires that the transducer must await for the echoes ("round trip") before transmitting another imaging pulse if there is to be no range ambiguity; PRF typically ranges from 1000–5000 pulses/s (1–5 kHz); PRF and hence improved frame rates possible when imaging at shallow depths
Read zoom	A postprocessing function that allows simple image magnification of an operator-defined region of interest within a stored image (no change in image resolution compared with "write zoom")
Region of interest (ROI)	Anatomical area of interest within ultrasound imaging plane
Rejection	Selection of amplification and processing threshold; removal of unwanted "noise"
RES	Regional expansion selection (*see* write zoom)
Resolution	Imaging detail; the ability to display image detail without blurring; axial, lateral, slice-thickness, temporal, and contrast resolution
Scan plane	Anatomical scan plane within range of transducer beam

Continued

TABLE 11.3 Echocardiography Instrumentation—cont'd

Scan sector	Pie-shaped image frame of anatomical scan plane
Sector size	*See* Sector width; FOV; scan angle plus image depth
Sector width	Pie-shaped image with scan sector sweep angle ± 45°; a wide scan sector (with increased line density) results in lower frame rates and temporal resolution
Smoothing	Image smoothing or softening; a postprocessing function
Spatial compounding	Technique for improving image quality by combining or averaging ultrasound images acquired from multiple insonation angles into a single image
Suppression	Removal of unwanted low-level echoes or acoustic "noise"
Sweep speed	To change speed at which the timeline is swept
Time-Gain Compensation	TGC; compensates for beam attenuation (loss of acoustic energy with increasing imaging depth); depth-dependent amplification of echoes using sliding controls on display panel (apply based on appearance of image display); also called depth-gain compensation (DGC), time varied gain, or variable swept gain
Trace	Measurement tool for tracing selected region of interest (e.g., circumferences and cross-sectional areas)
Transducer	The probe housing the piezoelectric elements; phased array transducers permits a wide range of view despite confinement to a small transducer "foot print" (e.g., the intercostal spaces or the esophageal lumen)
Transducer frequency	A fundamental characteristic of the ultrasound beam (measured in megahertz, MHz); for transthoracic and transesophageal echocardiography, typical values range 2–5 MHz and 5–7.5 MHz, respectively; modern transducers are capable of multihertz operation.
Write zoom	A preprocessing function to allow image magnification of operator-defined region of interest within an active image; improved image resolution achieved by rescanning of selected region (with increase in line density and pixels compared to "read zoom"); RES: Regional expansion selection
Zoom	Read zoom, write zoom

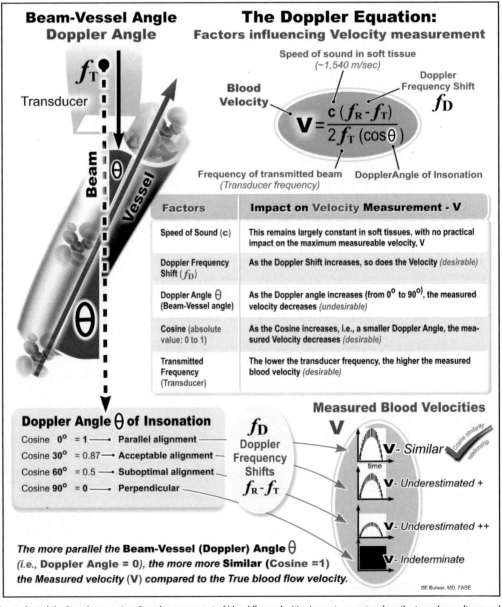

FIG. 11.9 The Doppler angle and the Doppler equation. Doppler assessment of blood flow velocities is most accurate when the transducer ultrasound beam is aligned parallel to the direction of blood flow (i.e., at a Doppler angle of zero degrees, 0°). The larger the Doppler angle (which means the less parallel the alignment), the greater is the underestimate of true velocity. *(Courtesy of Bernard E. Bulwer, MD, FASE.)*

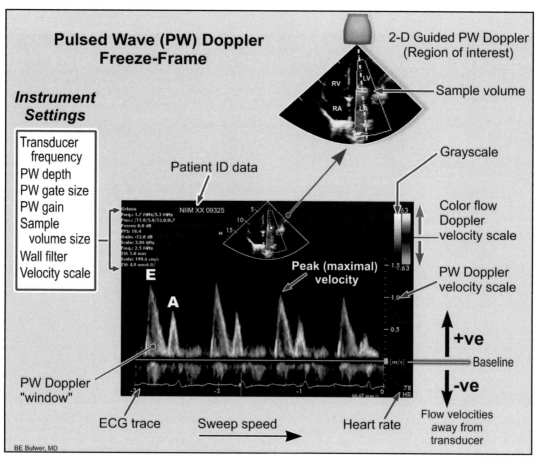

FIG. 11.10 Pulsed wave Doppler. The PW Doppler time-velocity spectral display shows a normal left ventricular filling or transmitral inflow pattern obtained from the apical four-chamber view. With PW Doppler imaging, optimal information is derived when close attention is paid to proper technique, including optimal transducer alignment (Doppler angle) as well as the appropriate instrument settings. *(Courtesy of Bernard E. Bulwer, MD, FASE.)*

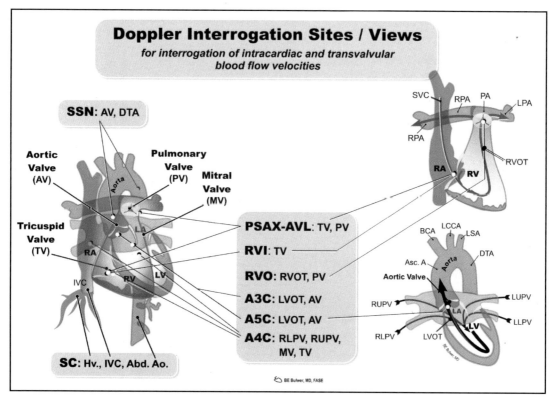

FIG. 11.11 Windows used for Doppler interrogation. Windows are chosen to maximize the alignment of the line of insonation with blood flow and to minimize the distance between the transducer and the region of interest. *A3C,* Apical 3 chamber; *A4C,* apical 4 chamber; *A5C,* apical 5 chamber; *Asc A,* ascending aorta; *AV,* aortic valve; *BCA,* brachio-cephalic artery; *DTA,* descending thoracic aorta; *IVC,* inferior vena cava; *LA,* left atrium; *LCCA,* left common carotid artery; *LLPV,* left lower pulmonary vein; *LPA,* left pulmonary artery; *LSA,* left subclavian artery; *LUPV,* left upper pulmonary vein; *LV,* left ventricle; *LVOT,* left ventricular outflow tract; *MV,* mitral valve; *PA,* main pulmonary artery; *PSA-AVL,* parasternal short axis at the level of the aortic valve; *PV,* pulmonic valve; *PVs,* pulmonary veins; *RA,* right atrium; *RLPV,* right lower pulmonary vein; *RPA,* right pulmonary artery; *RUPV,* right upper pulmonary vein; *RV,* right ventricle; *RVI,* right ventricular inflow tract view; *RVOT,* right ventricular outflow tract; *SC,* subcostal; *SSN,* suprasternal notch; *SVC,* superior vena cava; *TV,* tricuspid valve. *(Courtesy of Bernard E. Bulwer, MD, FASE.)*

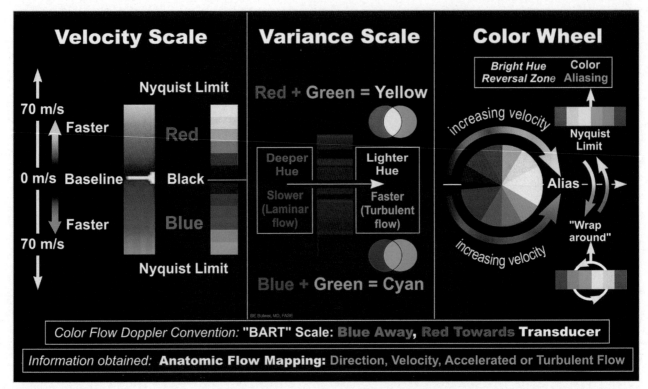

FIG. 11.12 Color Doppler concepts. The velocity scales are velocity reference maps that "translate" recorded colors into velocities. The standard display is the red-blue velocity "BART" scale shown on the left. The primary color assigned to a pixel is the mean velocity but the variation around that mean can be captured by superimposing a color-coded *(typically green)* measure of variance *(center panel)*. The right panel displays the concept of color aliasing *(wrap around)*. *(Courtesy of Bernard E. Bulwer, MD, FASE.)*

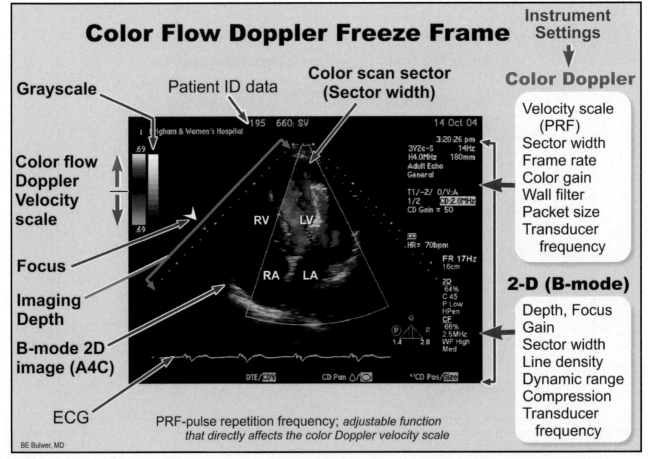

FIG. 11.13 Instrument control settings for color flow Doppler imaging. The annotations on the freeze frame pertain to important manual controls for *both* color flow Doppler and the two-dimensional B-mode image. *(Courtesy of Bernard E. Bulwer, MD, FASE.)*

BOX 11.1 Optimizing the Spectral Doppler (PW, CW) Examination

1. Optimize beam-vessel alignment: Minimize Doppler angle.
2. Use Color flow Doppler-guided placement of spectral Doppler cursor (PW/CW) ± Doppler sample volume (PW).
3. Avoid/correct aliasing: Adjust imaging window, baseline, and velocity scale settings to avoid aliasing on PW; switch to high PRF to increase aliasing velocity.
4. Adjust Doppler gain settings: Minimize noise and artifact.
5. Optimize wall filter settings: Minimize low frequencies (from vessel wall and valves) to optimize the appearance of spectral Doppler display.
6. Sample volume size—Gate length: Normally a sample volume of 2–5 mm is best for PW. Larger sample volumes diminish range specificity and broaden the Doppler spectrum.
7. Avoid or minimize Doppler artifacts—including aliasing, mirror imaging, shadowing, ghosting, cross-talk, beam width, and improper gain settings.

CW, Continuous-wave Doppler; *PRF,* pulsed-repetition frequency; *PW,* pulsed-wave Doppler.

BOX 11.2 Optimizing Color Flow Doppler Examination

1. Optimize the Doppler angle: parallel transducer beam-vessel alignment.
2. Increase the frame rate:
   a. Narrow the color scan sector width—this reduces the number or density of scan lines.
   b. Reduce the depth (distance) of color scan sector or region of interest—this increases the pulsed-repetition frequency (pulse repetition frequency).
3. Optimize color gain settings: Decrease gain to just above the point where image has black (color void) pixels.
4. Optimize color velocity scale setting. By convention, Nyquist limit should be 50–60 cm/s.
5. Avoid/minimize color Doppler artifacts: color aliasing, mirror image, improper color gain settings, shadowing, ghosting, beam width
6. Settings/variables with significant impact on color jet size in valvular heart disease assessment:
   a. Color gain
   b. Color velocity scale
   c. Transducer frequency

Suggested Reading

Hedrick, W. R., & Peterson, C. L. (1995). Image artifacts in real-time ultrasound. *Journal Diagnostics Medicine Sonog, 11,* 300–308.

Kisslo, J., Adams, D. B., & Belkin, R. N. (1988). *Doppler Color-Flow Imaging.* New York: Churchill Livingstone.

Lee, R. (1989). Physical principles of flow mapping in cardiology. In N. C. Nanda (Ed.), *Textbook of Color Doppler Echocardiography* (pp. 18–49). Philadelphia: Lea & Febiger.

Quiñones, M. A., Otto, C. M., Stoddard, M., et al. (2002). Doppler Quantification Task Force of the Nomenclature and Standards Committee of the American Society of Echocardiography. Recommendations for quantification of Doppler echocardiography: a report from the Doppler Quantification Task Force of the Nomenclature and Standards Committee of the American Society of Echocardiography. *Journal of the American Society of Echocardiography, 2,* 167–168.

Utilizing Contrast Echocardiography in Practice

Federico Moccetti, Jonathan R. Lindner

INTRODUCTION

Contrast echocardiography describes a set of specialized cardiovascular ultrasound techniques that rely on the administration of acoustically active contrast agents to complement standard imaging and Doppler echocardiography. Although there are many different types of acoustically active ultrasound contrast agents, those that are approved for clinical use are composed of gas-filled microbubbles encapsulated within a stabilizing exterior shell composed of surfactant materials, albumin, or biocompatible polymers (Fig. 12.1). The vast majority of microbubbles administered in humans are smaller than red blood cells, which allows their passage through the pulmonary circulation and distribution throughout the intravascular compartment after intravenous injection. For most forms of contrast ultrasound imaging, the signal from these agents is attributable largely to the linear and nonlinear oscillations of the microbubbles as they pass within the range of the acoustic imaging field. The type and magnitude of the ultrasound emission from microbubbles relates to acoustic variables (pressure, frequency, and pulse duration), microbubble size and concentration, and shell viscoelastic properties. The unique signature of microbubble oscillation is best detected by contrast-specific regimes, which have been described in Chapter 3, and is displayed as increased echogenicity or opacification.

In broad terms, contrast has been used in clinical practice either to better detect or characterize cardiovascular structures not well seen with noncontrast echocardiography, for example, endocardial-blood pool interfaces, or to detect physiologic or pathophysiologic features that cannot be evaluated with noncontrast echocardiography, for example, myocardial perfusion. Accordingly, the use of contrast during routine echocardiography has been advocated to improve diagnostic accuracy and confidence in specific patients or circumstances and to expand the role of echocardiography in applications where standard B-mode or Doppler echocardiography do not suffice.

In this chapter, we will discuss the clinical application of contrast ultrasound in a wide variety of circumstances where microbubble contrast agents have been proven to or theoretically can impact patient care. These applications will include the use of microbubbles for assessing (1) ventricular cavity size and function, (2) abnormal cardiovascular structures, (3) cardiovascular hemodynamics, and (4) tissue perfusion which

Shell	Gas	Size	Proprietary Name
Lipid/Surfactant	C_3F_8	1-3 μm	Definity
	C_4F_{10}	2 μm	Sonazoid
	SF_6	2-3 μm	Sonovue/Lumason
	Air	2-3 μm	Levovist
Albumin	C_3F_8	2-4 μm	Optison
Polymer (PLGA)	C_4F_{10}	2-3 μm	Imagify (AI-700)
Polymer/Albumin	Air	2-3 μm	Cardiosphere

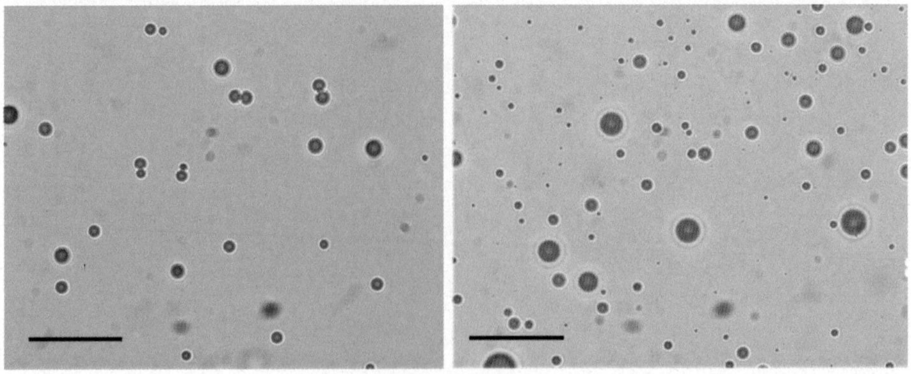

FIG. 12.1 Examples of ultrasound contrast agents that are or have been commercially produced for human use; not all agents have been approved by regulatory agencies for human use (Optison, Definity, and Lumason currently approved in the United States). The table provides data on microbubble composition and average mean diameter. The images illustrate examples of a relatively monodisperse *(left)* and a polydisperse *(right)* size distribution for two different microbubble agents, indicating that similar mean size does not necessarily indicate similar size distribution. *PLGA,* Poly-(D,L-lactide-co-glycolide).

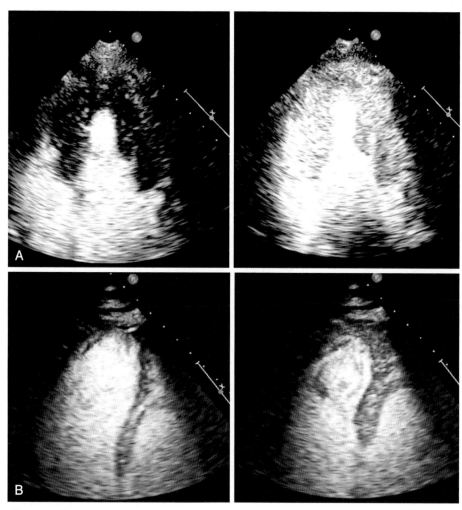

FIG. 12.2 **Examples of artifacts complicating interpretation of contrast echocardiography.** (A) End-systolic images in the apical four-chamber plane from a patient during dobutamine stress illustrating optimal contrast differential between the left ventricular cavity and myocardium *(left)* allowing easy identification of the endocardium and poor discrimination of the blood-myocardial interface *(right)* attributable to a combination of high microbubble concentration and hyperemic blood flow resulting in bright myocardial opacification. (B) Apical long-axis images from a patient obtained at end-diastole *(left)* and end-systole *(right)* illustrating rib shadowing of the mid to basal inferolateral segments.

relies on the detection of microbubbles as they transit the microcirculation (microvascular contrast echocardiography [MCE]).

LEFT VENTRICULAR OPACIFICATION

Endocardial Enhancement

Currently, the most common application of contrast echocardiography in clinical practice is to assess left ventricular (LV) function and regional wall motion when endocardial delineation is otherwise difficult. Despite advances in ultrasound imaging technology that have continuously improved image resolution and quality, the inability to adequately visualize the endocardial borders is still common. The intravenous administration of microbubbles in most subjects allows excellent discrimination between the LV blood pool and myocardium, thereby improving the ability to assess ventricular chamber dimensions and both global and regional systolic function (Videos 12.1 and 12.2).

Enhanced definition of the endocardial border is achieved by opacification of the LV cavity blood pool that provides contour recognition against the darker myocardium. Because only approximately 5%–10% of the mass of the myocardium is attributable to its microvascular blood volume (MBV)[1] the contrast signal in the myocardium is a small fraction of that within the LV cavity. An exception to this occurs when microbubble concentration is very high, well beyond saturation of the dynamic range for the blood pool, and the myocardial signal can approach that of the blood pool, making endocardial definition difficult (Fig. 12.2A). Very high concentration of microbubbles in the blood pool also causes

attenuation of the imaging beam, thereby producing shadowing of far field structures. Accordingly, left ventricular opacification (LVO) is generally performed with either small repetitive intravenous boluses of contrast or a continuous infusion of contrast at modest rates that result in full opacification of the blood pool without attenuation when imaged using low-power ultrasound to avoid microbubble destruction. Contemporary ultrasound imaging systems incorporate contrast-specific presets based on amplitude modulation or phase-inversion because of their ability to reliably produce high contrast signal and clear definition of the endocardial borders. However, the application of these algorithms can sometimes be disadvantageous when assessing regional wall motion during exercise or dobutamine stress due to the inherent reduction in frame rate with multipulse protocols, the production of "flash" artifact from tissue motion, and visualization of hyperemic myocardial perfusion at peak stress that can make differentiation of the border between myocardium and blood pool less clear. Although LVO is very effective at defining endocardial borders, it is important to recognize that, like all forms of imaging, the quality is affected by rib attenuation and beam-altering artifacts (see Fig. 12.2B, Video 12.3).

Assessing Left Ventricular Wall Motion and Systolic Function

Defining the LV endocardial borders is necessary for detecting the presence of wall motion abnormalities, assessing LV dimensions, and calculating left ventricular ejection fraction (LVEF). Endocardial definition is insufficient in up to 20%–30% of patients referred for stress

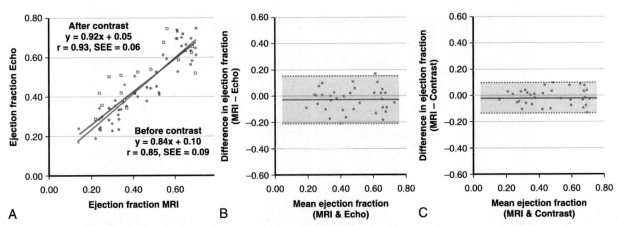

FIG. 12.3 Data illustrating better correlation of echocardiography with cardiac magnetic resonance imaging *(MRI)* for measuring left ventricular ejection fraction when left ventricular opacification (LVO) is performed with contrast in an unselected population. (A) Correlation between MRI and echocardiography ejection fraction *(squares = pre-contrast; diamonds = post-contrast)*, illustrating better correlation coefficient and smaller standard error for contrast LVO. Bland-Altman plots illustrate poorer agreement *(dashed lines)* for (B) noncontrast-enhanced echocardiography versus (C) contrast-enhanced. *(Adapted from Hundley WG, Kizilbash AM, Afridi I, Franco F, Peshock RM, Grayburn PA. Administration of an intravenous perfluorocarbon contrast agent improves echocardiographic determination of left ventricular volumes and ejection fraction: comparison with cine magnetic resonance imaging. J Am Coll Cardiol. 1998;32[5]:1426–1432.)*

echocardiography.[2] Poor echocardiographic windows are particularly a problem in subjects who are obese, suffer from chronic obstructive pulmonary disease, are on ventilators, or cannot be optimally positioned for imaging. LVO with contrast echocardiography provides an opportunity to improve endocardial border resolution. Studies using intravenously injected lipid or albumin encapsulated contrast agents have included both unselected patients and those with technically difficult conventional two-dimensional (2D) imaging.[3] These studies have unequivocally demonstrated that the use of contrast in both populations increases the number of interpretable studies, increases the number of interpretable LV segments with regard to evaluating wall motion, decreases interobserver variability, and increases reader confidence. The ability of contrast to transform an uninterpretable echocardiographic study into a diagnostic one appears to be particularly impactful in intensive care unit patients who have technically limited acoustic windows.[4,5] Interobserver variability for detecting regional wall motion abnormalities with contrast echocardiography has been shown in a multicenter study to be superior to that of cardiac magnetic resonance imaging (MRI), cine ventriculography, and noncontrast echocardiography.[6]

The range of clinical decisions that are based on a precise measurement of LV dimensions or LVEF continues to expand and evolve. Quantitative measurements are a component of patient selection for implantable defibrillators, cardiac resynchronization therapy, left-sided valve replacement/repair and for guiding optimal drug therapy with medications used for heart failure or cardiotoxic chemotherapeutic regimens. The gravity of the aforementioned decisions, both from the patient's perspective and based on the socioeconomic impact of the treatments, emphasizes the importance of reliable and reproducible measurements of LV volumes and LVEF. When using radionuclide or invasive left ventriculography or cardiac MRI as a gold standard, LVO with intravenous contrast administration has been shown to be more accurate and more precise than unenhanced images with regard to measuring LV volumes and LVEF even in a population not selected for difficult acoustic windows (Fig. 12.3). Contrast administration has been shown to consistently improve interobserver variability with regard to measurement of LV volumes or LVEF, particularly in patients with two or more adjacent poorly visualized segments,[4,6,7] and results in the lowest interobserver variability compared to cardiac MRI, noncontrast echocardiography,[4] and ventriculography.[4,9–16]

The cost effectiveness of using contrast echocardiography in selected patients has been examined in several studies. Although the cost of the contrast agent and additional time for preparing for and performing contrast echocardiography represent added costs, the added time may be minimized by imaging protocols that allow the decision to use contrast to be made early in the study, thereby eliminating the "struggle time" wasted when a sonographer tries unsuccessfully to improve unenhanced images. Another consideration in assessing the cost-effectiveness of contrast echocardiography is downstream costs of other diagnostic tests that

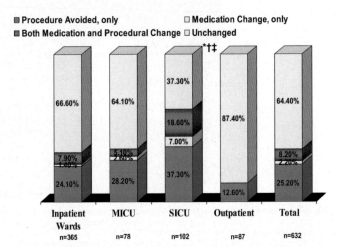

FIG. 12.4 Clinical impact of the use of contrast during echocardiography on patient management in a variety of inpatient and outpatient settings. The data do not reflect total impact since lack of any change in management does not necessarily indicate lack of impact. *MICU,* Medical intensive care unit; *SICU,* surgical intensive care unit. *P < .0001 versus inpatient ward; †P < .0001 versus outpatients; ‡P = .0004 versus MICU. *(From Kurt M, Shaikh KA, Peterson L, et al. Impact of contrast echocardiography on evaluation of ventricular function and clinical management in a large prospective cohort. J Am Coll Cardiol. 2009;53[9]:802–810.)*

must be used or inappropriate therapies that are used as a result of nondiagnostic echocardiograms. All studies performed to date examining cost-effectiveness have demonstrated that the reduction in downstream resource utilization makes the routine performance of contrast echocardiography in patients with technically limited windows an effective strategy.[5,13,17] Beyond just cost-savings, the ability to better understand regional and global LV function in inpatients and outpatients with technically difficult echocardiograms has been demonstrated to have an impact on management regarding changes in therapy or subsequent procedures performed (Fig. 12.4).[5] It should be recognized that in this type of analysis the lack of change in management does not necessarily indicate that the information did not impact patient care. It has been proposed that the superior information provided by contrast when image quality is otherwise limited is the reason for the finding of a significant one-third reduction in mortality in those receiving contrast in retrospective studies performed in critically ill patients undergoing echocardiogiography.[17]

Stress Echocardiography

Stress echocardiography has become a cornerstone in the noninvasive evaluation of patients with suspected coronary artery disease (CAD). When

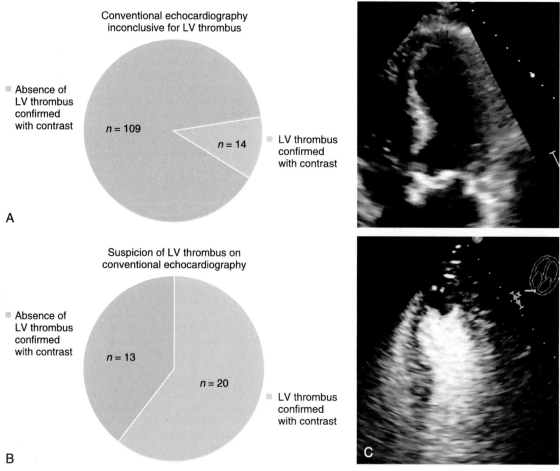

FIG. 12.5 Impact of contrast echocardiography for evaluation of thrombus. The pie charts represent data on reclassification of the diagnosis of left ventricular (LV) thrombus using contrast echocardiography for left ventricular opacification from 156 post-MI patients in whom noncontrast echocardiography was either (A) inconclusive or (B) suspicious but not diagnostic for thrombus. (C) End-systolic images from an apical four-chamber view illustrating the identification of an apical LV thrombus *(bottom panel)* that was not apparent on satisfactory quality noncontrast enhanced images *(top panel).* ([A and B] From Siebelink HM, Scholte AJ, Van de Veire NR, et al. *Value of contrast echocardiography for left ventricular thrombus detection postinfarction and impact on antithrombotic therapy.* Coron Artery Dis. 2009;20[7]:462–466.)

performed in appropriate pretest probability populations, the sensitivity of stress echocardiography for detecting obstructive epicardial disease is between 80% and 90%, while the specificity is just under 80%.[19] Conventionally, stress echocardiography relies on the detection of regional abnormalities and contractile reserve. Accordingly, optimal performance of stress echocardiography relies on the ability to see every segment, the ability to see every segment *well,* and a high level of reader confidence. Contrast echocardiography for LVO during stress has been shown to increase the number of interpretable segments, to increase subjective study quality, and to increase reader confidence.[10,21,22] LVO has a greater impact in those patients with technically difficult baseline images and when images are interpreted by less experienced readers.[7,22] The impact of LVO is particularly high in segments that most commonly suffer from poor endocardial discrimination, such as the basal lateral and basal inferior regions. The ability to ensure that the true LV apex is imaged and not foreshortened is also a valuable contribution of LVO. It has been advocated by some that contrast should be used in the majority of patients referred for stress echocardiography because of difficulties in being able to predict which patients who have adequate baseline images will have a deterioration in poststress image quality due to hyperventilation or excessive cardiac translation. However, this recommendation is tempered by the finding that the impact of using contrast is greatest in those with poor or marginal image quality at baseline.[22]

Left Ventricular Opacification for Masses and Miscellaneous Left Ventricular Abnormalities

Thrombus formation in the LV cavity can occur from several pathophysiological processes but most commonly occurs in the setting of ischemic LV dysfunction involving the anteroapical region. The presence of an LV thrombus on echocardiography is associated with a fivefold increased risk of an embolic complication after myocardial infarction (MI).[24–26] The ability to accurately detect thrombus not only impacts anticoagulation decisions but is also important for the evaluation of embolization risk in subjects being evaluated for percutaneous valve procedures that involve placement of large catheters in the LV or for placement of an apical inlet cannula for LV assist devices. The ability to detect thrombus by nonenhanced echocardiography depends largely on image quality. Moreover, the majority of LV thrombi occur at the apex that lies in the near field on apical views and is subject to artifacts from clutter, rib reverberation, power heterogeneity, and weak harmonic signal generation.[27,28] Accordingly, the prevalence of apical LV thrombus on nonenhanced echocardiography has varied widely,[29–32] and the sensitivity for detecting thrombus when using cine-MRI as a gold standard has been shown to be as low as 50%.[32] The diagnostic accuracy and interobserver variability for detecting LV thrombi with echocardiography has been shown to be markedly improved by LVO (Videos 12.4 and 12.5),[33–38] resulting in a level of accuracy similar to that achieved with cine-MRI.[39] The clinical impact of LVO for thrombus detection has been demonstrated in post-myocardial infarction patients who are at particularly high risk for thrombus formation. In patients whose noncontrast echocardiograms were either inconclusive or suspicious but not definitive for thrombus, LVO excluded thrombus and reversed recommendations for oral anticoagulation therapy in almost one-third of patients with suspected thrombus and detected thrombus in 11% of patients in whom noncontrast echo was inadequate for thrombus evaluation (Fig. 12.5).[40] An additional application of contrast in the post-MI setting is the delineation of incomplete myocardial rupture (pseudoaneurysm).

The role of contrast in establishing the diagnosis of hypertrophic cardiomyopathy is based on its ability to define endocardial borders permitting accurate measurement of regional myocardial thickness. The artifacts that are common in the near field pose problems in imaging the LV apex and lead to a missed diagnosis of hypertrophic cardiomyopathy in around 10% of patients with apical hypertrophic cardiomyopathy.[41] Both cardiac MRI and contrast-enhanced ultrasound have been shown to be extremely useful for diagnosing apical hypertrophic cardiomyopathy and differentiating it from apical foreshortening.[42–45] Moreover, a subset of patients with apical hypertrophic cardiomyopathy also present with localized apical aneurysms for which a variety of mechanisms have been proposed (Videos 12.6 and 12.7).[46] Accordingly, recent guidelines have advocated using contrast in the evaluation of suspected apical hypertrophic cardiomyopathy.[47]

Two other disease states that often have pathologic changes manifest at the LV apex are eosinophilic cardiomyopathy and LV noncompaction cardiomyopathy. Eosinophilic cardiomyopathy is often a progressive disease manifest by eosinophilic infiltration, myonecrosis, and finally fibrosis culminating in a restrictive cardiomyopathy. Superimposed thrombus is common.[48] Eosinophilic degranulation and myocyte necrosis both contribute to the loss of normal antithrombotic properties of the endocardium and release of prothrombotic substances. The ability of contrast to clearly visualize a filling defect involving the LV or right ventricular (RV) apex created by the inflammatory process and thrombosis facilitates the diagnosis of eosinophilic cardiomyopathy.[48] Moreover, the ability to perform myocardial perfusion imaging (see below) is often helpful for spatially delineating myocardium from thrombus, thereby differentiating this entity from a severe form of apical hypertrophic cardiomyopathy.

Left ventricular noncompaction cardiomyopathy (LVNC) has many different phenotypic manifestations and occurs secondary to the incomplete consolidation of the myocardial trabecular network that normally occurs by a gestational age of around 18 weeks. The result is a spongiform appearance to the myocardium that is usually regional, most often involving the apex and distal lateral walls. Mutations in several genes (*G4.5, ZASP,* α-dystrobrevin) have been implicated in this disease.[49] Several echocardiographic criteria for diagnosing LVNC and differentiating it from simply prominent LV trabeculation have been proposed.[50] Some of the major elements of these criteria are the systolic or diastolic ratio of noncompacted to compacted myocardium of 2:1, at least three major trabulecula, flow into trabecular recesses, and compacted myocardial thickness of less than 8 mm. The use of contrast has been shown to be helpful not only for delineating the presence of hypertrabeculation and intertrabecular flow but also for measuring the relative thickness of the compacted and noncompacted myocardial layers (Videos 12.8 and 12.9).[51,52]

CONTRAST ECHOCARDIOGRAPHY FOR DOPPLER SPECTRAL ENHANCEMENT

While an off-label use, enhancement of Doppler signals with echo contrast has been shown to be helpful in a number of scenarios, notably in providing better delineation of aortic stenotic and tricuspid regurgitant spectra, which, in turn, provide more definitive assessments of aortic stenosis and pulmonary artery pressure. The doses used for Doppler enhancement are typically low. See also Chapter 29.

SAFETY OF MICROBUBBLE CONTRAST AGENTS

A more complete review of the safety of microbubble contrast agents is presented in Chapter 2 of this text. Important safety-related issues that influence clinical use will be summarized here. A series of steps to evaluate microbubble safety have been taken as part of the process of regulatory approval for each of the contrast agents that are currently being marketed for use in contrast echocardiography. These studies include the evaluation of vital signs, hemodynamics, blood chemistries, blood counts, complement activation, and the rheologic behavior of contrast. The approval process has also required a demonstration that cavitation of these agents within approved ultrasound power guidelines does not produce any adverse bioeffects. Despite the demonstrated safety of these agents, in 2007, the United Sates Food and Drug Administration placed a "black box" warning on ultrasound contrast agents

based on adverse cardiovascular events that occurred in four critically ill patients (out of several million doses administered) and that were deemed to be possibly but not definitely related to contrast administration. This warning triggered several large registry studies demonstrating that severe cardiopulmonary reactions with lipid microbubbles are extremely rare, occurring at a rate of 0.01% of subjects receiving contrast agents.[53] Moreover, a propensity-matched study of hospitalized patients demonstrated that those receiving ultrasound contrast agents during echocardiography have a lower, not higher, mortality rate, possibly indicating improved care based on the information provided by the contrast-enhanced echocardiogram.[54] Studies examining the safety of ultrasound contrast agents in pulmonary hypertension and atrial shunts have also established the safety of microbubble contrast agents in these special populations in whom there was special concern with contrast administration as reflected in the US Food and Drug Administration (FDA)-mandated labeling.[55]

The serious reactions that are seen rarely with lipid-shelled microbubble agents are, similar to liposomal drugs, related to non-Ig E-related pseudoanaphylaxis from local complement activation (complement activation related pseudo-allergy [CARPA]). Because of this possibility, laboratories that administer contrast agents must be staffed by personnel with appropriate training in contrast use and treatment of hypersensitivity reactions. A somewhat more frequent, mostly nonserious reaction that has been reported with lipid-shelled microbubble agents is back or flank pain. Studies evaluating the mechanism of this reaction have pointed to nonobstructive retention of microbubbles within the renal glomeruli and subsequent production of mediators such as bradykinin that activate pain receptors.[56] These reactions generally resolve shortly after terminating the administration of the contrast agent.

Despite the demonstrated safety of ultrasound contrast agents, it should be noted that product inserts identify major contraindications to their use including previous hypersensitivity or reaction to the contrast agent or intracardiac right-to-left shunts. Other contraindications that vary between agents include pregnancy, lactation, pulmonary hypertension, and severe hepatic diseases.

General Recommendations for the Use of Contrast

The positive impact that contrast has been shown to have on both diagnostic accuracy and reader confidence in a wide variety of situations has led to societal recommendations regarding its use and the roles of the different healthcare providers in establishing policy regarding contrast use.[35] Although these documents provide strong evidence for the use of contrast in different clinical scenarios, specific recommendations for when to use contrast in an individual subject have been somewhat vague other than to recommend its use when there is inability to visualize a certain number of myocardial segments. The difficulty in providing firm recommendations stems from the wide variety of clinical questions that justify referral for echocardiography. Accordingly, it is reasonable to recommend the use of contrast based on two separate considerations that are depicted in Fig. 12.6: (1) will contrast have a major impact on answering the clinical question; and (2) what is the quality of noncontrast echocardiographic images? With this paradigm, the more liberal use of contrast is recommended for situations such as the exclusion of any wall motion abnormalities or the precise measurement of LV systolic function or size; whereas contrast is unlikely to aid in evaluating conditions such as mitral stenosis or the presence of a pericardial effusion.

The positive impact that contrast has on patient care has also resulted in specific recommendations for contrast policies as part of the process of accreditation of echocardiographic laboratories in countries such as the United States. Similarly, statements stating the need for training in the use of ultrasound contrast agents have been incorporated into the policies and guidelines for competency of trainees in adult cardiovascular medicine.[57]

MYOCARDIAL CONTRAST ECHOCARDIOGRAPHY

General Considerations

MCE refers to techniques where ultrasound contrast agents are used to assess microvascular perfusion or related parameters of physiologic

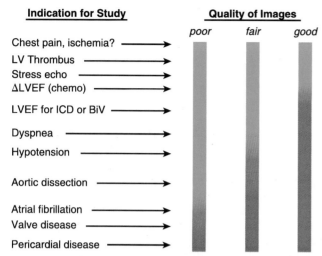

Indication for Study

FIG. 12.6 Considerations for determining the potential impact of contrast for left ventricular opacification during transthoracic echocardiography. The impact of contrast is influenced by both the indication for echocardiography and the quality of the noncontrast enhanced study. Green colors denote situations where contrast is likely to have an impact of diagnostic accuracy and/or confidence, whereas red colors denote situations where impact is low. *BiV*, Biventricular pacemaker; *ICD*, implantable cardioverter defibrillator; *LVEF*, left ventricular ejection fraction.

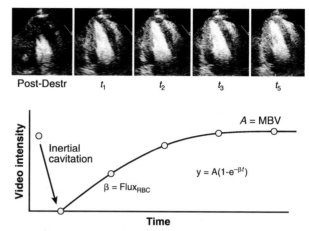

FIG. 12.7 Method for assessing myocardial perfusion with myocardial contrast echocardiography (MCE). The graph and end-systolic MCE images illustrate typical time-intensity data obtained after high-power ultrasound destruction of microbubbles with inertial cavitation within the imaging sector followed by low-power imaging of myocardial microvascular replenishment of microbubble signal. The time-intensity data are fit to a 1-exp function for calculation of the *A*-value reflecting microvascular blood volume (MBV) and the rate constant or *β*-value reflecting red blood cell (RBC) flux rate (Flux$_{RBC}$). *t*, Time.

importance. The ultrasound contrast agents that are conventionally used for LVO are pure intravascular tracers. Accordingly, the degree of signal enhancement in any tissue is proportional to the relative amount of functional (actively perfused) blood volume, providing that the contrast agent remains stable and is not destroyed through inertial cavitation. The actual relationship between the intensity of contrast enhancement within any tissue and microbubble intensity is also determined by the dynamic range and postprocessing algorithms of the imaging systems. When imaging the MBV within a tissue such as the myocardium, it is necessary that the concentration of microbubbles within the blood pool be well above the noise floor but still within the relatively linear or measurable portion of the microbubble concentration-contrast enhancement intensity relationship (below the dynamic range saturation point). When performing MCE, certain myocardial regions are particularly prone to attenuation artifact due to the intervening position of the RV or LV cavity, which generally possess a microbubble concentration that is 10–20-fold higher than that of myocardial tissue. The use of nontraditional echocacardiographic imaging planes can be helpful for overcoming this limitation.

Assessment of Myocardial Blood Volume

The blood volume of the coronary circulation in large mammals is approximately 12 mL of blood per 100 g of LV myocardium.[58] This blood volume is roughly evenly distributed in arteries, veins, and the microcirculation that is composed of capillaries and medium to small arterioles and venules. Anatomically, the bulk of the large-caliber arteries and veins reside on the epicardial surface. Approximately 80%–90% of the intramyocardial MBV is represented by the microcirculation, most of which is in the capillary compartment. Accordingly, myocardial signal enhancement during MCE represents primarily microbubbles within the microcirculation and is skewed toward the capillary compartment.

Quantification of Myocardial Blood Flow

Myocardial blood flow can be defined as the volume of blood transiting through tissue at a certain rate. The two parameters needed for this calculation can be determined with MCE. If one performs MCE without destroying or otherwise altering microbubble integrity, then signal enhancement at any given point in time represents relative MBV. The calculation of absolute MBV (mL/g) requires normalizing this intensity to that in the blood pool, most commonly the LV cavity, provided that the concentration of microbubbles in tissue and the LV cavity remains within the dynamic range of the concentration-intensity relationship.

For the measurement of myocardial microvascular blood flow, kinetic information is needed. This information is provided by first destroying microbubbles through inertial cavitation that is achieved by high-power, low-frequency ultrasound. The rate at which the signal reappears into the volume of myocardium in the imaging plane reflects microvascular flux rate of blood since microbubbles have microvascular behavior similar to that of erythrocytes.[59] Generally, this kinetic information can be achieved by one of two approaches. The first approach is to use a rapid series of high-power frames to destroy all microbubbles within the volume of the ultrasound sector. Low-power real-time imaging can then be used over the next 5 to 15 cardiac cycles to image microbubble reentry into the microcirculation (Fig. 12.7). End-systolic frames gated to the T-wave of the electrocardiogram (ECG) are ordinarily used for this analysis since the signal from large intramyocardial vessels is minimized by systolic contraction.[60] A second method for measuring flux rate is to perform image acquisition using only high-power ultrasound where microbubble signal from each frame is produced during inertial cavitation. Kinetic information is provided by progressively prolonging the interval between ultrasound frames to as long as 15 seconds between frames. This technique provides a high degree of contrast signal enhancement but requires more time than real-time low-power imaging and is technically more difficult to perform due to the need to maintain a constant imaging plane. The time (or pulsing interval) versus intensity relation can then be fit to a first-exponential function:

$$y = A\left(1 - e^{-\beta t}\right)$$

where y is intensity at time t, A is the plateau intensity representing MBV, and β is the rate constant of the curve which represents microvascular flux rate. The product of MBV and β represents myocardial blood flow and can be quantified in mL/min per gram tissue when MBV is normalized to the blood pool.[58,61,62] This approach to myocardial blood flow quantification is predicated on a constant concentration of microbubbles within the blood pool during imaging, which is best accomplished by a constant intravenous infusion of contrast.

Myocardial Viability

Large multicenter studies in subjects with ischemic LV dysfunction have raised questions regarding the utility of differentiating patients as either having or lacking myocardial viability in a binary fashion.[63] Yet information on myocardial viability in patients with recent MI or chronic CAD is still of interest to clinicians. The presence and extent of myocardial viability provides important information on prognosis and can help guide clinical decision making with regard to planning coronary revascularization on a territorial basis.[64–66]

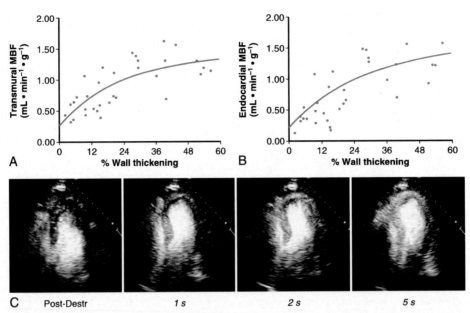

FIG. 12.8 Myocardial contrast echocardiography (MCE) for evaluating the effect of endocardial blood flow on resting left ventricular systolic function. The graphs were derived from a canine model of chronic ischemic cardiomyopathy and illustrate that radial wall thickening is reduced by a reduction in microsphere-derived transmural myocardial blood flow (MBF) (A) and that the strongest relation between wall thickening was with endocardial MBF (B). (C) MCE images obtained in the apical four-chamber plane from a patient with near akinesis of the distal anteroseptum and apex. The images taken at incremental times after the postdestructive frame illustrate hypoperfusion isolated primarily to the subendocardium. ([A and B] From Firoozan S, Wei K, Linka A, Skyba D, Goodman NC, Kaul S. A canine model of chronic ischemic cardiomyopathy: characterization of regional flow-function relations. Am J Physiol. 1999;276[2 pt 2]:H446–H455.)

MCE detects the presence and extent of viability by quantifying the spatial extent of an intact microcirculation. In general, the lower threshold of flow required to maintain myocyte viability is approximately 0.20–0.25 mL/min per gram (about 25% of the normal resting myocardial blood flow), below which myocellular necrosis occurs.[67,68] Flow must also be adequately spatially distributed at the capillary level, a factor that relies on the integrity of the distal portions of the coronary microcirculation. Accordingly, the presence of myocardial viability can be assessed by MCE imaging of MBV that reflects microvascular integrity. A simplified method for examining myocardial viability in this manner has used the absence of any enhancement after intravenous bolus injection of microbubbles to delineate nonviable tissue.[69–71] In patients with CAD and chronic LV dysfunction, the presence of *both* viability and ischemia, either at rest or during stress, is of key interest. This has led to the more common use of destruction-replenishment kinetics to simultaneously assess viability and hypoperfusion.[72,73] However, the approach of using MBV alone to reflect viability has been used as an effective approach in the setting of acute myocardial infarction to differentiate stunning from persistent hypoperfusion.[74,75]

Studies that have evaluated the performance of MCE in acute or chronic CAD have used several different definitions for viability. Defining myocardial viability by the recovery of resting function after revascularization has been used but is no longer thought to be appropriate, since wall thickening at rest is determined largely by the status of the endocardial layer, either endocardial viability or endocardial flow status (Fig. 12.8).[76–78] Even if recovery of function does not occur because of subendocardial or patchy scar, revascularization of viable mid-myocardial and epicardial segments can lead to preservation of contractile reserve during exercise, and is clinically beneficial for reducing symptoms of ischemia and heart failure, improving exercise capacity, and reducing the likelihood of remodeling and sudden cardiac death.[64,79–83]

In patients with chronic ischemic LV dysfunction, MCE has been demonstrated to provide information on the transmural distribution of viability that is similar to that provided by delayed enhancement on gadolinium-enhanced cardiac MRI.[84] Studies have also demonstrated that the spatial distribution and extent of myocardial viability as demonstrated with quantitative MCE correlate well with radionuclide single photon emission computed tomography (SPECT) techniques, and, in some studies, MCE has been reported to be superior to SPECT when using recovery of resting function as an outcome measure.[73,85–87] MCE has also been

shown to be at least as accurate as dobutamine stress echo for assessing myocardial viability.[75,88] Some studies have suggested greater sensitivity for resting MCE, which may be explained by the fact that the wall motion response during dobutamine stress is influenced not only by viability but also potentially by an ischemic response. Advantages of MCE imaging of microvascular integrity for the assessment of viability include low cost and ability to be performed at the bedside. However, acoustic attenuation from contrast in the LV cavity or from other anatomic structures can lead to signal loss and underestimation of viability in myocardial segments prone to these artifacts such as the basal segments on apical views.

Even with complete cessation of antegrade coronary flow, myocardial blood flow that is sufficient for maintaining viability can be provided by collateral perfusion in patients with either chronic CAD or acute myocardial infarction. MCE with destruction-replenishment imaging has been useful for detecting both the presence and adequacy of collateral flow. In this situation, the microvascular flux rate (β function or signal replenishment rate) provides information on the degree of microvascular perfusion that is provided by collaterals. The region that demonstrates any contrast enhancement, even if delayed, will reflect the spatial extent of the collateralized segment.[89] In the setting of acute ST-elevation MI, the presence of collateral flow has been demonstrated to predict a favorable return of resting LV function irrespective of the duration of coronary occlusion.[69] It should be mentioned, however, that the appearance of slow flow into the infarct segment can also represent reduced antegrade flow through the infarct-related artery.

In the early post-MI period, MCE can also provide early information on not only the success of reperfusion therapy but also the extent of myocardial salvage (post-infarct viability). The area lacking capillary perfusion predicts the extent of the definitive infarct zone and segments with poor microvascular perfusion after reperfusion will not have recovery of wall motion.[90–93] The presence of microvascular perfusion does not, however, guarantee recovery of contractile function in all patients, since infarction that is patchy or confined to the subendocardial region will often not have normokinesia.[69,72,91,92,94,95] Hence, segments with partial myocardial opacification on MCE but lacking recovery of wall motion following acute revascularization have been shown to have contractile reserve under low-dose dobutamine echocardiography.[69] It should be cautioned that because of hyperemia that occurs immediately after reperfusion of the infarct-related artery, MCE can underestimate the eventual infarct size when performed in the first several hours after epicardial artery recanalization.[94,96]

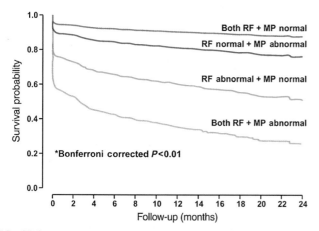

FIG. 12.9 Adjusted event-free (myocardial infarction, death and heart failure) survival in 1017 patients presenting to the emergency department with chest pain undergoing myocardial contrast echocardiography. Data are stratified according whether regional function *(RF)* and myocardial perfusion *(MP)* were normal or abnormal and comparisons made with Cox proportional hazards model. *(From Rinkevich D, Kaul S, Wang XQ, et al. Regional left ventricular perfusion and function in patients presenting to the emergency department with chest pain and no ST-segment elevation. Eur Heart J. 26[16]:1606-1611, 2005.)*

Myocardial Perfusion Imaging at Rest in Suspected or Known CAD

Because of its widespread availability and portability, including handheld echocardiographic imaging systems, resting 2D echocardiography is increasingly being used to rapidly evaluate patients who present to the emergency department with symptoms suspicious for angina. The use of echocardiography in this setting reflects the limitations of existing approaches (clinical history, ECG, cardiac enzymes) to either rapidly confirm or exclude myocardial ischemia. These limitations can lead to a delay in effective therapy or even inappropriate discharge of about 5% of patients with ongoing myocardial ischemia, resulting in high mortality risk.[97] Echocardiography can rapidly detect segmental wall motion abnormalities caused by either ongoing or recently resolved ischemia.[98,99] Aside from the detection of ischemic segmental LV dysfunction, echocardiography can identify other conditions that may be responsible for symptoms such as aortic, pericardial or valvular disease, or nonischemic cardiomyopathy.

When using regional wall motion on resting echocardiography to assess the patient with suspected ischemia, it is of great importance for the reader to visualize every myocardial segment well and to have a high level of confidence. Hence, as has already been noted, many recent studies have used ultrasound contrast agents to increase the accuracy for the detecting resting wall motion abnormalities.[100–102] The value of adding perfusion imaging when there is already a wall motion abnormality is based on the ability to identify the flow status as either (1) complete lack of perfusion, (2) hypoperfusion with some antegrade or collateral flow, or (3) stunning where perfusion has normalized but a wall motion abnormality persists (Videos 12.10–12.12). Perfusion imaging may also be helpful for discerning a pattern typical for conditions that may mimic acute coronary syndrome (ACS) such as stress cardiomyopathy[103] in which perfusion is normal despite a striking wall motion abnormality. For this reason, perfusion imaging with MCE has been shown to not only increase the predictive accuracy for the diagnosis of ischemia beyond clinical information, ECG, and early cardiac enzymes, but also to provide prognostic information on risk for short-term and long-term cardiac events (Fig. 12.9).[100,102,104,105] The high negative predictive value of normal wall motion and normal myocardial perfusion during or soon after symptom resolution has been suggested as a way for streamlining care and for cost-saving. It should be noted, however, that in patients who have had a history of prior cardiac events, the presence of a regional wall motion abnormality or perfusion defect may not have a high positive predictive value unless prior studies are available for comparison.[106] Likewise, the negative predictive value may suffer if there is a long delay between resolution of ischemic symptoms and imaging.

Even in those with recognized acute coronary syndromes, MCE perfusion imaging can provide information on the risk area (see Video 12.10).[107–109] The risk area is not necessarily equivalent to the perfusion territory of the infarct-related artery and is instead defined by the region destined to undergo necrosis unless recanalization is achieved. Although the clinical value of routine assessment of risk area has not been verified in clinical studies, risk area delineation has been shown to be of value in clinical trials testing the efficacy of therapies whose goal is microvascular salvage and reduction of infarct size.[110] MCE has also been used to assess the adequacy of revascularization in acute MI. Clinical surrogate markers for myocardial reperfusion include resolution of ST-segment elevation and angina, as well as ventricular arrhythmias such as accelerated idioventricular rhythm. These are poor surrogates for reperfusion and do not offer any quantitative or spatial information on myocardial salvage.[111] As mentioned previously in the section on myocardial viability, MCE is able to spatially and quantitatively assess the adequacy of microvascular reperfusion after revascularization. The importance of this issue is underscored by the knowledge that normal appearing flow on angiography in patients with acute MI does not necessarily indicate the absence of microvascular no reflow that occurs secondary to edema, microvascular obstruction with microthrombi, cellular debris, and inflammatory cells.[112–114]

Assessment of Myocardial Perfusion During Stress Testing

In experimental models of coronary artery stenosis, it has been shown that both the spatial extent and magnitude of change in MBV can be reliably assessed with MCE. In these studies, maximal hyperemia was achieved with vasodilator[115] or inotropic stress.[116] Imaging of MBV generally involves the simple visual assessment of contrast intensity either during bolus injection or continuous infusion of microbubbles without any destructive pulse sequence. Abnormalities in regional MBV during inotropic or vasodilator stress are thought to represent either lack of recruitment or active de-recruitment of microvascular units (depending on stenosis severity) produced by lower pre-capillary perfusion pressure during stress.[117] Similarly, clinical studies using bolus injection of microbubbles have demonstrated that abnormal MBV may be detectable both at rest and during vasodilator stress. With this approach, the spatial localization and physiologic relevance (fixed vs. reversible) of the perfusion defects are comparable to the information obtained with ^{99m}Tc-sestamibi single photon emission computed tomography.[86,87,118,119]

Low-power real-time perfusion imaging protocols without destructive pulse sequences detect defects that represent MBV rather than myocardial perfusion. Stress MCE assessment of myocardial perfusion by imaging MBV is limited by several factors. Most importantly, the relative reduction in MBV is not linearly related with the relative degree of reduction in myocardial blood flow.[117,120] Also, the measurement of MBV to detect hyperperfusion during hyperemia is subject to both attenuation in the far field and saturation of signal beyond the upper limit of the dynamic range.[61] The issue of saturation is especially relevant when administering microbubbles as bolus injections that often transiently produce very high blood pool concentrations.

Because of the limitations of using MBV alone to detect coronary stenoses, information in the temporal domain, namely the measurement of microvascular blood flux rate (β-value), has more commonly been used to detect the presence of stress-induced perfusion defects. Compared to MBV, changes in microvascular blood velocity have a closer correlation with changes in myocardial perfusion.[120] The stress-mediated increased microvascular flux rate during exercise, inotropic, or vasodilator stress is thought to represent reactivity of classic resistance arterioles.[117,120,121] In the presence of a coronary stenosis, both vasodilator reserve and pre-capillary microvascular pressure are reduced leading to slower capillary flux rate of RBCs.

The blood flow or simply microvascular flux rate (β-value) at rest and during stress can be quantified using first exponential functions and correlate well with microvascular blood flow measured by other methods such as radiolabeled microspheres, intracoronary flow wires, and positron emission tomography (Fig. 12.10).[62,122,123] A reduction in absolute β-reserve from rest to stress has been shown to provide high sensitivity for detecting significant coronary stenosis.[124] Quantitative MCE, and

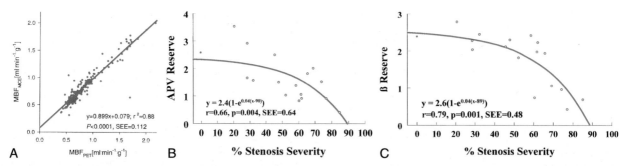

FIG. 12.10 Correlation of myocardial contrast echocardiography (MCE) perfusion imaging with other quantitative methods for assessing the severity of coronary artery disease. (A) Relation between positron emission tomography with ^{13}N-ammonia and MCE quantitative perfusion imaging of myocardial blood flow (MBF) in humans at rest and during hyperemic stress with adenosine. (B and C) Relationships between percent coronary stenosis by angiography and either coronary flow velocity reserve by intracoronary flow wire or β-reserve on MCE in patients referred for diagnostic coronary angiography undergoing vasodilator stress with intracoronary adenosine. ([A] From Vogel R, Indermühle A, Reinhardt J, et al. The quantification of absolute myocardial perfusion in humans by contrast echocardiography: algorithm and validation. J Am Coll Cardiol. 2005;45[5]:754–762. [B and C] From Wei K, Ragosta M, Camarano G, Coggins M, Moos S, Kaul S. Noninvasive quantification of coronary blood flow reserve in humans using myocardial contrast echocardiography. Circulation. 2001;103[21]:2560–2565.)

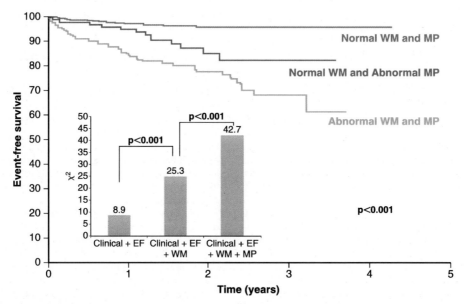

FIG. 12.11 Prognostic value of myocardial contrast echocardiography (MCE) during dobutamine stress is incremental to that of the wall motion response. The Kaplan-Meier survival curve demonstrates event-free survival (death, MI) in 788 patients undergoing dobutamine stress MCE for wall motion (WM) and myocardial perfusion (MP) and followed for a median of 20 months. The inset depicts the incremental values, expressed as χ^2 values in a model including clinical data, left ventricular ejection fraction, and dobutamine stress wall motion and MCE perfusion. (Adapted from Tsutsui JM, Elhendy A, Anderson JR, Xie F, McGrain AC, Porter TR. Prognostic value of dobutamine stress myocardial contrast perfusion echocardiography. Circulation. 2005;112[10]:1444–1450.)

in particular, β-reserve have also been shown to be highly sensitive for detecting the presence of multivessel CAD, which is a recognized weakness in other perfusion imaging techniques that rely on territorial heterogeneity in tracer uptake.[125]

A more common and practical approach has been to use a more simple semiquantitative visual analysis whereby normal resting perfusion is defined by a complete postdestructive signal replenishment time of four to five cardiac cycles at rest and one to two cycles during stress.[116,123,124,126,128] Clinical studies using a variety of stress approaches have shown that this approach produces at least comparable and often higher sensitivity and specificity for the detection of ischemia compared to radionuclide SPECT imaging.[128] A large multicenter trial enrolling over 600 subjects was an exception and demonstrated a much higher sensitivity of MCE versus SPECT for the detection of significant (>70%) and moderate (>50%) stenoses, but a lower specificity.[131] Higher sensitivity compared to SPECT may reflect both the ability of MCE to detect isolated subendocardial perfusion defects, which tend to be the earliest manifestation of obstructive CAD, and the fact that intensity on SPECT imaging with technetium-based agents largely reflects MBV.[128,132] Because of the quantitative or semiquantitative nature of MCE imaging, it has also been shown to be extremely sensitive for detecting the presence of multivessel CAD.[131–135]

Conventional stress echocardiography relies on the imaging of contractile reserve which is visually assessed by radial thickening. In general,

the evaluation of contractile reserve has performed well for the detection of significant CAD. However, the relationship between hyperemic blood flow during stress and radial thickening is not linear, and mild to moderate reductions in flow reserve may be manifest by very subtle abnormalities in wall motion.[136] Accordingly, the semiquantitative analysis of myocardial perfusion with MCE during stress has been shown to be superior to wall motion assessment with regards to sensitivity for the detection of stenosis (particularly for moderate rather than severe stenosis), and the detection of disease at a relatively lower work level.[133] It has also been shown to be superior to wall motion for determining the spatial extent of ischemia and for the detection of multivessel CAD.[131,135,138] Because the sensitivity of contractile reserve for the diagnosis of ischemia is particularly problematic in the presence of existing wall motion abnormalities at rest (such as from prior MI), perfusion may be particularly important in this setting. Because MCE directly evaluates myocardial microvascular perfusion, it is able to be used in stress imaging protocols that involve either exercise, inotropic agents such as dobutamine, or vasodilators.[119,139,140]

Because of its sensitivity and ability to accurately identify the true ischemic area, stress-rest MCE has been shown to provide valuable prognostic information, incremental to that provided by inotropic wall motion response, with regard to adverse clinical events (death, MI) as well as clinically indicated revascularization (Fig. 12.11).[141,142] Quantitative measurement of β-reserve on MCE has been shown to provide prognostic information that is superior to stress wall motion assessment for the prediction of death and acute coronary syndromes.[143]

Increasingly, it is being recognized that myocardial perfusion abnormalities can be the result of processes other than obstructive stenosis of the epicardial arteries. Functional abnormalities of the microcirculation or conditions that produce abnormalities in blood rheology at the capillary level can also produce abnormalities in microvascular perfusion during stress. Because of its ability to rapidly assess perfusion at the microvascular level, MCE has been used not only to detect the presence of microvascular dysfunction but also to assess the response to therapies.[70,110,111] Similarly, MCE performed in a population of asymptomatic patients with diabetes mellitus has been demonstrated to detect not only the presence of high risk obstructive CAD, but also the perfusion abnormalities from diffuse coronary narrowing or microvascular dysfunction.[144]

SUMMARY

Contrast echocardiography with commercially produced microbubble agents should be considered an essential component of a state-of-the-art echocardiography laboratory. It provides unique information for the interpreter that can be helpful in increasing the accuracy of diagnosis and for enhancing interpreter confidence. Clinical situations where the use of contrast for LVO is particularly useful include stress echo for the detection of CAD, quantitative measurement of LVEF, serial assessment of LV function, and the assessment for ventricular thrombi. Although not yet considered to be mainstream, MCE perfusion imaging has potential advantages for the bedside detection of myocardial viability or salvage and for enhancing the diagnosis of coronary artery disease or microvascular dysfunction.

Suggested Readings

Chahal, N. S., & Senior, R. (2010). Clinical applications of left ventricular opacification. *JACC Cardiovasc Imaging, 3*, 188–196.

Hoffmann, R., von Bardeleben, S., Kasprzak, J. D., et al. (2006). Analysis of regional left ventricular function by cineventriculography, cardiac magnetic resonance imaging, and unenhanced and contrast-enhanced echocardiography: a multicenter comparison of methods. *Journal of the American College of Cardiology, 47*, 121–128.

Kaufmann, B. A., Wei, K., & Lindner, J. R. (2007). Contrast echocardiography. *Current Problems in Cardiology, 32*, 51–96.

Mulvagh, S. L., Rakowski, H., Vannan, M. A., et al. (2008). American society of echocardiography consensus statement on the clinical applications of ultrasonic contrast agents in echocardiography. *Journal of the American Society of Echocardiography, 21*, 1179–1201.

Wei, K., Mulvagh, S. L., Carson, L., et al. (2008). The safety of deFinity and Optison for ultrasound image enhancement: a retrospective analysis of 78,383 administered contrast doses. *Journal of the American Society of Echocardiography, 21*, 1202–1206.

A complete reference list can be found online at ExpertConsult.com.

Echo On-Call: Echocardiographic Emergencies

Justina C. Wu

INTRODUCTION

Echocardiography can be used appropriately to diagnose and triage emergent situations. The life-threatening pathologies in which real-time assessment by echocardiography can be critical include pericardial tamponade, aortic dissection, acute myocardial infarction (MI), acute pulmonary embolus (PE), and cardiac trauma. These conditions may cause severe chest pain, dyspnea with hypoxia, hypotension, and ultimately cardiogenic and respiratory shock. Even in cases where the primary cause of a patient's deteriorating condition is unclear, such as isolated profound hypotension, the importance of echocardiography in rapidly assessing heart function and ruling out these critical abnormalities in an unstable patient cannot be understated.

This chapter is intended to be a guide to echocardiography in the acute scenario, that is, "echo on-call," or "STAT" requests. In these situations, the sonographer must quickly grasp (1) the clinical scenario, (2) the indication for the exam, that is, the specific question being asked, and (3) key pathologies that must be ruled in or out. If a specific pathology is found, the ensuing clinical management decisions may be beyond the scope of the specific sonographer and this text, but they are touched upon in the interests of facilitating rapid patient care.

CARDIOVASCULAR EMERGENCIES

Cardiogenic shock is heralded by profound hypotension and often respiratory failure. Specifically, systolic blood pressure falls below 80 mm Hg, with signs of end-organ insufficiency (cool extremities, altered mentation) and there is dyspnea, tachypnea, and hypoxia. This is a common and compelling scenario for emergency echocardiography.

From the broadest perspective, there are four very common acute life-threatening emergencies in which echocardiography may assist with diagnosis and/or triage: **MI** (and its related complications), **tamponade, aortic dissection,** and **PE**. Each has specific clinical settings, signs, and symptoms that would lead a clinician to suspect their occurrence in a given patient; although the sonographer may assess for echocardiographic signs of all in one exam, it is best to have an idea of the most likely suspected condition(s) to hasten the relevant imaging and patient care.

Acute MI and mechanical complications of MI are discussed fully in Chapters 18 and 19. For rapid reference, the most salient echocardiographic diagnoses are reproduced here in Table 13.1. To be clear, in a patient who clearly has acute symptoms of myocardial infarct and ST elevations on electrocardiogram (ECG), coronary angiography and urgent revascularization is the first-line treatment, and obtaining an echocardiogram to confirm wall motion abnormalities would only be an impediment to appropriate treatment. Once the patient is stabilized or revascularized, if acute decompensation occurs, the key findings to assess on echocardiography are detailed below.

Note that these mechanical complications tend to occur 5–14 days after the actual coronary artery occlusion. All represent varying degrees of tissue necrosis, of papillary muscle versus ventricular wall, due to hypoxia. They typically occur in patients who have had large infarcts, or delayed or unsuccessful revascularization. The mortality rate of all is high and depends on rapid identification, stabilization, and repair.

Acute Mitral Regurgitation (Flail Leaflet) (Fig. 13.1, Videos 13.1–13.3)

Mitral regurgitation (MR) may occur both acutely and chronically in patients with MI. When there is sudden hypotension and respiratory distress in the days after a large MI, one potential cause could be rupture of the papillary muscle trunk, tip, or chordae causing acute severe MR.

To assess for flail mitral valve:

1. Obtain a standard parasternal long-axis view showing the mitral valve. Ask:
   Do the mitral valve leaflet tips meet normally (i.e., touch each other just below the annulus)?
   Or does the tip of one prolapse or "flail" back into the left atrium in systole? (see Fig. 13.1 and Video 13.1)
2. Place a color Doppler sector over the mitral valve and left atrium. Ask:
   Is there a jet of MR (high velocity or turbulent speckled flow in systole)? In many cases, this will be directed eccentrically towards either the anterior or the posterior wall of the left atrium. Typically, a flail leaflet will direct the MR jet away, that is, in the opposite direction, from the damaged leaflet itself (refer to Fig. 19.2; see Videos 13.2 and 13.3).
3. Repeat two-dimensional (2D) imaging and color Doppler scans of the mitral valve in apical four-chamber and apical three-chamber windows. For technical reasons, it is not unusual for poor image quality to preclude an absolute determination of whether there is a flail leaflet or not, but an eccentric jet of brisk MR or a chordal structure oscillating in the left atrium proximal to the mitral valve (Videos 13.4 and 13.5) raises the strong possibility of ruptured mitral apparatus.

   The figures in this chapter show an example of posterior mitral leaflet flail. Examples of anterior mitral leaflet flail are shown in Chapter 19, Figs. 19.1 and 19.3, and Videos 19.1–19.5.

   Urgent management: Even the suspicion of flail mitral leaflet should generally trigger immediate cardiac surgical consultation. If needed, a transesophageal echocardiography (TEE) may be performed in the operating room (OR), or if the patient is in an intensive care unit with ventilator and pressor support providing enough stabilization, bedside TEE may be considered to confirm or refute the diagnosis. Pressors and an intraaortic balloon pump (IABP) may allow enough stabilization preoperatively to get the patient to the operating room.

TABLE 13.1 Echocardiographic Emergencies

	MECHANICAL	OTHER CAUSES
Complications of MI	Acute MR (ruptured papillary muscle)	Global LV failure
	VSD	RV failure/RV infarct
	Pseudoaneurysm	LVOT obstruction
	Free wall rupture	
	Hemopericardium and tamponade	
Tamponade	LV rupture or RV puncture	Pericarditis
	Postcardiac surgery	Malignant
	Aortic dissection	Renal
Aortic dissection	Traumatic (recent instrumentation, deceleration injury)	Spontaneous Aortic aneurysm
Pulmonary embolus		

LV, Left ventricle; *LVOT*, left ventricular outflow tract; *MI*, myocardial infarction; *MR*, mitral regurgitation; *RV*, right ventricle; *VSD*, ventricular septal defect.

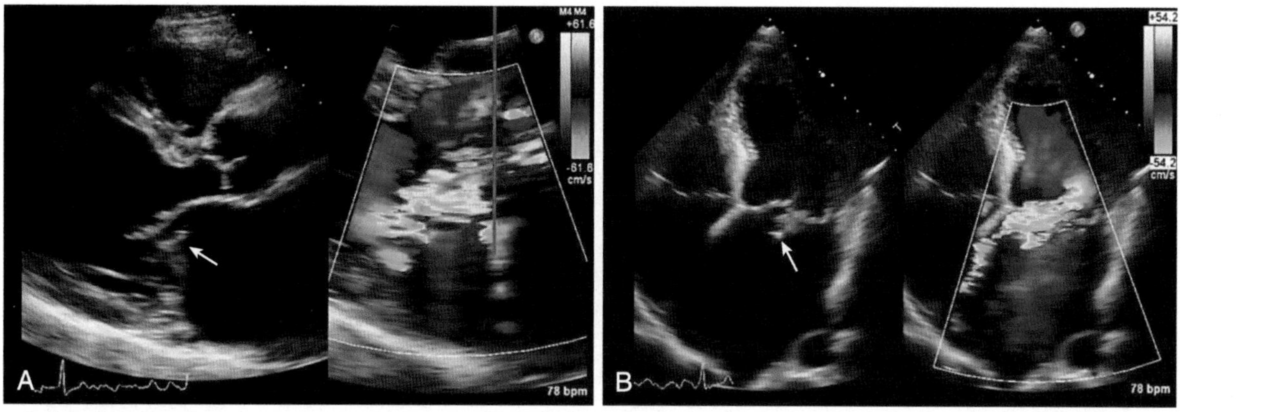

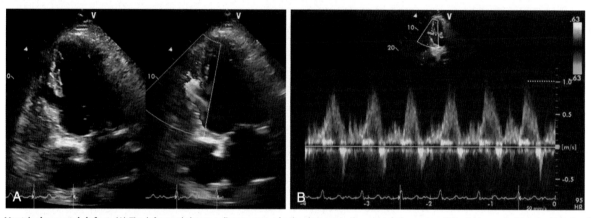

FIG. 13.1 Flail mitral leaflet. (A) Parasternal long-axis views of the mitral valve showing a flail posterior mitral valve leaflet *(arrow)* on the left, with corresponding color Doppler view of severe mitral regurgitation directed eccentrically in the opposite (anterior) direction. (B) Apical four-chamber views of the flail posterior mitral leaflet *(arrow)* and associated MR. See also Videos 13.1–13.3 .

FIG. 13.2 Ventricular septal defect. (A) The left panel shows a discrete area of echo dropout in the mid-inferior septum. The right panel with color Doppler demonstrates left-to-right flow through a large muscular VSD. (B) Flow velocities by PW Doppler are relatively low (<1.0 m/s), which is consistent with a large defect. The patient had suffered an IMI 2 weeks ago; at which time, cardiac angiography revealed totally occluded vein grafts to his right coronary artery.

Ventricular Septal Defect

Another cause of sudden hypotension and pulmonary edema in a patient in the peri- and post-MI period is rupture of the interventricular septum. This causes oxygenated blood to flow from the left to the right ventricle and mix with deoxygenated blood. Ventricular Septal Defects (VSDs) may occur in the anteroseptum (best seen in parasternal windows) due to anterior MIs or in the inferoseptum (best seen in apical four-chamber and subcostal windows) as a result of inferior MIs. Both types of VSDs may be screened for using parasternal short-axis windows. Using color Doppler is essential to detecting these ruptures, because the tissue discontinuity is often slit-like or serpentine and may not be readily visible on 2D imaging alone.

To assess for VSD:

1. Obtain a standard parasternal long-axis view showing the left ventricle (LV) and right ventricle (RV). Ask:

   Is the interventricular septum of normal thickness and contracting during systole?

2. Place a color Doppler window over the interventricular septum, particularly any akinetic sections or segments with echo drop-out.
   - Color flow from left to right penetrating through the septum indicates a VSD. (See Chapter 19, Fig. 19.4A and Video 19.6.)
   - Place a continuous wave (CW) Doppler cursor line through the color flow. If one measures the peak velocity of the CW Doppler flow envelope, the interventricular pressure gradient (ΔP) = 4 × peak gradient[2] (where peak gradient is expressed in m/s) (Fig. 13.2B; see also Fig. 13.3E, later).
   - The narrower the neck of the color flow and the higher the peak velocity of the flow, the smaller or more restrictive the VSD is.

3. Rotate the transducer clockwise 90 degrees and obtain parasternal short-axis windows of the LV and interventricular septum. Tilt the

transducer apically to sweep the imaging plane from base to apex. Look for akinetic areas or focal echo dropout. Turn the color Doppler sector to cover the interventricular septum, and similarly sweep from base to apex looking for color flow from left-to-right. (See Chapter 19, Fig. 19.4B and Video 19.7.)

4. In apical four-chamber view, examine the interventricular septum on 2D images, then position a color Doppler sector over the septum. Fig. 13.2 and Video 13.6 show an example of an inferoseptal VSD.

5. In subcostal four-chamber view, turn the color Doppler sector on and position it over the interventricular septum. Again, look for color flow through the septum from left to right.

   Urgent management: The treatment of choice is early surgical closure, which reduces mortality. Basal septal rupture is technically more difficult to repair fully, in part due to proximity to the mitral valve. In poor operative candidates, percutaneous closure may be considered (shown in Video 13.7).

Pseudoaneurysm

A pseudoaneurysm, or false aneurysm, is a locally contained rupture of all myocardial layers that is locally contained only by thrombus and pericardial adhesions. They typically have a narrow neck that allows blood flow to communicate freely with the left ventricular cavity and tend to grow and rupture.

To assess for pseudoaneurysm: The most common locations are the basal inferior or inferolateral (for inferior MIs) and apical segments (for anterior MIs). They can vary greatly in size from very small spaces to large fluid collections. (See Chapter 19, Fig. 19.5, and Video 19.8.) Thus look carefully with 2D imaging:

1. At the LV apex on apical four- and two-chamber windows, and

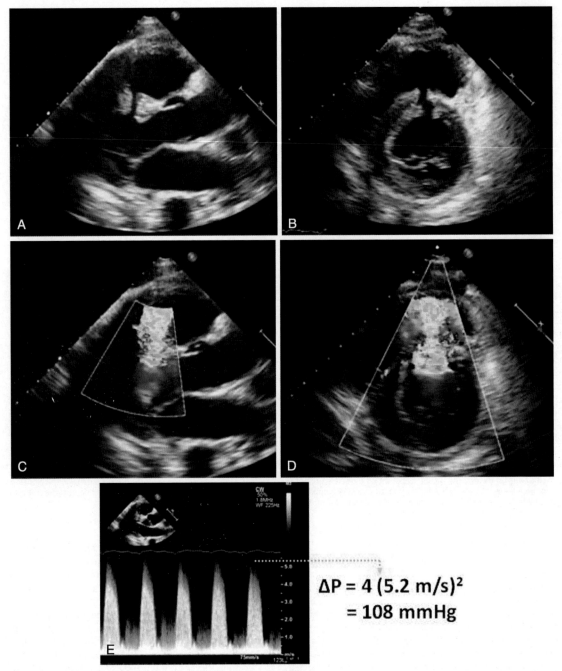

$$\Delta P = 4 \ (5.2 \ m/s)^2$$
$$= 108 \ mmHg$$

FIG. 13.3 Stab wound VSD. Transthoracic views on 2D (A and B) and color Doppler (C and D) of a VSD caused by knife attack in parasternal long-axis (A and C) and short-axis (B and D) views. E shows the calculation of interventricular pressure gradient by Bernoulli equation. The patient ultimately expired from RV rupture and VSD, despite attempts at emergent surgical repair.

2. At the basal inferior and inferolateral segments on parasternal and long-axis three- and two-chamber windows for any echo-free space.

3. If any echo-free or inhomogeneously echogenic space is seen, particularly if it appears to be bulging during systole, place a color Doppler sector over the area including the nearby ventricle and look for blood flow from the LV into the space (Video 13.8).

4. If the diagnosis is still uncertain and patient stable, the use of intravenous (IV) echocardiographic contrast can demonstrate flow into the pseudoaneurysm (see Chapter 19, Fig. 19.5B, and Video 19.9).

Urgent management: If echocardiography raises the possibility of pseudoaneurysm, but cannot confirm it or cannot distinguish it from aneurysm, cardiac MRI or LV angiography may be required for definite diagnosis. There is a 30%–45% risk of evolving to complete free wall rupture (below) and amortality rate up to 50%, so urgent surgery

to close or patches the rupture is considered the definitive therapy for pseudoaneurysms.

Free Wall Rupture

Complete rupture of the ventricular free wall is typically sudden and catastrophic, and rarely permits time for echocardiography. It may be suspected when acute cardiogenic shock follows a large unreperfused MI, especially if signs of tamponade or electromechanical dissociation are present. Fig. 19.6 and Video 19.11 show examples of a free wall rupture that rapidly evolved into complete rupture, tamponade with hemopericardium (see next section), and ultimately the demise of the patient. Immediate surgery is the only hope of surviving this with temporizing measures including fluids, inotropes, IABP, and/or peripheral ventricular assist devices utilized if needed to get the patient to surgery.

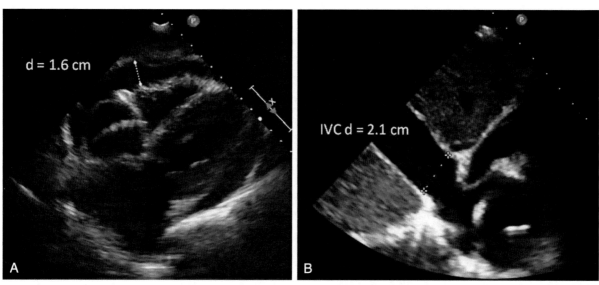

FIG. 13.4 Subcostal windows of (A) the heart four-chamber view, showing a pericardial effusion measuring 1.6 cm along the diaphragmatic *(inferior)* RV wall in diastole, and (B) the IVC that is high-normal in size at 2.1 cm. Full assessment would include monitoring over multiple cycles for normal (at least 50%) decrease in IVC diameter with inspiration.

Nonmechanical Causes of Cardiogenic Shock

If the above mechanical causes for cardiac shock, including tamponade, are not found on echocardiography, then one must consider other potential causes that may contribute, such as the following:

1. LV failure: This is illustrated by poor overall ejection fraction and may represent global hypokinesis, reinfarction, or infarct extension.
2. LV outflow tract obstruction: This is associated with a hyperdynamic base, upper septal hypertrophy and small LV outflow tract, and systolic anterior motion of the mitral valve. If these findings are noted, pulse wave (PW) and CW Doppler of the LV outflow tract should be performed, placing the sample volume at the area of highest velocity in the subaortic area (using the color Doppler window as a guide).
3. RV failure, which may be secondary to RV infarct (virtually always associated with inferior LV infarct and wall motion abnormalities) or PE (see later).

Tamponade

If fluid accumulates in the pericardium at high-enough pressure to impede cardiac filling, the clinical syndrome of hypotension and dyspnea due to decreased cardiac output known as tamponade will result. In the setting of a recent MI, tamponade may occur abruptly from free wall rupture as discussed above. In patients who have had recent coronary angiography and angioplasty, however, one should also consider an iatrogenic complication such as coronary artery dissection. Aortic dissection, either due to recent angiography or other causes (spontaneous, or trauma-induced), is another important cause of tamponade and sanguineous pericardial effusions. Also, patients who have just undergone pacemaker or automated implantable cardiac defibrillator (AICD) placement or RV biopsy are at risk for hemorrhaging into the pericardium. Oncology patients, particularly those with breast, lung, and hematologic malignancies as well as mesothelioma or melanoma, may present acutely or subacutely with a new hemodynamically significant pericardial effusion. Lastly, patients with severe renal failure may also develop significant pericardial effusions, although these do not accumulate rapidly.

Echocardiography is the foremost tool in evaluating for tamponade.[1] The sonographer must rapidly identify the size and distribution of the pericardial effusion, and its hemodynamic impact. Hemodynamically significant effusions will often (1) cause collapse of chambers of the heart, typically the right atrium and ventricle first, and (2) cause respirophasic flow variation in the atrioventricular valves (as well as the corresponding outflow tracts of the left and right heart) in opposing directions, as measured by peak flow velocities.

A quick but comprehensive overall protocol for assessing pericardial effusions is as follows:

1. Place ECG leads (and if time permits, a respirometer; alternatively, use the ECG baseline dial to manually indicate inspiration and expiration).
2. On supine patients, obtain a quick subcostal view to look for any pericardial fluid (Fig. 13.4). Since fluid tends to flow dependently, it often accumulates above the liver and anterior/inferior to the right heart. Fortuitously, this is also the position where a pericardiocentesis needle is targeted towards for drainage.
   - If fluid is present, begin a full evaluation from this window.
   - Note location and overall dimensions. In particular, it is useful to note the largest linear dimension (in centimeter), as well as the measurement anterior/inferior to the right heart, for planning future pericardiocentesis or other surgical therapies.
   - Two-dimensional images of four-chamber view (still subcostal) should be obtained, looking for indentation or collapse of the right atrium and/or RV (as well as left-sided chambers) (Video 13.9).
   - Show the inferior vena cava (IVC) over multiple beats (Fig. 13.4B): assess for size (>2.1 cm is dilated) and respirophasic size variation (normally the diameter reduces by 50% with inspiration). This will give a rough approximation of right atrial (RA) filling pressure. A dilated IVC that remains plethoric even in inspiration is a sign of markedly elevated central venous pressure that accompanies tamponade greater than 90% of the time.

If the patient is stable, one may then move to a standard sequence of echo views (parasternal and apical windows) as follows:

3. In the standard parasternal long-axis window, ensure there is enough depth (at least 18–20 cm) to detect both a pericardial and pleural effusion, since these collections are frequently mistaken for each other. A key landmark is the *descending thoracic aorta* that may be seen in a cross-section on the parasternal and occasionally on the apical four- and three-chamber windows section (Fig. 13.5; also refer to Fig. 33.2). *Pericardial effusions will stay close to the heart borders and insinuate between the aorta and the heart, respecting the pericardial reflections.*
4. In the windows above as well as apical four-chamber windows, assess for collapse of the right heart chambers (Fig. 13.6, see Videos 13.9–13.11). The right atrium, being at relatively low pressure particularly at end diastole, is often the first chamber to indent (see Video 13.9). This should be distinguished from normal RA contraction during atrial systole, however. The RV, particularly the anterior wall and RV outflow tract, is often sensitive to elevated intrapericardial pressure as well, particularly in early diastole when RV volume is low, as demonstrated on parasternal long-axis windows (see Video 13.11). M-mode may be used to illustrate the timing of collapse during diastole in any window (see Fig. 13.6B). The RV will collapse during the T wave on

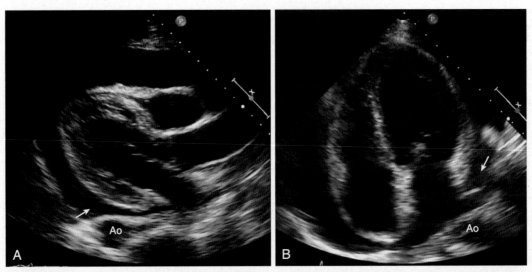

FIG. 13.5 Parasternal long-axis (A) and apical four-chamber (B) views of moderate-to-large pericardial effusions *(arrows)*. Note that effusions are anechoic spaces that closely hug the contours of the heart, interposing between the aorta and the lateral borders of the heart as the pericardial reflections. *Ao,* Descending thoracic aorta, a key landmark.

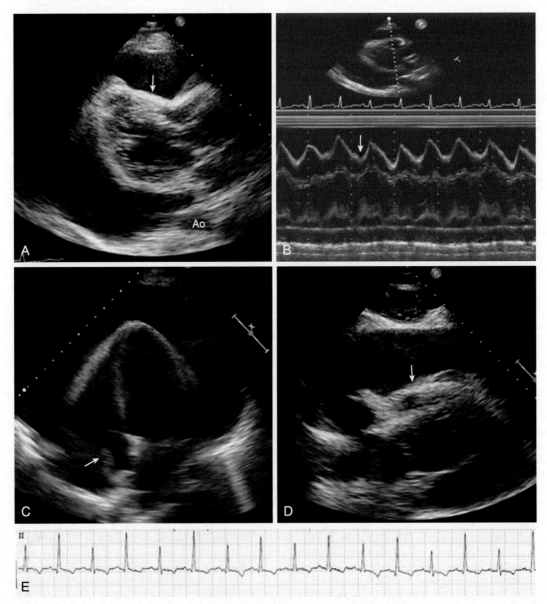

FIG. 13.6 **Tamponade with right heart chamber collapse.** (A) Anterior RV/RVOT collapse in diastole. *AO,* Aorta. (B) M-mode across the RVOT, illustrating the early diastolic inversion of the RVOT due to the large pericardial effusion. (C) Right atrial inversion. (D) RV collapse due to a large pericardial effusion with fibrin deposition along the inferior (diaphragmatic) wall of the RV. (E) Electrical alternans on ECG, which can often be seen on the echocardiogram ECG with large pericardial effusions as well. See also the corresponding Videos 13.9–13.11.

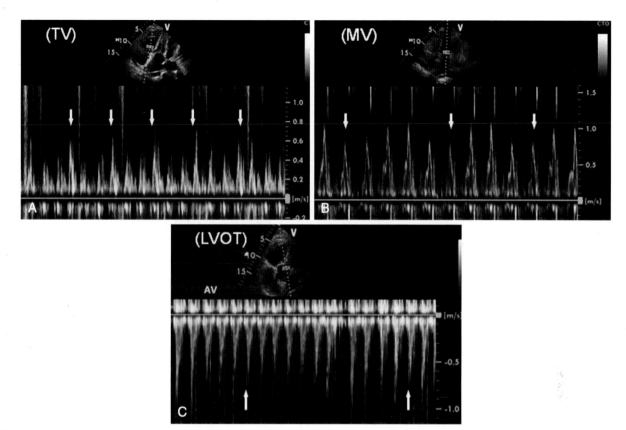

FIG. 13.7 Respirophasic variation in valvular inflow and outflow during tamponade. Right-sided, that is, tricuspid valve inflow (A) and pulmonic outflow flow velocities will increase with inspiration. Left-sided, that is, mitral valve (B) and LV outflow (C) flow velocities will decrease with inspiration. The variation in LVOT velocities is the echocardiographic sign of the clinical sign known as pulsus paradoxus (a >10 mm Hg drop in systolic blood pressures with inspiration). *Arrows* = inspiration.

the ECG or as the aortic leaflets are closed on M-mode. The RA will collapse during ventricular systole (atrial diastole).

5. Respirophasic flow illustrating interventricular dependence (Fig. 13.7).

A tense pericardial sac will limit the total volume of blood that the heart can accommodate. During inspiration, venous return to the right heart increases and causes an increase in flow (and hence peak flow velocities) in tricuspid valve inflow and right ventricular outflow tract (RVOT) outflow. The filling of the right heart forces the interventricular septum to shift leftwards, decreasing left heart filling. Thus, contrary to the right-sided patterns, mitral valve inflow and left ventricular outflow tract (LVOT) velocities decrease during inspiration. This is an exaggeration of the same slight respirophasic variation that exists in normal conditions. There is variation in the criteria adopted, but greater than 50% variation in tricuspid inflow velocities and greater than 25% variation in mitral inflow velocities is a common diagnostic standard considered to be indicative of a hemodynamically significant effusion. The drop in LVOT velocities with inspiration (see Fig. 13.7C) is the direct echocardiographic equivalent of the pulsus paradoxus (a >10 mm Hg drop in systolic blood pressure during inspiration). Respirophasic flow across the valves and outflow tracts alone should not be used to diagnose tamponade, but in the presence of chamber collapse and IVC plethora, the specificity for clinical tamponade is very high.

Caveats: The sensitivity and specificity of right-sided chamber collapse for clinical tamponade is relatively high in most clinical settings. In particular, RA inversion of at least 1/3 of the total cardiac cycle has proven to be very specific for clinically apparent tamponade. In theory, if there is significant pulmonary hypertension or RV dysfunction, the elevated intracavitary pressures may prevent RA and RV inversion from occurring despite elevated intrapericardial pressures (i.e., false-negative echocardiographic findings). Respirophasic variation in valvular flow, however, is not very specific and may be seen in patients with large swings in intrathoracic pressure for any reason (e.g., intubation, acute respiratory distress) similar to a pulsus paradoxus. Tamponade is emphatically a *clinical* diagnosis, and a patient may in fact be adequately compensated, without symptoms, despite echocardiographic signs of elevated intrapericardial pressures (i.e., not reaching a threshold for causing clinical tamponade). This can occur if the effusion has accumulated slowly over a long period of time.

Hemopericardium refers to frank blood or formed thrombus (pericardial hematoma) in the pericardium, and should immediately raise suspicion for LV rupture or aortic dissection. Examples are shown in Videos 13.12 and 19.12. Pericardial effusions may be localized, impinging on isolated areas of the heart. Although left atrial and even left ventricular regional collapse is rare, there are instances in which regional cardiac tamponade can occur (Videos 13.13 and 13.14). Typically, this occurs after cardiac surgery, pericardiotomy, or MI but can also present due to thoracic malignancies. Pericardial effusions may also be loculated with extensive fibrin stranding, which can cause effusive-constrictive physiology (i.e., persistent of interventricular interdependence even after fluid removal). Theoretically, thick fibrin strands extending from visceral to parietal pericardium might actually prevent the appearance of chamber collapse as well, again causing a false-negative interpretation of the echocardiogram.

Occasionally transthoracic echocardiography cannot reliably distinguish a pericardial from a pleural effusion, particularly if image quality or windows are very limited. In such cases, chest x-ray data can be very useful, demonstrating either cardiomegaly (usually present when there is at least 200 mL of pericardial fluid) or a left pleural effusion. Finally, if there is a pericardial effusion with discrepant or borderline echocardiographic indications of tamponade, it is reasonable to perform follow up echocardiograms to assess for evolution of the effusion and its clinical impact over time. Patients who are significantly hypovolemic, due to overdiuresis, volume removal through hemodialysis, dehydration, or hemorrhage, will be more prone to tamponade physiology even at relatively low pericardial volumes and pressures. An IV fluid bolus may be utilized to stabilize those patients who have only mildly elevated intrapericardial pressures without frank tamponade, but if signs of chamber collapse and respiratory variation in transvalvular flows remain and clinical symptoms develop, then true "low-pressure" tamponade is present.

Urgent management: Immediate management in general for tamponade often requires pericardiocentesis (generally the most rapid), which can only safely reach circumferential, anterior, and inferior effusions of at least 1 cm. Of note, pericardiocentesis is contraindicated if the effusion is due to myocardial rupture or aortic dissection, since theoretically decompression may extend the rupture or dissection.[2]

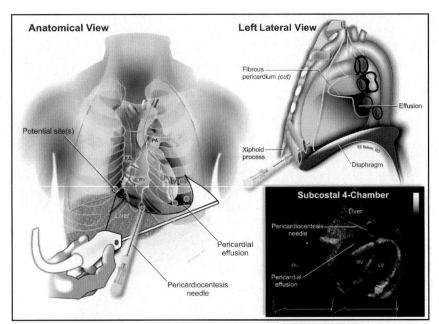

FIG. 13.8 Echo-guided pericardiocentesis. The subxiphoid approach to pericardiocentesis may be guided by echocardiography using a needle inserted next to the probe in the same plane. The *green circles* indicate several potential entry points to tap an effusion, but subxiphoid approach is commonly used, as it avoids coronary and thoracic arteries. The subcostal echocardiographic window is shown in the inset with the needle seen entering the pericardium. A small amount of agitated saline may be injected to document that the needle tip is in the pericardial sac. *(Courtesy of Bernard E. Bulwer, MD, FASE.)*

IV fluids are recommended in the interim to elevate intracavitary pressures beyond pericardial pressures. Effusions that are regionalized behind or lateral to the heart must be addressed by surgical drainage. Surgical washout of the pericardium may also be required for effusions that are highly fibrinous or loculated. For recurrent effusions, a pericardial window (surgical or percutaneous) may be considered.

Pericardiocentesis: Echocardiography can identify the optimal site of puncture for pericardiocentesis by identifying the largest fluid collection, measuring the distance from the chest wall to the effusion, and confirming needle placement within the pericardial sac. Although both anterior (parasternal) and subxiphoid approaches are possible for tapping the effusion, the subxiphoid approach is more commonly used, as there is less likelihood of lacerating a coronary artery (Fig. 13.8). Echocardiography may be done continuously during the procedure (using a sterile sheath for the transducer if done in a procedure room): the transducer is used in parasternal or subcostal windows to obtain an optimal view of the effusion, and the needle is introduced right next to the transducer. However, in practice, it can be technically difficult to maintain visualization of the needle tip in the same plane, and concurrent imaging is not usually necessary. An alternative approach is to obtain needle access, and then inject a small amount of agitated saline under ultrasound guidance to confirm that the tip is in the pericardial effusion. A pigtail catheter may then be inserted for continuous drainage and is generally retained until drainage has diminished to less than 25 mL in 24 hours. Repeat echocardiography should be performed to confirm no significant reaccumulation of the effusion.

Aortic Dissection

The possibility of aortic dissection is usually raised when a patient presents with acute severe chest pain that is sharp or radiates to the back or scapula. Accompanying syncope, a pulse deficit, neurologic deficits, or shock and tamponade are highly suggestive of this entity.[3] The dissection is initiated by a tear in the aortic intima, which allows a pressurized hematoma to accumulate within the aortic media.

On echocardiography, aortic dissection is identified by the finding of an intimal flap within the aorta. This will appear as a free undulating linear membrane that separates the aorta into a true and a false lumen (Fig. 13.9A; see also Fig. 34.15 and Videos 34.3 and 34.4). Dissections often occur within aneurysmal segments of the aorta (in spontaneous dissections) or at the aortic isthmus (in deceleration chest trauma). If the proximal root is involved, the dissection may extend proximally to the aortic valve, resulting in aortic regurgitation (see Fig. 13.9B and Videos 13.15 and 13.16) or even into a coronary artery causing a myocardial infarct. Separation of the tunica intima and the media can then propagate in linear, circumferential, or spiral patterns up and down the aorta. Pericardial effusions, most alarmingly hemopericardium, may be caused by aortic dissection within the pericardial sac as well.

Although limited segments of the aorta, the aortic root and valve, proximal and distal portions of the ascending aorta, the transverse arch, and skip portions of the descending thoracic and abdominal aorta, can be visualized on echocardiography (see Fig. 34.5), it remains a useful first tool in emergencies particularly for ruling out type A (ascending aorta) or arch dissections. To be thorough, the sonographer should also slide upwards or move up an interspace from the standard parasternal windows to try to visualize as much of the ascending aorta as possible. If a dissection flap is identified, one should try to track the tissue plane both proximally (towards the aortic valve) and distally along the aorta and into the aortic arch and great vessels (see Fig. 13.9A and C). Color Doppler is useful for delineating the flap, the true and false lumena, and distinguishing tissue flap from artifact. Rotating the transducer 90 degrees to show the cross-section of the aorta is also useful (see Fig. 13.9D); this will often distinguish a true flap from echo artifact (a curvilinear echodensity that does not respect aortic borders). If there is a true dissection, the intraaortic space that enlarges during systole will be the true lumen (see Fig. 34.5). The false lumen is often the larger overall of the two lumena and may be occupied by forming thrombus that will appear more echodense and static. With color Doppler one can occasionally identify entrance tears, with flow from the true to the false lumen (see Fig. 34.15F).

Transthoracic echocardiography cannot entirely exclude aortic dissection due to its technical limitations: if suspicion is high, one should go onto utilize TEE (covered in Chapter 34), cardiac tomography (CT) angiography or magnetic resonance angiography, which are all comparable for diagnostic accuracy in type A dissections.[4] TEE will be more informative regarding the aortic valve, coronary artery ostia, and hemodynamic significance of any pericardial effusion. It also has the advantage of being portable and obviating the need for nephrotoxic dyes. CT angiography and MR angiography are often utilized, because they can view the entirety of the dissection and the aorta and branches in all planes.

Urgent management: Cardiac surgery is indicated emergently for type A (DeBakey type I and II) aortic dissections, and the mortality of these emergencies is high and increases by the hour. If the aortic valve is involved and unsalvageable, a composite aortic valve replacement with

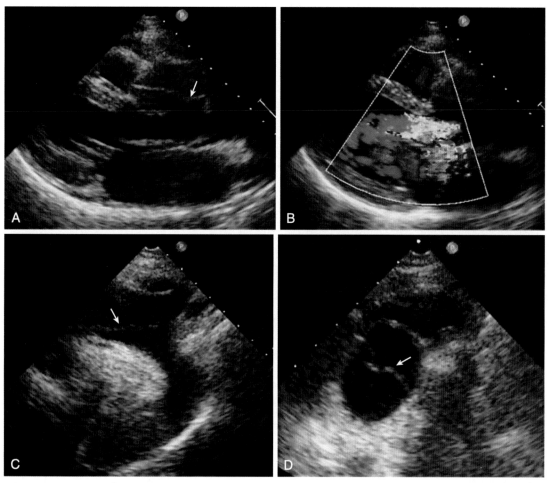

FIG. 13.9 Aortic dissection. The aortic root is aneurysmal in this patient with a type A aortic dissection. *Arrow* = dissection flap. (A) The flap is seen originating from the sinus of Valsalva and extending proximally into the aortic root, as well as (B) extending distally into the right brachiocephalic artery, causing decreased right brachial blood pressure. (C) The flap has extended into the aortic valve itself and prolapses into it, causing severe aortic insufficiency. (D) The ascending aorta in short axis, showing the dissection flap separating true and false lumen of nearly equal sizes.

conduit is necessary, as opposed to valve-sparing surgery with an interposed conduit. Details of the surgical options and echocardiographic considerations are presented in Chapter 34. Type B (descending aorta) dissections are often managed medically; as with surgical repair, there is a high risk of paralysis. However, impending rupture or other complications of type B dissections (malperfusion of end organs or limbs) may compel surgical or endovascular repair. The acute medical management of all aortic dissections is focused on lowering blood pressure and aortic shear forces with beta-blockers, as well as pain control.

Pulmonary Embolus

PE can present in a variety of ways, ranging from asymptomatic, to sinus tachycardia, to shock and sudden death. Most commonly, acute dyspnea, cough, and pleuritic chest pain are the presenting symptoms.

Echocardiography should not be used to rule out or screen for PE, as it is poorly sensitive. Rather, it can be used to assess for the sequelae of PE. In particular, it has utility in cases of submassive pulmonary emboli (i.e., acute PE with preserved systolic blood pressure >90 mm Hg), where it has a role in treatment algorithms and has prognostic value. If there is severe RV dysfunction, thrombolytics or embolectomy may be of clinical benefit.

On transthoracic echocardiography, the key findings of an acute PE are acute RV dilatation and dysfunction, the combination of which is termed "RV strain." For both echocardiography and CT, RV dilatation is defined as an RV/LV diameter ratio of greater than 0.9 on a four-chamber view. At least moderate-to-severe RV strain should be present before considering fibrinolysis. Although there may be diffuse RV hypokinesis, typically accompanied by a small, underfilled but normally contracting LV,

a distinctive pattern of wall motion abnormality is often recognized with acute PE, wherein there is marked dyskinesis of the mid RV free wall, but relative sparing of the apex and base (Fig. 13.10 and Video 13.17). This is also known as the "McConnell sign" (see Chapter 35, Fig. 35.11), and is highly specific for conditions in which pulmonary vascular resistance increases abruptly.

Serum biomarkers such as troponin, brain natriuretic peptide (BNP), or pro-BNP, may also be used as an indicators of RV strain.

If RV strain is present, one should take the opportunity to also examine the main pulmonary artery (PA) and branches in the parasternal short-axis view. Rarely, this can reveal an actual thrombus at the bifurcation or in one of the main branches (see Fig. 35.6 and Video 35.6). Thromboembolus in transit may also be visualized anywhere within the IVC and right heart (Video 13.18; see also Fig. 35.3 and Video 35.3). Long- and short-axis views of the heart can reveal the total extent of RV dilatation, and there may be flattening of the interventricular septum severe enough to produce a D-shaped LV consistent with RV pressure overload (see Fig. 35.18). PA pressures, as calculated from the tricuspid regurgitant peak flow velocity, may remain relatively normal unless there is preexisting pulmonary vascular disease.

The classic echocardiographic RV strain pattern is of lower sensitivity and have low negative predictive value in patients with long-standing pulmonary hypertension, such as those with chronic obstructive pulmonary disease (COPD) or chronic thromboembolic disease. However, if present in documented acute PE, RV dilatation or dysfunction is an independent predictor of adverse outcomes and short-term mortality even in hemodynamically stable patients.

Urgent management: For virtually all documented PEs, oxygenation, hemodynamic and ventilatory support as needed, and empiric

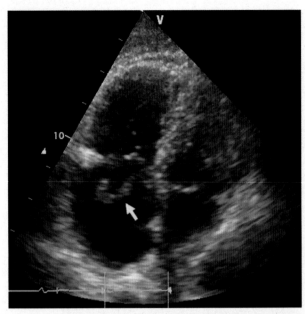

FIG. 13.10 Acute pulmonary embolus. This echocardiogram shows the RV strain pattern, or "McConnell sign," in which there is overall severe RV dilation and hypokinesis, with relatively preserved contractility at the apex but a hingepoint of dyskinesis at the RV free wall. A long serpentine thrombus in transit *(yellow arrow)* is noted oscillating in the right atrium, threatening to prolapse through the tricuspid valve into the right ventricle. See corresponding Video 13.18.

anticoagulation are the initial steps. For massive PE, defined as those with shock or persistent hypotension, immediate thrombolytic therapy and/or embolectomy are indicated. Fibrinolysis may be administered by systemic IV infusion, but catheter-directed fibrinolysis is a useful option for patients with high bleeding risk. For patients confirmed to have submassive PE, systemic fibrinolysis is not generally recommended due to a bleeding risk that may outweigh the benefit. However, catheter-directed reperfusion (which often combines ultrasound dispersion of clot with a low dose of intraarterial rtPA, such as in the EkoSonic endovascular system) appears successful in improving hemodynamics, reducing pulmonary hypertension and right heart strain, and improving survival in patients with both massive and submassive PE with less bleeding risk.[5] Low-risk PEs may be treated simply with anticoagulation.

By echocardiography, improvement in RV function can be seen by echocardiography within several days of successful treatment (reperfusion by either embolectomy or thrombolysis) of pulmonary embolism. Chapter 35 fully discusses the findings and implications of echocardiography in PE.

CODES AND SHOCK: WHERE DOES STAT ECHOCARDIOGRAPHY FIT IN?

Knowing the above-mentioned echocardiographic emergencies, comprising the mechanical complications of myocardial infarct, tamponade, aortic dissection, and PE, one can approach most code situations with confidence that specific events that require the appropriate interventions discussed above can be rapidly screened for by transthoracic echocardiography.

However, echocardiography is *not* routinely indicated in code situations, in large part because there are many life-threatening urgencies that simply cannot be diagnosed or addressed by this noninvasive approach and to a lesser extent because bedside echocardiography is not always immediately available. The major codes are listed in Table 13.2, and depending on the clinical scenario, echocardiography may or may not prove useful.

In cases of ventricular fibrillation (VF)/pulseless ventricular tachycardia (VT) or pulseless electrical activity (PEA) or asystolic arrest, if there is a history of recent MI, certainly one should scan quickly with mechanical complications of MI and tamponade in mind. Pulseless or asystolic arrests and certainly respiratory arrests may be caused by PE, but the differential diagnosis also includes aspiration and mucous plugging events. For any cardiac arrest or code, etiologies that would *not* be diagnosed by echocardiography include electrolyte imbalances (hypo- or hyperkalemia),

TABLE 13.2 Codes and the Role of Echo

	STAT ECHO HELPFUL TO RULE OUT	STAT ECHO NOT HELPFUL
VF/pulseless VT	Echo emergencies above	
PEA or asystole	PE Tamponade	
ACS and STEMI		Revascularization (angioplasty)
Bradycardia/tachycardia		Prior echo can indicate propensity for arrhythmia (e.g., LV scar, left atrial enlargement)
Respiratory arrest		Usually not helpful, may consider PE
Stroke		Not helpful acutely. Echo later could establish cardiac source of embolus.

ACS, Acute coronary syndrome; *PE,* pulmonary embolus; *PEA,* pulseless electrical activity; *STEMI,* ST elevation myocardial infarction; *VF,* ventricular fibrillation; *VT,* ventricular tachycardia.

TABLE 13.3 Types of Shock

	POTENTIAL ETIOLOGIES	ECHO FINDINGS
Cardiogenic	All echo emergencies above (mechanical) Cardiomyopathic Arrhythmic Severe aortic/mitral stenosis or regurgitation Severe restriction or constriction	See text
Obstructive	Pulmonary embolus Tamponade Aortic dissection LVOT obstruction Severe valvular stenosis Tension pneumothorax	See text
Hypovolemic	Dehydration Overdiuresis Bleeding (internal or external) Third spacing (low oncotic intravascular pressure)	Small hyperdynamic LV Collapsed IVC
Distributive	Sepsis/SIRS Metabolic acidosis (toxic-metabolic) Anaphylaxis Neurogenic, endocrine (adrenal, thyroid) shock Vasoplegia	LV systolic function may be normal, hyperkinetic, or hypokinetic

IVC, Inferior vena cava; *LV,* left ventricle; *LVOT,* left ventricular outflow tract; *SIRS,* systemic inflammatory response system.

hypoxia from airway obstruction or intrinsic lung processes, toxic or metabolic acidosis, tension pneumothorax, and hypothermia. Pneumothorax will almost definitely severely limits any ultrasound imaging of the heart, as air does not conduct ultrasound well and causes severe echo artifact. Seizures can mimic codes, but the patient's heart rate, blood pressure, and oxygenation are typically preserved.

For shock (prolonged hypotension and reduced tissue perfusion) in general, a quick mental checklist before echocardiography is even ordered should be done to consider the major causes (Table 13.3): hypovolemia (due to dehydration, overdiuresis, or internal/external bleeding), septic or distributive shock (often signaled by acidosis), obstructive shock (many of which are in fact cardiogenic), and of course cardiogenic shock.[6] Hypovolemic shock may manifest on echocardiography as a small underfilled LV (i.e., LV end-diastolic dimension <3.7 cm)

TABLE 13.4 Trauma: Potential Echo Findings

Blunt	Cardiac contusion or rupture "Commotio cordis" (structurally normal heart) Coronary artery injury Valve injury: prolapse/flail and associated regurgitation Tamponade Aortic injury: dissection flap, pseudoaneurysm, rupture
Penetrating	RV/LV free wall rupture, hemopericardium/hemothorax VSD Coronary artery or aortic/pulmonary artery laceration
Foreign body	Echobright object: intracavitary or intramyocardial Pericardial effusion Associated vegetation or abnormal flow

LV, Left ventricle; *RV,* right ventricle; *VSD,* ventricular septal defect.

that is hyperdynamic, accompanied by a small and collapsed IVC. Global LV or RV dysfunction would indicate that low cardiac output is certainly contributing to shock, and new focal wall motion abnormalities would strongly suggest an acute coronary artery obstruction. However, sepsis and acidosis are also associated with global LV hypokinesis, which often recovers when the systemic inflammatory response and metabolic derangements resolve. Obstructive shock (resistance to blood flow through the cardiovascular system) may be caused by tension pneumothorax but also by many of the same entities that ultimately lead to cardiogenic shock; these include acute PE and tamponade, and less frequently dynamic LVOT obstruction and critical aortic or mitral stenosis. The latter lesions may not be the sole cause of acute shock but can present progressively or contribute to shock when initiated by other causes. Echocardiography is generally not urgently indicated when a patient is septic or even bacteremic, since initial care will be dictated by empiric then tailored antibiotic therapy plus blood pressure support. In the course of the patient's workup, it is invaluable to survey for vegetations and the sequelae of endocarditis (particularly if prolonged fever failing antibiotics, congestive heart failure, systemic emboli, or atrioventricular conduction defects develop).

Lastly, as stated previously, echocardiography is not an appropriate tool to definitively rule out PE, although it can quickly determine RV size and function. It is not unusual for echocardiography to be technically challenging with poor image quality in the code situation, and if the patient stabilizes, further diagnostic imaging with other modalities including TEE and radiologic modalities should be considered. The exam selected is dependent upon the level of suspicion for specific pathologies and the patient's comorbidities and clinical presentation (see Chapter 48). Although TEE may be done at the bedside, it requires that the patient be hemodynamically stable enough to tolerate at least 15 minutes of imaging with a probe in the esophagus and be cooperative or appropriately sedated, and it may require or precipitate intubation in patients who are tenuous from a respiratory or neurologic standpoint.

TRAUMA

Traumatic injuries are the fifth leading cause of death in the United States. Trauma may present unique challenges for the echocardiographer, but there are circumstances in which ultrasound may play a key role. Trauma may be categorized as *blunt* force trauma; such as from a fall, motor vehicle accident (MVA), blast, or sport injury, versus *penetrating* trauma, in which an object such as a bullet or sharp object pierces the body. The two types are associated with different potential injuries to the heart, as summarized in Table 13.4. Potential mechanisms of injury are shown in Box 13.1. In general, for any trauma suspected to damage the heart, the initial survey on echocardiography should be to look for pericardial effusion/tamponade or aortic dissection, as these are of high mortality and require urgent surgery. Focused assessment with sonography for trauma (FAST) is an American Thoracic Society-recommended algorithm that many emergency rooms use for rapid assessment of thoracoabdominal trauma.[7] Of note, the general probe is not optimized for cardiac imaging, but it can be used to rule out life-threatening emergencies. However, in suspected cardiac trauma, a comprehensive echo is recommended as soon as feasible.

BOX 13.1 Blunt Trauma: Mechanisms of Injury

Direct pressure on myocardium (sudden decrease in thoracic anterior-posterior diameter)
Deceleration force → shearing
Increased intrathoracic pressure ("water ram" effect)
Contre-coup injury

Blunt Trauma

Blunt trauma to the chest is extremely common, particularly in MVAs. In the most severe cases, the direct impact can cause sternal and multiple rib fractures with resultant flail chest, as well as pulmonary contusion, and hemo- and/or pneumothorax. A direct blow or crush injury of the heart can cause damage in a number of ways. With respect to the myocardium, there can be simple concussion or contusion, typically of the anterior thin-walled RV. The RV is involved in 60%, LV in 30%, and both ventricles in 10% of cases.[8] Contusions are typically suspected when there are ECG ST elevations, elevated cardiac biomarkers, and transient tachyarrhythmias (which also raise the suspicion for acute coronary syndrome). On echocardiography, there can be diffuse hypokinesis or focal wall motion abnormalities, including focal RVOT hypokinesis, and RV dilatation (Fig. 13.11A and Video 13.19), and LV focal hypokinesis. Pericardial effusions may be associated. Although the complication rate is very low in patients with normal ECG and troponins, in one retrospective study, the presence of myocardial dysfunction on echo was associated with threefold higher mortality in patients with suspected cardiac contusion.[8,9] With severe impact, chamber rupture can occur, but these cases usually die on site with the findings described at autopsy. "Commotio cordis" is a term for sudden cardiac death occurring from a low-velocity (<40 mph) blow to the heart (such as a ball or a tackle during sports), which appears to be due to the impact occurring on the T wave upslope of the ECG, a vulnerable period that precipitates ventricular fibrillation. This is primarily an electrical accident, as the hearts are structurally normal.

Valve rupture has been reported in 6% of blunt cardiac injury cases. The aortic and mitral valve are more frequently involved and can lead to regurgitation and acute congestive heart failure requiring immediate surgery. An example of a traumatic flail aortic leaflet is shown in Fig. 13.11C and D and Video 13.20. In contrast, tricuspid and pulmonic valve flail may be unrecognized and asymptomatic for years. (Videos 13.21 and 13.22 show tricuspid valve chordal and leaflet rupture discovered early and late, respectively after accidents.)

Fig. 13.12 charts the direct and indirect complications of blunt cardiac injury in one meta-analysis. The figure shows that transient arrhythmias are the predominant outcome, which usually resolves within the first 48 hours. The other more malignant outcomes comprise less than 25% of the complications.[8]

Aortic dissection is one of the most lethal events to occur after MVAs. Unlike spontaneous dissections, traumatic aortic dissections most commonly occur at the aortic isthmus, that is, distal to the left subclavian artery. The reason is theorized to be that the descending thoracic aorta is tethered to the posterior thorax, but the portion proximal to the ligamentum arteriosum is more mobile. With rapid deceleration, such as a high velocity head-on impact, the heart and aortic arch lurch forward, exerting shear force at the transition zone of the aorta. Tears through the aortic wall layers to varying degrees may produce a dissection flap, aortic hematoma, partial rupture, or even complete transection at the isthmus.

Transthoracic echocardiography to visualize the aortic arch is technically possible in a stable patient, but more often than not in the acute setting, the presence of an obligate cervical collar to stabilize the neck makes this window inaccessible, and the obtained images may be of suboptimal quality. In an unstable patient, by TEE, the ascending aorta, arch, and descending aorta may be thoroughly inspected at the bedside or in the OR. *First, however, cervical neck stability must be ascertained.* If neurology or orthopedics is unable to clear the patient's neck in terms of stability and there are no other options for aortic imaging, the patient will need to have a cervical immobilizer in place during the entire exam. Intubation and sedation, and possibly even paralytics

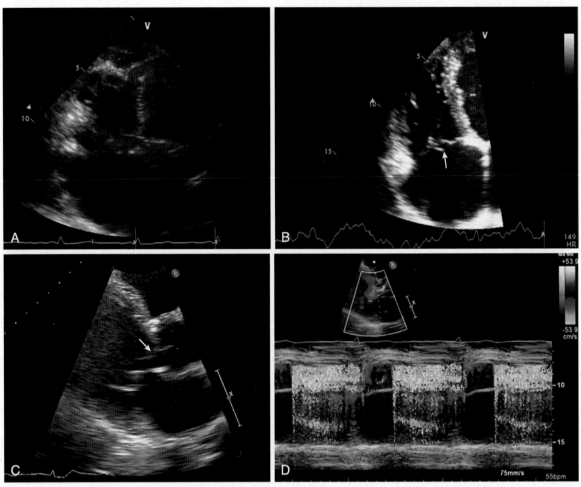

FIG. 13.11 Cardiac trauma causing contusion and valvular rupture. (A) Cardiac contusion, manifest as RV dilatation and focal dyskinesis of the RV free wall, seen after patient fell off a deck onto hard ground. (B) Tricuspid valve ruptured chord *(arrow)*. (C) Traumatic rupture causing aortic valve leaflet flail *(arrow)* and severe pandiastolic aortic insufficiency seen by color M-mode Doppler in D. See corresponding Videos 13.19–13.21.

Direct complications
- Arrhythmia (90% occur w/i 1st 48 h)
- Ventricular dysfunction (CHF, hypotension)
- Rupture (RV more common) → frequently lethal
- Aneurysm
- Papillary muscle dysfunction

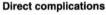
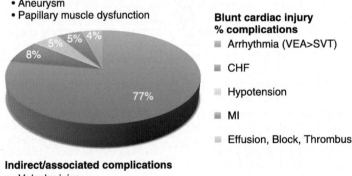

Blunt cardiac injury % complications
- Arrhythmia (VEA>SVT)
- CHF
- Hypotension
- MI
- Effusion, Block, Thrombus

Indirect/associated complications
- Valvular injury
- MI

FIG. 13.12 Complications seen after blunt cardiac injury. Self-resolving arrhythmias such as ventricular ectopy and SVTs account for approximately three-quarters of the clinical sequelae, and the remaining complications together are less than one-quarter. *(Data from Maenza RL, Seaberg D, D'Amico F. A meta-analysis of blunt cardiac trauma: ending myocardial confusion. Am J Emerg Med. 1996;14[3]:237–241.)*

may be required to safely perform the exam without risk of cervical spine injury and quadriplegia. Evidence of a dissection flap or even a free-floating aortic lumen within mediastinal hematoma can be seen by TEE (Video 13.23). Fig. 13.13 shows a CT angiogram of an aortic rupture (hematoma) that was treated urgently with an endovascular stent, which is visualized on follow-up transthoracic echocardiograms and CTs. A sudden new pericardial effusion accompanied by acute chest pain, particularly if there appears to be spontaneous echo contrast or thrombus forming within the fluid, should always raise suspicion for aortic dissection (see Video 13.12).

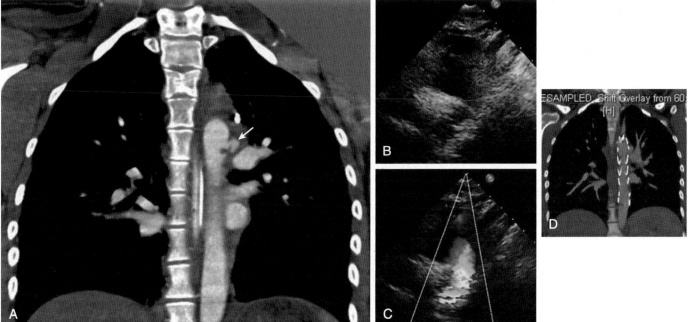

FIG. 13.13 Traumatic pseudoaneurysm of the aorta at the isthmus. Patient was an unrestrained female in a high-speed motor vehicle accident with multiple injuries. (A) By CTA, there is a 1.5-cm aortic pseudoaneurysm *(arrow)* with a narrow neck at the level of the ligamentum arteriosum, with a small amount of surrounding mediastinal hematoma and extravasation indicative of transection distal to the left subclavian origin. This area underwent endovascular stenting, with the subsequent TEE showing a well-seated endograft covering the disrupted aortic area. (B and C) Transthoracic suprasternal images of the aortic arch on 2D (B) and color Doppler (C) imaging, showing the area of the isthmus s/p endovascular stenting. (D) CT of the endovascular stent in the descending aorta.

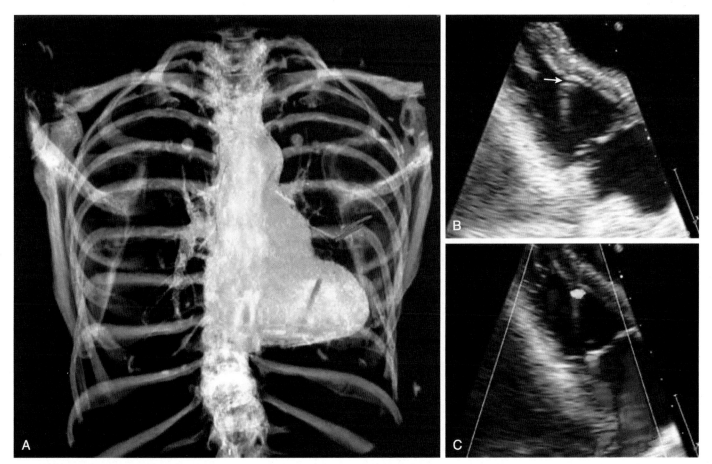

FIG. 13.14 Intramyocardial needle. (A) Three-dimensional (3D) CT reconstruction showing three sewing needles *(in red)* in the chest, one of which appears to be penetrating the heart. (B and C) Zoomed transthoracic views of the right heart showing the echobright needle tip in the interventricular septum with echo artifact cast into the RV. C shows a very focal jet of left-to-right interventricular flow around the needle. At surgery, the needle base was noted protruding from the anterior surface of the heart, where a small pericardial hematoma had collected, and intra-op TEE showed the needle penetrating the interventricular septum. It was simply pulled without incident, with no further VSD or pericardial bleeding noted on TEE.

Penetrating Trauma

In the United States, penetrating chest injuries are less common but more deadly than blunt trauma and are most often caused by gunshots and stabbings.[10] An initial FAST survey is usually performed to rule out hemopericardium, but repeat or dedicated cardiac imaging may be indicated if there are initial poor windows (e.g., due to large concurrent hemothorax or pneumomediastinum prior to chest tube insertion) and clinical signs suggestive of cardiac injury.

Penetrating trauma may cause chamber rupture (commonly the RV, as the anterior-most structure), VSDs, or laceration of the coronary arteries, aorta, or PA. There are cases where initially there is surprisingly no evident hemopericardium, presumably due to local pressure or containment at the site of penetration. Fig. 13.3 and corresponding Videos 13.24 and 13.25 show views of a stabbing victim's heart, in which a large VSD is found. RV laceration was also identified in the operating room, but attempts at emergent surgical repair failed, as the patient was already in deep cardiogenic shock.

Finally, there are foreign body injuries that are rarely reported with cases of bullet fragments, sewing needles, or migrated needle tips and device fragments found in and around the heart. These are usually incidentally picked up by x-ray or CT scans and confer a risk of infection, embolization, and erosion. Foreign bodies that are partially extracardiac appear to be at more risk for erosion and tamponade due to repetitive wounding and re-bleeding from the beating of the heart. Fig. 13.14 and the corresponding echo in Video 13.26 show sewing needles that were unknowingly imbedded in a patient's chest, with one of them found to be intramyocardial, invading the interventricular septum with a small localized pericardial hematoma. Surgical extraction is usually preferred, although if the foreign body is completely imbedded in the myocardium and there is no accompanying pericarditis or endocarditis, conservative observation only may be considered.

Late sequelae of cardiac trauma, both blunt and penetrating, are rare but can include LV aneurysms, VSDs, intracardiac fistulas, aorto-RA or RV fistulas, retained bullet emboli, valvular injury, and coronary artery-cameral fistulas.

Suggested Reading

Goldstein, S. A., Evangelista, A., Abbara, S., et al. (2015). Multimodality imaging of diseases of the thoracic aorta in adults: from the American Society of Echocardiography and the European Association of Cardiovascular Imaging Endorsed by the Society of Cardiovascular Computed Tomography and Society for Cardiovascular Magnetic Resonance. *Journal of the American Society of Echocardiography, 28*, 119–182.

Klein, A. L., Abbara, S., Agler, D. A., et al. (2013). American Society of Echocardiography clinical recommendations for multimodality cardiovascular imaging of patients with pericardial disease. *Journal of the American Society of Echocardiography, 26*, 965–1012.

Kutty, R. S., Jones, N., & Morrjani, N. (2013). Mechanical complications of acute myocardial infarction. *Cardiology Clinics, 31*, 519–531.

Marcolini, E. G., & Keegan, J. (2015). Blunt cardiac injury. *Emergency Medicine Clinics of North America, 33*, 519–527.

McLean, A. S. (2016). Echocardiography in shock management. *Critical Care, 20*, 275.

A complete reference list can be found online at ExpertConsult.com.

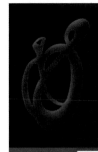

14 Assessment of Left Ventricular Systolic Function

Scott D. Solomon, Bernard E. Bulwer

INTRODUCTION

A major goal of the echocardiographic examination is the assessment of left ventricular (LV) structure and systolic function. This plays a critically important role in the diagnosis, risk evaluation, and management of patients with suspected or established cardiovascular disease. The left ventricle can be assessed qualitatively and quantitatively to define any alterations in cardiac size and geometry by using comprehensive measurements (Fig. 14.1). Established normal values are shown in Tables 14.1–14.3.

Echocardiography offers several methods for assessment of systolic function. Routine assessment of ventricular systolic function typically begins with a qualitative evaluation. However, more precise quantification

methods of global and regional ventricular systolic function are recommended. Linear and volumetric LV measures such as wall thicknesses, mass, and volumes remain clinically useful parameters supported by extensive data. These are based primarily on M-mode, two-dimensional (2D), and Doppler hemodynamic measures (Figs. 14.1 and 14.2).

Traditional M-Mode and 2D-derived measurements, such as left ventricular ejection fraction (LVEF), are still widely used but have important limitations. They are based on comparisons of frames and measures obtained at the beginning and end of the contractile cycle. They are load and heart rate–dependent and do not directly measure dynamic LV myocardial performance. Additionally, the geometric assumptions and derived LV measures have inherent inaccuracies. The advent of real-time

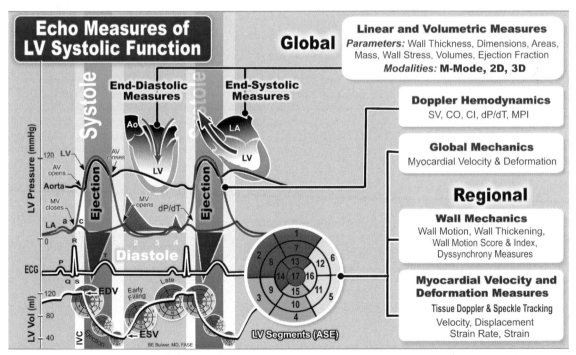

FIG. 14.1 Echocardiographic measures of ventricular systolic function can be categorized using established global and regional systolic function. Global ventricular function parameters include *linear and volumetric dimensions*, for example, wall thicknesses, ventricular areas, ventricular volumes. From these, traditional measures such as *left ventricular ejection fraction (LVEF) and LV mass* can be derived. Global hemodynamic measures of global ventricular function obtained on Doppler echocardiography includes stroke volume, cardiac output, rate of rise of pressures within the left ventricle during systole (d*P*/d*T*), and myocardial performance index (MPI) or Tei index. Regional measures of ventricular systolic function include qualitative assessment of regional wall motion, semiquantitative assessment of regional wall motion or wall motion score index (WMSI), tissue Doppler imaging (TDI) techniques to quantify systolic cardiac mechanics and deformation. Speckle tracking imaging (STI) techniques to quantify systolic cardiac mechanics and deformation. *ASE,* American Society of Echocardiography; *CI,* cardiac index; *CO,* cardiac output; d*P*/d*T,* rate of change of pressure during the isovolumetric contraction phase of systole; *IVC,* isovolumetric contraction; *LVEF,* left ventricular ejection fraction; *SV,* stroke volume; *TDI,* tissue Doppler imaging; *WMSI,* wall motion score index. (*Courtesy of Bernard E. Bulwer, MD, FASE.*)

TABLE 14.1 Normal Values for Two-Dimensional Echocardiographic Parameters of Left Ventricular Size and Function According to Gender

Parameter	MALE Mean ± SD	MALE 2-SD Range	FEMALE Mean ± SD	FEMALE 2-SD Range
LV internal dimension				
Diastolic dimension (mm)	50.2 ± 4.1	42.0–58.4	45.0 ± 3.6	37.8–52.2
Systolic dimension (mm)	32.4 ± 3.7	25.0–39.8	28.2 ± 3.3	21.6–34.8
LV volumes (biplane)				
LV EDV (mL)	106 ± 22	62–150	76 ± 15	46–106
LV ESV (mL)	41 ± 10	21–61	28 ± 7	14–42
LV volumes normalized by BSA				
LV EDV (mL/m^2)	54 ± 10	34–74	45 ± 8	29–61
LV ESV (mL/m^2)	21 ± 5	11–31	16 ± 4	8–24
LV EF (biplane)	62 ± 5	52–72	64 ± 5	54–74

BSA, Body surface area; *EDV*, end-diastolic volume; *EF*, ejection fraction; *ESV*, end-systolic volume; *LV*, left ventricular; *SD*, standard deviation.
From Lang RM, Badano LP, Mor-Avi V, et al. *Recommendations for cardiac chamber quantification by echocardiography in adults: an update from the American Society of Echocardiography and the European Association of Cardiovascular Imaging.* J Am Soc Echocardiogr. 2015;28(1):1–39.

TABLE 14.2 Reference Limits and Partition Values of Left Ventricular Mass and Geometry

	WOMEN Reference Range	WOMEN Mildly Abnormal	WOMEN Moderately Abnormal	WOMEN Severely Abnormal	MEN Reference Range	MEN Mildly Abnormal	MEN Moderately Abnormal	MEN Severely Abnormal
Linear Method								
LV mass (g)	67–162	163–186	187–210	≥211	88–224	225–258	259–292	≥293
LV mass/BSA (g/m^2)	*43–95*	*96–108*	*109–121*	*≥122*	*49–115*	*116–131*	*132–148*	*≥149*
LV mass/height (g/m)	41–99	100–115	116–128	≥129	52–126	127–144	145–162	≥163
LV mass/height$^{2.7}$ (g/m$^{2.7}$)	18–44	45–51	52–58	≥59	20–48	49–55	56–63	≥64
Relative wall thickness (cm)	0.22–0.42	0.43–0.47	0.48–0.52	≥0.53	0.24–0.42	0.43–0.46	0.47–0.51	≥0.52
Septal thickness (cm)	*0.6–0.9*	*1.0–1.2*	*1.3–1.5*	*≥1.6*	*0.6–1.0*	*1.1–1.3*	*1.4–1.6*	*≥1.7*
Posterior wall thickness (cm)	*0.6–0.9*	*1.0–1.2*	*1.3–1.5*	*≥1.6*	*0.6–1.0*	*1.1–1.3*	*1.4–1.6*	*≥1.7*
Two-Dimensional Method								
LV mass (g)	66–150	151–171	172–182	≥183	96–200	201–227	228–254	≥255
LV mass/BSA (g/m^2)	*44–88*	*89–100*	*101–112*	*≥113*	*50–102*	*103–116*	*117–130*	*≥131*

Bold italic values are recommended and best validated.
BSA, Body surface area.
From Lang RM, Bierig M, Devereux RB, et al. *Recommendations for chamber quantification: a report from the American Society of Echocardiography's Guidelines and Standards Committee and the Chamber Quantification Writing Group, developed in conjunction with the European Association of Echocardiography, a branch of the European Society of Cardiology.* J Am Soc Echocardiogr. 2005;18(12):1440–1463.

TABLE 14.3 Reference Limits and Partition Values of Left Ventricular Function

	WOMEN Reference Range	WOMEN Mildly Abnormal	WOMEN Moderately Abnormal	WOMEN Severely Abnormal	MEN Reference Range	MEN Mildly Abnormal	MEN Moderately Abnormal	MEN Severely Abnormal
Linear Method								
Endocardial fractional shortening (%)	27–45	22–26	17–21	≤16	25–43	20–24	15–19	≤14
Midwall fractional shortening (%)	15–23	13–14	11–12	≤10	14–22	12–13	10–11	≤9
Two-Dimensional Method								
Ejection fraction (%)	≥55	45–54	30–44	<30	≥55	45–54	30–44	<30

Bold italic values are recommended and best validated.
From Lang RM, Bierig M, Devereux RB, et al. *Recommendations for chamber quantification: a report from the American Society of Echocardiography's Guidelines and Standards Committee and the Chamber Quantification Writing Group, developed in conjunction with the European Association of Echocardiography, a branch of the European Society of Cardiology.* J Am Soc Echocardiogr. 2005;18(12):1440–1463.

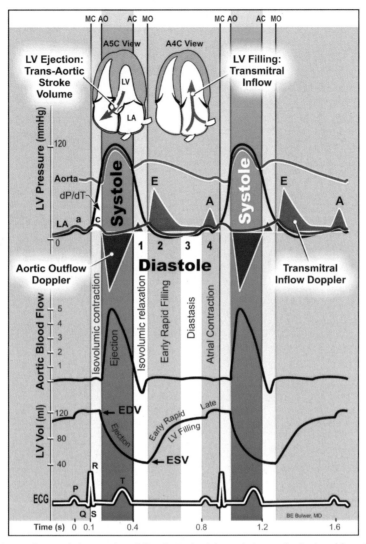

FIG. 14.2 The cardiac cycle with superimposed events during systole and diastole. During *left ventricular systole*, ejection of from the left ventricle, through the aortic valve, and into the aorta, occurs. These systolic events can be assessed on the echocardiographic views and Doppler measures depicted. *AC,* Aortic valve closure; *AO,* aortic valve opening; *IVSd,* interventricular septal diameter; *LV,* left ventricle; *MC,* mitral valve closure; *MO,* mitral valve opening. (*Courtesy of Bernard E. Bulwer, MD, FASE.*)

three-dimensional (3D) echocardiography, however, has overcome some of these inaccuracies. Nevertheless, continuing challenges such as endocardial border delineation remain.

Recent advances in cardiac deformation imaging, primarily using tissue Doppler and 2D speckle tracking imaging, has made possible the measurement of global and regional LV systolic mechanics. The additional insights they provide about regional LV contractile mechanics have been shown to be more sensitive measures of preclinical and clinical myocardial pathology. An increasing body of data indicates that they provide superior prognostic and incremental information over traditional systolic measures. LV deformation indices, such as velocities, displacement, strain, and strain rate, are now increasing employed in the comprehensive assessment of LV systolic function.

LEFT VENTRICULAR SYSTOLE: CARDIAC CYCLE AND HEMODYNAMICS

Measurements of the Left Ventricle

Measurements of the LV include linear, area, or volumetric measures (Figs. 14.1, 14.3, and 14.4–14.7). These methods are often complementary and best suited to characterize LV size, and many laboratories continue to record linear cavity measurements, a practice supported by the extensive data correlating these measures with outcomes in many disease states. Moreover, linear measures are subject to less variability than area- or volume-based measures and can therefore be more reliable when assessing changes over time.

Left Ventricular Structure: Size and Mass

LV volumes can be estimated using several formulas based on linear or 2D measurements based on the assumption that the LV approximates a prolate ellipsoid (see Fig. 14.5). These approaches are limited when ventricular geometry deviates substantially from normal, as is the case in patients with myocardial infarction (MI), where the LV can be substantially distorted. The single-plane or biplane Simpson method of disks is an approach that does not rely on rigid geometric assumptions and has been demonstrated to be the most accurate method (see Fig. 14.6). It involves identifying the endocardial border in the apical four- (A4C) and/or two-chamber (A2C) views with computerized assistance to measure the diameter of equally distributed slices along the ventricle. A cross sectional area is calculated from this diameter by assuming a circle if the single-plane method is used or an ellipse if two orthogonal planes are used. Although the Simpson method is usually more accurate than other methods of assessing ventricular volumes, precise identification of the endocardial border can be challenging when image quality is reduced. Moreover,

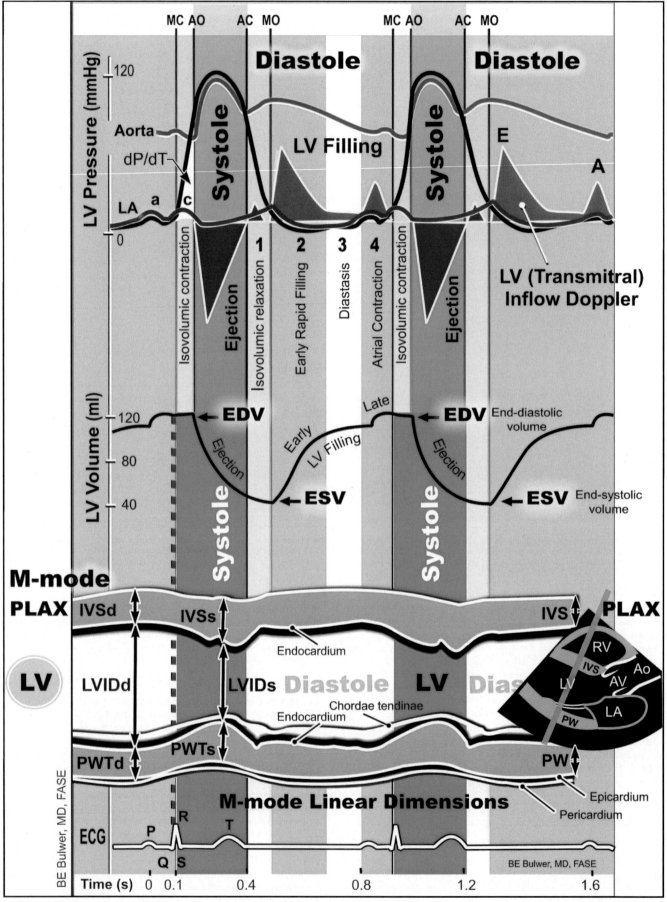

FIG. 14.3 The cardiac cycle and linear measures of left ventricle *(LV)* systolic function: Schema showing M-mode of the LV superimposed on the cardiac cycle. Note the timing of events. Compare with the Doppler hemodynamic profiles shown. *AC,* Aortic valve closure; *AO,* aortic valve opening; *MC,* mitral valve closure; *MO,* mitral valve opening. *(Courtesy of Bernard E. Bulwer, MD, FASE.)*

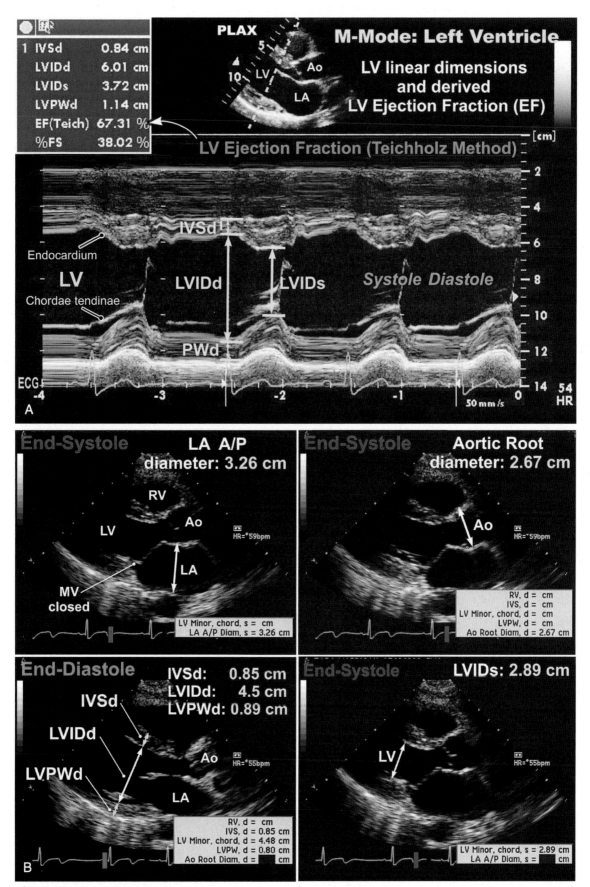

FIG. 14.4 (A and B) Linear measurements of the left ventricle *(LV)* on M-mode and two-dimensional (2D). M-mode is simple, reproducible, and provides excellent temporal resolution of the endocardial border. It retains utility in the assessment of LV dimensions (e.g., cavity size, wall thicknesses, and fractional shortening). Its reliability is diminished with abnormal LV geometry, even when guided two-dimensionally. Several formulas can be used to calculate volumes from M-mode–based ventricular cavity diameter measures. The primary method used is the Teichholz method [Teichholz formula: Volume = [7.0/(2.4 + LVIDd)] (LVIDd) 3]. This method is only useful, however, when ventricular geometry is relatively normal. The American Society of Echocardiography recommends two-dimensional measurements of linear dimensions using the leading-edge-to-leading-edge method as shown. *Ao,* Aorta; *LA,* left auricle; *LVIDd,* LV internal diameter at end diastole; *LVIDs,* LV internal diameter at end systole; *LVPWd,* LV posterior wall thickness at end diastole; *MV,* mitral valve; *RV,* right ventricle. *(Courtesy of Bernard E. Bulwer, MD, FASE.)*

Area-Length Geometric Models
for Calculating LV Volumes on 2D Echocardiography

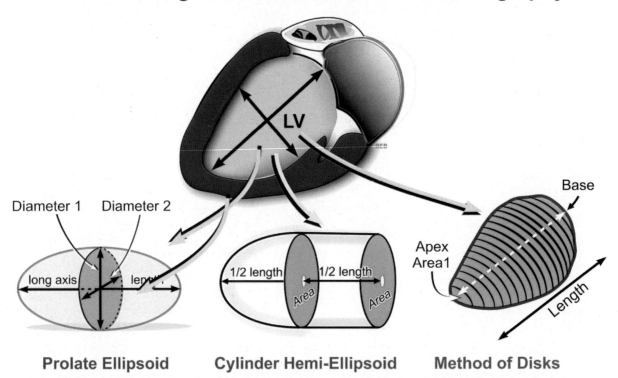

Prolate Ellipsoid   **Cylinder Hemi-Ellipsoid**   **Method of Disks**

FIG. 14.5 Linear and volumetric measurements EDV and ESV volumes by area × length methods. Area-length geometric models used to estimate LV volumes and ejection fraction by two-dimensional echocardiography require measurements of short-axis areas multiplied by long-axis lengths. When poor endocardial border delineation occurs, the area-length based methods (e.g., cylinder hemi-ellipse or bullet formula) can be employed to calculate end-diastolic and systolic volumes, and hence ejection fraction. The following formula is used: ($V = [5$ (Area) (Length)]/6). *LV*, Left ventricle. (*Courtesy of Bernard E. Bulwer, MD, FASE.*)

Biplane Method of Disks - Simpson's Rule

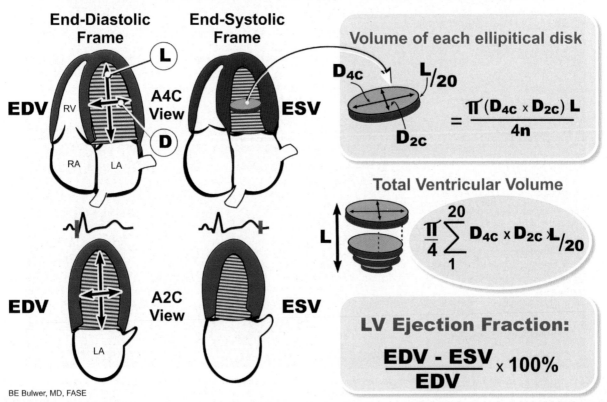

FIG. 14.6 The left ventricular ejection fraction (LVEF) using the Simpson's rule method of disks. The LVEF remains the most common and accepted method for assessing ventricular volumes, despite limitations, such as being volume and heart rate dependent *(see text)*. This method assumes that the ventricle is composed of a stacked series of elliptical disks. By knowing the major and minor diameters of each disk, an ellipse can be defined, and the area of each ellipse is then multiplied by the slice thickness. When these disks are summated, as in the formula, the overall volume of the ventricle can be determined. *A4C*, Apical four chamber; *A2C*, apical two chamber; *EDV*, end-diastolic volume; *ESV*, end-systolic volume. (*Courtesy of Bernard E. Bulwer, MD, FASE.*)

Quantitative Estimates of LVEF by 2D or 3D Echocardiography

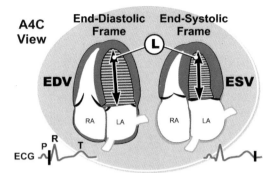

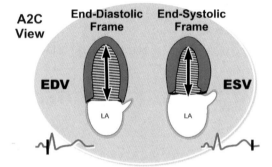

Measurements of **End-Systolic** and **End-Diastolic Volumes**
(**ESV**, **EDV**, and **LVEF** (*Biplane Simpson's Rule*)

Biplane Simpson's Method (2D)

1. In **A4C View**, Scroll through frames and select **End-Diastolic Frame** (start of R-wave on ECG or frame with largest LV volume, just before AV opens
2. Trace endocardial border from septal to lateral MV annulus and join ends with straight line for **EDV**
3. Measure **LV cavity length** (**L**) - apex to MV annulus
4. Scroll A4C video loop; choose **End-Systolic Frame** (end of T-wave on ECG, or smallest LV diameter - frame before MV opens) and Measure **ESV**
5. Repeat steps 1 to 4 above for **A2C View** measures
6. Auto-calculate **LVEF**

Semi-Automated LV Volumes-EF (3D)

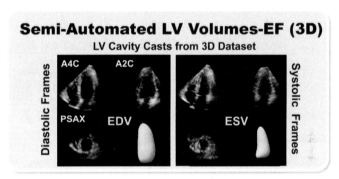

HR, Heart Rate   (*If no mitral regurgitation*)

$$LVEF = \frac{EDV - ESV}{EDV} \times 100\%$$

EDV - ESV = Stroke Volume (SV)
(*Normal **SV** = ~75-100 ml; Index to Body Wt*)

Cardiac Output = SV x HR

FIG. 14.7 Assessment of left ventricular ejection fraction (*LVEF*) by 2D and 3D echocardiography (*see text*). A4C, Apical four-chamber; A2C, apical two-chamber; LV, left ventricle. (*Courtesy of Bernard E. Bulwer, MD, FASE.*)

foreshortening of the ventricle in one of the apical views, which can occur simply by minor changes in the transducer angle, can dramatically reduce the measured volume and adversely affect volumetric estimations.

3D echocardiography has the potential to reduce some of the inherent limitations of 2D imaging (see Chapter 5) (see Fig. 14.7). LV mass may be calculated by using one of several formulas that take into account both wall thickness and chamber size (Fig. 14.8; see Table 14.3) These formulas have been validated in geometrically normal ventricles, but their accuracy is markedly reduced in the setting of altered ventricular geometry, such as following MI. LV hypertrophy is defined by the overall LV mass. In general, if LV diameter is not decreased, wall thickness of 12 mm or greater is usually indicative of LV hypertrophy (see Table 14.1). Both myocardial and valvular diseases can result in remodeling of the left ventricle and hence abnormal ventricular geometry. Categorization of ventricular geometry is based on relative wall thickness and the LV mass index (see Figs. 14.8 and 14.9). The specific pattern of ventricular is related to prognosis in a variety of diseases.

Assessment of Cardiac Function

The LVEF, calculated as the difference between end-diastolic volume and end-systolic volume divided by end-diastolic volume, remains the most commonly used method for assessing systolic function (see Fig. 14.7). It is one of the best-studied measures in cardiovascular medicine and has proved useful in diagnosis and risk stratification in a variety of cardiovascular diseases. Although accurate assessment of LVEF requires calculation from ventricular volumes, many echocardiography laboratories estimate LVEF visually.

Even though calculation of LVEF from volumes is preferred, the accuracy of this estimation is affected by image quality, endocardial border definition, ventricular geometry, and representative orthogonal imaging planes. When one or more of the aforementioned factors are suboptimal, visual estimation by experienced echocardiographers can be more accurate and sufficient for most clinical scenarios.

Other approaches are commonly used in addition to LVEF to assess systolic function. Stroke volume (SV) can be determined by subtracting end-systolic volume from end-diastolic volume (calculated as described earlier) or through hemodynamic Doppler-based methods (Figs. 14.10–14.12). Multiplying the velocity time integral (VTI) in the LV outflow tract (LVOT), assessed with pulsed wave Doppler on the A4C view, by the cross-sectional diameter at the same location (measured on the parasternal long-axis view) yields SV (see Fig. 14.10), which can be multiplied by the heart rate to obtain cardiac output.

Several other novel methods have been proposed for assessment of systolic function. The myocardial performance index, also known as the Tei index, is defined as the sum of isovolumic relaxation time and isovolumic contraction time divided by ejection time, and this method takes into account both systolic and diastolic performance, with a lower index being associated with better function (see Fig. 14.12). In adults, values of the LV index lower than 0.40 and right ventricle index lower than 0.30 are considered normal. This measure has been related to outcomes in a variety of conditions, including heart failure and following MI.

Doppler tissue imaging (DTI) can be used to assess myocardial contraction velocity, or S′ although this technique has proved more useful for assessment of diastolic function (Fig. 14.13).

Left Ventricular (LV) Mass

Two Methods validated for measurement of LV Mass
Method 1: Area x Length (**AL**) Formula
Method 2: Truncated Ellipsoid (**TE**) Model

These 2 methods are based on measurements of myocardial area at the mid-LV (papillary muscle level.

1. Trace Epicardium to obtain **Total LV Area** (A_1)
2. Trace Endocardium to obtain **LV Cavity Area** (A_2).
3. **Myocardial Area** (A_m) is the difference: **Total LV Area** (A_1) - **LV Cavity Area** (A_2).

$$A_m = A_1 - A_2$$

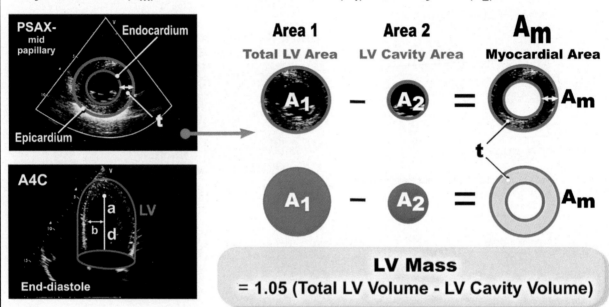

Area 1 — Total LV Area (A_1)
Area 2 — LV Cavity Area (A_2)
A_m — Myocardial Area

$$A_1 - A_2 = A_m$$

LV Mass
$$= 1.05 \text{ (Total LV Volume - LV Cavity Volume)}$$

t = mean wall thickness obtained from the *short-axis Epicardial* and *Cavity areas*.

BE Bulwer, MD, FASE

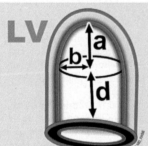

a: long or semi-major axis from widest minor axis radius to apex of the LV
b: short-axis radius (back calculated from the LV short-axis cavity area)
d: truncated semi-major axis from widest short-axis diameter to mitral anulus plane

Assuming a circular area, the **radius (b)**, *the short-axis radius of the LV*

$$b = \sqrt{\frac{A_2}{\pi}} \qquad t = \sqrt{\frac{A_1}{\pi}} - b$$

LV Mass (AL Formula) $= 1.05 \left\{ \left[\frac{5}{6} A_1 \, (a+d+t) \right] - \left[\frac{5}{6} A_2 \, (a+d) \right] \right\}$

LV Mass (TE Model) $= 1.05 \times \left\{ (b+t)^2 \left[\frac{2}{3}(a+1) + d - \frac{d^3}{3(a+t)^2} \right] - b^2 \left[\frac{2}{3}a + d - \frac{d^3}{3a^2} \right] \right\}$

Reference: Lang RM et. al. ASE/EAE-Recommendations for chamber quantification. J Am Soc Echocardiogr. 2005;12:1440-63

FIG. 14.8 The area-length method for using a cylinder hemi-ellipsoid of the left ventricle (LV) is the recommended method for measuring LV mass. It is a simple formula with easily obtainable measurements. End-diastolic measurements using c and apical four-chamber (A4C) views at the mid- or high-papillary muscle levels are made and then inserted into the equation as shown. *L1*, end-diastolic LV cavity length; *A1*, total planimetered PSAX area at the mid- or high-papillary muscle level; *A2*, LV cavity planimetered PSAX area; *Am*, myocardial "shell" area; *A_epi*, total planimetered PSAX area at the mid- or high-papillary muscle level; *A_endo*, LV cavity planimetered PSAX area; *b*, minor axis radius; *t*, wall thickness. (*Courtesy of Bernard E. Bulwer, MD, FASE.*)

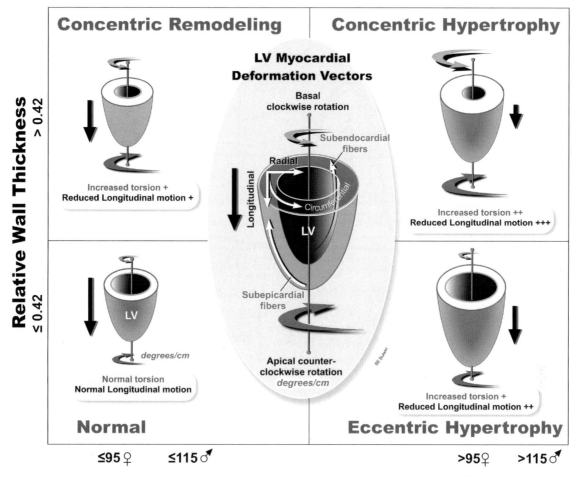

FIG. 14.9 Relative wall thickness and left ventricular mass index in normal and disease states, with superimposed LV myocardial deformation vectors *(see text)*. *LV,* Left ventricle. *(Courtesy of Bernard E. Bulwer, MD, FASE.)*

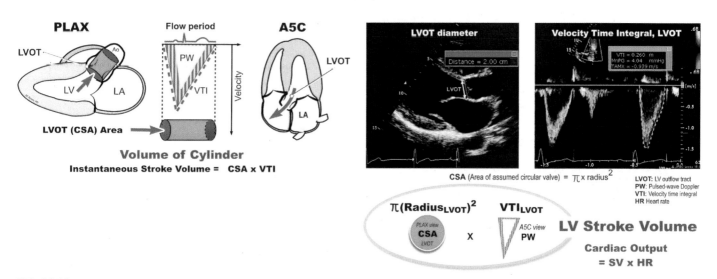

FIG. 14.10 Doppler-based method for assessment of left ventricular systolic function. Left ventricular (LV) stroke volume calculated at the LV outflow tract *(LVOT)*. Doppler echocardiography can be used to assess stroke volume. The cross-sectional area of the LVOT is multiplied by the velocity time integral *(VTI)* of flow at the same location to obtain the stroke volume. Typically, the LVOT diameter is measured in the parasternal long-axis *(PLAX)* view, and the LVOT Doppler is obtained in the apical five-chamber view *(A5C)*. *(See text.)* *(Courtesy of Bernard E. Bulwer, MD, FASE.)*

III

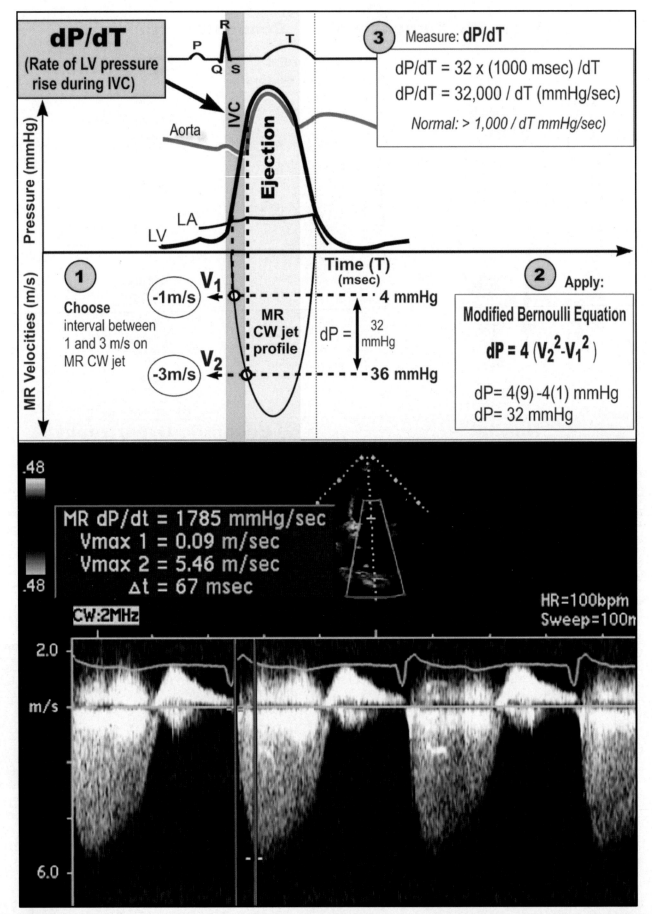

dP/dT
(Rate of LV pressure rise during IVC)

1 Choose interval between 1 and 3 m/s on MR CW jet

V_1 -1m/s 4 mmHg

V_2 -3m/s 36 mmHg

MR CW jet profile

$dP = 32$ mmHg

3 Measure: **dP/dT**

dP/dT = 32 x (1000 msec) /dT
dP/dT = 32,000 / dT (mmHg/sec)

Normal: > 1,000 / dT mmHg/sec

2 Apply:

Modified Bernoulli Equation

$$dP = 4\,(V_2^2 - V_1^2)$$

dP= 4(9) -4(1) mmHg
dP= 32 mmHg

MR dP/dt = 1785 mmHg/sec
Vmax 1 = 0.09 m/sec
Vmax 2 = 5.46 m/sec
Δt = 67 msec

HR=100bpm
Sweep=100n

CW:2MHz

FIG. 14.11 Doppler-based d*P*/d*T* as a measure of left ventricular systolic function. The rate of LV pressure rise (d*P*/d*T*) during the isovolumetric contraction *(IVC)* phase of systole is a useful measure of LV contractility. In patients with mitral regurgitation *(MR)*, estimates of d*P*/d*T* can be derived from the time interval it takes for the pressure to rise by 32 mm Hg (i.e., from 1 to 3 m/s). The Bernoulli equation is used to estimate LV pressures from the MR CW spectral Doppler velocities. *CW,* Continuous wave spectral Doppler; *LA,* left atrium; *LV,* left ventricle. *(Courtesy of Bernard E. Bulwer, MD, FASE.)*

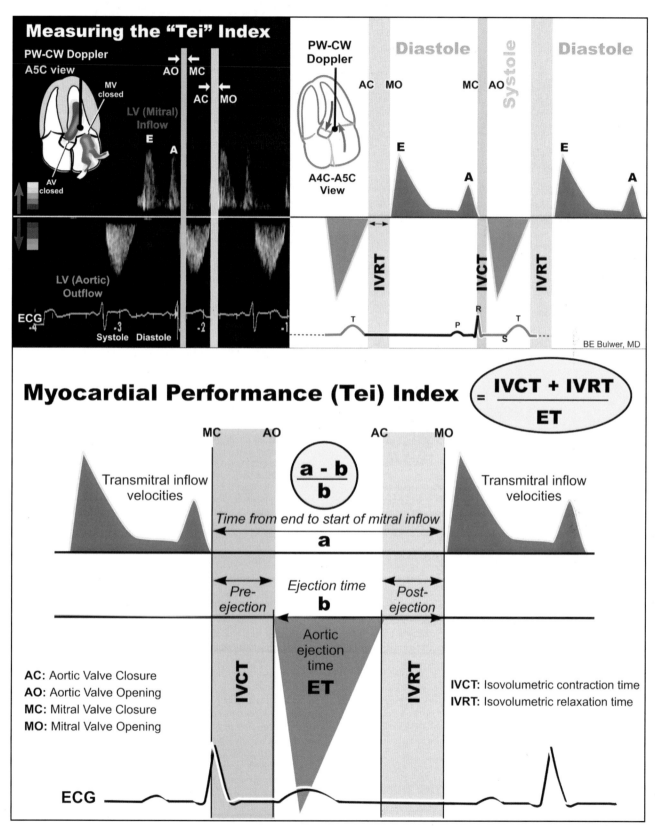

FIG. 14.12 The myocardial performance (Tei) index is a dimensionless index based on the sum of the isovolumetric contraction and relaxation times (*IVCT* and *IVRT*, respectively) divided by the ejection time *(ET)*. This index incorporates assessment of both systolic and diastolic function and has been related to prognosis in a variety of disease states. *A4C*, Apical four-chamber; *A5C*, apical five-chamber; *CW*, continuous wave spectral Doppler; *LV*, left ventricle; *PW*, pulsed wave. (*Courtesy of Bernard E. Bulwer, MD, FASE.*)

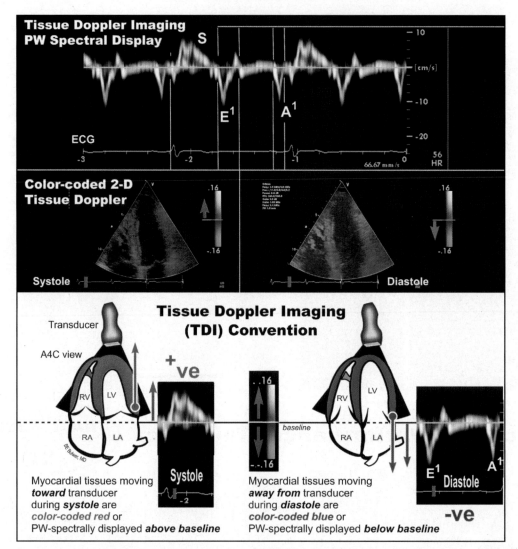

FIG. 14.13 Doppler tissue imaging or tissue Doppler imaging *(TDI)* as a measure of left ventricular systolic function. TDI employs Doppler principles to assess myocardial velocities. The Doppler sample volume placed at either the septal or lateral mitral annulus (MA) records longitudinal myocardial velocities during the cardiac cycle. This typically reveals three primary waveforms. The first is the S, representing the systolic contraction velocity; the second is E_1, representing the diastolic relaxation velocity during early mitral inflow; and the third is A_1, representing the late diastolic relaxation velocity during atrial contraction. The same TDI data can be color-coded (blue away-red toward transducer) to assess ventricular wall movements (color-coded two-dimensional tissue Doppler). *(Courtesy of Bernard E. Bulwer, MD, FASE.)*

The contractile mechanics of the LV myocardium—where a mere 13% shortening of the cardiac sarcomere (the contractile unit of the myocardium) results in some 20% longitudinal and circumferential shortening, and in excess of 40% radial thickening, resulting in the ejection of more than 60% of the LV end-diastolic volume—is attributable to the double-helical architecture of the LV myofibers (Fig. 14.14). LV systolic mechanics occurs along four principal cardiac vectors, longitudinal and circumferential shortening, radial thickening, and torsion (differential rotation). Quantification of the systolic mechanics of the LV along these principal vectors is the basis of cardiac deformation imaging in health and disease (Figs. 14.9 and 14.15).

GLOBAL MEASURES OF LEFT VENTRICULAR SYSTOLIC FUNCTION

Myocardial Strain Imaging

Myocardial deformation, or strain, imaging is a relatively novel yet promising method for assessment of cardiac function. Strain refers to the percent deformation between two regions and reflects shortening in myocardial muscle (see Fig. 14.15). Myocardial strain can be assessed by Doppler methods in which myocardial tissue velocities in multiple regions are integrated to obtain change in distance (Fig. 14.16). Doppler-based assessments of myocardial strain are relatively noisy and require dedicated acquisition during scanning, thus limiting their usefulness. In addition, Doppler-derived strain information is angle dependent.

In contrast, strain imaging based on speckle-tracking techniques has proved to be much more robust and reliable, although it has poorer temporal resolution than Doppler-based techniques do, thus limiting its use at high heart rates. Nevertheless, 2D methods have virtually replaced Doppler-based strain assessments for most applications. These techniques take advantage of the coherent speckle within the myocardial tissue signature to determine regions that are contracting versus those that are moving passively (Figs. 14.17 and 14.18).

Myocardial strain measures have been validated with sonomicrometry, and strain can be estimated in the longitudinal, circumferential, and radial directions by using the appropriate imaging plane (see Figs. 14.9 and 14.15). Speckle methods can also be used to assess ventricular twist and torsion or the wringing motion of the heart during contraction and relaxation (see Fig. 14.18).

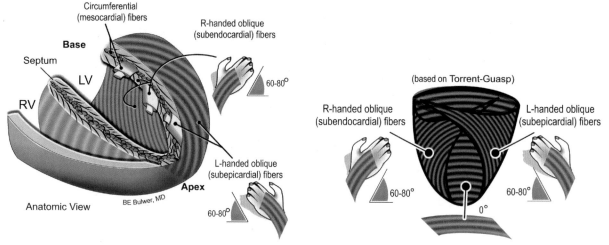

FIG. 14.14 The heart is described, using the Torrent-Guasp model, as single helical band wrapped in what can be described as a figure-of-eight arrangement. The myocardial architecture consists of three interwoven but macroscopically discernible layers. When viewed from the apex, the outer left ventricular myofibers of the myocardium, that is, the subepicardial layer are oriented in a left-handed oblique helical arrangement. These fibers assume a horizontal orientation in the middle layer, becoming oriented as right-handed oblique helical arrangement in the innermost subendocardial layer of the myocardium. *LV,* Left ventricle; *RV,* right ventricle. (*Courtesy of Bernard E. Bulwer, MD, FASE.*)

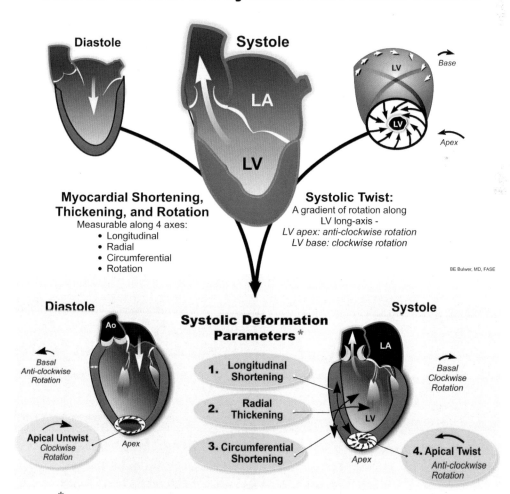

FIG. 14.15 Cardiac motion is complex, involving translational movements of the whole heart along with the diaphragm during respiration, as well as LV deformation, *shortening, thickening,* and *twisting* during systole. *Bottom panel:* Such myocardial deformation that can be measured along four axes using deformation imaging, speckle tracking imaging *(STI). Ao,* Aorta; *LA,* left auricle; *LV,* left ventricle. (*Courtesy of Bernard E. Bulwer, MD, FASE.*)

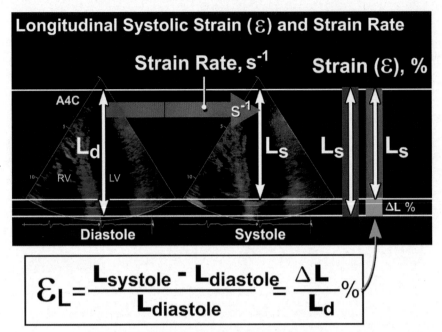

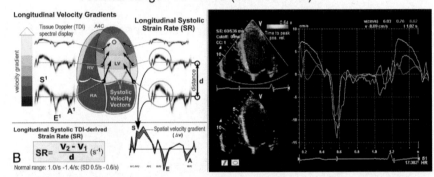

FIG. 14.16 Tissue Doppler imaging *(TDI)*-derived longitudinal systolic strain *(ε)* and strain rate *(SR)*. (A) During systole, the left ventricle *(LV)* shortens, thickens, and twists. *Above right:* Longitudinal systolic strain (ε_L) is the total amount of LV shortening that occurs during ventricular systole. It is a comparison of the diastolic length ($L_{diastole}$ or L_d) to the systolic length ($L_{systole}$ or L_s) and as represented in the equation *(below)*. *Above left:* The rate of this change in length, or the spatial velocity gradient, is the SR. (B) TDI can be used to assess myocardial velocity, as well as myocardial strain and SR using the apical four-chamber views. SR is derived directly from the velocity measured at two different points; strain represents the integration of SR with respect to time. The instantaneous A-velocity gradient exists from LV apex to base as measured by TDI, with higher velocities at the base compared to the relatively stationary apex. Note the color-coded velocity depiction and differential tissue Doppler velocities at different levels within the LV *(upper left panel)*. The difference or velocity gradient within two adjacent points within the sample volume of myocardium (during ventricular systolic shortening) can be quantified using a regression calculation from the velocity data obtained by TDI *(lower left panel and right panel)*. This spatial velocity gradient is called the SR, and the SR curve reflects the rate of longitudinal deformation or LV systolic shortening and lengthening during the cardiac cycle. By convention, SR shortening is negative during systole and positive during diastolic lengthening. The total amount of shortening or lengthening during the cardiac cycle or strain (S or ε) is obtained by the integration of this curve. *4AC,* Apical four-chamber; *RV,* right ventricle. *(Courtesy of Bernard E. Bulwer, MD, FASE.)*

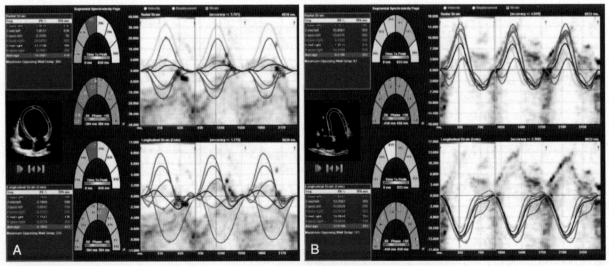

FIG. 14.17 Assessment of myocardial strain from the apical four-chamber view using a 2D-based speckle-tracking imaging technique. Average radial and longitudinal strain is calculated from six different regions in the ventricle. The waveforms depicted demonstrate both the timing and magnitude of peak strain in these regions. A shows a patient with cardiomyopathy before therapy with a cardiac resynchronization device. B shows the same patient after 12 months of CRT with dramatic improvement in ventricular synchrony.

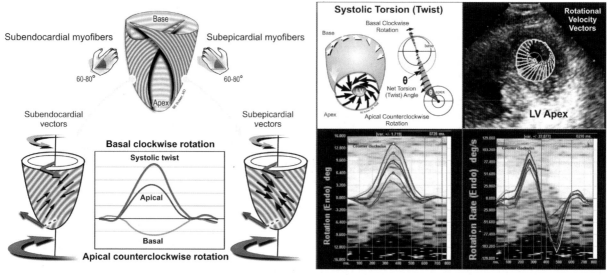

FIG. 14.18 Ventricular torsion (or twist) can be assessed by comparing the rotation occurring at the base of the heart with that occurring at the apex. Rotation at two locations can be assessed by speckle tracking echocardiography. Rotation and the rate of rotation can be assessed and displayed. *LV*, Left ventricle. *(Modified from Bulwer BE, Solomon SD. Assessment of systolic function. In: Solomon SD, ed. Atlas of Echocardiography. 2nd ed. Philadelphia: Current Science/Springer Science; 2009:63.)*

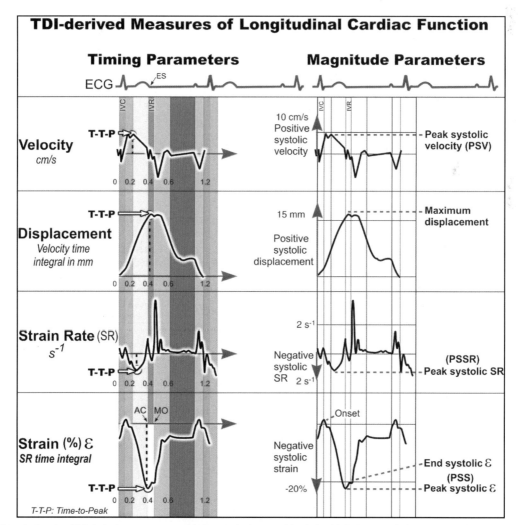

FIG. 14.19 Tissue Doppler imaging (TDI)-derived parameters, starting from top to bottom: (1) velocity, (2) displacement (velocity × time), (3) strain (ε), change in length-shortening or thickening, and (4) strain rate *(SR)* rate of myocardial deformation. Tissue velocities (by TDI) indicate myocardial motion but do not distinguish motion of healthy versus nonviable myocardium that moves along passively. Strain *(ε)* and SR measures can distinguish true contractile tissue motion from motion simply due to tethering. These measures have promising applications in patients with coronary artery disease. *AC*, Aortic valve closure; *ES*, end systole; *IVC*, isovolumetric contraction; *IVR*, isovolumetric relaxation; *MO*, mitral valve opening; *S*, peak systolic velocity. *(Courtesy of Bernard E. Bulwer, MD, FASE.)*

Longitudinal strain can be assessed with the A4C view, and global longitudinal strain has emerged as an important measure of cardiac performance that has been shown to add incremental value to standard measures such as the ejection fraction. Current equipment both assesses regional strain and calculates global longitudinal strain either by averaging regional strain or by determining the percent difference in the endocardial perimeter between systole and diastole. Longitudinal deformation reflects function of the subendocardial myocardial fiber bands primarily, whereas circumferential deformation, best assessed on short-axis views, may reflect the function of more epicardial layers (see Figs. 14.9 and 14.17).

Several diseases have been associated with a reduction in global longitudinal myocardial function as estimated by strain, including hypertension, diabetes mellitus, renal insufficiency, infiltrative cardiomyopathies, valvular heart disease, and hypertrophic cardiomyopathy (HCM). These measures also appear to predict survival or the development of heart failure in patients following MI and correlate with the burden of scar.

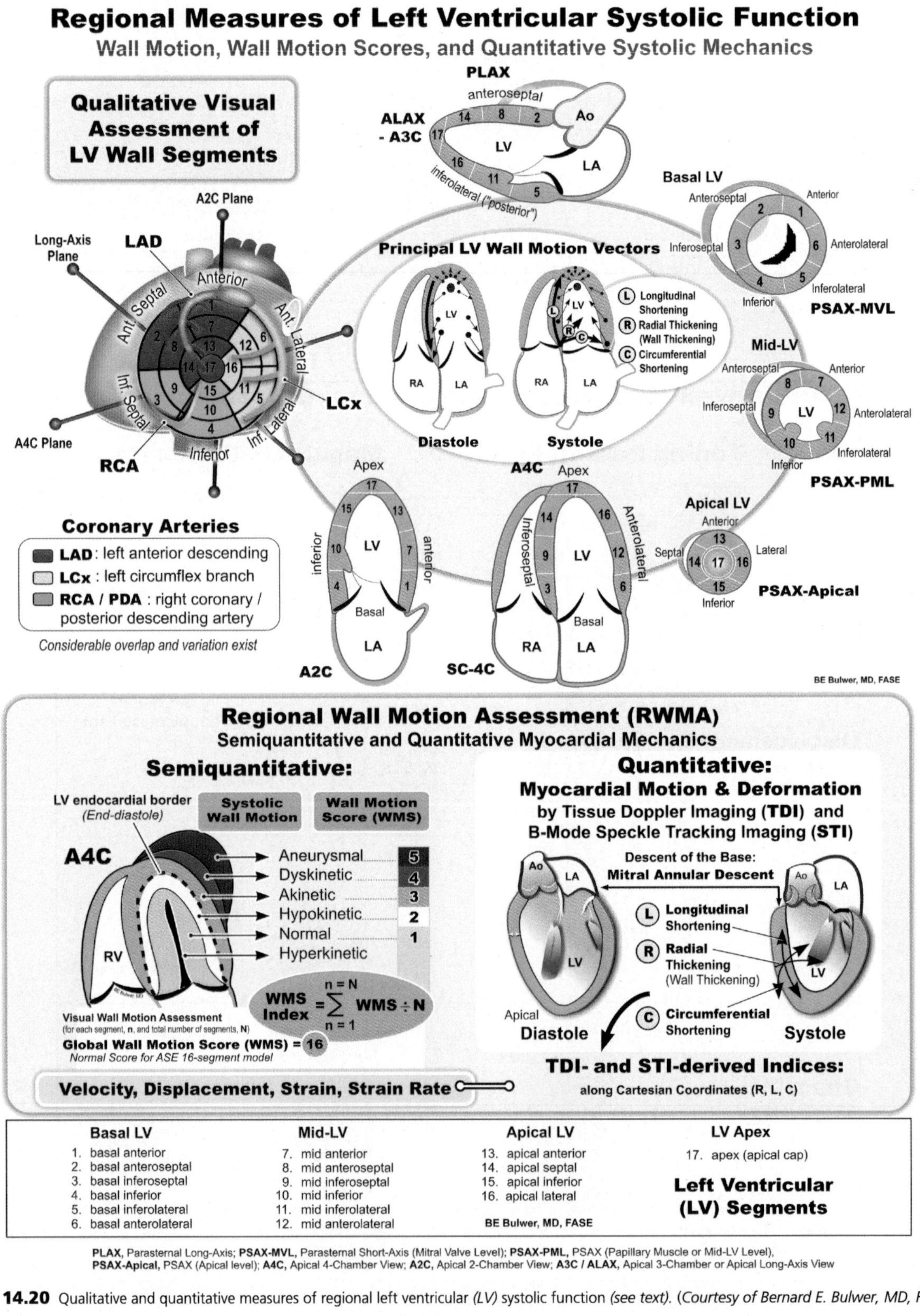

Regional Measures of Left Ventricular Systolic Function
Wall Motion, Wall Motion Scores, and Quantitative Systolic Mechanics

FIG. 14.20 Qualitative and quantitative measures of regional left ventricular (LV) systolic function (see text). (Courtesy of Bernard E. Bulwer, MD, FASE.)

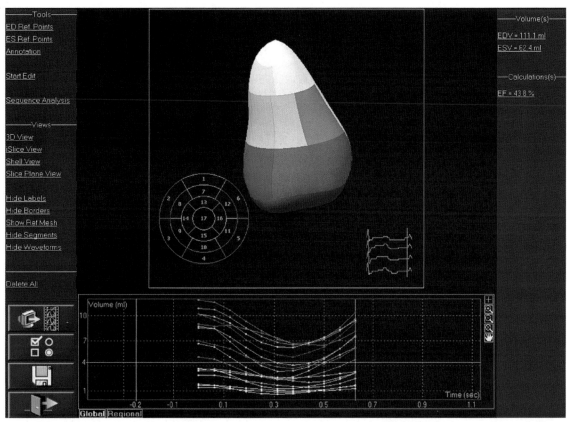

FIG. 14.21 Global and regional measures of left ventricular (LV) volumes can be quantified using novel three-dimensional speckle tracking techniques. Each LV segment depicted above *(upper panel)* can be tracked and its contribution to global left ventricular volumes and ejection fraction quantified and plotted *(lower panel)*.

Myocardial deformation imaging has been used recently for the evaluation of cardiac synchrony by assessing the time to peak strain (reflective of maximal contraction) across many cardiac regions. Both regional timing, reflecting synchrony, and myocardial peak strain, reflecting contractile function, have prognostic significance in patients undergoing cardiac resynchronization therapy (CRT) (Fig. 14.19; see Chapters 6, 15, and 25), and these data have been used to identify those who will benefit most from CRT.

In addition to assessment of global function, strain imaging can be used to assess and quantify regional function. Regional strain has been shown to correlate with the degree of myocardial scar in patients with ischemic heart disease (see Chapter 6) and in HCM (see Chapter 23). These measures can also be used to assess ischemia in the setting of stress echocardiography. An offshoot of myocardial strain imaging has been the quantitative assessment of ventricular twist and torsion (see Figs. 14.9 and 14.15). There are several limitations of strain imaging based on 2D echocardiography. First, myocardial deformation occurs in three dimensions and out-of-plane movement is lost. Second, these measures are subject to the same limitations as conventional ultrasound images, including frame rate and image quality. Finally, although deformation imaging is offered by most ultrasound vendors, as well as by several off-line systems, there is a lack of standardization in technique, data acquisition, and normal values among vendors. As strain imaging measures become standardized and these techniques become more refined and automated, their usefulness and applicability will increase.

REGIONAL MEASURES OF LEFT VENTRICULAR SYSTOLIC FUNCTION

Even though measures of global LV function provide quantification of overall cardiac performance and have prognostic value, regional function can vary substantially, such as in ischemic heart disease or other focal processes. Acute MI can cause regional wall motion abnormalities in a coronary distribution, with very specific myocardial regions being associated with specific coronary artery distributions (see Chapters 18, 19, and 20; Fig. 14.20). Regional wall motion may be assessed qualitatively or

semiquantitatively with a scoring system. The most popular current scoring system is based on a 17-segment model advocated by the American Society of Echocardiography (ASE) in which each segment is scored as normal (one point), hypokinetic (two points), akinetic (three points), or dyskinetic (four points) (Figs. 14.20 and 14.21). The wall motion score index (WMSI) is equal to the sum of these grades divided by the number of segments visualized, so a normokinetic ventricle should have a score of 1.0. A WMSI of 1.7 or higher is usually associated with the physical examination findings of heart failure. This score also has prognostic value, and a higher score is an independent predictor of mortality and morbidity, including increased hospitalization for heart failure, following MI.

The main goal of detecting regional myocardial dysfunction is to identify patients with coronary artery disease (CAD). Nevertheless, assessment of regional wall motion cannot easily distinguish between old and new wall motion abnormalities, although local myocardial thinning and increased brightness consistent with substantial scar tissue can be suggestive of chronic infarction. Typically, MI is associated with discrete regions of severe hypokinesis, akinesis, or even dyskinesis with a discernible "border" or hinge point. Regional wall motion abnormality can be apparent even within the first few minutes of acute MI, thus making assessment of regional wall motion particularly suited for diagnosis in the acute setting, for example, in patients with acute chest pain and equivocal abnormalities on the electrocardiogram (ECG) in whom a discrete regional wall motion abnormality might argue for early intervention (see Chapters 18 and 19). Although MI, either acute or old, is the most likely reason for regional wall motion abnormalities, other conditions such as myocarditis or sarcoidosis can affect the myocardium regionally, but not generally in a clear coronary distribution. Additionally, the LV dysfunction that can accompany valvular or hypertensive heart disease may also be regionally variable.

Assessment of regional wall motion is particularly important in stress echocardiography, in which induced regional wall motion abnormalities in the setting of exercise-induced or pharmacologic stress indicate myocardial ischemia. In stress echocardiography, regions are compared before and after stress in a

ASSESSMENT OF CARDIAC STRUCTURE AND FUNCTION

III

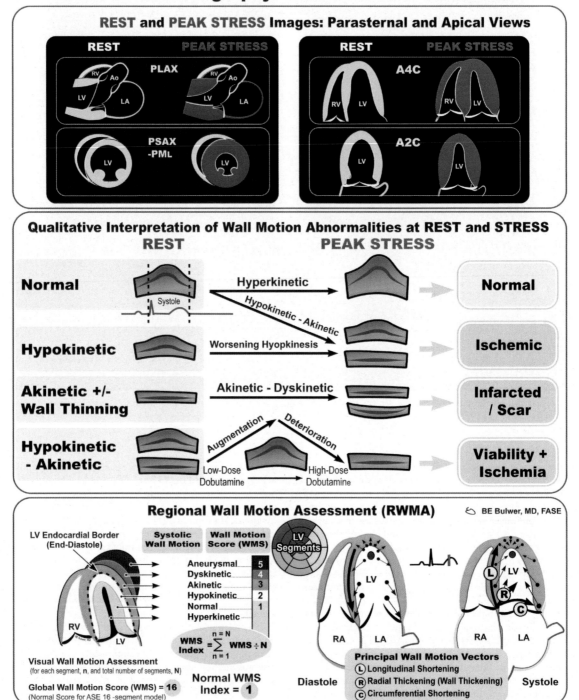

Stress Echocardiography and Wall Motion Assessment

REST and PEAK STRESS Images: Parasternal and Apical Views

Qualitative Interpretation of Wall Motion Abnormalities at REST and STRESS

Regional Wall Motion Assessment (RWMA)

FIG. 14.22 Regional wall motion assessment in stress echocardiography *(see text). A2C,* Apical two-chamber; *A4C,* apical four-chamber; *Ao,* aorta; *LA,* left auricle; *LV,* left ventricle; *PLAX,* parasternal long-axis; *PSAX,* parasternal short-axis; *PML,* papillary muscle; *RA,* right auricle; *RV,* right ventricle. *(Courtesy of Bernard E. Bulwer, MD, FASE.)*

side-by-side fashion, and wall segments with unchanged or worsening systolic function are compared qualitatively and scored (Fig. 14.22; see Chapter 27).

Suggested Reading

Buckberg, G. D., Weisfeldt, M. L., Ballester, M., et al. (2004). Left ventricular form and function: scientific priorities and strategic planning for development of new views of disease. *Circulation, 110,* e333–e336.

Kirkpatrick, J. N., Vannan, M. A., Narula, J., & Lang, R. M. (2007). Echocardiography in heart failure: applications, utility, and new horizons. *Journal of the American College of Cardiology, 50,* 381–396.

Lang, R. M., Badano, L. P., Mor-Avi, V., et al. (2015). Recommendations for cardiac chamber quantification by echocardiography in adults: an update from the American Society of Echocardiography and the European Association of Cardiovascular Imaging. *Journal of the American Society of Echocardiography, 28*(1), 1–39.

Lang, R. M., Bierig, M., Devereux, R. B., et al. (2005). Recommendations for chamber quantification: a report from the American Society of Echocardiography's Guidelines and Standards Committee and the Chamber Quantification Writing Group, developed in conjunction with the European Association of Echocardiography, a branch of the European Society of Cardiology. *Journal of the American Society of Echocardiography, 18,* 1440–1463.

Marwick, T. H. (2006). Measurement of strain and strain rate by echocardiography: ready for prime time? *Journal of the American College of Cardiology, 47,* 1313–1327.

Moore, C. C., Lugo-Olivieri, C. H., McVeigh, E. R., & Zerhouni, E. A. (2000). Three-dimensional systolic strain patterns in the normal human left ventricle: characterization with tagged MR imaging. *Radiology, 214,* 453–466.

Sengupta, P. P., Korinek, J., Belohlavek, M., et al. (2006). Left ventricular structure and function: basic science for cardiac imaging. *Journal of the American College of Cardiology, 48,* 1988–2001.

Tei, C., Ling, L. H., Hodge, D. O., et al. (1995). New index of combined systolic and diastolic myocardial performance: a simple and reproducible measure of cardiac function—a study in normals and dilated cardiomyopathy. *Journal of Cardiology, 26,* 357–366.

Thomas, J. D., & Popovic, Z. B. (2006). Assessment of left ventricular function by cardiac ultrasound. *Journal of the American College of Cardiology, 48,* 2012–2025.

Torrent-Guasp, F., Ballester, M., Buckberg, G. D., et al. (2001). Spatial orientation of the ventricular muscle band: physiologic contribution and surgical implications. *The Journal of Thoracic and Cardiovascular Surgery, 122,* 389–392.

15 Left Ventricular Diastolic Function

Patrycja Z. Galazka, Amil M. Shah

INTRODUCTION

Echocardiography plays a central role in the assessment of left ventricular (LV) diastolic function, which is often a challenging task for the clinician. Normal diastolic function allows for the LV to sufficiently fill and to generate the necessary stroke volume without exceeding certain pressure limits during filling. Diastolic dysfunction primarily results from increased resistance to ventricular filling, leading to an upward and leftward shift of the LV pressure volume relation, often during exercise or tachycardia.[1] The physiological hallmarks of LV diastolic dysfunction are impaired relaxation, loss of restoring forces, reduced diastolic compliance, and elevated filling pressure.[2] When LV and left atrial (LA) pressures start to increase, patients may develop dyspnea and/or pulmonary congestion. The assessment of diastolic function has become particularly relevant, as approximately half of patients with heart failure have normal or near normal ejection fraction (HFpEF),[3,4] a condition in which diastolic dysfunction is thought to be a key pathophysiologic mediator.[5,6] Diastolic function is multifaceted, and there is no one echocardiographic measure that fully captures diastolic dysfunction. However, by using a combination of different echocardiographic indexes, diastolic performance can be reasonably estimated in most patients.

WHAT IS DIASTOLIC FUNCTION AND DYSFUNCTION?

For normal cardiac performance, the LV should be able to eject an adequate stroke volume at arterial pressure (systolic function) and fill without requiring elevated LA pressure (diastolic function). Systolic and diastolic function must be adequate to meet the needs of the body both at rest and during stress.[1] Diastole denotes the portion of the cardiac cycle between aortic valve closure and subsequent mitral valve closure, during which time the myocardium does not generate force or shorten and returns to its unstressed length (Fig. 15.1). Diastolic function consists of both an early period of active relaxation, which is an adenosine triphosphate-dependent process that is also partially dependent on diastolic suction or restoring forces, and diastolic chamber compliance, which is operant throughout the diastolic period and determined by the elastic properties of the myocardium.[2] Traditionally, these two aspects of diastolic function were evaluated by invasive hemodynamic assessment: the isovolumic relaxation rate of pressure decline (tau) as a measure of active relaxation, and the LV diastolic pressure-volume relationship as a measure of compliance (Fig. 15.2).[6] Impairment in active relaxation results in prolongation of the tau, while decrease in LV diastolic compliance is reflected in an upward and leftward shift of the LV pressure-volume relationship (Fig. 15.3). Impairments in either or both of these components of LV diastolic performance can lead to slowed or incomplete LV diastolic filling, unless also accompanied by an increase in LA pressure. However, these methods are invasive, resource intensive, and not practical for routine or widespread clinical application.

Echocardiographic Measures of Diastolic Performance

Echocardiography allows for the noninvasive evaluation of LV diastolic performance and diastolic filling pressure with use of conventional two-dimensional (2D) imaging combined with spectral, tissue, and color Doppler. Several echocardiographic measures have been proposed as markers of diastolic performance.[7] In the following sections, we will review the measures routinely employed in the clinical evaluation of diastolic function and recommended by professional society guidelines.

Transmitral Doppler: E Wave Peak Velocity, A Wave Peak Velocity, and E/A Ratio

Pulsed wave spectral Doppler allows for the assessment of the instantaneous LA-to-LV pressure gradient throughout the diastolic period and characterization of patterns of LV diastolic filling (see Fig. 15.1).[8,9] Mitral inflow Doppler should be obtained from the apical four-chamber view with color flow imaging to optimally align the pulse wave sample volume (1–3 mm) between the tips of the mitral leaflets.[10] The E wave is the peak early filling velocity, a measure of the peak LA to LV diastolic pressure gradient, and is therefore influenced by LA pressure at mitral valve opening, minimal LV diastolic pressure, compliance of the LA, and the rate of LV relaxation.[10–12] The rate of decrease of velocity following the E wave is measured as the deceleration time (Fig. 15.4). The A wave is the velocity at atrial contraction (AC), which usually occurs after relaxation is completed, and is influenced by LV chamber compliance and the volume and contractility of the left atrium.[10] The normal mitral flow pattern (i.e., the height of the E wave and A wave, and the relationship between these) varies with loading conditions, age, and heart rate.[13–15] In a normal middle-aged subject, the E velocity is slightly larger than the A velocity, and the deceleration time is 200 ± 40 ms.[10] Mitral inflow E/A ratio and deceleration time (DT) have been used to define LV filling patterns as normal, impaired relaxation, pseudonormal, and restrictive filling,[16] which correspond to progressively higher filling pressure (Fig. 15.5). The

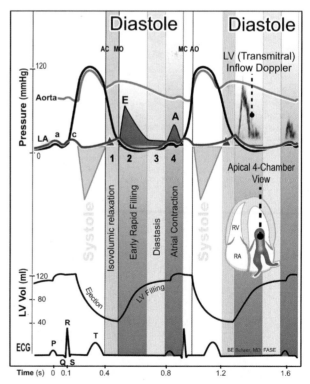

FIG. 15.1 Simultaneous representation of electrocardiography, left ventricular (LV; *black line*), left atrial (LA; *blue line*), and ascending aortic (Ao; *red line*) pressure, spectral Doppler of mitral inflow and left ventricular outflow tract outflow, and LV volumes. Diastole can be divided into four phases: isovolumic relaxation (IVR), rapid filling, diastasis, and atrial contraction (AC). *ECG,* Electrocardiogram; *RA,* right atrial; *RV,* right ventricle. *(Courtesy of Bernard E. Bulwer, MD, FASE.)*

age dependency of normal for these filling patterns cannot be overstated. The definitions provided below apply primarily to persons in middle age.

"Impaired relaxation," also termed mild or grade 1 diastolic dysfunction, is characterized by a transmitral flow pattern with a low E wave, high A wave, low E/A ratio, and a prolonged deceleration time.[10] These findings reflect a slower rate of decrease of LV early diastolic pressure, such that the duration of relaxation is prolonged into mid- or even late diastole, in the absence of elevation in LA pressure. As a result, early diastolic driving force across the mitral valve is reduced and the E wave is lower. There is a compensatory increase in transmitral flow at AC from the high residual atrial preload, resulting in a high A wave.

Worsening diastolic dysfunction is characterized by progressive decrease in the effective operative LV chamber compliance resulting in increased mean LV and LA diastolic pressures. A high LA pressure at the time of mitral valve opening and a large LA–LV gradient in early diastole results in a high E wave, shortened deceleration time, and higher E/A ratio, producing a pattern similar to a normal inflow pattern and termed "pseudonormalized."[10] Until the advent of tissue Doppler imaging (TDI; see later), distinguishing a normal from a "pseudonormal" pattern relied on pulmonary vein Doppler patterns (see below) and changes in the inflow pattern associated with the Valsalva maneuver, which decreases

preload during the strain phase. A decrease of 50% in the E/A ratio with Valsalva is highly specific for a pseudonormal filling pattern (Fig. 15.6).[17]

Finally, the restrictive filling pattern, due to advanced abnormality of LV compliance and markedly elevated LA pressure, is characterized by a high E wave, a short deceleration time, and a small A wave.[10] An E wave greater than twice the A wave amplitude or a deceleration time <150 ms identifies a restrictive pattern of filling.

Limitations to assessing LV filling patterns with peak E and A waves, and E/A ratio, include sinus tachycardia and first-degree atrioventricular (AV) block, which can result in partial or complete fusion of the E and A waves.[18] Also, as previously mentioned, age must be acknowledged when assessing diastolic function, as filling patterns in even healthy elderly persons at low risk for heart failure may resemble mild diastolic dysfunction in younger patients.[19–21] With increasing age, the mitral E velocity and E/A ratio decrease, while DT and A velocity increase.

Tissue Doppler Imaging e′

Tissue Doppler-based mitral annular early relaxation velocity (e′) is a measure of the rate of early diastolic lengthening of LV. As the change in length of the LV has a direct relationship with the change in volume of the LV, e′ is a correlate of the dV/dt and of tau.[22] As such, e′ reflects both

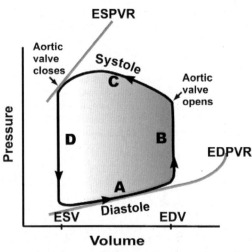

FIG. 15.2 Schematic representation of the normal left ventricular pressure volume relationship. *A,* Diastolic filling period which includes rapid filling, diastasis, and atrial contraction. *B,* Isovolemic contraction period. *C,* Systolic ejection period. *D,* Isovolumic relaxation period. *EDV,* End-diastolic volume; *EDPVR,* end-diastolic pressure-volume relationship; *ESV,* end-systolic volume; *ESPVR,* end-systolic pressure-volume relationship. (*From Ho CY. Echocardiographic assessment of diastolic function. In: Solomon SD, ed.* Essential Echocardiography: A Practical Handbook With DVD. *Totowa, NJ: Humana Press; 2007:119–132.*)

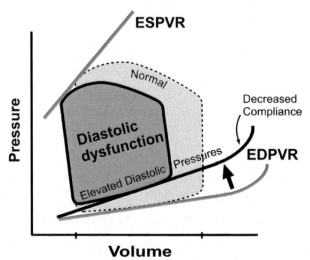

FIG. 15.3 Characteristic alteration in the left ventricular (LV) pressure-volume relationship characterizing isolated diastolic dysfunction. Decreased LV diastolic compliance is evidenced by an upward and leftward shift of the LV end-diastolic pressure-volume relationship. Note that the LV end-systolic pressure-volume relationship is unchanged, indicated preservation of systolic function. *EDPVR,* End-diastolic pressure-volume relationship; *ESPVR,* end-systolic pressure-volume relationship. (*From Ho CY: Echocardiographic assessment of diastolic function. In: Solomon SD, ed.* Essential Echocardiography: A Practical Handbook With DVD. *Totowa, NJ: Humana Press; 2007:119–132.*)

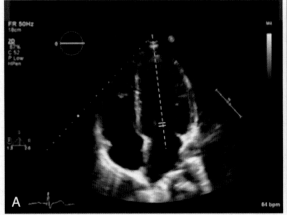
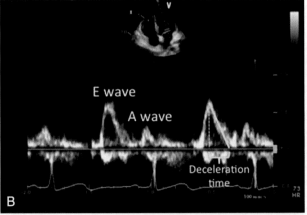

FIG. 15.4 Pulsed-wave Doppler assessment of mitral inflow. (A) Assessment occurs in the apical four-chamber view, with the pulsed-wave sample volume at the tip of the mitral leaflets in diastole. (B) Normal mitral inflow pattern showing the *E* wave (the peak early filling velocity), deceleration time (the rate of decrease of velocity following the E wave), and the *A* wave (the peak velocity at atrial contraction).

LV restoring forces and active relaxation. Lower e' is related to worse diastolic function in a monotonic fashion, and e' is therefore helpful in discerning normal from pseudonormal mitral inflow patterns as noted above (Fig. 15.7). As TDI measures the low-velocity, high-amplitude signal of myocardial tissue, high-velocity and low-amplitude signals of blood must be filtered. Annular velocities are typically measured at both the septal and lateral aspects of the mitral annulus in the apical four-chamber view (Fig. 15.8).[18] Similar to standard Doppler, the accuracy of tissue Doppler is dependent on a parallel angle of incidence of the ultrasound beam to myocardial motion. Therefore, the longitudinal motion of the LV must be optimally aligned with the ultrasound beam, and the tissue Doppler sample volume (typically 5–10 mm axial size) must be appropriately placed at the level of annulus. Septal e' is normally lower than lateral e'. Per American Society of Echocardiography (ASE) 2016 guidelines, the abnormal values are considered: septal $e' < 7$ cm/s and lateral $e' < 10$ cm/s.[18] These cutpoints are likely most relevant to a middle-aged population.

Despite early data to the contrary, e' is affected by both preload[23] and afterload.[24] However, in the context of LV systolic dysfunction, e' appears less load dependent than the transmitral velocities.[25] Importantly, similar to the E/A ratio, prominent age-associated changes in the e' have been repeatedly observed in population-based studies. Older age is associated with lower septal and lateral e' values, even among persons free of cardiovascular disease or risk factors.[19,21,26,27] At the writing of this chapter, it remains unclear whether these age-associated changes are prognostically benign or represent malignant cardiac senescence, although their presence even among persons at low clinical risk for incident cardiovascular disease perhaps suggests the former. Regardless, these age-related changes make interpretation of e' in the elderly particularly challenging, particularly as existing guideline recommendations for defining abnormal e' do not necessarily recognize these age-related differences.[18]

E/e' Ratio

The early diastolic transmitral flow by Doppler (E wave) reflects the early diastolic LA to LV pressure gradient and is therefore affected by both LA pressure and LV early diastolic relaxation. As e' is primarily a measure of early diastolic relaxation, dividing the E wave by e' (E/e' ratio) provides an estimate of LA pressure.[22] One advantage of E/e' ratio over the E/A ratio as an index of LV filling pressure is that it is monotonically related to LA pressure. Several studies have demonstrated robust correlation between E/e' ratio and invasively measured LV pressure in patients with heart failure.[28–30] However, several studies in patients with less pronounced abnormalities of LV filling pressure have failed to demonstrate a robust association of E/e' with LA pressure or pulmonary artery wedge pressure (PAWP) or of changes in E/e' with changes in PAWP.[23,31] Therefore, this measure is likely most useful in evaluating LV filling pressure when either clearly high or low.

As TDI e' is typically lower at the septal annulus than the lateral annulus, E/e' is normally lower when using the lateral e' compared to the septal e'. Per ASE 2016 guidelines, abnormal values for E/e' include: average E/e' ratio >14, lateral E/e' ratio >13, and septal E/e' ratio >15.[18] Importantly, conditions that alter either early diastolic transmitral flow (significant mitral regurgitation or stenosis, prior mitral repair or replacement) or e' (e.g., pericardial disease) make the E/e' ratio less reliable.

Left Atrial Size

Doppler-based measures reflect instantaneous pressure gradients and myocardial motion. In contrast, LA size is felt to be more stable over time, with LA enlargement reflective of chronic elevations in LA pressure and (in the absence of significant mitral valve disease) LV diastolic pressure.[10] LA size can be measured by the LA anterior-posterior dimension in the parasternal long axis view or the LA maximal volume using the biplane Simpson's method or the area-length method from the apical four-chamber and two-chamber views at end systole. As chamber size varies physiologically with body size, current guidelines favor the use of the LA volume indexed to body surface area as the primary measures of LA size in evaluating diastolic function. Per ASE 2016 guidelines, LA volume index >34 mL/m² is considered abnormal.[18]

Color M-Mode Propagation Velocity

In the setting of diastolic dysfunction, the rate of propagation of blood into the LV is diminished, a phenomenon that can evaluated by color M-mode Doppler echocardiography performed in the apical four-chamber view

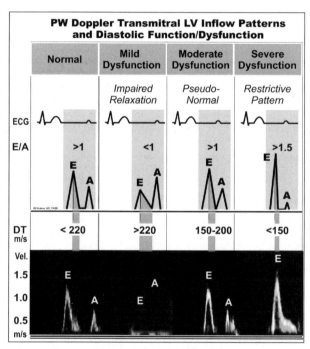

FIG. 15.5 Left ventricle diastolic filling patterns (normal, impaired relaxation, pseudonormal, and restrictive filling). See text for details. *ECG,* Electrocardiogram; *LV,* left ventricle; *PW,* pulsed wave. *(Courtesy of Bernard E. Bulwer, MD, FASE.)*

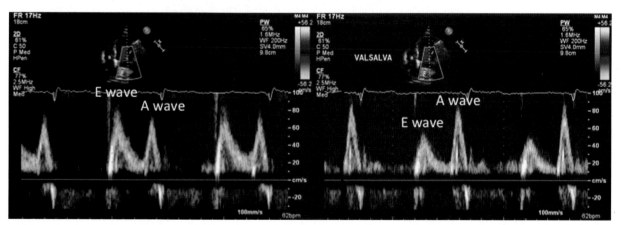

FIG. 15.6 Use of Valsalva maneuver to uncover pseudonormal left ventricular diastolic filling pattern. At baseline, *E/A* ratio is 1.1 *(left)* and decreases to 0.6 (impaired relaxation pattern; *right*) with Valsalva.

(Fig. 15.9).[32] Color M-mode Doppler recordings show the early diastolic LA to LV flow stream, the slopes of which are functions of the transit rate of intracardiac LV filling.[33] Color M-mode Doppler recordings exhibit a striking reduction in the slope of early filling with restrictive diastolic dysfunction and a milder reduction in the presence of impaired relaxation. Flow propagation velocity (Vp) is measured as the slope of the first aliasing velocity during early filling, measured from the mitral valve plane to 4 cm into the LV cavity.[18] Alternatively, the slope of the transition from no color to color can be measured. Vp >50 cm/s is considered normal.[34] In most patients with depressed LV ejection fraction (LVEF), Vp is reduced, and should other Doppler indices appear inconclusive, an E/Vp ratio >2.5 predicts PAWP >15 mm Hg with reasonable accuracy.[7] The Color M mode Doppler is not routinely used in patients with normal LV volume and LVEF, where Vp may be normal despite elevated LV filling pressure.[18]

Pulmonary Venous Flow

Primary measurements of pulmonary venous waveforms include peak systolic (S) velocity, peak anterograde diastolic (D) velocity, the S/D ratio, and the peak Ar velocity in late diastole (Fig. 15.10). Pulsed-wave Doppler of pulmonary venous flow is performed in the apical four-chamber view.[18] A 2–3-mm sample volume is placed 5 mm into the pulmonary vein for optimal recording of the spectral waveforms. In normal subjects, pulmonary venous recordings consist of forward systolic (S) and diastolic (D) flow velocities of approximately equal magnitudes, with a short, low-velocity flow reversal into the veins after atrial contraction (atrial reversal wave, Ar). In contrast, in patients with increased LA pressure and simultaneous impaired relaxation causing pseudonormalization, pulmonary vein Doppler demonstrates A wave reversal of increased duration and velocity, often with a diminished S wave (see Fig. 15.10).[33] Indeed, a pulmonary venous A flow reversal greater in duration than the duration of the forward transmitral A wave has been shown to indicate an elevated LV end-diastolic pressure, and the magnitude of the difference has been related to the magnitude of pressure elevation.[35] This occurs because in the setting of increased LV end-diastolic pressure, greater LV impedance favors reversed flow into the pulmonary veins rather than forward transmitral flow after atrial contraction. While this augmented flow reversal may manifest as a greater velocity, it is most reliably evidenced by a greater flow duration.

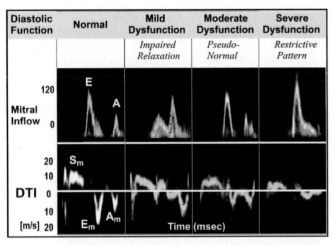

FIG. 15.7 Integration of Left ventricle (LV) diastolic filling pattern with tissue Doppler-based LV relaxation velocities. Tissue-Doppler e′ distinguishes normal from pseudonormal LV filling patterns. Unlike the E/A ratio, e′ demonstrates as monotonic association with diastolic dysfunction, such that worse diastolic function is associated with lower e′. Note: time scales are not the same for mitral inflow (diastolic period only) and Doppler tissue imaging (DTI) (full cardiac cycle). *(From Ho CY. Echocardiographic assessment of diastolic function. In: Solomon SD, ed. Essential Echocardiography: A Practical Handbook With DVD. Totowa, NJ: Humana Press; 2007:119–132.)*

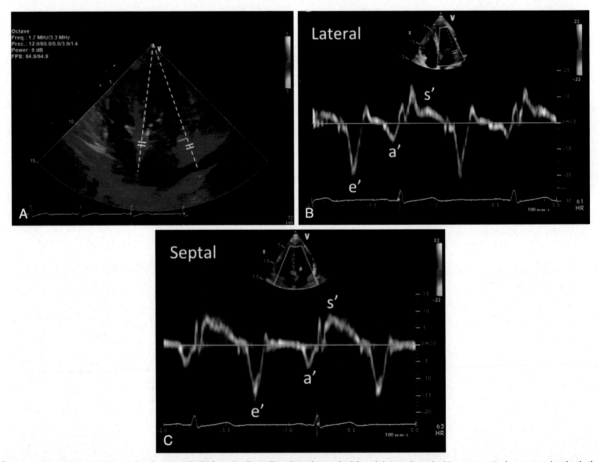

FIG. 15.8 Tissue Doppler acquisition of Left ventricle (LV) early diastolic relaxation velocities. (A) Annular velocities are routinely measured at both the septal and lateral aspects of the mitral annulus in the apical four-chamber view, with the tissue Doppler sample volume (typically 5–10 mm axial size) placed approximately at the level of annulus. The longitudinal motion of the LV must be optimally aligned with the ultrasound beam. Normal lateral (B) and septal (C) mitral annular tissue Doppler profile with e′ (peak early diastolic relaxation velocity), a′ (peak late diastolic velocity), and s′ (peak systolic velocity).

Published studies suggest that pulmonary venous flow can be obtained in 80% of ambulatory patients, though the feasibility is much lower in the intensive care unit setting.[36] Therefore, one of the important limitations in interpreting pulmonary venous flow is the difficulty in reliably obtaining high-quality recordings suitable for measurements.

Tricuspid Regurgitation Velocity

The peak tricuspid regurgitation velocity reflects the peak systolic right ventricle (RV) to right atrial (RA) pressure gradient and, when combined with an estimate of RA pressure, can be used to estimate RV systolic pressure and pulmonary artery (PA) systolic pressure in the absence of pulmonic stenosis. Per ASE 2016 guidelines, tricuspid regurgitation (TR) velocity >2.8 m/s is considered abnormal.[18] While the presence of pulmonary hypertension is not itself a measure of LV filling pressure or diastolic performance, group 2 pulmonary hypertension is a recognized complication of chronically elevated LA pressures. Therefore, in the absence of concomitant pulmonary vascular disease, the presence of pulmonary hypertension may be a secondary indicator of elevated LV filling pressure.[18] However, it is important to recognize that primary pulmonary vascular disease (e.g., group 1 pulmonary hypertension), pulmonary parenchymal disease (obstructive or restrictive, which can lead to group 3 pulmonary hypertension), and pulmonary thromboembolic disease all may coexist in patients with heart failure (HF) and are in the differential diagnosis of patients with dyspnea. Appropriate clinical judgment is therefore necessary before using the presence of pulmonary hypertension as an indicator of LV diastolic function.

Prognostic Relevance of Echocardiographic Measures of Diastolic Performance

Each of the key measures of diastolic function discussed previously has been associated with adverse prognosis across a range of cardiovascular disorders. Among heart failure patients with both reduced and preserved LVEF, short deceleration time, *e′* velocity, LAVi, and elevated PA systolic pressure are all predictive of adverse outcomes including mortality and hospitalization.[37–39] Doppler-based markers of elevated filling pressure, the *E/A* ratio, and *E/e′* ratio are also associated with HF hospitalization or death in HFrEF and HFpEF.[37,39] The *E/A* ratio, *e′*, and *E/e′* ratio are also predictive of incident HF in community-based studies.[16,40–42]

Grading Diastolic Function

Several schema have been employed to combine these individual measures of diastolic performance into an integrated diastolic grade. An early method employed in the Olmsted County study (Fig. 15.11) incorporated *E/A* ratio, DT, *E/e′* ratio, pulmonary venous flow pattern, and changes with Valsalva maneuver to grade diastolic function as normal, mild dysfunction (impaired relaxation), moderate dysfunction (pseudonormal), or severe dysfunction (restrictive filling).[16] Using this classification approach, these investigators have demonstrated the prognostic

relevance of worse diastolic grade[16] and longitudinal worsening of diastolic grade[40] for incident heart failure in a community-based sample. One limitation of this approach includes the need for multiple measures of diastolic function that may not be uniformly obtainable.

The American Society of Echocardiography (ASE) and European Association of Cardiovascular Imaging (EACVI) have also published guidelines for the integrated grading of diastolic dysfunction (Figs. 15.12 and 15.13).[7,18] The original guidelines from 2009 incorporated many of the same measures in their classification scheme,[7] while a recent update in 2016 aimed to simplify the approach to evaluation of diastolic function and increase the utility of these guidelines in daily clinical practice.[18] The approach recommended in these contemporary guidelines is presented in some detail later in the chapter. However, it is important to recognize that these recommendations are based largely on expert consensus and, as of the writing of this chapter, few prospective data with clinical outcomes can validate this approach.

Determining Diastolic Function in Patients With Normal Left Ventricle Systolic Function

In evaluating diastolic function, age and hemodynamic parameters, such as heart rate and blood pressure, must be considered, as they may significantly affect diastolic performance. Also, the quality of each parameter should be well assessed and, if inadequate, those parameters should not be used. The ASE/EACVI updated 2016 guidelines recommend four parameters be evaluated when determining diastolic function in patients with normal systolic function: TDI *e′*, *E/e′* ratio, LA volume index, and TR velocity.[18] LV diastolic function is considered normal if more than half of the available parameters are within the normal cutoff values, inconclusive if exactly half of the parameters do not meet the cutoff criteria, and abnormal if more than half parameters are abnormal. Fig. 15.12 demonstrates the recommended approach to determining LV diastolic function in patients with normal systolic function.[18]

Assessing Left Ventricle Filling Pressures and Diastolic Dysfunction Grade in Abnormal Systolic Function

In patients with reduced LVEF, diastolic function will be abnormal. The main reason for evaluating diastolic measures in these patients is to estimate LV filling pressure. Since mean left atrial pressure (LAP) correlates better with PAWP as compared to LV end-diastolic pressure (LVEDP), algorithms to estimate LV filling pressures assumes the estimation of mean LAP. ASE/EACVI guidelines recommend using mitral inflow velocities, mitral *e′* velocity, mitral *E/e′* ratio, LA volume index, and peak TR velocity (see Fig. 15.13).[18] In most cases, mitral inflow pattern including *E/A* ratio and peak *E* wave velocity should be sufficient to estimate LV filling pressure in patients with reduced LVEF. In patients with intermediate values for *E/A* ratio and *E* wave velocity, evaluation of additional measures of filling pressure, *E/e′* ratio, LAVi, and TR velocity is recommended. Notable situations in which this approach to estimating filling pressures is problematic include

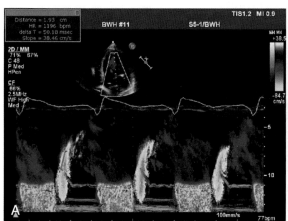
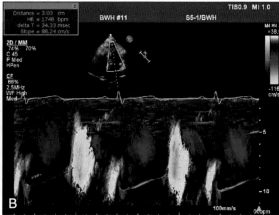

FIG. 15.9 Color M-mode. (A) Normal color M-mode Doppler with a slope of 88 cm/s in a patient with normal systolic and diastolic function. (B) Abnormal color M-mode Doppler with slope of 38.5 cm/s in a patient with history of severe left ventricular systolic dysfunction and restrictive physiology.

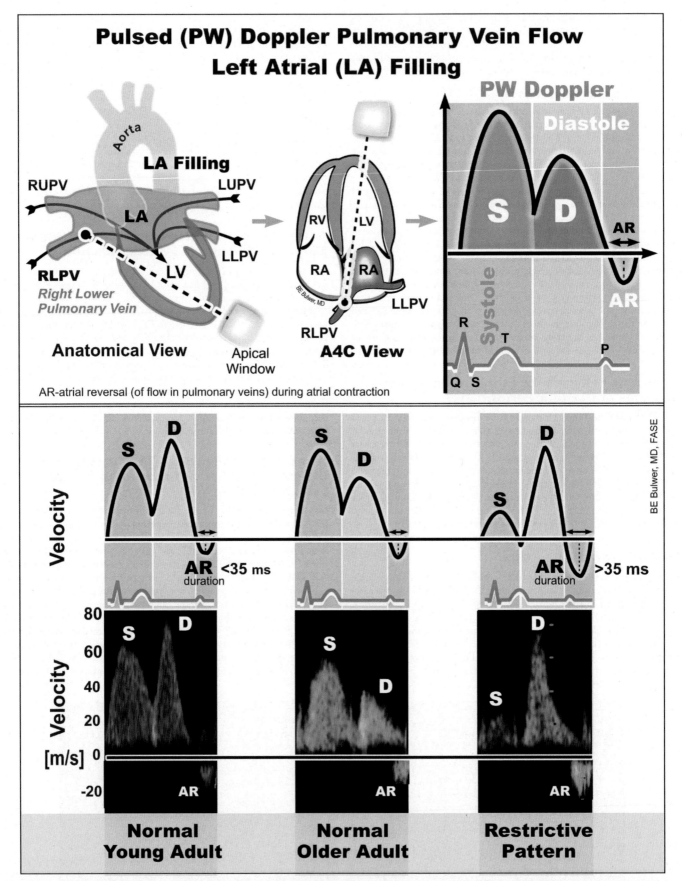

Pulsed (PW) Doppler Pulmonary Vein Flow
Left Atrial (LA) Filling

PW Doppler

Diastole

LA Filling

Aorta

RUPV   LUPV

LA

LLPV

RLPV

Right Lower Pulmonary Vein

LV

Anatomical View

Apical Window

RV   LV

RA   RA

LLPV

RLPV

A4C View

S   D

AR

AR

Systole

R   T   P

Q   S

AR-atrial reversal (of flow in pulmonary veins) during atrial contraction

Velocity

S   D

S   D

S

D

AR <35 ms
duration

AR
duration   >35 ms

Velocity

80

S   D

S

D

D

60

S

40

S

20

[m/s] 0

-20   AR   AR   AR

Normal Young Adult   **Normal Older Adult**   **Restrictive Pattern**

BE Bulwer, MD, FASE

FIG 15.10 Doppler assessment of pulmonary venous flow pattern. *Upper left panel,* Pulsed-wave Doppler of pulmonary venous flow is performed in the apical four-chamber view, with the sample volume (2–3 mm) placed ~5 mm into the pulmonary vein. *Upper right panel,* Pulmonary venous waveforms include *S* wave (peak systolic velocity), *D* wave (peak anterograde diastolic velocity), and Ar (late diastolic flow reversal at atrial contraction). *Bottom panel,* Pulmonary venous flow pattern and alterations in flow pattern with diastolic dysfunction. See text for details. *Ar,* Atrial reversal; *LA,* left atrial; *LLPV,* left lower pulmonary vein; *LUPV,* left upper pulmonary vein; *LV,* left ventricle; *RA,* right atrial; *RLPV,* right lower pulmonary vein; *RUPV,* right upper pulmonary vein; *RV,* right ventricle. *(Courtesy of Bernard E. Bulwer, MD, FASE.)*

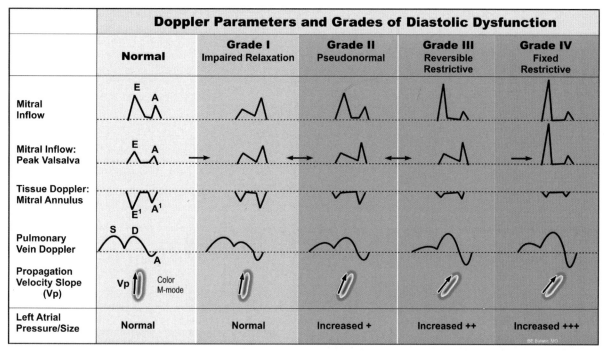

FIG. 15.11 Doppler criteria for classification of diastolic function. (*Courtesy of Bernard E. Bulwer, MD, FASE; Data from Redfield MM, Jacobsen SJ, Burnett JC, Jr, Mahoney DW, Bailey KR, Rodeheffer RJ. Burden of systolic and diastolic ventricular dysfunction in the community: appreciating the scope of the heart failure epidemic. JAMA. 2003;289(2):194–202.*)

atrial fibrillation, moderate or greater mitral valve calcification, moderate or greater mitral stenosis or regurgitation, prior mitral valve repair or replacement, LV assist devices, left bundle-branch block, and paced rhythms.[18]

Estimation of Left Ventricle Filling Pressures in Specific Patient Populations

Atrial Fibrillation

Atrial fibrillation is also often associated with diastolic dysfunction, and the presence and severity of diastolic dysfunction are independently predictive of first documented nonvalvular atrial fibrillation in the elderly.[43] However, assessing diastolic dysfunction in patients with atrial fibrillation can be difficult. Beat-to-beat variability in stroke volume results in significant associated variability in Doppler-based measures (E wave, e', E/e', DT), and the E/A ratio cannot be assessed due to the absence of the A wave. In addition, the specificity of LA enlargement for elevated LV filling pressures is lower, as ongoing arrhythmia and absent organized atrial activity itself may contribute to LA enlargement. It is crucial to average parameters over several cardiac cycles and to use matched R-R intervals. The DT (<160 cm/s) and TR peak velocity (>2.8 m/s) have been identified as particularly useful for assessing filling pressure in this context.[44,45]

AV Block and Pacing

Abnormally short PR interval (<120 ms) may result in early termination of atrial filling by LV contraction with resulting reduction in A wave amplitude and duration.[18] With an unusually long PR interval (typically >320 ms), diastolic mitral regurgitation may occur. These alterations in E and A velocities preclude accurate evaluation of filling pressure using mitral inflow Doppler.

Valvular Disease

Moderate to severe mitral annular calcification limits assessment of diastolic dysfunction, related to higher mitral inflow velocities due to mitral annular restriction and lower mitral annular velocities caused by decreased mitral annular motion.[46] Mitral stenosis separates LA pressure from LV diastolic pressure. Severe mitral regurgitation results in a larger volume of antegrade transmitral flow and associated elevation of E velocity. Regurgitation-associated elevation in LA systolic pressure results in a decrease in pulmonary venous systolic velocity, decreasing S/D ratio and systolic pulmonary flow reversal. Aortic stenosis should not hinder the assessment of diastolic dysfunction.

DIASTOLIC STRESS TESTING IN PATIENTS WITH NORMAL DIASTOLIC FUNCTION AT REST: IS THERE A ROLE?

Routine evaluation of diastolic dysfunction is performed at rest. However, patients frequently develop symptoms such as dyspnea only with exertion, and in a subset of patients, diastolic abnormalities may only be unmasked with exercise. Much interest has focused on the use of exercise echocardiography to noninvasively assess changes in LV filling pressure with exercise. These investigations have largely focused on changes in E wave, e', and E/e' ratio at rest and with exercise.[47] With exercise, E and e' are normally expected to increase proportionally such that the ratio remains constant.[48] Some studies have noted good correlation of changes in E/e' with changes in invasively measured LVEDP, with $E/e' > 13$ accurately identifying raised LVEDP (>15 mm Hg).[49] However, other studies have found no association between changes in E/e' and changes in invasively measured PAWP, calling into question the utility of this measure.[23,31] Differences in the hemodynamic response–based position (supine vs. upright) and exercise modality (cycle ergometry vs. treadmill), differential behavior of the primary diastolic measures (E, e', E/e' ratio) in different patient populations, and difficulties in ascertainment due to E-A fusion at higher heart rates are all important limitations in the application and interpretation of a "diastolic stress test." Therefore, while exercise echocardiography holds promise for the evaluation of exercise-induced elevations in LA pressure, further evaluation for feasibility, accuracy, and diagnostic utility is necessary.

CONCLUSION

Echocardiography is the most common modality employed clinically to assess LV diastolic function. Several measures reflecting LV diastolic properties are routinely available, including transmitral Doppler flow pattern, tissue Doppler early relaxation velocities, and LA size. These measures are prognostic of adverse outcomes across a range of cardiovascular disorders. However, context must be accounted for in interpreting these measures, including age, rhythm, and concomitant cardiac pathology, and no one echocardiographic measure fully captures diastolic dysfunction. However, by using a combination of different echocardiographic indexes, diastolic performance can be reasonably estimated in most patients.

For patients with normal LVEF:

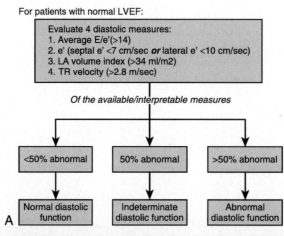

Evaluate 4 diastolic measures:
1. Average E/e'(>14)
2. e' (septal e' <7 cm/sec *or* lateral e' <10 cm/sec)
3. LA volume index (>34 ml/m2)
4. TR velocity (>2.8 m/sec)

Of the available/interpretable measures

<50% abnormal	50% abnormal	>50% abnormal

Normal diastolic function	Indeterminate diastolic function	Abnormal diastolic function

A

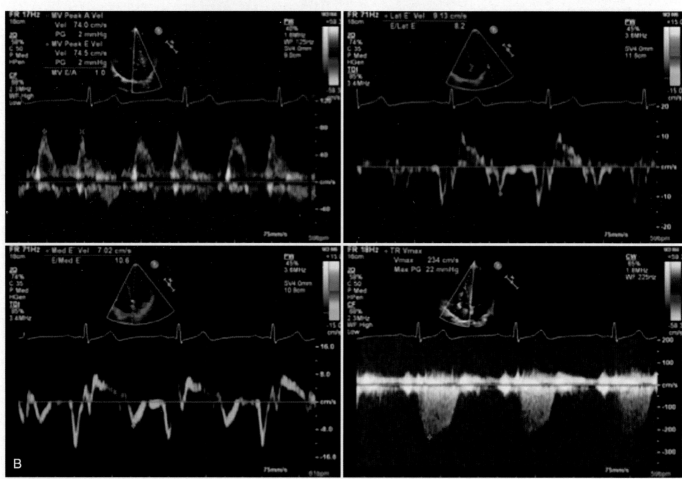

B

FIG. 15.12 American Society of Echocardiography (ASE) and European Association of Cardiovascular Imaging (EACVI) Guideline recommendations for diagnosing diastolic dysfunction. (A) Proposed algorithm proposed by the Guidelines. (B) Example of a patient with normal diastolic indices (septal *e'* >7 cm/s, lateral *e'* >10 cm/s, average *E/e'* ratio <14 cm/s, and peak TR velocity <2.8 m/s). *LA,* Left atrial; *TR,* tricuspid regurgitation. ([A] Adapted from Nagueh SF, Smiseth OA, Appleton CP, et al. Recommendations for the evaluation of left ventricular diastolic function by echocardiography: an update from the American Society of Echocardiography and the European Association of Cardiovascular Imaging. J Am Soc Echocardiogr. 2016;29(4):277–314.)

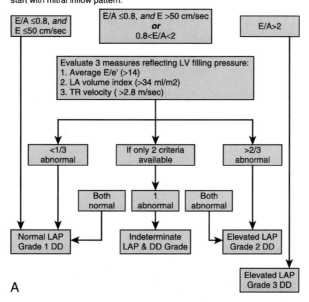

For patients with reduced LVEF,
start with mitral inflow pattern:

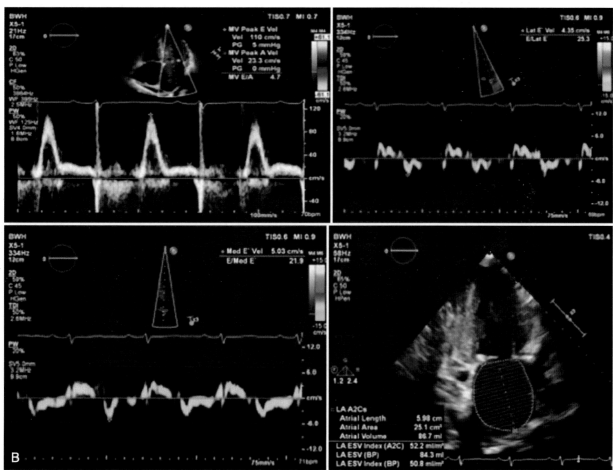

FIG. 15.13 American Society of Echocardiography (ASE) and European Association of Cardiovascular Imaging (EACVI) Guideline recommendations for evaluating LV filling pressure in patients with reduced LVEF. (A) Proposed algorithm proposed by the guidelines. (B) Example of a patient with Grade III diastolic dysfunction (*E/A* ratio >2; also supportive are E wave deceleration time ~140 cm/s, *E/A* ratio >2, *E/e′* ratio >20, and severe left atrial enlargement). *LA*, Left atrial; *LV*, left ventricle. (*[A] Adapted from Nagueh SF, Smiseth OA, Appleton CP, et al. Recommendations for the evaluation of left ventricular diastolic function by echocardiography: an update from the American Society of Echocardiography and the European Association of Cardiovascular Imaging. J Am Soc Echocardiogr. 2016;29[4]:277–314.*)

Suggested Readings

Kane, G. C., Karon, B. L., Mahoney, D. W., et al. (2011). Progression of left ventricular diastolic dysfunction and risk of heart failure. *JAMA: The Journal of the American Medical Association, 306,* 856–863.

Nagueh, S. F., Appleton, C. P., Gillebert, T. C., et al. (2009). Recommendations for the evaluation of left ventricular diastolic function by echocardiography. *Journal of the American Society of Echocardiography, 22,* 107–133.

Redfield, M. M., Jacobsen, S. J., Burnett, J. C., Jr., et al. (2003). Burden of systolic and diastolic ventricular dysfunction in the community: appreciating the scope of the heart failure epidemic. *JAMA: The Journal of the American Medical Association, 289,* 194–202.

A complete reference list can be found online at ExpertConsult.com.

16 Assessment of Right Ventricular Structure and Function

Judy R. Mangion

INTRODUCTION

The assessment of right ventricular (RV) structure and function is one of the most critical roles of echocardiography, often impacting the diagnosis, management, and prognosis of patients with suspected cardiovascular disease. Historically, the echocardiographic assessment of diseases affecting the RV has lagged behind that of the left ventricle, despite knowledge demonstrating that diseases affecting the right heart have been shown to have the same clinical consequences of those affecting the left heart.[1-4] More recently, the assessment of RV structure and function has been an active area of investigation. The geometry of the RV is very complex, even in normal subjects, and even more complex in diseased states, which makes it especially difficult to assess with two-dimensional (2D) echocardiographic techniques. The RV myocardium is thin-walled and has a circumferential arrangement of myofibers in the subepicardium and longitudinal fibers in the endocardium (Fig. 16.1). It assumes a flattened pear-shaped appearance folded over the left ventricle and consists of three components: (1) an inlet portion consisting of the tricuspid valve, chordae tendineae, and papillary muscles; (2) a trabecular apical myocardium; and (3) an infundibulum or conus, which encompasses the smooth walled RV outflow tract beneath the pulmonic valve (Fig. 16.2).[6] The need for

careful and comprehensive echocardiographic evaluation of RV systolic function occurs in multiple clinical settings, including suspected RV cardiomyopathy, inferior wall myocardial infarction, atrial and ventricular septal defects, complex congenital heart disease, as well as valvular heart disease. Systolic dysfunction of the RV is also frequently observed in acute pulmonary embolism, pulmonary hypertension, and arrhythmogenic right ventricular dysplasia (ARVD), as well as in intraoperative settings.[7-9] Despite the obvious need for accurate quantitative information, the assessment of RV systolic function is frequently more difficult to obtain due to the irregular crescent shape of this chamber, making quantitative assessment based on geometric remodeling especially challenging, although newer technologies have attempted to overcome these challenges.

CLINICAL ASSESSMENT OF RIGHT VENTRICULAR ANATOMY AND FUNCTION

Today, in the majority of clinical settings, the assessment of RV anatomy and systolic function by echocardiography is still most often performed qualitatively with 2D techniques and relies on the scanning ability of the sonographer and trained interpretive eye of the

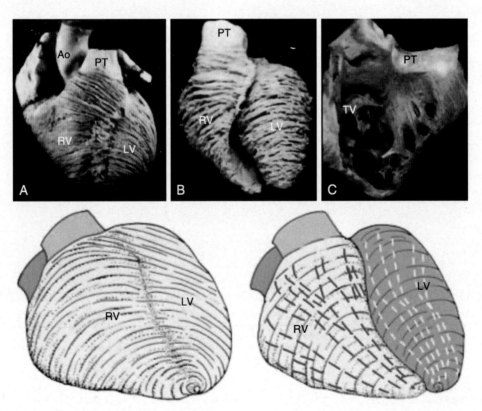

FIG. 16.1 Gross anatomic specimens of the right ventricle (RV) demonstrating circumferential arrangement of subepicardial myofibers (A and B) and longitudinal arrangement of myofibers in the subendocardium (C). *Ao,* Aorta; *LV,* left ventricle; *PT,* pulmonary trunk; *TV,* tricuspid valve. (*Courtesy of Bernard E. Bulwer, MD, FASE.*)

echocardiographer.[10] There is, however, increasing demand for more quantitative assessments of RV structure and function, and newer technologies, including RV strain and three-dimensional (3D) imaging of the right ventricle, have made the quantitative assessment of RV structure and systolic function more efficient, easy to obtain, and reproducible.[11]

The ability to accurately assess global and regional RV systolic function with echocardiography requires continuous practice and attention

to detail, with frequent correlation of coronary anatomy, other imaging tests, and pathologic findings. Knowledge of coronary flow to the RV and the use of multiple echocardiographic views to ensure that the entire RV is visualized are essential.

It is especially important to recognize that RV systolic dysfunction may be regional in the setting of coronary artery disease as well as other clinical scenarios, such as pulmonary embolism. Standard transthoracic apical views tend to optimize visualization of the left

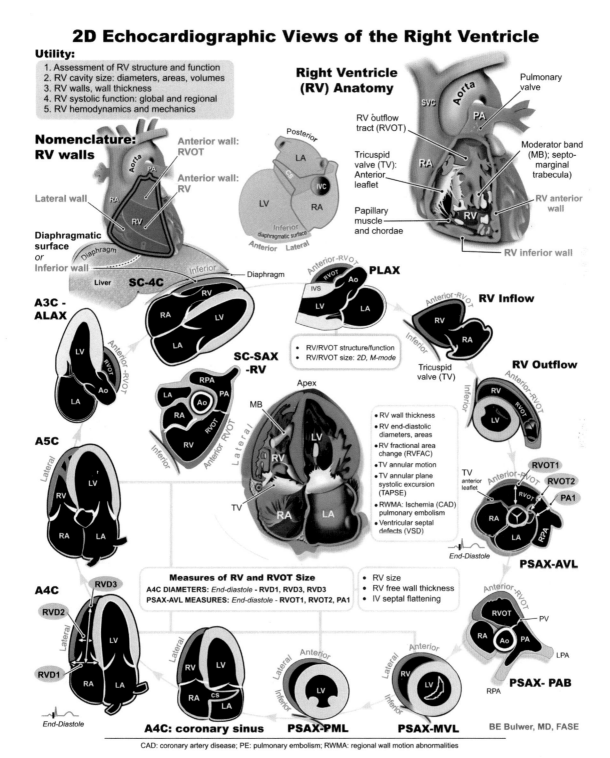

FIG. 16.2 Anatomy of the right ventricle (RV). The RV has three distinct parts, an inlet component including the tricuspid valve, chordae tendineae, and papillary muscles; an apical trabecular component including the apical myocardium; and an infundibular or outlet component, which includes the smooth RV outflow tract up to the pulmonic valve. *Ao,* Aorta; *IVS,* interventricular septum; *LA,* left atrial; *LV,* left ventricle; *PA,* pulmonary artery; *PLAX,* parasternal long axis; *PV,* pulmonic valve; *RA,* right atrial; *RPA,* right pulmonary artery. (*From Bulwer BE, Solomon SD, Janardhanan R. Echocardiographic assessment of ventricular systolic function. In: Solomon SD, ed. Essential Echocardiography: A Practical Handbook With DVD. Totowa, NJ: Humana Press; 2007:89–118.*)

ventricle, and the transducer may need to be moved more laterally to optimize visualization of the RV. Since the RV myocardium is thin, measurement of wall thickening is usually not practical, and endocardial excursion alone must be evaluated. The interventricular septum is also frequently flattened in the setting of RV systolic dysfunction, and this creates challenges to the accurate assessment of systolic function. Despite these challenges, a complete evaluation of the RV should be a routine part of every comprehensive echo study, and with practice, overall accuracy will improve.

Coronary Flow to the Right Ventricle

The echocardiographer must think about RV anatomy in the context of coronary flow to the RV. Coronary flow to the RV is unique in that it occurs in both systole and diastole.[12] The right coronary artery (RCA) provides predominant flow, supplying the lateral wall through acute marginal branches, and it also supplies the posterior wall and posterior interventricular septum through the posterior descending artery. The anterior wall of the RV is supplied by the conus artery branch of the RCA and by branches of the left anterior descending artery (Fig. 16.3).[13,14]

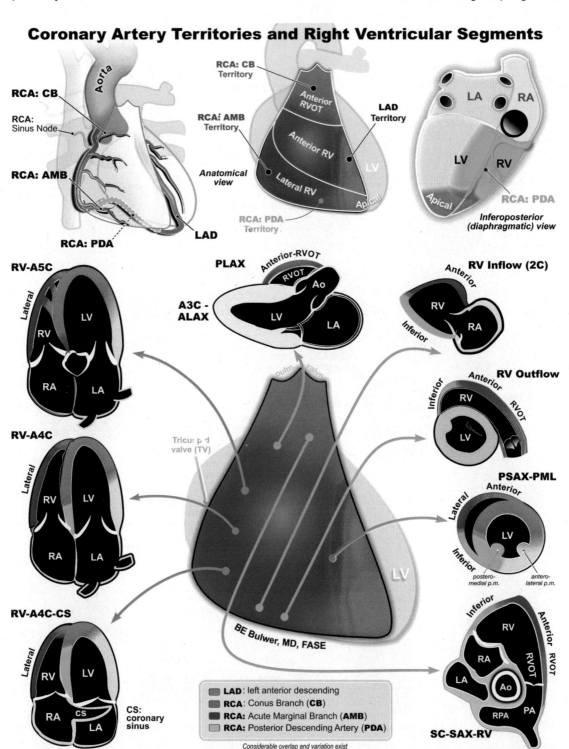

FIG. 16.3 Coronary flow to the right ventricle (RV). This is a postmortem specimen from a patient with a dominant right coronary artery (RCA), which occurs in 90% of the population. Here the posterior descending artery and posterior left ventricular branches originate from the RCA. The RCA supplies the predominant flow to the RV. The conus branch of the RCA and branches of the LAD supply the anterior wall of the RV, while the marginal branches of the RCA supply the lateral wall of the RV. The posterior descending branch (PDA) supplies the posterior wall of the RV and the posterior interventricular septum. *ALAX*, Apical long axis; *AMB*, acute marginal branch; *Ao*, aorta; *CB*, conus branch; *LA*, left atrial; *LAD*, left anterior descending; *LV*, left ventricle; *PDA*, posterior descending artery; *PML*, posterior medial; *RA*, right atrial. (*Courtesy of Bernard E. Bulwer, MD, FASE.*)

Right Ventricular Structure as Assessed by Two-Dimensional Echocardiography

The initial evaluation of global systolic performance of the RV includes measurement of the linear dimensions of the RV cavity (Fig. 16.4). A quick qualitative assessment of RV size is readily accomplished from the apical four-chamber view. In this view, the mid-cavity diameter of the RV should be smaller than the left ventricle. Quantitative measurements of the RV must be assessed from multiple views according to established protocols, as outlined in the recently published American Society of Echocardiography guidelines for chamber quantification, which include the assessment of RV size and systolic function, with new reference limits for RV chamber size, taking into account both gender and body surface area.[11]

RV anatomy must be thought of in segmental terms, just like the left ventricle. The segments of the RV are subdivided into an anterior wall, inferior wall, lateral wall, and RV outflow tract (Fig. 16.5). A segmental approach to the evaluation of RV systolic function begins with each of the standard 2D transthoracic views. In the parasternal long-axis view, the RV outflow tract is visualized. In the parasternal short-axis view, the anterior free wall, lateral free wall, and inferior free wall of the RV are visualized. In the RV inflow view, the anterior free wall and inferior free wall of the RV are visualized. In the standard apical four-chamber view, the lateral free wall and RV apex are visualized. In the subcostal four-chamber view, the inferior free wall of the RV or diaphragmatic surface of the RV is visualized (Videos 16.1–16.5). It should be emphasized that the standard apical four-chamber view optimizes the visualization of the left ventricle. To optimize the visualization of the RV, the transducer needs to be moved more laterally. This avoids dropout of the lateral free wall of the RV and RV apex (Figs. 16.6 and 16.7; Videos 16.6 and 16.7).

The extent of RV regional wall motion abnormalities has been shown to correlate with the site of coronary occlusion (Videos 16.8–16.11). Gemayel et al. studied 25 patients with clinical evidence of RV infarction, who underwent echocardiography and coronary angiography, and reported that RV infarction may be missed by echocardiography in approximately 20% of patients, when the RCA occlusion is distal, if the subcostal four-chamber view of the right ventricle is not adequately obtained, and, as a result, the inferior free wall of the right ventricle, supplied by the posterior descending branch, is not visualized. In such patients, in the apical four-chamber view, the lateral free wall of the right ventricle contracts normally, while the inferior free wall of the right ventricle, best seen in the subcostal view, will be akinetic (Fig. 16.8; Videos 16.12 and 16.13).[15]

Contrast Echocardiography for Right Ventricular Opacification

Echocardiographic contrast agents capable of opacifying the left ventricle and improving endocardial border definition following intravenous injection are valuable but are historically underutilized tools in echocardiography.[16] Recent data suggests the use of contrast echo in climbing again, and in 2015, contrast echo comprised 4.5% of the number of echo studies.[17] Despite the improvement in ability to improve the accuracy and reproducibility of echocardiographic structure and function, they are even less likely to be utilized to facilitate RV endocardial border definition.

Intravenous saline contrast is a less expensive tool that can also be used to facilitate visualization of the RV, although its effects last only seconds, whereas the echo contrast agents last several minutes. Imaging the RV with echo contrast agents requires slower injection of the contrast media to avoid attenuation artifact and requires optimizing transducer position for visualizing the RV (Fig. 16.9; Video 16.14). Otherwise, these agents are administered using the same ultrasound machine contrast presets as for the left ventricle. The recently US Food and Drug Administration (FDA)-approved contrast agent, *Lumason* (sulfur hexaflouride lipid A microspheres), appears to have advantages over other available contrast agents for assessing the RV due to substantially less attenuation artifact.

The American Society of Echocardiography has published both a consensus statement on the clinical applications of ultrasonic contrast agents and echocardiography, as well as guidelines for the cardiac sonographer in the performance of contrast echocardiography, both of which expertly describe how to best implement the use of these agents.[18,19] The vast majority of patients who can benefit from echo contrast can be reassured that these agents are extremely safe, and in fact safer than other agents used in alternative imaging studies, such as computed tomography scans, cardiac magnetic resonance imaging (MRI), nuclear cardiology scans, or coronary angiography. In general, echo contrast should not be administered intraarterially or in patients with known right-to-left or bidirectional shunts or in patients with a known history of allergy to perflutren or sulfur hexafluoride. The risk for serious cardiopulmonary reactions may be increased among patients with unstable cardiopulmonary conditions (acute myocardial infarction, acute coronary artery syndromes, worsening or unstable congestive heart failure, or serious ventricular arrhythmias). In the event of a hypersensitivity reaction to echo contrast (1 in 10,000), the infusion of contrast should be stopped immediately, and intravenous (IV) saline should be administered at 200 mL/h. Epinephrine (1:1000) should be administered at a dose of 0.1 mg subcutaneous or intramuscular every 5–10 minutes as needed up to four doses. Diphenhydramine should be administered 50 mg IV or IM once and methylprednisolone 40 mg IV should also be administered once.

Quantitative Assessment of Right Ventricular Systolic Function

Methods for quantitatively assessing RV systolic function with echocardiography have not traditionally been widely applied in clinical practice; however, newer technologies have recently become more automated, and quantitative assessment has become easier to obtain and more reproducible. As knowledge regarding the prognostic significance of RV systolic function has become more widespread, the demand for quantitative assessment will undoubtedly increase. Efforts have been hampered by the RV's geometrically complex structure, which is irregular, asymmetric, crescentric, and truncated in shape. The RV has reduced amplitude of normal contraction compared to the left ventricle, and the RV outflow tract comprises 25% of the entire volume of the RV.[20] Until relatively recently, echocardiography has been able to provide only planar 2D images.

One method that has been frequently used to quantify RV systolic function in clinical trials is fractional area change, and the RV area is traced at end diastole and end systole in the apical four-chamber view. The end-systolic area is subtracted from the end-diastolic area and then this value is divided by the end-diastolic area (Fig. 16.10). Normal values are 49 + 7 ± 7% or >35%.[11] An advantage of this method is that measurements are not squared. Nevertheless, these measurements are preload and afterload dependent.

Other quantitative 2D methods for assessing RV systolic function with echocardiography include a tricuspid annular plane systolic

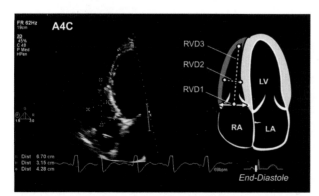

FIG. 16.4 Linear measurements of the right ventricle cavity are obtained from the apical four-chamber view and include basal and mid-cavity diameters as well as maximal long-axis diameters. *LA*, Left atrial; *LV*, left ventricle; *RA*, right atrial. (*Courtesy of Bernard E. Bulwer, MD, FASE.*)

Right Ventricle Walls: Nomenclature and Echocardiographic Views

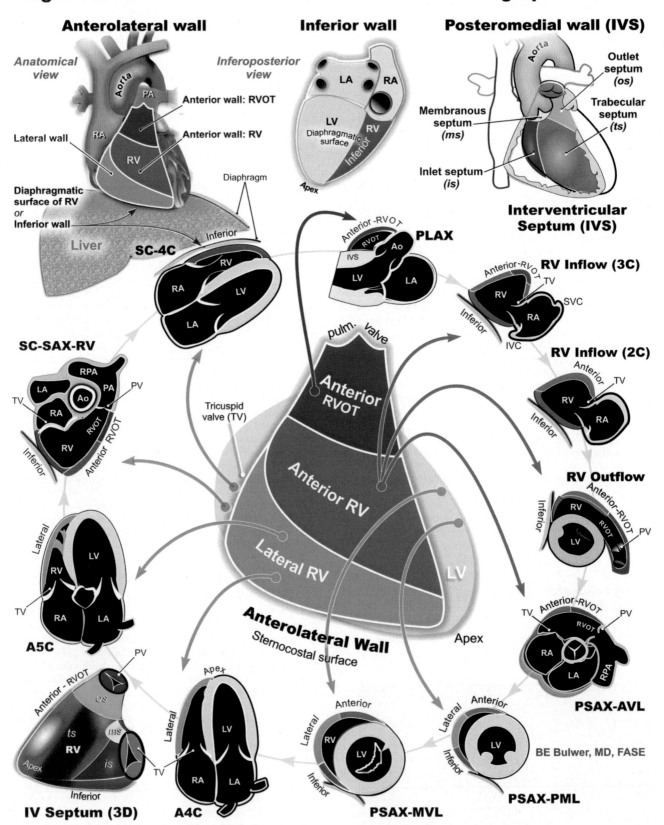

FIG. 16.5 Diagram illustrating right ventricle (RV) anatomy in segmental terms. The RV is subdivided into an anterior wall *(top, solid dots)*, inferior wall *(bottom, solid)*, lateral wall *(criss-cross)*, and right ventricular outflow tract (RVOT, *hollow dots*). *Ao*, Aorta; *LA*, left atrial; *LV*, left ventricle; *RA*, right atrial; *RV*, right ventricle; *RVOT*, right ventricle outflow tract; *TV*, tricuspid valve. *(Courtesy of Bernard E. Bulwer, MD, FASE.)*

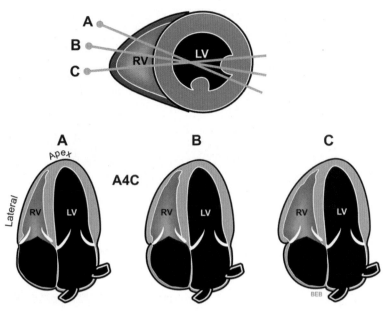

FIG. 16.6 In the apical four-chamber view, the lateral free wall is visualized. The transducer should be placed at the level of the tricuspid annulus to avoid underestimation of right ventricular size. *A*, Transducer above TV annulus; *B*, trasducer slightly above TV annulus; *C*, transducer at TV annulus (correct position); *LV*, left ventricle; *RV*, right ventricle. (*Courtesy of Bernard E. Bulwer, MD, FASE.*)

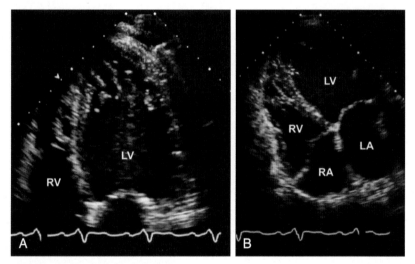

FIG. 16.7 The standard apical four-chamber view (A) optimizes visualization of the left ventricle (LV). To optimize visualization of the right ventricle (RV) you need to move the transducer more laterally, as this case illustrates (B). *LA*, Left atrial; *RA*, right atrial.

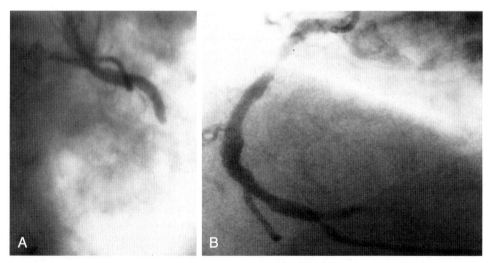

FIG. 16.8 Note the proximal occlusion of the right coronary artery in this patient (A). A more proximal right coronary artery (RCA) occlusion indicates a more extensive right ventricle (RV) infarction. (B) In contrast, the site of RCA occlusion in this patient is distal. This illustrates the importance of subcostal views in diagnosing RV infarction when the RCA occlusion is distal.

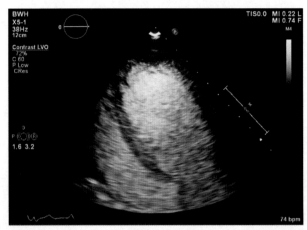

FIG. 16.9 Apical four-chamber view demonstrating ultrasound contrast enhancement of the right ventricle and left ventricle. The window should be optimized to enhance visualization of the right ventricle by moving the transducer more laterally. The contrast agent should be given slowly to avoid attenuation artifact.

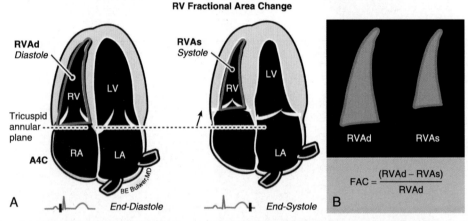

FIG. 16.10 **Quantification of right ventricle (RV) systolic function by measuring fractional area change.** The RV area is measured in end diastole (A) and end systole (B). The end-systolic area is subtracted from the end-diastolic area, and then this value is divided by the end-diastolic area. *LA,* Left atrial; *LV,* left ventricle; *RA,* right atrial; *RV,* right ventricle. (*Courtesy of Bernard E. Bulwer, MD, FASE.*)

excursion (TAPSE) in the apical four-chamber view and pulsed tissue Doppler S′ measurements (Fig. 16.11). These described the apex to base shortening of the right ventricle and provide an assessment of global RV systolic function. There are significant challenges associated with these measurements. Marked regional differences exist in the extensive fiber shortening within the right ventricle, with apical trabeculations making locating endocardial borders difficult. Furthermore, chamber orientation varies considerably between patients, and preload, afterload, and ventricular performance all affect these measurements.[20] Normal values for TAPSE is 24+ or –3.5 mm or >17 mm, and normal values for pulsed tissue Doppler S wave is 14.1 ± 2.3 or >9.5 cm/s.[11]

RV dP/dT may also provide useful information regarding RV systolic function, and may be calculated by using continuous wave Doppler of the tricuspid regurgitant jet; using a similar approach as that used for measuring left ventricular dP/dT, only the calipers are placed differently at 1 and 2 m/s or 12/T (T = time in seconds) with values measured in mm Hg/s (Fig. 16.12). In general, the normal range is 255 ± 17.5.[20, 21] It should be noted that values for RV dP/dT are influenced by the presence of pulmonary hypertension, and they are less reliable in this setting.

The Tei Index or myocardial performance index is a quantitative method for assessing RV systolic function, which is highly feasible in patients with poor image quality, providing accurate quantification of RV systolic function despite complex geometry. This calculation is the sum of the isovolumic contraction time and isovolumic relaxation time divided by the RV ejection time. It can be measured by measuring the tricuspid valve opening time and RV ejection time using pulsed wave Doppler of the tricuspid regurgitant jet and pulmonary outflow velocities (Fig. 16.13) or Tissue Doppler of the RV free wall at the level of the tricuspid annulus

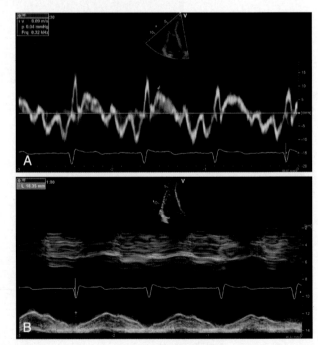

FIG. 16.11 Tricuspid annular plane systolic excursion (TAPSE) measurement (A) and Tissue Doppler S′ (B) is performed in the apical four-chamber view. The m-mode cursor is placed from the RV apex to RV base and the degree of excursion is measured from end-diastole to systole for TAPSE. The pulsed tissue Doppler cursor is placed at the lateral aspect of the tricuspid annulus for Tissue Doppler S′. In this example, both TAPSE and Tissue Doppler S′ measurements are normal.

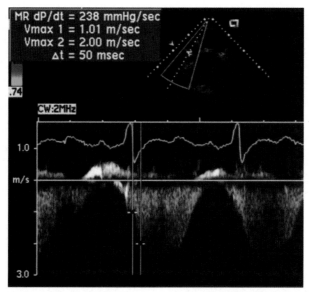

FIG. 16.12 Measurement of RV d*P*/d*T* from Doppler of the tricuspid regurgitant jet. Calipers are placed at 1 and 2 m/s and values are measured in mm Hg/s.

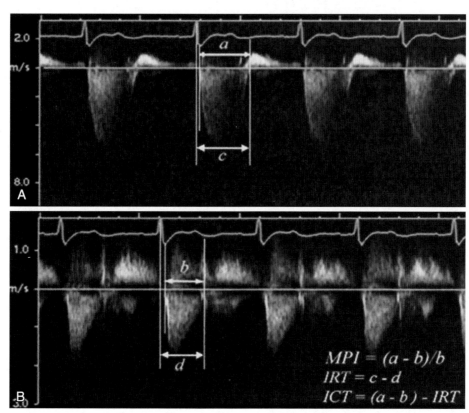

FIG. 16.13 (A and B) Measurement of the myocardial performance index with Doppler of the tricuspid regurgitant jet and pulmonary outflow tract velocities.

(Fig. 16.14). Tissue Doppler is a form of pulsed Doppler that measures low-frequency high-amplitude signals that return from tissue. This measurement is low dependent. Normal pulsed Doppler myocardial performance index (MPI) values are 0.26 ± 0.085 or >0.43. Normal tissue Doppler MPI values are 0.38 ± 0.08 or >0.54.[11] The myocardial performance index is not validated in patients with heart block or in patients with arrhythmias. It is unreliable when right atrial pressure is elevated. An easier to measure and reproducible quantitative assessment of RV longitudinal systolic function is the pulsed tissue Doppler S wave. Normal pulsed Doppler S wave of the right ventricle values are 14.1 ± 2.3 cm/s or >9.5 cm/s.[11]

Newer approaches to assessing RV systolic function include strain and strain rate imaging. Strain imaging measures the deformation

of the myocardium and strain rate imaging measures the rate of the deformation of the myocardium (Fig. 16.15). These measurements have the advantage of being load independent. They can be derived from Doppler tissue imaging techniques, in which case they are angle dependent. They can also be derived from speckle tracking imaging techniques, which measure changes in the position of myocardial speckles in relation to each other at various times in the cardiac cycle. Speckle tracking allows strain and strain rate data to be derived that are load independent as well as translational and angle independent. The challenge in making these measurements for the RV is that it is very thin-walled, while the septum is a hybrid structure. Published values tend to be higher and more heterogeneous when compared with similar

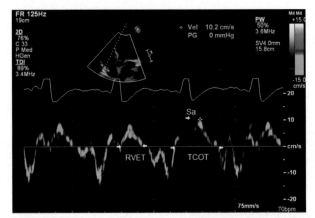

FIG. 16.14 Measurement of the myocardial performance index with Tissue Doppler at the tricuspid valve annulus in the apical four-chamber view.

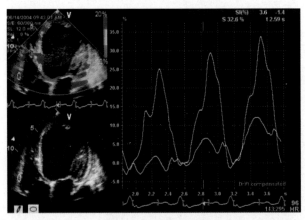

FIG. 16.15 Strain imaging of the right ventricular myocardium obtained from the base of the lateral free wall of the right ventricle in the apical four-chamber view.

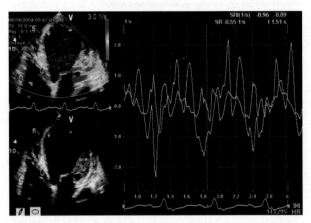

FIG. 16.16 Strain rate imaging of the right ventricular myocardium obtained from the base of the lateral free wall of the right ventricle in the apical four-chamber view.

measurements for the left ventricle.[22–30] Strain data is thought to be more clinically useful than strain rate data due to the inherent noise observed in strain rate tracings (Fig. 16.16). Normal valves for RV free wall 2-D strain are –29 ± 4.5% or <–20%.[11]

Three-Dimensional Imaging of the Right Ventricle

Real time 3D echocardiography is currently available for both transthoracic and transesophageal imaging. These methods a more accurate and reproducible than 2D methods and clinically or especially useful in

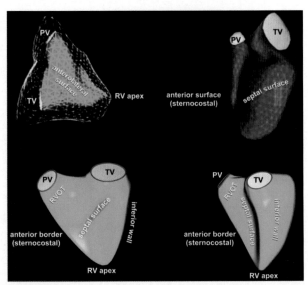

FIG. 16.17 The three-dimensional reconstruction of the right ventricle illustrating its complex geometry. *RV,* Right ventricle; *RVOT,* right ventricle outflow tract; *TV,* tricuspid valve.

patients with advanced heart failure, congenital heart disease, pulmonary embolism and pulmonary hypertension as well as RV dysplasia.[31–33] The complex geometry of the right ventricle makes it ideally suited for 3D analytic methods (Fig. 16.17). Qualitatively, 3D echo provides a method for imaging the entire right ventricle. Quantitatively, 3D echocardiographic measurements are usually made off-line and have tended to be tender specific, with a few exceptions.

3D echo continues to rapidly evolve with both transthoracic and transesophageal echocardiography techniques. Image quality continues to improve and single beat acquisitions of moving 3D images of the RV are now available, which avoids stitching artifacts, and may also be used in the setting of arrhythmia.

Similar to other echocardiographic techniques, the acquisition of accurate 3D volumes of the right ventricle relies heavily on the scanning abilities of the sonographer. RV volumes are best acquired from the apical four-chamber transducer location with a transducer moved more laterally and more anteriorly with a dilated RV, and in some situations, the transducer may need to be moved up the space. In more technically difficult patients, RV volumes may need to be acquired from a sub-xiphoid location. The three standard planes of the right ventricle that need to be visualized in their entirety before acquisition include the coronal or short-axis plane, sagittal or two-chamber plane, and four-chamber views. A large enough volume size must be obtained, and it is critical for the sonographer to recognize technically difficult situations and challenges that may prohibit when the total was used.

Once the volume datasets are acquired and downloaded, the echocardiographer can make quantitative volume measurements off-line with special RV volume software (available from Tomtec) on a 3D echo workstation. The image is optimized by adjusting brightness and contrast and the center of the tricuspid and mitral valves are marked as landmarks. The initial contours are confirmed and the automated software now automatically traces both end-diastolic and end-systolic measurements in the coronal, sagittal and four-chamber planes (Fig. 16.18). These measurements can then be adjusted if necessary. Beutel (mathematic dynamic 3D model) analysis generates a casting of the RV volume filling and squeezing, with generation of a volumetric curve and calculation of RV ejection fraction. Published normal reference values for RV volumes and ejection fractions with real-time 3D echo now exist.[34] Normal RV ejection fraction by 3D methods is 58 ± 6.5 % or >45%.[11] Several studies have now shown a quantitative 3D echo assessment of RV volumes and systolic function have correlated well with cardiac MRI in both adults and children, as well as patient's with complex congenital heart disease, while 3D echo clearly has advantages over cardiac MRI with respect to portability, cost-effectiveness, and patient tolerability.[35–38]

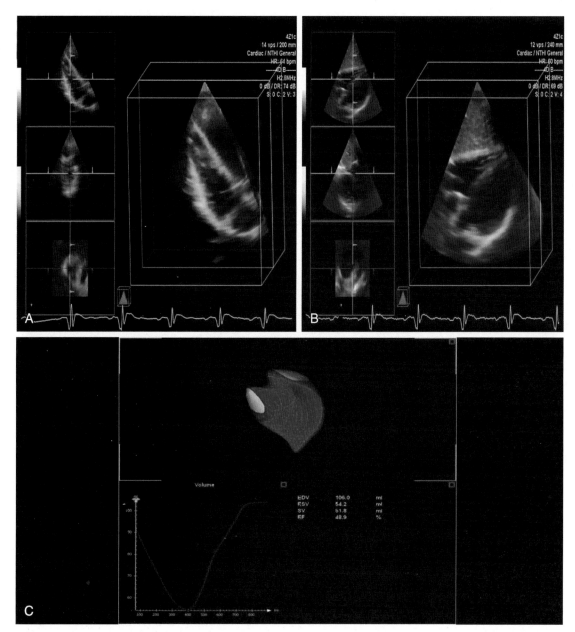

FIG. 16.18 Real-time three-dimensional imaging of the right ventricle (RV). RV volumes are best acquired from the apical four-chamber transducer location (A), and in more technically difficult patients, RV volumes may need to be acquired from the subxiphoid position (B). The coronal (short-axis), sagittal (two-chamber), and four-chamber views must all be visualized and traced in end-diastole and end-systole. Beutel mathematical analysis can then generate a casting of the RV volume with generation of a volumetric curve (C).

SUMMARY

The structure of the RV is complex, and needs to be described in segmental terms, similar to the left ventricle. Coronary flow to the RV mostly occurs from the RCA and its marginal and posterior descending artery branches, and by branches of the LAD. The prognostic importance of RV systolic function has been shown to be just as significant as left ventricular systolic function. As a result, the demand for more quantitative assessment of RV systolic function by echocardiography is increasing. Quantitative methods for assessing RV structure and function with 2D Doppler, tissue Doppler, 2D strain, and 3D echocardiography exist, are constantly improving, with more automated and reproducible features, and correlate well with cardiac MRI. Although in the past the right ventricle was described as the "forgotten chamber," it

is now a leading subject of investigation and technological innovation in the field of echocardiography and cardiovascular medicine.

Suggested Reading

Lang, R. M., Badano, L. P., Mor-Avi, V., et al. (2015). Recommendations for cardiac chamber quantification by echocardiography in adults: an update from the American Society of Echocardiography and the European Association of Cardiovascular Imaging. *Journal of the American Society of Echocardiography*, 28, 1–39.e14.

Tamoborini, G., Marsan, N., Gripari, P., et al. (2010). Reference values for right ventricular volumes and ejection fraction with real-time three-dimensional echocardiography: evaluation in a large series of normal subjects. *Journal of the American Society of Echocardiography*, 23, 109–115.

Zornoff, L. A., Skali, H., Pfeffer, M. A., et al. (2002). Right ventricular dysfunction and risk of heart failure and mortality after myocardial infarction. *Journal of the American College of Cardiology*, 39, 1450–1455.

A complete reference list can be found online at ExpertConsult.com.

Assessment of the Atria

Deepak K. Gupta

INTRODUCTION

With each cardiac cycle, the left and right atria act as reservoirs, conduits, and pumps for blood traveling from the pulmonary and systemic veins into the ventricles. Normally functioning atria are compliant, with the ability to accommodate dynamic changes in intravascular volume without pathologic increases in pressure and are active pumps with the ability to enhance ventricular filling and cardiac output. Atrial structure and function can be characterized by echocardiography, which provides diagnostic and prognostic information.

LEFT ATRIUM

Structure

The left atrium is located superior to the left ventricle, posterolateral to the right atrium, posterior to the aortic root, and anterior to the esophagus. The left atrium receives the pulmonary veins, has an appendage, and directs blood into the left ventricle through the mitral valve. With conventional two-dimensional (2D) transthoracic echocardiography, the left atrium should be visualized from the parasternal, apical, and subcostal views. However, inherent to the limitations of 2D imaging, no single view completely characterizes the shape and size of the left atrium. Therefore it is recommended that multiple views from standard imaging planes be obtained to more completely visualize the left atrium with careful attention to focus on the structure of interest, optimize endocardial border definition, and avoid foreshortening.

Quantification of left atrial size by transthoracic echocardiography has advanced from M-mode and 2D linear measurements to 2D and three-dimensional (3D) volumes. Compared with linear measures, volumes more accurately quantify left atrial size and perform better as prognostic markers.[1,2] Left atrial volumes obtained with 3D imaging are similar to those obtained from cardiac computed tomography (CT) or magnetic resonance imaging (MRI).[3,4] However, the lack of widespread clinical availability, standardization, and normative data from 3D echocardiography has led the American Society of Echocardiography to currently recommend 2D left atrial volumetric assessment by transthoracic echocardiography.[5] Characterization of left atrial size by transesophageal echocardiography is limited to semiquantitative assessment, because the entire left atrium usually does not fit within the image. However, transesophageal echocardiography is superior to transthoracic echocardiography for imaging of the left atrial appendage, interatrial septum, and pulmonary veins.

Quantification of 2D left atrial volume is performed from the transthoracic apical four- and two-chamber views. In each of these views, the left atrial endocardial borders are traced at end ventricular systole just before mitral valve opening when the left atrium is at its maximal size. A modified Simpson's (method of disks) biplane volume can then be calculated (Fig. 17.1).[5] Alternatively, the area (cm^2) and lengths (cm) of the left atrium can be measured in each view with volume calculated as $(0.85 \times \text{Area}_{4c} \times \text{Area}_{2c})/\text{length}$, where the shorter length of the major axis from the four- or two-chamber view is used.[6,7] With either the biplane Simpson's or area-length approach, it is recommended that left atrial volume be indexed to body surface area to account for gender differences, with the upper limit of normal for both men and women being less than 34 mL/m^2 (Table 17.1).[5] If volumetric assessment from the apical views cannot be obtained, then the 2D linear anterior-posterior length from the parasternal long-axis view can be used to size the left atrium. This measure is the distance between the posterior edge of the aortic root and the posterior wall of the left atrium, timed at the end of ventricular systole in the cardiac cycle.[5,8]

Left atrial size is a barometer for left-sided filling pressures, with enlargement typically correlating with chronically elevated left ventricular end-diastolic pressure, and/or pulmonary capillary wedge pressure.[6,9,10] Therefore left atrial enlargement (>34 mL/m^2) is a central component of the algorithm for the echocardiographic assessment of left ventricular filling pressures and diastolic dysfunction.[11] However, left atrial enlargement also occurs in the setting of mitral valve disease, atrial fibrillation, and intracardiac shunts, such that the presence of these conditions must be considered when assessing left ventricular filling pressures and diastolic function. Left atrial enlargement has been consistently demonstrated to be a powerful predictor of adverse cardiovascular outcomes, including incident atrial fibrillation, stroke, heart failure, and death.[1,12–25] Importantly, the prognostic information carried in left atrial size is independent of clinical factors, left ventricular size, and ejection fraction.

Function

While not commonly clinically reported on transthoracic echocardiography, quantification of left atrial function from conventional 2D and Doppler imaging as well as speckle tracking and 3D echocardiography is garnering increased attention. Atrial function is typically described in three phases: reservoir, conduit, and pump (Fig. 17.2).[26,27] The atrial reservoir phase corresponds to ventricular systole (atrial relaxation) when the mitral valve is closed and the left atrium expands due to venous return and descent of the mitral annulus towards the left ventricular apex. The conduit (passive emptying) phase begins with ventricular diastole when the mitral valve opens and blood flows through the atrium into the ventricle. The pump (active emptying) phase coincides with atrial contraction and is completed with the onset of ventricular systole, when the reservoir phase starts again. Overall left atrial function (emptying fraction) can be quantified from the largest and smallest left atrial volumes.[27] Using 2D or 3D volumetric measurements, overall and phasic atrial function can be calculated with the following formulas:

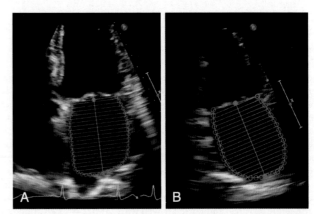

FIG. 17.1 Measurement of left atrial volume on transthoracic echocardiography. In the apical four-chamber (A) and apical two-chamber (B) views, the endocardial borders of the left atrium are traced, with exclusion of the pulmonary veins and appendage. The biplane method of disks method is the recommended by the American Society of Echocardiography.

TABLE 17.1 Quantification of Left and Right Atrial Size by 2D Transthoracic Echocardiography

			NORMAL	MILD	MODERATE	SEVERE
Left atrium	Volume index (mL/m²)	Men	16 to <34	34 to <41	41 to ≤48	>48
		Women	16 to <34	34 to <41	41 to ≤48	>48
	A-P diameter (cm)	Men	3.0 to <4.0	4.0 to <4.6	4.6 to <5.2	≥5.2
		Women	2.7–3.8	3.8 to <4.2	4.2 to <4.7	≥4.7
Right atrium[a]	Volume index (mL/m²)	Men	18 to <32	—	—	—
		Women	15 to <27	—	—	—

[a]Threshold values for defining severity of right atrial enlargement have not been established.

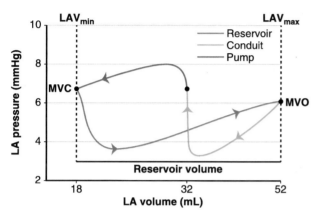

FIG. 17.2 Left atrial phasic function according to the pressure-volume relationship. The reservoir phase corresponds to ventricular systole when the mitral valve is closed, allowing the atrium to fill with blood. The conduit phase begins with mitral valve opening and corresponds to early ventricular diastole. The pump phase follows atrial contraction in late diastole. *LA,* Left atrium; *LAV,* left atrium volume; *MVC,* mitral valve closure; *MVO,* mitral valve opening. *(From Abhayaratna WP, Fatema K, Barnes ME, et al. Left atrial reservoir function as a potent marker for first atrial fibrillation or flutter in persons ≥65 years of age. Am J Cardiol. 2008;101(11):1626–1629.)*

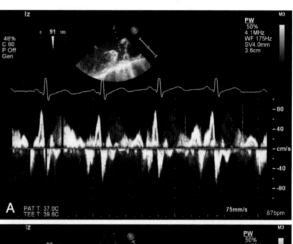

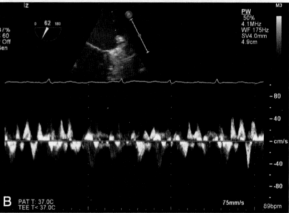

FIG. 17.4 Left atrial appendage emptying velocities on transesophageal echocardiography. Pulse wave spectral Doppler at the orifice of the left atrial appendage demonstrates normal emptying velocities in sinus rhythm (A) and reduced velocities (<40 cm/s) in atrial fibrillation (B).

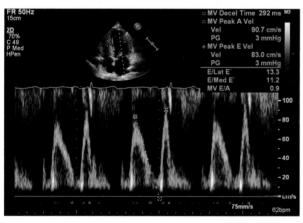

FIG. 17.3 Transmitral spectral Doppler demonstrating left ventricular inflow. The E and A waves are measures of atrial conduit and pump function, respectively.

Overall by emptying fraction: (LA max vol – LA min vol)/LA max vol
Conduit by passive emptying fraction: (LA max vol – LA pre A vol)/LA max vol.
Pump by active emptying fraction: (LA pre A vol – LA min vol)/LA pre A vol.
Reservoir by expansion index: (LA max vol – LA min vol)/LA min vol.
Blood flow Doppler can also be used to assess left atrial function. Early diastolic blood flow (conduit phase) from the left atrium into the left ventricle can be measured with pulse wave spectral Doppler at the tips of the mitral valve leaflets as the E wave. From this same Doppler tracing, atrial pump function can be quantified from the A wave peak velocity and velocity time integral, which coincides with the electrocardiographic P wave and atrial contraction (Fig. 17.3).[28] Pulse wave spectral Doppler of the pulmonary veins can also reveal an A wave, which can be used to

characterize atrial contractile function. In contrast to blood flow Doppler, which is driven by pressure gradients between two chambers, pulse wave tissue Doppler of the mitral annulus provides information regarding the mechanical properties of the myocardium. The late diastolic A prime velocity of the mitral annular tissue Doppler signal is also a measure of left atrial contraction.[29,30] In atrial fibrillation, the spectral Doppler and tissue Doppler A waves are absent.

Assessing left atrial function has informed understanding of thromboembolic risk in atrial fibrillation. Using Doppler imaging, electromechanical dissociation of the left atrium has been demonstrated to occur following electrical cardioversion of atrial fibrillation to sinus rhythm.[31] Similarly, patients with amyloidosis may have markedly reduced atrial contractile function despite electrocardiographic sinus rhythm.[32] Spectral Doppler has also been used to interrogate blood flow velocities in the left atrial appendage during transesophageal echocardiography, with values below 34 cm/s associated with greater risk of atrial fibrillation recurrence and stroke (Fig. 17.4).[33]

Recently, speckle tracking echocardiography has been applied to study left atrial function (Fig. 17.5).[34–36] Patients with a history of paroxysmal atrial fibrillation but sinus rhythm during echocardiography have impaired left

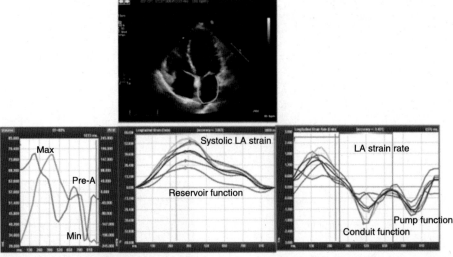

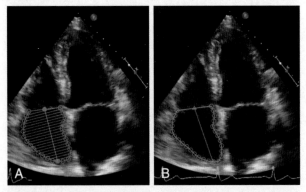

FIG. 17.5 Speckle tracking echocardiography of the left atrium. The endocardial border of the left atrium is traced and then tracked over the cardiac cycle, generating time volume as well as longitudinal systolic strain and strain rate curves, corresponding to the three phases (reservoir, conduit, and pump) of atrial function. (*From Santos AB, Kraigher-Krainer E, Gupta DK, et al. Impaired left atrial function in heart failure with preserved ejection fraction. Eur J Heart Fail. 2014;16(10):1096–1103.*)

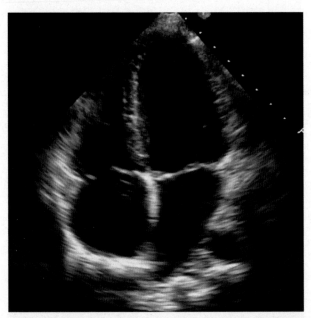

FIG. 17.6 Measurement of right atrial volume on transthoracic echocardiography. In the apical four-chamber view, the endocardial borders of the right atrium are traced, allowing calculation of the volume by either the method of disks (A) or area-length (B).

atrial function, suggesting a more chronic atrial myopathy.[36] Furthermore, despite the correlation between left atrial size and function, recent studies demonstrate that left atrial function can be impaired even in the absence of left atrial enlargement.[36] In small studies, functional impairments of the left atrium appear to offer additional prognostic information beyond left atrial size for the prediction of adverse cardiovascular outcomes.[37–39]

RIGHT ATRIUM

The right atrium is located superior to the right ventricle and anteromedial to the left atrium. The right atrium receives the vena cava and coronary sinus, has an appendage, and directs blood into the right ventricle through the tricuspid valve. With conventional 2D transthoracic echocardiography, the right atrium should be visualized from the parasternal, apical, and subcostal views. As compared with the left atrium, there is less data regarding quantification of right atrial size and function. However, analogous to the left atrium, enlargement of the right atrium may reflect right ventricular dysfunction, tricuspid valve disease, atrial fibrillation, and/or intracardiac shunts. The American Society of Echocardiography currently recommends quantifying right atrial size using a single plane volumetric measure (either method of disks or area-length [0.85 × area^2/length]) obtained from the apical four-chamber view (Fig. 17.6). This volume should be indexed to body surface area with the upper limits of normal being 32 mL/m^2 in men and 27 mL/m^2 in women.[5] When quantification of right atrial size cannot be performed, semi-quantitative assessment of right atrial size can be provided in relation to left atrial size. If the right atrium appears larger than the left atrium, this is indicative of right atrial enlargement. Right atrial enlargement is typically a marker of right ventricular dysfunction and elevated right-sided pressures. Right atrial

FIG. 17.7 Lipomatous hypertrophy of the interatrial septum. Note the thickened echobright interatrial septum with a "dropout" in the region of the fossa ovalis. (*Image courtesy of Benjamin F. Byrd III, MD, Vanderbilt University School of Medicine.*)

pressure is conventionally estimated from the size and respirophasic collapse of the inferior vena cava. Another indicator of elevated right atrial pressure includes bowing of the interatrial septum from right to left. However, right atrial function has not been well studied by echocardiography.[40]

THE INTERATRIAL SEPTUM AND CONGENITAL ABNORMALITIES OF THE ATRIA

The interatrial septum is a thin structure best visualized by transesophageal echocardiography but is also readily seen on transthoracic imaging, particularly in the subcostal view. The interatrial septum should by interrogated with 2D, color Doppler, and if clinically indicated, agitated saline ("bubble") contrast. Abnormalities of the interatrial septum include lipomatous hypertrophy, patent foramen ovale, aneurysm, and atrial septal defects (primum, secundum, and sinus venosus).

Lipomatous hypertrophy of the interatrial septum is typically a benign condition acquired with advancing age. It is due to fatty infiltration of the superior and inferior segments of the interatrial septum, with sparing of the fossa ovalis, producing a "dumbbell" appearance in the apical four-chamber and/or subcostal views (Fig. 17.7; Video 17.1).[41]

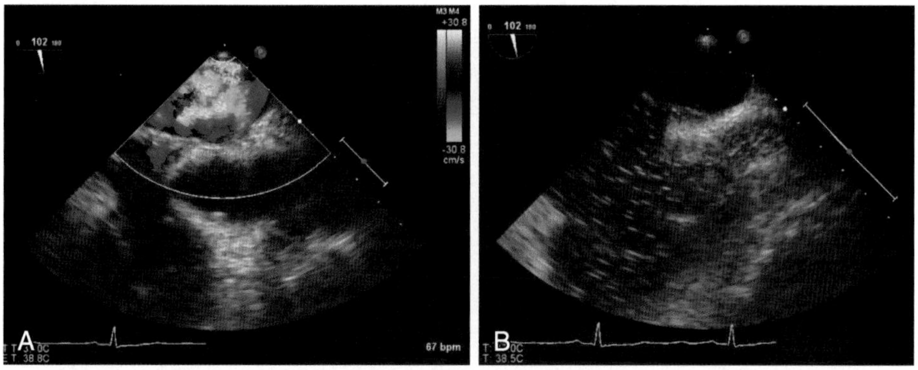

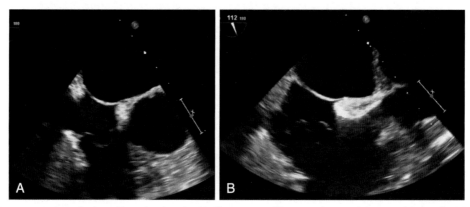

FIG. 17.8 Patent foramen ovale on transesophageal echocardiography. From the mid-esophageal perspective, the interatrial septum can be visualized. (A) Color flow Doppler demonstrates a left-to-right shunt. (B) Agitated saline "bubble" contrast demonstrates right-to-left shunting originating from the site of the patent foramen ovale.

FIG. 17.9 Chiari network on transesophageal echocardiography. Note the thin filamentous and fenestrated structure that extends across the right atrium. (*Images courtesy of Michael T. Baker, MD, Vanderbilt University School of Medicine.*)

A patent foramen ovale results from failed fusion of the primum and secundum septum, and may be present in 25%–30% of the adult population (Fig. 17.8; Videos 17.2 and 17.3). It is generally visualized as a small left-to-right shunt with color Doppler or as a right-to-left shunt detected with injection of agitated saline into a peripheral vein that crosses into the left atrium within three to four cardiac cycles following the appearance of "bubbles" in the right heart.[42] Given that left atrial pressure normally exceeds right atrial pressure, the detection of a patent foramen ovale using agitated saline can be enhanced by using maneuvers to increase right atrial pressure, such as Valsalva, coughing, or applying abdominal pressure. The prevalence of a patent foramen ovale or atrial septal defect may approach 75% when the interatrial septum is aneurysmal, defined as a hypermobile septum with >1 cm of maximal deviation from the plane of interatrial septum. The combination of interatrial septal aneurysm and patent foramen ovale has also been associated with an increased risk for thromboembolism.[43] Atrial septal defects are typically larger and may be described as primum, secundum, or venosus defects. For a detailed description of the echocardiographic assessment of atrial septal defects, please see Chapter 43.

Other congenital remnants commonly visualized in the right atrium include the Eustachian valve and Chiari network.[44,45] The Eustachian valve is a normal variant due to incomplete regression of the inferior portion of the right sinus venosus valve present in utero that directs blood from the inferior vena cava across the atrial septum into the left atrium. Depending on the extent of regression, the Eustachian valve may be seen as a rigid linear structure protruding near the orifice of the inferior vena cava to a near complete band of tissue across the right atrium, known as cor triatriatum dexter. An unrecognized Eustachian valve may sometimes be confused with an atrial septal defect due to changes in blood flow patterns. A Chiari network is a fine membranous highly mobile and fenestrated structure that represents the embryologic valve of the right sinus venosus (Fig. 17.9; Videos 17.4 and 17.5). While benign, a Chiari network can also be confused with a vegetation or thrombus.

BOX 17.1 Atrial Masses

Myxoma
Thrombus
Sarcoma
Rhabdomyoma
Melanoma
Adrenocortical cancer
Thyroid carcinoma
Renal cell carcinoma
Hepatoma
Breast cancer
Lymphoma
Fibroelastoma

ATRIAL MASSES

In day-to-day clinical practice, the most frequent consideration for atrial masses is thrombi as a source for systemic or pulmonary thromboembolism. Less common causes of atrial masses are myxoma, sarcoma, rhabdomyoma, fibroelastoma, renal cell carcinoma, thyroid tumor, melanoma, and adrenal cell carcinoma (Box 17.1). Lung and breast cancer and lymphoma can cause pericardial studding that may even infiltrate the myocardium of the atria and ventricles.

Transthoracic echocardiography has relatively poor sensitivity for detection of atrial appendage thrombus, and in particular, left atrial appendage thrombus. Transesophageal echocardiography is the preferred modality for excluding atrial thrombus, particularly in patients undergoing cardioversion from atrial fibrillation. The left atrial appendage is typically a multilobed structure that should be visualized across many planes in the mid to upper esophageal view (Fig. 17.10). The left atrial appendage contains pectinate muscles that should be differentiated from thrombus. In addition, the left atrial appendage lies in close proximity

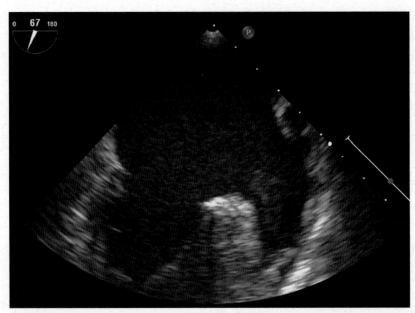

FIG. 17.10 Left atrial appendage thrombus on transesophageal echocardiography. A heterogeneous echodensity is present within the body of the left atrial appendage.

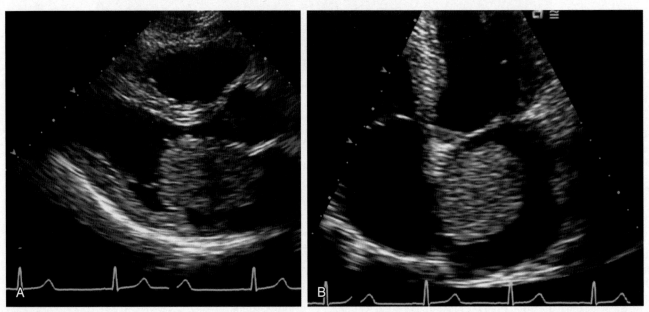

FIG. 17.11 Left atrial myxoma. (A) Parasternal long-axis view of large atrial myxoma prolapsing across the mitral valve. (B) Apical 4 chamber view of the same atrial myxoma attached to the interatrial septum. (*Images courtesy of Lisa Mendes, MD, Vanderbilt University School of Medicine.*)

to the left superior pulmonary vein and is separated by a ridge of tissue that is sometimes confused for thrombus. Color and pulse-wave spectral Doppler can aid in the identification and differentiation of the pulmonary veins and left atrial appendage. The right ventricle also has an appendage that is heavily trabeculated and best visualized with transesophageal echocardiography focused on the right atrium near the entry of the vena cava. Thrombi can also form on intracardiac devices, of which the most common are pacemaker leads and indwelling catheters, although the echocardiographic differentiation of device-related thrombus versus vegetation is difficult and often depends upon the clinical scenario.

Atrial myxomas are the most common primary tumor of the heart (Fig. 17.11; Videos 17.6 and 17.7).[46] These typically arise from the left atrial side of the interatrial septum but can also been seen in the right atrium. While considered a benign tumor, large myxomas may cause obstruction to atrial and ventricular filling and may be sources

for thromboembolic events. The other tumors that have been reported in the atria are much less common and are covered elsewhere (see Chapters 37 and 39).

Suggested Reading

Lang, R. M., Badano, L. P., Mor-Avi, V., et al. (2015). Recommendations for cardiac chamber quantification by echocardiography in adults: an update from the American Society of Echocardiography and the European Association of Cardiovascular Imaging. *Journal of the American Society of Echocardiography, 28*, 1–39.e14.

Pritchett, A. M., Jacobsen, S. J., Mahoney, D. W., Rodeheffer, R. J., Bailey, K. R., & Redfield, M. M. (2003). Left atrial volume as an index of left atrial size: a population-based study. *Journal of the American College of Cardiology, 41*, 1036–1043.

Takemoto, Y., Barnes, M. E., Seward, J. B., et al. (2005). Usefulness of left atrial volume in predicting first congestive heart failure in patients > or = 65 years of age with well-preserved left ventricular systolic function. *The American Journal of Cardiology, 96*, 832–836.

Tsang, T. S., Abhayaratna, W. P., Barnes, M. E., et al. (2006). Prediction of cardiovascular outcomes with left atrial size: is volume superior to area or diameter? *Journal of the American College of Cardiology, 47*, 1018–1023.

A complete reference list can be found online at ExpertConsult.com

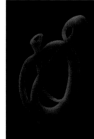

ECHOCARDIOGRAPHY FOR DISEASES OF THE MYOCARDIUM

18 | Acute Myocardial Infarction
Justina C. Wu

INTRODUCTION

Acute myocardial infarction (MI), the classic "heart attack," is caused by the sudden loss of blood flow and oxygenation to the heart muscle due to complete occlusion of a coronary artery. The risk factors, clinical presentation, and serial changes in electrocardiogram (ECG) and serologic markers as myocardium is damaged are well known. For the physician and technologist, echocardiography often plays a critical role in the early diagnosis and management of the patient, but it should be used judiciously.

In the setting of suspected acute MI, echocardiography is appropriate to evaluate (1) a patient with acute chest pain, with suspected MI but a nondiagnostic ECG (particularly if the scan can be performed during pain), (2) a patient who has had recent chest pain and other features or laboratory markers indicative of ongoing myocardial infarction who is currently chest pain–free, and (3) to evaluate for a suspected complication of MI such as myocardial or valve disruption, right or left heart failure, or tamponade (see Chapter 19).[1] Importantly, when a patient's symptoms and ECG are clearly indicative of an ongoing acute MI, there is no need to obtain an echo in the acute setting, when the focus should be on progression towards definitive therapy (i.e., opening the coronary artery). Atypical symptoms, as may occur in women, those with diabetes, or the elderly, may benefit from an echocardiogram early on when there is sufficient suspicion. The following section addresses considerations in imaging a patient in the setting of acute MI (0–48 hours after presentation), focusing primarily on diagnosis, ventricular function, and recognition of critical complications.

ESTABLISHING THE DIAGNOSIS, EXTENT, AND LOCATION OF MYOCARDIAL INFARCTION

When a coronary artery is occluded, echocardiography will demonstrate changes in the left ventricular (LV) myocardial wall motion within 30 seconds, even before chest pain or ECG changes occur.[2] Instead of a normokinetic area, myocardium that is starved of oxygen will thicken to a lesser degree and become hypokinetic.

There are five degrees of myocardial wall motion (Table 18.1): *normokinesis, hyperkinesis, hypokinesis, akinesis,* and *dyskinesis.* Normokinetic motion is the systolic thickening of the ventricular wall, usually increasing by at least 30%–50% due to shortening of the myocardial cells that

are arranged in concentric spirally oriented layers around the barrel and apex of the left ventricle. Videos 18.1 and 18.2 show normal parasternal long and short-axis views of the left ventricle with normokinesis of all segments. Hyperkinesis (unusually brisk or exaggerated thickening) is seen when the left ventricle is adapting overall to increased demand, such as in exercise, stress, or hyperadrenergic states. In cases where there is recent focal LV dysfunction, the remaining uninjured myocardial segments may become hyperkinetic as a compensatory mechanism for maintaining overall stroke volume and cardiac output.

Videos 18.3 through 18.6 show examples of these varying degrees of kinesis. The latter three types of wall motion, hypokinesis, akinesis, and dyskinesis (see Videos 18.3, 18.4, and 18.5 respectively), are indicative of dysfunctional myocardium and hence termed "wall motion abnormalities (WMA)." Hypokinetic segments thicken less than 30% in systole and indicate dysfunctional myocardium. Akinetic segments do not thicken at all. Dyskinetic segments actually bulge away from the LV center in systole. If there is a large area of both myocardial thinning (<6 mm in thickness) and dyskinesis, this implies that there is an extensive fibrotic scar that has replaced functioning myocardium, and these areas are deemed aneurysmal (see Video 18.6). The most severe degrees of dysfunction (akinesis and dyskinesis) occur with prolonged injury, as ischemic myocardium can no longer contract, die, and become replaced by fibrocytes. Oftentimes, the presence of preserved remaining normo- or hyperkinetic myocardium surrounding a discrete wall motion abnormality can create *hinge points*, which better delineate the poorly contractile segments (see Video 18.4).

There are various classification schemes assigning numerical values to these types of segmental WMAs, with 1 representing normal or hyperkinetic segments and 5 representing the most dysfunctional aneurysmal segments. The sum of these scores for a 17-segment model will give a quantitative assessment of overall LV systolic function.

Importantly, the degree of kinesis is primarily an indicator of full-thickness myocardial contractility at the indicator segment. Taken without clinical context, a hypo- or akinetic segment may indicate any state along the spectrum that includes acute ischemia, subendocardial or subepicardial injury, stunned myocardium (i.e., reperfused but still not fully functioning cells), and hibernating (chronically underperfused, barely metabolically active but still viable) myocardium to completed transmural infarct. Additional techniques and agents may be required to distinguish

TABLE 18.1 Wall Motion Assessment

WALL MOTION TYPE	THICKENING	TISSUE	WALL MOTION SCORE (ASE MODEL)
Hyperkinetic	>50%	Compensatory/hyperadrenergic state	—
Normokinetic	30%–50%	Normal perfusion and function	1
Hypokinetic	<30%	Ischemic or nontransmural infarct	2
Akinetic	None	Transmural infarct (or stunned or hibernating)	3
Dyskinetic	Bulges outwards (paradoxically)	Infarcted and fibrosed	4
Aneurysmal	Thinned and bulges outwards	Extensive infarct/fibrosed area	5

among these states (see Chapters 12 and 27). Myocardial dysfunction due to other causes than hypoxia may also cause WMA.

As a caveat, there is a "fake-out" wall motion abnormality termed "pseudodyskinesis."[3] This is the apparent systolic paradoxical bulging of the entire inferior ventricular wall in systole, best seen on short-axis windows, which can be misinterpreted to be true dyskinesis (Video 18.7). In fact, slowing the playback speed of the loop to carefully inspect the actual thickening between the epicardium and endocardium will reveal that the inferior wall is flattened (distorting the normal circular cross-sectional shape of the left ventricle) in diastole by external compression from the abdominal organs. In systole, it assumes the usual circular profile and hence gives the appearance that the wall is bulging radially outwards in systole. Pseudodyskinesis is frequently observed in patients with liver failure and ascites.

The coronary artery that is occluded will dictate which ventricular segments have abnormal function.[4] For reference, the normal coronary tree as it relates to the entire heart, particularly the left ventricle, is shown by 3D computed tomography (CT) angiography in Fig. 18.1, with the corresponding 360-degree view in Video 18.8.

On echocardiography, for the purposes of standardization, the left ventricle is divided along the long axis into quadrants of anterior, inferior, septal, and lateral walls. The septal and lateral walls may be further bisected into anterior and inferior sectors. There is also segmentation in the orthogonal short-axis plane into thirds (basal, midventricular, and apical) with an additional single distal apical cap segment. The cumulative result is the 17-segment model espoused by the American Society of Echocardiography and most other cardiac imaging modalities (Fig. 18.2 and Video 18.9). Superimposing the normal coronary artery distribution onto this model gives the usual coronary supply to each segment.

In general, the more coronary arteries affected or the more proximal the occlusion is in a coronary artery, the more extensive the myocardial territory will be affected. Optimally, both long- and short-axis images of the heart should be inspected, from base to apex, in multiple windows to evaluate all segments. In addition to mapping the WMA to the corresponding coronary artery, the astute sonographer should be aware of patterns of myocardial infarction and their associations with other complications such as valvular disease and other sequelae in the acute and subacute setting.

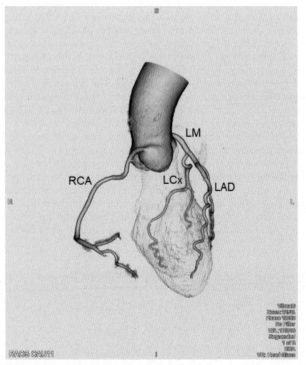

FIG. 18.1 The normal coronary artery tree. 3D computed tomography angiogram of normal coronary artery anatomy. *LAD,* Left anterior descending artery; *LCx,* left circumflex artery; *LM,* left main artery; *RCA,* right coronary artery. The left ventricle is displayed in light gray.

PATTERNS OF MYOCARDIAL INFARCTION BY CORONARY ARTERY TERRITORY

Anterior Myocardial Infarcts (Left Anterior Descending Territory)

The left anterior descending (LAD) coronary artery supplies a major portion of the left ventricle. Typically, the LAD branches off the left main (LM) coronary artery. Its diagonal (D) branches perfuse the entire anterior wall, and its septal branches supply the anterior 2/3 of the septum (red area shaded in Fig. 18.2). The LAD itself continues distally and may wrap around the tip of the LV to supply the apex. An example of an acute LAD infarct on echocardiography is shown in Video 18.10. A proximal LAD infarct will affect the entire anterior and anteroseptal wall from base to apex. Typically such a lesion, if not revascularized, will compromise overall LV systolic function and reduces the overall left ventricular ejection fraction to at least 35%–40%. Clinically, this leads to hypotension directly due to a drop in forward cardiac output as well as congestive heart failure. By comparison, a mid- or distal LAD infarct would be expected to cause mid-to-apical WMA, with the basal LV segments spared or even hyperkinetic.

Lateral Myocardial Infarcts (Left Circumflex Territory)

The left circumflex (LCx) artery is the other major branch of the LM coronary artery. The LCx proper runs in the atrioventricular groove and perfuses the lateral wall via its obtuse marginal (OM) branches that extend longitudinally towards the apex. Hence, an acute proximal LCx or OM occlusion will cause segmental WMA in the anterolateral and inferolateral segments (shaded yellow in Fig. 18.2). This is typically best seen on parasternal and apical 3 and 4 chamber windows (see Video 18.11). The remaining distal LCx supplies the LV inferior wall via posterolateral branches. The LCx terminates in a posterior descending artery (left PDA); in approximately 15% of the population termed "left-dominant," the left PDA supplies the distal inferior wall. In patients with codominant circulation, a right PDA supplied by the right coronary artery (RCA) may also contribute to the distal inferior wall blood supply. Importantly, LCx lesions are notorious for being electrocardiographically "silent," that is, not manifest on ECGs; hence, echocardiography is an important adjunctive tool to detect LCx ischemia in a patient with suspicious symptoms and no obvious ECG changes.

Anterolateral Myocardial Infarcts (Left Main Territory)

Complete occlusion of the LM coronary artery is an uncommon but catastrophic event due to the sudden drop in cardiac output incurred by widespread anterior and lateral ischemia. Hence, any LM coronary stenoses of 50% or greater are clinically considered severe (in comparison with ≥70% in the other epicardial coronary arteries as the definition of severe stenosis). Imaging should not be pursued in the acute presentation due to profound cardiogenic shock and the need to intervene emergently. Intra-aortic balloon pump and urgent coronary artery bypass grafting (CABG) or high-risk LM angioplasty are the only definitive therapies in this potentially lethal event.

Inferior Myocardial Infarcts

The RCA usually has its own origin from the right sinus of Valsalva, which can occasionally be seen on standard transthoracic windows (Fig. 18.3 and Video 18.12) when it takes off anteriorly. It travels anteriorly around the right atrioventricular groove at the base of the heart. Its proximal branches, termed acute marginal branches, supply the right ventricle. Once it reaches the interventricular groove, the posterior descending branch (right PDA) descends in the posterior interventricular groove towards the apex and supplies the inferior 1/3 of the interventricular septum as well as the inferior left ventricle in approximately 85% of the general population, which are "right-dominant." (This area is shaded green in Fig. 18.2.) The remainder of the RCA may travel farther along the left atrioventricular groove and is termed the right posterolateral ventricular (right PLV) branch. In most individuals, this is a minor branch, but there

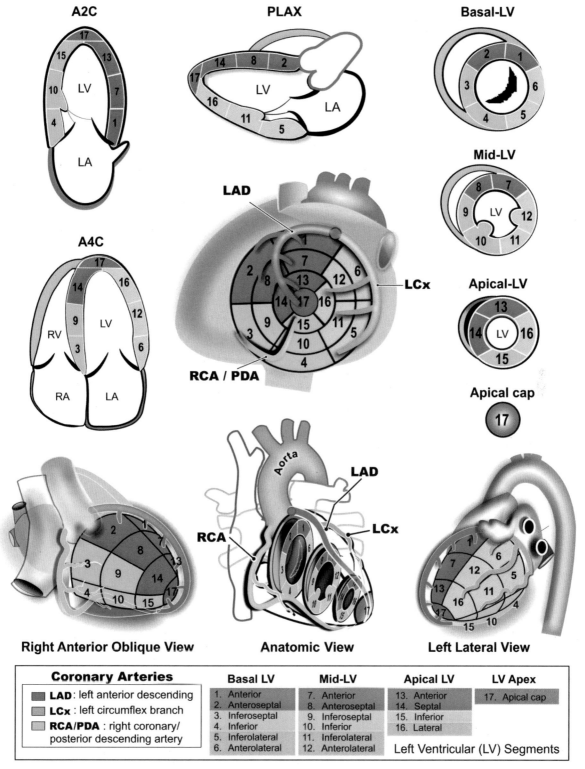

FIG. 18.2 Standardized 17 segment model of the left ventricle with nomenclature and corresponding coronary artery territories. (*Courtesy of Bernard E. Bulwer, MD, FASE; Modified from Bulwer BE, Rivero JM, eds.* Echocardiography Pocket Guide: The Transthoracic Examination. *Burlington, MA: Jones & Bartlett Learning; 2011, 2013:131.*)

is a small fraction of patients that have "super right dominant" circulation in which the right PLV is large and supersedes the territory usually supplied by the LCx, which in turn is small and vestigial.

The magnitude of the effect of an RCA infarct depends on the distance of the acute occlusion from the origin and the dominance of the vessel: a proximal occlusion can cause both right ventricular (RV) infarct in addition to LV inferior infarct and hence cardiogenic shock, whereas a more distal occlusion would cause a smaller area of isolated inferoseptal

and inferior LV dysfunction. Videos 18.13 shows an example of a typical basal inferior infarct due to occlusion in the mid RCA. Videos 18.14 and 18.15 are examples of a higher RCA occlusion, with ensuing RV infarct. In Video 18.15, note the diffusely hypokinetic right ventricle, the so-called T-sign manifest on short-axis windows (see also Fig. 18.4), as well as the accompanying inferoseptal and inferior LV hypokinesis. Other signs of RV dysfunction, such as decreased tricuspid annular systolic excursion, can be visualized directly or quantitatively displayed using tissue Doppler. RV infarct is virtually always accompanied by inferior myocardial infarct and should be suspected when inferior ST segment ECG changes are accompanied by hypotension; the hypotension is often exacerbated by conditions that further drop preload, such as nitrates or diuresis. Conversely, a more distal RCA occlusion proximal to the R. (right) PDA can cause isolated inferoseptal and inferior injury with*out* RV involvement. Super right-dominant individuals are more likely to suffer more myocardial injury, with more inferolateral myocardial dysfunction than would otherwise be anticipated without knowledge of their coronary artery configuration.

URGENT CONSEQUENCES OF ACUTE MYOCARDIAL INFARCTION

This section has focused on myocardial infarct patterns regarding coronary artery distributions, but aside from the myocardium directly affected by the occluded artery, there are other consequences that may be present in the acute phase and diagnosed by echocardiography. These are often heralded by hemodynamic deterioration, seemingly out of proportion to the extent of affected myocardium. The most common complications in the acute setting are mentioned here, but a more comprehensive discussion ensues in Chapter 19. In addition, the treatment of MI by urgent revascularization may also lead to unintended adverse consequences, which echocardiography can easily detect.

Papillary Muscle Dysfunction and Mitral Regurgitation

The mitral valve should be surveyed for the presence of mitral regurgitation. If there is significant mitral regurgitation, possible causes to consider include

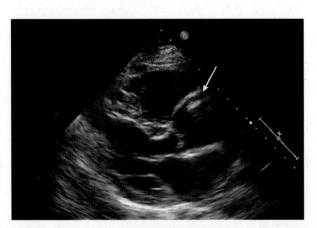

FIG. 18.3 Anterior takeoff of the right coronary artery (RCA; a normal finding). The proximal RCA *(arrow)* is seen originating from the right sinus of Valsalva and running anteriorly and parallel to the aortic root for its initial course.

papillary muscle dysfunction and/or leaflet disruption. Of the two papillary muscles, the anterolateral one tends to supply primarily the anterior leaflet; it receives a dual blood supply from both the LAD (via diagonal branches) and LCx. Therefore, mitral regurgitation due to papillary muscle dysfunction or chordal disruption is rare unless there is an extremely large infarct or preexisting chronic disease. In contrast, the posteromedial papillary muscle is supplied solely by the R. PDA (in right-dominant patients); thus, it is not uncommon to see inferior infarcts accompanied by mitral regurgitation due to hypoxic injury to and dysfunction of this papillary muscle. If revascularization is successful in avoiding permanent necrosis of the muscle or valvular apparatus, then this secondary, or functional, mitral regurgitation can resolve entirely following revascularization. (See Video 18.16, which shows ischemic mitral regurgitation provoked by demand ischemia during a stress echocardiogram. In this instance, stenting of the culprit RCA lesion led to complete resolution of the mitral regurgitation.) Cases in which there is actually disruption of the chordae or leaflets are discussed later (see Chapter 19).

Myocardial disruption, that is, ventricular septal defects (VSDs), pseudoaneurysms, and free wall rupture are all rare early in the course of MI, since they require extensive tissue necrosis to arise. VSDs are the most common defect detected. They are typically detected on echo by color flow Doppler showing a jet crossing the septum from left to right ventricle and less commonly by actual discontinuity of the tissue. VSDs associated with anterior MIs are usually located towards the apex, whereas inferior infarctions often involve the basal inferior septum. The rarer and more severe myocardial defects are discussed later. Pseudoaneurysms are contained ruptures, and they are more often detected in the inferior wall, late after MI. Free wall rupture, if captured at all on echocardiography before the patient expires, results in blood flowing freely into the pericardium and thorax. This manifests as tamponade and cardiogenic shock.

We briefly mention arrhythmias in the setting of acute MI here, primarily for the purposes of placing them in the context of the myocardial infarct patterns they accompany. Anterior MIs may be associated with lethal rhythms such as ventricular fibrillation or polymorphic ventricular tachycardia (due to widespread). Monomorphic ventricular tachycardia, however, implies that there is reentrant circuit, caused by scar from prior myocardial infarct that may be revealed as a large akinetic, thinned, or dyskinetic area. Inferior MIs may be accompanied by bradyarrhythmias and/or atrioventricular (AV) block, since the proximal RCA gives rise to the sinoatrial node branch in 60% of patients, and the dominant RCA also gives rise to the AV nodal branch at the crux of the heart near the origin of the PDA. Inferior MIs are also often associated with high vagal tone, which can contribute to bradycardia and hypotension. Lastly, atrial fibrillation is not uncommon in both situations, presumably due to high adrenergic state and potentially accompanying elevated LV filling pressures.

In today's environment, patients often receive revascularization of acute coronary syndromes so rapidly that the imaging of the heart often occurs after the symptoms and coronary blockage have resolved. Post-angioplasty complications that can arise include aortic dissection, tamponade, and coronary artery dissection. Coronary artery dissection may be

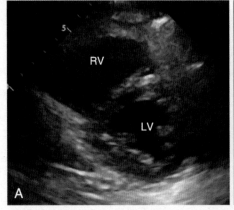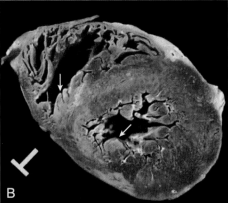

FIG. 18.4 **The "T" sign, caused by hypokinesis of both the inferior right ventricle (RV) and adjacent inferior and inferoseptal left ventricle (LV) segments, supplied by an occluded right coronary artery.** (A) Short-axis transthoracic view at the midpapillary muscle level, and (B) gross pathology of the heart cut and oriented in the same section, with the light tan areas *(arrows)* demonstrating infarcted left ventricle inferoseptum, inferior wall and posterior papillary muscle, and right ventricle.

self-limited and/or treated by stenting. If the artery is not occluded, it may not be apparent on echocardiography. However, if actual perforation of the coronary artery has occurred, an intramyocardial hematoma may be visible on echocardiogram where it appears as a discrete area of myocardial swelling and increased homogeneous echodensity (almost mimicking a tumor), which may expand over time, together with focal hypokinesis. There may be associated pericardial effusion.

LIMITATIONS TO ECHOCARDIOGRAPHY IN THE ACUTE SETTING

The above classic presentations of MI by coronary artery territory may be altered in patients with preexisting coronary artery disease (CAD). Patients with prior flow-limiting CAD or MIs usually develop collateral vessels, which can mitigate the extent of myocardial dysfunction in a given coronary artery territory. For example, it is very common to visualize only basal inferior hypokinesis, with sparing of the apical inferior segments, in an acute inferior MI when the patient has had time to develop collaterals from the LAD or LCx. Patients who have had CABG for LM or ostial LAD occlusions are often observed to have long-standing residual hypokinesis at the basalmost interventricular septum, with contractility improved distal to where the bypass graft (often a left internal mammary artery, or LIMA) touches down on the LAD. Comparing current images with any available prior echocardiogram can be helpful to delineate truly new versus preexisting myocardial dysfunction.

The endocardium and subendocardial layers are the least perfused regions of the heart and most vulnerable to damage by ischemia. Echocardiography alone may underdiagnose subendocardial infarcts (those limited to the innermost layer of the myocardium, as opposed to transmural infarcts). In other words, overall wall thickening may appear normal even though there is cardiac ischemia.

In practice, if echo images are poor with respect to endocardial definition, or if not all windows on the heart are obtainable, the sensitivity of transthoracic echo for detecting WMA obviously suffer. For instance, the presence of extensive mitral annular calcification can cause acoustic shadowing and render analysis of basal inferolateral wall motion difficult. Subendocardial ischemia is often better revealed by myocardial contrast and/or dobutamine stress testing (see Chapter 27). Hence, complete testing with serial ECGs and cardiac biomarkers is still required to truly rule out an acute coronary syndrome.

Patients who are chest pain–free at the time of imaging may in fact have had an acute coronary syndrome (with spontaneous or intermittent reperfusion) or significant stable CAD that is only manifest when their myocardial demands outstrip the limited supply. Hence, even when acute infarction is ruled out, further stratification of coronary artery patency via stress testing or even angiography may be warranted depending on the clinical setting.

Suggested Reading

Douglas, P. S., Garcia, M. J., Haines, D. E., et al. (2011). ACCF/ASE/AHA/ASNC/HFSA/HRS/SCAI/SCCM/SCCT/SCMR 2011 Appropriate Use Criteria for Echocardiography. A Report of the American College of Cardiology Foundation Appropriate Use Criteria Task Force, American Society of Echocardiography, American Heart Association, American Society of Nuclear Cardiology, Heart Failure Society of America, Heart Rhythm Society, Society for Cardiovascular Angiography and Interventions, Society of Critical Care Medicine, Society of Cardiovascular Computed Tomography, and Society for Cardiovascular Magnetic Resonance Endorsed by the American College of Chest Physicians. *Journal of the American College of Cardiology*, 57, 1126–1166.

Rallidis, L. S., Makavos, G., & Nihoyannopoulos, P. (2014). Right ventricular involvement in coronary artery disease: role of echocardiography for diagnosis and prognosis. *Journal of the American Society of Echocardiography*, 27, 223–229.

Sechtem, U., Achenbach, S., Friedrich, M., Wackers, F., & Zamorano, J. L. (2012). Non-invasive imaging in acute chest pain syndromes. *European Heart Journal Cardiovasc Imaging*, 13, 69–78.

Yosefy, C., Levine, R. A., Picard, M. H., Vaturi, M., Handschumacher, M. D., & Isselbacher, E. M. (2007). Pseudodyskinesis of the inferior left ventricular wall: recognizing an echocardiographic mimic of myocardial infarction. *Journal of the American Society of Echocardiography*, 20, 1374–1379.

A complete reference list can be found online at ExpertConsult.com.

19 Mechanical Complications of Myocardial Infarction

Justina C. Wu

INTRODUCTION

There is a short list of structural complications of which every cardiologist and sonographer must be aware that may arise in the subacute period after myocardial infarct (MI), that, within the first week (Box 19.1). These are caused by necrosis of the heart muscle, and are frequently lethal if not caught early enough and repaired. The mechanical complications are: acute mitral regurgitation (MR), ventricular septal defect (VSD), pseudoaneurysm, free wall rupture, and tamponade. In any patient with sudden hypotension, chest pain, congestive heart failure or hypoxia post-MI, or electromechanical dissociation, there must be a high index of suspicion for these entities. The incidence of these complications has cumulatively decreased to less than 1% since primary percutaneous coronary intervention has become standard treatment for acute MI, but when they do occur, mortality is high.[1] Echocardiography with color flow Doppler is a crucial tool for bedside diagnosis and differentiation of these complications.

ACUTE MITRAL REGURGITATION

The appearance of a new large color jet of MR after MI, particularly if turbulent (as indicated by a multicolored signal) or directed eccentrically against the left atrial wall, should prompt the sonographer to search for structural abnormalities of the mitral apparatus (Fig. 19.1 and Videos 19.1 and 19.2). As mentioned previously in Chapter 18, the diagonal branches of the left anterior descending (LAD) and the left circumflex artery (LCx) both supply the anterolateral papillary muscle, but the posterior descending artery (PDA; usually a branch of the right coronary artery [RCA]) alone supplies the posteromedial papillary muscle. For this reason, posteromedial papillary muscle rupture is far more common (6–12 times more), and RCA infarcts have the highest incidence of acute MR. For the most part, the anterolateral papillary muscle connects via chordae tendinae to the anterior leaflet and the posteromedial papillary muscle connects to the posterior leaflet. Rupture of the papillary muscle trunk, heads, or chordae will cause the associated leaflet tip to flail backward into the left atrium (LA), with consequent MR in a jet that is directed *away* from that leaflet onto the opposing wall (Fig. 19.2). Hence, infarct of the posteromedial papillary muscle will cause posterior leaflet flail, which directs the jet anteroseptally. (Clinically, the sudden presence of a new murmur in the aortic area could be a telltale sign.) Infarct of the anterolateral papillary muscle, which would require extensive damage in both diagonal and LCx territories, would cause MR directed posteriorly (where the MR murmur might only be detected if the patient's back was auscultated).

Depending on the extent and duration of hypoxemia, the level of injury may involve the entire papillary muscle, or be more limited to one or more papillary muscle heads, tips, or chordae. In reality, there is variation in the chordal fan configuration, with occasional overlap and crossover between the papillary muscle heads and chordae tendinae (see Chapter 39, Fig. 39.2.) Hence there are instances in which inferior infarcts can lead to anterior leaflet flail, or conversely, anterior infarcts can cause posterior mitral leaflet flail. In these cases a smaller segment of leaflet, such as the tip only, is usually involved.

A patient's echocardiographic windows may be poor in the setting of acute shock due to mitral valve disruption caused by multiple factors such as suboptimal patient positioning, volume overload, and tachycardia. Furthermore, poor cardiac contractility overall or a wide open mitral valve will also theoretically diminish the left ventricular (LV)-LA pressure differences and cause the MR color Doppler jet to appear less impressive. A very eccentric jet that hugs the left atrial wall and escapes the usual transducer planes of insonation may also cause underdetection of MR. Hence, even if transthoracic echo windows are poor and nondiagnostic, *if the clinical scenario strongly suggests acute MR, one should pursue*

transesophageal echocardiography while the patient is being treated supportively and surgical consultation is underway (i.e., without delaying either). Fig. 19.3 shows an entire head of the anterior papillary muscle that has ruptured, which can be seen on the corresponding Video 19.3 and 19.4 (transthoracic echocardiogram [TTE] 2D and color views, of suboptimal image quality as might be obtained in real life, but showing a very eccentric mitral regurgitant jet) and subsequent transesophageal echocardiogram (TEE) confirming flail mitral valve in Video 19.5.

VENTRICULAR SEPTAL DEFECT

The LAD septal branches supply the anterior two-thirds of the interventricular septum, and the remaining inferior portion is supplied by the PDA. VSDs occurring after MI are typically detected by a color flow Doppler jet penetrating from the left to right ventricle. VSDs may be described as simple in type, which means a direct perforation through both sides of the septum at the same level, or complex, with multiple serpiginous tracts through the septum. VSDs caused by anterior MIs tend to be simple and arise more apically (Fig. 19.4A and Video 19.6), whereas VSDs in the setting of inferior MIs are often more complex and involve the basal portions of the septum (see Fig. 19.4B and Video 19.7). The latter tissue defects may also (rarely) extend to involve the adjacent inferior and right ventricular wall. Inferobasal defects are difficult for the surgeon to reach and repair by virtue of their location, complex configuration, and thin myocardial walls.

The actual width and extent of the VSD may not be readily apparent on echocardiography as an actual defect or discontinuity in the muscle layer, except in large cases. The area of the defect may simply appear akinetic, or thinned, as opposed to a discrete area of echo dropout in the muscular septum. Careful "sweeping" of the transducer plane with color Doppler by tilting the transducer systematically through short-axis and long-axis planes may be required to detect and localize smaller VSDs. Using continuous-wave (CW) Doppler collinearly with the color jet, one can obtain the peak velocity difference between the left and right ventricles. This difference is inversely proportional to the size of the defect: smaller (restrictive) VSDs will have high gradients, and the larger (nonrestrictive) VSDs will display lower gradients. If one documents the patient's systolic blood pressure (SBP) at the time of study (which should equal LV systolic pressure in the absence of aortic stenosis), then the right ventricular systolic pressure (RVSP) may be calculated as:

$$RVSP = SBP - 4 \times (\text{maximal interventricular pressure gradient in m/s})^2$$

Intuitively from the above, it can be reasoned that the large VSDs with lower interventricular pressure gradients will have higher RVSPs, that is, more tendency toward pulmonary hypertension. With the larger

> **BOX 19.1 Mechanical Complications of Acute Myocardial Infarction**
>
> Acute mitral regurgitation (papillary muscle rupture)
> Ventricular septal defect
> Pseudoaneurysm
> Free wall rupture
> Tamponade
> Other potential factors contributing to cardiogenic shock post-AMI
>   LV failure
>   LV outflow tract obstruction
>   RV failure: RV infarct, pulmonary embolus

AMI, Acute myocardial infarction; *LV,* left ventricular; *RV,* right ventricular.

VSDs, however, the Bernoulli equation may become a less accurate model due to the nonlimiting nature of the defect to flow.

VSDs can occur within fewer than 24 hours post-MI (post-percutaneous coronary intervention),[1] and often precipitate cardiogenic shock. Patients who have had extensive infarcts, delayed or poor revascularization, and who are smaller, elderly, or female are at higher risk of developing a VSD.[2] If undetected, continued interventricular shunting can eventually cause right-sided pressure overload. This in turn leads to pulmonary hypertension and right heart failure, causing the amount of left-to-right shunting to paradoxically decline over time. Treatment is generally surgery to reconstruct the septum (often along with coronary artery bypass graft [CABG]), but overall mortality remains high.[3] In cases where the surgical risk is prohibitive, percutaneous closure with a device, using echocardiographic guidance, can be a useful alternative for reducing shunting.[4]

There have been rare cases of *intramyocardial dissecting hematomas* occurring as a rare complication of MI. These may occur in the septum, lateral wall, or even the apex and are thought to represent a subacute form of cardiac hemorrhage and rupture that is still confined within the spiral layers of the myocardium.[5]

PSEUDOANEURYSM

A pseudoaneurysm is a ventricular free wall perforation that is locally contained. Unlike a true aneurysm (see Chapter 20), in which there is thinning of the myocardium but preservation of the endocardium and epicardium, a pseudoaneurysm is defined as a discrete disruption in all three layers of the heart, with the contents of the left ventricle locally contained by adhesions and the adjacent remaining pericardium (Fig. 19.5A).

Most pseudoaneurysms are found after inferior MIs, and less commonly in the lateral or apical regions. On echocardiogram, they appear as echo-free chambers or spaces adjacent to and continuous with the LV cavity. The most frequent site of occurrence is the basal inferior or inferolateral wall, although pseudoaneurysms can also arise at the LV apex after LAD occlusion (see Fig. 19.5 and Videos 19.8 and 19.9).

In reality, pseudoaneurysms cannot always be definitely distinguished from true aneurysms on echocardiography, but some studies have shown certain characteristics to be more indicative of pseudoaneurysms: A narrow neck, specifically less than 50% of the maximum diameter of the aneurysm itself, ragged edges with an abrupt transition from normal to thinned walls, and turbulent bidirectional flow by Doppler (Video 19.10) have been associated more with pseudoaneurysms. Intravenous (IV) echocardiographic contrast can be helpful in defining pseudoaneurysms (see Fig. 19.5B and Videos 19.8 and 19.9). If the patient is stable and there is doubt as to the existence of extent of pseudoaneurysm, cardiac magnetic resonance imaging (MRI) or alternatively angiography with LV gram can also be confirmatory.

Pseudoaneurysms are overall relatively rare, but portend poor prognosis (mortality rate of 21%–50% in most case series).[6] They may present with congestive heart failure, angina, ventricular arrhythmia, or embolization. Pseudoaneurysms that occur a few days after acute MI are quite unstable and prone to rupture. The mean time to diagnosis of pseudoaneurysm is generally in the range of 6 months. Surprisingly, some pseudoaneurysms may be found relatively late, even years, after MI in asymptomatic patients. Even with surgical treatment, which consists of direct closure or a pericardial patch, mortality remains high.

Aside from pseudoaneurysms and true LV aneurysms, there are a limited number of differential diagnoses of a discrete echo-free space adjacent to the left ventricle. If the patient is post-CABG, a coronary artery or bypass graft aneurysm may present similarly. In younger patients without a history of MI, rare congenital abnormalities such as LV diverticuli or an accessory left ventricle could be considered.[7]

FREE WALL RUPTURE

Free wall rupture is a devastating complication post-MI. Due to its acuity of presentation and rapid mortality, this event is rarely captured on echocardiography. The findings include an acute pericardial effusion in association with a discrete focal wall motion abnormality. Typically there is thinning in the area of the involved section. The actual point of rupture may not be easy to demonstrate without actual surgical exploration, due to the slit-like nature of many defects. However, there are cases in which discontinuity or even dissection into the infarcted area are directly demonstrated on ultrasound by color Doppler flow. IV echocardiographic contrast may be useful in demonstrating flow from the left ventricle to the pericardium in the small cases. Obviously, this should never impede immediate surgical consultation, and should only be considered if diagnosis is unclear and the patient appears clinically

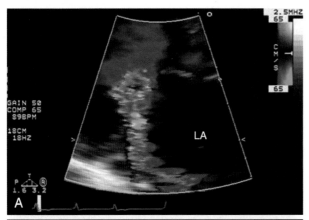

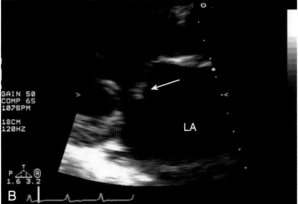

FIG. 19.1 Acute mitral regurgitation due to flail mitral leaflet. (A) Color Doppler jet showing a turbulent and eccentric posteriorly directed "wall-hugging" jet of mitral regurgitation on parasternal long-axis view. (B) 2D parasternal long-axis view of the same valve, showing the anterior mitral valve leaflet tip *(arrow)* flailing back into the left atrium in systole. See also corresponding Videos 19.1 and 19.2.

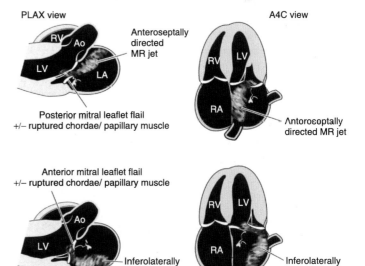

FIG. 19.2 Mitral valve flail schematic. In general, flail of a mitral valve leaflet directs the mitral regurgitant (MR) flow toward the opposite direction. Anterior leaflet flail (as in the preceding Fig. 19.1) will cause an eccentric jet of posteriorly directed MR, and posterior leaflet flail will give rise to inferolaterally directed MR. *Ao,* Aorta; *LA,* left atrium; *LV,* left ventricular; *RA,* right atrium; *RV,* right ventricular. *(Courtesy of Bernard E. Bulwer, MD, FASE; From Solomon SD, Wu J, Gillam L. Echocardiography. In: Mann DL, Zipes DP, Libby P, et al., eds. Braunwald's Heart Disease: A Textbook of Cardiovascular Medicine. 10th ed. Philadelphia: Elsevier; 2015, 179–260.)*

stable (Fig. 19.6 and Video 19.11). The consequent pericardial effusion may be echolucent or have cloudy swirling echodensities due to early organizing fibrin within the hemopericardium (Fig. 19.7 and Video 19.12).

LV wall rupture has historically been reported to be most frequently detected within 5 days post-MI. Similar to other mechanical complications, the incidence has decreased as reperfusion therapies have improved, to less than 2% of ST elevation MIs.[8,9] In many series it is more frequent than septal or papillary muscle rupture. The most common site of LV rupture is debatable: the anterior wall site is the most common site found in autopsies, but there may be selection bias due to more frequent anterior MIs and inability to tolerate such large infarcts. Risk factors are similar to those for other mechanical complications, including female gender, hypertension, delayed or no reperfusion, extensive or anterior MI, poor collateral circulation to the infarcted area, and no prior history of MI. The clinical

presentation is usually abrupt cardiogenic shock with tamponade and electromechanical dissociation. Pericardiocentesis in this setting is somewhat controversial (due to the theoretic risk of increasing LV intracavitary pressure and thus enlarging the tear), but may provide temporary stabilization. If the rupture is identified expeditiously enough, surgery is the only potentially life-saving option (with a mortality rate of up to 33%), although temporary support with an intraaortic balloon pump (IABP), left ventricular assist device (LVAD), and even extracorporeal membrane oxygenation (ECMO) have been used adjunctively in addition to surgery.

TAMPONADE

There are pericardial complications that can arise from MI. Tamponade post-MI may arise from free wall rupture as discussed earlier, or as an iatrogenic complication of cardiac catheterization or surgery. Cardiac catheterization may inadvertently cause aortic dissection or coronary artery dissection.

The presence of a new echolucent or fibrinous pericardial effusion post-MI is always of concern for the previously noted causes. Frank hemopericardium has a distinctive appearance on echocardiography, with shimmering vague echodensities within the pericardial sac (see Fig. 19.7 and Video 19.12), and should prompt immediate surgical consultation, with the presumed source of bleeding being either the heart itself or the aorta. In cases where there is intermittent or "stuttering" bleeding into the pericardium, adhesions and fully organized thrombus may also be found within the pericardium. Lastly, post-CABG or other heart surgeries, a formed clot may accumulate anterior to the heart and cause right ventricular (RV) compression. Such cases may be missed because fully organized clots often have an even, homogenously echodense appearance and can be mistaken for anterior mediastinal tissue, RV myocardium, or pericardial fat.

Large pericardial effusion may also be caused by inflammation (peri-infarct pericarditis, postcardiac injury syndrome, or Dressler syndrome), but tend to occur more gradually over time. Hence, effusions from these causes are far less likely to cause hemodynamic embarrassment in the acute period post-MI unless they become acutely hemorrhagic.

OTHER CAUSES OF CARDIOGENIC SHOCK AFTER MYOCARDIAL INFARCTION

Hypotension and cardiogenic shock may also ensue from severe loss of global myocardial contractility due primarily to the infarct itself. In fact, circulatory failure from severe LV dysfunction accounts for most (78%) of the deaths due to shock following MI.[10] This is particularly true if the patient cannot be revascularized, has had multiple infarcts in the past, or has recurrent ischemia. Not only left, but also right ventricular failure, due to RV infarcts or pulmonary embolus, can accompany and exacerbate overall heart failure. Rarely, left ventricular outflow tract (LVOT) obstruction can occur in patients with distal LAD infarcts with compensatory hyperkinesis of the basal left ventricle, particularly in patients with focal upper septal or asymmetric septal hypertrophy. This will contribute to a drop in cardiac output post-MI, and blood pressure may paradoxically and dramatically drop after inotropes, IABP, and vasodilators in these patients.[11]

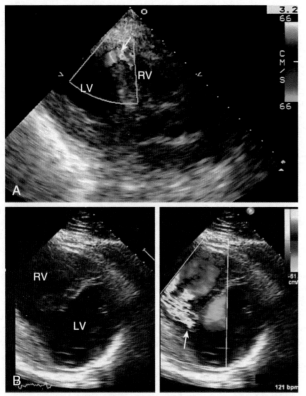

FIG. 19.4 Post-infarct ventricular septal defect. (A) Anteroseptal ventricular septal defect (VSD) of the simple type, on parasternal long-axis window with a color Doppler jet revealing left-to-right flow through the distal interventricular septum. See also corresponding Video 19.6. (B) Inferoseptal VSD seen as echo dropout in the tissue of the basal inferoseptum on subcostal short-axis windows *(left panel)*, and left-to-right flow by color Doppler *(right panel, arrow)*. See also corresponding Video 19.7. *LV,* Left ventricular; *RV,* right ventricular.

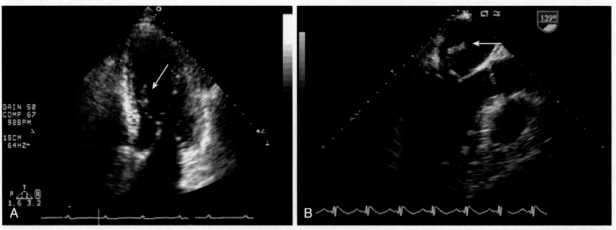

FIG. 19.3 Transthoracic echocardiogram (TTE) showing an entire trunk of the anterior papillary muscle *(arrow)* that has ruptured, in apical four-chamber view on TTE (A), and three-chamber view on transesophageal echocardiogram (B). See also corresponding Videos 19.3 and 19.4.

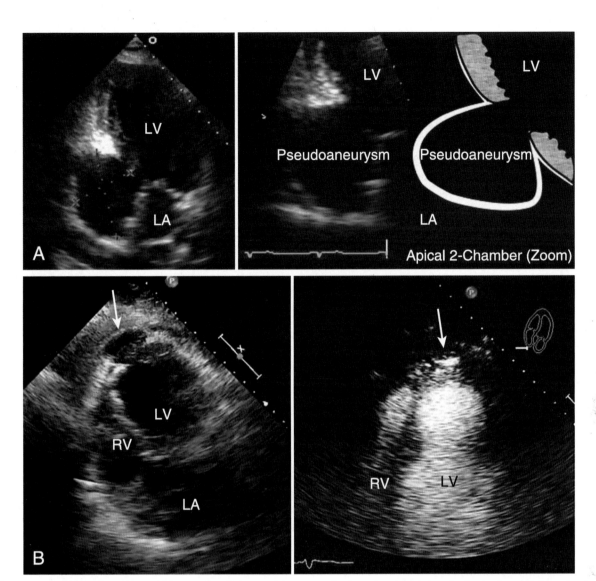

FIG. 19.5 Left ventricular pseudoaneurysms. (A) A large basal inferior pseudoaneurysm (by *green dotted* crosshairs to be 6 × 4 cm), on apical two-chamber view. Note the narrow neck and ragged edges of the pseudoaneurysm. The schematic in the *right upper panel* shows the layers of the heart disrupted with local containment of blood by adjacent pericardium and tissue. (B) A smaller apical pseudoaneurysm *(arrow)* on apical four-chamber view. The *right panel* demonstrates extravasation of intravenous echocardiographic contrast outside of the left ventricle (LV) into the previous echo-free space. See also corresponding Videos 19.8 and 19.9. *LA,* Left atrium; *RV,* right ventricular.

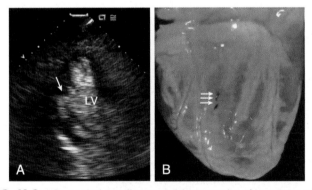

FIG. 19.6 Left ventricular wall rupture. (A) Extravasation of intravenous echo contrast from the left ventricular (LV) cavity through a slit-like orifice *(arrow)* into the pericardium inferolaterally, on this apical three-chamber view. (B) Posterior view of the heart, showing a linear myocardial rupture *(arrows)*. See also corresponding Video 19.11. (*A, Courtesy of Judy Mangion, MD, Brigham and Women's Hospital; B, Courtesy of Dr. Robert Padera, MD, PhD, Brigham and Women's Hospital.*)

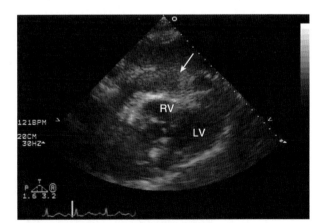

FIG. 19.7 Hemopericardium *(arrow),* on subcostal four-chamber view. See also corresponding Video 19.12.

Suggested Reading

Davis, N., & Sistino, J. J. (2002). Review of ventricular rupture: key concepts and diagnostic tools for success. *Perfusion, 17,* 63–67.

Dias, V., Cabral, S., Gomes, C., et al. (2009). Intramyocardial dissecting haematoma: a rare complication of acute myocardial infarction. *European Journal of Echocardiography, 10,* 585–587.

Güvenç, R. Ç., & Güvenç, T. S. (2016). Clinical presentation, diagnosis and management of acute mitral regurgitation following acute myocardial infarction. *Journal Acute Disease, 5,* 96–101.

Kutty, R. S., Jones, N., & Morrjani, N. (2013). Mechanical complications of acute myocardial infarction. *Cardiology Clinics, 31,* 519–531.

A complete reference list can be found online at ExpertConsult.com.

20 Long-Term Consequences and Prognosis After Myocardial Infarction

Justina C. Wu, Scott D. Solomon

INTRODUCTION

Substantial changes in cardiac structure can occur in the months to years following a completed myocardial infarct (MI), particularly if the culprit coronary artery supplied a large territory or flow was not rapidly restored. These changes may be clinically silent as they evolve, but with time can lead to extensive morbidity and mortality, including increased risk of developing heart failure and sudden cardiac death (SCD). Most of the pharmacologic, electrophysiologic, and interventional therapies indicated following MI are targeted toward prevention or amelioration of these complications. Both common and rare long-term complications after MI are summarized in Box 20.1. Most of these complications occur more commonly after large transmural infarcts, where revascularization was unsuccessful.

Echocardiography is appropriately used for the initial evaluation of ventricular function following an acute coronary syndrome (ACS), but is also very useful during the recovery phase to guide therapy (see Chapter 47).[1] For the chronic care of patients with coronary artery disease, deterioration in clinical status or physical exam (without a clear precipitating change in medication or diet), or intent to initiate or change therapy because of clinical status change is also grounds for a cardiac ultrasound. Echocardiography can also supply much prognostic data with respect to patient trajectory and outcomes.

LEFT VENTRICULAR SCAR AND ANEURYSM

A transmural infarct will result in a myocardial scar, seen on echocardiography as an akinetic or dyskinetic segment with thinning and increased echoreflectivity. One or more segments may be large and weak enough to form an aneurysm. An aneurysm is a discrete outpouching of the ventricle with preservation of all three heart layers (endocardium, residual myocardium, and epicardium). They tend to develop at either the basal inferior wall or at the left ventricular (LV) apex, and can grow to a size that rivals that of the adjacent chambers (Fig. 20.1 and Videos 20.1 and 20.2). Because there is no acute mechanical disruption of tissue, the transition from normal myocardium to aneurysm tends to be smooth and gradual, the outpouching may be relatively shallow, and flow by color Doppler tends to be laminar and nonturbulent (in contrast to pseudoaneurysms, as discussed in Chapter 19). The presence of the large aneurysmal area alters LV geometry and diminishes cardiac output. Attempts to improve the remodeling by surgically resecting or excluding aneurysmal and marginally viable surrounding areas (i.e., partial left ventriculectomy, or Batista operation) have shown limited benefits and a high overall failure rate, and thus is rarely recommended today. Aneurysms need to be distinguished from pseudoaneurysms, which are confined free wall ruptures, have a much worse prognosis, and represent a surgical emergency (see Chapter 19).

Flow within an aneurysm is frequently sluggish, as evidenced by spontaneous echo contrast, which can be more prominent and swirl locally

BOX 20.1 Long-Term Complications of Myocardial Infarction

Common Complications
LV scar and aneurysm
LV thrombus
LV remodeling (ischemic cardiomyopathy)
Functional (secondary) ischemic mitral regurgitation

Rare Complications
Chronic pericardial disease (constriction)
Saphenous vein graft aneurysms and pseudoaneurysms, status post CABG

CABG, Coronary artery bypass graft; *LV*, left ventricular.

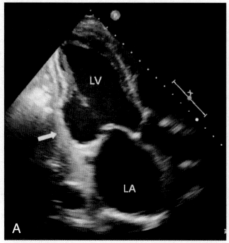
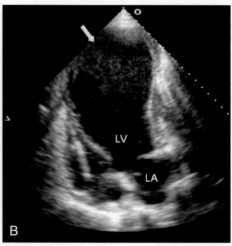

FIG. 20.1 Left ventricular aneurysms. (A) Inferobasal left ventricular aneurysm *(arrow)*, on apical three-chamber view. Note the thinning, increased reflectivity, and dyskinesis (outward bulge in systole) of the basal inferolateral segment. See also the corresponding Video 20.1. (B) Giant apical left ventricular aneurysm on apical four-chamber view. An 8-cm true aneurysm *(arrow)* is noted bulging from the apex and distal lateral wall of the left ventricle. Features typical of such aneurysms include a wide neck, smooth tapering of the walls, which contain all three tissue layers, and spontaneous echo contrast consistent with sluggish blood flow within the aneurysmal pouch. A pacemaker/automatic implantable cardioverter-defibrillator wire is present in the right heart. See also corresponding Video 20.2. *LA,* Left atrium; *LV,* left ventricle.

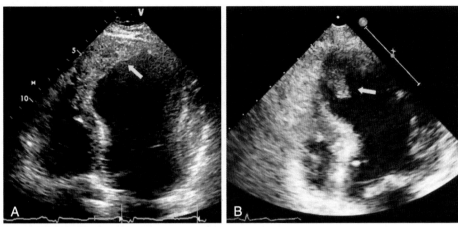

FIG. 20.2 Left ventricular apical thrombi. (A) A flat immobile mural thrombus *(arrow)* is layered within the aneurysmal left ventricular (LV) apex. (B) A 2-cm mobile finger-like thrombus *(arrow)* is seen protruding from an akinetic LV apex. See also corresponding Videos 20.3 and 20.4.

(see Video 20.2) within the aneurysm. If the patient is not anticoagulated, this will predispose to formation of LV thrombus. The presence of extensive myocardial scarring, which conducts electrical impulses poorly, can also pave the way for reentrant arrhythmias such as ventricular tachycardias (VTs). VTs due to scars tend to be monomorphic, have sudden onset, and can cause symptoms that range from palpitations to sudden loss of consciousness, and even SCD. For this reason, after large MIs, echocardiography is used to evaluate for global depression of left ventricular ejection fraction (LVEF), one of the criteria used for determining the need to implant an automatic implantable cardioverter-defibrillator (AICD) for primary and secondary prevention of SCD (generally indicated if LVEF is ≤35%). In cases where a ventricular tachyarrhythmia has already occurred or recurs post-MI, echocardiography is also useful for gross localization of areas likely to have slow conduction and for ruling out LV thrombi prior to a planned VT ablation. The presence of mobile thrombus is an absolute contraindication to catheter ablation, because it can be dislodged by catheter manipulations, induction of VT, or repeated cardioversions. If a laminated (immobile) mural thrombus is visualized, some electrophysiologists may consider VT ablation after the patient has been anticoagulated at therapeutic levels (conventionally with warfarin for 4 weeks prior to procedure). In high-risk cases, some centers use intracardiac echocardiography (ICE) with electroanatomic mapping systems to avoid inadvertent catheter entry into the thrombus. The ablation procedure itself can induce complications of thromboembolism or cardiac perforation leading to tamponade.[2]

LEFT VENTRICULAR THROMBUS

Formed thrombus may be detected in the left ventricle within 24 hours after MI, and most are formed within the first 1–2 weeks after MI.[3] The incidence is estimated to be 8%–15% in patients with acute anterior MI (treated with percutaneous coronary intervention and dual antiplatelet therapy). Patients with large anterior MIs, LVEF of less than 40%, and severe akinesis or dyskinesis are at high risk of LV thrombus. They most frequently occur in the region with the most severe wall motion abnormality, and hence are most often at the apex. Approximately 11% occur at the septum and 3% at the inferolateral wall.

Thrombi appear as discrete homogeneously echogenic deformable masses abutting the endocardial border, invariably next to an akinetic or dyskinetic segment. They are termed mural thrombi when they are fixed, flattened (i.e., parallel to the endocardial surface), and adhere closely to the endocardium. Other thrombi may protrude more prominently into the LV cavity and be more mobile (Fig. 20.2 and Videos 20.3 and 20.4). Of note, serial echocardiography on untreated patients has shown that the morphology of LV thrombi can change markedly over the first several months post-infarct.[3]

Although the specificity (>90%) of transthoracic echocardiography for detection of thrombus is good, the sensitivity ranges from only 30% to 60% in routine echocardiograms performed without echocardiographic contrast, when compared with delayed enhancement cardiac magnetic resonance

imaging (MRI) as a gold standard.[4] However, if performed specifically to evaluate for possible LV thrombus with echo contrast, echocardiography has a good negative predictive value (91%) and positive predictive value is approximately 93%.[5] Accuracy is highly dependent on pretest probability, image quality, and the size and type of thrombus (the mural type being more difficult to detect than smaller protuberant thrombi). For echocardiograms that are inconclusive, the use of intravenous echocardiographic contrast increases sensitivity. In contrast to its primary role in detecting thrombi in the left atrium and appendage, transesophageal echocardiography has less sensitivity in detecting LV thrombus, because the LV apex is in the far field on transesophageal echocardiogram (TEE) windows.

The larger and more mobile thrombi, particularly if they reside near hinge points with hypercontractile myocardium, may be more likely to embolize.[6] Persistent thrombi tend to become more compact, less mobile, and more echodense. Warfarin is currently the recommended treatment of LV thrombus. With anticoagulation, LV thrombi resolve in almost 50% of patients by 1 year and approximately 85% by 2 years of follow-up. The optimal duration of therapy remains unclear: although the risk of embolization decreases over time, as the thrombus resolves or organizes further, there may be residual risk, particularly if large wall motion abnormalities remain.

LEFT VENTRICULAR REMODELING (ISCHEMIC CARDIOMYOPATHY)

After MI, changes in left ventricular structure may not be limited to the infarcted area. The left ventricle as a whole can begin to expand in size and mass, in a process termed ventricular remodeling. In the broadest context, left ventricular remodeling can be defined as an increase in left ventricular volume in response to a physiologic or pathologic state, such as chronic ischemia or chronic volume overload.

On echocardiography, left ventricular diameters and volumes will increase. If the left ventricular wall thickness remains the same or increases, overall LV mass will increase (i.e., hypertrophy occurs). This pattern of enlargement is known as *eccentric hypertrophy* (Fig. 20.3). On echocardiography, a ratio termed the *relative wall thickness* (RWT), in combination with the total LV mass, allows one to characterize the type of hypertrophy (see Chapter 22). RWT (Fig. 20.4) is simply the ratio of the summed wall thicknesses of opposing sections (interventricular septum and posterior wall) over the LV end-diastolic diameter.

$$RWT = \frac{(IVSd + PWd)}{LVEDd}$$

These measures are conventionally taken from the parasternal long-axis window on M-mode or 2D-echocardiography in diastole. The RWT also provides an objective way to distinguish eccentric hypertrophy (in which RWT is conventionally defined as ≤0.42) from concentric hypertrophy (RWT ≥ 0.42), the latter being a type of hypertrophy and

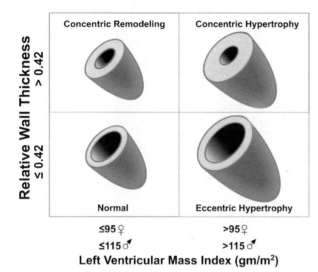

FIG. 20.3 Left ventricular remodeling and ischemic dilated cardiomyopathy. Cardiac hypertrophy is defined as an increase in overall left ventricular (LV) mass, or a shift to the models on the right side of this chart (reference cutoffs for males and females are shown on the X axis). If LV wall thickness increases without an overall increase in total cardiac mass, then concentric remodeling *(upper left model)* has occurred. If the cardiac mass increases due to thickened walls, the process is termed concentric hypertrophy *(upper right)*. If cardiac mass increases primarily because of LV dilation, then eccentric hypertrophy *(lower right)* has occurred. Calculation of relative wall thickness is in the next figure. *(Modified from Konstam MA, Kramer DG, Patel AR, Maron MS; Udelson JE. Left ventricular remodeling in heart failure: current concepts in clinical significance and assessment. JACC Cardiovasc Imaging. 2011;4(1):98–108.)*

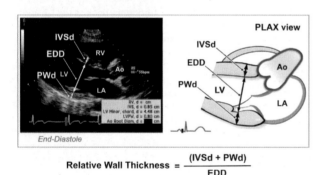

$$\text{Relative Wall Thickness} = \frac{(IVSd + PWd)}{EDD}$$

FIG. 20.4 Relative wall thickness calculation. This parameter is calculated simply from the standard measures taken from M-mode or 2D measurements at the base of the heart (at end-diastole). *EDD,* End-diastolic diameter; *IVSd,* interventricular septal thickness; *AO,* Aorta; *LA,* left atrium; *LV,* left ventricle; *PWd,* posterior wall thickness; *RV,* right ventricle. *(Courtesy of Bernard E. Bulwer, MD, FASE.)*

remodeling that arises after chronic pressure overload, which classically occurs in aortic stenosis or coarctation.

Concomitant changes in both geometry and function of the left ventricle frequently accompany remodeling. Border zones adjacent to recent infarcted areas can develop wall motion abnormalities (a process termed "infarct expansion"), but even areas relatively remote from the original infarct may become hypokinetic despite preserved epicardial coronary artery flow. The pathophysiology underlying these changes is complex, but is postulated to be initiated by increased myocardial load, which causes increased interstitial fibrosis and a further diminution in cardiomyocytes, which in turn decreases overall contractility and relaxation of the ventricle.

With more extensive remodeling, the heart often becomes more globular in shape. The change in shape may be measured by the *sphericity index* (Fig. 20.5). In normal hearts, the length (long-axis dimension) of the left ventricle is usually at least 1.5× greater than the width (short-axis dimension). Hearts that have remodeled after MI may have ratios that approach 1.0 (i.e., the ratio of a sphere).

From a hemodynamic standpoint, the previously discussed changes may initially help increase cardiac output, but in time the accompanying changes can have negative consequences and are a harbinger of poorer prognosis (see Prognosis section later). Severely dilated ventricles often

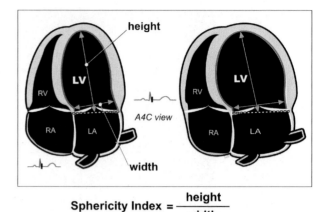

$$\text{Sphericity Index} = \frac{\text{height}}{\text{width}}$$

FIG. 20.5 Sphericity calculation. The left model shows a normal heart with its elliptical shape, and the right model shows a heart that has become more spherical in shape. Sphericity is calculated as the left ventricular (LV) height (length in apical four-chamber view from the mitral annulus to the endocardium at the LV apex) divided by the width (measured at the base of the heart in many studies, but more accurately measured at the widest portion of the heart, which is often the midventricular level). Both measurements are done at end-diastole. *(Courtesy of Bernard E. Bulwer, MD, FASE.)*

manifest with a combination of one or more of the following features, in addition to increased RWT and sphericity: very low ejection fraction, spontaneous echo contrast, dyssynchrony, and reduced aortic and mitral leaflet excursion. If the Doppler mitral inflow pattern reveals evidence of restrictive physiology, this portends a worse prognosis than earlier forms of diastolic dysfunction. The clinical correlates of these echocardiographic findings are frequent congestive heart failure symptoms and low exercise tolerance.

FUNCTIONAL (SECONDARY) MITRAL REGURGITATION

Functional, or secondary, mitral regurgitation is leakage of the valve that is fundamentally due to LV systolic dysfunction and remodeling (Videos 20.5 and 20.6). When the LV dysfunction is due to coronary artery disease, it is termed ischemic mitral regurgitation. Unlike acute ischemic mitral regurgitation, which is caused by papillary muscle rupture and flail leaflet, in functional ischemic mitral regurgitation the mitral apparatus is structurally intact but its geometry and the balances between opening and closing forces are altered in a way that prevents effective closure (see Chapter 28).

Many factors are known to contribute to functional mitral regurgitation (Fig. 20.6). Among the most important are tethering of the mitral leaflets and chordae, which are pulled both in the inferolateral direction by the increasingly spherical ventricle and in the apical direction by overall LV enlargement. The bases of the papillary muscles are displaced by this change in geometry and papillary muscle dysfunction, which contributes to suboptimal angulation of the chordae and restricted leaflet closure. Inferior and inferolateral infarcts, in particular, are strongly associated with functional mitral regurgitation because the RCA alone supplies the inferomedial papillary muscle and posterior leaflet. Reduced contractility of the left ventricle as a whole also means that the closing forces that contribute to pushing the mitral leaflets closed from "behind" are diminished. Mitral annular dilation from an enlarged left ventricle and left atrium, as well as insufficient mitral leaflet area to compensate for the enlarged orifice, may also play a role in further exacerbating the mitral regurgitation.

The sum of these changes, together with increased volume from the mitral regurgitation itself, which causes yet more chamber expansion and displacement of papillary muscles, appear to generate a cycle whereby "MR begets more MR." The effective regurgitant orifice area (EROA) is one key quantitative measure of mitral malcoaptation, which has a direct correlation with mortality in ischemic cardiomyopathy.[7] EROA is calculated from color and spectral Doppler measurements (see Chapter 28) and a value ≥0.20 cm² (and a regurgitant volume ≥30 mL or regurgitant fraction ≥50%) is indicative of severe secondary mitral regurgitation.

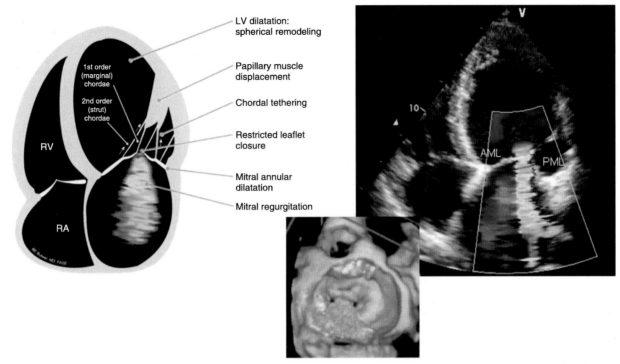

FIG. 20.6 **The multiple factors that interplay to cause functional (secondary) mitral regurgitation.** Restricted leaflet closure due to tethering and mitral annular dilation are thought to be the most important influences. Note how the posterior leaflet (PML) is held back and prevented from coapting fully with the anterior leaflet (AML). *Inset:* Three-dimensional transesophageal echocardiogram view from the atrial aspect, showing the mitral regurgitant jet hugging the posterior wall. See also corresponding Videos 20.5 and 20.6. *LV,* Left ventricular. *(Illustration from Solomon SD, Wu J, Gillam L. Echocardiography. In: Mann DL, Zipes DP, Libby P, et al., (eds).* Braunwald's Heart Disease: A Textbook of Cardiovascular Medicine. *10th ed. Philadelphia: Elsevier; 2015.)*

RARE COMPLICATIONS OF MYOCARDIAL INFARCTION

The complications noted previously are very common long-term sequelae of MI. In addition, there are complications that are far more unusual and encountered quite infrequently. If the MI is associated with acute pericarditis (i.e., Dressler syndrome, seen more frequently in transmural infarcts), some individuals may go on to develop a chronic constrictive pericarditis. Pericarditis may also occur infrequently after coronary artery bypass graft (CABG) as part of postcardiac injury syndrome (PCIS), at a rate of 0.2%–0.3% (see Chapter 33).

There is another pathology that is rarely encountered in the decades following CABG: weakness in the walls of saphenous vein grafts (SVGs), which leads to the development of SVG aneurysms and pseudoaneurysms. SVG aneurysms are defined as a dilation of the SVG of at least 1.5× the normal vessel diameter. They may initially be small and only detected during coronary angiography. However, over time these can grow to impressive sizes (>10 cm) and be detected as large, echolucent, or heterogeneous echogenic masses on echocardiography and radiography, typically adjacent to the right heart. They may exert mass effect on adjacent vessels or grafts or form fistulas. They may also thrombose and embolize distally, causing chest pain and infarcts. There is risk of outright graft rupture, which can essentially form a false aneurysm or cause hemothorax.[8]

PROGNOSIS AFTER MYOCARDIAL INFARCTION

After an acute MI, echocardiography can assist in assessing the prognosis for (1) patients at risk for recurrent ischemia and heart failure, and (2) overall risk of morbidity and mortality. LVEF is one of the most important predictors of overall morbidity and mortality after acute MI and is used as a surrogate endpoint in most major clinical trials of medical and procedural interventions.[9] As LVEF declines, the rate of SCD increases. Based on current evidence, the incidence of SCD at an LVEF of less than 35% is low enough to consider AICD implantation for primary (i.e., no known history of ventricular tachycardia/ventricular fibrillation [VT/VF]) prevention in selected patients with intraventricular conduction delay and heart failure.[10] It is important to recognize that functional recovery of

stunned myocardium can occur after reperfusion, leading to an improvement in LVEF when measured as early as 3–5 days after revascularization. In cases of rapid reperfusion, full recovery of function can occur within 2 weeks. For this reason, it is generally recommended that one wait at least 40 days post-acute MI, or as long as 3 months after CABG or percutaneous revascularization, then re-evaluate LVEF prior to making a decision on AICD implantation for primary prevention. Reduced global longitudinal and circumferential strain have emerged as important risk indicators for death or heart failure post-MI. A high degree of dyssynchrony, quantitated by the same technique, is also a risk factor. In addition to LVEF, overall LV size (as assessed by LV end-diastolic volume and diameter) and sphericity are important prognostic indicators. Other measures that are independently predictive of heart failure in patients with stable coronary artery disease (CAD) include: increasing left ventricular mass index (LVMI >90 g/m^2), a pseudonormalized or restrictive pattern of diastolic dysfunction, a left ventricular outflow tract (LVOT) velocity-time integral (VTI$_{lvot}$) of less than 22 mm, and left atrial volume index (LAVI) greater than 29 mL/m^2.[11] As noted previously, the presence of mild or greater mitral regurgitation is also an independent predictor of cardiac mortality and heart failure or recurrent MI.[7,9]

The wall motion score index (WMSI) may be a more discriminatory measure than LVEF (as measured by echocardiography or nuclear methods) in predicting cardiac events, in particular rehospitalization for heart failure. On resting echocardiography, WSMI greater than 1.7 that persists after treatment for MI suggests a substantial (>20%) perfusion defect and increased risk of complications. In stress echocardiography, a WMSI greater than 1.7 at peak stress and EF less than 45% are independent markers of patients at high risk for recurrent MI or cardiac death. When there is a question of whether revascularization will improve akinetic but viable areas, dobutamine or contrast echocardiography may delineate the extent of myocardium that is hibernating (hypocontractile yet viable and still perfused; see Chapter 27).

It should be noted that wall motion abnormalities are indicative of focal myocardial dysfunction but are not entirely specific for atherosclerosis-related MI. Vasospasm, inflammation or fibrosis due to myocarditis, swelling from intramural hematoma or edema, Takotsubo cardiomyopathy (apical ballooning syndrome), and any focal myocardial insult are

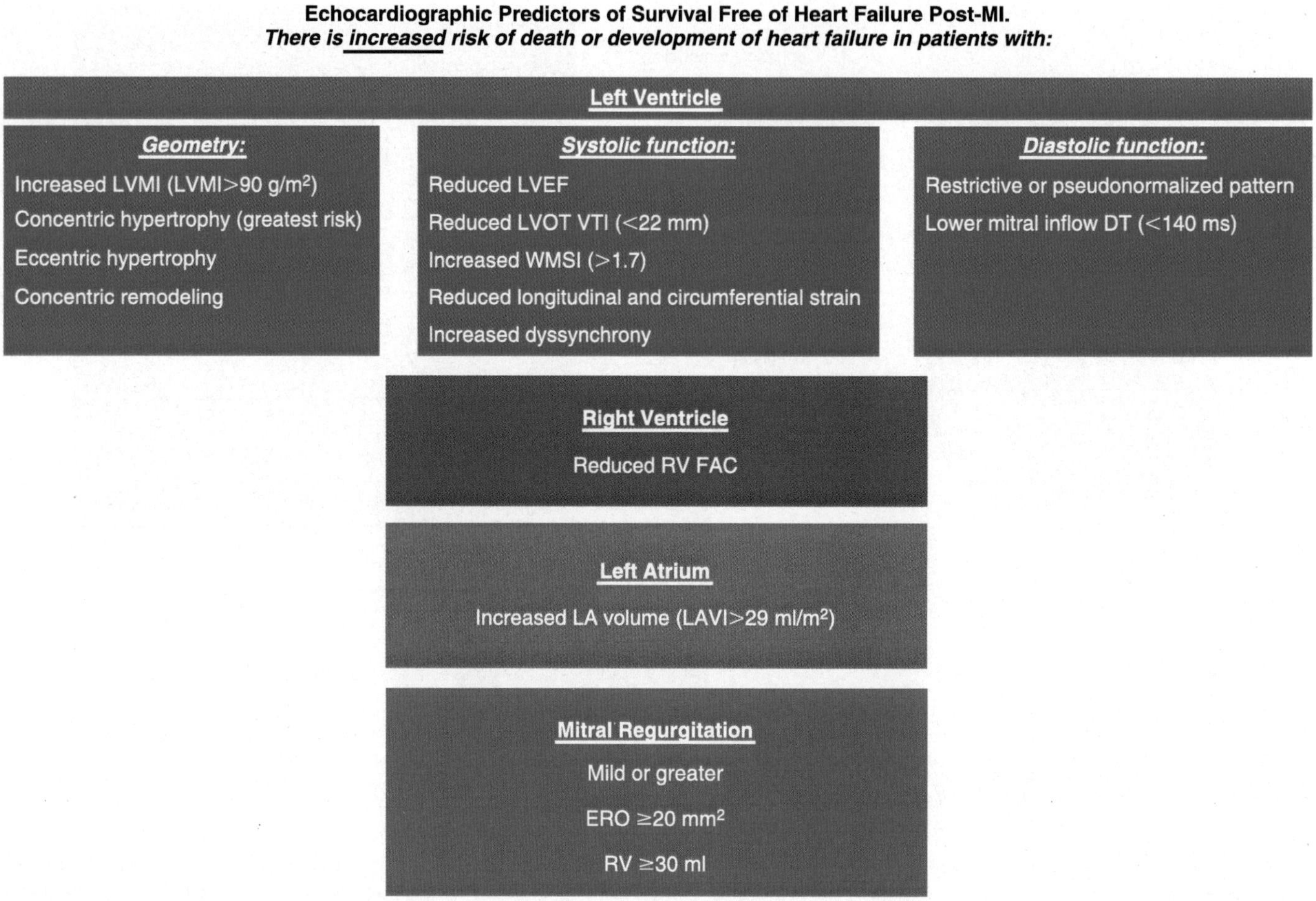

Echocardiographic Predictors of Survival Free of Heart Failure Post-MI.
There is increased risk of death or development of heart failure in patients with:

Left Ventricle

Geometry:

Increased LVMI (LVMI>90 g/m²)

Concentric hypertrophy (greatest risk)

Eccentric hypertrophy

Concentric remodeling

Systolic function:

Reduced LVEF

Reduced LVOT VTI (<22 mm)

Increased WMSI (>1.7)

Reduced longitudinal and circumferential strain

Increased dyssynchrony

Diastolic function:

Restrictive or pseudonormalized pattern

Lower mitral inflow DT (<140 ms)

Right Ventricle

Reduced RV FAC

Left Atrium

Increased LA volume (LAVI>29 ml/m²)

Mitral Regurgitation

Mild or greater

ERO ≥20 mm²

RV ≥30 ml

FIG. 20.7 Echocardiographic predictors of death or heart failure post-MI. *DT,* Deceleration time; *ERO,* effective regurgitant orifice; *LAVI,* left atrial volume index; *LVEF,* left ventricular ejection fraction; *LVMI,* left ventricular mass index; *LVOT,* left ventricular outflow tract; *VTI,* velocity time index at the left ventricular outflow tract; *RV FAC,* right ventricular fractional area change; *RV,* regurgitant volume; *WMSI,* wall motion score index.

also causes of wall motion abnormality. A comprehensive synthesis of the history, clinical, and physical exam findings, and ECG together with appropriate cardiac imaging will allow one to narrow down the differential diagnoses and pursue appropriate therapy.

Similarly, although LVEF and the echocardiographic prognostic indicators discussed earlier (and shown in Fig. 20.7) are each independent predictors of poor outcome after MI, the patient's overall clinical condition—including comorbidities such as diabetes and renal failure—has been shown to "weight" some factors. For instance, a mild reduction in LVEF in a diabetic patient post-MI appears to correlate with a higher impact on the risk of death or heart failure, when compared with that of a nondiabetic patient with the same LVEF.[12] Thus, the wealth of information that the standard echocardiographic exam provides in addition to LVEF, taken in context with the patient's other clinical data (including age, comorbidities, New York Heart Association [NYHA] status, and biomarkers) can provide more accurate risk assessment and a more informed platform from which to base clinical decisions post-MI.[12]

Suggested Reading

Cikes, M., & Solomon, S. D. (2016). Beyond ejection fraction: an integrative approach for assessment of cardiac structure and function in heart failure. *European Heart Journal, 37,* 1642–1650.

Delewi, R., Zijlstra, F., & Piek, J. J. (2012). Left ventricular thrombus formation after acute myocardial infarction. *Heart, 98,* 1743–1749.

Lancellotti, P., Zamorano, J. L., & Vannan, M. A. (2014). Imaging challenges in secondary mitral regurgitation: unsolved issues and perspectives. *Circulation Cardiovascular Imaging, 7,* 735–746.

Silbiger, J. J. (2011). Mechanistic insights into ischemic mitral regurgitation: echocardiographic and surgical implications. *Journal of the American Society of Echocardiography, 24,* 707–719.

A complete reference list can be found online at ExpertConsult.com.

21 Echocardiography in Heart Failure

Scott D. Solomon, Elke Platz, Justina C. Wu

Heart failure (HF) is a clinical syndrome characterized by fatigue, breathlessness, and edema caused by an abnormality of heart function. While the etiologies of HF differ, and HF can occur with reduced or preserved ejection fraction, or with low or high cardiac output, all forms of HF share a basic pathophysiology: the inability to provide adequate cardiac perfusion to the body at rest or with exertion or to only do so at the expense of elevated cardiac filling pressures. Clinically HF is characterized by a specific constellation of signs and symptoms (Box 21.1), and several of which must be present for the diagnosis. The Framingham HF criteria have further categorized signs and symptoms of HF into major and minor criteria and require that one major and two minor criteria be fulfilled to make the diagnosis (Box 21.2).

Echocardiography plays a central role in the diagnosis and management of patients with HF (Fig. 21.1). It is the primary method for assessment of left ventricular ejection fraction (LVEF), which is used to distinguish HF with reduced ejection fraction (HFrEF) from HF with preserved ejection fraction (HFpEF), a crucial determination because evidenced-based therapies only exist for the former. Echocardiography can also help to distinguish among the different types and the potential etiologies of HF and can be useful to identify specific causes of HD, such as sarcoidosis, amyloidosis, hypertrophic cardiomyopathy, or primary valvular abnormalities, some of which might be amenable to specific targeted therapies. Moreover, dilatation of the heart itself results in functional mitral regurgitation, which is both a marker of HF severity and may itself be amenable to therapeutic intervention. In addition, right ventricular function and left atrial (LA) size have incremental prognostic value in HF, and assessing these chambers has become crucial to the assessment of the HF patient.

ASSESSMENT OF CARDIAC STRUCTURE AND FUNCTION

Assessment of Ejection Fraction

Assessment of cardiac structure and function is an essential step in the evaluation of patients with HF. Determination of ejection fraction (see Chapter 14) is essential to categorizing the patient as having HFrEF, or HFpEF. An LVEF of 40% or less is generally considered evidence of "reduced" ejection fraction. The definition of what constitutes "preserved" ejection fraction has been debated; some have proposed that "preserved" be used generically for any ejection fraction over 40%, while others believe true HFpEF only begins with LVEF > 45% or even 50%. The 2016 European Society of Cardiology (ESC) Heart Failure Guidelines recently suggested that HF with LVEF in the range from 40% to 49% be termed "Heart Failure with Mid-Range Ejection Fraction" (HFmrEF) (Table 21.1).[1] This categorization has not been adopted by other guidelines. The crucial reason to assess ejection fraction in patients with HF is that evidenced-based therapies exist for patients with HF and rEF, including angiotensin converting enzyme (ACE) inhibitors, angiotensin receptor blockers (ARBs), angiotensin receptor neprilysin inhibitors (ARNIs), beta-blockers, and mineralocorticoid receptor antagonists. These therapies are not indicated in patients with LVEF > 40%, for which no specific treatment other than relief of symptoms is currently approved. Several methods used to assess LVEF are outlined in Chapter 14.

Echocardiographic measures of cardiac structure and function have been shown to have prognostic value in HF. Although LVEF has been the most studied and is a potent predictor of outcome in HF, it is certainly not the only predictor (Fig. 21.2), and measures of both systolic and diastolic function have been related to outcomes in heart failure. Measures

of left ventricular size, such as end-diastolic and end-systolic volumes also relate to outcomes.

Determination of Heart Failure Etiology

HF can be caused by numerous diseases that impair or influence cardiac function, which, while distinct, can lead to similar signs and symptoms (Table 21.2). While evidenced-based therapies in HFrEF are typically utilized irrespective of etiology, understanding the etiologic factors contributing to HF can be extremely useful on an individual patient basis, and echocardiography can be helpful in the determination of etiology. Patients whose HF is due to a prior myocardial infarction (see Chapter 20) will typically have evidence of regional wall motion abnormalities in a coronary artery distribution. Previously infarcted regions can be thin, severely hypokinetic, akinetic, or even aneurysmal. Occasionally, patients with profound ongoing ischemia can have global left ventricular dysfunction (hibernating myocardium). Hibernating myocardium may be distinguishable from irreversible left ventricular dysfunction with dobutamine echocardiography in which augmented function may be apparent at low doses of dobutamine, and dysfunction may be apparent at higher doses due to ischemia (see Chapter 27).

Regional wall motion abnormalities can also be present in other forms of cardiomyopathy leading to HF, including sarcoidosis or Chagas' disease and abnormalities of mechanical conduction, such as bundle branch blocks. Sarcoidosis should be considered when regional wall motion

---

BOX 21.1 Signs and Symptoms of Heart Failure

SYMPTOMS	SIGNS
Shortness of breath	Elevated jugular venous pressure
Fatigue	Third heart sound (gallop)
Reduced exercise tolerance	Rales on auscultation
Orthopnea	Radiographic cardiomegaly
Paroxysmal nocturnal dyspnea	Hepatojugular reflex
Edema	Hepatomegaly
Weight loss > 4.5 lbs in response to treatment	Pleural effusion
	Tachycardia

BOX 21.2 Framingham Criteria for the Diagnosis of Heart Failure

MAJOR CRITERIA	MINOR CRITERIA
Acute pulmonary edema	Ankle edema
Cardiomegaly	Dyspnea on exertion
Hepatojugular reflex	Hepatomegaly
Neck vein distention	Nocturnal cough
Paroxysmal nocturnal dyspnea or orthopnea	Pleural effusion
Pulmonary rales	Tachycardia (heart rate >120 beats per minute)
Third heart sound (S3 gallop rhythm)	

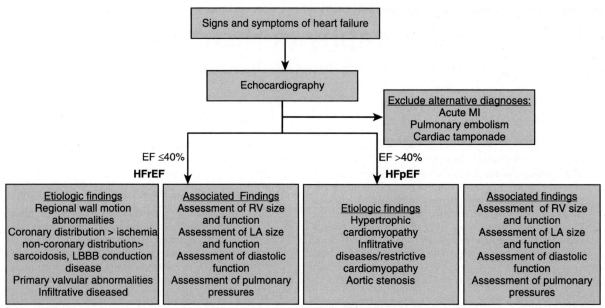

FIG. 21.1 Role of echocardiography in heart failure. *EF,* Ejection fraction; *HFpEF,* heart failure with preserved ejection fraction; *HFrEF,* heart failure with reduced ejection fraction; *LA,* left atrial; *LBBB,* left bundle branch block; *RV* right atrial.

TABLE 21.1 2016 ESC Categorization of Heart Failure

TYPE OF HF		HFrEF	HFmrEF	HFpEF
CRITERIA	1	Symptoms ± Signs[a]	Symptoms ± Signs[a]	Symptoms ± Signs[a]
	2	LVEF <40%	LVEF 40%–40%	LVEF ≥50%

	3	—	1. Elevated levels of natriuretic peptides[b]:
			2. At least one additional criterion:
			  a. relevant structural heart disease (LVH and/or LAE).
			  b. diastolic dysfunction
				1. Elevated levels of natriuretic peptides[b]:
				2. At least one additional criterion:
				  a. relevant structural heart disease (LVH and/or LAE).
				  b. diastolic dysfunction

[a]Signs may not be present in the early stages of HF (especially in HFpEF) and in patients treated with diuretics.
[b]BNP > 35 pg/mL and/or NT-proBNP > 125 pg/mL.
BNP, B-type natriuretic peptide; *HF,* heart failure; *HFmrEF,* heart failure with mid-range ejection fraction; *HFpEF,* heart failure with preserved ejection fraction; *HFrEF,* heart failure with reduced ejection fraction; *LAE,* left atrial enlargement; *LVEF,* left ventricular ejection fraction; *LVH,* left ventricular hypertrophy; *NT-proBNP,* N-terminal pro-B type natriuretic peptide.
From Ponikowski P, Voors AA, Anker SD, et al. 2016 ESC Guidelines for the diagnosis and treatment of acute and chronic heart failure: the task force for the diagnosis and treatment of acute and chronic heart failure of the European Society of Cardiology (ESC). Developed with the special contribution of the Heart Failure Association (HFA) of the ESC. Eur Heart J. 2016;37(27):2129–2200.

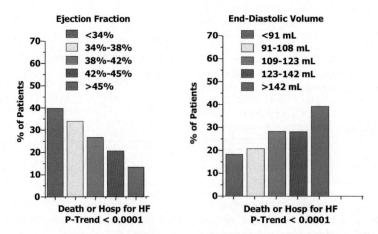

FIG. 21.2 Relationship between ejection fraction and end-diastolic volume and the composite outcome of death or development of heart failure following myocardial infarction. *HF,* Heart failure. (*Adapted from Solomon SD, Skali H, Anavekar NS, et al. Changes in ventricular size and function in patients treated with valsartan, captopril, or both after myocardial infarction. Circulation. 2005;111(25):3411–3419.*)

TABLE 21.2 Etiologies of Heart Failure

Diseased Myocardium		
Ischemic heart disease	Myocardial scar	
	Myocardial stunning/hibernation	
	Epicardial coronary artery disease	
	Abnormal coronary microcirculation	
	Endothelial dysfunction	
Toxic damage	Recreational substance abuse	Alcohol, cocaine, amphetamine, anabolic steroids
	Heavy metals	Copper, iron, lead, cobalt
	Medications	Cytostatic drugs (e.g., anthracyclines), immunomodulating drugs (e.g., interferons monoclonal antibodies such as trastuzumab, cetuximab), antidepressant drugs, antiarrhythmics, nonsteroidal antiinflammatory drugs, anesthetics.
	Radiation	
Immune-mediated and inflammatory damage	Related to infection	Bacteria, spirochetes, fungi, protozoa, parasites (Chagas disease), rickettsiae, viruses (HIV/AIDS)
	Not related to infection	Lymphocytic/giant cell myocarditis, autoimmune diseases (e.g., Graves disease, rheumatoid arthritis, connective tissue disorders, mainly systemic lupus erythematosus), hypersensitivity and eosinophilic myocarditis (Churg-Strauss).
Infiltration	Related to malignancy	Direct infiltrations and metastases
	Not related to malignancy	Amyloidosis, sarcoidosis, hemochromatosis (iron), glycogen storage diseases (e.g., Pompe disease), lysosomal storage diseases (e.g., Fabry disease)
Metabolic derangements	Hormonal	Thyroid diseases, parathyroid diseases, acromegaly, GH deficiency, hypercortisolemia, Conn disease, Addison disease, diabetes, metabolic syndrome, pheochromocytoma, pathologies related to pregnancy and peripartum
	Nutritional	Deficiencies in thiamine, L-carnitine, selenium, iron, phosphates, calcium, complex malnutrition (e.g., malignancy, AIDS, anorexia nervosa), obesity
Genetic abnormalities	Diverse forms	HCM, DCM, LV noncompaction, ARVC, restrictive cardiomyopathy (for details see respective expert documents), muscular dystrophies and laminopathies
Abnormal Loading Conditions		
Hypertension		
Valve and myocardium structural defects	Acquired	Mitral, aortic, tricuspid and pulmonary valve diseases
	Congenital	Atrial and ventricular septum defects and others (for details see a respective expert document)
Pericardial and endomyocardial pathologies	Pericardial	Constrictive pericarditis Pericardial effusion
	Endomyocardial	HES, EMF, endocardial fibroelastosis
High output states		Severe anemia, sepsis, thyrotoxicosis, Paget disease, arteriovenous fistula, pregnancy
Volume overload		Renal failure, iatrogenic fluid overload
Arrhythmias		
Tachyarrhythmias		Atrial, ventricular arrhythmias
Bradyarrhythmias		Sinus node dysfunctions, conduction disorders

ARVC, Arrhythmogenic right ventricular cardiomyopathy; *DCM,* dilated cardiomyopathy; *EMF,* endomyocardial fibrosis; *GH,* growth hormone; *HCM,* hypertrophic cardiomyopathy; *HES,* hypereosinophilic syndrome; *HIV/AIDS,* human immunodeficiency virus/acquired immune deficiency syndrome; *LV,* left ventricular.
From Ponikowski P, Voors AA, Anker SD, et al. 2016 ESC Guidelines for the diagnosis and treatment of acute and chronic heart failure: The task force for the diagnosis and treatment of acute and chronic heart failure of the European Society of Cardiology (ESC). Developed with the special contribution of the Heart Failure Association (HFA) of the ESC. Eur Heart J. 2016;37(27):2129-2200.

abnormalities are apparent but are not present in a coronary distribution, as specific treatments exist for cardiac sarcoidosis. Patients with wall motion abnormalities due to bundle branch block, specifically left bundle branch block, especially when there is no specific evidence or history of infarction, can have further deterioration of systolic function and ventricular dilatation due to inefficient contraction. Cardiac resynchronization therapy (CRT) has been shown to be beneficial when dilation or dysfunction is severe in patients with left bundle branch block.

Evaluation of cardiac chamber wall thickness can also point to specific etiologies and diagnoses. Increased wall thickness on echocardiography can be suggestive of hypertrophic cardiomyopathy (Chapter 23), infiltrative heart disease such as amyloidosis or glycogen storage diseases (Chapter 24), chronic kidney disease (Video 21.1; see also Chapter 41), or hypertensive heart disease. Distinguishing among these causes can be critical, as targeted therapies are available for some of these specific HF etiologies.

ASSESSMENT OF VALVULAR FUNCTION IN HEART FAILURE

Heart failure can be caused by primary abnormalities of cardiac valves. Aortic stenosis can lead to pressure-overload hypertrophy and, in the end stage, failure of the left ventricle (see Chapter 29). Aortic regurgitation can lead to severe dilatation of the left ventricle (see Chapter 29) secondary to the massive volume load imposed by an incompetent aortic valve. Mitral regurgitation, from any etiology, can similarly lead to HF by volume overload of the left ventricle, resulting in progressive dilatation and dysfunction, as well as contributing to elevation in LA pressures (see Chapter 28). While mitral stenosis typically will not result in left ventricular dilatation or dysfunction, the elevated LA pressure that results from mitral stenosis leads to elevated pulmonary venous pressures with resulting symptoms similar to HF secondary to left ventricular dysfunction and ultimately right HF. Right-sided valvular abnormalities, including both disorders of the pulmonary and tricuspid valves (see Chapter 30), can lead to right ventricular failure (see Chapter 16), with symptoms that typically include edema or anasarca, and ultimately renal and hepatic dysfunction secondary to high venous pressures.

MITRAL REGURGITATION IN HEART FAILURE

Mitral regurgitation can be caused by either primary processes (such as prolapse, flail, or valve degeneration due to endocarditis), or can be functional, that is, secondary to ventricular dilatation and apical displacement of the papillary muscles that occur as the ventricle remodels (see Chapters 20 and 28). Primary mitral regurgitation, when severe, will lead to volume overload and left ventricular dysfunction over a long period of time. There is considerable debate over timing of cardiac surgery in such patients. When signs and symptoms of HF have developed, the ventricular dysfunction is generally considered irreversible, although correction of the valvular abnormality, either with surgery or some of the newer percutaneous approaches, can retard or prevent further deterioration. Patients with primary mitral regurgitation should be followed with periodic assessment of ventricular size, function, and a quantitative measure of mitral regurgitation severity (see Chapter 28). Functional mitral regurgitation occurs when the ventricle dilates for any number of reasons, including myocardial infarction, and is usually a result of both annular dilatation and apical displacement of the papillary muscles. This results in tethering of the chordal structures and mitral leaflets. In functional mitral regurgitation, the regurgitant jet is central in origin (Videos 21.2 and 21.3), although leaflet tethering can eventually lead to an eccentric downstream direction (Video 21.4). Functional mitral regurgitation can further contribute to dilatation and dysfunction of the ventricle, and this can be amenable to surgical repair (using annuloplasty rings or replacements). Percutaneous approaches are already approved for treating primary (organic) mitral regurgitation and are being tested in clinical trial for functional mitral regurgitation, using devices that either bring the leaflets together or reduce mitral annular size. Functional mitral regurgitation is an independent risk factor for adverse outcomes in HF (Fig. 21.3).[2]

Patients with HF and mitral regurgitation should have full quantitative assessment of mitral regurgitant severity, including assessment of effective orifice area and regurgitant fraction by proximal isovelocity surface area (PISA) techniques (see Chapter 28). Moreover, the pulmonary veins should be assessed for potential flow reversal. In patients with moderate mitral regurgitation, serial assessment can determine when a patient is worsening and may encourage earlier consideration for intervention.

DOPPLER ASSESSMENT IN PATIENTS WITH HEART FAILURE

In addition to assessment of cardiac structure and traditional measures of cardiac function, such as ejection fraction, Doppler echocardiography can provide additional important functional information, and Doppler tissue imaging can be used to assess both systolic and diastolic function (see Chapters 14 and 15). For example, stroke volume and cardiac output can

be calculated by multiplying the left ventricular outflow tract area by the velocity time integral of flow in the same location. The mitral regurgitant jet velocity can be used to calculate dP/dT, a measure of contractile function (see Chapter 14). Mitral annular contraction and relaxation velocity can be measured easily with Doppler tissue imaging (see Chapter 1). Diastolic function is typically assessed by these methods (see Chapter 15). Left ventricular filling pressures can be estimated by dividing the standard mitral inflow E-wave by the mitral annual relaxation velocity (E'), resulting in a measure that has been shown to correlate with filling pressures,[3] E/E'. While this measure correlates reasonably well with invasively measured filling pressures, whether this technique is sufficiently robust to use for management of patients with HF remains controversial (Fig. 21.4).[4] Nevertheless, an increase in E/E' to >15 is considered evidence of elevated left ventricular filling pressures and can be helpful in the diagnosis. Patients with restrictive cardiomyopathies will usually demonstrate abnormalities of mitral inflow with very short mitral deceleration time (see Chapter 24), generally less than 140 ms. This finding can be nonspecific (for instance, patients with dilated cardiomyopathies can also have very short deceleration time), but it is indicative overall of restrictive physiology and overall poor outcome in HF.

Because pulmonary hypertension is frequent in patients with left-sided heart disease, assessment of tricuspid regurgitation velocity allows for estimation of pulmonary systolic pressures, which has incremental prognostic importance in patients with HF. In patients with pulmonary hypertension secondary to left-sided heart disease (i.e., type 2 pulmonary hypertension), pulmonary pressures can improve with adequate HF therapy.

ASSESSMENT OF LEFT ATRIAL AND RIGHT VENTRICULAR FUNCTION

The importance of the right ventricle and left atrium in patients with HF has been overlooked for some time. Both of these chambers represent "barometers" of left-sided function as left ventricular filling pressures are "transmitted" retrograde to the LA and right atrial (RV). LA dilatation can occur dynamically in the setting of elevated filling pressures and assessment of LA size is an important component of the echocardiographic exam in patients with HF (see Chapter 17). LA size and changes in LA size have been related to HF severity and prognosis and are closely related to other measures of HF severity, such as N-terminal pro-B type natriuretic peptide (NT-proBNP). The right ventricle responds to increased left-sided pressures by reduction in apparent function. Because the normal RV is used to low afterload generally, the RV is a thin-walled structure that cannot easily accommodate increases in load, either due to increases in pulmonary vascular resistance (as occurs in chronic obstructive pulmonary disease, primary pulmonary hypertension or even acute pulmonary embolism) or due to elevation in left-sided pressures. In these cases, the RV begins to dilate and dysfunction occurs. Reduction in RV function has been shown to be an independent predictor of outcome in patients with HF (Fig. 21.5).[5] There are several methods used for assessment of RV function (see Chapter 16), including fractional area change and tricuspid annular plane systolic excursion (TAPSE), both of which

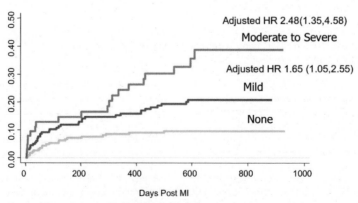

FIG. 21.3 Relationship between mitral regurgitation and the composite outcome of death or heart failure hospitalization following myocardial infarction (MI). *HR*, Heart rate. (*Adapted from Amigoni M, Meris A, Thune JJ, et al. Mitral regurgitation in myocardial infarction complicated by heart failure, left ventricular dysfunction, or both: prognostic significance and relation to ventricular size and function. Eur Heart J. 2007;28(3):326–333.*)

worsen with worsening left-sided heart disease. Assessment of RV function is especially important in patients being considered for left ventricular assist device (LVAD) therapy (see below).

ASSESSMENT OF VENTRICULAR SYNCHRONY

CRT can reduce HF hospitalizations and death in appropriate patients, typically those with reduced left ventricular function and wide QRS, as demonstrated in several outcomes trials.[6,7] The use of CRT has also been associated with marked improvement in echocardiographic parameters such as end-diastolic and end-systolic volume, ejection fraction, right ventricular function and LA size.[8] Most decisions regarding appropriateness for CRT are based on electrocardiogram (ECG), QRS width, and bundle branch morphology, as well as left ventricular systolic function. Patients with an indication for permanent pacemaker, in whom pacing is expected for a significant proportion (>50%) of their lifetime, are also candidates for CRT, since prolonged RV pacing has been shown to cause decrement in LV systolic function over time. The utility of echocardiographic assessment of ventricular synchrony in identifying patients who would benefit from CRT has been controversial. In the past, several methods using tissue Doppler and local strain measurements were proposed for assessing synchrony (as discussed in Chapter 25).[9–11] Many of these may be markers of prognosis after CRT but have proven not to be robust enough to be routinely used in clinical practice. In a large randomized outcomes trial, both ventricular synchrony and contractile function determined by echocardiography identified patients with increased likelihood of benefit from CRT.[9] However, whether these techniques can or should be used to identify patients who will most benefit from CRT remains controversial, since a multicenter study of echocardiographic assessment in CRT failed to show a benefit for echocardiographic assessment of mechanical synchrony using multiple older measures.[10]

DEFORMATION IMAGING IN HEART FAILURE

Myocardial deformation or strain imaging has evolved to become a sensitive method for assessment of cardiac function (see Chapter 14). Strain refers to the percent deformation between two regions, that is, shortening in myocardial muscle in systole or lengthening in diastole (see Fig. 14.16). Myocardial strain can be assessed by Doppler methods in which myocardial tissue velocities are integrated to obtain the change in distance between points, but these are relatively noisy, require dedicated acquisition, and are angle dependent. In contrast, strain imaging based on 2D speckle-tracking techniques appears more robust and reliable; hence, it has virtually replaced Doppler-based strain assessments for most applications. The technique has been validated by sonomicrometry and takes advantage of the coherent speckle within the myocardial tissue signature to determine regions that are contracting versus those that are moving passively. Strain can be measured in the longitudinal, circumferential, and radial directions by using the appropriate imaging plane (see Fig. 14.15).

Current equipment can assess regional strain and then calculate global longitudinal strain either by averaging regional strain values or by determining the percent difference in the endocardial perimeter between systole and diastole. Longitudinal deformation reflects function of the subendocardial myocardial fiber bands primarily, whereas circumferential deformation, best assessed on short-axis views, may reflect the function of more epicardial layers. An example of strain obtained in the longitudinal plane is shown in Video 21.5. Many echo machine packages now use the data obtained from multiple planes to automatically calculate global strain.

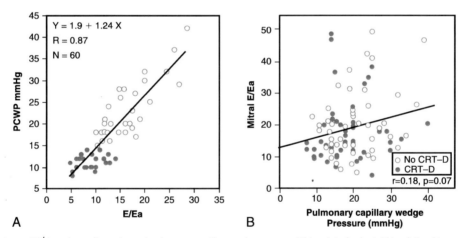

FIG. 21.4 Relationship between E/E′ by echocardiography and pulmonary capillary wedge pressure (A) in original cohort. This relationship was not as clear in patients with acute decompensated heart failure (B). (B, From Mullens W, Borowski AG, Curtin RJ, Thomas JD, Tang WH. Tissue Doppler imaging in the estimation of intracardiac filling pressure in decompensated patients with advanced systolic heart failure. Circulation. 2009;119(1):62–70.)

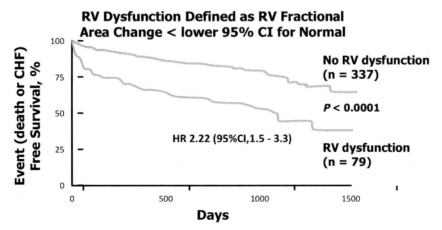

FIG. 21.5 Right atrial (RV) dysfunction is an independent predictor of death or heart failure hospitalization following myocardial infarction. (Modified from Zornoff LA, Skali H, Pfeffer MA, et al. Right ventricular dysfunction and risk of heart failure and mortality after myocardial infarction. J Am Coll Cardiol. 2002;39(9):1450–1455.)

Global strain, particularly longitudinal strain (GLS, or the relative change in length of myocardium during systole averaged over all walls), has emerged as an important measure of cardiac performance that has been shown to add incremental predictive value to standard measures such as the ejection fraction. Several diseases have been associated with a reduction in GLS, including hypertension, diabetes mellitus, renal insufficiency, infiltrative and hypertrophic cardiomyopathies, and valvular heart disease. This measure also appears to predict survival or the development of HF in patients following myocardial infarction (MI). Global strain measurements are also useful in assessing the effect of cardiotoxic chemotherapies on individual patients over time (Chapter 42).

Myocardial deformation imaging has been used for the evaluation of cardiac synchrony by assessing the time to peak strain (maximal contraction) across many cardiac regions. Both regional timing, reflecting synchrony, and myocardial peak strain, reflecting contractile function, have prognostic significance in patients undergoing CRT, and may be used to stratify those who will benefit most from CRT. Fig. 14.17 is an example of the improvement in ventricular synchrony, which may be demonstrated by speckle-tracking strain data.

In addition to assessment of global function, strain imaging can be used to assess and quantify regional function. Regional strain correlates with the degree of myocardial scar in patients with ischemic heart disease and in hypertrophic cardiomyopathy (HCM). An offshoot of myocardial strain imaging has been the quantitative assessment of ventricular twist and torsion or the wringing motion of the heart during contraction and relaxation (see Fig. 14.18).

There are currently several limitations to strain imaging based on 2D echocardiography. These measures are subject to the same limitations as conventional ultrasound images, including frame rate and image quality, with limited time resolution at high heart rates. Second, myocardial deformation occurs in three dimensions, and any out-of-imaging plane movement may not be captured accurately. Finally, the technique, data acquisition and calculations, and normal values are not yet standardized among the many vendors. Until this is achieved, it is highly recommended that the same vendor equipment and software be used to follow strain in a given patient. As strain techniques become more standardized, refined, and automated, their usefulness and applicability will increase.

ASSESSMENT AFTER ORTHOTOPIC HEART TRANSPLANT

Echocardiography is utilized both for determining that cardiac structure and function are normal in a potential heart donor and for monitoring for rejection in cardiac transplant recipients. After an uncomplicated orthotopic heart transplant, the "normal" transplanted heart should be nearly identical to a normal untransplanted heart with normal left ventricular size, wall thickness, and systolic function. In the early stages, the right ventricle may appear slightly enlarged and can be significantly hypokinetic, especially early postoperatively. In patients who have undergone the standard Shumway technique of transplantation, the resultant atria are very enlarged and deformed due to the retained upper portion of the dilated native heart. In these patients, the anastomosis between donor and recipient hearts may be visible as a thickened ridge that encircles the atria (see Fig. 39.4 C and D). The ridge can be mistaken for thrombus by inexperienced observers. Newer surgical methods retain no recipient myocardium (in the procedure of total atrioventricular transplantation) or only a limited cuff of LA wall with pulmonary vein ostia (in the bicaval technique) and thus preserve more normal atrial architecture with relatively inapparent suture lines. In the "normal" transplanted heart, there is often slight paradoxical septal motion, anterior motion of the septum in systole, and slight decrease in septal systolic thickening, which persists in the postoperative state. Over time, due in part to distortions in atrial geometry, supraventricular arrhythmias, and repeated endomyocardial biopsies causing incidental damage to the tricuspid valve, significant tricuspid and mitral regurgitation as well as atrial thrombi may develop in the allograft heart.

Cardiac allograft dysfunction may occur due to many reasons: acute rejection, coronary artery vasculopathy, myocardial fibrosis, acute myocarditis from opportunistic infections, or tachycardia-mediated cardiomyopathy. Echocardiography may detect the downstream effects of these

pathologic mechanisms. Acute cellular rejection, which causes edema and interstitial infiltrates in the myocardium, has been shown to cause detectable increases in LV wall thickness and mass, systolic dysfunction, and Doppler indices of elevated LA pressure and restrictive physiology (increased E wave velocities, decreased isovolumic relaxation time and mitral deceleration time), but these changes are not sensitive or specific enough to rely upon for routine clinical screening. Speckle tracking and assessment of LV torsion may have higher predictive accuracy (92%) and thus may have a potential role in serial monitoring for rejection,[11] but wider validation and outcome-based studies are required. Currently, the gold standard for detecting acute rejection remains endomyocardial biopsy, but echo has an appropriate supplementary role in monitoring for rejection and other complications following transplant.

For detecting cardiac allograft vasculopathy (CAV), coronary intravascular ultrasound (IVUS) is the gold standard, although coronary angiography is more routinely used for practical reasons. Among noninvasive imaging techniques, echocardiography is the most widely investigated and utilized. The presence of depressed LVEF or focal wall motion abnormalities on a *resting* echocardiogram is relatively specific (>80% in multiple studies) for CAV but of poor (<50%) sensitivity. Some centers utilize dobutamine stress echocardiography (DSE), which is preferential to exercise stress, since denervation of the allografted heart blunts the heart-rate response to exercise. Meta-analysis of the published data (small studies of <110 patients) on the accuracy of DSE indicate a mean specificity of 88%, and a sensitivity of 72%. The use of longitudinal strain rate imaging or myocardial echo contrast with DSE may increase the sensitivity, but again, more validation is needed. For prognostic purposes, however, a normal DSE has been shown to have a high negative predictive value for adverse cardiac events (0.6% incidence) over short-term follow-up. Conversely, worsening of serial DSEs confers increased risk compared with a stable DSE. Currently, DSE (as well as single-photon emission computed tomography [SPECT] imaging) is considered by the International Society of Heart and Lung Transplantation[12] as possibly useful (Class IIa, level of evidence B) in transplant recipients who are unable to undergo invasive evaluation. Some centers utilize DSE to minimize the exposure of transplant patients to coronary angiography, although currently no noninvasive imaging modality is sufficiently accurate to supplant it.

ASSESSMENT OF VENTRICULAR ASSIST DEVICES

The advent and increasing use of a variety of ventricular assist devices (VADs) for both bridge and destination therapy has mandated that echocardiography play an integral role in assisting with the optimal selection of patients for left and right VADs, implantation, optimization, and trouble-shooting (see Chapter 26). All LVADs work by unloading the ventricle, that is, removing some or all of the inflow and pumping it to the aorta. Echocardiography is useful in the evaluation of the patient *preoperatively* for VAD implant and for evaluating left but also right ventricular function.[13,14] If right ventricular failure is too severe, as may be indicated by a number of parameters such as right ventricular fractional area change, TAPSE, RV Tei index (see Chapter 16), there will be insufficient preload to fill the VAD and LV. The incidence of right HF is 20%–30% in patients implanted with an isolated LVAD, and a preoperative RV FAC <20% is associated with RV failure upon LVAD device activation. In addition, echocardiography (transthoracic echocardiography [TTE] and/or transesophageal echocardiography [TEE]) can identify aortic insufficiency, intracardiac shunting, left ventricular or LA appendage thrombi, or structural problems with inflow and outflow site cannulation such as excessive necrosis or atherosclerotic plaque, which are detrimental to proper LVAD function. *Intraoperatively*, TEE is used to ensure proper LV apical coring, deairing, cannula position, and to reassess RV function upon initial startup of the LVAD. Extreme RV failure may also mandate the placement of a right ventricular assist device.

Postoperatively, the echocardiogram may be used to identify causes of LVAD dysfunction and fine-tune its operation. When the LVAD is working properly, the ventricle should be "decompressed," that is, smaller than its original dilated size, with the interventricular septum in a neutral position. The aortic valve in a completely decompressed heart stays completely closed throughout the cardiac cycle. Thickening and fusion of the aortic valve may occur over time, particularly in nonpulsatile LVADs; growing experience with these continuous flow devices support a rationale for adjusting flow settings to permit at least occasional aortic valve opening (i.e., on a 1:3 cyclic ratio) to avoid this valvulopathy and associated aortic regurgitation. Enlargement of the LV, distension of the interventricular septum rightwards, and rising estimated pulmonary artery systolic pressure are signals of a relatively underfunctioning device that may be due to inadequate pump rate, worsening ventricular function, aortic regurgitation, volume overload, or systemic factors (e.g., sepsis). If the left ventricle appears small and the interventricular septum is shifted leftwards, this indicates that there is inadequate preload to the ventricle and factors such as RV failure, pulmonary embolus, tamponade, hypovolemia (e.g., bleeding), or inflow cannula obstruction should be sought. Obstruction may be caused by LV thrombus, a papillary muscle or chorda, or bending or slippage of the cannular or outflow graft. Such abnormalities may be demonstrated by 2D echo or by increased velocities and turbulence seen with Doppler evaluation at the cannula/graft orifices (see Fig. 26.4 and Video 26.4 for examples). The LVAD inflow cannula should be visible at the apex, and the outflow graft/cannula can occasionally be detected by angling into the ascending aorta with a right parasternal view. Occasionally, positional kinks in the LVAD cannulae or the aortic outflow graft, which tend to occur in smaller patients, can be demonstrated by scanning the patient in supine, sitting, and standing positions.

There are also percutaneously implanted VADs (PVADs) that provide partial support for the LV. Echocardiography can confirm position of the cannulas in the appropriate position across the interatrial septum (in the case of the TandemHeart PVAD, see Video 26.2) (CardiacAssist, Pittsburgh, Pennsylvania) or the aortic valve/LVOT (for the Impella™, see Video 26.3). Chapter 26 discusses comprehensive VAD assessment.

ECHOCARDIOGRAPHY IN THE CONTEXT OF OTHER DIAGNOSTIC MEASURES IN HEART FAILURE

Echocardiography is only one of a number of diagnostic tests that are typically used to assess patients with HF that includes a detailed medical history, physical examination, electrocardiography, and assessment of circulating biomarkers including BNP or NT-proBNP (Fig. 21.6). In addition, other imaging tests, such as cardiac magnetic imaging, cardiac computed tomography (CT), or nuclear imaging, can be used in place of or in addition to echocardiography (Table 21.3; see also Chapters 22 and 48). In addition, patients with HF, particularly HFrEF, are at increased risk for intracardiac thrombus due to stagnation of blood. Thrombus can occur in the atria, especially when atrial fibrillation coexists, or in the ventricle, particularly when there are akinetic regions, and can be visualized by echocardiography (see Chapter 38). When thrombus is suspected, use

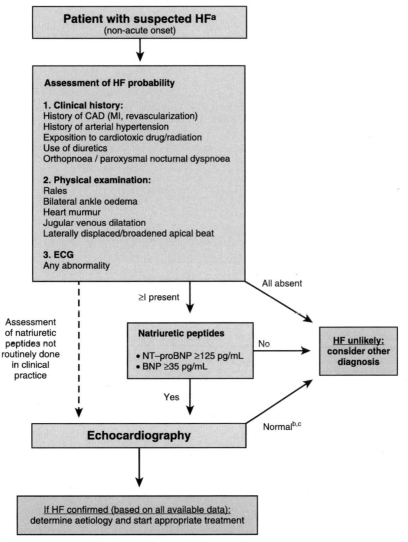

FIG. 21.6 Role of echocardiography in the diagnosis of heart failure. *BNP*, B-type natriuretic peptide; *CAD*, coronary artery disease; *HF*, heart failure; *MI*, myocardial infarction; *NT-proBNP*, N-terminal pro-B type natriuretic peptide. [a]Patient reporting symptoms typical of HF (see Box 21.1). [b]Normal ventricular and atrial volumes and function. [c]Consider other causes of elevated natriuretic peptides. (*From Ponikowski P, Voors AA, Anker SD, et al. 2016 ESC Guidelines for the diagnosis and treatment of acute and chronic heart failure: the task force for the diagnosis and treatment of acute and chronic heart failure of the European Society of Cardiology (ESC). Developed with the special contribution of the Heart Failure Association (HFA) of the ESC. Eur Heart J. 2016;37(27):2129–2200.*)

TABLE 21.3 Recommendations for Cardiac Imaging in Patients with Suspected or Established Heart Failure

RECOMMENDATIONS	CLASS[A]	LEVEL[B]	REF[C]
TTE is recommended for the assessment of myocardial structure and function in subjects with suspected HF to establish a diagnosis of HFrEF, HFmrEF, or HFpEF.	I	C	
TTE is recommended to assess LVEF to identify patients with HF who would be suitable for evidence-based pharmacological and device (ICD, CRT) treatment recommended for HFrEF.	I	C	
TTE is recommended for the assessment of valve disease, right ventricular function, and pulmonary arterial pressure in patients with an already established diagnosis of HFrEF, HFmrEF, or HFpEF to identify those suitable for correction of valve disease.	I	C	
TTE is recommended for the assessment of myocardial structure and function in subjects to be exposed to treatment which potentially can damage myocardium (e.g., chemotherapy).	I	C	
Other techniques (including systolic tissue Doppler velocities and deformation indices, i.e., strain and strain rate), should be considered in a TTE protocol in subjects at risk of developing HF to identify myocardial dysfunction at the preclinical stage.	IIa	C	
CMR is recommended for the assessment of myocardial structure and function (including right heart) in subjects with poor acoustic window and patients with complex congenital heart diseases (taking account of cautions/contraindications to CMR).	I	C	
CMR with LGE should be considered in patients with dilated cardiomyopathy to distinguish between ischemic and non-ischemic myocardial damage in case of equivocal clinical and other imaging data (taking account of cautions/contraindications to CMR).	IIa	C	
CMR is recommended for the characterization of myocardial tissue in case of suspected myocarditis, amyloidosis, sarcoidosis, Chagas disease, Fabry disease non-compaction cardiomyopathy, and hemochromatosis (taking account of cautions/contraindications to CMR).	I	C	
Noninvasive stress imaging (CMR, stress echocardiography, SPECT, PET) may be considered for the assessment of myocardial ischemia and viability in patients with HF and CAD (considered suitable for coronary revascularization) before the decision on revascularization.	IIb	B	Allman et al., 2002; Ling et al., 2013; Bonow et al., 2011
Invasive coronary angiography is recommended in patients with HF and angina pectoris recalcitrant to pharmacological therapy or symptomatic ventricular arrhythmias or aborted cardiac arrest (who are considered suitable for potential coronary revascularization) to establish the diagnosis of CAD and its severity	I	C	
Invasive coronary angiography should be considered in patients with HF and intermediate to high pretest probability of CAD and the presence of ischemia in noninvasive stress tests (who are considered suitable for potential coronary revascularization) to establish the diagnosis of CAD and its severity.	IIa	C	
Cardiac CT may be considered in patients with HF and low to intermediate pretest probability of CAD or those with equivocal noninvasive stress tests to rule out coronary artery stenosis.	IIb	C	
Reassessment of myocardial structure and function is recommended using noninvasive imaging: • In patients presenting with worsening HF symptoms (including episodes of AHF) or experiencing any other important cardiovascular event; • In patients with HF who have received evidence-based pharmacotherapy in maximal tolerated doses, before the decision on device implantation (ICD, CRT); • In patients exposed to therapies which may damage the myocardium (e.g., chemotherapy) (serial assessments).	I	C	

[a]Class of recommendation.
[b]Level of evidence.
[c]References supporting recommendations:
Allman KC, Shaw LJ, Hachamovitch R, Udelson JE. Myocardial viability testing and impact of revascularization on prognosis in patients with coronary artery disease and left ventricular dysfunction: a meta-analysis. J Am Coll Cardiol. 2002;39(7):1151–1158.
Bonow RO, Maurer G, Lee KL, et al. Myocardial viability and survival in ischemic left ventricular dysfunction. N Engl J Med. 2011; 364(17):1617–1625.
Ling LF, Marwick TH, Flores DR, et al. Identification of therapeutic benefit from revascularization in patients with left ventricular systolic dysfunction inducible ischemia versus hibernating myocardium. Circ Cardiovasc Imaging. 2013;6(3):363–372.
AHF, Acute heart failure; CAD, coronary artery disease; CMR, cardia magnetic resonance; CRT, cardiac resynchronization therapy; CT, computed tomography; HF, heart failure; HFpEF, heart failure with preserved ejection fraction; HFmrEF, heart failure with mid-range ejection fraction; HFrEF, heart failure with reduced ejection fraction; ICD, implantable cardioverter-defibrillator; LGE, late gadolinium enhancement; LVEF, left ventricular ejection fraction; PET, positron emission tomography; SPECT, single-photon emission computed tomography; TTE, transthoracic echocardiography.
Modified from Ponikowski P, Voors AA, Anker SD, et al. 2016 ESC Guidelines for the diagnosis and treatment of acute and chronic heart failure: the task force for the diagnosis and treatment of acute and chronic heart failure of the European Society of Cardiology (ESC). Developed with the special contribution of the Heart Failure Association (HFA) of the ESC. Eur Heart J. 2016;37(27):2129–2200.

of either high-frequency transducers or intracardiac contrast (Chapter 12) can be helpful in improving visualization.

LUNG ULTRASOUND IN HEART FAILURE

Recently, the sonographic assessment of patients with known or suspected HF has been expanded to include examination of the lungs and pleural space for the detection of pulmonary edema and pleural effusions. Lung ultrasound (LUS) can be performed with either standard ultrasound equipment or pocket devices with similar accuracy, typically with a phased array or curvilinear transducer within 2–5 minutes.[15] An overview of the technique is provided in Table 21.4. LUS allows quantification of vertical "B-lines" (Fig. 21.7) that, when present, provide a graded measure of extravascular lung water with high interrater reproducibility after as little as 30 minutes training.[16] "B-lines" on LUS are hyperechoic reverberation artifacts that are thought to stem from fluid filled or otherwise thickened interstitial spaces in the lungs. They arise from the pleural line, extend to the far field of the ultrasound

TABLE 21.4 Overview of Lung and Pleural Ultrasound Techniques in Heart Failure

	PULMONARY CONGESTION/EDEMA	PLEURAL EFFUSIONS
Ultrasound system	High-end, portable or pocket device	High-end, portable or pocket device
Transducer	Phased array or curvilinear	Phased array or curvilinear
Imaging depth	~18 cm	Variable
Scan areas	Anterior and lateral chest, both hemithoraces	Lateral chest at level of diaphragm
Number of areas (zones) on each hemithorax	(2 to) 4	1
Patient positioning	Sitting or supine	
Pathologic findings	Multiple B-lines (hyperechoic, vertical lines arising from the pleural line)	Anechoic fluid collection above the diaphragm; loss of mirror image artifact; visualization of thoracic spine

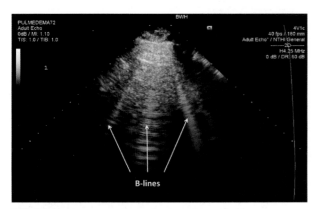

FIG. 21.7 B-lines on lung ultrasound indicative of pulmonary congestion.

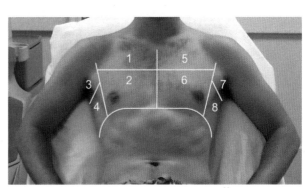

FIG. 21.8 Zones 1–8 used for the lung ultrasound examination. (*From Platz E, Meerz AA, Jhund PS, et al. Dynamic changes and prognostic value of pulmonary congestion by lung ultrasound in acute and chronic heart failure: a systematic review.* Eur J Heart Fail. *2017 May 30. [Epub ahead of print]*)

screen, and move back and forth during respiration. Horizontal artifacts ("A-lines") can be seen in normal lung and are not pathologic. LUS can be performed with the patient sitting or supine, however, for serial examinations, patient positioning and ultrasound clip length should be kept constant, since both may impact the number of B-lines.[16] While a number of different scanning methods have been described, a current, international guideline recommends the sonographic investigation of eight anterior and lateral chest zones (four on each hemithorax) (Fig. 21.8). An abbreviated protocol employing with six zones (three on each hemithorax) has also reported high diagnostic accuracy for the detection of pulmonary edema in acute HF, and as few as two "positive" zones (with ≥3 B-lines) may provide prognostic information in patients hospitalized for acute HF. A number of quantification methods for B-lines have been reported that are count- or score-based. All are based on totaling the maximum number of B-lines in one intercostal space per chest zone. Count based methods sum the number of B-lines across all zones, whereas score based methods consider one zone positive if at least three B-lines are visualized in one intercostal space.

Utility of Lung Ultrasound in Heart Failure

Pulmonary congestion is a common and important finding in acute HF. Traditionally, pulmonary edema and pleural effusions have been assessed through patients' symptoms (dyspnea), physical examination, and chest radiography. However, these signs and symptoms are insensitive for the diagnosis of acute HF and are difficult to quantify. In undifferentiated patients presenting to the emergency department, the detection of ≥3 B-lines on LUS in ≥2 intercostal spaces bilaterally has demonstrated higher sensitivity (85.3%, 95% CI 82.8–87.5) than rales on auscultation (62.3%, 95% CI 60.8–63.7) or pulmonary edema on chest x-ray (56.9%, 95% CI 54.7–59.1) for the diagnosis of acute HF in a meta-analysis (Fig. 21.9).[17] In a recent Italian multicenter study of >1000 patients presenting to emergency departments with undifferentiated dyspnea, use of LUS compared with a standard clinical assessment resulted in a net reclassification improvement of 19.1% (95% CI 14.6–23.6).[18] Moreover, higher numbers of B-lines are associated with higher levels of natriuretic peptides in both acute and chronic HF. LUS has recently been shown to be a good predictor of death or rehospitalization for HF

in patients with chronic HF.[19] Whether LUS findings provide incremental diagnostic value beyond natriuretic peptides in all or certain subsets of patients with suspected acute HF is unclear and warrants further investigation.

Recent data suggest that B-lines cannot only be detected in patients with acute HF but also in ambulatory patients with chronic HF, both in those with reduced and preserved ejection fraction. These data indicate that patients with HF may demonstrate a spectrum of pulmonary congestion rather than a binary finding (presence of absence of pulmonary edema) limited to acute HF. Higher degrees of pulmonary congestion on LUS in patients with chronic HF are associated with echocardiographic markers of cardiovascular risk, including higher LV mass index, LA volume index, estimated systolic pulmonary artery pressure and, in one study, with E/E′. In ambulatory HF patients (NYHA class II-IV), an increased number of B-lines may be detected with a pocket ultrasound device in one-third of patients even in the absence of crackles on auscultation in 80% of these patients.[19]

Limitations of Lung Ultrasound

Despite the high diagnostic accuracy for identifying pulmonary edema in patients with suspected acute HF, it is important to be aware that B-lines can be found in other conditions, such as interstitial lung disease, acute respiratory distress syndrome, pulmonary contusions, and pneumonitis. It is, thus, essential that clinicians interpret LUS findings in the clinical context. Furthermore, large pleural effusions may interfere with the quantification of B-lines, especially in the more caudal chest zones.

Assessment of Pleural Effusions

In addition to the assessment of pulmonary congestion by B-lines, the presence of pleural effusions may be examined laterally at the level of the diaphragm. If there is a pleural effusion, the normally visible mirror image artifact caused by the diaphragm is absent; instead, an anechoic fluid collection can be visualized above the diaphragm (Fig. 21.10). The presence of a pleural effusion usually allows for visualization of the thoracic spine. Pleural effusions can also be seen on standard echocardiographic views

ECHOCARDIOGRAPHY FOR DISEASES OF THE MYOCARDIUM

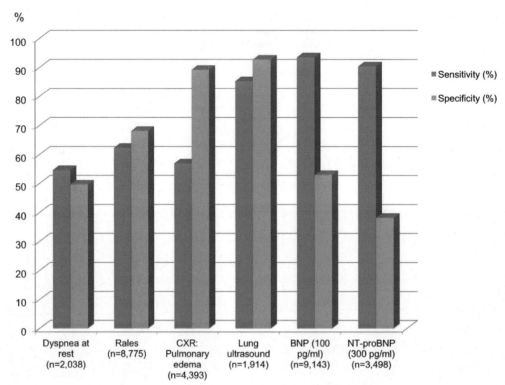

FIG. 21.9 Sensitivity and specificity of various measures of pulmonary congestion in heart failure. *BNP*, B-type natriuretic peptide; *CXR*, chest x-ray; *NT-proBNP*, N-terminal pro-B type natriuretic peptide. *(Adapted from Martindale, JL, Wakai A, Collins, SP, et al. (2016). Diagnosing acutre heart failure in the emergency department: a systematic review and meta-analysis.* Academic Emergency Medicine, 23, 223-242.)

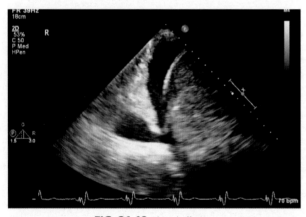

FIG. 21.10 Pleural effusion.

(e.g., the parasternal long axis view) and should be differentiated from pericardial effusions (see Chapter 33). Pleural effusions on ultrasound can be detected in approximately one quarter to one-third of patients with acute HF.[7,8] Although they may be clinically relevant in individual patients, their diagnostic and prognostic importance in acute HF is less clear than that of B-lines.

Suggested Reading

Cikes, M., & Solomon, S. D. (2016). Beyond ejection fraction: an integrative approach for assessment of cardiac structure and function in heart failure. *European Heart Journal, 37*(21), 1642–1650.

Gorscan, J., 3rd., & Tayal, B. (2017). Newer echocardiographic techniques in cardiac resynchronization therapy. *Heart Failure Clinics, 13*(1), 53–62.

Omar, A. M., Bansal, M., & Sengupta, P. P. (2016). Advances in echocardiographic imaging in heart failure with reduced and preserved ejection fraction. *Circulation Research, 119*(2), 357–374.

Patel, M. R., White, R. D., Abbara, S., et al. (2013). 2013 ACCF/ACR/ASE/ASNC/SCCT/SCMR appropriate utilization of cardiovascular imaging in heart failure: a joint report of the American College of Radiology Appropriateness Criteria Committee and the American College of Cardiology Foundation Appropriate Use Criteria Task Force. *Journal of the American College of Cardiology, 61*(21), 2207–2231.

Picano, E., & Pellikka, P. A. (2016). Ultrasound of extravascular lung water: a new standard for pulmonary congestion. *European Heart Journal, 37*(27), 2097–2104.

A complete reference list can be found online at ExpertConsult.com.

22 Dilated Cardiomyopathies

Maja Cikes

INTRODUCTION

Dilated cardiomyopathy (DCM) is predominantly diagnosed according to echocardiographic features that include left ventricular or biventricular dilation and reduced systolic function. Current classification schemes from major heart societies exclude primary ischemic heart disease or abnormal loading conditions (such as hypertension or valvular disease) that may cause a similar impairment in global systolic function.[1,2] Clinically, the term *ischemic cardiomyopathy* is frequently used to refer to the myocardial dysfunction caused by coronary artery disease (see Chapter 20) and is a leading cause of heart failure in the developed world. Whereas significant valvular disease is usually readily apparent on echocardiography, the exclusion of ischemic heart disease causing secondary left ventricular (LV) failure requires additional investigation, since the regional wall motion abnormalities suggestive of ischemic heart disease can also be noted in DCM. Many of the underlying diseases such as myocarditis, tachycardia-induced cardiomyopathy, peripartum cardiomyopathy (PPCM), as well as toxic-metabolic and other diseases with multiorgan system involvement (Box 22.1) share a similar end-stage phenotype characterized by left ventricular dilatation, reduced systolic function, and other common features that will be covered here. Other types of DCM (Box 22.2) such as Takotsubo cardiomyopathy, arrhythmogenic cardiomyopathy (ACM), noncompaction, and sarcoidosis typically manifest more disease-specific features in addition to overall LV dilatation. In addition, overlap of the aforementioned underlying etiologies may occur in a single patient, and a precisely defined diagnosis may occasionally only be revealed by genetic testing.

DCM is a chronic disease that requires follow-up of the structural changes and functional impairment of the heart. Some of these cardiomyopathies, notably Takotsubo, tachycardia-mediated, and postpartum states, can improve and even resolve completely with treatment and/or time. In the context of the clinical status of the patient and the patient's comorbidities, echocardiography often plays a crucial role in guiding further management of patients with DCM and their prognostication.

COMMON FEATURES OF DILATED CARDIOMYOPATHIES

Left Ventricular Dilation and Systolic Functional Impairment

The principal hallmark of DCM is **left ventricular cavity dilation**, although enlargement of other cardiac chambers also often occurs. Left ventricular cavity enlargement is usually quantified by measuring increased LV end-diastolic and end-systolic dimensions and volumes. Although the myocardial walls may be either of normal thickness or thinned, the total **left ventricular mass is increased** due to the overall increase in LV size. Furthermore, **measures of LV systolic function** such as fractional shortening, ejection fraction, stroke volume, and cardiac output are typically **reduced** (Fig. 22.1).

It should be emphasized that, although the stroke volume is reduced in most cases, LV cavity dilation may initially serve to compensate by restoring stroke volume (measured on echocardiography as the difference between the LV end-diastolic and end-systolic volume). Namely, a larger ventricle can eject much more volume than a smaller one, even with the same amount of contraction (i.e., segmental deformation) (Fig. 22.2). Hence, the final cardiac output may be initially preserved despite impairment in ejection fraction (measured as the stroke volume

divided by LV end-diastolic volume). Restoration of stroke volume by ventricular dilatation is an integral part of the process of LV remodeling in the adaptation to changes in contractility and loading conditions. Thus, (1) in DCM, although inherent myocardial dysfunction and diminished myocardial contractility is the primary defect, ventricular dilation may enable the generation of the same amount of stroke volume with less deformation, and (2) in volume overload states (e.g., valvular regurgitation, such as functional mitral regurgitation), an increased amount of stroke volume is required and may be generated (with the same amount of contractility) by an LV that dilates to adapt (see Fig. 22.2).[3] Indeed, preservation of stroke volume (as well as an increase in heart rate) to maintain overall cardiac output may explain why the severity of symptoms can remain relatively low despite notably impaired left ventricular ejection fraction (LVEF), despite the fact that the latter correlates strongly with prognosis.[4] Conversely, symptoms of congestive heart failure are more directly related to elevated LV filling pressures (see below). Fig. 22.1 and Video 22.1 provide an example of two patients with severely dilated left ventricles and severely reduced LVEF but different LV stroke volumes, atrial sizes, and functional class.

Based on the described principles of remodeling, the left ventricular shape changes with disease progression from the typical elongated shape to a more globular one. A simple measurement that can quantify this is the **sphericity index**, defined as the ratio of the LV length and width (Fig. 22.3). A normal sphericity index is greater than 1.6; in DCM, this is generally **reduced**, implying pathologic remodeling with notable cavity dilation (see also Fig. 20.5 in Chapter 20).

BOX 22.1 Possible Causes of the Dilated Cardiomyopathy Phenotype, Predominantly Without Characteristic Findings on Echocardiography, Which May Suggest the Etiology of the Disease

Infectious myocarditis (viral including HIV, Chagas, Lyme)
Peripartum
Tachycardia-mediated
Drugs (most common: chemotherapeutics)
Toxins and overload: excess alcohol intake; cocaine, amphetamines, ecstasy (MDMA); iron overload
Nutritional deficiency (e.g., carnitine, selenium, thiamine, zinc, copper deficiencies)
Endocrinologic disorders (hypo- and hyperthyroidism, diabetes mellitus, Cushing/Addison disease, pheochromocytoma, acromegaly)
Immune-mediated diseases: systemic lupus erythematosus (SLE), antiheart antibodies (AHA), Kawasaki disease, Churg-Strauss syndrome
Neuromuscular disorders (e.g., Duchenne/Becker, Emery-Dreifuss muscular dystrophies)
Mitochondrial disorders

HIV, Human immunodeficiency virus; *MDMA,* 3,4-Methylenedioxymethamphetamine.
Data from Elliott P, Andersson B, Arbustini E, et al. Classification of the cardiomyopathies: a position statement from the European Society of Cardiology Working Group on Myocardial and Pericardial Diseases. *Eur Heart J.* 2008;29: 270–276; Maron BJ, Towbin JA, Thiene G, et al. Contemporary definitions and classification of the cardiomyopathies: an American Heart Association Scientific Statement from the Council on Clinical Cardiology, Heart Failure and Transplantation Committee; Quality of Care and Outcomes Research and Functional Genomics and Translational Biology Interdisciplinary Working Groups; and Council on Epidemiology and Prevention. *Circulation* 2006;113:1807–1816.

Several features of DCM are manifest and quantifiable on **m-mode echocardiography** (see Chapter 2): LV and right ventricular (RV) cavity enlargement, changes in wall thickness and calculated LV mass, as well as reduced segmental wall thickening are classically recognizable on m-mode as signs of LV dilation and poor systolic performance. Poor aortic valve opening with premature closure can be noted in the setting of reduced stroke volume. Due to LV dilatation, the mitral leaflet echoes are often distanced to greater than 1.0 cm of the mitral E-point from the interventricular septum (see Fig. 2.16).[5] A characteristic pattern of decreased mitral leaflet opening and an occasional "b-notch" indicative of markedly elevated LV end-diastolic pressure are shown in Fig. 2.15 in Chapter 2. Impairment in LV systolic function can also be assessed on apical windows by **reduced mitral annular planar systolic excursion (MAPSE)** (Fig. 22.4). A MAPSE less than 10 mm (usually averaged from 2 to 4 point measurements spaced around the mitral annulus) is indicative of reduced longitudinal LV motion.[5]

BOX 22.2 Possible Causes of the Dilated Cardiomyopathy Phenotype, Often With Characteristic Findings on Echocardiography, Which May Suggest the Etiology of the Disease

Arrhythmogenic cardiomyopathy
Takotsubo (stress) cardiomyopathy
Left ventricular noncompaction
Sarcoidosis

Data from Elliott P, Andersson B, Arbustini E, et al. Classification of the cardiomyopathies: a position statement from the European Society of Cardiology Working Group on Myocardial and Pericardial Diseases. *Eur Heart J.* 2008;29: 270–276; Maron BJ, Towbin JA, Thiene G, et al. Contemporary definitions and classification of the cardiomyopathies: an American Heart Association Scientific Statement from the Council on Clinical Cardiology, Heart Failure and Transplantation Committee; Quality of Care and Outcomes Research and Functional Genomics and Translational Biology Interdisciplinary Working Groups; and Council on Epidemiology and Prevention. *Circulation* 2006;113:1807–1816.

Similarly to reduced MAPSE, impaired motion of the base of the heart towards the more stationary apex (expressing the **longitudinal function of the LV**) can be quantified by **Doppler Tissue Imaging S' (systolic) velocity** or more advanced parameters of myocardial deformation, such as systolic strain, which is often expressed as **global longitudinal strain** (Fig. 22.5) or less frequently as systolic strain-rate (see Chapter 6), all of which will typically be **reduced** in DCM.

Finally, **Doppler echocardiography** may be used in the hemodynamic assessment of LV systolic function: in addition to volumetric measurements of stroke volume and cardiac output, these calculations can also be performed using the continuity of flow equation (see Chapter 1). Multiplication of the cross-sectional area and the time velocity integral of the left ventricular outflow tract (LVOT) will provide the calculation of **left ventricular stroke volume** (Fig. 22.6), which is **typically reduced** in advanced DCM. The **change of pressure over time (d*P*/d*t*)** can be measured when a sufficient mitral regurgitation envelope (recorded by continuous wave Doppler) is present and will also be **reduced** in most patients with DCM (Fig. 22.7). This noninvasive parameter has shown good correlation with values measured by cardiac catheterization and has been associated with worse prognosis when less than 600 mm Hg/s.[5] For more details on the assessment of LV systolic function, please refer to Chapter 14.

Dilated cardiomyopathies that develop due to processes affecting the heart more globally, such as genetic DCM, postmyocarditis, postpartum, and toxic/metabolic etiologies, mostly present with **diffuse LV hypokinesis**. However, diseases such as sarcoidosis, stress cardiomyopathy, ACM, and some postmyocarditis states may affect the heart in a more regional pattern, with a predilection for certain hypokinetic or akinetic areas (see Chapter 41). Wall motion abnormalities that do not follow any specific coronary artery territory are often the clue that a true (nonischemic) cardiomyopathy exists. Also, the basal segments of the ventricular walls are often the last segments to remain normokinetic in DCM.

The severe impairment in contractility leading to akinetic or dyskinetic areas and cavity dilation creates a nidus for the **formation of**

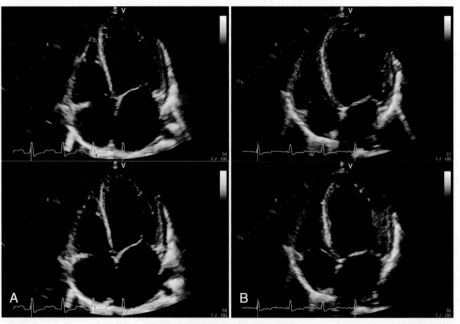

FIG. 22.1 Apical four-chamber views from two patients with dilated cardiomyopathy. (A) End-diastolic (*upper panel*) and end-systolic (*lower panel*) frames from a patient with dilated cardiomyopathy (DCM) and New York Heart Association (NYHA) functional class IV, referred for left ventricular assist device (LVAD) implantation. The biplane left ventricle (LV) end-diastolic and end-systolic volume indices are measured at 147 and 126 mL/m², respectively, indicating severe LV dilation. The calculated stroke volume is reduced at 48 mL, and the ejection fraction by the Simpson's biplane method is 14%. Both atria are also severely enlarged: the left atrial volume is 76 mL/m² (indexed to body surface area [BSA]), and the right atrial volume is 64 mL/m². See Video 22.1 (*left panel*) for the corresponding moving images. (B) End-diastolic (*upper panel*) and end-systolic (*lower panel*) frames from a patient with DCM and NYHA class II, presenting in regular heart failure clinic follow-up. The biplane end-diastolic and end-systolic volume indices are measured at 121 and 90 mL/m², respectively, also indicating a severely dilated LV. The calculated stroke volume, however, is preserved at 68 mL, while the ejection fraction by Simpson's biplane method is 26%. In this patient, there was only mild to moderate left atrial (LA) enlargement: the left atrial volume is 34 mL/m², and the right atrial volume indexed to BSA is 12.6 mL/m². See corresponding Video 22.1 (*right panel*). (A and B) Although there is severe LV dilation and severe LVEF reduction in both these examples, the calculated stroke volume of the patient in (B) is virtually normal, as opposed to the patient in (A). In addition to a preserved stroke volume, there is only initial LA dilation in the patient in (B), suggestive of potentially lower LV filling pressures and accounting for a better functional class. See further text for additional figures comparing these two patients.

intracardiac thrombi, which are predominantly mural and most frequently occurring in the apex of the LV (Fig. 20.2, Fig. 38.8 and corresponding Video 38.4, and Fig. 38.9).[6] Spontaneous echo contrast may also be seen, mainly within the cavity of the LV.

Elevation of Left Ventricular Filling Pressures

Although the severity of LV dysfunction expressed by LVEF relates to prognosis, its correlation with symptom severity is poor. Symptoms of congestive heart failure in patients with DCM relate better to the filling pressures of the left ventricle, which can be well assessed noninvasively by Doppler echocardiography (see Chapter 21).[7] Some degree of diastolic dysfunction nearly always accompanies the reduced systolic function in DCM. However, the severity of impairment of diastolic dysfunction does not necessarily correlate to the impairment of systolic function (and vice versa). With regard to symptoms, patients with an impaired relaxation pattern seen in the Doppler trace of mitral inflow will often tend to have dyspnea falling within the lower New York Heart Association functional classes, whereas higher grades of dyspnea are often associated with pseudonormal filling or even more frequently with restrictive filling patterns (Fig. 22.8).[8] One of the main features of restrictive filling is a very short deceleration time of the E wave, which has also been proven as a reliable harbinger of poor prognosis in DCM patients.[9,10] Of note, higher grades of diastolic dysfunction will most often be accompanied by predominantly diastolic flow in the pulmonary venous waveforms, which is also indicative of markedly increased left atrial (LA)/LV filling pressures. Initiation of diuretic and vasodilator therapy may reduce LV filling pressures and thus improve the pattern of transmitral flow as well as the functional class of the patient.[1]

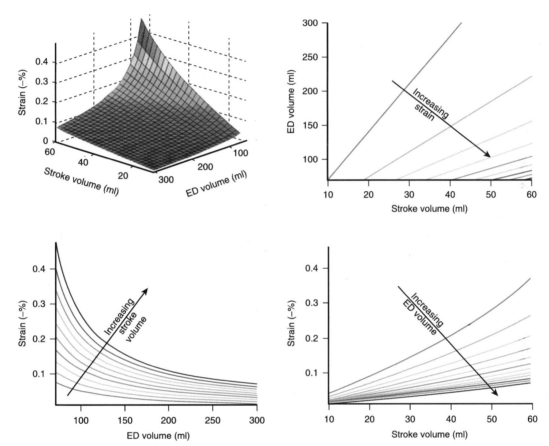

FIG. 22.2 Relation of ventricular size, stroke volume, and deformation. Ventricular size is expressed as end-diastolic volume (ED volume), and deformation is expressed as strain. (*From Bijnens B, Cikes M, Butakoff C, Sitges M, Crispi F. Myocardial motion and deformation: what does it tell us and how does it relate to function? Fetal Diagn Ther. 2012;32[1–2]:5–16, with permission from S. Karger AG, Basel.*)

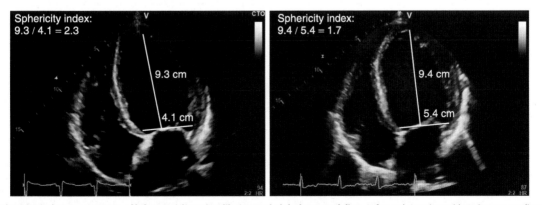

FIG. 22.3 The sphericity index as a measure of left ventricle cavity dilation and globular remodeling. *Left panel,* A patient with peripartum cardiomyopathy (a disease that may be of short duration and may remit) with a greater, i.e., more normal, or nonspherical, sphericity index of 2.3. Conversely, the *right panel* shows a patient with long-standing dilated cardiomyopathy and a low sphericity index of 1.7, suggesting a spherically remodeled left ventricle. (See also Fig. 20.5.)

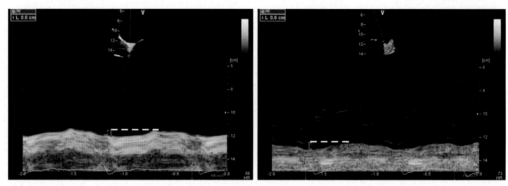

FIG. 22.4 **Mitral annular planar systolic excursion assessed from mitral annular motion by m-mode echocardiography.** Mitral annular planar systolic excursion (MAPSE) *(red mark)*, a simple measure of longitudinal left ventricular motion is severely reduced in this patient with dilated cardiomyopathy. The medial (septal) MAPSE is measured on the *left panel*, and lateral MAPSE is measured in the *right panel*. The MAPSE measurements are typically averaged, and a value less than 10 mm is considered abnormal.

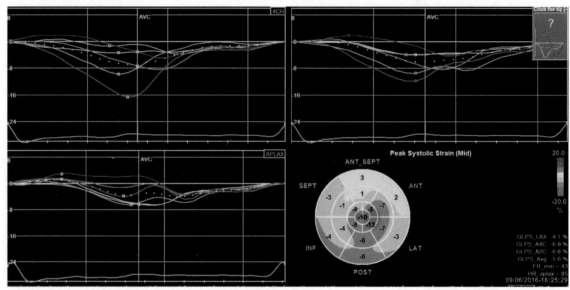

FIG. 22.5 **Global longitudinal strain (GLS) assessed by two-dimensional Speckle Tracking echocardiography.** Global longitudinal strain (GLS) is a more advanced measure of longitudinal left ventricular deformation, which is also severely reduced in this example of a patient with dilated cardiomyopathy (the same patient as Fig. 22.1B). *4CH*, Apical 4-chamber view; *ANT*, anterior wall; *ANT_SEPT*, anteroseptal wall; *APLAX*, apicla long axis view; *AVC*, aortic valve closure; *INF*, inferior wall; *LAT*, lateral wall; *POST*, posterior wall; *SEPT*, septum.

Left Atrial Dilation

An increase in LV filling pressures, discernable from the mitral inflow pattern, will over time lead to **left atrial dilation**, which can be quantified by an enlargement in LA diameter on 2D or M-mode echocardiography, or more precisely an enlargement in LA area and/or volume, measured by tracing the LA cavity in one or preferably two imaging planes (see Fig. 22.1). For clinical purposes, it is best to index the measured LA area and volumes to the body surface area of the patient. In some patients, LA enlargement is also accompanied by an impairment in LA function, which can easily be noticed on the mitral inflow pattern as a minimal or absent A wave. The frequent occurrence of atrial fibrillation in markedly enlarged atria denotes the intricate relation between abnormal atrial morphology and function.

Right Heart Dilation and Functional Impairment

Right heart chambers may also exhibit **dilation and/or functional impairment** in the setting of DCM. Primarily, this may be caused by the disease affecting the myocardium of both ventricles. Furthermore, a sustained increase in LV filling pressures may over time lead to pulmonary hypertension, which may in turn induce right ventricular overload, dilation, and functional impairment. The assessment of **RV size** is predominantly based on the measurement of its end-diastolic diameters (either in the parasternal long-axis view, or most frequently by measuring the widest diameter of the RV cavity in the apical four-chamber

view, as in Fig. 16.4). Furthermore, **RV area and volumes** can also be measured, but due to the complex crescent-shaped geometry of the RV, these measurements are often unreliable when obtained with 2D echocardiography. Several measures of **RV function** may be seen to decline when the RV becomes myopathic: a **decrease in fractional area change (FAC)** to ≤35%, or **reduced tricuspid annular planar systolic excursion (TAPSE)** to ≤16 mm and/or a **reduced Doppler tissue imaging (DTI) S′** of the tricuspid annulus to ≤10 cm/s, reflecting impaired shortening of the RV myocardium in the longitudinal directions, may all be detected in patients with DCM affecting the right heart (Fig. 22.9).

Pulmonary artery pressures can be assessed noninvasively by measuring the peak velocity, that is, peak gradient of the tricuspid regurgitation jet by Doppler echocardiography, applying the simplified Bernoulli equation (see Chapter 1), and adding in estimated right atrial pressure to sum up the total RV systolic pressure.

Impaired RV function and elevated pulmonary artery pressures are well-known determinants of poor outcomes in patients with heart failure, including those with DCM.[11,12] Thus, the evaluation of right heart morphology and function, as well as the assessment of pulmonary artery pressures should not be neglected in patients with DCM.[13] If implantation of a ventricular assist device (VAD) is being considered, a comprehensive assessment of right heart function is important for anticipation of potential severe right heart failure postoperatively (see Chapter 26). Further details on the assessment of RV structure and

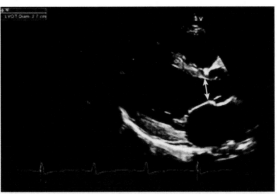

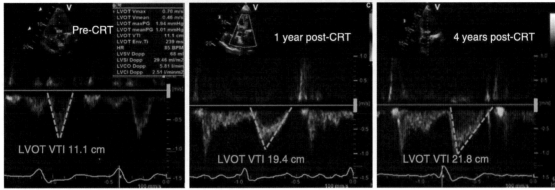

FIG. 22.6 Doppler-based calculation of left ventricular stroke volume. According to the continuity of flow equation, the stroke volume is calculated as left ventricular outflow tract cross sectional area (LVOT CSA) × left ventricular outflow tract velocity time integral (LVOT VTI), which in this example (the same patient as Fig. 22.1B) gives a left ventricular (LV) stroke volume of 68 mL (*lower left panel*, baseline). As SV decreases with disease progression, the LVOT VTI becomes reduced. **Changes in LVOT VTI with heart failure treatment (lower panels):** LVOT VTI measurements in a patient before cardiac resynchronisation therapy (CRT) implantation (*lower left panel*), 1 year after CRT implantation (*lower middle panel*) and 4 years after CRT implantation (*lower right panel*). This patient was a responder to resynchronization therapy in whom a clear increase in the LVOT VTI can be seen after CRT device implantation and during further follow-up. Also, note the change in the shape of the LVOT Pulsed wave Doppler trace: the trace is symmetric and triangular with a late peak during the low cardiac output state before CRT; it becomes more asymmetric with an early peak with improved LV function.

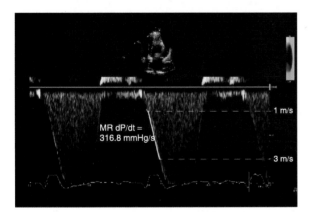

FIG. 22.7 The change of pressure over time (d*P*/d*t*) measured from a continuous wave Doppler trace of mitral regurgitation with a very low value in a patient with dilated cardiomyopathy.

function as well as pulmonary hypertension are covered in Chapters 16 and 36, respectively.

Functional Mitral Regurgitation

Within the context of pathological LV remodeling in DCM, an increase in LV spherical remodeling occurs, resulting in lateral and apical displacement of the papillary muscles. In addition to mitral ring dilation that parallels LV cavity dilation, papillary muscle displacement leads to poor mitral leaflet coaptation and is the main mechanism underlying **secondary (functional) mitral regurgitation** (see Fig. 28.10). Progression of mitral regurgitation is yet another harbinger of worse prognosis in DCM patients. Finally, severe mitral regurgitation causes marked volume overload and further dilation of the LV, which may in turn increase the calculated LVEF, thus concealing the actual underlying grave impairment in LV systolic function.

ARRHYTHMOGENIC CARDIOMYOPATHY

ACM is a genetically determined cardiomyopathy characterized by fibrofatty replacement of myocardial tissue. This disease was formerly known as "Arrhythmogenic right ventricular dysplasia/cardiomyopathy;" however, the term ACM is currently preferred as it is now recognized that LV involvement, either in the form of biventricular disease or purely LV involvement, can occur in up to 76% of patients.[1,14] The diagnostic approach to ACM encompasses findings from echocardiography and/or magnetic resonance imaging (MRI), RV biopsies, and multiple electrocardiographic criteria (Box 22.3).[15] There are also a growing number of genetic abnormalities that have been linked with the disease.

Establishing the diagnosis of ACM can be complicated by the three phases of disease, particularly during the first subclinical phase in which imaging studies are typically negative, yet sudden cardiac death may still occur. The second phase of disease is notable primarily for the absence of obvious RV abnormalities or signs and symptoms of RV failure and the onset of symptomatic ventricular arrhythmias (often symptomatic). The third phase of disease is characterized by severe RV dilatation and aneurysm formation due to progressive fibrofatty replacement, with clinically overt RV failure. LV dilation and failure may emerge during this phase or at a later stage of disease.[1] Of note, some overlap may be present in the phenotype of patients with DCM and ACM, particularly in ACM cases with biventricular or predominantly LV involvement.

The two-dimensional echocardiographic findings that are currently enlisted among the diagnostic criteria for ACM are regional RV akinesia, dyskinesia, or aneurysm accompanied by dilation of the right ventricular outflow tract (RVOT) measured at end diastole in the parasternal long- or short-axis view or reduced FAC (see Box 22.3). The sensitivity of the major criteria listed in Box 22.3, in addition to the aforementioned wall motion criteria, varies between 55% and 75% with a common specificity value of 95%.[15] The variability in sensitivity may well be due in part to the stage of disease presentation and expression. Examples of patients with ACM are given in Figs. 22.10 and 22.11 and the corresponding Videos 22.2 to 22.4.

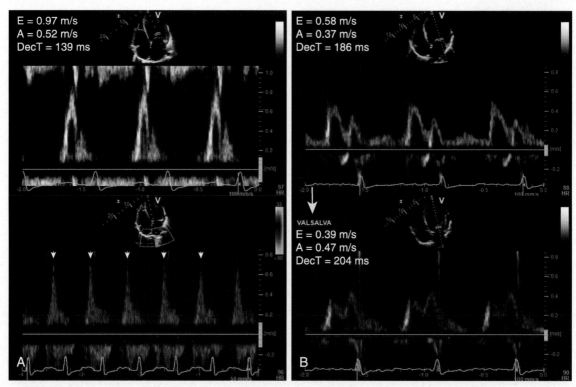

FIG. 22.8 Transmitral flow **(A, *upper panel* and B)** and pulmonary vein flow **(A, *lower panel*)** patterns in the assessment of left ventricle filling pressures. The images in (A) are taken from the same patient with New York Heart Association (NYHA) functional class IV symptoms imaged in Fig. 22.1A. Note that there is a restrictive filling pattern ([A] *upper panel*) and predominant diastolic flow on the traces of pulmonary vein flow ([A] *lower panel, white arrowheads*). (B) Shows transmitral flow of the patient in NYHA class II (presented in Fig. 22.1B), taken during normal breathing ([B] *upper panel*) and during a Valsalva maneuver ([B] *lower panel*). The reversibility of the flow to an impaired relaxation pattern suggests that the *upper panel* in fact represents pseudonormal filling.

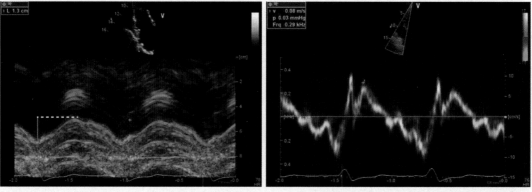

FIG. 22.9 Tricuspid annular planar systolic excursion (TAPSE) *(left panel, red mark)* and Doppler tissue imaging S′ *(right panel)* as additional measures of right ventricular systolic function. In this case, both are mildly reduced in a patient with dilated cardiomyopathy.

LEFT VENTRICULAR NONCOMPACTION

The American Heart Association Statement on the definitions and classification of the cardiomyopathies has defined left ventricular noncompaction (LVNC) as a genetic cardiomyopathy characterized by a "spongy" morphological appearance of the LV myocardium.[16] However, the classification of the cardiomyopathies by the European Society of Cardiology questioned whether LVNC is a distinct cardiomyopathy or a structural feature common to various cardiomyopathies, and so the issue continues to be under debate.[2] Some studies have found that up to 30% of adult patients presenting with heart failure of any cause, and even some athletes, have significantly increased LV trabeculations.[17] Indeed, LVNC has been recognized as an isolated entity in left ventricles that are otherwise of normal structure and function, but also in association with various types of cardiomyopathies as well as with congenital heart disease.[1] Some phenotypes may represent variable expressivity of a genetic disease or alternatively an epiphenomenon related to increased preload. These

issues highlight the importance and the difficulty of establishing agreed-upon criteria for LVNC.

Given the above, at present for practical purposes, the diagnosis of the LVNC phenotype is predominantly based on echocardiography and MRI. In contrast to most forms of dilated cardiomyopathies, the diagnostic criteria for LVNC do not require the assessment of LV size and function but are predominantly determined by the ratios of compacted and noncompacted myocardium obtained at end diastole or end systole (Box 22.4).[18] The noncompacted segments tend to involve the (mid and) apical portion of the LV walls and must measure at least twice the thickness of the compacted layers (NC:N ratio of at least 2:1 by most criteria) to fulfill diagnostic criteria; some of the criteria also require the presence of deep intertrabecular recesses with evidence of communication with the ventricular cavity.[18] Examples of two patients with LVNC are given in Fig. 22.12 as well as in Videos 22.5 and 22.6.

BOX 22.3 Revised Task Force Criteria for the Diagnosis of Arrhythmic Cardiomyopathy

Diagnostic Terminology for Revised Criteria
- Definite diagnosis: 2 major or 1 major and 2 minor criteria or 4 minor criteria from different categories
- Borderline: 1 major and 1 minor or 3 minor criteria from different categories
- Possible: 1 major or 2 minor criteria from different categories

I. Global and/or Regional Dysfunction and Structural Alterations
Major
By two-dimensional echocardiography:
  Regional RV akinesia, dyskinesia, or aneurysm *and* one of the following (end diastole):
    Parasternal long-axis view of the RVOT (PLAX) ≥32 mm (≥19 mm/m²)
    Parasternal short-axis view of the RVOT (PSAX) ≥36 mm (≥21 mm/m²)
    or
    Fractional area change <33%
By MRI:
  Regional RV akinesia, dyskinesia, or dyssynchronous RV contraction *and* one of the following: Ratio of RVEDV to BSA ≥110 mL/m² (male) or ≥100 mL/m² (female) *or* RVEF ≤40%
By RV angiography:
  Regional RV akinesia, dyskinesia, or aneurysm

Minor
By two-dimensional echocardiography:
  Regional RV akinesia or dyskinesia and one of the following (end diastole):
    PLAX RVOT ≥29 to <32 mm (≥16 to <19 mm/m²)
    PSAX RVOT ≥32 to <36 mm (≥18 mm to <21 mm/m²)
    or
    Fractional area change >33% to ≤40%
By MRI:
  Regional RV akinesia, dyskinesia, or dyssynchronous RV contraction *and* one of the following: Ratio of RVEDV to BSA ≥100 to <110 mL/m² (male) or ≥100 to <110 mL/m² (female) *or* RVEF <40% to ≤45%

II. Tissue Characterization of Wall
Major
Residual myocytes <60% by morphometric analysis (or <50% if estimated), with fibrous replacement of the RV free wall myocardium in at least 1 sample, with or without fatty replacement of tissue seen on endomyocardial biopsy

Minor
Residual myocytes 60%–75% by morphometric analysis (or 50%–65% if estimated) with fibrous replacement of the RV free wall myocardium in at least 1 sample and with or without fatty replacement of tissue seen on endomyocardial biopsy

III. Repolarization Abnormalities
Major
Inverted T waves in the right precordial leads (V_1, V_2, and V_3) or beyond in individuals >14 years of age (in the absence of complete right bundle branch block QRS ≥120 ms)

Minor
Inverted T waves in leads V_1 and V_2 in individuals >14 years of age (in the absence of complete right bundle branch block) or in V_4, V_5, or V_6
Inverted T waves in leads V_1, V_2, V_3, and V_4 in individuals >14 years of age in the presence of complete right bundle branch block

IV. Depolarization/Conduction Abnormalities
Major
Epsilon wave (reproducible low-amplitude signals between the end of the QRS complex to the onset of the T wave) in the right precordial leads (V_1 to V_3)

Minor
Late potentials by signal-averaged ECG in at least 1 of 3 parameters in the absence of a QRS duration ≥110 ms on standard ECG
Filtered QRS duration ≥114 ms
RMS voltage of terminal 40 ms <20 µV
Terminal activation duration of the QRS ≥55 ms measured from the nadir of the S wave to the end of the QRS complex, including R′, in V_1, V_2, or V_3 in the absence of complete right bundle branch block

BSA, Body surface area; *ECG*, electrocardiogram; *RVEDV*, RV end-diastolic volume; *RVEF*, RV ejection fraction; *RVOT*, RV outflow tract.
From Falk RH, Hershberger RE: The dilated, restrictive, and infiltrative cardiomyopathies. In Mann D, Zipes D, Libby P, Bonow R. Braunwald's Heart Disease, 10th ed. Philadelphia: Elsevier, 2014. Modified from Marcus FI, McKenna WJ, Sherrill D, et al. Diagnosis of arrhythmogenic right ventricular cardiomyopathy/dysplasia: proposed modification of the task force criteria. *Eur Heart J.* 2010;31(7):806–814.

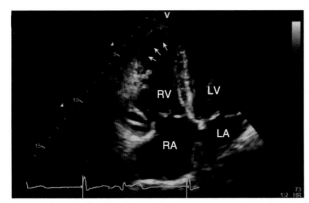

FIG. 22.10 Apical four-chamber view focused on the right ventricle in a patient with arrhythmogenic cardiomyopathy. The right ventricular (RV) cavity is dilated with a thinned free wall with notable trabeculations, akinetic in the mid-apical thirds with a clear aneurysm formed in the apical third of the RV free wall *(arrows)*. (Also see Video 22.2 for a cine-loop of this image). *LA*, Left atrium; *LV*, left ventricle; *RA*, right atrium.

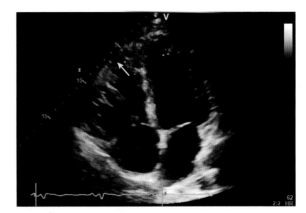

FIG. 22.11 Apical four-chamber view in a patient with arrhythmogenic cardiomyopathy and biventricular involvement. The right ventricular (RV) cavity is dilated with notable trabeculations and an aneurysm *(arrow)* of the hypocontractile RV free wall. (Also see Video 22.3 for a cine-loop of this image, which also shows reduced left ventricular systolic function, and Video 22.4 for an echocardiogram of the patient's sister who was also affected by arrhythmogenic cardiomyopathy.)

BOX 22.4 Echocardiographic and Magnetic Resonance Imaging Diagnostic Criteria for Left Ventricular Noncompaction

Echocardiographic Criteria

Chin et al. (California criteria)[a]
- LVNC is defined by an X/Y ratio ≤0.5
- These criteria evaluate trabeculae at the LV apex on the parasternal short-axis and apical views and by using the LV free wall thickness at end diastole

Jenni et al. (Zurich criteria)[b]
- Bilayered myocardium consisting of a thin C layer and a much thicker NC layer with deep endomyocardial recesses: NC/C > 2
- Predominant location of the pathology is midlateral, midinferior, and at the apex
- Evidence of intertrabecular recesses filled with blood from the LV cavity
- Acquisition of image views: short axis with measurement of the NC/C ratio performed at end systole

Stöllberger and Finsterer (Vienna criteria)[c]
- Four or more trabeculations protruding from the LV wall located apical to the papillary muscles and visible in one imaging plane
- Trabeculations with the same echogenicity as myocardium and synchronous movement with ventricular contractions
- Perfusion of the intertrabecular recesses from the LV cavity
- Acquisition of images in the apical four-chamber view, atypical views to obtain the best-quality image for differentiation between false chords, aberrant bands, and trabeculations

Paterick et al. (Milwaukee criteria)[d]
- Evaluation of trabeculation sizes (NC myocardium) in relation to C wall thicknesses in multiple imaging windows and at different ventricular levels throughout the cardiac cycle
- Identification of the bilayered myocardium (C and NC) in short-axis views at the mid and apical levels and in the apical two- and four-chamber and apical long-axis views
- Thicknesses of the C and NC sections of the myocardium are best measured in short-axis views at end diastole, with an NC/C ratio >2 being diagnostic of LVNC

Magnetic Resonance Criteria

Petersen et al.[e]
- Ratio between NC and C layers >2.3 at end diastole

Jacquier et al.[f]
- Trabeculated LV mass >20% of global LV mass (measurements made at end diastole)

C, Compacted; NC, noncompacted; X, distance from the epicardial surface to the trough of the trabecular recess; Y, distance from the epicardial surface to the peak of the trabeculation.

[a]Chin TK, Perloff JK, Williams RG, Jue K, Mohrmann R. Isolated noncompaction of left ventricular myocardium. A study of eight cases. *Circulation.* 1990;82(2):507–513.

[b]Jenni R, Oechslin E, Schneider J, Attenhofer Jost C, Kaufmann PA. Echocardiographic and pathoanatomical characteristics of isolated left ventricular non-compaction: a step towards classification as a distinct cardiomyopathy. *Heart.* 2001;86(6):666–6671.

[c]Stöllberger C, Finsterer J. Left ventricular hypertrabeculation/noncompaction. *J Am Soc Echocardiogr.* 2004;17(1):91–100.

[d]Paterick TE, Umland MM, Jan MF, et al. Left ventricular noncompaction: a 25-year odyssey. *J Am Soc Echocardiogr.* 2012;25(4):363–375.

[e]Petersen SE, Selvanayagam JB, Wiesmann F, et al. Left ventricular non-compaction: insights from cardiovascular magnetic resonance imaging. *J Am Coll Cardiol.* 2005;46(1):101–105.

[f]Jacquier A, Thuny F, Jop B, et al. Measurement of trabeculated left ventricular mass using cardiac magnetic resonance imaging in the diagnosis of left ventricular non-compaction. *Eur Heart J.* 2010;31(9):1098–1104.

From Falk RH, Hershberger RE: The dilated, restrictive, and infiltrative cardiomyopathies. In Mann D, Zipes D, Libby P, Bonow R. Braunwald's Heart Disease. 10th ed. Philadelphia: Elsevier, 2014. Modified from Paterick TE, Umland MM, Jan MF, et al. Left ventricular noncompaction: a 25-year odyssey. *J Am Soc Echocardiogr.* 2012;25(4):363–375.

TACHYCARDIA-INDUCED CARDIOMYOPATHY

Prolonged periods of tachycardia may result in tachycardia-induced cardiomyopathy that may present with preserved or reduced LVEF. The latter forms of tachycardia-induced cardiomyopathy show structural and functional overlap with DCM, and indeed may, in some cases, be an overlapping condition. A common clinical scenario is that of a patient with subclinical DCM developing atrial fibrillation with a rapid ventricular response, which becomes permanent and further worsens the cardiomyopathy, leading to overt heart failure. However, the diagnosis of tachycardia-induced cardiomyopathy can only be established retrospectively when improvement in ventricular function occurs after correction of the underlying arrhythmia (most often atrial arrhythmias, but also very frequent premature ventricular complexes [PVCs] or recurrent nonsustained ventricular tachycardia).[19,20] To adequately document the improvement of systolic function, for example, after cardioversion to sinus rhythm after atrial fibrillation, it is appropriate to measure LV function early after cardioversion (due to less reliable LVEF measurements in high beat-to-beat variability frequently encountered in atrial fibrillation) and 3–6 months thereafter.[1] Typically, the improvement of LV function can be noted within 3–6 months, whereas mild LV cavity dilation may remain in some cases. Videos 22.7 and 22.8 provide an example of a patient with tachycardia-induced cardiomyopathy induced by atrial flutter (see Video 22.7) in whom right atrial cavotricuspid isthmus ablation provided resolution of the arrhythmia and recovery of LV systolic function (see Video 22.8).

PERIPARTUM CARDIOMYOPATHY

PPCM is a form of DCM that is defined by the development of systolic heart failure towards the end of pregnancy or in the months following delivery (typically in the last month of pregnancy or during the 6 months after child birth), which cannot be attributed to a specific cause (Box 22.5).[14,21] The LVEF is usually below 45% and may or may not be accompanied with LV dilation.[2] The disease is often associated with older age, multiparity, multiple fetal pregnancies, hypertension (with or without preeclampsia), and Afro-Caribbean ethnicity, while other risk factors include autoimmunity, fetal microchimerism, viral infections, and malnutrition. There also appears to be a genetic basis to the disease.[1,14] The signs and symptoms of heart failure develop during pregnancy or after delivery; and while the disorder progresses more rapidly than other forms of DCM (e.g., genetic DCM, LVNC, or ACM) in the majority of cases, recovery is also more likely to occur.[1] Recurrence of the disease is likely related to the degree of recovery from the original episode: women with a normal LVEF at the onset of a second pregnancy are less likely to experience a recurrent episode of PPCM.[1]

According to a recent position statement by the Heart Failure Association of the European Society of Cardiology Working Group on Peripartum Cardiomyopathy, cardiac imaging (most widely performed by echocardiography) is indicated promptly in any peripartum woman presenting with symptoms and signs suggestive of heart failure.[21] Cardiac imaging establishes the diagnosis and provides prognostic information, should PPCM be proven. Namely, an LV end-diastolic diameter greater than 60 mm or an LVEF less than 30% predict poor recovery of LV function.[21] When imaging PPCM, it is also important to rule out potential LV thrombus formation, particularly in cases with severely depressed LVEF. An example of a patient with PPCM is given in Fig. 22.13 and Videos 22.9 and 22.10.

TAKOTSUBO CARDIOMYOPATHY

Takotsubo cardiomyopathy, also termed stress-induced cardiomyopathy, is a reversible form of cardiomyopathy with acute development. Although variable in presentation, the most frequent clinical features may mimic an acute myocardial infarction and include acute-onset chest pain, ST-segment changes, and regional LV dysfunction. Acute obstructive coronary artery disease as a causal factor, particularly in older individuals, typically must be excluded by coronary or computed tomography angiography before concluding the diagnosis. The majority (nearly 90%) of the cases presenting with this form of cardiomyopathy occur in females, most of whom are over 50 years old.[22] The onset of symptoms is frequently preceded by an emotional or physical stress, such as bereavement, surgery, or asthma exacerbation; a presumptive trigger is identifiable in the majority of cases.[1]

The echocardiographic examination reveals distinct wall motion abnormalities, which most frequently affect the LV apex with compensatory hyperkinesia of the basal LV segments. Hence, this cardiomyopathy

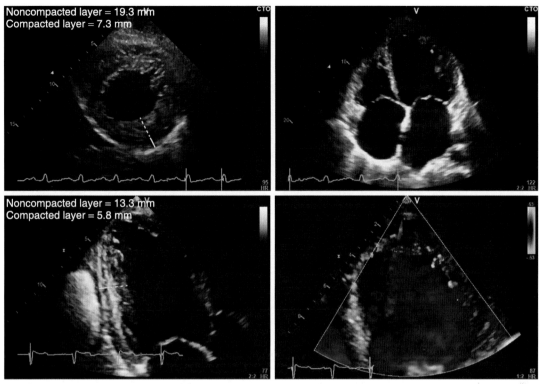

FIG. 22.12 Parasternal short-axis *(upper left panel)*, apical four-chamber view *(upper right panel)*, apical long-axis *(lower left panel)* and apical four-chamber view with a focus on the left ventricle *(lower right panel)* in two patients with left ventricular noncompaction. *Left panels:* A bilayered myocardium composed of a thin compacted layer *(full yellow line)* and a markedly thicker noncompacted layer *(dashed yellow line)* with deep endomyocardial recesses. Note that the measurements are performed in end systole. *Right panels:* Apical four-chamber views showing the deep endomyocardial recesses filled with blood from the left ventricular cavity. (Also see Videos 22.5 and 22.6 for cine-loops of these images.)

BOX 22.5 Causes of New or Exacerbated Heart Failure in the Peripartum Period

PPCM
Preexisting familial or idiopathic DCM
Human immunodeficiency virus-related cardiomyopathy
Cocaine-induced heart disease
Preexisting valve disease
Hypertensive heart disease
Pregnancy-associated myocardial infarction
Pulmonary embolism
Preeclampsia
Tachycardia-associated cardiomyopathy (from pregnancy-associated supraventricular tachycardia)

DCM, Dilated cardiomyopathy; *PPCM,* peripartum cardiomyopathy.
Data from Sliwa K, Hilfiker-Kleiner D, Petrie MC, et al. Current state of knowledge on aetiology, diagnosis, management, and therapy of peripartum cardiomyopathy: a position statement from the Heart Failure Association of the European Society of Cardiology Working Group on Peripartum Cardiomyopathy. *Eur J Heart Fail.* 2010;12(8):767–778.

---

is also termed "apical ballooning syndrome" (Fig. 22.14 and Videos 22.11 and 22.12), and was named after the Japanese octopus trap of the same shape, narrow neck and round bottom, that the LV assumes on the left ventriculogram in the left anterior oblique projection (which is analogous to echocardiographic parasternal long-axis views). In atypical forms of stress cardiomyopathy, other segments of the LV myocardium such as the base can also be affected by hypo- or akinesia (Video 22.13). In a recent registry, the apical Takotsubo form predominated in more than 80% of cases, midventricular wall motion abnormalities in approximately 15%, and basal and other focal forms in a minority of cases.[22] Regardless, the wall motion abnormalities cannot be attributed to a single coronary artery distribution. It is common for the preserved LV segments to become hyperdynamic in the acute setting. In fact, another echocardiographic feature that may be recognized in patients with Takotsubo

cardiomyopathy is the development of a left ventricular intracavity (mid-cavity or LVOT) gradient that may occur due to flow obstruction at the papillary muscle level or due to systolic anterior motion (SAM) of the mitral valve, which is similar to hypertrophic obstructive cardiomyopathy. Importantly, Takotsubo cardiomyopathy is characterized by full recovery of LV function within several weeks from presentation (see Video 22.12). However, the episodes may recur (at a rate of 1.8% per patient/year) even 10 years after the initial event.[22] Cases of inverted Takotsubo cardiomyopathy with akinetic basal portions of the LV and a hyperdynamic apex have been described as well, as imaged in Video 22.13. Of note, a similar finding and time course may be seen in some patients with documented myocardial infarction, which has been fully revascularized, in which ventricular function fully recovers on a follow-up echocardiogram, a phenomenon commonly referred to as myocardial "stunning."[6]

ALCOHOLIC CARDIOMYOPATHY

Excessive intake of alcohol, usually implying a history of drinking substantially for a minimum of 5 years, has been proven to induce cardiotoxic effects, which may present in the form of DCM.[1] Importantly, alcohol abuse is the leading cause of nonischemic DCM in industrialized countries, accounting for approximately 50% of the affected patients.[1] Moreover, alcoholism is associated with hypertension, which may lead to further deterioration of this acquired cardiomyopathy.

Replacement fibrosis, which is one of the underlying mechanisms of myocardial involvement in chronic alcoholism, affects both myocardial systolic and diastolic function. Diastolic dysfunction is often present in asymptomatic alcoholics that exhibit evidence of LV hypertrophy with preserved ejection fraction (EF) by echocardiography in as many as half of such patients, and 30% of asymptomatic individuals with chronic excessive alcohol intake have LV systolic dysfunction on echocardiography.[23] The course of the disease largely depends on further drinking habits: abstinence from alcohol may lead to reversal of myocardial involvement, while the condition may progress to DCM and overt heart failure with continuation of excessive alcohol

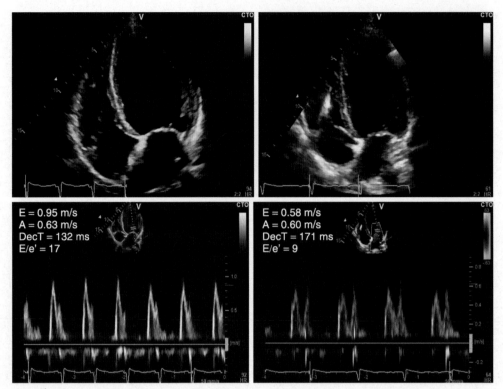

IV

FIG. 22.13 Apical four-chamber view and transmitral pulsed-wave Doppler traces from a patient with peripartum cardiomyopathy at presentation *(left panel)* and at 6-month follow-up *(right panel)*. At presentation, 2 days after delivery, the patient presented with symptoms corresponding to New York Heart Association (NYHA) functional class III and treatment with optimal medical therapy for heart failure was initiated. At presentation, the left ventricle (LV) was severely dilated with severely reduced left ventricular ejection fraction (LVEF) (Simpson biplane LVEF 28%) and a moderately enlarged left atrium (LA volume indexed to body surface area (BSA) 35 mL/m^2), while the RV size and function were still within normal limits *(upper left panel)*. The transmitral flow revealed a restrictive filling pattern *(lower left panel)*. Six months after childbirth, the patient had only slight dyspnea at exertion. On echocardiography, the LV had returned to a normal size with now mildly reduced systolic function (LVEF 42 %), and the left atrial size had also normalized *(upper right panel)*. The transmitral filling has at this point corresponded to an impaired relaxation pattern *(lower right panel)*. (Also see Videos 22.9 and 22.10 for cine-loops of this patient's images.)

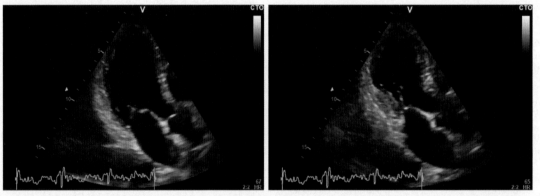

FIG. 22.14 Apical long-axis view at end diastole *(left panel)* and end systole *(right panel)* in a patient with Takotsubo cardiomyopathy. Note that in the end-systolic frame, there is only inward motion of the basal segments of the inferolateral wall and anteroseptum, while the mid and apical segments remain akinetic. (See Videos 22.11 and 22.12 for cine-loops of this patient's images at baseline and at 6 weeks follow-up.)

intake. Data from a large community-based study have confirmed specific alterations in cardiac structure and function with increasing alcohol intake: in both sexes, increased alcohol intake was associated with larger LV diameters (but not volumes) in both systole and diastole, as well as larger LA diameters. The individuals within the subgroup of highest alcohol intake (≥14 drinks/week) were more prone to moderate-severe diastolic dysfunction. In men, an association with greater LV mass, higher E/E' ratio, and TAPSE was determined per alcohol consumption category, while women exhibited lower LVEF and a tendency towards impaired LV global longitudinal strain per consumption category; even moderate alcohol intake was associated with modest impairment in systolic function, possibly increasing the risk of alcoholic cardiomyopathy.[24]

CARDIOMYOPATHY IN CHAGAS DISEASE

Chagas disease is a protozoal infection caused by *Trypanosoma cruzi*, which infects target organs, including the heart. In association with the activation of the immune system, such infection impairs myocardial function, which may present as DCM. Although formerly endemic in rural areas of Central and South America, it should also be suspected as a potential cause of nonischemic cardiomyopathy in the developed world where its incidence is increasing because of immigration of infected individuals.

Affected patients often remain asymptomatic during the acute phase of infection, while possible findings involving the cardiovascular system may include nonspecific electrocardiogram (ECG) changes, first-degree atrioventricular block, or cardiomegaly on chest x-ray, while the clinical presentation may correspond to myocarditis. If present, the symptoms of disease resolve spontaneously in the majority of patients. The chronic form of Chagas disease will become apparent in approximately 30%–40% of these patients, typically 5–15 years after the parasitic infection, while the remaining 60%–70% of these patients will not develop chronic Chagas disease (but will remain seropositive).[25] Antitrypanosomal treatment is recommended, particularly in the acute phases of disease; however, its effects are dubious in advanced heart failure when the structural derangement of the myocardium may already be irreversible.

The chronic form of Chagas disease involves more typical manifestations, partly detectable by echocardiography. These manifestations occur due to the ensuing derangement of myocardial structure and function and may include the destruction of the conduction system, myocardial fibrosis, ventricular dilatation, thinning of the apex of the heart as well as the formation of apical thrombi. Clinically, patients may present with heart failure, arrhythmias, or heart blocks (both atrioventricular or bundle branch blocks), as well as thromboembolic events.[25]

CHEMOTHERAPY-INDUCED CARDIOMYOPATHY

For the effects of chemotherapeutics on the development of DCM, refer to Chapter 42.

Suggested Reading

Arbustini, E., Narula, N., Dec, G. W., et al. (2013). The MOGE(S) classification for a phenotype-genotype nomenclature of cardiomyopathy: endorsed by the World Heart Federation. *Journal of the American College of Cardiology, 62*, 2046–2072.

Cikes, M., & Solomon, S. D. (2016). Beyond ejection fraction: an integrative approach for assessment of cardiac structure and function in heart failure. *European Heart Journal, 37*, 1642–1650.

Elliott, P., Andersson, B., Arbustini, E., et al. (2008). Classification of the cardiomyopathies: a position statement from the European Society of Cardiology Working Group on myocardial and pericardial diseases. *European Heart Journal, 29*, 270–276.

Mann, D. L., & Felker, G. M. (Eds.). (2015). *Heart failure: a companion to Braunwald's heart disease* (3rd ed.). Philadelphia: Elsevier.

Maron, B. J., Towbin, J. A., Thiene, G., et al. (2006). Contemporary definitions and classification of the cardiomyopathies: an American Heart Association Scientific Statement from the Council on Clinical Cardiology, Heart Failure and Transplantation Committee; Quality of Care and Outcomes Research and Functional Genomics and Translational Biology Interdisciplinary Working Groups; and Council on Epidemiology and Prevention. *Circulation, 113*, 1807–1816.

A complete reference list can be found online at ExpertConsult.com.

23

Hypertrophic Cardiomyopathy

Sara B. Seidelmann, Sheila M. Hegde, Carolyn Y. Ho

INTRODUCTION

Hypertrophic cardiomyopathy (HCM) is characterized by unexplained myocardial hypertrophy, that is, hypertrophy that has developed in the absence of other attributable etiology, myocyte disarray, and myocardial fibrosis (Fig. 23.1). In large part, through cardiac imaging and molecular research, our understanding of the pathophysiology, epidemiology, and prognosis of HCM in the last several decades has rapidly advanced. Echocardiography is an essential tool for examining the morphologic diversity, dynamic remodeling, hemodynamic changes, and complex disturbances of cardiac function associated with HCM. Current American Society of Echocardiography (ASE) Guidelines recommend an initial comprehensive echocardiographic evaluation of all patients with or suspected of having HCM (Table 23.1), including the assessment of cardiac structure, systolic and diastolic function, pulmonary artery pressures, valvular function, and dynamic outflow evaluation.[1]

This chapter reviews the echocardiographic evaluation and findings in HCM relevant to patient care and clinical investigation. Echocardiography is often the key to establishing the diagnosis of HCM and describing morphologic variants; characterizing natural history and heterogeneous phenotypic expression; evaluating pathophysiology, including obstructive physiology and diastolic abnormalities; and guiding therapeutic interventions including surgical septal myectomy and alcohol septal ablation

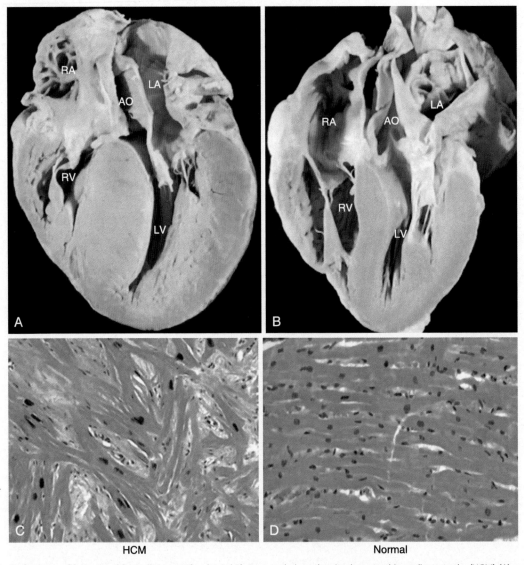

HCM   Normal

FIG. 23.1 Pathologic features of hypertrophic cardiomyopathy. (A and B) Gross pathology showing hypertrophic cardiomyopathy (HCM) (A) as compared to normal cardiac morphology (B). (C and D) Histologic sections stained with hematoxylin and eosin demonstrate myocyte disarray, where myocytes are oriented at bizarre and variable angles to each other, as well as increased myocardial fibrosis (C), the pathognomonic features of HCM. In contrast, normal myocardium demonstrates a very orderly arrangement of myocytes (D). *AO,* Aorta; *LA,* left atrium; *LV,* left ventricle; *RA,* right atrium; *RV,* right ventricle. (*Courtesy of Dr. Robert Padera, Department of Pathology, Brigham and Women's Hospital, Boston, MA.*)

TABLE 23.1 American Society of Echocardiography 2011 Recommendations for Parameters to Be Assessed During Echocardiographic Evaluation of Hypertrophic Cardiomyopathy

Cardiac Morphology	Presence of hypertrophy and its distribution; report should include measurements of LV dimensions and wall thickness (septal, inferior, and anterior) and location of maximal wall thickness
	RV hypertrophy and whether RV outflow dynamic obstruction is present
	LA volume indexed to body surface area
Cardiac Function	LV ejection fraction
	LV diastolic function (comments on LV relaxation and filling pressures)
Valvular Function	Mitral valve and papillary muscle evaluation, including the direction, mechanism, and severity of mitral regurgitation; if needed, TEE should be performed to satisfactorily answer these questions
	Estimation of pulmonary artery systolic pressure
Assessment of Obstruction	Dynamic obstruction at rest and with Valsalva maneuver; report should identify the site of obstruction and the gradient
Management Considerations	TEE is recommended to guide surgical myectomy and TTE or TEE to guide alcohol septal ablation
	Screening at-risk family members for the presence of disease is recommended

LA, Left atrium; *LV,* left ventricular; *RV,* right ventricular; *TEE,* transesophageal echocardiography; *TTE,* transthoracic echocardiography.
Adapted from Nagueh SF, Bierig SM, Budoff MJ, et al. American Society of Echocardiography clinical recommendations for multimodality cardiovascular imaging of patients with hypertrophic cardiomyopathy: endorsed by the American Society of Nuclear Cardiology, Society for Cardiovascular Magnetic Resonance, and Society of Cardiovascular Computed Tomography. J Am Soc Echocardiogr. 2011;24(5):473–498.

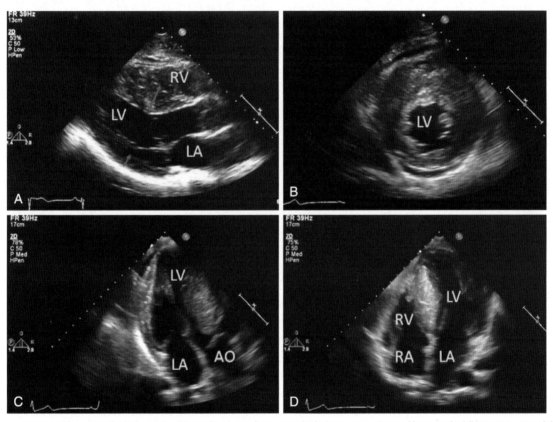

FIG. 23.2 **Asymmetric septal hypertrophy in hypertrophic cardiomyopathy.** Images displaying asymmetric septal hypertrophy (all images are at end diastole). (A) Parasternal long-axis view. *Red arrows* demonstrate wall thickness asymmetry between the interventricular septum and the posterior wall. (B) Short-axis view at the papillary muscle level, showing marked hypertrophy of the ventricular septum. (C) Apical three-chamber view. (D), Apical four-chamber view. *AO,* Aorta; *LA,* left atrium; *LV,* left ventricle; *RA,* right atrium; *RV,* right ventricle; calibration marks = 1 cm.

SARCOMERE GENE MUTATIONS CAUSE HYPERTROPHIC CARDIOMYOPATHY

HCM is often familial and is in fact the most common inherited cardiomyopathy. Genetic studies on families with HCM helped to establish the paradigm that HCM is a disease of the sarcomere and is caused by autosomal dominant mutations in genes that encode contractile proteins. The sarcomere is the functional unit of contraction of the myocyte and acts as the molecular motor of the heart. Over 1400 mutations have been identified in 11 different components of the sarcomere apparatus.[2] Mutations in the cardiac isoforms of β-myosin heavy chain (*MYH7*), myosin binding protein C (*MYBPC3*), and troponin T (*TNNT2*) are the

most frequent, together accounting for over 90% of cases where a genetic mutation has been identified.[3] Genetic testing of known HCM disease genes (predominantly sarcomere genes) typically detects mutations in ~30% of patients with HCM. However, if a family history of HCM is also present, the yield of genetic testing increases to ~60%.[3]

CARDIAC MORPHOLOGY

Cardiac morphology in HCM is typically notable for small left ventricular volumes with variable location and degree of hypertrophy. Although asymmetric septal hypertrophy (resulting in reversed septal curvature) is most common and classic (Fig. 23.2 and Videos 23.1 and

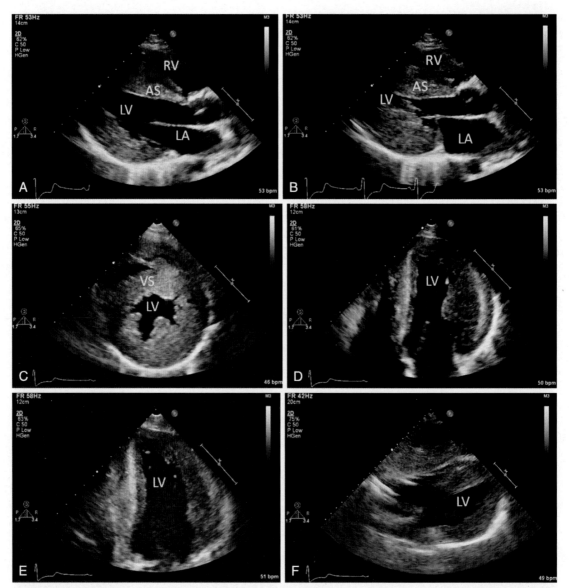

FIG. 23.3 **Concentric variant hypertrophic cardiomyopathy.** Images showing diffuse wall thickening involving substantial diffuse concentric hypertrophy. (A) Parasternal long-axis view (diastolic). (B) Parasternal long-axis view (systolic) showing LV midcavitary obliteration during systole. (C) Short-axis view at the papillary muscle level, showing global hypertrophy. (D) Apical four-chamber view demonstrating significant anterolateral hypertrophy and RV hypertrophy. (E) Apical two-chamber view. (F) Subcostal view. *AS,* Anteroseptal wall; *LA,* left atrium; *LV,* left ventricle; *RV,* right ventricle; *VS,* ventricular septum; calibration marks = 1 cm.

23.2), hypertrophy can involve any left ventricle (LV) segment and may be focal or concentric (Fig. 23.3). In classic HCM, in addition to the asymmetric hypertrophy at the basal septum, the left ventricular cavity often has a narrow crescentic shape (Video 23.3). Apical hypertrophy is a well-described morphologic variant of HCM (Fig. 23.4) in which hypertrophy occurs below the level of the papillary muscles in the distal portion of the LV chamber. As such, apical HCM is not associated with left ventricular outflow tract (LVOT) obstruction but may instead cause dynamic obstruction within the mid-to-distal ventricle. The LV often resembles the shape of a spade in diastole (see Fig. 23.4B and Video 23.4). First reported in Japan[4] and hence also referred to as "Yamaguchi variant," the prevalence of apical variant HCM appears to be higher in individuals of Japanese versus Western descent (13%–25% vs. 1%–2%).[5] A family history of HCM and disease-causing sarcomere gene mutations are rarely identified in patients with apical HCM,[6] suggesting that it is a different subtype of disease. While early studies suggested a more benign prognosis for apical HCM, a broad spectrum of clinical outcomes has been described.[7]

Septal morphology is predictive of the presence of sarcomere mutations. The likelihood of positive genetic testing is highest in patients with classic reversed septal curvature, and lowest in patients with a sigmoidal septum (focal upper septal thickening, Fig. 23.5).[8,9] Consistent correlations between the distribution of left ventricular hypertrophy (LVH) and clinical outcomes have not been established. Furthermore, even within families with HCM who share the same underlying sarcomere mutation, LV morphology is often varied.[10]

Cardiac morphology may occasionally not be adequately assessed by echocardiography due to suboptimal visualization of the LV apex, free wall, or endocardial/epicardial borders. In these cases, echocardiographic contrast administration or cardiac magnetic resonance (CMR) imaging should be considered to clarify the LV geometry (Fig. 23.6). Similarly, apical aneurysm (Fig. 23.7 and Video 23.5) is not only a rare consequence associated with obstructive HCM of any morphology that may be visualized with standard echocardiographic techniques, but may also require color Doppler interrogation or LV cavity opacification by echocardiographic contrast to aid with proper identification. The consequences of apical aneurysms are unclear, but they have been suggested to be associated with sudden death, progressive heart failure, and thromboembolic complications in a small patient series.[11,12]

Standard septal and posterior dimensions, as well as maximum wall thickness and its location, determined after inspecting all

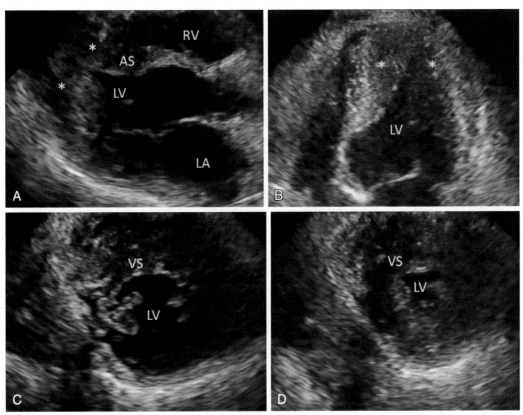

FIG. 23.4 Apical variant hypertrophic cardiomyopathy. Apical hypertrophy is a well-described morphologic variant of hypertrophic cardiomyopathy (HCM). Hypertrophy occurs below the level of the papillary muscles, in the distal portion of the LV chamber. As such, apical HCM does not result in left ventricular outflow obstruction. (A) Parasternal long-axis view. (B) Apical four-chamber view showing hypertrophy of the apical segments. (C) Parasternal short-axis view at the papillary muscle level, without significant hypertrophy. (D) Parasternal short-axis view at the apical level, showing hypertrophy of the apical segments. *AS*, Anteroseptal wall; *LA*, left atrium; *LV*, left ventricle; *RV*, right ventricle; *VS*, ventricular septum; *, apical segments with focal hypertrophy.

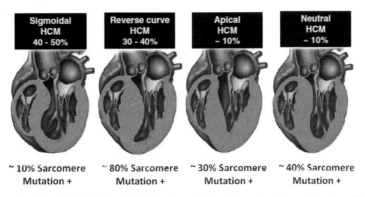

FIG. 23.5 Septal morphologies in hypertrophic cardiomyopathy. Illustration demonstrating different septal morphologies and their relation to likelihood that a sarcomere mutation will be identified with genetic testing. (*Modified from Binder J, Ommen SR, Gersh BJ, et al. Echocardiography-guided genetic testing in hypertrophic cardiomyopathy: septal morphological features predict the presence of myofilament mutations. Mayo Clin Proc. 2006;81(4):459–467.*)

imaging views, should be reported (see Table 23.1). In general, in the absence of another etiology for LV hypertrophy (i.e., pressure overload or infiltrative processes), a septal wall thickness (IVSd) ≥15 mm or a septal:posterior wall thickness ratio ≥1.3 support a diagnosis of HCM. Modified diagnostic criteria should be considered when evaluating relatives of HCM patients, recognizing the much higher *a priori* risk for HCM in the family members of patients with diagnosed disease. As summarized in Table 23.2,[13,14] more subtle abnormalities, particularly borderline or mild LVH, carry greater significance in this context. Other suggestive features that a sarcomere mutation is present include diastolic abnormalities (decreased early myocardial relaxation velocities, e′, by tissue Doppler interrogation)[15–17] and electrocardiographic changes (Q waves and marked repolarization changes such as ST segment depression and T wave inversion; see Fig. 23.6D).[18] Lastly, left atrial (LA) enlargement, measured by

anteroposterior linear dimensions or more accurately by volume, appears to be a marker for disease severity and is increased in patients with higher New York Heart Association (NYHA) classes.

Other incidental findings on echocardiography are common in classic HCM. The aortic leaflets tend to close early in midsystole as mitral-septal contact occurs, which can be observed particularly clearly on M-mode (Fig. 23.8). M-mode also can clearly diagram the systolic anterior motion (SAM) of the mitral leaflets in systole (refer to Fig. 23.13C later). Two-dimensional imaging of the LV may reveal an area of echogenicity and fibrotic thickening at the point of the repetitive SAM-mitral septal contact, which correlates with pathologic findings of a friction plaque. Mitral leaflets are occasionally elongated and/or chordal structures more slack, which may predispose or contribute to SAM. The mitral regurgitation (MR) engendered by SAM is characteristically posteriorly directed (see later).

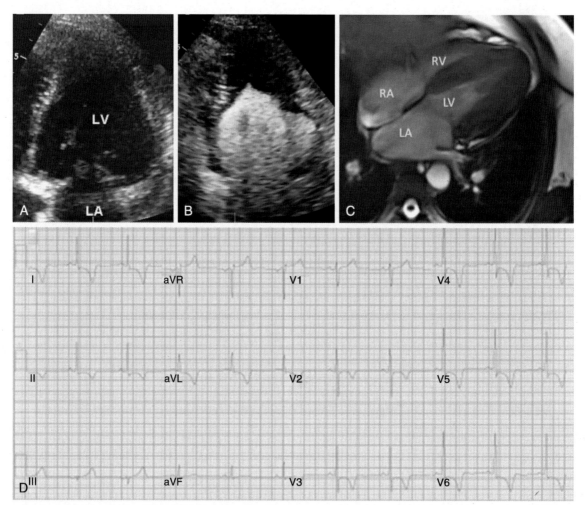

FIG. 23.6 Multimodality imaging to aid in characterizing apical hypertrophic cardiomyopathy. (A) Apical four-chamber view demonstrating apparently normal wall thickness but poor visualization of the apical endocardium. (B) Echocardiographic contrast provides definition of the typical "spade shaped" appearance of the left ventricle and apical wall thickening. (C) Cardiac magnetic resonance four-chamber image diagnostic of apical variant hypertrophic cardiomyopathy (HCM), demonstrating mid to apical segmental hypertrophy not readily apparent by standard echocardiography. (D) Marked precordial T-wave inversion on electrocardiogram are often associated with apical variant HCM. *LA,* Left atrium; *LV,* left ventricle; *RA,* right atrium; *RV,* right ventricle. I, II, III, aVR, aVL, V1-V6; Standard 12-lead ECG leads.

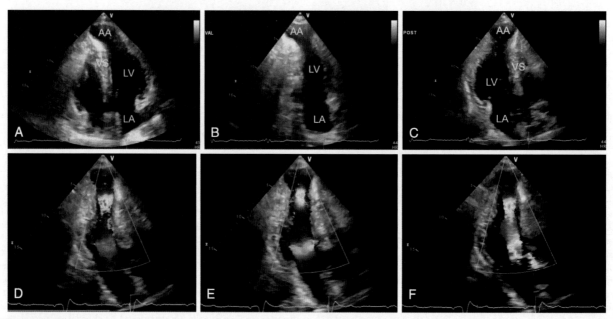

FIG. 23.7 Apical aneurysm formation in hypertrophic cardiomyopathy. Apical images illustrating a large left ventricle apical aneurysm. (A–C) Apical four-, two-, and three-chamber views demonstrating the apical aneurysm. (D–F) Apical three-chamber view with color Doppler flow showing flow during early diastole, end diastole, and midsystole.

LEFT VENTRICULAR SYSTOLIC AND DIASTOLIC FUNCTION

In most cases of HCM, LV ejection fraction is normal or hyperdynamic. However, there is a subset of patients with severe hypertrophy and restrictive physiology, in which LV end-diastolic volumes become reduced,

TABLE 23.2 Modified Criteria to Diagnose Hypertrophic Cardiomyopathy in Adult Members of Affected Families

	MAJOR CRITERIA	MINOR CRITERIA
Echocardiography	Maximal LV wall thickness ≥13 mm	Anterior septum or posterior wall ≥12 mm
		Posterior septum or free wall ≥14 mm
		SAM
		Redundant MV leaflets
Electrocardiography	Voltage criteria for LVH Pathologic Q waves	Complete BBB or (minor) interventricular conduction defect (in LV leads)
	T wave inversion • Leads I and aVL (≥3 mm) • V3–V6 (≥3 mm), or • II, III, aVF (≥5 mm) ST segment deviation >1 mm	

A diagnosis of HCM is suggested in the presence of one major criterion; two minor echocardiographic criteria or one minor echocardiographic and two minor electrocardiographic criteria.

BBB, Bundle branch block; *HCM,* hypertrophic cardiomyopathy; *LV,* left ventricular; *LVH,* left ventricular hypertrophy; *MV,* mitral valve; *SAM,* systolic anterior motion of the mitral valve.

Adapted from Michels M, Soliman OI, Phefferkorn J, et al. Disease penetrance and risk stratification for sudden cardiac death in asymptomatic hypertrophic cardiomyopathy mutation carriers. Eur Heart J. 2009;30(21):2593–2598.

thereby compromising stroke volume despite vigorous LV ejection fraction. Approximately 2%–5% of HCM patients progress to end stage or "burnt out" HCM; about 50% of those affected presenting early, in the first four decades of life.[19] This rare complication of HCM is characterized by a progression from a hypertrophied, nondilated, and hyperdynamic LV to a ventricle with systolic dysfunction (LV ejection fraction <50%). Approximately half of these patients also develop left ventricular cavity enlargement and regression of wall thickness (as illustrated in Fig. 23.9). The clinical course of end-stage HCM can vary but is typically highly unfavorable. Advanced heart failure therapies, including cardiac transplantation or mechanical support (left ventricular assist device), are considered when standard medical therapy for systolic heart failure is no longer effective.

Patients with clinically overt HCM typically demonstrate diastolic abnormalities by both standard Doppler interrogation of mitral inflow and tissue Doppler imaging (TDI). However, Doppler methods (see Chapter 15) are also useful for evaluating cardiac dysfunction earlier in the subclinical phases. Studies on sarcomere gene mutation carriers have shown that reduced early diastolic relaxation velocity (e' on TDI), indicative of impaired relaxation, may occur before overt LV hypertrophy (Fig. 23.10).[15–17] Although these findings help to understand the fundamental biology of HCM, there is no threshold value for e' that can discriminate at-risk mutation carriers from healthy relatives.

These studies suggest that diastolic abnormalities are a primary or early manifestation of the underlying sarcomere mutation itself in HCM, rather than simply being a consequence of LV hypertrophy or myocardial fibrosis. The etiology of diastolic dysfunction in preclinical HCM is incompletely characterized, but animal studies suggest decreased rates of actin-myosin cross-bridge detachment, and decreased rates of calcium reuptake into the sarcoplasmic reticulum may play a role.[20,21] Myocardial fibrosis, while often detected by CMR in patients with HCM and overt hypertrophy, is not presently detectable by standard echocardiography.

Speckle-tracking echocardiography is a newer echocardiographic technology that may additionally help characterize LV systolic and diastolic abnormalities in HCM. Speckle tracking capitalizes on the naturally occurring speckled appearance of the myocardium to provide an angle-independent, objective assessment of myocardial deformation, or *strain.*

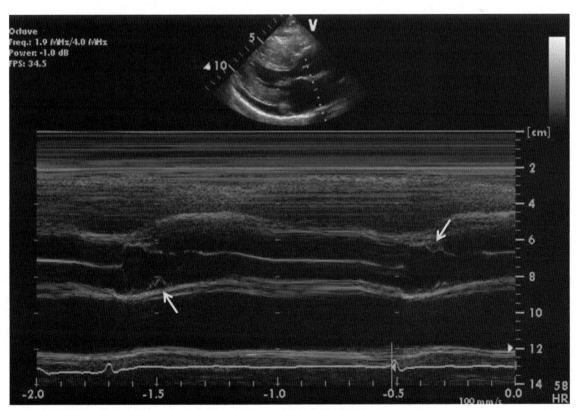

FIG. 23.8 Aortic valve M-mode in hypertrophic cardiomyopathy. M-mode imaging across the aortic valve shows early closure in late systole. Note that there is also midsystolic notching *(arrows)* and a coarse flutter to the aortic valves in mid-to-late systole. *AA,* Apical aneurysm; *LA,* left atrium; *LV,* left ventricle; *RV,* right ventricle; *VS,* ventricular septum.

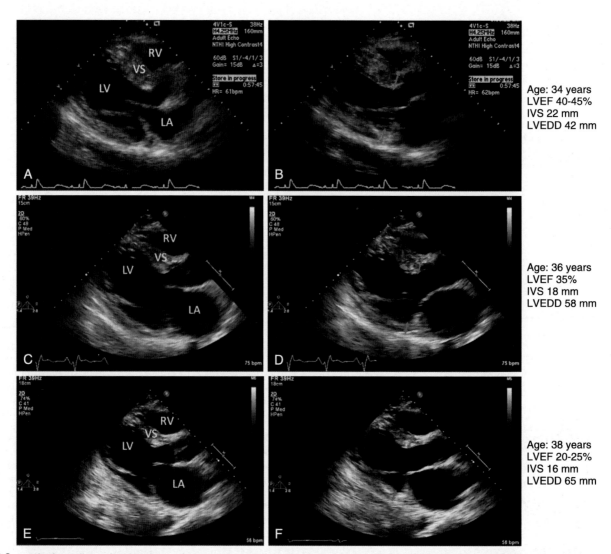

Age: 34 years
LVEF 40-45%
IVS 22 mm
LVEDD 42 mm

Age: 36 years
LVEF 35%
IVS 18 mm
LVEDD 58 mm

Age: 38 years
LVEF 20-25%
IVS 16 mm
LVEDD 65 mm

FIG. 23.9 Serial echocardiography identifies evolution to the end-stage phenotype of hypertrophic cardiomyopathy. Progression from a hypertrophied left ventricle (LV) to end-stage hypertrophic cardiomyopathy (HCM) is demonstrated in this series of images in a patient with familial HCM due to a *MYH7* mutation and diagnosed at 6 months of age. Images on left (A, C, E) are diastolic and on the right (B, D, F) are systolic. (A and B) Parasternal long-axis views at age 34 years. (C and D) Parasternal long-axis views at age 36 years demonstrates reduction in left ventricular ejection fraction (LVEF), regression of left ventricular hypertrophy (LVH), and new LV cavity dilation. (E and F) Parasternal long-axis views at age 38 years demonstrate further reduction in LVEF, regression of LVH, and cavity dilation. Heart transplantation was required soon thereafter. *IVS*, Intraventricular septum; *LA*, left atrium; *LVEDD*, left ventricular end-diastolic dimension; *RV*, right ventricle; *VS*, ventricular septum.

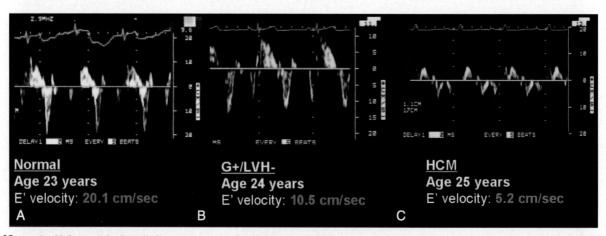

Normal
Age 23 years
E' velocity: 20.1 cm/sec

G+/LVH-
Age 24 years
E' velocity: 10.5 cm/sec

HCM
Age 25 years
E' velocity: 5.2 cm/sec

FIG. 23.10 Impaired left ventricle diastolic function precedes the development of left ventricular hypertrophy in family members with sarcomere gene mutations. (A) Tissue Doppler imaging (TDI) showing normal left ventricle (LV) relaxation in a 23-year-old healthy relative who does not carry the family's mutation and who has normal wall thickness. (B) TDI showing impaired LV relaxation in a 24-year-old that is gene positive but with normal wall thickness. (C) TDI showing impaired LV relaxation in a 25-year-old with phenotypic hypertrophic cardiomyopathy.

Septal longitudinal strain

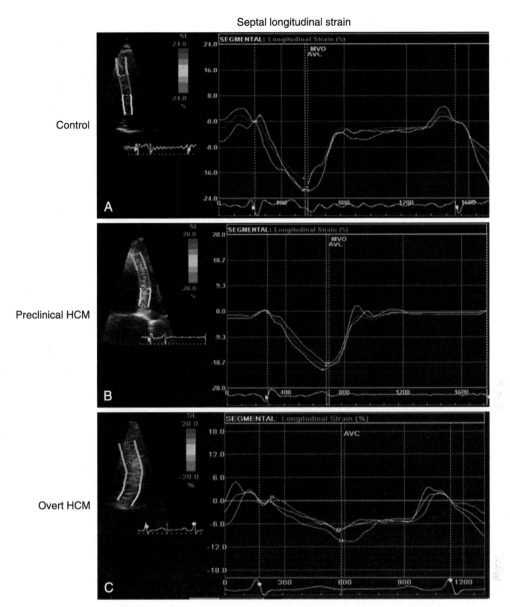

FIG. 23.11 Left ventricle strain imaging. Representative septal longitudinal strain *(left)* tracings from two-dimensional echocardiographic strain analysis in control (A) preclinical sarcomere mutation carriers (Gene+/LVH–) (B) and overt hypertrophic cardiomyopathy (HCM) (C) subjects demonstrating a reduction of longitudinal strain in HCM, but preserved strain in preclinical individuals. Measurements are taken from the interventricular septum. Tracings from the basal, mid, and apical segments are represented by different colors.

Recent studies have shown that there is a reduction in longitudinal strain in patients with HCM;[22,23] in contrast, longitudinal strain appears to be preserved in sarcomere mutation carriers with normal LV wall thickness (Gene+/LVH–; Fig. 23.11). Compared with control subjects, patients with HCM may also have increased circumferential strain.[24] Speckle-tracking technology is also being used to study more subtle changes in LV function, such as the differences in the rate and pattern of LV twisting and untwisting in patients with HCM. However, given the lack of clear segmental reference values and the need for more standardization of the technology, strain analysis has not yet been routinely incorporated in the echocardiographic evaluation of HCM patients. The relationship between the diastolic and strain parameters and implications for the clinical course of HCM are still being established.

DEVELOPMENT OF HYPERTROPHIC CARDIOMYOPATHY

The penetrance or clinical expression of an underlying gene mutation is age dependent, and LV wall thickness is typically normal throughout early childhood. Adolescence and young adulthood is the stereotypical time period for hypertrophic remodeling to occur. For example,

echocardiographic assessment of LV wall thickness may be normal during childhood but can increase rapidly at the time of phenotypic conversion (Fig. 23.12).[25] For this reason, longitudinal echocardiographic evaluation of all family members at risk for HCM is critical. If genetic testing has identified a definitively pathogenic mutation that is confirmed to be the cause of HCM in the family, serial echocardiographic follow up can be limited to those relatives who have inherited the causal mutation. Relatives who do not carry the pathogenic gene mutation are not at increased risk for developing HCM and do not require longitudinal follow-up, although evaluation should be pursued if there is clinical change.

LEFT VENTRICULAR OUTFLOW OBSTRUCTION AND MITRAL VALVE ABNORMALITIES

LV outflow obstruction (defined as a peak instantaneous Doppler outflow gradient of gradient ≥30 mm Hg at rest or with provocation) is a prominent feature of HCM (Fig. 23.13). A variety of predisposing functional and anatomic abnormalities are commonly seen in HCM, including septal hypertrophy, small LV outflow tract, hyperdynamic left ventricular function, and elongated mitral leaflets and/or slack chordal structures. These abnormalities can create altered hydrodynamic forces in the LV

Time (months)	Baseline	12	18	24	36
Age (years)	9	10	11	11	12

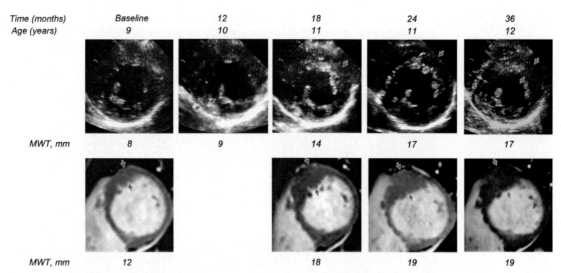

| MWT, mm | 8 | 9 | 14 | 17 | 17 |

| MWT, mm | 12 | | 18 | 19 | 19 |

FIG. 23.12 Phenotypic progression of hypertrophic cardiomyopathy in early years. These images show the evolution of hypertrophic cardiomyopathy (HCM) in a female carrying a pathogenic myosin heavy chain mutation. Echocardiographic images are in *top row*, and corresponding cardiac magnetic resonance (CMR) images at the same time points are in bottom row. Maximal left ventricular wall thickness (MWT) in millimeters is indicated below each image. At age 9 years, echocardiogram suggested borderline focal septal hypertrophy that appeared more prominent on CMR (CMR maximal left ventricle wall thickness of 12 mm involving 1 segment). Echocardiogram 12 months later showed no definitive change. Echocardiography and CMR 18 months later showed an increase in basal septal hypertrophy to 14 mm (by echo) and 18 mm (by CMR, involving three segments). There was no late gadolinium enhancement. Twenty-four months later, echocardiography and CMR showed localized hypertrophy, measuring up to 17–19 mm (z-score 10.9), then little change thereafter up to 36 months. Thus, much of the progression in hypertrophy occurred over years 9–11 of age.

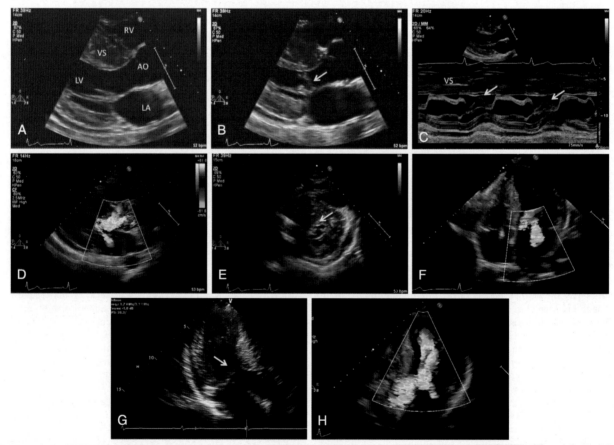

FIG. 23.13 Left ventricle outflow obstruction and mechanisms of systolic anterior motion. (A–H) Still-frame images that illustrate typical systolic anterior motion (SAM) showing the anterior mitral leaflet as it makes septal contact, producing mechanical impedance to left ventricle (LV) outflow and mitral regurgitation. (A) Parasternal long-axis view in diastole. (B) Parasternal long-axis view in midsystole showing typical SAM in which the anterior mitral leaflet bends acutely *(arrows)*, becoming almost perpendicular to the LV outflow tract in systole, resulting in localized septal contact and obstruction to flow (see Video 23.1). (C) M-mode depiction of mitral valve motion demonstrating anterior motion of the mitral valve and septal contact in midsystole *(arrows)*. (D) Parasternal long-axis image in midsystole with color Doppler demonstrating turbulent flow in the LV outflow tract due to systolic anterior motion and posteriorly directed mitral regurgitation (see Video 23.2). (E) Parasternal short-axis image in midsystole showing that the typical anterior motion of the mitral valve occurs in the center of the anterior mitral valve leaflet *(arrow* demonstrates septal contact). (F) Apical four-chamber view in midsystole with color Doppler demonstrating turbulent flow in the LV outflow tract and mitral regurgitation. (G and H) Apical three-chamber view in midsystole demonstrating elongated mitral leaflets, particularly the anterior mitral leaflet, and producing LV outflow obstruction from SAM *(single arrow)*, as shown by the accompanying color Doppler image. *AO,* Aorta; *LA,* left atrium; *LV,* left ventricle; *RV,* right ventricle; *VS,* ventricular septum.

outflow tract contributing to SAM(see Fig. 23.13) of the mitral valve, the predominant mechanism of LV outflow tract obstruction. Obstruction at rest has been identified in about 35% of patients with HCM.[26] Decreased LV cavity size and tachycardia can precipitate or provoke the development of obstructive physiology, as seen with exercise, Valsalva maneuver, or volume depletion.

Notably, because the LVOT obstruction can be latent and is inherently dynamic due to variations in loading conditions, careful evaluation for *provocable* obstruction is a crucial component of the echocardiographic evaluation of patients with HCM. Provocative maneuvers include maneuvers that decrease preload (i.e., Valsalva maneuver, sudden standing), decrease afterload, or increase contractility. Exercise is the most physiologic and clinically relevant provocation. Formal exercise echocardiography is used not only to identify dynamic obstruction, but also to assess functional capacity and blood pressure response to exercise (a component of sudden death risk assessment). LV outflow obstruction, either resting or provocable, may contribute to symptoms of heart failure and exercise intolerance, and obstruction has also been associated with adverse cardiovascular outcomes such as progression to severe heart failure and heart failure death.[27]

On echocardiography, one may characterize the location, mechanism, and severity of obstruction using pulse-wave (PW) and continuous-wave (CW) Doppler. The protocol is described in Fig. 23.14. It is important to distinguish Doppler signal from the LV outflow tract from the jet of MR (see Fig. 23.14 and Video 23.6), which may be mistaken for it. The Doppler envelope of LVOT obstruction typically has a profile that peaks in late systole, often described as dagger- or beak-shaped. In contrast, the MR Doppler envelope has a more bullet-shaped pattern, with a very rapid early rise to peak at the onset of systole and broader profile (see Fig. 23.14E). Whereas the peak of LVOT obstruction varies, the peak velocity of the MR signal is usually 4–5 m/s, corresponding to the LV-LA gradient in patients with preserved systolic function. At the bedside, the sonographer may find that the apical three-chamber views sometimes allows for more distinct angular separation of the posteriorly directed MR jet, from the anteriorly directed LVOT jet. In addition to quantification of the peak gradient, two dimensional and M-mode images can further characterize the mechanism of obstruction, broadly distinguishing dynamic

outflow tract obstruction related to SAM of the mitral valve from mid-cavity obstruction due to systolic cavity obliteration.

MR is regularly associated with SAM due to leaflet malcoaptation as the mitral valve moves towards and contacts the septum in midsystole (see Fig. 23.13 and Video 23.1). The dynamic cause of SAM was previously assumed to be due to the Venturi mechanism (where high velocity flow in the LVOT drags the leaflet into the LVOT), but there is evidence that in fact the midseptal bulge creates flow lines that actually *push* the underside of the protruding mitral leaflet into the septum.[28] The degree and duration of SAM-septal contact relates directly to the magnitude of the outflow gradient.[13] Owing to the anterior displacement of the mitral apparatus and distorted leaflet closure, MR caused by SAM is directed posteriorly and typically at least mild-to-moderate in degree. MR that is more centrally, or anteriorly, directed suggests intrinsic mitral valve disease (e.g., myxomatous changes with mitral valve prolapse, anomalous chordal structures, mitral annular calcification, or abnormal papillary muscles) and should prompt careful scrutiny of valvular morphology and function, potentially with transesophageal echocardiography.

TREATMENT OF HYPERTROPHIC CARDIOMYOPATHY

Medical therapy for HCM focuses on reducing LVOT obstruction and maximizing cardiac output by avoiding volume depletion, vasodilation, and tachycardia. Atrial fibrillation may not be well tolerated due to associated tachycardia and loss of atrial kick, so restoration of sinus rhythm should be attempted; if not, ventricular rates should be adequately controlled with medications.[28] Patients with LVOT obstruction with peak instantaneous Doppler outflow gradients ≥50 mm Hg and limiting symptoms despite maximal medical therapy are candidates for invasive septal reduction therapy, such as surgical myectomy or alcohol septal ablation.[29]

Septal myectomy is a surgical procedure used to treat LVOT obstruction in HCM that involves resecting the septum below the aortic valve to the point of mitral leaflet-septal contact (Fig. 23.15 and Video 23.7). When performed by an experienced operator, outflow tract obstruction is abolished or substantially reduced in the vast majority of patients,

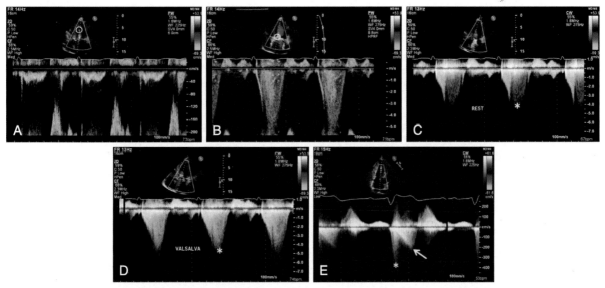

FIG. 23.14 Spectral Doppler mapping of left ventricle outflow tract gradient. Pulse (PW) and continuous-wave (CW) Doppler can be used to quantify and localize the intraventricular pressure gradient between the left ventricle (LV) cavity and outflow tract produced by systolic anterior motion (SAM) as follows: (A) Interrogation begins with PW Doppler (circled sample volume) in the mid-LV cavity on apical five-chamber view. (B) Advance the sample volume cursor to the outflow tract to identify the position of flow velocity acceleration, typically occurring at the position of maximal SAM-septal contact. At this point, flow velocities may exceed the Nyquist limit for PW Doppler, and aliasing will be seen. Switching to HPRF (high pulse repetition frequency) or CW Doppler will allow measurement of these higher velocities. (C) Continuous-wave Doppler identifies the peak instantaneous outflow gradient of 4.1 m/s *(asterisk)*, predicting a peak LVOT gradient of 66 mm Hg at rest using the modified Bernoulli equation. (D) Valsalva maneuver increases peak velocity *(asterisk)* increases to 4.9 m/s (correlating with a peak instantaneous gradient 96 mm Hg). (E) Doppler signal from the LV outflow tract versus the jet of mitral regurgitation (MR). The waveform of mitral regurgitation begins immediately at the onset of systole, during isovolumic contraction, (corresponding to the onset of the QRS complex) with a rapid increase in peak velocity (4.0 m/s; *asterisk*). The early portion of the MR envelope *(asterisk)* is seen here. In contrast, the late-systolic peaking signal from the LV outflow tract can be seen embedded within the MR signal (2.0 m/s; *arrow*). Two-dimensional and color flow Doppler imaging can typically be used to differentiate the signals from these two jets.

associated with improvement of exercise capacity and symptoms. Elimination of SAM and normalization of mitral valve coaptation also reduces MR after the procedure, often without the need for additional procedures on the mitral valve. Complications are rare but include the creation of a ventricular septal defect (VSD) due to excessive resection, coronary-cameral fistulas, complete heart block, and rarely, aortic insufficiency due to surgical manipulation of the aortic valve while gaining access to the interventricular septum. Long-term outcomes following surgical myectomy are excellent with improvements in symptoms, exercise capacity, and survival compared to nonoperated patients with obstruction.[30]

Alcohol septal ablation is the deliberate creation of a "controlled" septal myocardial infarction to force remodeling and thinning of upper septum, thereby alleviating SAM and LV outflow obstruction (Figs. 23.16 and 23.17). The procedure has been associated with effective reduction in gradients, improvement in symptoms, exercise tolerance, and oxygen consumption. The technique consists of the cannulation and isolation of a septal perforator coronary artery that supplies the region of the septum most involved in SAM and outflow tract obstruction. This is usually identified as the region of actual mitral-septal contact during SAM on echocardiogram. Then, 100% ethanol is injected to cause a controlled infarct (transmural in 75% of cases) and ultimately enlargement of the LVOT (Video 23.8). Contrast echocardiography guidance is essential

during the procedure to assist in targeting the appropriate septal perforator branch for injection and reducing the likelihood of potential complications.[31,32] Relative thinning and hypokinesis of the injected septal segment are expected in subsequent echocardiograms, and the extent may be predicted by using contrast. Contrast use also appears to confer a higher rate of procedural success and lower rate of complications such as complete heart block. The major advantage of alcohol septal ablation is its noninvasive nature. Although results can be immediate, it may also take up to 3 months to see optimal reduction of outflow tract gradient and MR, presumably due to a slower remodeling process. Disadvantages or risks include those similar to surgical myectomy such as complete heart block (in 8–10% of cases), left anterior descending (LAD) coronary artery dissection or fistula, pericardial effusion, inadvertently large infarction from leak of ethanol to another coronary vessel, and ventricular tachyarrhythmias. Due to the risk of creating a VSD, patients with basal septal wall thickness ≤15 mm are not candidates for alcoholic septal ablation.

In some cases—<2% of patients after surgical resection but up to 10% after alcohol ablation—there is insufficient reduction of LVOT gradients or recurrent symptomatic LVOT obstruction, and the septal reduction by either technique may be repeated. For ethanol ablation, insufficient LVOT gradient reduction is associated more with nontransmural (as opposed to transmural) infarcts. Surgical myectomy

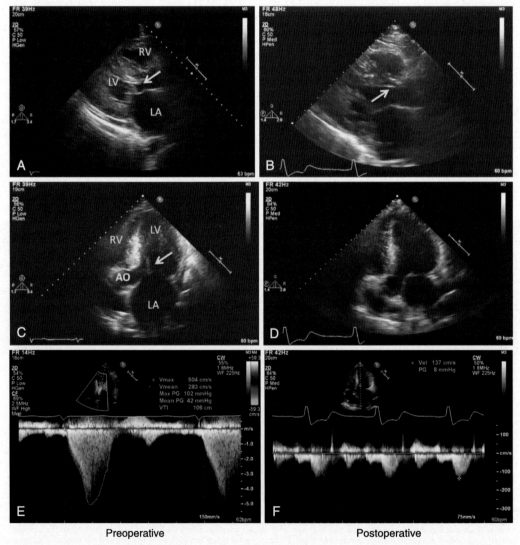

Preoperative   Postoperative

FIG. 23.15 Images before and after surgical septal myectomy. (A) *Preoperative*: Parasternal long-axis view shows marked hypertrophy of the septum and systolic anterior motion of the mitral valve (systolic anterior motion [SAM]; *arrow*). (B) *Postoperative*: Parasternal long-axis view shows a myectomy "notch" *(arrow)* representative of the portion of the upper septum that was resected, resulting in an increase of the cross sectional area of the left ventricle outflow tract, ultimately, eliminating SAM and left ventricular outflow tract (LVOT) obstruction. See also Video 23.7. (C) *Preoperative*: Apical five-chamber view showing hypertrophy of the ventricular septum and SAM *(arrow)*. (D) *Postoperative*: Apical five-chamber view showing resection of the basal ventricular septum and resolution of SAM. (E) *Preoperative*: Apical five-chamber view with continuous-wave Doppler showing a peak LVOT velocity of 5.0 m/s. (F) *Postoperative*: Apical five-chamber view with continuous wave Doppler showing a reduction in peak LVOT velocity to 1.4 m/s post resection. *AO*, Aorta; *LA*, left atrium; *LV*, left ventricle; *RV*, right ventricle; *VS*, ventricular septum.

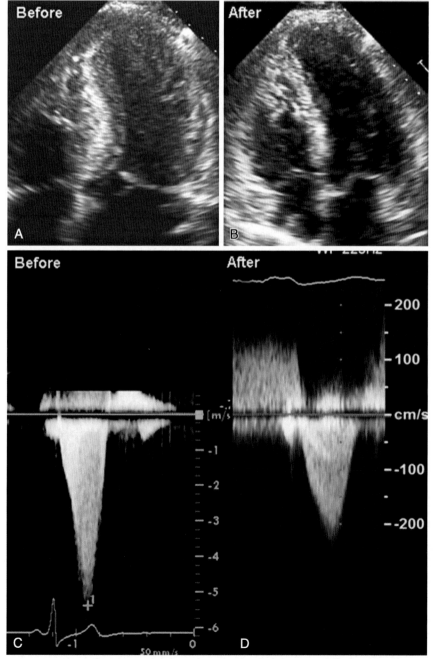

FIG. 23.16 Alcohol septal ablation. (A) Baseline apical four-chamber view identifies the area of maximal SAM-septal contact to target for ablation *(arrow)*. (B) Intracoronary injection of echocardiographic contrast is used to verify that the identified septal perforator branch supplies the target area of the ventricular septum, at the site of maximal systolic anterior motion (SAM)-septal contact. The region supplied by the injected septal branch is highlighted by the contrast agent manifest as an echogenic signal created by the accumulation of contrast within the myocardium *(arrow)*. Contrast defines the site of potential ablation and determines if infarction size will be too large or involve unintended structures such as the right ventricle. (C) After defining the site of potential ablation, alcohol is injected into the selected septal perforator branch, targeting the region of the septum that is highlighted by intracoronary contrast and seen as an intensely echobright signal from the alcohol collection within the myocardium *(arrow)*. *VS,* Ventricular septum. See also Video 23.8.

FIG. 23.17 Hemodynamic effects of successful alcohol septal ablation. (A and C) *Before Ablation*: Mid-systolic apical four-chamber view demonstrates severe systolic anterior motion (SAM) with prolonged septal contact (A) and a resting gradient of 100 mm Hg (C). (B and D) *Post-Ablation*: Two months following septal ablation, the proximal septum is notably thinner with resolution of SAM (B) and a resting gradient of 20 mm Hg (D).

TABLE 23.3 Clinical Features Suggestive of Pathological Left Ventricular Hypertrophy/Hypertrophic Cardiomyopathy in Athletes With Left Ventricular Wall Thickness Between 13 and 16 mm

Symptoms	Unexplained syncope—particularly exertional
	Palpitations
	Shortness of breath disproportionate to the performed exercise
	Dizziness
	Chest pain
Family history	HCM in a first-degree relative
Demographics	Age <16 years old
	Female sex
	Participation in purely isometric sport
	Small body surface area
Echocardiography	Left ventricular wall thickness ≥ 16 mm
	Apical, asymmetric septal or mixed pattern hypertrophy
	Left ventricular cavity diameter in end diastole ≤ 51 mm
	Presence of SAM of the mitral valve leaflet and associated LV outflow obstruction
	Septal E′ ≤ 11 cm/s
12-lead ECG	Pathological Q-waves
	ST segment depressions
	Deep T-wave inversions in the lateral leads
Cardiac MRI	Apical, asymmetric septal or mixed pattern hypertrophy
	Significant myocardial fibrosis with gadolinium enhancement
Detraining	Failure of regression of LV hypertrophy within a 3-month time frame of deconditioning

HCM, Hypertrophic cardiomyopathy; *LV*, left ventricular; *SAM*, systolic anterior motion.
Data from Rawlins J, Bhan A, Sharma S. Left ventricular hypertrophy in athletes. Eur J Echocardiogr. 2009;10(3):350–356; Sheikh N, Papadakis M, Schnell F, et al. Clinical profile of athletes with hypertrophic cardiomyopathy. Circ Cardiovasc Imaging. 2015;8(7):e003454.

versus alcohol septal ablation have been compared in studies out to 10 years, and survival appears similar regardless of medical, alcohol ablation, or septal myectomy treatment. Without longer-term studies or randomized trials, the advantages and risks of each procedure need to be weighed on an individual basis. Finally, the treatment of concomitant mitral valve disease and SAM is generally avoided with the presumption that reducing septal hypertrophy will resolve the issue, but in a small minority of cases mitral annuloplasty, replacement, or even more recently, percutaneous Mitraclip implantation has been investigated in patients with underlying and contributing mitral pathology.

USING ECHOCARDIOGRAPHY IN THE DIFFERENTIAL DIAGNOSIS OF HYPERTROPHIC CARDIOMYOPATHY

Athlete's Heart

Intense athletic training can result in cardiac remodeling, including increased LV wall thickness that can be difficult to distinguish from HCM. Athletic remodeling does not typically result in severe (>20 mm) LV hypertrophy,[33] and even highly trained athletes display normal or only mildly increased LV wall thickness (≤15 mm). However, approximately 2% of elite athletes have LV wall thickness 13–16 mm, falling into a morphologic "gray zone" where physiological hypertrophy and pathologic HCM overlap.[34] Differentiating the benign state of

athlete's heart from HCM is important, as HCM carries the potential for increased risk of sudden death with vigorous physical activity,[34,35] as well as important implications for family members. As summarized in Table 23.3, echocardiographic findings can aid in discriminating pathologic from physiologic hypertrophy. Findings suggestive of HCM include LVH in which asymmetry is prominent, the anterior ventricular septum is spared, or the region of predominant thickening involves the posterior septum or LV free wall; small LV cavity size < 51 mm;[36] abnormal LV diastolic function; marked LA dilatation; and no reduction in LVH with detraining.[34,35] Athletes, on the other hand, particularly in the endurance sports, are known to frequently develop left (and right) ventricular dilatation, of variable degree, along with the milder symmetric increases in wall thickness, with left ventricular ejection fraction (LVEF) typically in the low-normal range (~50%). Furthermore, diastolic function as measured by standard flow Doppler are normal or even supranormal (higher e′ velocities and transmitral $E/A > 2$) in athletes, and speckle-based local and global longitudinal strain parameters are also generally higher. Often, exercise testing to document exercise capacity and presence/lack of induced gradients, cardiac MRI, and even a period of detraining may be undertaken to discriminate the athlete's heart from HCM.

Focal Upper Septal Hypertrophy

Focal upper septal hypertrophy (also referred to as sigmoid septum, septal bulge, and discrete upper septal hypertrophy) is a common morphological subtype of HCM. It is seen often particularly in elderly, hypertensive individuals, in whom it is likely a manifestation of acquired remodeling from hypertensive heart disease and not an inherited or primary cardiomyopathy. In patients with and without HCM, age appears to increase the angulation between the long axis of the LV and the aorta, accentuating the focal bulge of the upper septum as it protrudes into the LVOT, particularly in small elderly women. Sarcomere mutations are rarely identified in isolated individuals with focal upper septal thickening. In this clinical context and in the absence of family history, this entity is highly unlikely to represent genetic HCM, and extensive family screening is typically not warranted.[37]

Infiltrative and Metabolic Cardiomyopathies

Very rare genetic conditions can also lead to myocardial infiltration or altered metabolism, resulting in increased LV wall thickness that appears grossly very similar to the left ventricular hypertrophy seen in sarcomere HCM. These are rare even among patients referred for unexplained HCM and includes mutations in non-sarcomeric proteins, such as the gene encoding the γ2 regulatory subunit of the adenosine monophosphate-activated protein kinase or AMP-activated protein kinase (PRKAG2) and that encoding lysosome-associated membrane protein 2 (LAMP-2). PRKAG2 mutations are inherited in autosomal dominant fashion and cause the accumulation of vacuoles filled with glycogen-associated products in skeletal muscle and cardiomyocytes. Unlike sarcomere HCM, myofibrillar disarray and fibrosis is not seen pathologically, and ventricular preexcitation (i.e., Wolff-Parkinson-White syndrome) and conduction system defects are highly prevalent. Another rare metabolic disease, Danon disease (also called glycogen storage disease IIB), is caused by a semidominant mutation in the protein (LAMP-2; Fig. 23.18).[38] This typically causes a hypertrophic phenotype in males, but frequently a dilated cardiomyopathy in females, and is also associated with preexcitation (in 75% of patients), skeletal muscle weakness, and mental retardation.

Cardiac amyloidosis (Fig. 23.19) and Fabry disease (Fig. 23.20) are more prevalent infiltrative cardiomyopathies due to mutations in other proteins, leading to adult-onset restrictive cardiomyopathy and concentric increases in myocardial thickness (see Chapter 24). Fabry disease is a lysosomal storage disorder due to an X-linked mutation causing deficiency of the lysosomal enzyme alpha-galactosidase A (agal-A). Cardiac amyloidosis is caused by the extracellular deposition of amyloidogenic proteins (see later and Chapter 24) and encompasses three forms: AL (primary light-chain), ATTR (transthyretin), and AA (secondary, serum amyloid A protein) amyloidosis.

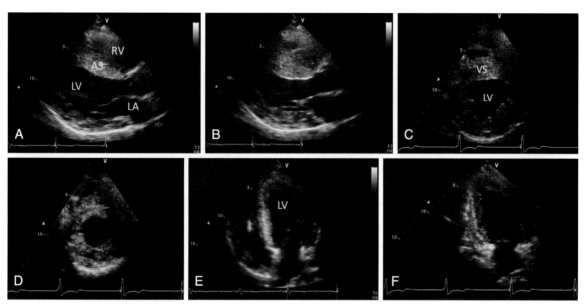

FIG. 23.18 Danon disease. Parasternal images from a 21-year-old patient with a LAMP2 mutation causing Danon disease, a lysosomal storage disease that clinically mimics hypertrophic cardiomyopathy (HCM). Note the severe, diffuse thickening of the left ventricle (LV) walls with a maximal LV septal wall thickness of 21 mm. (A) Parasternal long-axis view (in diastole). (B) Parasternal long-axis view (in systole). (C) Short-axis view: At the papillary muscle level, all segments of the LV wall are hypertrophied. (D) Parasternal short-axis view at the apical level. (E), Apical four-chamber view. (F) Apical two-chamber view. *AS,* Anteroseptal wall; *LA,* left atrium; *RV,* right ventricle; *VS,* ventricular septum.

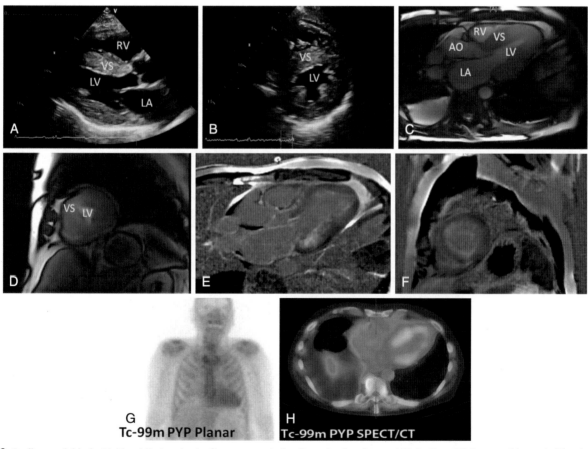

FIG. 23.19 Cardiac amyloidosis. Multimodality imaging is often necessary in the diagnosis of cardiac amyloidosis. (A and B) Parasternal long-axis (A) and short-axis (B) echocardiographic images showing echobright, marked, diffuse left ventricular hypertrophy, with a maximal wall thickness of 18 mm. (C and D) Cardiac magnetic resonance imaging (MRI) five-chamber (C) and short-axis (D) views demonstrating diffuse left ventricle (LV) hypertrophy. (E and F), Cardiac MRI demonstrating transmural late gadolinium enhancement and abnormal blood-pool gadolinium kinetics, consistent with cardiac amyloidosis. (G and H) ^{99m}Technetium-pyrophoshate (^{99m}Tc-PYP) with planar whole body imaged *(top)* and single-photon positive emission computed tomography (SPECT/CT, *bottom,* transaxial chest CT image in *gray scale,* and ^{99m}Tc-PYP image in *color*) demonstrates diffuse myocardial retention of ^{99m}Tc-PYP, consistent with transthyretin-related cardiac amyloidosis. *AO,* Aorta; *AS,* anteroseptal wall; *LA,* left atrium; *LV,* left ventricle; *RV,* right ventricle; *VS,* ventricular septum. *(G and H Courtesy of Sharmila Dorbala MD, MPH, Brigham and Women's Hospital, Boston, MA.)*

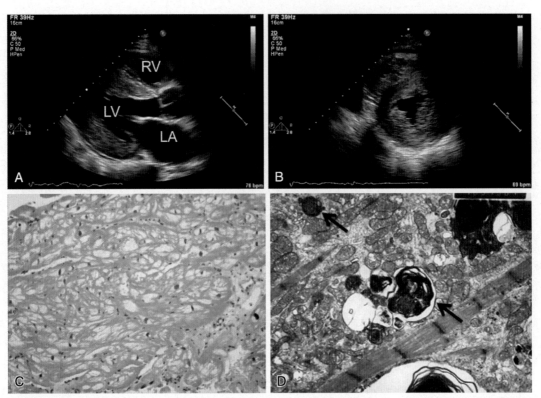

FIG. 23.20 Fabry disease. (A and B) Parasternal views showing concentric left ventricular hypertrophy and an echobright appearance to the myocardium in a male patient with Fabry disease. (C) Hematoxylin and eosin staining demonstrating typical vacuolated cardiomyocytes (100× magnification). (D) Electron micrograph demonstrating characteristic lamellar bodies (arrows) within a cardiomyocyte. *AS,* Anteroseptal wall; *LA,* left atrium; *LV,* left ventricle; *RV,* right ventricle; *VS,* ventricular septum. (*C and D Courtesy of Robert F. Padera MD, PhD, Brigham and Women's Hospital, Boston, MA.*)

HCM and infiltrative cardiomyopathies may be difficult to distinguish by echocardiography alone. Particularly striking concentric hypertrophy, biatrial enlargement, and an echo-bright "scintillating" appearance to the myocardium are clues that an infiltrative process rather than typical HCM may be present. Prominent findings in male patients/family members and lack of father to son transmission are clues that an X-linked condition such as Danon or Fabry disease is present. Young age and conduction abnormalities (progressive atrioventricular block, atrial fibrillation, ventricular preexcitation) are important clinical clues in diagnosing disorders secondary to *PRKAG2 or LAMP2* mutations (see Fig. 23.18), whereas older/elderly onset disease is suggestive of cardiac amyloidosis. Of the types of cardiac amyloidosis, transthyretin amyloidosis (mutated or wild-type) is stereotypically seen in elderly men, and AL amyloidosis is associated with plasma cell dyscrasias such as multiple myeloma (see Fig. 23.19).

Multimodality imaging, including cardiac MRI and nuclear scans, can play a key role in establishing the correct diagnosis, differentiating sarcomeric HCM from some of its phenocopies. (99m)Technetium-pyrophosphate scintigraphy (^{99m}Tc-PYP) can help to establish the correct diagnosis of either mutant or wild-type transthyretin-related amyloidosis,[39,40] aiding the clinician in ruling in amyloidosis and ruling out HCM (see Fig. 23.19G and H). However, pyrophosphate scans cannot be used to assist in the diagnosis of AL amyloidosis.

Myocardial biopsy and enzyme activity testing may be required to provide the ultimate diagnosis when infiltrative cardiomyopathies are suspected, as demonstrated in Fig. 23.20, where histology aided in the definitive diagnosis of Fabry disease. Establishing the correct diagnosis has critical implications for the management of both the patient and their family. For example, enzyme replacement therapy is available for Fabry disease while chemotherapy may be appropriate for managing AL amyloidosis. Disease-modifying therapies are under development for cardiac amyloidosis caused by mutant or wild-type transthyretin, as well as other

forms of genetic heart disease. As such, precision and accuracy in diagnosis willplay an increasingly important role in clinical management in the future. In addition, if a nongenetic etiology can be confirmed, the patient's family is not at risk and can be relieved from the burden of serial clinical evaluation and the potential for disease development.

CONCLUSION

Echocardiographic imaging has played a central role in furthering our understanding of the pathophysiology, epidemiology, and prognosis of HCM. This imaging modality is well suited to evaluate disease progression and to provide pertinent information—with regard to morphology, hemodynamic changes, and dynamic assessment of cardiac structure and function—to guide clinicians in the management of HCM. When assessing individuals with unexplained cardiac hypertrophy, echocardiography must be considered in the context of individual demographics, clinical and familial history, electrocardiogram, laboratory findings, and, at times, in conjunction with complementary imaging modalities, such as cardiac MRI and nuclear imaging, to reach a final diagnosis.

Suggested Reading

Afonso, L. C., Bernal, J., Bax, J. J., & Abraham, T. P. (2008). Echocardiography in hypertrophic cardiomyopathy: the role of conventional and emerging technologies. *JACC Cardiovascular Imaging, 1,* 787–800.

Nagueh, S. F., Bierig, S. M., Budoff, M. J., et al. (2011). American Society of Echocardiography clinical recommendations for multimodality cardiovascular imaging of patients with hypertrophic cardiomyopathy: endorsed by the American Society of Nuclear Cardiology, Society for Cardiovascular Magnetic Resonance, and Society of Cardiovascular Computed Tomography. *Journal of the American Society of Echocardiography, 24,* 473–498.

Silbiger, J. J. (2016). Abnormalities of the mitral apparatus in hypertrophic cardiomyopathy: echocardiographic, pathophysiologic, and surgical insights. *Journal of the American Society of Echocardiography, 29,* 622–639.

Wasfy, M. M., & Weiner, R. B. (2015). Differentiating the athlete's heart from hypertrophic cardiomyopathy. *Current Opinion in Cardiology, 30,* 500.

A complete reference list can be found online at ExpertConsult.com.

Restrictive and Infiltrative Cardiomyopathies

Vikram Agarwal, Rodney H. Falk

INTRODUCTION

Restrictive cardiomyopathy (RCM) refers to either an idiopathic or a systemic myocardial disorder in the absence of underlying atherosclerotic coronary artery disease, valvular disease, congenital heart disease, or systemic hypertension, which is characterized by abnormal left ventricular filling, and is associated with normal or reduced left ventricle (LV) and right ventricle (RV) volumes and function.[1] The term is not precise, but it incorporates infiltrative and fibrotic cardiac pathology, which are dealt with in this chapter. While the majority of patients with infiltrative and fibrotic cardiomyopathies develop a restrictive filling pattern, especially in the later stages of the disease, it is important to differentiate the pathology from a restrictive filling *pattern,* which can be associated with other types of heart disease, such as dilated cardiomyopathy. In patients with dilated cardiomyopathy the restrictive filling pattern is often a reversible phenomenon, related to worsening heart failure, and morphologically the ventricle is dilated, usually with severe reduction in ejection fraction. Although the clinical presentation of RCM may be similar to dilated cardiomyopathy, the nondilated, stiff ventricles often result in highly sodium-sensitive heart failure symptoms, associated in the late stage of the disease with a low cardiac output due to the small stroke volume. Because of the restriction to diastolic filling and an associated impaired ability to augment cardiac output at higher heart rates, these patients may also present with symptoms of exercise intolerance.

Diastolic dysfunction in the presence of preserved left ventricular ejection fraction (LVEF) is the key component of pathophysiology of RCM. Initial stages of RCM demonstrate preserved LVEF with noncompliant walls that impair the normal diastolic filling of the ventricle. This restriction can be isolated to either ventricle, or show biventricular involvement. Biventricular volumes are either normal or reduced. Over a period of time, the chronically elevated LV diastolic pressure leads to increased atrial size, which may be considerable. Although severe biatrial enlargement without valve disease is a classic finding of RCM, this is a nonspecific feature, as it may occur in other conditions, particularly if associated with long-standing atrial fibrillation. In later stages of the disease, as the compliance of the LV decreases, a small change in LV volume is associated with a steep rise in LV pressure. A reduced ejection fraction may occur in the very late stages of the disease. It is important to recognize that, although the left ventricle may show diastolic dysfunction with a normal ejection fraction, longitudinal systolic function may be significantly impaired, and thus a normal ejection fraction should not be considered synonymous with normal systolic function (Videos 24.1 and 24.2).

SPECTRUM OF RESTRICTIVE CARDIOMYOPATHY

RCM can be considered as either "primary" RCM or RCM secondary to other conditions such as infiltrative disorders and storage disorders. **Infiltrative disorders** primarily affect the interstitial space of the myocardium, whereas **storage diseases** are associated with deposits within the cardiac myocytes. In addition, endomyocardial involvement, leading to restriction, may occur in a variety of uncommon conditions (Box 24.1).

Diagnosis of Restrictive Cardiomyopathy

Due to the varied pathophysiology and clinical manifestations of the underlying systemic process, a systematic approach, beginning with a comprehensive history and detailed systemic evaluation, can help guide further management. Among patients with suspected idiopathic and familial RCM, a comprehensive family history should be obtained, as the condition is increasingly being recognized as familial. Clinical screening of first-degree relatives should be considered, and abnormalities, if present, may include hypertrophic and dilated cardiomyopathy. Comprehensive genetic screening should also be considered, particularly if family members with suspicious cardiac abnormalities are identified.

ECHOCARDIOGRAPHY IN RESTRICTIVE CARDIOMYOPATHY

Cardiac imaging plays a pivotal role in establishing the diagnosis of RCM. Despite the availability of multiple cardiac imaging options, including cardiac magnetic resonance (CMR) imaging and nuclear cardiology, echocardiography remains the initial imaging method of choice among patients with suspicion of RCM. Echocardiography not only assesses the anatomy and function of the cardiac chambers, but it can also provide vital clues to the diagnosis of the underlying etiology. The first step in cardiac assessment when interpreting an echocardiogram in suspected restrictive heart disease involves a thorough evaluation of the overall and regional anatomy of the left ventricle with regard to underlying wall thickness, altered myocardial texture, and wall motion abnormality. LV mass assessed by using three-dimensional (3D) echocardiogram is more reproducible, and mirrors the mass obtained by cardiac MR more closely. Similarly, while the quantitative assessment of overall left ventricular volumes and systolic function assessment are usually performed using the biplane method of disks (modified Simpson's rule), the use of 3D-based volumes and ejection fraction, when feasible and available, is encouraged since it does not rely on underlying geometric assumptions leading to superior accuracy and reproducibility. Nevertheless, two-dimensional (2D) echocardiography can give extremely useful diagnostic information, and the use of contrast for better delineation of the endocardium when two or more contiguous LV endocardial segments are poorly visualized in apical views improves accuracy and reduces inter-reader variability of LV functional analyses. In "primary" RCM, ventricular wall thickness is usually normal, whereas the myocardium in patients with cardiac amyloidosis is usually thickened, and may show increased echogenicity. It is also important to evaluate the right ventricular wall thickness and function, as involvement of right ventricle may have prognostic significance in a number of diseases.

Doppler Features

Diastolic functional assessment of myocardium plays an important role in the diagnosis of RCM. In the early stages of restrictive heart diseases, the myocardial relaxation (e′) is reduced, resulting in septal e′ less than 7 cm/s and lateral e′ less than 10 cm/s (Fig. 21.1A and B). In early stages of the disease, the mitral inflow pulse-wave Doppler shows an abnormal relaxation pattern, is characterized by an E/A ratio of ≤0.8, an increased mitral inflow E-wave deceleration time (≥240 ms), and an increased isovolumic relaxation time (>90 ms). At this stage of the disease, the left atrium is usually normal or mildly dilated in size, and the patient is rarely symptomatic. As this pattern is common in older patients in the general population, it is nondiagnostic even in a gene-positive patient. With progression of disease, the mitral inflow pulse wave Doppler pattern shows pseudonormal filling pattern, where the E/A ratio is 0.8–2, and this ratio reverses with Valsalva maneuver. Due to the elevated left ventricular filling pressures, there is an increase of the E/e′ ratio (≥10) and the left atrial volume index is elevated, ≥34 mL/m². There is also a reversal in the pulmonary vein Doppler velocity pattern, with gradual blunting of the systolic wave and dominance of the diastolic wave (S/D <1, while normal S/D is >1; see Fig. 24.1C and D). With further deterioration of

ventricular compliance, advanced diastolic dysfunction develops, characterized by a restrictive filling pattern, namely an E/A ratio greater than 2, and a short (<160 ms) transmitral E wave deceleration time due to rapid equalization of atrioventricular pressures (<160 ms). As the left ventricular compliance decreases further, the diastolic filling pattern becomes irreversible, which can be demonstrated by the lack of reversibility of E/A ratio with Valsalva maneuver.

A major limitation of using these traditional Doppler echocardiographic features is their lack of specificity. In addition, there are significant limitations to acquisition and interpretation of these measurements in patients with underlying atrial fibrillation and in patients with significant mitral valvular disease (including ≥ moderate mitral regurgitation and stenosis, or mitral valve repair or mitral valve replacement).

Speckle Tracking

Speckle tracking tissue Doppler echocardiography can assess cardiac mechanics, including global and regional myocardial deformation, which can differentiate active wall thickening from passive motion. It allows detection and quantification of subclinical LV and RV systolic dysfunction, even when the global and segmental LV ejection fraction appears preserved. An important strength of this technique is that myocardial deformation or strain can be assessed in different spatial directions, including radial, circumferential, longitudinal, and transverse directions, as the technique is angle-independent. Reduction in echocardiographic measures of myocardial deformation parameters may be a sign of early myocardial dysfunction, and these measures have now been well validated for several clinical conditions, including cardiac amyloidosis (see Video 24.1) and postchemotherapy. Speckle tracking has also been shown to provide greater accuracy than LV ejection fraction in predicting adverse cardiac events in patients with heart failure.

Speckle tracking also possesses the ability to identify different patterns of changes in cardiac mechanics produced by various diseases, and can thus help to facilitate the diagnosis. For example, apical sparing is a pattern of

---

BOX 24.1 Cardiac Diseases Associated With Restrictive Pathophysiology

Primary RCM
- Idiopathic and familial RCM
- Mitochondrial cardiomyopathy

Infiltrative Diseases
- Amyloidosis
- Mucopolysaccharoidoses (Hurler syndrome, Gaucher disease)

Storage Diseases
- Anderson-Fabry disease
- Glycogen storage disorders
- Hemochromatosis (may present with restrictive or, more commonly, dilated phenotype)

Endomyocardial Involvement
- Endomyocardial fibrosis and Löffler endocarditis
- Carcinoid syndrome
- Postradiation
- Postchemotherapy
- Lymphoma
- Scleroderma
- Churg-Strauss syndrome
- Pseudoxanthoma elasticum

RCM, Restrictive cardiomyopathy.

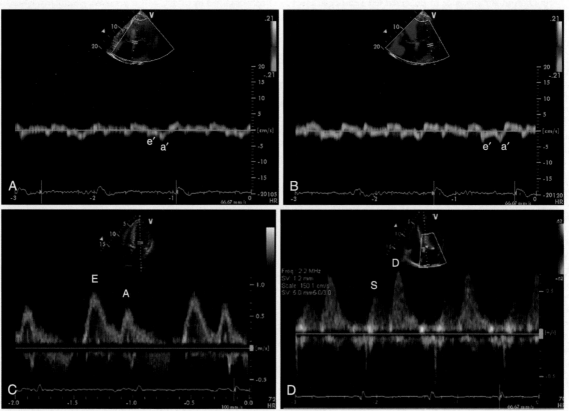

FIG. 24.1 Reduced tissue Doppler in a patient with underlying cardiac amyloidosis demonstrating reduced septal (A) and lateral (B) e′ velocities. The patient also demonstrated pseudonormal mitral inflow pattern (C), but the pulmonary vein Doppler pattern demonstrates reduced diastolic predominance with systolic blunting, consistent with increased left atrial pressure (D). *A*, Atrial component of transmitral Doppler flow; *a′*, atrial component of myocardial lengthening; *D*, pulmonary vein diastolic flow; *E*, early transmitral Doppler flow; *e′*, early myocardial relaxation velocity; *S*, pulmonary vein systolic flow.

regional differences in deformation seen in cardiac amyloidosis, where the longitudinal strain in the basal and middle segments of the left ventricle is more severely impaired compared with strain values in apical segments. This can help distinguish cardiac amyloidosis from other conditions that cause true left-ventricular hypertrophy, such as hypertensive heart disease and Fabry disease.

CARDIAC AMYLOIDOSIS

Cardiac amyloidosis is an infiltrative cardiomyopathy, which in some forms has a toxic component. It is the most commonly encountered cause of restrictive cardiac disease. The term "amyloid" refers to proteinaceous material derived from misfolded products of a variety of precursor proteins. This abnormal protein is deposited in the extracellular space of all chambers of the heart, including the coronary vasculature, and alters the tissue structure and function. Cardiac dysfunction in the form of diastolic and systolic dysfunction, conduction system disturbances, and ischemia are a result of not only direct tissue infiltration, but also due to the toxic effect of the circulating precursor proteins, especially the immunoglobulin light chain amyloidosis (AL). Several different forms of amyloidosis are recognized, with the type of amyloidosis being defined by the precursor protein. The four most common precursor proteins associated with cardiac amyloidosis are abnormal light chains produced by a plasma cell dyscrasia (AL amyloidosis), amyloid derived from wild-type transthyretin (ATTRwt) or mutant TTR (familial ATTR amyloidosis, ATTRm), and localized atrial amyloid deposits derived from atrial natriuretic peptide. In secondary amyloidosis the deposits are derived from the inflammatory protein serum

amyloid A, but the heart is rarely involved. Of these different types of cardiac amyloidosis, the AL and transthyretin (TTR) form of amyloidosis are the most common forms to involve the heart.

Cardiac amyloidosis should be suspected in a patient with a thick left ventricular wall with nondilated ventricle, normal or near-normal ejection fraction, and a normal LV cavity size in the absence of a history of poorly controlled hypertension (Fig. 24.2). In AL amyloidosis low QRS voltage pattern and pseudoinfarction pattern may be present on the electrocardiogram (ECG), but voltage is often normal in TTR amyloidosis.[2] Especially in ATTR, wall thickness may approach or exceed 20 mm—this is very rarely seen in hypertensive heart disease. Once the diagnosis of cardiac amyloidosis is entertained, advanced echocardiographic techniques, including speckle strain imaging, can be used, as can several other imaging modalities. However, since the therapy and prognosis of cardiac amyloidosis differs among the different types, the diagnosis has to be eventually confirmed histologically, which often requires endomyocardial biopsy and special staining.

On 2D echocardiography, other features of infiltrative cardiomyopathy can be appreciated: symmetric increased LV and RV wall thickness, sometimes with increased echogenicity; speckled or granular sparkling appearance; normal or small ventricular cavity size; and diffuse valvular and interatrial septum thickening, with biatrial enlargement (see Fig. 24.2 and Video 24.3). A small pericardial effusion is often present, but hemodynamically significant effusion is rare. It is important to recognize that the increased ventricular wall thickness in patients with cardiac amyloidosis is due to infiltration with amyloid, and not true hypertrophy as in patients with systemic hypertension or aortic stenosis. Hence the use of "left ventricular hypertrophy" to describe the

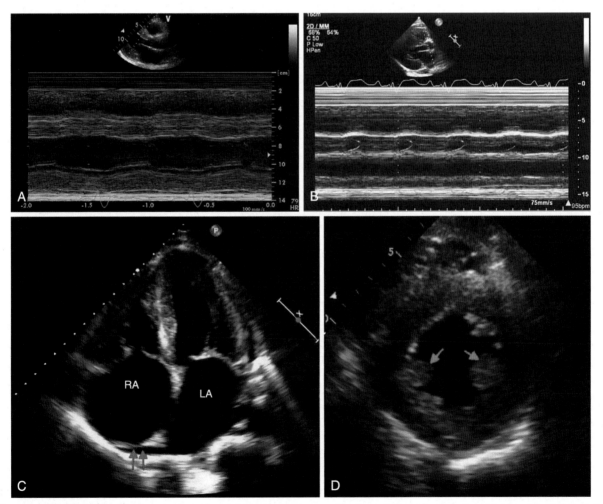

FIG. 24.2 M mode through the left ventricle in a patient with underlying transthyretin type of cardiac amyloidosis, demonstrating thickening of the right end left ventricular walls (A). (B) M mode through the aortic valve which demonstrates reduced duration of opening of the leaflets of aortic valve, with gradual aortic valve closure demonstrating reduced cardiac output. (C) Four-chamber apical view with dilated left atrium (LA) and right atrium (RA), with a small pericardial effusion (red arrows). (D) Characteristic thickening of the papillary muscle demonstrating infiltration of the papillary muscle (green arrows).

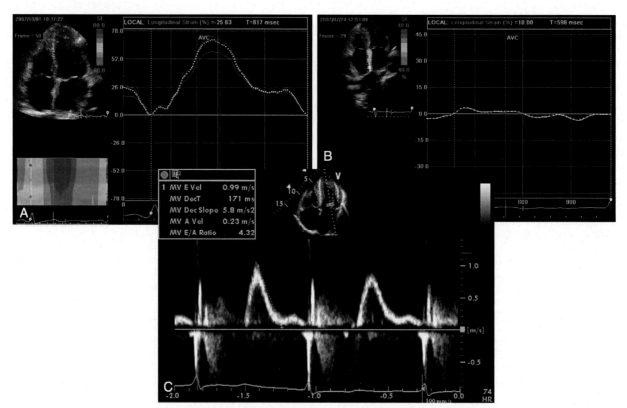

FIG. 24.3 **Atrial failure in cardiac amyloidosis, demonstrated by speckle tracking.** (A) Shows the normal strain pattern of the atrial septum—note the greater than 60% increase in length during atrial filling representing the reservoir function, the shortening after the mitral valve opens shortly after aortic valve closure (AVC), and the further shortening to baseline associated with atrial contraction after a short period of diastasis (contractile function). In contrast, (B) shows atrial septal strain in a patient with cardiac amyloidosis. There is virtually no reservoir function (due to the very stiff atrium) or contractile function despite the patient being in sinus rhythm. The atrium simply acts as a conduit. (C) Shows the corresponding transmitral Doppler with very small A wave and normal mitral deceleration time.

increased left ventricular wall thickness is inappropriate. Although the left ventricle almost never dilates in cardiac amyloidosis, the right ventricle may demonstrate dilation late in the disease, most likely due to an underlying combination of increased afterload from pulmonary hypertension and intrinsic right ventricular systolic dysfunction due to infiltration. Atrial function may be severely impaired, due to the infiltration of atrial wall with amyloid protein (Fig. 24.3), and thromboembolism may occur even in the presence of underlying sinus rhythm (Fig. 24.4). LV[3] and RV tissue Doppler imaging,[4] and strain imaging of the right and left ventricles (longitudinal 2D strain) are very sensitive for the early identification of cardiac amyloidosis, even with a near-normal LV ejection fraction.[3] Cardiac amyloidosis demonstrates a specific pattern of longitudinal strain characterized by worse longitudinal strain in the mid and basal ventricle with relative sparing of the apex. This pattern can help distinguish cardiac amyloid from true ventricular hypertrophy of hypertensive heart disease and hypertrophic cardiomyopathy.[5] When the strain pattern is color coded, a typical "bulls eye" appearance pattern is noted (see Video 24.1).

Multiple echocardiographic parameters have been associated with worse prognosis in patients with underlying cardiac amyloidosis. Increased LV wall thickness is inversely related to long-term survival and is strongly correlated with the severity of chronic heart failure.[6] RV involvement, including increased RV thickness (≥7 mm),[7] dilation,[8] systolic dysfunction, and reduced RV longitudinal strain, are associated with advanced disease and portend a worse prognosis. On Doppler echocardiography, a deceleration time ≤150 ms has been shown to be a predictor of cardiac death (Table 24.1).[7]

Cardiac MRI is a powerful diagnostic tool in cardiac amyloidosis. Cardiac amyloidosis is associated with short subendocardial T1 times and a distinctive pattern of diffuse subendocardial and mid-myocardial delayed gadolinium late enhancement, which also involves the atrium in many cases (Fig. 24.5).[9] This diffuse subendocardial pattern is more common than patchy focal delayed enhancement patterns, which gradually progresses to transmural involvement as the disease progresses. T1

mapping is useful to assess extracellular volume, which is often present prior to the development of left ventricular wall thickening and late gadolinium enhancement. However, a considerable number of patients with cardiac amyloidosis have a contraindication to MRI because of either an implanted pacemaker or a contraindication to gadolinium because of a reduced glomerular filtration rate associated with renal amyloid or with low cardiac output.

Radionuclide imaging of ATTR cardiac amyloidosis with bone imaging agents (Tc-99m pyrophosphate or Tc-99m 3,3-diphosphono-1,2-propanodicarboxylic acid [DPD]) is a valuable sensitive and specific technique. The reason for the avid cardiac uptake is not fully understood but if equal to, or greater than, rib uptake is sensitive for both ATTRwt and ATTRm cardiac amyloidosis.[10]

MITOCHONDRIAL CARDIOMYOPATHY

Mitochondrial disease is a maternally inherited condition with multiple phenotypes. Cardiomyopathy may be a prominent feature, and is often characterized by an appearance similar to an infiltrative cardiomyopathy such as amyloidosis. Mitochondrial encephalomyopathy, lactic acidosis, and stroke-like episodes (MELAS) are some of the more common syndromes, and are associated with a mitochondrial DNA mutation A3243G. The same mutation is responsible for maternally inherited diabetes, deafness, and cardiomyopathy. An example of this condition is seen in Videos 24.4 and 24.5.

ENDOMYOCARDIAL FIBROSIS AND LÖFFLER (EOSINOPHILIC) ENDOCARDITIS

Endomyocardial fibrosis (EMF) is probably the most common cause of RCM, and it is estimated to affect more than 10 million people worldwide. It is endemic in tropical and subtropical Africa, Asia, and South America, and is an important cause of heart failure. The rate of occurrence of EMF peaks twice; the first peak occurs during the second

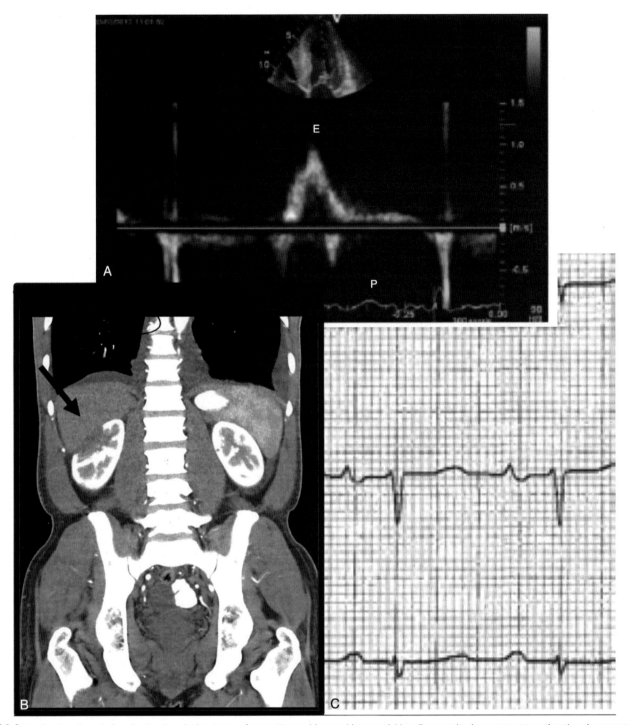

FIG. 24.4 Cardiac thromboembolism despite sinus rhythm: images from a 48-year-old man with an amyloid cardiomyopathy due to mutant transthyretin, who presented with flank pain. (A) Shows transmitral Doppler with an absent A wave despite sinus rhythm (C). (B) Shows embolic infarction of right kidney *(arrow)*. *E,* Transmitral E wave; *P,* P wave of ECG.

decade, and the second during the fourth decade of life. While the exact underlying etiology and pathological mechanism of the disease remains unknown, several conditions share the main morphological characteristic of fibrosis of the endocardial layer, predominantly in the apical region. Although no unifying hypothesis for this pathology has emerged, the inciting factor, for example, parasitic infections, autoimmune disorders, and hematologic malignancies, precipitate an initial necrotic phase similar to Löffler endocarditis, which clinically manifests with fever, facial and periorbital swelling, urticaria, eosinophilia, and pancarditis. After the development of this initial acute phase, the disease alternates between active episodes and stable periods. As the disease progresses, there is an intermediate thrombotic stage which is associated with the formation of thrombi in the left and right ventricle. Finally,

months to years later there is the development of endocardial fibrosis. This fibrotic process predominantly involves the left and right ventricular apices, and the inflow tract of both the ventricles. This leads to a significant reduction in the size of the ventricular cavities. Gradually this extends to the chordae, and the atrioventricular valves, which leads to tethering of the valve leaflets, causing mitral and tricuspid regurgitation. In some cases, there can be associated endocardial calcification and pericardial effusion. The extensive fibrosis not only causes diastolic dysfunction with restrictive filling pattern, but there is also reduction in the size of the ventricular cavities, resulting in marked reduction of ventricular stroke volumes.

The typical echocardiographic findings of EMF include endomyocardial plaques with apical obliteration of ventricular cavity with

TABLE 24.1 Echocardiographic Features of Cardiac Amyloidosis

PARAMETERS	COMMENTS
Increased myocardial echogenicity	• When present it provides a clue to the diagnosis of cardiac amyloidosis, but is neither sensitive nor specific, and not quantitative
Increased LV and RV wall thickness	• Due to amyloid infiltration of the interstitial space • Related to the burden of amyloid disease • Global distribution, can help differentiate from hypertrophic cardiomyopathy
Decreased LV end-diastolic volumes	• Reduced stroke volume despite near normal LVEF
Typically preserved or mildly reduced LVEF	• LVEF may decrease in end-stage disease
Doppler and tissue Doppler abnormalities	• Initial stages with impaired LV relaxation and increased deceleration times • Advanced stages of disease with restrictive filling pattern and reduced deceleration times • High E/e′ suggests increased left atrial pressures • Reduced amplitude A wave may be due to poor atrial function with higher risk of thrombus formation
Increased left and right atrial volumes	• A common feature • Atrial strain can be significantly reduced
LS in the left ventricle is impaired and worse at the base and mid-ventricular regions when compared with the apex	• Specific patterns of LV LS may differentiate amyloid from aortic stenosis and hypertrophic cardiomyopathy • LS is sensitive and precedes LV systolic dysfunction, and may be impaired even with normal LV wall thickness
Reduced RV myocardial velocities on tissue Doppler imaging, reduced tricuspid annular plane excursion, and reduced RV LS	• Impaired TAPSE and RV LS are early, but nonspecific, indicators of cardiac involvement in patients with systemic AL amyloidosis • RV LS may be an independent predictor of cardiac death
Valve thickening	• Nonspecific
Pericardial effusion	• Common but nonspecific
Interatrial septal thickening	• Characteristic feature of cardiac amyloidosis, but present in <50%.
Papillary muscle	• Thickened and prominent papillary muscles
Dynamic LV outflow tract obstruction	• Rare • LV LS pattern and CMR to distinguish from hypertrophic cardiomyopathy

AL, Amyloid light-chain; *CMR,* cardiac magnetic resonance; *LS,* longitudinal strain; *LV,* left ventricular; *LVEF,* LV ejection fraction; *RV,* right ventricular; *TAPSE,* tricuspid annular plane excursion.

a cleavage plane between the area of fibrosis and the myocardium, severe atrial dilation, normal sized or mild ventricular dilation, and thickening of the inferolateral or anteroseptal walls of the left ventricle with predominantly left sided and right sided involvement, respectively. Depending upon the underlying stage of the disease process, ventricular thrombi, tricuspid regurgitation, tethering of the posterior mitral valve leaflet, and associated mitral regurgitation may also be seen. The aortic and pulmonary valves are usually spared. In patients with suspicion of EMF, it is important to distinguish the echocardiographic features from other conditions that may mimic this condition, including apical dyskinesis with apical thrombus, left ventricular noncompaction, and apical hypertrophic cardiomyopathy.

Eosinophilic endocardial disease (Löffler syndrome) is an RCM found in some patients with underlying hypereosinophilic syndrome, in which there is an elevated eosinophil count of greater than 1500/mL for at least 1 month. This directly causes organ damage or dysfunction. The causes of elevated eosinophils can be due to (1) primary (neoplastic) cause, such as stem cell, myeloid or eosinophilic neoplasm, (2) secondary (reactive) cause due to over-production of eosinophilopietic cytokines from causes such as parasitic infection and T cell lymphoma, and (3) idiopathic cause. The underlying pathophysiology is due to the degranulation of the elevated eosinophil count, which causes endocardial damage followed by fibrosis. The underlying chain of events which leads to cardiac damage is similar to EMF as discussed previously and the echocardiographic appearance is similar. As with EMF, there is an initial acute inflammatory stage, followed by an intermediate thrombotic stage, and finally the fibrotic stage. Both the right and left ventricles can be affected (Fig. 24.6, Videos 24.6 and 24.7).

IDIOPATHIC RESTRICTIVE CARDIOMYOPATHY

Idiopathic RCM is a rare and poorly characterized entity, which has been described in individuals from infancy to late adulthood, and usually carries a poor prognosis, especially in children. Genetic studies have demonstrated that RCM is not a single entity, but is instead a heterogeneous group of disorders, in which the disease-causing mutation can be identified in ≥60% of cases.[11] The genetic mutations can present with a spectrum of cardiac phenotypes, including HCM, dilated cardiomyopathy, or left ventricular noncompaction. Echocardiographic screening of first-degree relatives is recommended in all cases of RCM. Mutations in sarcomere protein genes (cardiac troponin I, Troponin T, alpha cardiac actin, and beta-myosin heavy chain) are an important cause of apparently idiopathic RCM. Although the underlying pathophysiology is still not clear, increased myofilament sensitivity to calcium, which causes severe diastolic impairment, is thought to have a central role. Associated skeletal myopathy may also be present. The echocardiographic features of this disease are consistent with overall features of RCM as described earlier, including a typical pattern of biatrial enlargement, and nondilated ventricles with a normal LV ejection fraction and LV wall thickness (Video 24.8).

MUCOPOLYSACCHARIDOSES

Mucopolysaccharidoses are a group of inherited lysosomal storage diseases that results in progressive systemic deposition of partially degraded or undegraded glycosaminoglycans in the absence of the functional enzymes that contribute to their usual degradation. This can affect all the somatic organs of the body, and cardiac involvement is a common finding in this condition. Patients affected by this disorder may demonstrate multiple phenotypic features, including growth retardation, dysmorphic facial characteristics, skeletal and joint deformities, and central nervous system involvement, including developmental disabilities, among others.

Cardiac involvement has been reported in all types of mucopolysaccharidoses syndromes. However, it is a common and early feature with type I, II, and VI mucopolysaccharidoses. The deposition of the undegraded glycosaminoglycans in the myocardium leads to hypertrophy of both the right and left ventricular walls, with development of RCM. In addition, there is significant cardiac valve thickening with associated dysfunction, which is more severe for left-sided than for right-sided valves. Mitral valve is affected more commonly then the aortic valve, with the mitral valve leaflets developing a cartilage-like appearance with marked thickening, particularly of the edges. The mitral valve subvalvular apparatus is also affected with shortening of the chordae tendineae and thickening of the papillary muscles. Collectively, there is significant restriction of the mobility of the mitral

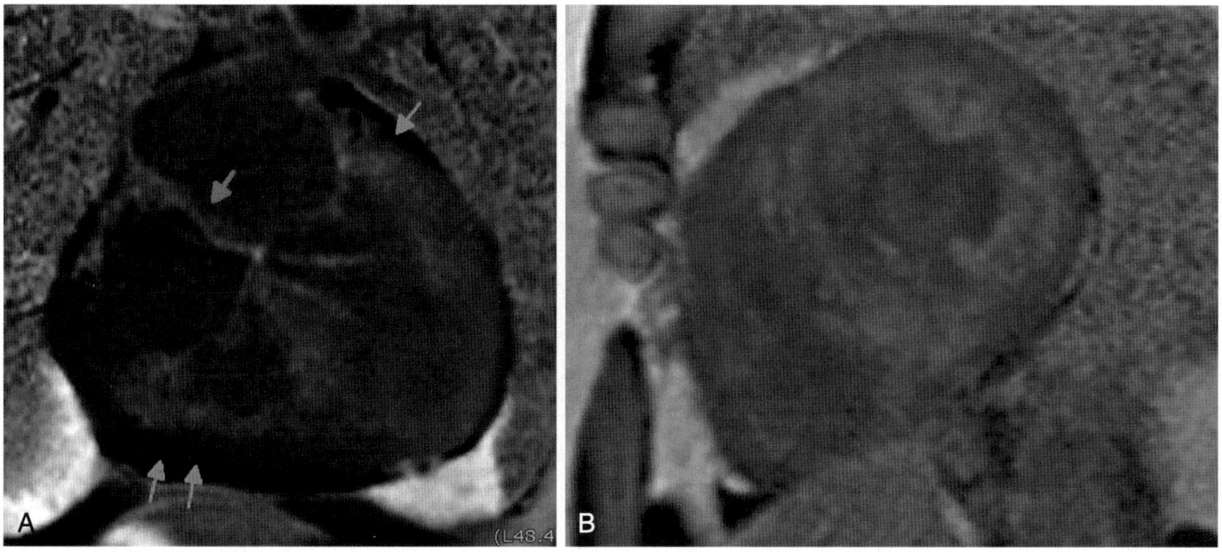

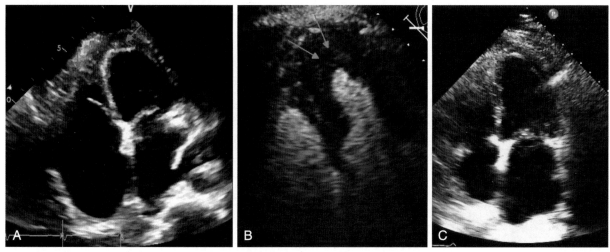

FIG. 24.5 Typical cardiac magnetic resonance imaging features in patient with transthyretin cardiac amyloidosis, showing characteristic late gadolinium enhancement of the interatrial septum (A, *red arrow*), and diffuse transmural LGE in the left ventricular myocardium, including the papillary muscle (B). (A) Also demonstrates a small pericardial effusion *(green arrows)*.

FIG. 24.6 Löffler endocarditis: apical four-chamber view showing endomyocardial fibrosis along both ventricular apices *(red arrows)*, extending all the way to the posterior mitral valve leaflet *(yellow arrow)*, with biatrial enlargement (A). (B) Contrast echocardiography in the apical four-chamber view with layering left ventricular apical clot at left ventricular apex in patient with hypereosinophilia *(green arrows)* and congestive heart failure. (C) Resolution of the left ventricular apical clot after 6 months of anticoagulation.

valve leaflets, and resulting regurgitation is seen more commonly than stenosis. Although the cardiac involvement with mucopolysaccharidoses can be well assessed with echocardiogram, the underlying skeletal deformities like pectus excavatum can cause technical challenges in obtaining adequate images.

ANDERSON-FABRY DISEASE

Anderson-Fabry disease is an X-linked disorder caused by deficiency of lysosomal enzyme alpha-galactosidase A, resulting in progressive intracellular accumulation of glycosphingolipids in different tissues, including skin, kidneys, vascular endothelium, ganglion cells of peripheral nervous system, and heart. Cardiac involvement is characterized by progressive left-ventricular hypertrophy, which mimics the morphologic and clinical features of hypertrophic cardiomyopathy, but tends to be symmetric (Fig. 24.7). It has been suggested that Anderson-Fabry disease may account up to 2%–4% of patients with unexplained left ventricular hypertrophy. Patients with Anderson-Fabry disease demonstrate lysosomal inclusions within myofibrils and vascular structures, with variable degrees of underlying fibrosis. The accumulation of these

lysosomal inclusions leads to cellular dysfunction, which activates common signaling pathways leading to hypertrophy, apoptosis, necrosis, and fibrosis. Fibrosis has been shown to be the major component of increased left ventricular mass, while the intracellular accumulation of glycosphingolipids by themselves contributes only 1%–2% of the increased left ventricular mass.

More than 50% of patients with Anderson-Fabry disease have a cardiomyopathy. These patients may also demonstrate characteristic electrocardiographic features including a short PR interval, abnormalities of conduction, LV hypertrophy, and atrial or ventricular enlargement (Fig. 24.8).[12] Typically, there is concentric left ventricular hypertrophy, commonly with an end diastolic left ventricular wall thickness greater than 15 mm, although patients with normal left ventricular wall thickness have also been reported.[13] Unlike hypertrophic cardiomyopathy, these patients usually do not demonstrate left ventricular outflow tract obstruction (Video 24.9). Although LVEF usually remains normal until the late stage of the disease, early resting regional wall motion abnormalities, particularly of the inferolateral wall, may be seen. Due to the significant amount of underlying fibrosis, the diastolic function is impaired in the early stages of the disease.[14] Global longitudinal strain, as well as regional

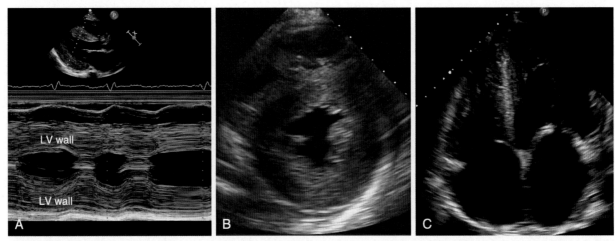

FIG. 24.7 (A) M mode in a patient with Fabry disease with severe thickness of the left and right ventricular walls. (B) and (C) Short-axis and four-chamber view in the same patient. Note the concentric left ventricular hypertrophy (LVH), in contrast with the asymmetric LVH usually seen in hypertrophic cardiomyopathy.

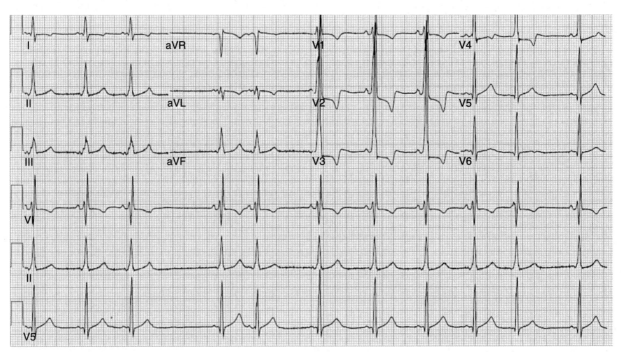

FIG. 24.8 Electrocardiogram in a patient with Anderson-Fabry disease showing sinus rhythm with occasional atrial premature contractions. There is also left ventricular hypertrophy, with shortened PR interval, and ventricular preexcitation, best seen in the leads III and aVF.

longitudinal strain especially of the inferolateral wall, may be impaired prior to reduction of LVEF. The end stage of Anderson-Fabry cardiomyopathy is characterized by intramural replacement fibrosis, which may also be limited to the basal inferolateral wall of the left ventricle.

GLYCOGEN STORAGE DISEASES

Glycogen storage diseases are disorders of metabolism caused by enzyme defects that affect glycogen synthesis or degradation within muscles, liver, heart, and other cell types. Over 15 different types of glycogen storage disease have been identified, and these diseases have variable cardiac involvement.

Pompe disease or glycogen storage disease type II (GSD II) occurs due to an α-1,4-glucosidase deficiency, characterized by progressive deposition of glycogen in all tissues, most notably cardiac, skeletal, and smooth muscles. The classic form of Pompe disease is the infantile onset form, with symptoms developing prior to 1 year of age with underlying hypertrophic cardiomyopathy. About 75% of patients with the

classic infantile form of Pompe disease die before 12 months of age. The late onset form of Pompe disease include childhood-, juvenile-, and adult-onset subgroups, which typically present with muscle weakness and respiratory failure without cardiac manifestations. However, since Pompe disease is a continuum of clinical manifestations with varying degrees of organ involvement, there are many cases which do not fit into the two categories described above.[15] Although the cardiac involvement among adults with Pompe disease is not as striking as among the infantile form, there have been occasional descriptions of isolated thickening of the left ventricle.

Danon disease or glycogen storage disease type IIb (GSD IIb) is a rare X-linked disorder due to lysosome-associated membrane protein 2 (LAMP2) deficiency. Since it is an X-linked disorder, males usually develop symptoms before age 20, whereas female carriers manifest cardiomyopathy during adulthood. It is clinically characterized by the triad of ventricular hypertrophy, skeletal myopathy, and variable intellectual disability. Other manifestations include the presence of ventricular preexcitation (Wolff-Parkinson-White syndrome, short

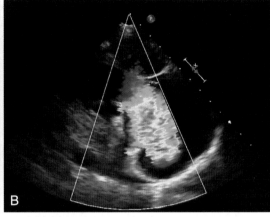

FIG. 24.9 Tricuspid valve in a patient with underlying carcinoid syndrome. (A) Right ventricular inflow view, which shows a dilated right atrium (RA) with a dilated right ventricle (RV), and a noncoapting tricuspid valve that is frozen in a semiopen and semiclosed position *(arrow)*. (B) There is resulting severe tricuspid regurgitation, which demonstrates laminar flow on color Doppler.

PR interval and delta waves), increased creatinine kinase, and ophthalmic abnormalities. All patients develop cardiomyopathy, which is the most severe and life-threatening manifestation. The cardiomyopathy is progressive with marked symmetrical increase in left ventricular wall thickness (>20 mm), and typically manifests with preserved ejection fraction and normal cavity dimensions early in the course of disease, which later progresses to dilated cardiomyopathy in about 10% of the affected males.[16] On CMR imaging, Danon disease most commonly has a subendocardial pattern of late gadolinium enhancement, whereas classical hypertrophic cardiomyopathy demonstrates patchy late gadolinium enhancement with subepicardial and midwall distribution.

IRON OVERLOAD CARDIOMYOPATHY

Iron overload cardiomyopathy results from the accumulation of iron in the myocardium. The primary form of iron overload is termed hereditary or primary hemochromatosis, an autosomal disorder which affects the genes encoding proteins involved in iron metabolism, and also causes increased intestinal iron absorption. Hereditary hemochromatosis is associated with the classic triad of liver cirrhosis, diabetes mellitus, and skin pigmentation. Secondary iron overload or hemosiderosis is mainly caused by the considerably high parenteral iron administration and is primarily observed in association with transfusion-dependent hereditary or acquired anemias, such as thalassemia and sickle cell disease.

Two phenotypes of iron overload cardiomyopathy have been identified: (1) the dilated phenotype, which is characterized by a process of left ventricular remodeling leading to chamber dilatation and reduced LVEF; and (2) the less common restrictive phenotype, characterized by diastolic left ventricular dysfunction with restrictive filling pattern, preserved LVEF, pulmonary hypertension, and subsequent right ventricular dilatation. However, in the early stages of the disease in both phenotypes, echocardiography detects diastolic dysfunction. With gradual progression of the disease, the echocardiogram may demonstrate either a reduced LVEF, or restrictive filling pattern, or a combination of both. In some hemoglobinopathies with associated anemia there is a high output state. This may mask early LV systolic dysfunction, but may be associated with abnormality of diastolic function. In advanced stages of the disease, the right ventricular function may be impaired with development of pulmonary hypertension. Although echocardiography has the potential to identify early pathophysiology due to iron overload, it is not sensitive enough to reveal actual iron deposition in tissues. T2* magnetic resonance imaging is the best way for early detection of iron overload in patients with suspicion of iron overload cardiomyopathy. T2* assessment can also be used to assess response to therapy as T2 relaxation time has a linear correlation with the total iron content in the heart.

CARCINOID SYNDROME

Carcinoid tumors typically arise from derivatives of the embryological gastrointestinal tract, with the majority of such tumors arising from the small intestine, while some may arise from the lungs. Carcinoid heart disease, which has been estimated to affect at least 20% of patients with metastatic carcinoid syndrome, is a paraneoplastic syndrome caused by tumor-derived vasoactive substances, such as serotonin, histamine, tachykinins, kallikrein and prostaglandin.[17] Although it is predominantly a valve disorder, it can affect the cardiac chambers. The assessment of cardiac involvement in patients with underlying carcinoid is important as patients with cardiac involvement have a significantly worse prognosis when compared to those without cardiac involvement. Depending upon the primary location of the systemic carcinoid tumor, either the right or left side of the heart is predominantly involved. If the primary tumor is an intestinal carcinoid, the right heart will be predominantly involved, and if (less commonly) the primary tumor is a bronchial carcinoid, the left heart will be predominantly involved. The left side of the heart may also be involved in the presence of an intestinal carcinoid if there is an interatrial shunt, which allows the passage of the vasoactive substances to the left side of the heart without being deactivated in the pulmonary circulation.

The two primary features of carcinoid heart disease are mural plaques and valvulitis, with regurgitation and stenosis of the affected valves. The mural plaques produced in this condition appear along the valvular or endocardial surface, and typically appear to have a "stuck-on" appearance, without destruction of the underlying valvular architecture.[17] The appearance of the affected valves appears similar to chronic rheumatic valvular heart disease, with leaflet thickening and retraction, mild focal commissural fusion, and chordal thickening.

On echocardiogram, the tricuspid valve is affected in approximately 90% of patients with cardiac involvement (Fig. 24.9). The earliest changes are thickening of the valve leaflets and subvalvular apparatus. Gradual loss of the normal concave curvature of the tricuspid valve leaflets leads to mild tricuspid regurgitation. With gradual worsening of the disease, the leaflets and the subvalvular apparatus become fixed and retracted, and the noncoapting tricuspid valve leaflets appear frozen in semi-open/semi-closed state, resulting in severe tricuspid regurgitation (Videos 24.10 and 24.11). When evaluating the tricuspid valve on echocardiogram it is important to note that in advanced disease with worsening insufficiency, the regurgitant jet flow becomes laminar and color Doppler may underestimate the severity of regurgitation. In such cases, careful attention should be paid to the continuous wave Doppler profile which may demonstrate a "dagger shaped pattern" with an early peak pressure and rapid decline, as opposed to the typical parabolic regurgitation profile (Fig. 24.10).[17] In contrast to the tricuspid valve which usually shows isolated insufficiency, involvement of the pulmonary valve most commonly results

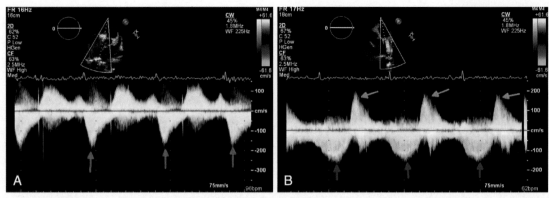

FIG. 24.10 Continuous-wave spectral Doppler profiles through tricuspid and pulmonic valves in a patient with underlying carcinoid syndrome. (A) Tricuspid valve demonstrating a low-velocity jet with triangular jet profile indicating severe tricuspid regurgitation jet *(red arrows)*. (B) Pulmonic valve demonstrating both pulmonic stenosis *(blue arrows)*, and triangular profile of pulmonic regurgitant jet demonstrating rapid deceleration *(green arrows)*.

in mixed regurgitation and stenosis.[17] It has been hypothesized that the smaller diameter of the pulmonary valve annulus as compared to the tricuspid valve annulus leads to increased incidence of stenosis. Similar to the tricuspid valve, when the left-sided valves (mitral valve > aortic valve) are involved, regurgitation is commoner than stenosis. In patients with predominant right-sided involvement due to severe underlying valvulopathy, the right-sided cardiac chambers may become progressively dilated and hypokinetic.

POSTRADIATION THERAPY AND CHEMOTHERAPY-RELATED CARDIAC DYSFUNCTION

Radiation exposure to the thorax is associated with substantial risk for the subsequent development of cardiovascular disease. There are a number of possible cardiovascular complications following radiation treatment, including pericardial disease, cardiomyopathy, coronary artery disease, valvular disease, cardiomyopathy, and vasculopathy. Radiation-induced fibrosis occurs in the myocardium and the pericardium, due to extensive collagen deposition. This leads to reduced distensibility of both the myocardium and pericardium, resulting in myocardial diastolic dysfunction, constrictive pericarditis or a combination of both. There may also be valvular involvement, especially of the left-sided valves, due to fibrotic thickening, valvular retraction, and late calcification of the valves and the surrounding myocardium. The extent of valvular abnormality may vary from mild valve leaflet thickening to hemodynamically significant stenosis and regurgitation. Echocardiography typically demonstrates normal left ventricular wall thickness, abnormal left ventricular filling parameters as assessed by transmitral Doppler flow pattern, and impaired diastolic function assessed by tissue Doppler. These myocardial findings may be associated with valvular calcification, and, in many patients, features of pericardial constriction.[18]

Chemotherapy-related cardiac dysfunction is a frequent complication of some classes of chemotherapeutic agents. While the cardiac effects of the anthracycline class of agents and trastuzumab is well established, the effects of other newer agents are still being evaluated. Anthracyclines cause type I chemotherapy-related dysfunction, an irreversible and dose-dependent process, mediated by oxidative stress.[19] Trastuzumab-induced myocardial dysfunction results from inhibition of the ErbB2 pathway, is not related to the cumulative dose, and is usually reversible. Although ejection fraction is commonly used to assess cardiotoxic effects of chemotherapy, it has considerable inter- and intraobserver variability when measured by 2D echocardiography. Volumetric assessment using 3D echocardiography does not rely on geometric assumptions and is superior to 2D evaluation. Unfortunately, a reduction in ejection fraction caused by chemotherapy probably represents severe myocardial damage and

myocardial strain imaging can detect much LV dysfunction at a much earlier stage, thereby permitting dose reduction or cessation, if feasible. Peak left ventricular systolic global strain has demonstrated the most prognostic value with ongoing treatment, and relative reduction by 10%–15% is a useful predictor of cardiotoxicity early during the course of treatment. Diastolic function is also affected by chemotherapy, and should be assessed serially.

Cyclophosphamide cardiotoxicity, although rare, is an example of acute myocardial dysfunction characterized by both severe systolic and diastolic dysfunction. It is frequently fatal and associated with myocardial edema and hemorrhage.[20] On echocardiography, the LV walls are thickened due to edema, with a nondilated hypokinetic left ventricle and impaired diastolic function. There may be an associated acute reduction in electrocardiographic voltage, so that the picture mimics an infiltrative cardiomyopathy. An example is shown in Videos 24.12–24.15.

SYSTEMIC SCLEROSIS

Progressive systemic sclerosis is a chronic multisystem disease characterized by microangiopathy, fibrosis of the skin and internal organs, and autoimmune disturbances. Recent studies have suggested that clinical evidence of myocardial disease may be seen in 20%–25% of patients with systemic sclerosis, but this is often mild. Cardiac involvement can generally be divided into direct myocardial effect due to the underlying microvascular dysfunction and recurrent small vessel vasospasm, and the indirect effect of other organ involvement (i.e., pulmonary hypertension or renal crisis). This direct cardiac toxicity leads to vascular obliteration, with resulting fibrosis and inflammation, which manifests as a myriad of clinical features such as myositis, cardiac failure, cardiac fibrosis, coronary artery disease, conduction system abnormalities, and pericardial disease.[21] The earliest signs of cardiac involvement are manifest in the form of impaired diastolic function. Although a decrease in left and right ventricular ejection fractions is seen much later in the course of the disease, myocardial strain imaging can detect reduction in systolic function prior to the drop in ejection fraction.

PSEUDOXANTHOMA ELASTICUM

Pseudoxanthoma elasticum is a rare autosomal recessive connective tissue disorder characterized by the mineralization and fragmentation of elastic fibers in the skin, retina, and cardiovascular system. Although the usual cardiovascular manifestations are caused by accelerated atherosclerosis, patients with pseudoxanthoma elasticum may also demonstrate atrial and ventricular endocardial thickening and calcification (Fig. 24.11), diastolic dysfunction, atrial enlargement, and RCM.[22]

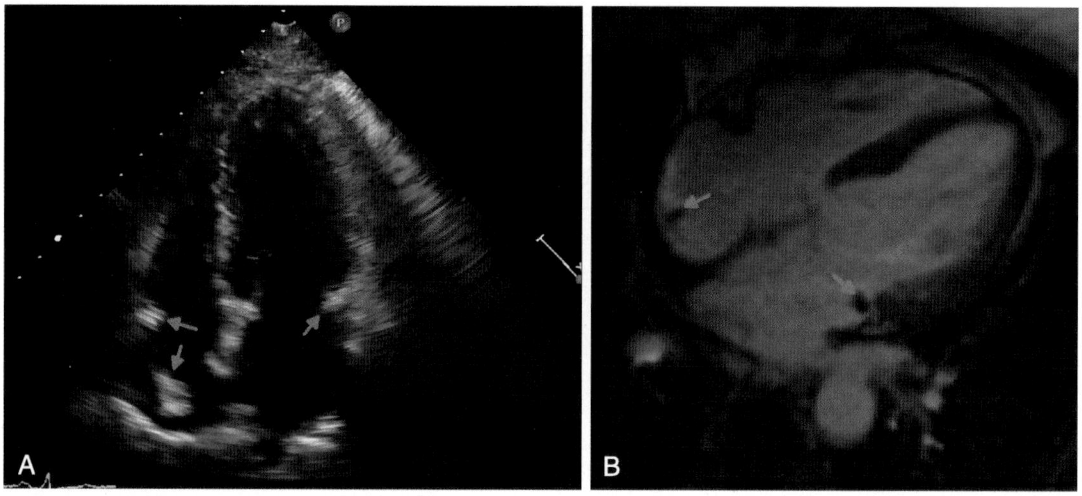

FIG. 24.11 Pseudoxanthoma elasticum: endocardial calcification involving both the atria, with the mitral and tricuspid annular calcification in patient with underlying pseudoxanthoma elasticum on apical four-chamber view in a transthoracic echocardiogram (A), and cardiac magnetic resonance imaging (B).

Suggested Reading

Falk, R. H., & Quarta, C. C. (2015). Echocardiography in cardiac amyloidosis. *Heart Failure Reviews, 20*(2), 125–131.

Falk, R. H., Quarta, C. C., & Dorbala, S. (2014). How to image cardiac amyloidosis. *Circulation Cardiovascular Imaging, 7*(3), 552–562.

Mankad, R., Bonnichsen, C., & Mankad, S. (2016). Hypereosinophilic syndrome: cardiac diagnosis and management. *Heart, 102*(2), 100–106.

Seward, J. B., & Casaclang-Verzosa, G. (2010). Infiltrative cardiovascular diseases: cardiomyopathies that look alike. *Journal of the American College of Cardiology, 55*(17), 1769–1779.

A complete reference list can be found online at ExpertConsult.com.

25 Echocardiography in Assessment of Cardiac Synchrony

John Gorcsan III

INTRODUCTION

Electromechanical association in a normal heart results in synchronous regional left ventricular (LV) contraction. Differences in the timing of regional contraction may be associated with the failing human heart. Interest in echocardiographic assessment of synchrony began with applications for pacing therapy, in particular cardiac resynchronization therapy (CRT).[1–5] CRT, also known as biventricular pacing, was an important advance in treatment of heart failure (HF) patients with reduced ejection fraction (EF) and electrical dispersion recognized by widened electrocardiographic (ECG) QRS complexes. Although CRT often results in improvement in symptoms, LV reverse remodeling, and prolonging life, one-third to one-half of patients do not appear to benefit and are referred to as nonresponders.[6,7] Several investigators have observed that differences in LV regional timing referred to as dyssynchrony can be measured by a variety of echocardiographic techniques.[8–11] Interest in measuring regional timing of LV contraction increased with the advent of tissue Doppler imaging (TDI) and speckle tracking strain measures.[3,9,11] Many reports have documented that patients with widened QRS complexes have variable degrees of mechanical dyssynchrony at baseline before CRT (Fig. 25.1).[3–5,8,11–15] It was observed that patients with measurable dyssynchrony at baseline before CRT had a much more favorable response to CRT than patients who lacked baseline dyssynchrony. Accordingly, there was anticipation that measures of timing of regional contraction by echocardiographic methods would play a role in improving patient selection for CRT. However, the field advanced to reveal that mechanical dyssynchrony was more complicated than originally thought, and current clinical guidelines focus exclusively on ECG criteria.[16,17] This chapter will review the progress in understanding of mechanical dyssynchrony, define the current state of the art, and project potential future clinical applications of assessing cardiac synchrony.

ECHOCARDIOGRAPHIC METHODS TO ASSESS DYSSYNCHRONY

Normal LV mechanical activation results in peak contraction occurring at the same time. Videos 25.1 and 25.2, using three-dimensional (3D) echocardiographic strain, demonstrate normal contraction. The classic LV dyssynchrony pattern responsive to CRT is observed with a typical left bundle branch block (LBBB) consisting of early contraction of the septum followed by delayed posterior contraction. Videos 25.3 and 25.4, using 3D echocardiographic strain, demonstrate a typical LBBB contraction pattern. There have been many echocardiographic approaches to define dyssynchrony. The most common methods have been a variety of means to measure regional contractions in the LV. The majority of the literature has focused on methods to measure peak-to-peak regional events representing contraction or the variations in regional contraction, expressed as standard deviation (Table 25.1). A simple approach has been to measure the time difference in peak sepal velocity to peak lateral wall velocity using TDI, including color-coded time to peak velocity (Fig. 25.2).[3,9] Another tissue-Doppler-based method was to assess the standard deviation in time-to-peak velocities from 12 segments in three standard apical views, introduced by Yu et al. and known as the Yu Index. A more complex method of tissue Doppler cross-correlation was introduced and associated with response to CRT.[10] A simpler approach to dyssynchrony has been the "septal flash" (visual rapid inward and outward

septal motion in the preejection period) assessed by routine M-mode or color-tissue Doppler M-mode and used as a marker of CRT response.[18,19] Speckle tracking methods to assess regional contraction from radial, circumferential, and longitudinal strain have been used frequently and continue to gain in popularity.[3,11,20] The original application of speckle tracking strain for dyssynchrony analysis was radial strain from the midventricular short-axis view (Fig. 25.3).[11] The original approach was to measure the time delay in peak-to-peak septal to posterior wall strain at baseline before CRT. CRT patients who had a peak-to-peak radial strain delay greater than 130 ms had a more favorable response to CRT compared to those who did not.[11,13] The standard deviation in longitudinal strain peaks has been associated with response to CRT.[21,22] Alternate approaches include measuring delayed LV ejection delay, which is the result of regional dyssynchrony. Both LV preejection time and interventricular mechanical delays have been associated as markers for CRT response.[8] The preejection delay has been defined as an increase in time from onset of QRS complex to onset of LV ejection using pulsed Doppler placed in the LV outflow tract. Interventricular mechanical delay is a related index defined as the time difference in LV preejection time and right ventricular preejection time.[8] More recent approaches have been to evaluate the mechanical contraction pattern associated with electrical delay in radial and longitudinal strain curves. A major advance in understanding has come from computer simulations of the electromechanical substrate responsive to CRT and quantification of these mechanical events as the systolic stretch index (SSI), described in more detail later.[23] A similar approach came from observing a typical LBBB contraction pattern in longitudinal strain curves consisting of early contraction of the septum (before ejection) followed by delayed posterior contraction (after aortic value closure).[11,20] In addition, more simple visual assessments of apical rocking resulting from early septal shorting followed by late lateral wall contraction was also associated with favorable response to CRT (Video 25.5).[19] Many of the original dyssynchrony approaches have been criticized by the Predictors of Response to Cardiac Resynchronization Therapy (PROSPECT) study, which was an observational study of echocardiographic markers and response to CRT.[24] The results of this study

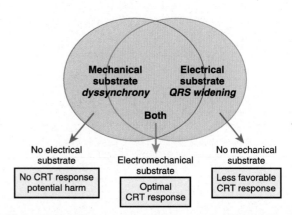

FIG. 25.1 A hypothetical scheme of electrical substrate identified by QRS widening and mechanical substrate identified by regional contraction delay by imaging methods as it relates to cardiac resynchronization therapy (CRT). The electromechanical substrate with elements of both electrical and mechanical delays is associated with the optimal response to CRT.

were affected by an overly simplistic interpretation of mechanical dyssynchrony, variability in methods, and lack of a unified echocardiographic approach. There were significant associations of several markers of baseline dyssynchrony with favorable LV reverse remodeling after CRT.[24] However, sensitivity and specificity were considered to be too low, and variability in these measurements considered to be too high to influence patient selection. The current role measures of dyssynchrony remain as markers of prognosis after CRT rather for patient selection.[16,17] Further work on the potential utility of these measures to influence patient selection for CRT continues to be ongoing.

TABLE 25.1 Measures of Echocardiographic Dyssynchrony

METHOD	MEASUREMENT	MARKER FOR CRT RESPONSE
Interventricular Mechanical Delay LV outflow track and RV outflow tracks	Time difference between RV preejection and LV preejection	≥40 ms
Tissue Doppler Longitudinal Velocity Apical 4-chamber view (2 sites)	Time from peak septal to peak lateral wall velocity	≥65 ms
Tissue Doppler Yu Index Apical, 4-, 2-, and 3-chamber views (12 sites)	Standard deviation of 12-site peak velocity measures	≥33 ms
Septal Flash Parasternal views: M-mode or color tissue Doppler M-mode	Brief inward and outward motion of the septum early during preejection	Presence or absence
Speckle tracking radial strain Mid ventricular short-axis view	Time difference in peak septal to peak posterior wall strain	≥130 ms
Tissue Doppler cross-correlation of myocardial acceleration Apical 4-chamber view	Maximum activation delay from opposing septal and lateral walls	>35 ms
Visual Assessment of longitudinal strain pattern of typical left bundle branch Apical 4-chamber view	(1) Early septal peak shortening; (2) early stretching in lateral wall; (3) lateral wall peak shortening after aortic valve closure	All three criteria
Apical Rocking Apical 4-chamber view	Visual movement of apex toward septum early during preejection, followed by lateral motion of apex during ejection	Presence or absence
Systolic Stretch Index Radial Strain Mid-ventricular short-axis view	Posterolateral prestretch (before aortic valve opening) + Septal systolic stretch (to aortic valve closure)	≥9.7 %

CRT, Cardiac resynchronization therapy; LV, left ventricular; RV, right ventricular.

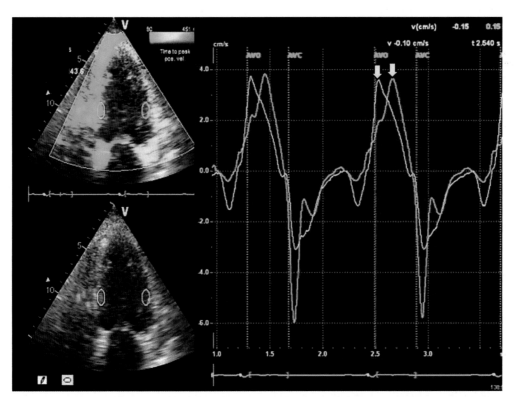

FIG. 25.2 Tissue Doppler longitudinal velocity from an apical four-chamber view in a patient with traditional peak-to-peak mechanical dyssynchrony. Echocardiographic images appear on the left, and time-velocity curves on the right. Regions of interest are placed in the septum (yellow curve) and lateral wall (turquoise curve). The time to peak velocity is color-coded in the upper left panel (green as early and yellow as later). There is a 90-ms peak-to-peak delay (arrow) from septal to lateral wall in longitudinal velocity between aortic valve opening (AVO) and aortic valve closure (AVC).

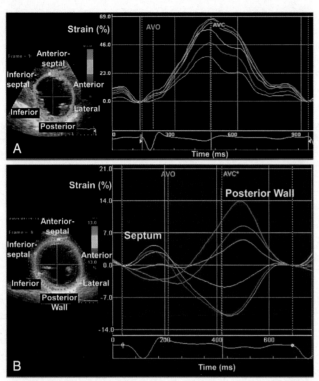

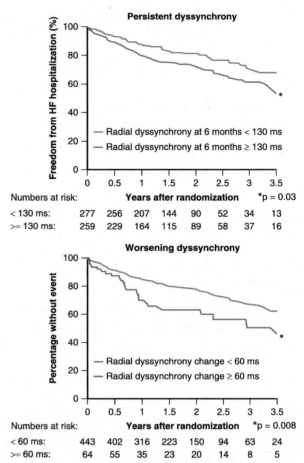

FIG. 25.3 Examples of speckle tracking radial strain from the mid-ventricular short-axis view with six color-coded time-strain curves. (A) Is from a normal volunteer demonstrating synchronous contraction. (B) Is from a patient with left bundle branch block with strain curves representing dyssynchrony associated with response to cardiac resynchronization therapy. The septal segments contract early before aortic valve opening and are associated with stretching of the posterior wall. The posterior wall contraction is delayed and reaches peak contraction after aortic valve closure associated with stretching of the septum. The peak-to-peak approach was to measure the time difference from peak septal strain to peak posterior wall strain.

FIG. 25.4 Kaplan-Meier plots of patients in the EchoCRT randomized trial who had narrow QRS width, echocardiography dyssynchrony, and reduced ejection fraction. Patients are included who had follow-up dyssynchrony analysis at 6 months. *Top:* Patients with persistent dyssynchrony reached the end-point of heart failure hospitalization more often than patients with improved dyssynchrony. *Bottom:* Patients with worsened dyssynchrony reached the end-point of heart failure (HF) hospitalization more often than patients with no worsening. These findings were not associated with cardiac resynchronization therapy (CRT)-On or CRT-Off randomization. (*Modified from Gorcsan J 3rd, Sogaard P, Bax JJ, et al. Association of persistent or worsened echocardiographic dyssynchrony with unfavourable clinical outcomes in heart failure patients with narrow QRS width: a subgroup analysis of the EchoCRT trial.* Eur Heart J. 2016;37[1]:49-59.)

NEW UNDERSTANDING OF MECHANICAL DYSSYNCHRONY

Enthusiasm for mechanical dyssynchrony to be used for patient selection resulted in two prospective randomized clinical trials of CRT in HF patients with narrow QRS width (<130 ms) selected by echocardiographic mechanical dyssynchrony. The first was the ReThinQ trial which enrolled 172 patients with QRS width less than 130 ms and used tissue Doppler peak-to-peak measures of contraction delay.[25] This trial failed to show any benefit to these patients with LV reverse remodeling at 6 months as the outcome variable. The larger more definitive trial was Echocardiography Guided Cardiac Resynchronization Therapy (EchoCRT), which enrolled and randomized 809 reduced EF HF patients with QRS less than 130 ms and either tissue Doppler longitudinal velocity peak-to-peak delay of ≥80 ms or speckle tracking radial strain septal to posterior wall peak-to-peak delay of ≥130 ms.[26] EchoCRT also failed to show benefit in the primary endpoint of HF hospitalization or death. Surprisingly, there was an increase in mortality in EchoCRT patients randomized to CRT-On versus the control group randomized to CRT-Off.[26] These trials brought new insight for peak-to-peak measures of dyssynchrony as markers of contractile heterogeneity that are not associated with favorable response to CRT as in patients with widened QRS complexes. Combining previous studies of dyssynchrony and CRT response with the narrow QRS CRT trials resulted in changing concepts of dyssynchrony and CRT response.

Subsequently, more recent EchoCRT substudy analysis revealed that peak-to-peak echocardiographic dyssynchrony in patients with narrow QRS complexes can be a marker of unfavorable clinical outcome.[27] There were 614 patients in the EchoCRT study (EF ≤35%, QRS <130 ms) who had baseline and 6-month echocardiograms. All patients were required to have baseline dyssynchrony by tissue Doppler longitudinal velocity peak-to-peak delay ≥80 ms or radial strain septal to posterior wall peak-to-peak delay ≥130 ms for randomization in the EchoCRT trial. In this substudy, the measures of tissue Doppler peak-to-peak longitudinal velocity delay and speckle tracking radial strain peak-to-peak septal to posterior wall delay were reassessed at 6-month follow-up. Remarkably, 25% of patients improved either longitudinal or radial dyssynchrony at 6 months, regardless of randomization to CRT-Off or CRT-On. The associated improvement in dyssynchrony was hypothesized to be related to improvements in LV function associated with pharmacological therapy, as 97% of patients in both groups were on beta-blocker therapy and 95% were on angiotensin converting enzyme inhibitors or angiotensin II receptor blockers. Using the same predefined criteria for significant dyssynchrony at baseline, as at 6 months, persistent dyssynchrony was associated with a significantly higher primary endpoint of death or HF hospitalization (hazard ratio [HR] = 1.54, 95% confidence interval [CI] 1.03–2.30, P = .03). In particular, persistent dyssynchrony at 6 months was associated with the secondary endpoint of HF hospitalization (HR = 1.66, 95% CI 1.07–2.57, P = .02; Fig. 25.4). These observations were similar in patients randomized to CRT-Off as well as CRT-On and were not associated with CRT treatment. Furthermore, HF hospitalizations were also associated with both worsening longitudinal dyssynchrony, defined as an increase in peak-to-peak delay from baseline ≥30 ms (HR = 1.45, 95% CI 1.02–2.05, P = .037), and worsening radial dyssynchrony, defined as an increase in peak-to-peak delay from baseline ≥60 ms (HR = 1.81, 95% CI 1.16–2.81, P = .008). Worsening dyssynchrony was

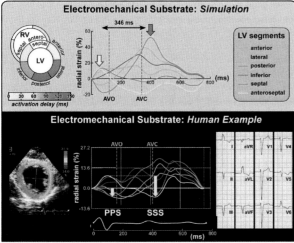

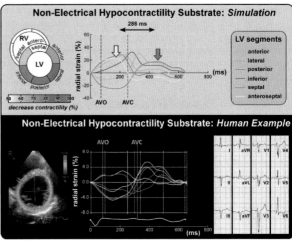

FIG. 25.5 *Top:* A computer simulation of progressive electrical delay and radial strain curves in six color-coded segments representing the electromechanical substrate responsive to cardiac resynchronization therapy. The arrows demonstrate a 346-ms peak-to-peak delay in septal to posterior wall strain. The early septal contraction before aortic valve opening (AVO) is associated with posterior wall *(purple curve)* stretching below the zero baseline. The posterior wall delayed contraction is associated with stretching of the septal segments *(yellow and red curves)*. AVC, Aortic valve closure. *Bottom:* The echocardiogram from a patient with reduced ejection fraction and QRS duration of 132 ms before cardiac resynchronization therapy (CRT). The radial strain curves resemble the simulation with early septal contraction associated with posterolateral prestretch (PPS) at 13.3% and later posterior wall contraction associated with septal systolic stretch (SSS) at 15.9%. The systolic stretch index (PPS + SSS) was high at 29.2%, indicating a favorable electromechanical substrate for CRT response. *(Modified from Lumens J, Tayal B, Walmsley J, et al. Differentiating electromechanical from non-electrical substrates of mechanical discoordination to identify responders to cardiac resynchronization therapy.* Circ Cardiovasc Imaging. *2015;8[9]:e003744.)*

FIG. 25.6 *Top:* A computer simulation of dyssynchrony from a nonelectrical substrate that is not responsive to cardiac resynchronization therapy. There are progressive decreases in segmental contractility of the posterior wall without significant electrical delay and radial strain curves in six color-coded segments. The arrows show a 286-ms peak-to-peak delay in septal to posterior wall strain. This simulation demonstrates how peak-to-peak dyssynchrony can exist from contractile heterogeneity without significant electrical delay, such as in a patient with a narrow QRS complex. *Bottom:* The echocardiogram from a patient with reduced ejection fraction and QRS duration of 130 ms before cardiac resynchronization therapy (CRT). The radial strain curves demonstrate minimal early posterolateral prestretch (PPS) at 2.7% with most of stretch occurring during ejection. There is also minimal septal systolic stretch (SSS) at 1.8%. The systolic stretch index (PPS + SSS) was low at 4.5%, indicating a substrate that is unresponsive to CRT response. AVO, Aortic valve opening; AVC, aortic valve closure. *(Modified from Lumens J, Tayal B, Walmsley J, et al. Differentiating electromechanical from non-electrical substrates of mechanical discoordination to identify responders to cardiac resynchronization therapy.* Circ Cardiovasc Imaging. *2015;8[9]:e003744.)*

associated with unfavorable clinical outcomes, in particular for HF hospitalizations, in both CRT-Off and CRT-On groups, unrelated to the randomization arm. These findings suggested that echocardiographic dyssynchrony is a new prognostic marker in HF patients with reduced left ventricular ejection fraction (LVEF) and narrow QRS width, Since these associations were similar in CRT-On and CRT-Off groups, these observations suggested that tissue Doppler or radial strain peak-to-peak dyssynchrony may possibly be a marker for unfavorable LV mechanics and myocardial disease severity in patients with narrow QRS width.

MYOCARDIAL SUBSTRATES OF SYNCHRONY AND DISCOORDINATION

Further understanding of the mechanisms of mechanical dyssynchrony without a significant electrical delay came from computer simulations of the cardiovascular system. Using the CircAdapt system, Lumens et al. programed progressive degrees of electrical delay coupled with computer simulations of segmental LV strain.[23] The characteristics of the electromechanical substrate responsive to CRT were documented to include early septal contraction causing stretching of the posterior-lateral walls before aortic valve opening (posterolateral prestretch or PPS) followed by delayed posterolateral contraction causing septal stretch (systolic septal stretch or SSS) (Fig. 25.5). From these components, the SSI was calculated as SSI = PPS + SSS as a marker for the electromechanical substrate responsive to CRT. The previous terms of systolic prestretch have been revised to PPS and systolic rebound stretch revised to SSS as felt to be more accurate descriptors. A computer simulation was then performed varying regional contractility, but no electrical delay. Peak-to-peak delays in radial strain were simulated with contractile heterogeneity, but no significant electrical delay, which resulted in peak-to-peak delays as observed in humans with narrow QRS widths (Fig. 25.6). Regional scar was then simulated by decreasing contractility and increasing passive stiffness (which are mechanical properties of myocardial scar). Peak-to-peak delays in radial strain associated with scar were measured without electrical delay (Fig. 25.7).[23] These simulations represented the typical patients who were enrolled in the narrow QRS CRT trials (RethinQ or EchoCRT) with

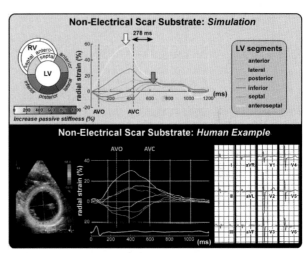

FIG. 25.7 *Top:* A computer simulation of dyssynchrony from scar with progressive increases in passive stiffness along with segmental hypocontractility in the posterior wall without significant electrical delay and radial strain curves in six color-coded segments. The arrows show a 278-ms peak-to-peak delay in septal to posterior wall strain. This simulation demonstrates how peak-to-peak dyssynchrony can exist from scar without significant electrical delay, such as in a patient with a narrow QRS complex who will not respond to cardiac resynchronization therapy. *Bottom:* The echocardiogram from a patient with transmural posterior infarction, reduced ejection fraction, and QRS duration of 130 ms before cardiac resynchronization therapy (CRT). The radial strain curves demonstrate peak-to-peak dyssynchrony, but minimal early posterolateral prestretch (PPS) at 1.2% with most of stretch occurring during ejection. There is minimal septal systolic stretch (SSS) at 2.8%. The systolic stretch index (PPS + SSS) was low at 4.0%, indicating a substrate that is unresponsive to CRT response. AVO, Aortic valve opening; AVC, aortic valve closure. *(Modified from Lumens J, Tayal B, Walmsley J, et al. Differentiating electromechanical from non-electrical substrates of mechanical discoordination to identify responders to cardiac resynchronization therapy.* Circ Cardiovasc Imaging. *2015;8[9]:e003744.)*

peak-to-peak dyssynchrony but no QRS widening.[25,26] Examining the differences in these strain patterns, differences in the nonelectrical contractile heterogeneity or scar substrates were that they were lacking significant posterolateral prestretch or septal systolic stretch, which was, in contrast, seen in the electromechanical substrate responsive to

CRT. There is mechanistic support of the deleterious effects of stretch on myocardial function with stretch near the start of cardiac tension development substantially increasing twitch tension and mechanical work production, whereas late stretches decrease external work.[28] The mechanical phenomenon with LBBB of septal contraction and lateral

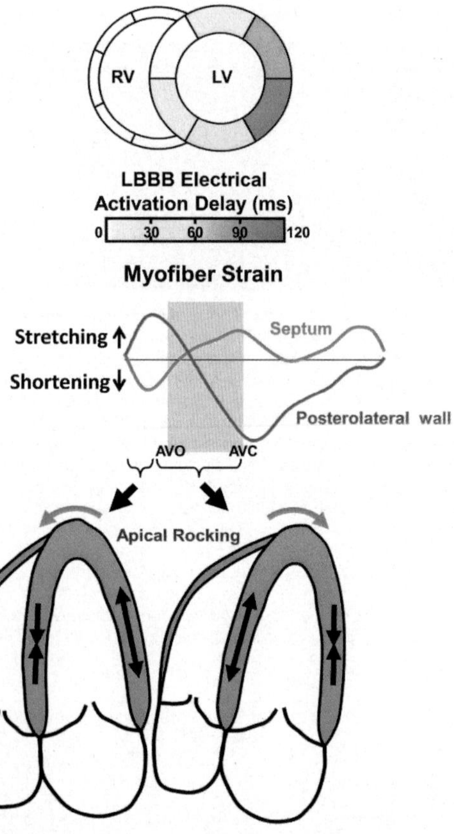

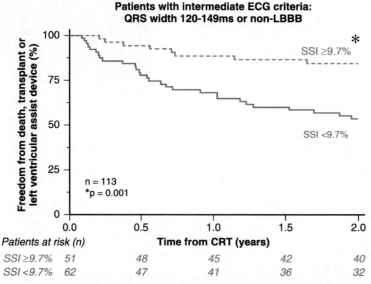

FIG. 25.8 A computer simulation of electrical activation delay with left bundle branch block (LBBB) demonstrating shortening and stretching of left ventricular septum and posterior-lateral wall that may explain the mechanism of apical rocking observed with LBBB. (*Modified from Gorcsan J 3rd, Lumens J. Rocking and flashing with RV pacing: implications for resynchronization therapy. JACC Cardiovasc Imaging. 2016;16:30811–30817.*)

wall prestretch followed by lateral wall contraction and septal stretch appears to be related to apical rocking, which is a visual marker associated with response to CRT response (Fig. 25.8; see Video 25.5).[19,28a]

Following the computer simulations, the predictive value of SSI was then tested in a series of 191 patients who underwent CRT (all had QRS duration ≥120 ms; LVEF ≤35%). SSI was determined from mid-LV short-axis views radial strain analysis. Patients with lower SSI less than 9.7% had significantly more HF hospitalizations or deaths over 2 years after CRT (HR = 3.1, 95% CI 1.89–5.26, $P < .001$), and more deaths, heart transplants, or LV assist devices (LVAD; HR = 3.57, 95% CI 1.81–6.67, $P < .001$).[23] Current clinical guidelines advocate CRT as a Class I indication in patients with LBBB morphology and QRS width greater than 150 ms. Presently, there is less clinical certainty for CRT utilization for patients with intermediate ECG criteria: QRS 120–149 ms or non-LBBB morphologies, where CRT are Class IIa or Class IIb indications.[16,17] Accordingly, analysis of SSI was tested in a subgroup of 113 patients with these intermediate ECG criteria. SSI less than 9.7% was independently associated with significantly more HF hospitalizations or deaths (HR = 2.44, 95% CI 1.27–4.35, $P = .004$), and more deaths, heart transplants or LVADs (HR = 3.70, 95% CI 1.67–8.33, $P = .001$) (Fig. 25.9). These data suggest that SSI can identify the electromechanical substrate responsive to CRT and differentiate from nonelectrical causes of peak-to-peak dyssynchrony, such as contractile heterogeneity or scar that is not responsive to CRT. Furthermore, SSI can be additive to ECG criteria in patients with QRS width 120–149 ms or non-LBBB in its association with outcomes following CRT.

LACK OF SYNCHRONY AND RISK FOR VENTRICULAR ARRHYTHMIAS

The assessment of LV synchrony has been extended to be used as a marker for arrhythmia risk. A multicenter study of 569 patients greater than 40 days after acute myocardial infarction included longitudinal strain echocardiography and follow-up for serious ventricular arrhythmias.[29] There were 268 patients with ST-segment elevation myocardial infarction and 301 with non-ST-segment elevation myocardial infarction. The peak longitudinal strain from three standard apical views and the time from the ECG R-wave to peak negative strain were assessed in each segment. Peak strain dispersion was defined as the standard deviation from these 16 segments, reflecting contraction heterogeneity (Fig. 25.10). Ventricular arrhythmias, defined as sustained ventricular tachycardia or sudden death during a median 30 months

FIG. 25.9 Kaplan-Meier plots of cardiac resynchronization therapy (CRT) patients with intermediate electrocardiographic (ECG) criteria (QRS 120–149 ms or nonleft bundle branch block) grouped by baseline systolic stretch index (SSI) above and below 9.7%. The freedom from death, heart transplant, or left ventricular assist device was significantly greater (*P* = .001) after CRT in patients with SSI ≥9.7%. These data support SSI as identifying the electromechanical substrate responsive to CRT in these patients with intermediate ECG criteria. (*Modified from Lumens J, Tayal B, Walmsley J, et al. Differentiating electromechanical from non-electrical substrates of mechanical discoordination to identify responders to cardiac resynchronization therapy. Circ Cardiovasc Imaging. 2015;8[9]:e003744.*)

(interquartile range: 18 months) of follow-up, occurred in 15 patients (3%). Mechanical dispersion was increased (63 ± 25 ms vs. 42 ± 17 ms, $P < .001$) in patients with arrhythmias compared with those without. Mechanical dispersion was an independent predictor of arrhythmic events (per 10-ms increase, HR: 1.7; 95% CI: 1.2–2.5; $P < .01$). Importantly, mechanical dispersion was a marker for arrhythmia risk in patients with LVEFs greater than 35% ($P < .05$), whereas LVEF was not ($P = .33$). A combination of mechanical dispersion and global longitudinal strain showed the best positive predictive value for arrhythmic events (21%; 95% CI: 6%–46%). In another important study, 94 patients with nonischemic cardiomyopathy were studied by speckle-tracking longitudinal strain echocardiography.[30] Global longitudinal strain was calculated as the average of peak longitudinal strain from a 16-segments and peak strain dispersion was defined as the standard deviation of time to peak negative strain from 16 LV segments. These 94 patients were followed for a median of 22 months (range, 1–46 months), where 12 patients (13%) had experienced arrhythmic events, defined as sustained ventricular tachycardia or cardiac arrest. As expected, LVEF and global longitudinal strain were reduced in the nonischemic cardiomyopathy patients with arrhythmic events compared with those without (28 ± 10% vs. 38 ± 13%, $P = .01$, and −6.4 ± 3.3% vs. −12.3 ± 5.2%, $P < .001$, respectively). Patients with arrhythmic events had significantly increased mechanical dispersion (98 ± 43 vs. 56 ± 18 ms, $P < .001$). Mechanical dispersion was found to predict arrhythmias independently of LVEF (HR, 1.28; 95% CI, 1.11–1.49; $P = .001$).[30]

Tissue Doppler cross-correlation analysis was also used as a measure of lack of synchrony after CRT-defibrillator therapy (CRT-D) associated with ventricular arrhythmias. In a two-center study, 151 CRT-D patients (New York Heart Association functional classes II–IV, EF ≤35%, and QRS duration ≥120 ms) were prospectively studied by tissue Doppler cross-correlation analysis of myocardial acceleration curves from the basal segments in the apical views.[31] Cross-correlation assessments were performed at baseline and 6 months after CRT-D implantation. Patients were divided into four subgroups on the basis of dyssynchrony at baseline and follow-up after CRT-D. Outcome events were predefined as appropriate anti-tachycardia pacing, shock, or death over 2 years. There were 97 patients (64%) with cross-correlation dyssynchrony at baseline and 42 (43%) had persistent dyssynchrony at 6 months. Among the 54 patients with no dyssynchrony at baseline, there were 15 (28%) who had onset of new cross-correlation dyssynchrony after CRT-D. In comparison with the group with improved cross-correlation dyssynchrony, patients with persistent dyssynchrony after CRT-D had a substantially increased risk for ventricular arrhythmias (HR, 4.4; 95% CI, 1.2–16.3; $P = .03$) and ventricular arrhythmias or death (HR, 4.0; 95% CI, 1.7–9.6; $P = .002$) after adjusting for other covariates. Similarly, patients with newly developed cross-correlation dyssynchrony after CRT-D had increased risk for serious ventricular arrhythmias (HR, 10.6; 95% CI, 2.8–40.4; $P = .001$) and serious ventricular arrhythmias or death (HR, 5.0; 95% CI, 1.8–13.5; $P = .002$). These studies combine to demonstrate the promising clinical utility of tissue Doppler cross-correlation or speckle tracking strain dispersion as risk markers for ventricular arrhythmias in patients with a range of cardiac diseases.

DYSSYNCHRONY ASSOCIATED WITH RIGHT VENTRICULAR PACING

The original randomized controlled clinical trials for CRT did not include patients who have received right ventricular (RV) pacing for bradycardia indications and, accordingly, upgrade to RV pacing was not originally in the guidelines for CRT. Echocardiographic applications of speckle tracking strain analysis have made contributions to our understanding of mechanical activation with RV pacing.[32] Tanaka et al. used three-dimensional strain imaging to demonstrate that LBBB has early basal septal mechanical activation with later posterior wall activation (Fig. 25.11).[33] In comparison, RV pacing demonstrated early apical septal mechanical activation with later posterior wall activation (Fig. 25.12; Videos 25.6 and 25.7). Both scenarios of LBBB and RV apical pacing

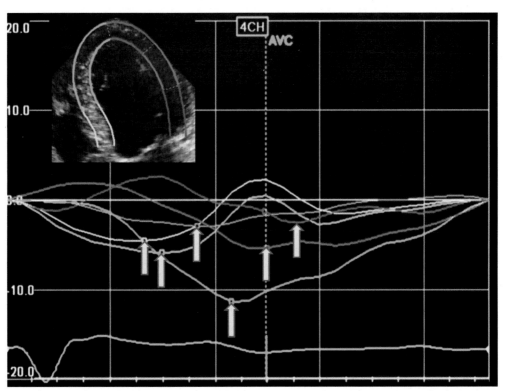

FIG. 25.10 An echocardiographic four-chamber view with regions of interest placed on the left ventricular walls and six color-coded segmental longitudinal strain curves. The *arrows* demonstrate differences in time to peak longitudinal strain, consistent with a patient with longitudinal peak strain dispersion. An increase in peak longitudinal strain dispersion has been associated with risk for ventricular arrhythmias.

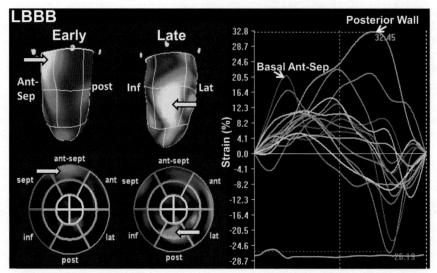

FIG. 25.11 **Three-dimensional strain images of a patient with intrinsic left bundle branch block.** Three-dimensional strain images are at the *top left* with polar maps at the *bottom left*, and time-strain curves from a 16-segment model appear on the *right*. Images show early mechanical activation of the basal septum and late activation of the mid-posterior wall *(arrows)*, associated with septal stretch. *LBBB,* Left bundle branch block.

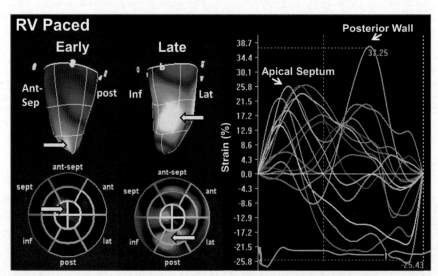

FIG. 25.12 Three-dimensional strain images of a patient with right ventricular (RV) pacing who subsequently underwent an upgrade to resynchronization therapy. Three-dimensional strain images are at the *top left* with polar maps at the *bottom left*, and time-strain curves from a 16-segment model appear on the *right*. Images show early mechanical activation of the apical septum and late activation of the mid-posterior wall *(arrows)*, associated with septal stretch.

can be associated with dyssynchronous regional contraction and stretch in the opposing walls, which has been associated with LV remodeling.[32] Several groups have shown that patients with reduced EF and RV pacing can receive clinical benefits from CRT.[34–36] A recent study of 135 patients compared 85 with native wide LBBB greater than 150 ms to 50 with RV pacing who underwent CRT.[36] At baseline the LV contraction pattern was determined using speckle tracking echocardiography in the apical four-chamber view. Although both patient groups received benefit, patients with RV pacing were found to have a significantly favorable long-term outcome compared to LBBB (HR = 0.36 95% CI 0.14–0.96; *P* = .04). Both LBBB and RV pacing groups demonstrated typical dyssynchronous contraction patterns. These data combine to support echocardiographic assessment of synchrony to guide support for CRT upgrade in patients with reduced EF and RV pacing.

FUTURE APPLICATIONS OF ECHOCARDIOGRAPHIC SYNCHRONY

In summary, interest in echocardiographic assessment of mechanical synchrony and dyssynchrony has remained high for over 15 years.

Great advances in understanding of mechanical dyssynchrony have occurred, in particular, a new appreciation of confounding variables that affect regional contraction synchrony and potential means to identify the electromechanical substrate of CRT response. However, the current role of echocardiographic measures of dyssynchrony remain as prognostic markers and further work is required (Box 25.1). In a unifying hypothesis for the role of measuring mechanical dyssynchrony for CRT (Fig. 25.13), a large body of literature has supported that patients who have widened QRS complexes but no measurable mechanical dyssynchrony have a less favorable response to CRT. The mechanistic basis for this association remains unknown. Electromechanical association exists at the cellular and myofiber level, so the reason for electrical dispersion (QRS widening) with no measurable mechanical dyssynchrony by current techniques remains a topic for future investigation. A new understanding of mechanical dyssynchrony in narrow QRS width patients from contractile heterogeneity or regional scar has shown that this interaction was more complicated than originally thought. We have learned that CRT in narrow QRS patients with mechanical dyssynchrony and reduced EF is not beneficial and may be harmful. Among patients with QRS widening,

BOX 25.1 Clinical Utility of Echocardiographic Measures of Synchrony

Established Roles
- As marker for prognosis after cardiac resynchronization therapy.
- As marker for prognosis in other cardiac diseases.

Potential Future Roles
- As an adjunct to ECG to improve patient selection for cardiac resynchronization therapy.
- As an adjunct to ejection fraction to improve patient selection for defibrillator implantation.

ECG, Electrocardiographic.

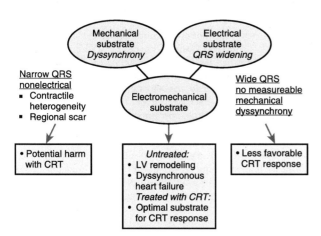

FIG. 25.13 A diagram of the proposed interaction between electrical delay (QRS widening) and mechanical delay (dyssynchrony) in myocardial substrates. The electromechanical substrate contains minimal elements of both electrical and mechanical properties associated with response to cardiac resynchronization therapy (CRT). *LV,* Left ventricular.

it appears that systolic stretch is a mechanical marker for LV remodeling that can respond favorably to CRT. Specifically, prestretch of posterolateral free wall before aortic valve opening and subsequent septal stretch appear to be important markers for CRT response, in particular with patients in whom the QRS pattern is of intermediate criteria (120–149 ms width or non-LBBB). Understanding and clinical applications of echocardiographic measures of dyssynchrony have changed considerably over the last decade and will continue to evolve with advances in greater understanding.

Suggested Reading

Ahmed, M., Gorcsan, J., 3rd, Marek, J., et al. (2014). Right ventricular apical pacing-induced left ventricular dyssynchrony is associated with a subsequent decline in ejection fraction. *Heart Rhythm, 11*(4), 602–608.

Gorcsan, J., 3rd, Abraham, T., Agler, D. A., et al. (2008). Echocardiography for cardiac resynchronization therapy: recommendations for performance and reporting—a report from the American Society of Echocardiography Dyssynchrony Writing Group endorsed by the Heart Rhythm Society. *Journal of the American Society of Echocardiography, 21*(3), 191–213.

Gorcsan, J., 3rd, Sogaard, P., Bax, J. J., et al. (2016). Association of persistent or worsened echocardiographic dyssynchrony with unfavourable clinical outcomes in heart failure patients with narrow QRS width: a subgroup analysis of the EchoCRT trial. *European Heart Journal, 37*(1), 49–59.

Lumens, J., Tayal, B., Walmsley, J., et al. (2015). Differentiating electromechanical from non-electrical substrates of mechanical discoordination to identify responders to cardiac resynchronization therapy. *Circulation Cardiovascular Imaging, 8*(9), e003744.

Risum, N., Tayal, B., Hansen, T. F., et al. (2015). Identification of typical left bundle branch block contraction by strain echocardiography is additive to electrocardiography in prediction of long-term outcome after cardiac resynchronization therapy. *Journal of the American College of Cardiology, 66*(6), 631–641.

A complete reference list can be found online at ExpertConsult.com.

26 Echocardiography in Assessment of Ventricular Assist Devices

Deepak K. Gupta

INTRODUCTION

Mechanical circulatory support is increasing in the acute and chronic management of heart failure patients. Both short-term and longer-term support ventricular assist devices (VADs) are in clinical use. Echocardiography may help guide patient selection as well as placement, optimization, and surveillance of these devices. This chapter will focus on the role of echocardiography in the evaluation and management of the patient who may need or has a left ventricular assist device (LVAD), in particular, the longer-term surgically implanted continuous flow devices.

TYPES OF VENTRICULAR ASSIST DEVICES

Short-Term Ventricular Assist Devices

For acute or short-term mechanical circulatory support, several devices are currently available. The intraaortic balloon pump (IABP) is the "original" short-term VAD and is frequently used for very short-term support in shock, often during revascularization procedures. It augments left ventricle (LV) output via balloon deflation in systole (decreasing afterload), and improved coronary perfusion by inflation during diastole. On transthoracic echocardiography, it can be viewed on parasternal long-axis and subcostal windows within the thoracic and abdominal aorta (Video 26.1). Percutaneously placed VADs (PVADs) that are Food and Drug Administration (FDA) approved include the TandemHeart (CardiacAssist, Inc., Pittsburgh, Pennsylvania) and Impella system (Abiomed Inc., Danvers, Massachusetts). The TandemHeart is an extracorporeal centrifugal pump that draws blood out of the body through an inflow cannula positioned in the left atrium (Video 26.2) (access via femoral vein and transseptal puncture) and delivers blood through an outflow cannula positioned in a femoral artery. The Impella is a catheter-based system that contains a microaxial continuous flow pump at its distal end and outflow cannula more proximally. The Impella catheter is placed via a femoral or axillary artery retrograde across the aortic valve such that the distal cannula lies in the LV and proximal outflow port lies in the ascending aorta (Video 26.3). Echocardiographic imaging is useful prior to PVAD placement to identify contraindications to their use; for example, left atrial or left ventricular thrombus, severe aortic or mitral stenosis (Impella), or severe aortic regurgitation. Echocardiography may help guide placement of these devices, and assess proper catheter position and stability: the TandemHeart catheter should cross the interatrial septum, with the perforated end residing in the left atrium only. Prolapse of the perforated segment into the right atrium would result in desaturated venous blood being drawn in to the LVAD. The Impella catheter should be seen traversing the left ventricular outflow tract (LVOT) into the aortic root and ascending aorta. Serial echocardiography may also be used to assess the ventricular response to mechanical unloading.

Surgically implanted short-term extracorporeal VADs include the Thoratec Paracorporeal Ventricular Assist Device and CentriMag (Thoratec Corp., Pleasanton, California), which are pneumatically driven pulsatile and centrifugal continuous flow pumps, respectively. Similar to the TandemHeart, these devices have inflow cannulas placed in the chamber proximal to the failing ventricle (i.e., the left atrium), which draw blood out of the body via an extracorporeal pump and then into an outflow cannula that is surgically implanted into the vessel distal to the failing ventricle (i.e., the aorta). Echocardiography is used for preimplant

evaluation and postimplant surveys for complications and/or myocardial recovery.

Long-Term Surgically Implanted Ventricular Assist Devices

The two currently FDA-approved continuous-flow left VADs are the HeartMate II (Thoratec Corp., Pleasanton, California) and heartware ventricular assist device Ventricular Assist System (Heartware International Inc., Framingham, Massachusetts). The HeartMate II is approved for both bridge to transplantation and destination therapy, while the Heartware device is approved for bridge to transplantation. Both devices have an inflow cannula implanted near the LV apex, a mechanical impeller, and outflow graft to the ascending aorta. The axillary flow impeller for the HeartMate II is implanted subdiaphragmatically, whereas the centrifugal flow Heartware impeller is intrapericardial (Fig. 26.1A, B). The impeller location influences echocardiographic imaging because of the shadowing and artifact produced, as described later. The remainder of this chapter will focus on long-term surgically implanted LVADs, with regard to echocardiographic imaging needed when planning for LVAD, during LVAD implantation, and post-LVAD placement.

PLANNING FOR A LEFT VENTRICULAR ASSIST DEVICE

A number of considerations regarding cardiac structure and function inform the decision and planning for implantation of an LVAD. Most patients with suspected or known heart failure will have had one or more echocardiograms prior to the initiation of a formal evaluation for or the decision to implant an LVAD. Consequently, in a patient with suspected or known heart failure, it is important to perform a comprehensive transthoracic echocardiogram that will allow the health care team to appropriately evaluate a patient's candidacy and suitability for a LVAD if one is needed. Several parameters of cardiac structure and function are of particular relevance to this decision making (Table 26.1).

Left Ventricular Structure and Function

Severe left ventricular dysfunction, typically an ejection fraction less than 25%, is required to be a candidate for an LVAD. Therefore, the accurate quantification of left ventricular volumes at end diastole and systole is necessary using the biplane method of disks to allow calculation of left ventricular ejection fraction. Left ventricular size, measured on the parasternal long-axis view as the end-diastolic diameter, may also factor into the assessment of a patient's candidacy for LVAD, as pre-LVAD end-diastolic diameters less than 6.3 cm may be associated with an increased risk of postoperative morbidity and mortality.[1] The presence of left ventricular, particularly apical, thrombus, will also impact surgical planning, approach, and procedure. Evaluation of left ventricular function, size, and thrombus may be facilitated by the use of echocardiographic contrast agents.[2]

Right Ventricular Structure and Function

Right ventricular size and systolic function, as well as tricuspid regurgitation, should be assessed on pre-LVAD echocardiography. Right

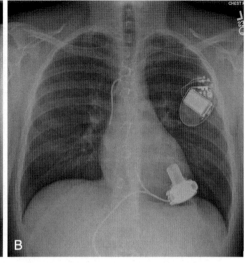

FIG. 26.1 Chest x-rays of continuous flow left ventricular assist devices. (A) HeartMate II. Note the subdiaphragmatic position of the axillary flow pump, which limits subcostal echocardiographic views. (B) Heartware. Note the apical (intrapericardial) position of the centrifugal flow pump, which limits apical echocardiographic views.

TABLE 26.1 Key Features of Cardiac Structure and Function to Be Evaluated on Pre-Left Ventricular Assist Device Echocardiography

STRUCTURE	PRE-LVAD EVALUATION	IMPLICATION
Left ventricle	Function	Indication for LVAD, LVEF typically <25%
	Size	LVEDD <6.3 cm associated with worse post-LVAD outcomes
	Thrombus	May cause obstruction of LVAD inflow cannula or emboli
Right ventricle	Size and function	Enlargement and dysfunction associated with worse post-LVAD outcomes May indicate need for biventricular mechanical support
Septum	Shunt	May result in post-LVAD hypoxemia or paradoxic emboli
Aortic valve	Regurgitation	Attenuates LV unloading and systemic delivery of blood post-LVAD
	Mechanical prosthesis	Increased thrombosis risk post-LVAD
Mitral valve	Stenosis	Impaired filling of LVAD
Tricuspid valve	Regurgitation	Indicator of right ventricular dysfunction and worse post-LVAD outcomes
	Stenosis	Impairment to filling left heart and LVAD
Pulmonic valve	Regurgitation	Indicator of right ventricular dysfunction
	Stenosis	Impairment to filling left heart and LVAD
Aorta	Dilation, plaque, dissection	May impact outflow graft cannulation site
Endocarditis	Valves or devices	Active infection is a contraindication to LVAD placement
Thrombus	Left atrial or ventricular	May embolize causing LVAD obstruction or systemic emboli

LV, Left ventricular; *LVAD,* left ventricular assist device; *LVEF,* left ventricular ejection fraction; *LVEDD,* left ventricular end diastolic diameter.

ventricular dilation and dysfunction may influence medical and surgical management decisions regarding the need for biventricular support rather than LVAD alone, perioperatively, and more long term.[3] A preoperative RV fractional area change (RVFAC) of less than 20% is associated with RV failure upon LVAD device activation. Additionally, right ventricular dysfunction and other clinical factors (such as dependence on inotropes, or elevated liver function tests) are markers of worse prognosis post-LVAD implantation. Currently, however, there is no single right ventricular parameter or clinical factor that accurately differentiates patients who will have a better or worse prognosis.[4,5]

Valves

Valvular lesions that may potentially impair LVAD function are critical to identify and treat prior to or at the time of LVAD implantation. Moderate or severe mitral stenosis impairs left ventricular filling and, therefore, flow into the LVAD inflow cannula. Similarly, right-sided valvular stenosis will also impair filling of the left heart and LVAD

inflow. In contrast, aortic stenosis, regardless of severity, typically does not impair LVAD function, as the outflow cannula bypasses the LVOT and aortic valve.

Careful attention must be given to the presence, mechanism, and severity of aortic regurgitation prior to LVAD implantation. Aortic regurgitation attenuates left ventricular unloading and systemic delivery of blood in the setting of an LVAD due to the creation of a loop of blood that travels through the LVAD inflow cannula, pump, then outflow graft into the ascending aorta, where it falls back into the LV through the regurgitant aortic valve. Significant regurgitation of right-sided valves is also a concern of pre-LVAD, as this may be a marker of right ventricular dysfunction, which is associated with a worse prognosis post-LVAD. Following LVAD implantation, tricuspid regurgitation could worsen due to changes in right ventricular geometry and tricuspid valve anatomy that result from over-decompression of the LV and shifting of the interventricular septum. Mitral regurgitation, however, typically improves as a result of an LVAD placement because of decompression of the LV both with

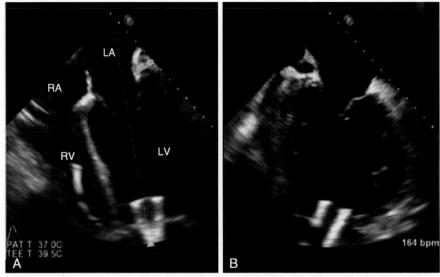

FIG. 26.2 Intraoperative transesophageal echocardiography demonstrating proper positioning of the left ventricular assist device inflow cannula. (A) Mid-esophageal four-chamber view. (B) Mid-esophageal two-chamber view. *LA,* Left atrium; *LV,* left ventricle; *RA,* right atrium; *RV,* right ventricle. (*From Stainback RF, Estep JD, Agler DA, et al. Echocardiography in the management of patients with left ventricular assist devices: recommendations from the American Society of Echocardiography.* J Am Soc Echocardiogr. *2015;28[8]:853-909.*)

regard to size, resulting in better mitral valve leaflet coaptation, and decline in pressures.

A mechanical aortic valve also needs to be identified pre-LVAD implantation and converted to a bioprosthetic valve at the time of LVAD placement to limit the risk of aortic valve thrombosis. Since LVAD outflow bypasses the native LVOT, a mechanical aortic valve would not open sufficiently in the setting of an LVAD and therefore be likely to thrombose. This is less of an issue for mechanical mitral valves, as the forward flow from left atrium to LV is maintained by the LVAD.

Endocarditis

Active infection is a contraindication to LVAD implantation; therefore, lesions suspicious for endocarditis, whether on valves or indwelling devices such as pacemaker/defibrillator leads or catheters, must be carefully evaluated.

Aorta

Since the LVAD outflow graft is typically implanted into the ascending aorta, attention should be given to the presence of aortic pathology, such as dilation, plaque, and dissection.

Congenital Heart Disease

Right-to-left shunts, such as a patent foramen ovale, atrial and ventricular septal defects, need to be identified prior to LVAD implantation because decompression of the left side of the heart by the LVAD may increase right-to-left shunting and sequelae, such as hypoxemia and paradoxic emboli. The evaluation for shunts is typically performed on the intraoperative transesophageal echocardiogram at the time of LVAD implantation. Detection of shunts is enhanced with agitated saline ("bubble") contrast.[6]

INTRAOPERATIVE

Preimplantation

An intraoperative transesophageal echocardiogram should be performed prior to LVAD implantation to identify any pathology that may impact proper LVAD function that has not been identified or has changed compared with preoperative transthoracic echocardiograms. The comprehensive transesophageal echocardiographic evaluation should include assessment of left and right ventricular structure and function, valves, aorta, and the atrial and ventricular septum, with particular attention to

aortic regurgitation, right ventricular function, tricuspid regurgitation, shunts, and thrombi.

Implantation and Activation of Left Ventricular Assist Device

Near the apex of the LV a core of myocardium is removed to allow placement of the LVAD inflow cannula. Consequently, air enters the LV, prompting the need for deairing maneuvers prior to completion of the surgery. Continuous transesophageal echocardiogram (TEE) monitoring of the pulmonary veins, left heart chambers, LVAD inflow cannula, and outflow graft, as well as aorta, are needed to guide the de-airing maneuvers.

When the LVAD is activated, transesophageal echocardiography may help identify acute complications that include shunt, aortic regurgitation, right ventricular dysfunction, and/or malpositioning of the LVAD inflow cannula and outflow graft. With decompression of the left side of the heart by the LVAD, a shunt may be more easily detected, and therefore, a repeat agitated saline ("bubble") contrast study should be performed. Similarly, the presence, duration, and severity of aortic regurgitation may be more readily visualized when the LV is decompressed. Whether and to what extent the aortic valve opens with each cardiac cycle should also be evaluated by two-dimensional (2D) and M-mode imaging. Right ventricular dysfunction is not uncommon following cardiac surgery and this may be transient or represent worsening of chronic dysfunction. Excessive LVAD speeds may also cause right ventricular dysfunction through distortion of the right ventricular geometry and tricuspid valve structure induced by shifting the interventricular septum leftward.

Transesophageal echocardiography can also help visualize positioning of the LVAD inflow cannula and outflow graft, during implantation, once the LVAD is activated and at different speed settings, and following closure of the chest. The LVAD inflow cannula is implanted near the apex and is typically directed towards the mitral valve without interfering with the subvalvular apparatus (Fig. 26.2). While some angulation towards the septum may occur, excess angulation or proximity to the septum may be problematic acutely or chronically as an impediment to LVAD filling or a trigger for ventricular arrhythmias (Video 26.4). Doppler interrogation of the inflow cannula should reveal continuous laminar low velocities (≤1.5 m/sec) directed into the LVAD with slight systolic and diastolic variation, but without regurgitation (Fig. 26.3).[7,8] High velocities may indicate mechanical obstruction along the path of blood flow into the LVAD inflow cannula. This may be caused by obstruction due to the septum, papillary muscles or mitral chordae, or thrombi either at the mouth of or within the inflow cannula. Doppler signals can typically be obtained on the HeartMate II device, but the pericardial position of the Heartware

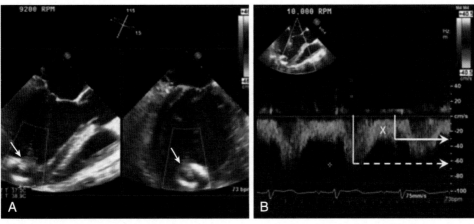

FIG. 26.3 Color (A) and spectral (B) Doppler interrogation of left ventricular assist device inflow on transesophageal echocardiography. The lack of aliasing in the color Doppler signal suggests unobstructed laminar flow. The spectral Doppler tracing shows systolic augmentation of inflow *(dotted arrow)* above the continuous inflow observed in diastole *(solid arrow)*. *(From Stainback RF, Estep JD, Agler DA, et al. Echocardiography in the management of patients with left ventricular assist devices: recommendations from the American Society of Echocardiography. J Am Soc Echocardiogr. 2015;28[8]:853-909.)*

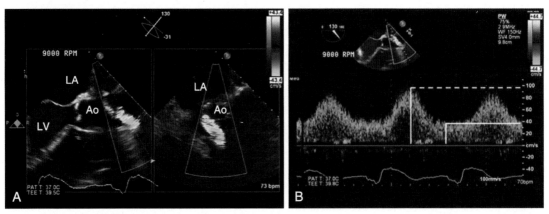

FIG. 26.4 Color (A) and spectral (B) Doppler interrogation of left ventricular assist device outflow in the ascending aorta by transesophageal echocardiography. The spectral Doppler tracing shows systolic augmentation of inflow *(dotted line)* above the continuous inflow observed in diastole *(solid line)*. *Ao,* Aorta; *LA,* left atrium; *LV,* left ventricle. *(From Stainback RF, Estep JD, Agler DA, et al. Echocardiography in the management of patients with left ventricular assist devices: recommendations from the American Society of Echocardiography. J Am Soc Echocardiogr. 2015;28[8]:853-909.)*

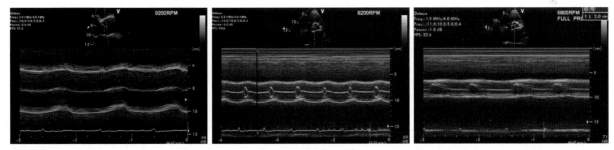

FIG. 26.5 Aortic valve opening assessed by M-mode during speed changes in a patient with a HeartMate II left ventricular assist device. As the speed decreases from 9200 to 6800 rpm, the left ventricle is less unloaded and aortic valve opening increases in duration.

device interferes with Doppler signals and often precludes interpretable tracings, particularly when the cannula is present within the imaging window. The body of the outflow graft as it courses along the right ventricle and the anastomosis with the ascending aorta near the right pulmonary artery are usually visualized on TEE. Doppler interrogation should reveal continuous and laminar low velocities with slight systolic and diastolic variation (Fig. 26.4). Increases in velocity to greater than 2.0 m/s should raise suspicion for outflow obstruction, for example by thrombus or kinking of the apparatus.

POSTIMPLANT

The post-LVAD transthoracic echocardiography imaging protocol typically includes a comprehensive 2D, M-Mode, and Doppler study

similar to what would be done pre-LVAD for a heart failure patient, with the addition of images to characterize the LVAD inflow cannula and outflow graft. Transthoracic imaging of the LVAD inflow cannula and velocities can usually be obtained in patients with a HeartMate II device, but is more difficult in patients with Heartware devices because of interference and shadowing induced by apical intrapericardial position of the pump. The outflow graft at its aortic anastomosis can be visualized from a high left parasternal long-axis imaging window, while the body of the graft can be visualized in the right parasternal view.

The aortic valve is particularly important to evaluate on post-LVAD echocardiography. Aortic valve opening by 2D and M-mode imaging should be assessed on each study as it provides important information regarding LVAD and native ventricular function (Fig. 26.5). A closed aortic valve may reflect appropriate or possibly over-decompression of the LV. However, an aortic valve that remains closed with every cardiac cycle may be at risk for aortic root thrombosis (Video 26.5), cusp thickening/fusion, as well as aortic regurgitation (Video 26.6).[10–13] Whether the optimal LVAD speed setting is one that leads to complete closure of the aortic valve or intermittent opening remains controversial and may change in an individual patient over time.[9] Alternatively, the aortic valve may be closed because of surgical or percutaneous treatment of a regurgitant aortic valve at the time of or following LVAD implantation.[14,15] In contrast, an aortic valve that opens fully with every cardiac cycle may indicate insufficient decompression due to LVAD dysfunction, as in pump thrombosis, or conversely, may suggest improvement in native left ventricular function. These two scenarios should clinically present in different ways, with the former patient likely having symptomatic heart failure, while the latter should not. Left ventricular function should also differentiate these patients, with the former having more severely depressed function, and the latter likely having normal to mildly reduced function.

The indications for post-LVAD echocardiography include evaluation for complications and assessment for reverse remodeling or improvement in native left ventricular function. The timing of post-LVAD echocardiography may be driven by chronic surveillance in a stable patient and acute changes in clinical condition. For chronic surveillance in a stable asymptomatic patient, transthoracic echocardiography is recommended by the American Society of Echocardiography to occur postoperatively at 2 weeks, 1, 3, 6, and 12 months, and then every 6–12 months thereafter.[9] Surveillance images are typically obtained only at the baseline LVAD speed setting, unless unexpected findings are visualized prompting the need for speed changes.

Changes in clinical status of a LVAD patient may also warrant evaluation by echocardiography. Conditions in LVAD patients in which echocardiography may be helpful diagnostically include worsening heart failure, syncope, hypotension or hypertension, arrhythmias, fever, anemia, stroke or systemic emboli, bleeding, renal failure, and/or cardiac arrest. A summary of selected post-LVAD complications and echocardiographic findings is shown in Table 26.2. An example of post-LVAD pericardial effusion causing tamponade is shown in Video 26.7. An example of the LVAD outflow graft (extending from the outflow cannula in the ascending aorta) kinking and causing increased flow velocities is shown in Fig. 26.6 and Video 26.8. In some cases, particularly small patients, changes in position may alter the geometry of the LVAD hardware with respect to the heart, and dynamic echocardiography performed in the positions that bring on symptoms should be considered.

Dynamic or speed-change echocardiography (also known as "ramp" or "optimization") protocols with imaging at baseline LVAD speed and following increases or decreases in speed may be necessary in symptomatic patients or asymptomatic patients based upon findings on surveillance echocardiography, lab results (e.g., anemia and hemolysis), or those experiencing LVAD alarms. For example, if an LVAD patient presents in heart failure and the LV is found to be dilated, with a rightward-shifted interventricular septum and severe mitral regurgitation, then an increase in LVAD speed may be necessary not only to help decompression, but also to evaluate if there is LVAD dysfunction, as in pump thrombosis. Conversely, if an LVAD patient presents with symptoms of orthostasis and syncope and the LVAD inflow cannula is found to be abutting a leftward-shifted interventricular septum (i.e., a "suction-down" effect), then a decrease in LVAD speed may be necessary. Specific optimization and ramp protocols vary by center. In general, these protocols require an experienced sonographer as well as a member of LVAD team that has expertise in image interpretation and decision algorithms regarding LVAD speed changes based upon the echocardiographic findings in the context of the clinical scenario. Key parameters to follow include left and right ventricular size and systolic function, the frequency of aortic valve opening, the position of the interventricular septum, and any significant valvular regurgitation as well as estimated PA systolic pressures. Confirmation of therapeutic anticoagulation on the day of echocardiography is important given the risk of pump thrombosis and emboli, particularly with reduction in LVAD speeds. Additionally, speed changes should not be made if aortic root or intracardiac thrombus is identified on images obtained at the baseline speed.

Post-LVAD echocardiography may also be indicated to assess for reverse remodeling and recovery of native myocardial function, albeit

TABLE 26.2 Left Ventricular Assist Device-Related Complications and Associated Echocardiographic Findings

COMPLICATION	ECHOCARDIOGRAPHIC FINDINGS
Pericardial effusion (± tamponade)	RV compression Respirophasic changes in flow Reduced right-sided stroke volume and output
Heart failure due to insufficient LV unloading	Increased LV size Aortic valve opening Increased left atrial size Increased transmitral Spectral Doppler E velocity Increased transmitral E/A Increased E/e′ Shortened E wave deceleration time Increased mitral regurgitation Increased right ventricular systolic pressure
Heart failure due to RV failure	Increased RV size Decreased RV systolic function High right atrial pressure (IVC dilation, bowing of interatrial septum to left) Leftward position of interventricular septum (possibly due to high LVAD speed) Increased tricuspid regurgitant flow Reduced RV stroke volume and output Reduced LVAD inflow and outflow velocities (<0.5 m/s) with severe RV failure
Excessive LV unloading or underfilled LV	Small LV size (< 3 cm) Small LA size Leftward position of interventricular septum
LVAD suction	Small LV size or LVAD inflow cannula abutting myocardium (typically septum) Ventricular ectopy
Aortic insufficiency	Dilated LV Aortic regurgitant jet to LVOT height >46% Aortic regurgitant jet vena contract ≥3 mm Reduced RV stroke volume despite normal to increased LVAD flow
Mitral regurgitation	Primary: due to LVAD inflow interference with mitral apparatus Secondary (Functional): due to insufficient LV unloading by LVAD
Intracardiac thrombus	Left ventricular or LVAD associated Aortic root (particularly with closed aortic valve) Atrial
Inflow-cannula abnormality	Obstruction due to myocardium, mitral apparatus, or thrombus Malpositioning High inflow velocities (>1.5 m/s) and/or aliasing (turbulent flow) on color Doppler Severely reduced LVAD inflow velocities suggestive of pump thrombosis
Outflow-graft abnormality	Obstruction due to kink or thrombosis High outflow velocities (>2 m/s) near obstruction Low or absent outflow velocities if pulsed wave Doppler interrogated away from obstruction No change in LV size or RV stroke volume with increases in LVAD speed
Hypertensive emergency	Reduction in aortic valve opening Increase in LV size Increase in mitral regurgitation
Pump malfunction/pump arrest	Reduced LVAD inflow and outflow graft flow velocities Aortic valve opening despite increase in LVAD speed Increased mitral regurgitation Increased tricuspid regurgitation Pump arrest (off): diastolic flow reversal of flow through LVAD into LV Increase in LV size

IVC, Inferior vena cava; *LA*, left atrium; *LV*, left ventricle; *LVOT*, left ventricular outflow tract; *RV*, right ventricle.

Adapted from Stainback RF, Estep JD, Agler DA, et al. Echocardiography in the management of patients with left ventricular assist devices: recommendations from the American Society of Echocardiography. J Am Soc Echocardiogr. 2015;28[8]:853-909.

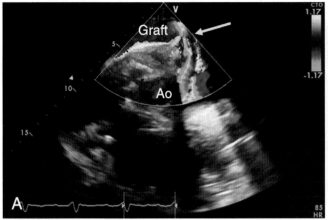 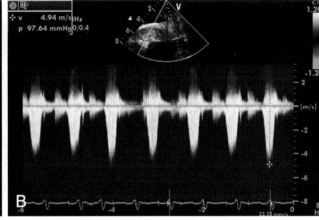

FIG. 26.6 Left ventricle outflow graft kink. (A) Shows a high parasternal transthoracic echocardiogram of the ascending aorta (Ao) with left ventricular outflow tract cannula and graft, showing an acute kink *(arrow)* in the graft obstructing outflow. This causes turbulence on color Doppler and severely increased peak flow velocities as shown on spectral Doppler in (B). See also corresponding Video 26.8.

this is an infrequent event.[16] Due to poor acoustic windows and artifact induced by the LVAD inflow cannula, apical images for assessment of LV volumes are limited. Therefore, quantification of LV size in LVAD patients is typically taken as the internal diastolic dimension from the parasternal long-axis view.[9] Native left ventricular ejection fraction is also difficult to assess post-LVAD implantation. If sufficient quality apical images are obtainable to make reliable measures of end-diastolic and systolic volumes, then ejection fraction should be quantified. In the absence of interpretable apical images, other options for assessing left ventricular function include fractional area change as determined from parasternal short-axis images at the level of papillary muscles, the Quinones method, or fractional shortening obtained from the parasternal long-axis images.[17–20] All of these methods are limited by assumptions regarding regional and global wall motion and synchrony. A constellation of parameters that may indicate reverse remodeling and recovery include palpable pulse with measurable pulse pressure, aortic valve opening with each cardiac cycle even at relatively high LVAD speeds, normal position of the interventricular septum, and reduction in left ventricular size and improvement in ejection fraction compared with preimplantation images. To more completely assess native cardiac function, LVAD speeds should be turned down incrementally towards minimal settings (HeartMate II = 6000 RPM and Heartware 1800 RPM) with imaging to identify when net neutral flow occurs through the LVAD. If at low speed there is evidence of substantial reverse remodeling and improvement in left ventricular function, then the patient may be a candidate for LVAD explantation. Provocative maneuvers, such as exercise, pharmacologic stress testing, or volume loading, can be performed with or without echocardiographic imaging and invasive hemodynamics at minimum LVAD

speed to further assess left ventricular functional reserve and the patient's candidacy for explantation. Following the low-speed study, the LVAD settings should be returned to baseline.

CONCLUSIONS

Mechanical circulatory support is increasing in the acute and chronic management of heart failure patients. Echocardiography may help guide patient selection as well as placement, optimization, and surveillance of these devices. Understanding the anatomic configuration of an LVAD within a patient's body and how this influences image acquisition and interpretation is important. LVAD echocardiography requires experienced sonographers, cardiologists, and members of the heart failure/LVAD team that are able to integrate the clinical scenario and echocardiographic data to inform management decisions. Standardization of imaging protocols, particularly for surveillance and dynamic (speed-change, or "ramp") echocardiography, may aid in defining the diagnostic and prognostic information gained from echocardiography in the LVAD patient population.

Suggested Reading

Ammar, K. A., Umland, M. M., Kramer, C., et al. (2012). The ABCs of left ventricular assist device echocardiography: a systematic approach. *European Heart Journal Cardiovascular Imaging, 13*, 885–899.
Estep, J. D., Stainback, R. F., Little, S. H., Torre, G., & Zoghbi, W. A. (2010). The role of echocardiography and other imaging modalities in patients with left ventricular assist devices. *JACC Cardiovasc Imaging, 3*, 1049–1064.
Stainback, R. F., Estep, J. D., Agler, D. A., et al. (2015). Echocardiography in the management of patients with left ventricular assist devices: recommendations from the American Society of Echocardiography. *Journal of the American Society of Echocardiography, 28*, 853–909.

A complete reference list can be found online at ExpertConsult.com.

27 Stress Echocardiography and Echo in Cardiopulmonary Testing

Mário Santos, Amil M. Shah

INTRODUCTION

Ischemic Cascade

Myocardial ischemia is classically characterized by a consistent, time-sequenced series of events known as the "ischemic cascade" (Fig. 27.1), which form the physiologic basis for greater sensitivity of stress testing with imaging (including echocardiography) compared to electrocardiography alone. The imbalance between oxygen demand and supply driven by heterogeneity in coronary flow initially results in metabolic changes, followed by abnormal mechanical function, and ultimately electrocardiographic changes and symptoms of angina.[1]

Stress Protocols

Exercise Protocols

Either exercise or pharmacologic stress agents can be used to increase myocardial oxygen demand. In general, exercise stress should be preferentially employed in any patient able to exercise given the wealth of prognostic and diagnostic information provided by functional capacity, heart rate response and recovery, blood pressure response, and electrocardiography. Symptom-limited exercise can be performed using a treadmill or cycle ergometer. In general, treadmill exercise is more widely available, allows for the attainment of greater maximal oxygen consumption (VO_{2max}), and is more physiologic, but has the disadvantage of allowing for imaging only after exercise, which limits the number of images that can be acquired and fails to record echo parameters at peak exercise when hemodynamics are maximally affected (Table 27.1). The semisupine cycle ergometer with a tilting table permits acquisition of images during each stage of the exercise protocol, including peak exercise. Initial workload and increases in workload are usually adjusted to each patient's expected functional capacity (10–25 W increase every 2–3 minutes). However, in patients who are not used to the cycle ergometer, VO_{2max} is expected to be lower than with treadmill exercise. Compared to the cycle ergometer, treadmill tests tend to demonstrate 10%–15% higher VO_{2max}, 5%–20% higher peak heart rate, and more frequent ST segment changes.[2] The contraindications for performing exercise echocardiography are the same as those for classical exercise testing.[3]

A standard set of echocardiographic images is obtained in the resting state, prior to exercise initiation, and either immediately postexercise (treadmill testing) or at peak exercise (cycle ergometer testing). Standard imaging views include: (1) parasternal long axis view; (2) parasternal short axis at the left ventricle (LV) base; (3) parasternal short axis at the mid-ventricular level; (4) apical 4-chamber; (5) apical 2-chamber; and (6) apical 3-chamber views. For treadmill testing, imaging is performed with the patient in left lateral decubitus position preexercise and immediately postexercise. As with standard exercise testing, achieving a peak heart rate of at least 85% of age-predicted maximal heart rate is considered a diagnostic workload.[4] As ischemia can rapidly resolve following the cessation of exercise, images should be acquired within 60 seconds of exercise termination.[5] With cycle ergometer stress, imaging is typically performed at rest, submaximal exercise (~25 W), peak exercise, and during recovery.

Pharmacologic Stress Protocols

Although either dobutamine or vasodilator agents can be used with echocardiography, dobutamine is the preferred and most commonly used agent for pharmacologic stress echocardiography. Dobutamine increases myocardial oxygen demand by increasing contractility primarily at lower doses and primarily heart rate at higher doses. In a standard dobutamine stress echocardiogram, dobutamine is infused at 5, 10, 20, 30, and 40 mcg/kg per minute, with the subsequent administration of atropine in 0.25–0.50 mg doses to a total of 2.0 mg to achieve a peak heart rate of 85% age-predicted maximal heart rate. Indications for test termination include (1) achievement of 85% of age-predicted maximal heart rate; (2) new or worsening wall motion abnormalities involving at least two segments; (3) significant arrhythmia; (4) hypotension; (5) severe hypertension; or (6) intolerable symptoms. Although rare, given the potential for serious risks, clinical judgment is essential in selecting patients appropriate for stress testing, as is careful monitoring by appropriately trained staff pre-, during, and posttesting.[6] For dobutamine stress tests in particular, beta-blocking agents (e.g., metoprolol, esmolol) should be available if necessary to treat potential atrial or ventricular tachyarrhythmias, severe hypertension, or angina.

Assessment of Ischemia

Image Interpretation

Regardless of the stress modality, interpretation of the echocardiographic images is based on assessment of the excursion and thickening of each myocardial segment at rest and with stress, along with changes in left ventricular ejection fraction (LVEF) and LV size with stress (Table 27.2). American Society of Echocardiography (ASE) Guidelines recommend use of the 16-segment model (or 17 segments with inclusion of the apical cap if comparison with other imaging modalities is anticipated) to evaluate segmental motion (Fig. 27.2).[7] Wall motion is classified as: (1) normal [resting] or hyperkinetic [stress]; (2) hypokinetic defined as preservation of thickening and inward systolic endocardial excursion but not to the extent of normal segments; (3) akinetic defined as absence of wall thickening or inward systolic endocardial excursion; and (4) dyskinetic defined as wall thinning and outward motion of the myocardial segment in systole (see Table 27.2). The normal response to stress is for all segments to become hyperkinetic. Based on segmental wall motion at rest and with

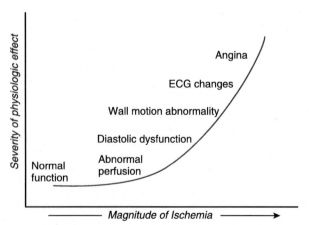

FIG. 27.1 The ischemic cascade. *ECG,* Electrocardiography.

TABLE 27.1 Comparison Between Treadmill and Semisupine Exercise Testing

	STRESS MODALITY	ADVANTAGES	DISADVANTAGES
Exercise	Treadmill	More physiological Widely available	Allows imaging only pre- and postexercise
	Semisupine	Allows imaging during each stage of an exercise protocol, both at lower workloads and at peak exercise	Lower expected maximal oxygen consumption Patient adaptation
Pharmacologic	Dobutamine	Allows for assessment in patients unable to exercise Allows for imaging at each stage of dobutamine infusion, both low and high dose	No data on functional capacity or exercise performance Risk of atrial and ventricular arrhythmias

TABLE 27.2 Classification of Regional Wall Motion

	WALL MOTION SCORE[a]	DEFINITION
Normal	1	Normal thickening and inward systolic endocardial excursion
Hypokinetic	2	Thickening and inward systolic endocardial excursion but not to the extent of normal segments
Akinetic	3	Absence of wall thickening or inward systolic endocardial excursion
Dyskinetic	4	Wall thinning and outward motion of the myocardial segment in systole

[a]Wall Motion Score Index (WMSI) is calculated as the sum of the segmental wall motion scores (using the 17-segment model) divided by the number of segments assessed.

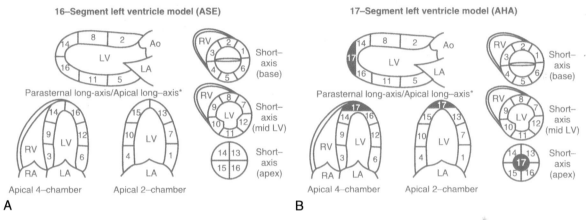

FIG. 27.2 Segmentation models of the left ventricle. (A) 16-segment model; (B) 17-segment model. *AHA,* American Heart Association; *Ao,* aorta; *ASE,* American Society of Echocardiography; *LA,* left atrium; *LV,* left ventricle; *RA,* right atrium; *RV,* right ventricle; *, also termed apical 3-chamber view. (*From Bulwer BE, Solomon SD, Janardhanan R. Echocardiographic assessment of ventricular systolic function. In: Solomon SD, ed.* Essential Echocardiography: A Practical Handbook with DVD. *Totora, NJ: Humana Press; 2007: 89–119.*)

TABLE 27.3 Image Interpretation of Stress Echocardiography for Ischemia Assessment[a]

DIAGNOSIS	REST	STRESS
Normal	Normal	Hyperkinetic
Ischemia	Normal	Worsens to hypokinetic, akinetic, or dyskinetic
Ischemia	Hypokinetic	Worsens to akinetic or dyskinetic
Infarct	Hypokinetic, akinetic or dyskinetic	No change
Viable	Akinetic	Improves to hypokinetic or normal

[a]See text for further discussion.

stress, each segment can be classified as normal, ischemic, infarcted, or viable (Table 27.3). An ischemic response is characterized by worsening contractility of at least two contiguous segments (Fig. 27.3). Infarction is characterized by resting dysfunction that fails to improve with stress. Using the 17-segment model, the Wall Motion Score Index (WMSI) is one method to quantify the global ventricular burden of ischemia and/or infarction. Segments are scored as 1 (normal [rest], hyperkinetic [stress]), 2 (hypokinetic), 3 (akinetic), and 4 (dyskinetic) at rest and at stress. The WMSI is calculated as the sum of segmental scores divided by the number of visualized segments. Moderate-severe ischemia is considered present when three or more newly dysfunctional segments are observed

with stress.[8] Additional potential etiologies for lack of a hyperkinetic response that must be considered during image interpretation include: (1) low workload including low heart rate secondary to beta-blocker use; (2) prolonged delay in image acquisition following test termination; and (3) severe hypertensive response to stress. Variability in image quality is the main limitation of stress echocardiography. The use of echo contrast to enhance endocardial border delineation in patients with poor acoustic windows can improve the diagnostic performance of the test and should be considered when two or more endocardial segments cannot be visualized at rest.[9]

Changes in global LV function and size are also important for test interpretation. Normally, LVEF should increase and become hyperdynamic with stress. With the treadmill, exercise is normally accompanied by a decrease in LV diastolic and systolic volumes. Increase in LV volume with stress is a high-risk finding in this context, associated with multivessel ischemia (Fig. 27.4). Of note, increase in LV cavity size is not necessarily an abnormal finding with supine cycle ergometry, given the associated preload recruitment.

The sensitivity and specificity of stress echocardiography for the detection of coronary artery disease is approximately 80%.[10] Patients with an intermediate probability of coronary disease will benefit most from stress echocardiography. Diagnostic performance is superior to exercise electrocardiography alone, and similar to nuclear perfusion stress testing. Studies suggest the stress echocardiography has a slightly lower sensitivity but better specificity compared to nuclear perfusion stress testing.[11] As noted previously, the risk of a false positive result is increased in

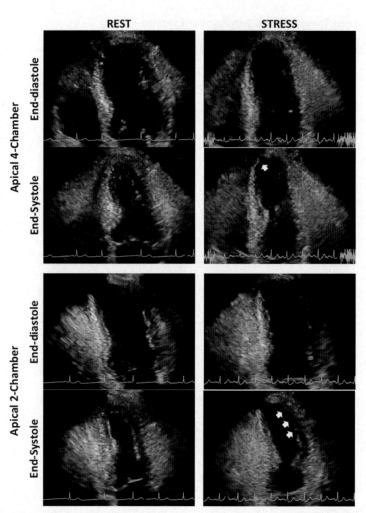

FIG. 27.3 Example of a treadmill stress echocardiogram demonstrating an inducible wall motion abnormality involving the mid and apical anterior segments. *Arrows* indicate segments of regional hypokinesis induced with exercise.

the presence of abnormal septal motion due to left-bundle branch block and a hypertensive response to exercise, while low workload, beta-blocker use, and prolonged delay in poststress image acquisition increase the risk of a false-negative result.

In addition to providing diagnostic information, stress echocardiography also provides important prognostic information. In patients with suspected coronary artery disease across a range of pretest probability, stress echocardiography provides incremental prognostic value beyond clinical, electrocardiographic, and resting echocardiographic variables.[12] A negative stress echocardiogram is associated with a rate of myocardial infarction or cardiac death similar to age-matched controls (<1%/year), suggesting that additional testing and intervention is unnecessary.[13] Similarly, among patients with known coronary artery disease, including prior revascularization, an abnormal stress echocardiogram is independently associated with a twofold greater risk of adverse outcomes.[14] Additional prognostic information is provided by the pharmacologic dose or exercise workload that elicits the ischemic response, the affected coronary territory (left anterior descending vs. left circumflex or right coronary), the presence of multivessel wall motion abnormalities, the peak WMSI, the LVEF and end-systolic volume changes during stress, and the time necessary for recovery of the stress-induced abnormalities.[7]

Assessment of Viability

Dobutamine stress echocardiography is a useful tool for the assessment of viability in patients with resting LV dysfunction and segmental wall motion abnormalities. Myocardium with reversible contractile dysfunction (e.g., with revascularization) is termed viable. Echocardiographic evaluation of viability typically involves assessment of dysfunctional LV segments at rest, low-dose dobutamine (typically 5–20 mcg/kg per

minute), and if necessary, high-dose dobutamine (typically 30–40 mcg/kg per minute). The presence of myocardial viability is suggested by an improvement of function in at least two segments during dobutamine infusion (Table 27.4), whereas no improvement in contractility suggests nonviable myocardium. The biphasic response is characterized by an early improvement in contractility at low-dose dobutamine, which then worsens with high-dose dobutamine, and suggests both viability and ischemia. Improvement in contractility at low-dose dobutamine is the more sensitive pattern for viability, whereas the biphasic response is the most specific and most predictive of functional improvement with revascularization.[7]

Similar to ischemic evaluation, when compared to nuclear imaging assessments of viability, dobutamine stress echocardiography demonstrates lower sensitivity, but higher specificity.[15] Older data suggest a sensitivity and specificity of 75%–90% to predict LV functional recovery with revascularization. Poor image quality, concomitant use of beta-blockers, and variable interobserver agreement—particularly in the face of several resting dysfunctional myocardial segments—are the main limitations of stress echocardiography.

Emerging Echocardiographic Approaches to the Assessment of Ischemia and Viability

Advances in echocardiographic imaging techniques promise to further improve the performance of stress echocardiography for the evaluation of myocardial ischemia and viability. Considerable interest has focused on the use of echo contrast for the evaluation of myocardial perfusion,[16] 2D speckle tracking-based assessments of strain to quantify segmental LV deformation at rest and with stress,[17] and 3D imaging approaches to improve the quality and rapidity of image acquisition at

REST | STRESS

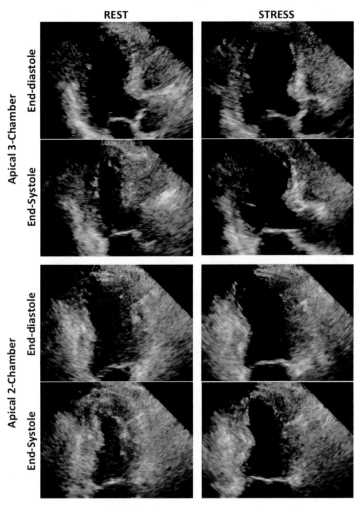

Apical 3-Chamber

End-diastole

End-Systole

Apical 2-Chamber

End-diastole

End-Systole

FIG. 27.4 **Example of a treadmill stress echocardiogram demonstrating left ventricle end-systolic enlargement with stress.** These findings are suggestive of multi-vessel coronary artery disease and were accompanied by a poststress reduction in left ventricle ejection fraction in this patient.

TABLE 27.4 **Image Interpretation of Dobutamine Stress Echocardiography for Viability Assessment[a]**

DIAGNOSIS	REST	LOW-DOSE DOBUTAMINE	HIGH-DOSE DOBUTAMINE
Viable	Abnormal	Improves	Improves further
Viable[b]	Abnormal	Improves	Worsens
Not viable	Abnormal	No change	—
Ischemic	Abnormal	Worsens	—

[a]See text for further discussion.
[b]Biphasic response.

rest and—particularly—post stress.[18] Although all of these hold promise, none have matured to the point of clinical implementation at this time and are not recommended by current guidelines.[5]

UTILITY OF EXERCISE ECHOCARDIOGRAPHY BEYOND ISCHEMIA

The utility of exercise echocardiography extends beyond the evaluation of coronary artery disease. Assessing the cardiovascular response to a stressor (e.g., exercise) can also be used to unmask the presence of, and to assess the severity of, valvular heart disease, heart failure (HF), hypertrophic cardiomyopathy (HCM), and pulmonary hypertension (PH). Resting echocardiography does not fully capture the dynamic nature of these diseases, which are influenced by loading conditions and changes in cardiac output. In addition to this advantage, exercise echocardiography can assess ventricular reserve, which is an important prognostic marker

in cardiovascular diseases. In clinical settings outside of coronary disease evaluation, there is no data comparing the performance of treadmill versus semisupine bicycle protocols in exercise echocardiography (see Table 27.1). Furthermore, exercise protocols can also be adapted to the specific aim of the testing (see section on heart failure with preserved ejection fraction [HFpEF]).

Valvular Disease

In general, the goal of performing exercise echocardiographic assessment in patients with valvular heart disease is to (1) clarify symptom etiology in nonsevere valve disease, (2) rule out the presence of symptoms in patients with severe valve disease, or (3) identify predictors of adverse events or rapid disease progression in asymptomatic severe valve disease. In addition to information on the presence of exertional symptoms, blood pressure response to exercise, or complex ventricular arrhythmias, exercise echocardiography will report on (1) parameters related to the affected valve, (2) the left ventricular contractile reserve, and (3) the hemodynamic consequences (pulmonary arterial pressure, left ventricular filling pressure) during exercise.

In the following subsections, we describe the most relevant exercise echocardiographic assessments for individual valvular lesions (Table 27.5). However, it is important to be cognizant of the limitations of the studies in this field in appropriately interpreting and acting upon the information given by this exam. These include small sample size, single center design, exclusion of patients with more severe disease, and the inclusion of aortic valve replacement (AVR) as an outcome for tests assessing aortic valve disease. "High-risk" echo findings on exercise echocardiography should always be comprehensively weighed with the clinical

TABLE 27.5 Primary Imaging Measures of Interest With Exercise Echocardiography for Indications Beyond Ischemia Evaluation[a]

—	LVEF	TR VELOCITY	MEAN TRANSVALVULAR GRADIENT	OTHER
Aortic stenosis	✓	✓	✓	
Aortic regurgitation	✓			
Mitral stenosis		✓	✓	
Mitral regurgitation	✓	✓		Measures of MR severity (EROA, RVol)
Hypertrophic cardiomyopathy		✓		Dynamic LVOT gradient, SAM MR severity
Pulmonary arterial hypertension		✓		LVOT VTI
Heart failure with preserved ejection fraction		✓		Diastolic measures: (E wave, septal and lateral e')

[a]See text for further discussion.

EROA, Effective regurgitant orifice area; *LV*, left ventricle; *LVEF*, left ventricle ejection fraction; *LVOT*, left ventricle outflow tract; *MTAG*, mean transaortic gradient; *MTMG*, mean transmitral gradient; *MR*, mitral regurgitation; *RVol*, regurgitant volume; *SAM*, systolic anterior motion of the mitral valve; *TAPSE*, tricuspid annulus plane systolic excursion; *TR*, tricuspid regurgitant; *VTI*, velocity-time integral.

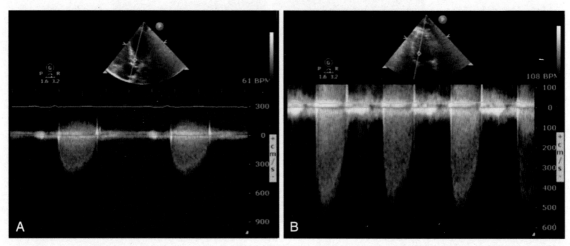

FIG. 27.5 **Assessment of transaortic gradients by exercise echocardiography.** Mean transaortic gradient at rest ([A] 50 mm Hg) and at peak exercise ([B] 70 mm Hg) of an asymptomatic patient with severe aortic stenosis.

features and resting echocardiography findings. The timing of exercise-induced changes in transvalvular gradients and pulmonary artery pressure should be also considered, because abnormalities at low workloads provide valuable evidence in favor of more advanced valvular disease.

Aortic Stenosis
Valve-Related Parameters

Exercise-associated changes in the peak and mean transaortic gradients among patients with high-gradient severe aortic stenosis (AS) have been associated with subsequent cardiac events (Fig. 27.5). In 69 asymptomatic severe AS patients, an increase in mean transaortic pressure gradient greater than 18 mm Hg was an independent predictor of developing symptoms or having a cardiac-related event (HF hospitalization, aortic valve replacement, or cardiac death).[19] These findings were replicated in an independent study showing that in 135 severe AS patients with normal LV function and normal exercise testing (no symptoms, no arrhythmias, and normal blood pressure response to maximal exercise), those with an increase in mean transaortic gradient by 18–20 mm Hg had an almost fourfold increased risk of cardiac-related events at a mean follow-up of 20 months (cardiovascular death, aortic valve replacement due to symptoms, or LV systolic dysfunction).[20] An increase in mean transaortic pressure gradient above 18–20 mm Hg was prognostic beyond clinical data, resting echocardiography findings, and exercise testing performance.

Left Ventricle Function

Limited contractile reserve (absence of an increase of at least 5% in LVEF) during exercise indicates more advanced valvular disease, and it is associated with an increased risk of cardiac events, including death.[21]

Exercise-Induced Pulmonary Hypertension

In at least one study, an increase of systolic pulmonary artery pressure above 60 mm Hg was associated with a twofold increase in the risk of cardiac events (aortic valve replacement motivated by symptoms or LV systolic dysfunction, and cardiac death) in asymptomatic patients with severe AS and preserved LVEF, after adjusting for age, sex, and resting and exercise-induced changes in mean transaortic pressure gradient.[22]

Clinical Significance

The European Society of Cardiology (ESC)/European Association for Cardio-Thoracic Surgery (EACTS) guidelines give a class IIb recommendation for AVR based on an increase of mean transaortic pressure gradient by more than 20 mm Hg.[23] American College of Cardiology/American Heart Association (ACC/AHA) guidelines do not endorse the use of any of these exercise echocardiographic parameters in clinical decision making.[24]

Low-Flow, Low-Gradient Aortic Stenosis With Preserved Left Ventricle Ejection Fraction

The use of low-dose dobutamine stress echocardiography in the assessment of low-flow, low-gradient severe AS with reduced LVEF is discussed in detail elsewhere. In contrast to low-flow, low-gradient AS with reduced LVEF, stress echocardiography with dobutamine is less useful in patients with preserved LVEF because the latter are thought to have reduced LV compliance as opposed to reduced contractility, the mechanistic target of dobutamine. In addition, these patients often have small LV cavities due to concentric remodeling, and may therefore be at greater risk of hemodynamic deterioration during dobutamine infusion.

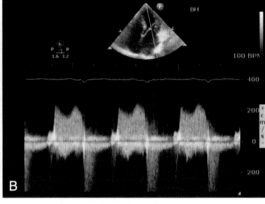

FIG. 27.6 Exercise echocardiography for the assessment of pulmonary pressure with exercise in mitral regurgitation. Pulmonary artery systolic pressure at rest ([A] TR velocity 3.06 m/s peak gradient 38 mm Hg) and at peak exercise ([B] TR velocity 4.19 m/s, peak gradient 70 mm Hg) in an asymptomatic patient with a severe mitral regurgitation.

In theory, exercise-induced hemodynamic changes (decreased LV afterload and increased LV preload) might be more appropriate to increase the transaortic flow (stoke volume) and allow for re-examination of the peak transvalvular velocities and gradients to assess for the presence of true stenosis in these patients. However, to date, relatively little data exist regarding the use of exercise echocardiography for this indication and the feasibility of this approach needs to be tested in larger series.[25,26] Currently, exercise echocardiography in this specific subset of AS patients is not the standard of care, nor is it endorsed by professional society guidelines.

Aortic Regurgitation

Little data exist on the role of exercise echocardiography in aortic regurgitation (AR). In patients with borderline resting echocardiographic parameters of LV structure and function, assessing the LV contractile reserve may aid the in decision making regarding surgical treatment, although studies have been inconsistent. Wahi et al.[27] studied 61 patients with asymptomatic or minimally symptomatic severe AR and found that the failure to augment LVEF during exercise was a predictor of aortic valve replacement, postsurgery LVEF, and decline in LVEF among patients treated conservatively. In contrast, Kusunose et al.[28] did not find LVEF changes during exercise to be an independent prognostic marker after excluding patients who underwent aortic valve replacement in the first 3-month period after the exercise echocardiography (to minimize the influence of test results on clinical decision making). In this study of 159 consecutive asymptomatic patients with isolated moderately severe or severe AR, resting LV and right ventricular (RV) strain and exercise tricuspid annulus plane systolic excursion (TAPSE) were the only independent predictors of cardiac events (aortic valve surgery and all-cause death).

Mitral Stenosis
Valve-Related Parameters

Limited data on the role of *exercise* echocardiography in mitral stenosis (MS) is available. In 53 patients with rheumatic MS undergoing dobutamine stress echocardiography, the increase in mean transmitral gradient (MTMG) was an independent predictor of cardiac adverse events (hospitalizations, acute pulmonary edema, or supraventricular arrhythmias) at 61 months of mean follow-up, irrespective of the presence of symptoms, resting mitral valve area or pulmonary artery systolic pressure (PASP).[29] At peak exercise, an MTMG greater than 18 mm Hg had a sensitivity of 90% and a specificity of 87% to detect events (Fig. 27.6).

Exercise-Induced Pulmonary Hypertension

In 48 asymptomatic patients with significant MS, an increase in PASP of more than 90% of its resting value in the early phase of exercise (60 W), but not the peak PASP, was associated with increased risk of developing dyspnea or of requiring mitral valve intervention.[30] Notably, this study showed no association between MS severity and resting PASP with the development of dyspnea during exercise.

Clinical Significance

The MS patients who benefit most from exercise echocardiography evaluation are those with a discrepancy between the severity of MS at rest and exertional symptoms, which are often difficult to interpret. The limitations of the existing data only permit recommendation for closer follow-up of patients exhibiting the described high-risk exercise echocardiographic features. Nevertheless, in symptomatic patients with mild MS (mitral valve area [MVA] > 1.5 cm²), the presence of exercise-induced PH and an increase in MTMG can be used to consider early referral for percutaneous valvuloplasty (ACC/AHA guidelines, class IIb).[24]

Mitral Regurgitation
Valve-Related Parameters

Exercise echocardiography can help evaluate exercise-induced worsening of mitral regurgitation (MR) severity using quantitative measures based on the proximal isovelocity surface area (PISA) method. For example, in 61 asymptomatic patients with moderate to severe primary MR, worsening of MR defined by an increase in the effective regurgitant orifice area of more than 10 mm² and regurgitant volume greater than 15 mL during exercise was independently associated with reduced symptom-free survival (shortness of breath, angina, dizziness, or syncope with exertion).[31] Notably, in this study, the extent of MR worsening during exercise did not correlate with the MR severity on resting echocardiography.

Left Ventricle Function

Absence of LV contractile reserve with exercise, defined by a change in LVEF or using more novel measures of LV deformation such as strain, appear to predict worse outcomes in severe MR. Of 115 patients with at least moderate degenerative MR and no LV dysfunction or dilation, those with absent contractile reserve (defined as an increase of LV global longitudinal strain ≥2%) had a 1.6-fold increased risk of cardiac events (cardiovascular death, HF hospitalization, and mitral valve surgery due to symptoms). Contractile reserve defined as an exercise-induced LVEF increase of more than 4% did not relate to prognosis in this study. In contrast, Lee et al. demonstrated that in 71 patients with moderately severe to severe isolated MR, the absence of contractile reserve (defined as an LVEF increase of >4%) or an end-systolic volume index greater than 25 cm²/m² at peak exercise were both associated with postoperative LV dysfunction after mitral valve surgery or progressive LV dysfunction in medically treated patients.[32,33] Differences in the study populations and endpoints might explain these differences.

Exercise-Induced Pulmonary Hypertension

Exercise-induced PH and associated RV dysfunction are each predictive of adverse outcomes in severe MR (Fig. 27.7). In 78 patients with at least moderate degenerative MR, 46% demonstrated exercise-induced PH (PASP > 60 mm Hg during maximal exercise), and exercise-induced PH was an independent predictor of symptom onset during a 2-year follow-up (3.4-fold increased risk).[34] In MR patients, an exercise-induced PASP greater than 60 mm Hg also predicts postoperative outcomes such

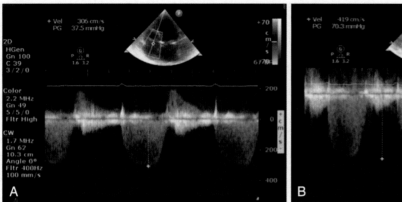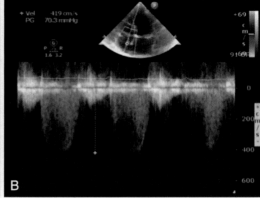

FIG. 27.7 Assessment of mean antegrade transmitral gradient by exercise echocardiography in mitral stenosis. Mean transmitral gradient at rest ([A] 10 mm Hg at a heart rate of 84 bpm) and at peak exercise ([B] 20 mm Hg at a heart rate of 100 bpm) in a patient with moderate mitral stenosis.

as the occurrence of atrial fibrillation, stroke, cardiac-related hospitalization, or death.[35] Concomitant with exercise-induced PH, the presence of exercise-induced right ventricular dysfunction defined by a TAPSE less than 19 mm was an independent predictor of time to surgery in 196 patients with isolated moderate to severe MR.[36]

Clinical Significance

In asymptomatic patients with severe primary MR and preserved LVEF, exercise-induced increase in PASP (class IIb in ESC/EACTS guidelines),[23] and possibly also MR severity and absence of LV contractile reserve, can be used to identify a subset of high-risk patients who may benefit from early intervention.

Secondary Mitral Regurgitation

Exercise echocardiography can help in the management of patients with LV systolic dysfunction and out-of-proportion symptoms (exertional dyspnea, acute pulmonary edema with no obvious cause) because resting MR severity does not predict the magnitude of exercise-induced increase of MR.[37] In 161 patients with chronic ischemic HF and at least mild MR, an exercise-induced increase in effective regurgitant orifice area (EROA) greater than 13 mm[2] predicted mortality and HF hospitalizations.[38] Exercise-induced increases in EROA or PASP were also independently associated with the occurrence of pulmonary edema.[39] Considering the prognostic significance of an exercise-induced increase of MR, ACC/AHA guidelines suggest that MR worsening and PASP increase during exercise echocardiography might be useful for the management of patients with moderate MR undergoing coronary surgical revascularization (class IIa).[24]

Hypertrophic Cardiomyopathy

Exercise echocardiography is a useful tool to assess symptoms in HCM. The exercise intolerance in HCM can be multifactorial, involving the interplay of diastolic dysfunction, dynamic left ventricle outflow tract (LVOT) obstruction, mitral regurgitation, and myocardial ischemia, among others (Fig. 27.8). The identification of the culprit mechanism is clinically relevant as treatment options differ substantially. In HCM, exercise echocardiography demonstrates better sensitivity than Valsalva maneuver or nitrates in elucidating pathophysiological mechanisms.[40,41] On the other hand, dobutamine stress echocardiography is not recommended in HCM because it can be poorly tolerated by causing midcavity obliteration, which can also make evaluation of dynamic LVOT obstruction challenging.[42] Cardiac imaging during exercise on a treadmill has the advantage of using a more physiological body position (orthostatic) associated with greater preload reduction than supine exercise.[43] If the image acquisition is done post-peak after the patient assumes a supine position, the delay in imaging should be minimized.[44] The LVOT gradients captured by a semisupine cycle ergometry protocol, which might have an intermediate preload change between upright and supine positions, correlates with those from the postexercise supine position.[45] In symptomatic HCM patients, exercise echocardiography has an established role

in identifying a provocable dynamic LVOT gradient and/or worsening MR. In asymptomatic patients, the role of this assessment is debatable because the prognostic impact of an exercise-induced LVOT obstruction is uncertain.[46,47]

Pulmonary Arterial Hypertension

Pulmonary arterial hypertension (PAH) is characterized by a progressive narrowing of the pulmonary vessels, which causes an increase in pulmonary vascular resistance and, subsequently, an increase of pulmonary arterial pressure. The early detection of PAH is challenging because early symptoms are vague and nonspecific. However, early diagnosis prompts early treatment and is associated with improved survival.[48] Resting echocardiography has limited diagnostic accuracy for early PAH.[49] Exercise echocardiography might be useful (1) to diagnose PAH at a subclinical stage of the disease, (2) to identify patients at a high risk of developing PAH, and (3) to better predict the future course of patients with established PAH.

Increases in pulmonary artery pressure with exercise are related to both the increase in cardiac output and pulmonary vascular reserve (i.e., the ability of the increased blood flow to distend and recruit pulmonary vessels). Relatively modest reductions in pulmonary vascular reserve may only be unmasked when the pulmonary circulation is stressed by the exercise-induced augmentation of cardiac output. Therefore, PH manifested during exercise that was unapparent at rest, in an asymptomatic subject with risk factors for developing pulmonary vascular disease, might represent PAH at a subclinical stage or signal a patient at high-risk of developing PAH.[50] Another potential utility of exercise echocardiography is in patients with overt PAH, in whom right ventricular functional reserve may be a useful prognostic marker given the prognostic importance of right ventricular function in this population.[51]

Several exercise protocols (6-minute walk test, treadmill testing, two-step test, and cycle ergometers), with different levels of effort (maximal and submaximal) and different body positions during image acquisition (upright, supine, semisupine), have been used to assess the pulmonary vascular response to exercise. The echocardiographic parameters of interest are the peak tricuspid regurgitation jet velocity to estimate PASP, and the LVOT diameter and time-velocity integral to estimate cardiac output. Most studies assign a constant value to right atrial pressure (e.g., 5 mm Hg) or assume it to be zero to estimate PASP. Right heart catheterization and cardiac magnetic resonance imaging are the gold-standard methods to evaluate pulmonary hemodynamics and RV function, respectively. However, exercise echocardiography also appears to be an accurate tool for this purpose.[52]

The PASP cutoff value used to define PH varies between studies (40, 45, or 50 mm Hg). The major limitation of using PASP to assess the pulmonary vascular response to exercise is the flow-dependent nature of this measure. For a higher cardiac output, the PASP will be physiologically higher. Nevertheless, a PASP higher than 50 mm Hg is not expected during maximal exercise in patients at high risk for developing PAH,[53] which might be the best cutoff to screen for PAH

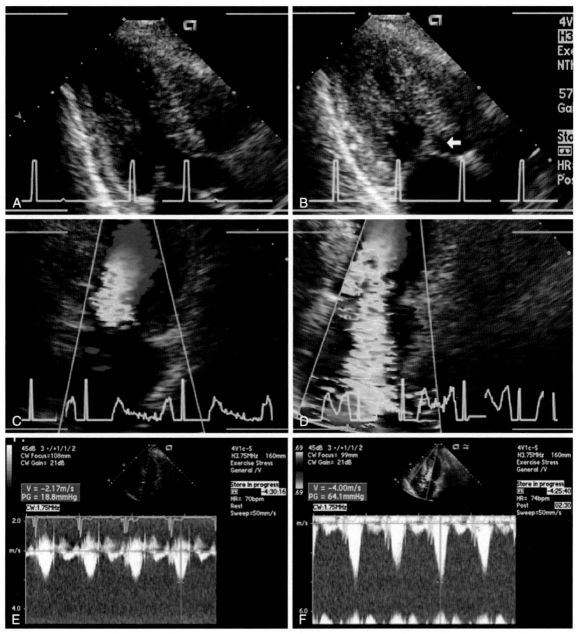

FIG. 27.8 Exercise echocardiography assessment of hypertrophic cardiomyopathy. Mild systolic anterior motion of the mitral valve is noted at rest (A), which becomes more prominent with exercise (B). Only trace mitral regurgitation is noted at rest (C), which becomes moderate to severe in exercise (D). A modest left ventricle outflow tract gradient is noted at rest ([E] peak velocity 2.17 m/s, peak instantaneous gradient 19 mm Hg), which becomes more severe with exercise ([F] peak velocity 4.00 m/s, peak instantaneous gradient 64 mm Hg).

given the lower expected false-positive rate. To overcome the limitations inherent in the flow dependency of PASP, the mean pulmonary arterial pressure to cardiac output (mPAP/CO) relationship is a more informative parameter for assessing the pulmonary circulation during exercise.[54] It has been shown that there is a linear relationship between these variables, with values greater than 3 mmHg/L per minute being a signal of an abnormal pulmonary vascular response to exercise.[55] The mPAP can be derived from PASP using the Chemla formula: mPAP = 0.61 × PASP + 2.[56] The mPAP/CO slope can be calculated from a simple linear model using the resting, submaximal, and maximal echocardiographic measurements of PASP and CO. Alternatively, two simpler ways of assessing the relationship between these two measurements is to use the PASP and CO only at peak exercise (mPAP/CO max) or calculate the change from resting to peak (ΔmPAP/ΔCO). Relating PASP to workload (in watts) could also be an accurate and simpler way of identifying patients with abnormal pulmonary vascular response to exercise.[52]

Most studies enrolled asymptomatic patients predisposed to develop PAH, such as those with scleroderma, with the aim of identifying subclinical PAH or patients at higher risk of developing PAH. In patients with connective tissue disease, one-third had PH due to elevated left ventricle filling pressures, which can only be assessed by right heart catheterization.[57] In patients with connective tissue disease, mPAP/CO change after a 6-minute walk test independently predicted the development of PAH over a median follow-up of 32 months.[58] In contrast, among patients with established PAH, increase in PASP with exercise may indicate RV functional reserve, and an increase greater than 30 mm Hg was independently associated with a better prognosis in patients with PAH and chronic thromboembolic PH.[51]

Despite the strong pathophysiological rationale, the role of exercise echocardiography in the assessment of PAH is not yet firmly established. An increased PASP or mPAP/CO change during exercise might help in detecting subclinical or high-risk patients for developing PAH. In contrast, among patients with established PAH, an increase greater than 30 mm Hg in PASP is associated with a better prognosis as it indicated RV functional reserve.

Heart Failure With Preserved Ejection Fraction

HFpEF affects half of HF patients and is challenging to diagnose because patients can have normal or only mildly impaired diastolic function at rest.[59] Diastolic stress testing aims to detect changes in LV diastolic function and its hemodynamic consequences during exercise, because many HFpEF patients have reduced diastolic reserve due to blunted augmentation in myocardial relaxation causing increased LV filling pressure during exercise.[60] Patients who may benefit most from this test are those with unexplained exertional symptoms, preserved LVEF, and mild alterations in diastolic function at rest.

Several exercise protocols have been used. One protocol[61] involves a semisupine bicycle exercise with submaximal intensity aiming to reach a heart rate of 110–120 bpm to avoid fusion of the transmitral E and A waves. A ramp protocol with low baseline (e.g., 15 W) and incremental workload (e.g., 5 W), changing to a steady load when the heart rate goal is achieved,[61] may be the best option for patients referred for this testing because they are often older adults, have reduced functional capacity, and have several comorbidities. The main echocardiographic variables of interest for each exercise stage are mitral inflow E-wave peak velocity, mitral annular tissue Doppler velocities (medial and lateral e′), and peak TR velocity. Several other parameters (mitral flow propagation velocity, pulmonary venous flow, isovolumic relaxation time, among others) have also been described to assess diastolic functional reserve but their feasibility during exercise and clinical significance is less established.[61] According to recent ASE and European Association of Cardiovascular Imaging (EACVI) guidelines,[62] diastolic stress testing is abnormal when all of the following are present: (1) average E/e′ greater than 14 or septal E/e′ ratio greater than 15 with exercise; (2) peak TR velocity greater than 2.8 m/s with exercise; and (3) baseline septal e′ velocity less than 7 cm/s or, if only lateral velocity is acquired, baseline lateral e′ less than 10 cm/s. The test is normal when both (1) the average or septal E/e′ ratio is less than 10 with exercise; and (2) the peak TR velocity is less than 2.8 m/s with exercise. The test is considered indeterminate otherwise.

Despite the clear and attractive pathophysiological rationale, the lack of validation of diastolic stress test with respect to both diagnostic accuracy and prognostic value make the clinical significance of this test unclear.

Simultaneous Use of Exercise Echocardiography and Cardiopulmonary Exercise Testing

Cardiopulmonary exercise testing (CPET) is a useful tool to assess patients with a wide range of cardiopulmonary diseases exhibiting exertional intolerance, providing rigorous quantification of the functional impairment that is both diagnostic and provides prognostic value.[63] However, CPET provides limited insight into the potential mechanisms limiting the exercise capacity. Simultaneous exercise echocardiography can help in this respect, through assessments of left[64] and right[65] ventricular contractile reserve, valvular function,[66] intraventricular gradients,[67] and diastolic function.[68] The combination of both exams can also potentially provide information about abnormalities in peripheral oxygen extraction causing exertional dyspnea.[69] Despite these recognized synergies between exercise echocardiography and CPET, logistic complexity and limited data regarding the incremental value of this combined approach explain its current limited applicability.

Suggested Reading

Erdei, T., Smiseth, O. A., Marino, P., & Fraser, A. G. (2014). A systematic review of diastolic stress tests in heart failure with preserved ejection fraction, with proposals from the EU-FP7 MEDIA study group. *European Journal of Heart Failure*, 16, 1345–1361.

Henri, C., Piérard, L. A., Lancellotti, P., Mongeon, F. P., Pibarot, P., & Basmadjian, A. J. (2014). Exercise testing and stress imaging in valvular heart disease. *Canadian Journal of Cardiology*, 30, 1012–1026.

Magne, J., Pibarot, P., Sengupta, P. P., Donal, E., Rosenhek, R., & Lancellotti, P. (2015). Pulmonary hypertension in valvular disease: a comprehensive review on pathophysiology to therapy from the HAVEC Group. *JACC Cardiovascular Imaging*, 8, 83–99.

Maréchaux, S., Hachicha, Z., Bellouin, A., et al. (2010). Usefulness of exercise-stress echocardiography for risk stratification of true asymptomatic patients with aortic valve stenosis. *European Heart Journal*, 31, 1390–1397.

Reant, P., Reynaud, A., Pillois, X., et al. (2015). Comparison of resting and exercise echocardiographic parametrs as indicators of outcomes of hypertrophic cardiomyopathy. *Journal of the American Society of Echocardiography*, 28, 194–203.

A complete reference list can be found online at ExpertConsult.com.

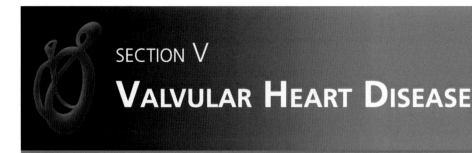

VALVULAR HEART DISEASE

28 Mitral Valve Disease

Romain Capoulade, Timothy C. Tan, Judy Hung

INTRODUCTION

Approximately 2.5% of the general US population suffers from significant valvular heart disease. Mitral valve disease (MVD) constitutes one of the most prevalent forms and is associated with significant cardiovascular morbidity and mortality.[1–3] Furthermore, the prevalence of MVD increases exponentially with age reaching up to 10% in patients older than 75 years.[1] Typically, MVD can be classified into mitral regurgitation (MR) and mitral stenosis (MS), which have a prevalence in the general US population of around 1.7% and 0.1%, respectively.[1] MR can be further subdivided into primary MR (i.e., due to intrinsic mitral valve [MV] apparatus abnormalities) or secondary MR (i.e., as a consequence of other cardiac diseases, such as myocardial infarction and/or dilation). Similarly, MS can be broadly subdivided into two main groups based on the two most common etiologies of MS: rheumatic and calcific (or degenerative) MS.

Echocardiography plays an important role in the diagnosis and management of MVD. This noninvasive and relatively accessible imaging tool allows assessment of MV structure and hemodynamics, which guide clinical management and decision making. In addition to standard transthoracic echocardiography (TTE), transesophageal echocardiography (TEE) may also provide valuable and complementary information on the anatomy of the MV and the underlying etiology of anatomic abnormalities, particularly in MR. Additionally, recent technological advances, such as three-dimensional (3D) echocardiography, have increased the value and scope of echocardiography by improving its ability to define anatomy and function.

The aim of this chapter is to provide a comprehensive review of MVD and the role of echocardiography in this context. Hence, this chapter will include a description of the anatomy of the MV and the standard echocardiographic views of the MV apparatus, followed by an overview of the common MV lesions and their echocardiographic features.

MITRAL VALVE ANATOMY

The MV apparatus is a complex structure that includes the mitral annulus, two leaflets, and associated chordae tendineae and papillary muscles (PMs; Fig. 28.1).[4] The mitral annulus is a D-shaped fibromuscular ring to which the MV leaflets are anchored. It is elliptical and has a saddle shape, which is the optimal configuration for leaflet coaptation and for minimizing leaflet stress.[5–10] The anteromedial portion of the mitral annulus shares a common wall with the aortic annulus and is called the intervalvular fibrosa. Because the intervalvular fibrosa is more rigid than the fibrous attachment of the posterior annulus, dilation of the mitral annulus typically occurs posteriorly (see Fig. 28.1).

The two leaflets of the MV are known as the anterior leaflet (which is typically the leaflet with the larger area), and the posterior leaflet. Each leaflet is also typically divided into three segments (scallops): anterolateral (A1 and P1), middle (A2 and P2), and posteromedial (A3 and P3)

based on the Carpentier classification with the leaflets limited by commissures (see Fig. 28.1).[11] Leaflet redundancy (i.e., larger leaflet surface area than MV annulus area) is needed to allow coaptation and avoid valve incompetence.[12]

Chordae tendineae extend from the PMs and attach to the ventricular surface of the mitral leaflets (see Fig. 28.1). They serve to allow coaptation and prevent leaflet prolapse or flail. The chordae tendineae can also be divided into three types: the primary (marginal) chordae, which attach at the free edge of the leaflets and provide the support to allow for leaflet coaptation, preventing prolapse and flail; the secondary (basal) chordae attach the leaflets to the left ventricle (LV) and help optimize ventricular function; and the tertiary chordae, which attach to the base of the posterior leaflet, also provide structural support.

There are typically two PMs located within the LV, known as the anterolateral and posteromedial PMs. They are attached to the leaflets via the chordae, and play a role in the regulation of normal valve function.

ECHOCARDIOGRAPHIC VIEWS OF THE MITRAL VALVE

MVD can arise due to the disruption or malfunction of any the different components of the MV apparatus. Hence, accurate diagnosis of MV pathology requires a comprehensive and systematic assessment of the MV apparatus including the individual anatomical components, determination of the severity of the MV dysfunction using Doppler and imaging techniques, and assessment of the impact of the MV lesion on ventricular and atrial structure and function and on hemodynamics, notably pulmonary artery pressures.[13–16] Frequently, this may require integration of 2D multiplanar and 3D imaging of the MV apparatus, from both TTE and TEE images.[13–16]

Transthoracic Echocardiography

TTE is considered the standard of care for the primary assessment of the MV. MV anatomy can be evaluated using multiple 2D views (Fig. 28.2A and B): standard imaging of the MV by TTE should include parasternal long axis, basal short axis, and apical two-, three-, and four-chamber views.[15,16] Nonstandard or off-axis views and subcostal images may also be needed to fully interrogate the valve with the goal of identifying each of the leaflet scallops and/or identifying localized abnormalities as may be encountered in endocarditis. Segmental MV anatomy can be identified in transthoracic views. Parasternal long-axis views show the middle segments (A2, P2) of the mitral leaflets. Short-axis views of the MV display the entire leaflets in a medial-to-lateral orientation from left to right. The apical four-chamber view display is more variable depending on the degree to which the probe is angled posteriorly or anteriorly, but typically shows A2 with variable portions of A1 and A3 and P1 or P2 near the transition from one scallop to another (see Fig. 28.2C). The apical two-chamber view shows the MV across the coaptation line and includes

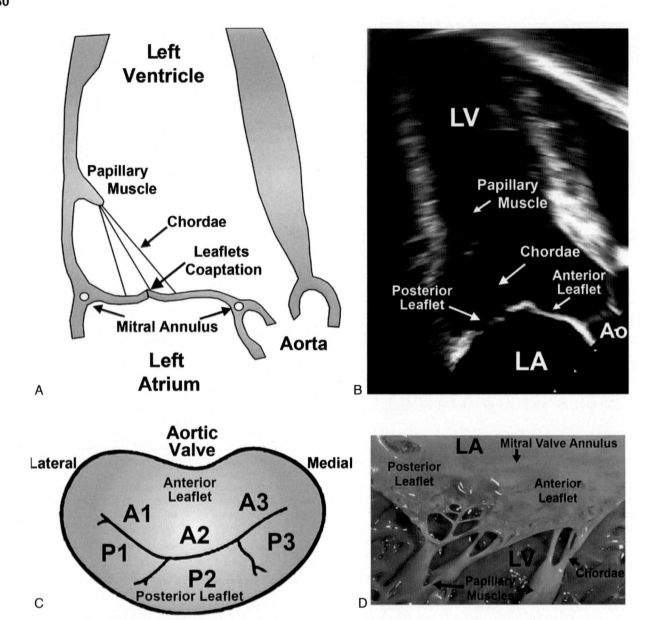

FIG. 28.1 Schematic representation of the normal mitral valve apparatus (A) and related echocardiographic apical three-chamber view (B), standard segmentation of the mitral valve leaflets in a short-axis view (C), and an anatomic pathological view of the mitral valve apparatus (D). *Ao,* Aorta; *LA,* left atrium; *LV,* left ventricle.

a portion of the P3 and P1 scallops along with A2 (see Fig. 28.2C). The apical long-axis view displays the A2 and P2 scallops, similar to the parasternal long-axis view (see Fig. 28.2C). Integrating imaging and Doppler information from each of these 2D views should provide a thorough anatomic and functional evaluation of the MV.[15,16]

Transesophageal Echocardiography

Although TTE is used as the primary tool to assess and quantify MVD, TEE provides complementary imaging, especially if TTE windows are technically difficult. In addition, due to the TEE transducer proximity to the left atrium, TEE is particularly suited to define MV anatomy and function with the precision needed to guide surgical decision making.[15–17]

Standard TEE imaging to visualize the MV includes four mid-esophageal views (Fig. 28.3A) and multiple transgastric views including the short-axis view (see Fig. 28.3B) that uniquely shows all scallops of both leaflets.[15,16] Slight modifications of each of the mid-esophageal views are needed to ensure that all scallops are visualized from this window.

Like the TTE apical four-chamber view, the mid-esophageal view at 0 degrees has a display of the scallops that varies depending on the degree to which the probe is anteflexed or retroflexed, but typically shows A2

(or A1 if anteflexed, A3 if retroflexed) and P2 (or P1 if anteflexed, P3 if retroflexed near the transition from one scallop to another). The mid-esophageal view at approximately 60 degrees shows the MV across the coaptation line (the transcommissural view) and includes a portion of the P3 and P2 along with A2 floating in the middle. Manually rotating the probe (as opposed to changing the angle) can result in views that show only the anterior or posterior leaflets. The mid-esophageal view at 90 degrees displays P3 and A1 with variable portions of the A3 and A2 scallops. The mid-esophageal view at 120 degrees shows A2 and P2 (see Fig. 28.3C). Note the impact of manual changes in the position of the probe anteflexion/retroflexion, right/left flexion, and mediolateral rotation, which can vary the scallops seen in individual views.

3D TEE can provide views that are not possible with 2D TEE, and by showing both complete leaflets simultaneously, eliminate some of the ambiguity inherent in 2D TEE imaging. Specifically, 3D TEE can display the "surgeon's view" (Fig. 28.4A) in which the MV is viewed enface from the left atrial aspect.[18] Additionally, MV clefts and the MV commissures can be better displayed with 3D compared to 2D TEE.[18] Recent advances in 3D echo imaging and advanced analytic techniques have greatly improved image resolution and the quantitative assessment of the valve. 3D imaging can now be used to provide robust and quantitative evaluation of MV anatomy including assessment of each component of

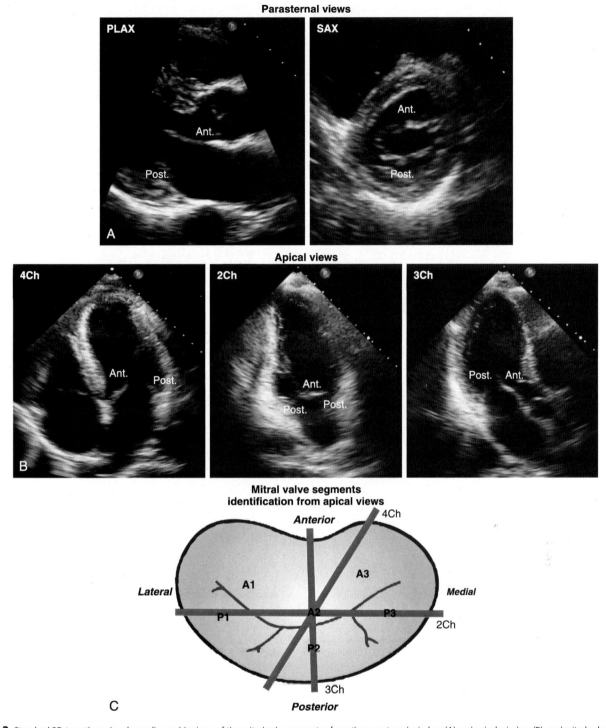

FIG. 28.2 Standard 2D transthoracic echocardiographic views of the mitral valve apparatus from the parasternal window (A) and apical window (B), and mitral valve segments captured from the apical views (C). *2Ch,* Apical two-chamber; *3Ch,* apical three-chamber; *4Ch,* apical four-chamber; *Ant.,* anterior leaflet; *PLAX,* parasternal long axis; *Post.,* posterior leaflet; *SAX,* short axis. See text for further details.

the MV (see Fig. 28.4B). 3D has thus rapidly become part of the standard TEE evaluation of the MV.[19]

Doppler evaluation (spectral and color [2D and 3D]) complements the anatomic characterization of the MV by providing functional information including the localization of the mitral regurgitant jets.

MITRAL REGURGITATION

MR is classically subdivided into two broad categories with distinct underlying mechanisms: primary MR or secondary MR.[13,14] Primary MR encompasses MVD in which there is a structural abnormality of the leaflets and/or associated chords. In contrast, in secondary MR, the MV leaflets are essentially normal but the LV is dysfunctional and distorted due to ischemic or myopathic remodeling resulting in leaflet tethering and incomplete closure of the mitral leaflets. Box 28.1 summarizes common etiologies for primary and secondary MR. The differentiation between these types of MVD is necessary because management, particularly surgical decision making, is dependent on the underlying etiology of the MV dysfunction.[13,14] A Carpentier classification of the mechanisms of MR that is based on leaflet mobility has also been proposed (Table 28.1 and Fig. 28.5). Type I is defined by normal leaflet motion but with annular dilation, leaflet perforation, or cleft; Type II is defined by excessive

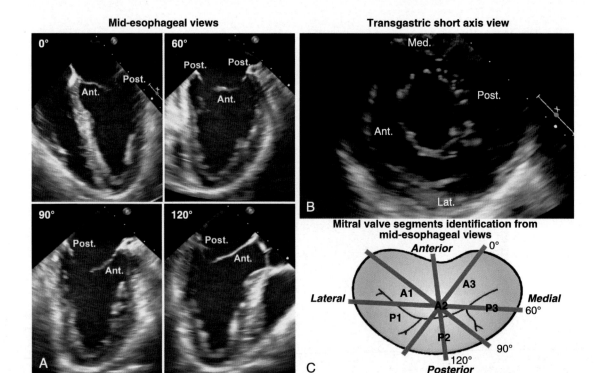

Mid-esophageal views

0° Ant. Post. Post.

60° Post. Post. Ant.

90° Post. Ant.

120° Post. Ant.

A

Transgastric short axis view

Med.

Post.

Ant.

Lat.

B

Mitral valve segments identification from mid-esophageal views

Anterior 0°

Lateral A1 A3 *Medial* 60°

A2 P3

P1

P2 90°

120°

Posterior

C

FIG. 28.3 Standard 2D transesophageal echocardiographic views of the mitral valve apparatus from mid-esophageal window (A) and transgastric window (B), and mitral valve segments captured from the mid-esophageal views (C). *Ant.,* Anterior leaflet; *Med.,* medial; *Lat.,* lateral; *Post.,* posterior leaflet. See text for further details.

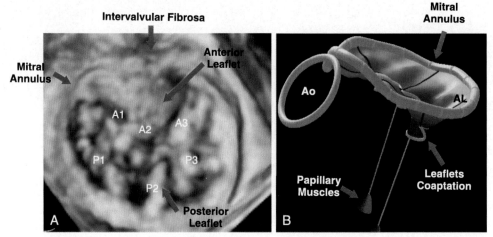

Intervalvular Fibrosa

Mitral Annulus

Mitral Annulus

Anterior Leaflet

A1 A2 A3

P1 P3

P2

A

Posterior Leaflet

Ao

AL

Papillary Muscles

Leaflets Coaptation

B

FIG. 28.4 3D transesophageal echocardiography evaluation of the mitral valve apparatus with the 3D surgeon's view (A) and 3D mitral valve quantitative modeling (B). *AL,* Anterolateral; *Ao,* aorta. See text for further details.

BOX 28.1 Common Etiologies for Primary and Secondary Mitral Regurgitation

Primary Mitral Regurgitation
Degenerative
    Mitral valve prolapse spectrum
    Annular calcification
    Nonspecific thickening
Infectious (endocarditis with vegetation, perforation, or
    chordal rupture)
Inflammatory (collagen-vascular diseases)
Rheumatic
Radiation-induced
Drug-induced (e.g., anorectic drugs)
Congenital
    Mitral valve cleft
    Mitral valve parachute
    Mitral arcade
    Supravalvular mitral ring

Secondary Mitral Regurgitation
Ischemic left ventricular dysfunction
Nonischemic cardiomyopathy
Atrial fibrillation

TABLE 28.1 Carpentier's Surgical Classification of Mitral Regurgitation Dysfunction

TYPE	LEAFLET MOTION	LESIONS	ETIOLOGY
I	Normal	Annular dilation Leaflet perforation	Atrial Fibrillation Endocarditis Dilated cardiomyopathy
II	Excessive	Elongated/ruptured chordae Elongated/ruptured papillary muscle	Degenerative valve disease Endocarditis Trauma Ischemic cardiomyopathy
IIIa	Restrictive (diastole and systole)	Leaflet thickening/retraction Leaflet calcification Chordal thickening/retraction/fusion Commissural fusion	Rheumatic heart disease Carcinoid heart disease Calcific mitral valve Radiotherapy Inflammatory disease
IIIb	Restrictive (systole)	Left ventricle dilation/aneurism Papillary muscle displacement Chordae/leaflet tethering	Ischemic cardiomyopathy Dilated cardiomyopathy

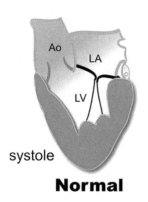

Normal

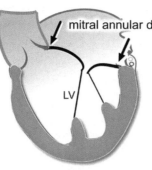
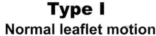

Type I
Normal leaflet motion

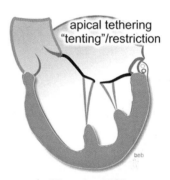

Type I
Normal leaflet motion

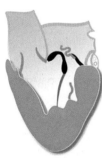

Type II
Excessive leaflet motion
(Prolapse/Flail)

Type IIIa
Restrictive leaflet motion
(diastole and systole)

Type IIIb
Restrictive leaflet closure
(systole)

FIG. 28.5 The Carpentier classification system of mitral regurgitation is based on leaflet motion. Type I is defined by normal leaflet motion but with annular dilation, leaflet perforation, or cleft; Type II is defined by excessive leaflet motion (i.e., mitral valve prolapse or flail) and elongated/ruptured chordae or papillary muscles; Type IIIa is defined by diastolic and systolic restrictive leaflet motion and leaflet or chordal thickening/calcification with or without commissural fusion such as occurs with rheumatic mitral valve disease; Type IIIb is defined by systolic restrictive leaflet motion and left ventricular dilation/aneurysm, papillary muscle displacement, and chordal tethering (secondary or functional mitral regurgitation). *Ao,* Aorta; *LA,* left atrium; *LV,* left ventricle. *(Courtesy of Bernard E. Bulwer, MD, FASE.)*

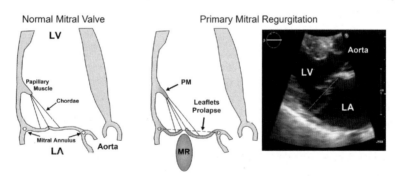

FIG. 28.6 Schematic representation (i.e., apical three-chamber view) of the mitral valve apparatus in the presence of mitral valve prolapse as compared to normal mitral valve geometry *(left and middle panels)*, and the echocardiographic parasternal long-axis *(right panel)* showing that the billowing leaflets extend more than 2 mm above an annular plane defined by the insertion of the leaflets *(dashed line)*. *LA,* Left atrium; *LV,* left ventricle; *MR,* mitral regurgitation; *PM,* papillary muscle.

leaflet motion (i.e., MV prolapse or flail) and elongated/ruptured chordae or PMs; Type IIIa is defined by diastolic and systolic restrictive leaflet motion and leaflet or chordal thickening/calcification with or without commissural fusion such as occurs with rheumatic MVD; and Type IIIb is defined by systolic restrictive leaflet motion and left ventricular dilation/aneurysm, PM displacement, and chordal tethering (secondary or functional MR). The clear distinctions among the different categories of MR can only be achieved by comprehensively assessing the anatomy and function of the MV to define underlying mechanisms.

Primary Mitral Regurgitation

The most common cause of primary MR in developed countries is MV prolapse or flail (Carpentier type II). Prolapse is defined as leaflet

billowing by more than 2 mm above the annular "plane" during systole (Fig. 28.6).[20] This assessment is typically made in the parasternal long-axis view, which displays the highest points of the saddle-shaped annulus. The diagnosis of prolapse should not be made exclusively from the apical four-chamber view, which shows lower (more apical) points on the annulus. MV prolapse spans a spectrum from minimum prolapse of the leaflets into the left atrium to diffuse leaflet thickening and redundancy. Flail leaflet is part of the MV prolapse spectrum and is defined as occurring when the leaflet becomes everted and loses its normal convex shape with the leaflet tip seen within the left atrium (Fig. 28.7). Flail leaflet is caused by disruption of the primary (marginal) chordae such that effective coaptation is no longer present.

Clinically important MV prolapse/flail typically presents as two types (Fig. 28.8): Barlow disease and fibroelastic deficiency.[21,22] Barlow disease

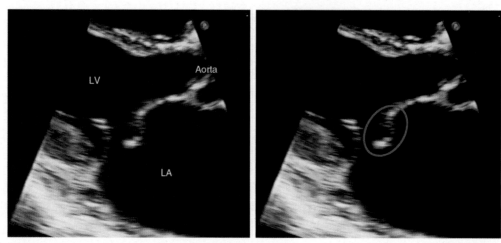

FIG. 28.7 Echocardiographic view of an anterior leaflet mitral valve flail *(red circle)* in the parasternal long-axis view. *LA,* Left atrium; *LV,* left ventricle.

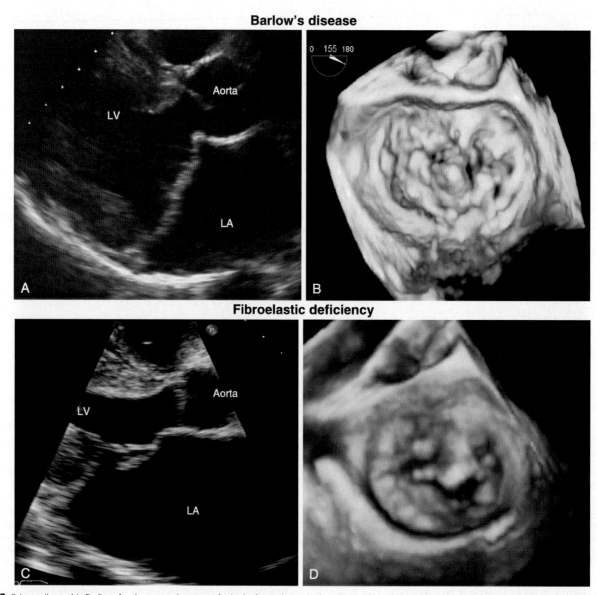

FIG. 28.8 Echocardiographic findings for the two major types of mitral valve prolapse: Barlow disease (A and B) and fibroelastic deficiency (C and D), in the parasternal long-axis view (A and C) and 3D surgeon's view (B and D). Note that for Barlow disease (A and B), 2D and 3D images come from two different patients and that, in addition to diffuse prolapse, there is a flail P2 scallop. In the example with fibroelastic deficiency, there is a flail A2 scallop with multiple ruptured chordae, whereas the remaining scallops appear normal. *LA,* Left atrium; *LV,* left ventricle.

is an infiltrative disease characterized by excessive myxomatous tissue associated with mucopolysaccharide accumulation that can affect one or both leaflets, and chordae.[23–25] In Barlow disease, there is thickening of the leaflets leading to redundant valvular tissue (see Fig. 28.8A and B; Video 28.1) and frequently elongated or ruptured chordae.[21,23,25] Patients with Barlow disease are usually diagnosed in young adulthood and typically present with bileaflet and multisegmental prolapse with or without flail scallops (see Fig. 28.8A and B; Video 28.1). In contrast, in fibroelastic deficiency, which is the most common form of degenerative MR in the MV prolapse spectrum, the loss of mechanical valve integrity due to abnormal connective tissue structure and function is the most common finding. Patients with fibroelastic deficiency are usually identified in their 60s and typically present with localized and unisegmental prolapse or flail (see Fig. 28.8C and D; Video 28.2). However, clear distinction between these two entities is difficult because it has been suggested that they constitute the different ends of a disease spectrum with some valves not demonstrating the typical appearance of Barlow disease but having myxoid infiltration on histopathological exam.

Infective endocarditis with leaflet vegetation and fenestration (Carpentier Type I) is an important cause of primary MR associated with significant morbidity and mortality. The mechanism of MR with infective endocarditis is initially an inflammation of the valve leaflets causing a valvulitis, which is seen as nonspecific thickening on echocardiography, although in many cases, thickening is not evident. Valvulitis results in inefficient or incomplete coaptation of the leaflets and MR. Subsequently, as the inflammatory response progresses, valve tissue is destroyed and vegetation forms on the valve leaflets. The destruction of valve tissue, often signaled by the development of vegetation, may also result in MR (Fig. 28.9; Video 28.3). In some cases, an aneurysm or perforation of the leaflets or chordal rupture can develop (see Fig. 28.9; Video 28.3). The role of echocardiography in endocarditis is also discussed in Chapter 40.

Secondary Mitral Regurgitation

The mechanism of secondary MR is mainly a consequence of abnormal leaflet tethering forces due to LV or annular distortion and dysfunction rather than valvular abnormalities (Carpentier Type IIIB). Hence the mitral leaflets appear "normal" in secondary MR. Altered LV geometry results in PM displacement, which in turn is associated with increased leaflet tethering, resulting in the apical displacement of the coaptation zone and incompetence of the MV (Fig. 28.10).[26–32] Tethering of the mitral leaflets is central to the pathophysiology of secondary MR and predominates even if there is large heterogeneity in the manifestation of the secondary MR.[26,29–31] The displacement of the PM alters the force and direction of the tension exerted on the chordae preventing complete coaptation between apically displaced leaflets.[29,33,34] Coaptation is further impeded by reduced closing forces as a result of LV systolic dysfunction. Hence, secondary MR is characterized by a significantly tented valve with restricted closure of the valve leading to incomplete mitral leaflet closure (Figs. 28.10 and 28.11; Video 28.4). Annular dilation contributes to incomplete mitral leaflet closure and, less commonly, may be the sole cause of secondary MR (Carpentier Type I, see Fig. 28.5). In secondary MR, MV dysfunction should be understood and interpreted in relation to LV geometry and function and not as intrinsic MV abnormalities.

Two distinct entities of secondary MR can be defined according to the underlying cause of the LV geometric alteration: ischemic and nonischemic MR. Ischemic MR refers to mitral regurgitation that occurs as a result of left ventricular remodeling and dysfunction due to coronary artery disease (CAD). The most common mechanism of ischemic MR is characterized by increased MV tethering as a consequence of acute or chronic regional or global LV dilation/dysfunction and altered PM geometry.[35–37] According to the distribution of CAD and the location of the ischemic myocardium, the resulting severity of MR can vary significantly:[31,37,38] even a small ischemic portion of the myocardium can lead to significant MR with preserved overall LV ejection fraction, while

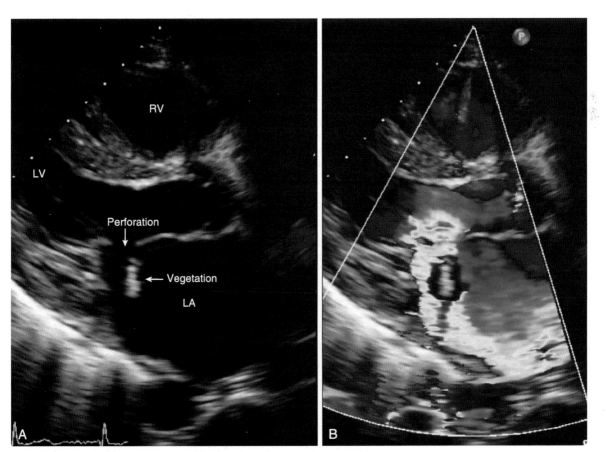

FIG. 28.9 Mitral valve vegetation and perforation (A) and associated mitral regurgitation (B) caused by infective endocarditis (parasternal long-axis view). *LA,* Left atrium; *LV,* left ventricle; *RV,* right ventricle.

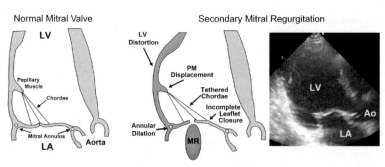

FIG. 28.10 Schematic representation (i.e., apical three-chamber view) of mitral valve apparatus geometry. *Left panel* depicts normal geometry, whereas the *middle panel* depicts secondary mitral regurgitation. In this example, distortion of the left ventricle (LV) wall underlying the papillary muscle, due to ischemia (i.e., infarction) or cardiomyopathy, results in lateral displacement of the papillary muscle. This leads to tethered chordae with incomplete mitral leaflet closure and mitral regurgitation (MR). Annular dilation also contributes to incomplete leaflet closure as do reduced closing forces due to LV systolic dysfunction. The corresponding echocardiographic apical three-chamber view is shown in the *right panel. Ao,* Aorta; *LA,* left atrium; *PM,* papillary muscle.

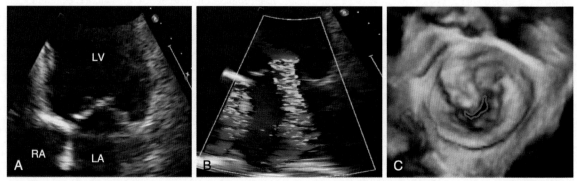

FIG. 28.11 Echocardiographic findings in secondary mitral regurgitation: tethered mitral valve leaflets in apical four-chamber view (A) and associated mitral regurgitation (B), as well as 3D tethered mitral valve in surgeon's view (C). A visible regurgitant orifice *(red line)* is seen in systole. *LA,* Left atrium; *LV,* left ventricle; *RA,* right atrium.

global LV dilation resulting from multiple infarcts could also result in MR of similar severity. In the case of nonischemic MR, the pathophysiology is similar with the exception of the root cause of the LV abnormalities (see Fig. 28.10): remodeling of the LV causes displacement of the PM(s), which increases tethering and malcoaptation of the leaflets).[28,34] In the nonischemic subset of patients with secondary MR, there is usually more homogeneous dilation of the LV but fundamentally, the mechanism is similar to that when the ventricular abnormalities are ischemic.

Less commonly, annular dilation alone without LV dilation or dysfunction can be the mechanistic cause of secondary MR.[32,39,40] This typically occurs in the setting of atrial fibrillation with concomitant annular dilation and dysfunction and can be associated with significant MR.

Assessment of the Degree of Mitral Regurgitation Severity

Assessment of MR severity is essential for clinical decision making due to the strong relationship between the severity of MR and patient outcomes.[13,14,35,41] The American Society of Echocardiography and European Association of Echocardiography (now Cardiovascular Imaging) recommend an integrated approach to the quantitation of MR incorporating semiquantitative measures such as the height of the peak mitral E wave, vena contracta diameter and pulmonary venous flow patterns, and quantitative methods that can derive regurgitant volume and fraction (Table 28.2). The peak E velocity reflects the initial diastolic gradient between the left atrium and LV and increases when MR has resulted in elevation of left atrial pressure and increased early transmitral diastolic flow. E wave height greater than 1.2 mps has been reported in the setting of severe MR.

The vena contracta is the narrowest region of a color jet just distal to the anatomic regurgitant orifice. It is best measured in zoom mode in the parasternal long-axis view or apical views. Cutoffs are: mild, less than 0.3; moderate, 0.3–0.6; and severe, greater than 0.7 cm. In the European guidelines, particularly for secondary MR where the vena contracta is typically ovoid instead of round, it has been suggested that the vena contracta

TABLE 28.2 Doppler-Echocardiographic Parameters to Determine Degree of Mitral Regurgitation Severity

	PRIMARY MITRAL REGURGITATION	SECONDARY MITRAL REGURGITATION
Mild	No MR jet or small central jet area <20% LA on Doppler Small vena contracta 0.3 cm	No MR jet or small central jet area <20% LA on Doppler Small vena contracta <0.30 cm
Moderate	Central jet MR 20%–40% LA or late systolic eccentric jet MR Vena contracta <0.7 cm Regurgitant volume <60 mL Regurgitant fraction <50% ERO <0.40 cm²	ERO <0.20 cm² Regurgitant volume <30 mL Regurgitant fraction <50%
	Angiographic grade 1–2+	
Severe	Central jet MR >40% LA or holosystolic eccentric jet MR Vena contracta ≥0.7 cm Regurgitant volume ≥60 mL Regurgitant fraction >50% ERO ≥0.40 cm² Angiographic grade 3–4+	ERO ≥0.20 cm² Regurgitant volume ≥30 mL Regurgitant fraction ≥50%

Note that not all Doppler echocardiographic parameters are present in each patient. *ERO,* Effective regurgitant orifice; *LA,* left atrium; *MR,* mitral regurgitation. *Data from Nishimura RA, Otto CM, Bonow RO, et al. 2014 AHA/ACC guideline for the management of patients with valvular heart disease: executive summary. A report of the American College of Cardiology/American Heart Association Task Force on Practice Guidelines. J Am Coll Cardiol. 2014;63(22):2438–2488.*

measurements from the apical four- and two-chamber views be averaged with 0.8 cm as a cutoff for severe MR.

Pulmonary venous flow patterns reflect the impact of the MR jet on flow into the left atrium. With severe MR, there is systolic flow reversal of the pulmonary venous flow pattern. Although a color flow jet area indexed to the

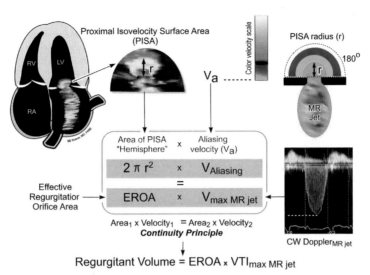

FIG. 28.12 Measurements of the effective regurgitant orifice area and regurgitant volume as determined by the proximal isovelocity surface area (PISA) method. See text for details. *CW*, Continuous-wave; *LV*, left ventricle; *MR*, mitral regurgitation; *RA*, right atrium; *RV*, right ventricle. *(Courtesy of Bernard E. Bulwer, MD, FASE.)*

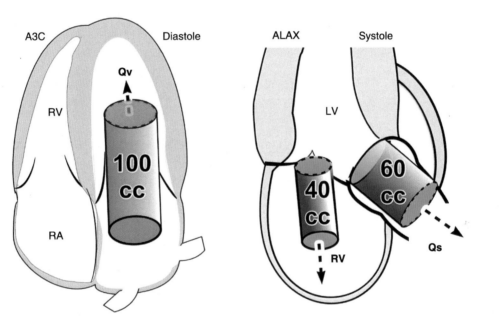

FIG. 28.13 Schematic representing the principle that transmitral flow (or left ventricle [LV] stroke volume) represents the sum of regurgitant volume and forward transaortic stroke volume. See text for details. *(Courtesy of Bernard E. Bulwer, MD, FASE.)*

left atrial area has been used to quantitate MR, its use is discouraged in the current European guidelines. Although the color jet size approach is easy, it is influenced by machine settings and underestimates severity with eccentric jets and overestimates severity with non-holosystolic MR. Importantly, the color jet area is simply not equivalent to the regurgitant volume.

Quantitation of regurgitant volume and effective regurgitant orifice area (EROA) is possible with the proximal isovelocity surface area (PISA) approach, which is based on the concept of acceleration of flow proximal to the regurgitant orifice (Fig. 28.12). Application of this technique requires zooming in on the color jet and baseline shifting in the direction of the jet to optimize the hemisphericity of the PISA shell, the point at which flow reaches the Nyquist limit with the resultant shift in the color display. The distance from the vena contracta to the shell (PISA radius) is combined with measurements taken from the continuous-wave (CW) Doppler MR spectrum to provide EROA and regurgitant volume (see Fig. 28.12). The PISA method is limited in situations where the assumption of a hemispheric PISA shell and circular regurgitant orifice is invalid, as may be encountered with eccentric jets due to degenerative MR as well as many cases of functional/ischemic MR. In non-holosystolic MR, the EROA calculated with the PISA approach will overestimate severity

because it reflects the maximum, not an average EROA. It is also limited in the setting of multiple jets.

The quantitative Doppler approach (Fig. 28.13) uses the continuity equation to provide an alternative method of calculating regurgitant volume and can also provide the regurgitant fraction (= regurgitant volume/LV stroke volume). It is the only method that is well suited to multiple jets. This method calculates forward stroke volume as flow across a nonstenotic, nonregurgitant reference valve, typically the aortic valve and subtracts this from either the total antegrade flow across the MV or the LV stroke volume. Antegrade flow across the MV is calculated by assuming that the orifice is circular with the diameter measured from the four-chamber view and calculation of the cross-sectional area as (π * $(d/2)^2$), or that it is oval, incorporating the diameters from the four- and two-chamber views. The velocity time integral from the pulsed Doppler spectral recording taken at the annulus, not at the leaflet tips, is combined with the mitral cross-sectional area to yield antegrade transmitral flow.

The major limitation of the quantitative Doppler technique lies in the assumption of planar circular (or oval) mitral orifice geometry in calculating transmitral flow. The use of left ventricular stroke volume calculated from echo-measured LV volumes compared with aortic outflow has been suggested as an alternate approach. The advent of 3D echo has provided methods for direct planimetry of regurgitant orifices and optimized assessment of nonhemispherical PISA shells, but these methods are not yet widely used clinically.

It is important to recognize that functional and, to a lesser degree, MR of other etiologies is afterload dependent and determination of severity must take into account left ventricular systolic pressure. Clinical decision making based on severity determinations made under general anesthesia is to be avoided because anesthesia is associated with a predictable fall in systemic vascular resistance and may dramatically reduce the degree of regurgitation.

Although current imaging guidelines indicate that many of the parameters used to assess the severity of MR apply regardless of MR etiology, the 2014 ACC/AHA Guidelines for Management of Patients with Valvular Disease[13] suggest that the quantitative cut-points defining severity of MR based on PISA are different depending on the underlying etiology of the MR (i.e., primary or secondary MR), a recommendation that has been controversial.[14,16,42] For primary MR, the cutoff values for EROA and regurgitant volume for severe MR are 0.4 cm² and 60 mL

respectively. For secondary MR, the cutoff values are 0.2 cm² and 30 mL for EROA and regurgitant volume respectively. This difference in cutoff values depending on etiology is based on the prognostic importance of mild or greater secondary MR.[14,35] However, there are important considerations in applying a lower EROA standard for secondary MR. First, the prognostic data are based on retrospective analyses and subject to selection bias.[42,43] Second, EROA and regurgitant volume values are affected by underlying LV end-diastolic volume, ejection fraction, and the pressure gradient between the LV and left atrium, and can thus result in lower EROA values for secondary MR.[42] Finally, a hemispherical assumption tends to underestimate the EROA and regurgitant volume. This underestimation is exacerbated to a greater extent in secondary MR due to the more elliptical shape of the regurgitant orifice in secondary MR.[44,45]

MITRAL STENOSIS

The two most common etiologies of MS are rheumatic MS and calcific (or degenerative) MS. Rheumatic MS is more frequently encountered in developing countries and may affect young and middle-aged patients,

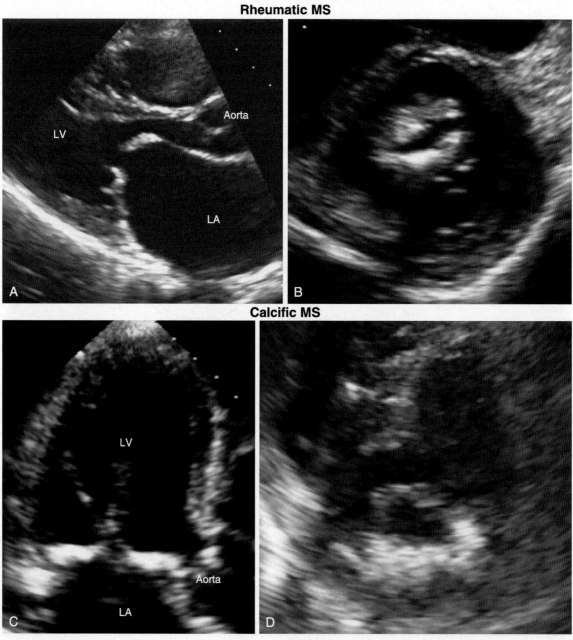

FIG. 28.14 Echocardiographic findings for the two most common etiologies of mitral valve stenosis: rheumatic mitral stenosis in parasternal long- and short-axis views (A and B) and calcific (or degenerative) mitral stenosis in apical three-chamber and parasternal short-axis views (C and D). *LA*, Left atrium; *LV*, left ventricle; *MS*, mitral stenosis.

particularly women.[3,46,47] Calcific MS is a degenerative disease associated with other cardiac risk factors (i.e., hypertension, atherosclerosis, kidney failure, etc.) and mostly affects older patients in industrialized countries.[1,2,46,48]

Rheumatic Mitral Stenosis

The development of rheumatic MS is the result of streptococcus infection leading to rheumatic fever.[3,46] Rheumatic MS is mainly characterized by commissural fusion resulting in reduced leaflet mobility (Fig. 28.14A and B). Leaflet thickening and fibrosis, as well as chordal shortening are also frequent in rheumatic MS, but their hemodynamic consequences are heterogeneous. Echocardiographic features are (see Fig. 28.14A and B) (1) doming of the anterior leaflet, where the narrowest orifice occurs at the leaflet tips; (2) posterior leaflet immobility; (3) fusion of the commissures resulting in a "fish mouth" appearance of the MV orifice; and (4) thickening, calcification, and shortening of the subvalvular chords, which extends to the PMs in severe cases. Rheumatic disease may also be associated with MR (Carpentier Type IIIA; see Fig. 28.5).

Morphological features of the MV as assessed by echocardiography have been shown to predict the success of percutaneous mitral valvulotomy (PMV).[49] A common scoring system used for this purpose, the Wilkins Score, is based on four echo-defined morphological features of the mitral valve apparatus: leaflet mobility, leaflet thickening, leaflet

calcification, and subvalvular thickening (Table 28.3).[49] Each morphological feature is assigned a score from 0 to 4 for a total score ranging from 0 to 16 (see Table 28.3). The higher the number, the worse the outcome of PMV with scores of 8 or below favoring successful PMV.[49]

The development of severe MR is an important determinant of morbidity and mortality following PMV. Calcification of the commissures has been shown to be a predictor of severe post-PMV MR.[50] However, assessment of morphological features using the Wilkins score and commissural calcification to predict post-PMV MR is semiquantitative, subject to observer variability, and less reliable for scores in the midrange. A recent study examined the prognostic value of commissural area and leaflet displacement, which are quantitative echocardiographic measures that combine functional and morphological features of the Wilkins Score and commissural calcification (Fig. 28.15). An alternative scoring system (the Nunes score) based on four morphological features including commissural area, leaflet displacement, mitral valve area (MVA), and subvalvular involvement has demonstrated improved accuracy for predicting PMV success and development of severe MR compared to the Wilkins score and commissural calcium.[48] Low scores (0–3) out of a total of 11 are associated with favorable PMV outcome, both in regard to MVA achieved and MR development. A commissural area ratio of greater than 1.25 or leaflet displacement of less than 12 mm is associated with poor PMV success.[51] Fig. 28.16 shows TTE findings of a patient with a high Nunes score.

TABLE 28.3 Wilkins Score Grading in Mitral Valve Stenosis

GRADE	LEAFLET MOBILITY	LEAFLET THICKENING	LEAFLET CALCIFICATION	SUBVALVULAR THICKENING
1	Highly mobile valve with only leaflet tips restricted	Leaflets near normal in thickness (4–5 mm)	A single area of increased echo brightness	Minimal thickening just below the mitral leaflets
2	Leaflet mid and basal portions have normal mobility	Mid-leaflets normal considerable thickening of margins (5–8 mm)	Scattered areas of brightness confined to leaflet margins	Thickening of chordal structures extending up to one-third of the chordal length
3	Valve continues to move forward in diastole, mainly from the base	Thickening extending through the entire leaflet (5–8 mm)	Brightness extending into the midportion of the leaflets	Thickening extending to the distal third of the chords
4	No or minimal forward movement of leaflets in diastole	Considerable thickening of all leaflet tissue (>8–10 mm)	Extensive brightness throughout much of the leaflet tissue	Extensive thickening and shortening of all chordal structures extending down to the papillary muscles

According to the above criteria, each morphological feature of the mitral valve is assigned a score from 0 to 4 for a total Wilkins score ranging from 0 to 16.
Adapted from Wilkins GT, Weyman AE, Abascal VM, Block PC, Palacios IF. Percutaneous balloon dilatation of the mitral valve: an analysis of echocardiographic variables related to outcome and the mechanism of dilatation. Br Heart J. 1988;60(4):299–308.

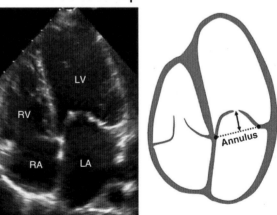

FIG. 28.15 Measurements of the two quantitative echocardiographic parameters integrated in the Nunes score to predict success of percutaneous mitral valvulotomy: commissural area ratio (*left*; from parasternal short axis) and maximal apical leaflet displacement (*right*; from apical four-chamber). The commissural area ratio is calculated as follows. The mitral valve area was first outlined by tracing the inner margin of the leaflets from the parasternal short-axis view. Second, the ventricular (outer) surface of the leaflets was traced, and the area between the two tracings was recorded. The major diameter of the outer border was then measured, and its midpoint was determined. A line perpendicular to the major dimension passing through this point (the minor dimension) was then drawn, and the leaflet area on either side of the minor dimension was measured. The symmetry of commissural thickening was then quantified as the ratio between the leaflet areas on either side of the minor dimension. Because the ratio between the areas was used rather than absolute values, variation in receiver gain settings should have limited influence on the ratio. Apical displacement of the leaflets was measured in the apical four-chamber view as the distance from the mitral annulus to the midportion of the leaflets at their point of maximal displacement from the annulus (doming height) in diastole. The midportion of the leaflet was taken as the end of the height measurement to account for variation in leaflet calcification. *LA*, Left atrium; *LV*, left ventricle; *RA*, right atrium; *RV*, right ventricle. *(From Nunes MC, Tan TC, Elmariah S, et al. The echo score revisited: impact of incorporating commissural morphology and leaflet displacement to the prediction of outcome for patients undergoing percutaneous mitral valvuloplasty. Circulation. 2014;129[8]:886–895.)*

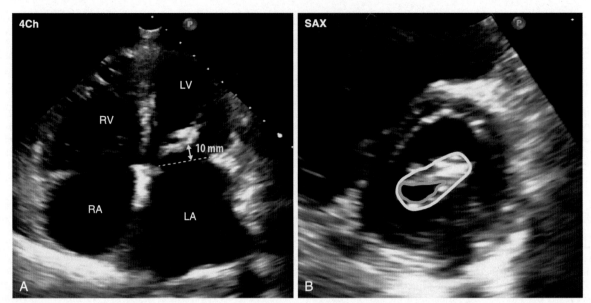

FIG. 28.16 **Example of a high Nunes score.** Transthoracic echocardiography showing a decreased maximal leaflet displacement (10 mm, *yellow arrow*; A) and a high commissural area ratio (>1.25; B). *4Ch,* Apical four-chamber; *LA,* left atrium; *LV,* left ventricle; *RA,* right atrium; *RV,* right ventricle; *SAX,* short axis.

Calcific Mitral Stenosis

This degenerative disease is characterized by nonrheumatic calcification of the MV apparatus.[52] In older patients, mitral annular calcification is often encountered, and in some cases can extend to the mitral leaflets (see Fig. 28.14C and D). The calcification and thickening starts at the mitral annulus and extends into the leaflet bodies, resulting in a narrowed mitral orifice. The leaflet tips and commissures are typically not affected or involved late in the process, in contrast to rheumatic MS. Traditional cardiovascular risk factors, such as female gender, age, diabetes, hypertension, CAD, and chronic kidney disease, are associated with annular calcification and, by extension, calcific MS.

Assessment of the Degree of Mitral Stenosis Severity

A comprehensive assessment of the MV leaflets and associated apparatus (i.e., leaflet thickening, mobility and calcification, commissural fusion, and chordal abnormalities) is essential to determine the underlying pathophysiology of MS: rheumatic or calcific MS.[15] The assessment of MS severity is also essential for therapeutic decision making in patients with MS.[13,14] Echocardiographic indices that are typically used for the assessment of the severity of MS include MVA, mean transvalvular mitral velocities (or gradients), and diastolic pressure half-time (PHT; Table 28.4; Fig. 28.17).[13–15] However, it should be noted that for calcific MS, there are no validated approaches to assessing MVA.

MVA is an important parameter for the assessment of rheumatic MS severity[13–15] and can be derived using a number of methods. Transvalvular mitral velocities (or gradient) and PHT (mainly used to determine MVA) are complementary parameters in rheumatic disease and play a more important role in calcific disease.[13–15] Transvalvular velocities, which are strongly dependent on transvalvular mitral flow, frequently underestimate the severity of MS in patients with low cardiac output.[53]

MVA is measured clinically by two methods (see Fig. 28.17): (i) direct 2D or 3D guided planimetry and (ii) PHT. Alternate methods include the continuity equation or PISA method but these are less well validated and less commonly used.[15] The planimetry method requires that the MVA be imaged at the leaflet tips in the parasternal short-axis view (see Fig. 28.17). 3D imaging can help guide the plane to the tips of the leaflets to ensure that the narrowest MV orifice is measured (see Fig. 28.17).[54,55]

MVA derived from the PHT is based on an empirically derived formula: MVA = 220/PHT. However, PHT is affected by altered LV compliance and is inaccurate in situations in which diastolic filling is not exclusively due to transmitral flow such as aortic regurgitation. The presence of aortic regurgitation results in a more rapid increase in LV

TABLE 28.4 Doppler-Echocardiographic Parameters to Determine Degree of Mitral Stenosis Severity

	MILD MS	MODERATE MS	SEVERE MS
Trans-mitral flow velocities	Normal velocities	Increased velocities	Increased velocities
Mitral valve area	—	>1.5 cm^2	≤1.5 cm^{2a}
Diastolic pressure half-time	—	<150 ms	≥150 ms^b

^{a}Very severe MS if mitral valve area ≤1.0 cm^2.
^{b}Very severe MS if diastolic pressure half-time ≥220 ms.
Note that not all Doppler echocardiographic parameters are present in each patient.
MS, Mitral stenosis.
Data from Nishimura RA, Otto CM, Bonow RO, et al. 2014 AHA/ACC guideline for the management of patients with valvular heart disease: executive summary. A report of the American College of Cardiology/American Heart Association Task Force on Practice Guidelines. J Am Coll Cardiol. *2014;63(22):2438–2488; Baumgartner H, Hung J, Bermejo J, et al. Echocardiographic assessment of valve stenosis: EAE/ASE recommendations for clinical practice.* Eur J Echocardiogr. *2009;10(1):1–25.*

pressure than would occur due to transmitral flow alone, thereby providing a misleadingly short PHT that will overestimate the MVA. Reduced ventricular compliance will similarly affect PHT. In addition, it can be difficult to measure PHT in the setting of atrial fibrillation with varying R-R intervals and the method has been shown to be invalid in the early postvalvuloplasty period. The PHT may be difficult to calculate when the mitral inflow Doppler spectrum has a biphasic contour and, importantly, it has not been validated for calcific MS or for prosthetic valves.

Although the continuity equation or PISA method to determine MVA is not used routinely, these may provide an alternate measure of MVA when planimetry or PHT is unclear.[15] In the PISA approach, MVA = $(\Pi r^2)(V_{aliasing})/(Peak\ V_{mitral}) \times \alpha/180$, where α is the angle formed by the doming cusps, or a simplification of this equation, where α is assumed to be 100 degrees (Fig. 28.18). A continuity-based method has also been proposed where MVA = $\Pi\ (D_{LVOT}/2)^2(VTI_{LVOT}/VTI_{MV})$, where D is the diameter of the left ventricular outflow tract measured in the parasternal long-axis view.

An integrative approach is important to define the degree of MS severity. The strengths and weaknesses of each approach should also be considered. Ultimately, the measurements of MVA should be consistent with transvalvular velocities (or gradient).[15]

Radiation-Associated Mitral Valve Disease

Radiation-associated MVD occurs following mediastinal radiation for treatment of certain malignancies such as Hodgkin lymphoma. As

3D-Guided MVA planimetry

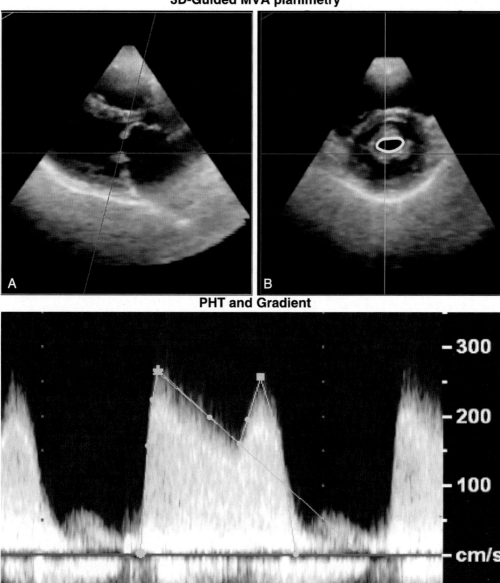

PHT and Gradient

FIG. 28.17 Measurements of the main quantitative parameters used to determine the degree of mitral stenosis: 3D guided mitral valve area by planimetry (*yellow circle*; A and B), and pressure half-time and mitral valve gradient (C). *MVA*, Mitral valve area; *PHT*, pressure half-time.

regimens reduce radiation dose and use shielding that minimizes cardiac radiation exposure, the incidence of radiation-associated MVD should decrease. The pathophysiology of radiation-induced MVD is felt to be due to direct radiation damage to MV tissue, resulting in a cascade of inflammatory changes with eventual fibrosis and calcification. The echocardiographic features are diffuse thickening and calcification of the mitral leaflets and subvalvular region leading to reduced mobility. Commonly, mixed MV dysfunction is present with both MS and MR.[56,57]

CONGENITAL MITRAL VALVE DISORDERS

Congenital anomalies of the MV represent a spectrum of lesions affecting different components of the MV apparatus. Mitral cleft, parachute, and supravalvular ring are the most frequently encountered congenital lesions.

Mitral Valve Cleft

Mitral cleft is characterized by the division of one leaflet, usually the anterior leaflet of the MV (Fig. 28.19A and B; Video 28.5). Congenital mitral

clefts may be isolated or occur in combination with atrioventricular canal septal defects.[58-62] The presence of mitral cleft is frequently associated with MR, which can be severe in 50% of cases.[63]

Mitral Valve Parachute

MV parachute is characterized by the attachment of chordae to a single PM (or fused PM). This PM is usually located centrally and receives all the chordae from both leaflets but may be eccentric and have multiple heads (see Fig. 28.19C and D; Video 28.6). The chordae are also typically short and thickened, resulting in restriction of leaflet motion and stenosis of the valve with varying degrees of severity.

Mitral Arcade

Mitral arcade results from lack of development of the mitral chordae leading to an "arcade" or hammock-like appearance of the mitral chordae. Functionally, the chordae are thickened or absent, and leaflets appear to attach directly to the PMs, resulting in MS.

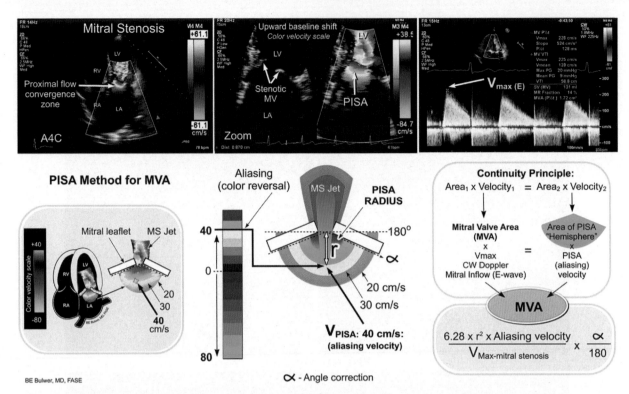

PISA Method for MVA

BE Bulwer, MD, FASE

∝ - Angle correction

Continuity Principle:

$$Area_1 \times Velocity_1 = Area_2 \times Velocity_2$$

Mitral Valve Area (MVA) × Vmax CW Doppler Mitral Inflow (E-wave) = Area of PISA "Hemisphere" × PISA (aliasing) velocity

MVA

$$\frac{6.28 \times r^2 \times Aliasing\ velocity}{V_{Max-mitral\ stenosis}} \times \frac{\propto}{180}$$

FIG. 28.18 Schematic of the proximal isovelocity surface area (PISA) approach to calculating the mitral valve area (MVA). MVA = $(\Pi r^2)(V_{aliasing})/(Peak\ V_{mitral}) \times \alpha/180$, where α is the angle formed by the doming cusps. *(Courtesy of Bernard E. Bulwer, MD, FASE.)*

MV Cleft

MV Parachute

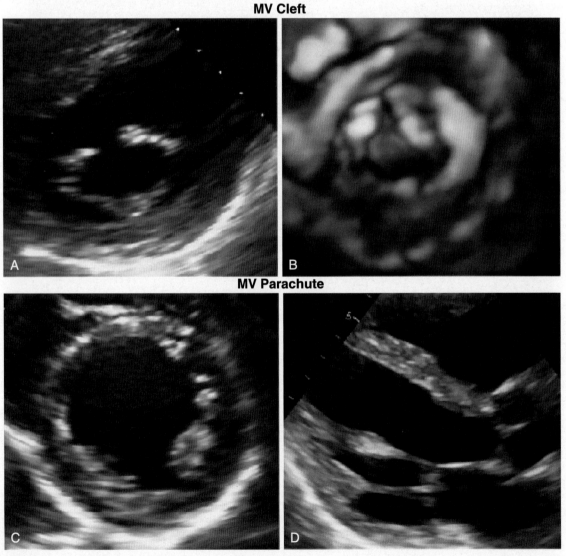

FIG. 28.19 Echocardiographic findings for mitral valve (MV) cleft in short-axis and 3D surgeon views (A and B) and MV parachute in parasternal short- and long-axis views (C and D).

Supravalvular Mitral Ring

A supravalvular mitral ring is a fibrous membrane originating above the mitral annulus but not directly attached to the MV apparatus, resulting in supra-annular stenosis of the MV.

CONCLUSION

MVD is associated with significant cardiovascular morbidity and mortality.[1–3] With aging of the population, the prevalence of MVD will increase exponentially. Echocardiography is the primary imaging modality for the assessment of MV anatomy and function and plays a critical role for clinical decision making for MVD.

Suggested Reading

Grayburn, P. A., Carabello, B., Hung, J., et al. (2014). Defining "severe" secondary mitral-regurgitation: emphasizing an integrated approach. *Journal of the American College of Cardiology, 64*(25), 2792–2801.

Lancellotti, P., Moura, L., Pierard, L. A., et al. (2010). European Association of Echocardiography recommendations for the assessment of valvular regurgitation. Part 2: mitral and tricuspid regurgitation (native valve disease). *European Journal of Echocardiography, 11*(4), 307–332.

Lang, R. M., Tsang, W., Weinert, L., Mor-Avi, V., & Chandra, S. (2011). Valvular heart disease: the value of 3-dimensional echocardiography. *Journal of the American College of Cardiology, 58*(19), 1933–1944.

Nishimura, R. A., Otto, C. M., Bonow, R. O., et al. (2014). 2014 AHA/ACC guideline for the management of patients with valvular heart disease: a report of the American College of Cardiology/American Heart Association Task Force on Practice Guidelines. *Journal of the American College of Cardiology, 63*(22), 2438–2488.

Zoghbi, W. A., Enriquez-Sarano, M., Foster, E., et al. (2003). Recommendations for evaluation of the severity of native valvular regurgitation with two-dimensional and Doppler echocardiography. *Journal of the American Society of Echocardiography, 16*(7), 777–802.

A complete reference list can be found online at ExpertConsult.com.

29 Aortic Valve Disease

Linda D. Gillam

INTRODUCTION

Aortic valve (AV) disease is the most common valve disease in developed countries. Aortic stenosis (AS), which is most often due to calcification and degeneration of congenitally normal tricuspid valves, affects approximately 1.5 million people in the United States with a prevalence that increases with age. While hemodynamically significant AS (moderate or severe) is unusual before the age of 65, in those aged 65–74 the prevalence is approximately 1%, increasing to 3%–5% of those over the age of 75. Aortic sclerosis, arguably a precursor to AS, is even more common, affecting 40% of those over the age of 75, and, while not hemodynamically significant, it is associated with an increased risk of stroke, myocardial infarction, and death, even with adjustment for traditional cardiovascular risk factors.

In those under the age of 70, AS is most typically based on a bicuspid AV, often with superimposed calcific changes. Bicuspid AV is one of the most common forms of congenital heart disease, affecting 0.5%–0.8% of the population, and occurring more commonly in men. Rheumatic valve disease is a less common cause of AS and there are rare cases of AS due to endocarditis, Fabry disease, lupus, ochronosis, hyperuricemia, and Paget's disease.

Aortic regurgitation (AR) may be due to a primary valvular problem or loss of support as a result of aortic root or annular dilatation. A less common cause is aortic dissection with prolapse of the intimal flap. The most common valvular abnormality is bicuspid AV with less common causes being endocarditis, rheumatic disease, aortic sclerosis, connective tissue disease, anorectic drug toxicity, radiation, antiphospholipid syndrome, subaortic stenosis, ventricular septal defect, and systemic inflammatory disorders. Moderate to severe AR has a reported prevalence of 0.5% in the US population.

Echocardiography plays an important role in the diagnosis and management of AV disease with the introduction of transcatheter AV replacement greatly expanding its role in guiding treatment. Both transthoracic echocardiography (TTE) and transesophageal echocardiography (TEE) and, increasingly, three-dimensional (3D) techniques are essential tools. This chapter covers the use of echocardiography in the comprehensive evaluation of the AV, with the objectives of assessing the nature, severity and etiology of valve dysfunction (stenosis and/or regurgitation), the anatomic changes responsible for this dysfunction, and, where possible, the disease process that has resulted in these anatomic changes. Importantly,

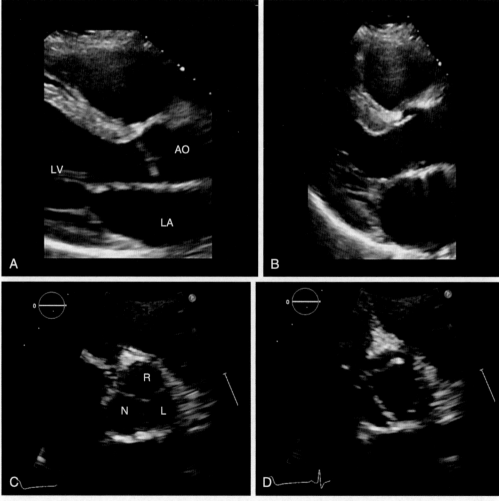

FIG. 29.1 Parasternal long-axis (A and B) and short-axis (C and D) echocardiograms showing the normal appearance of the aortic valve in diastole (A and C) and systole (B and D). *Ao,* Aorta; *L,* left coronary cusp; *LA,* left atrium; *LV,* left ventricle; *N,* noncoronary cusp; *R,* right coronary cusp.

echo also provides important information concerning secondary changes in cardiac anatomy and function, notably those of the left ventricle.

NORMAL AORTIC VALVE ANATOMY AND COMMON CONGENITAL ANOMALIES

The normal AV consists of three symmetric cusps that are supported by the aortic annulus and extend into the aortic root. The right and left coronary cusps lie within the sinuses of Valsalva that give rise to the corresponding coronary arteries with the remaining cusp termed the noncoronary cusp. The ideal views for assessing AV anatomy are the parasternal short- and long-axis views (Fig. 29.1, Videos 29.1 and 29.2) and their comparable views on transesophageal echocardiography. The short-axis view shows all three cusps that create a triangular-shaped orifice when open and have a Y-shaped appearance when closed. The long axis typically displays the right and noncoronary cusps that flatten against the walls of the aortic root when normally open and meet centrally without prolapse below the plane of the aortic annulus with normal closure. The long-axis view can be angulated to show the right and left coronary cusps. Doppler evaluation employs these views as well as the apical three- and five-chamber, suprasternal and right parasternal views, all of which ensure that Doppler interrogation is parallel to flow.

The most common congenital abnormalities of the AV result from failures of cusp development and include, in order of decreasing frequency, bicuspid, unicuspid, and quadricuspid valves (Fig. 29.2, Videos 29.3–29.8). Bicuspid valves can be distinguished based on the position of

the coronary arteries to the line of closure. When both coronaries arise on the same side, the commissure is termed horizontal while, with a vertical commissure, the coronaries arise on opposite sides. The newer alternative nomenclature systems reflect which commissures are absent or exist as raphes (vestigial commissures) or the spatial orientation of the commissure (right-left or anterior-posterior). Right-left fusion with a raphe is the most common.[1,2] A discussion of the clinical implications of bicuspid valve classification is beyond the scope of this chapter.

Because of the inability of bicuspid valves to open fully, the systolic orifice of a bicuspid AV is oval when seen in short axis while the long-axis view demonstrates protrusion of one or both cusp tips into the aortic lumen (doming; see Fig. 29.2 and Videos 29.3 and 29.4). While classically bicuspid AVs have a single line of closure, many such valves have an echogenic ridge or raphe that represents a vestigial commissure. The closed appearance of such valves may be indistinguishable echocardiographically from a tricuspid valve. Thus, bicuspid AV is an echocardiographic systolic diagnosis. Unicuspid valves typically have circular openings that may be central or asymmetrically positioned, while quadricuspid valves have a cloverleaf-like appearance in systole and cross-like appearance in diastole (see Fig. 29.2 and Videos 29.5–29.8).

Congenital abnormalities of the left ventricular outflow track include subaortic membranes characterized by linear echoes extending from the anterior mitral leaflet to the septum (Fig. 29.3, Video 29.9) or fibromuscular tunnels in which there is an echogenic ridge extending into the left ventricular outflow track. The presence of subaortic systolic turbulence should prompt

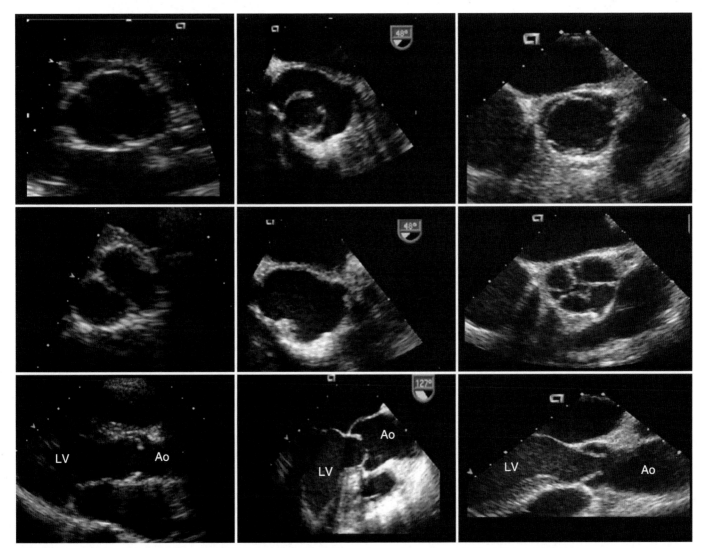

FIG. 29.2 Congenital abnormalities of the aortic valve with (top to bottom) systolic short-axis, diastolic short-axis, and systolic long-axis views. *Left panels:* bicuspid aortic valve. *Middle panels:* unicuspid unicommissural aortic valve. *Right panels:* quadricuspid aortic valve. *Ao,* Aorta; *LV,* left ventricle. (From Solomon SD, Wu J, Gillam L. Echocardiography. In: Mann DL, Zipes DP, Libby P, et al., eds. Braunwald's Heart Disease: A Textbook of Cardiovascular Medicine. *10th ed. Philadelphia: Elsevier; 2015:179–260.*)

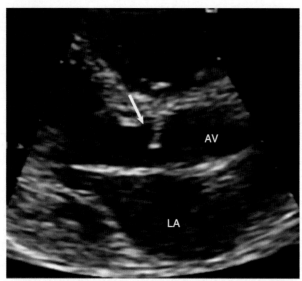

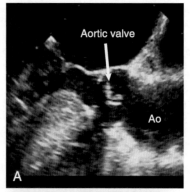

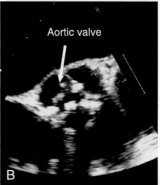

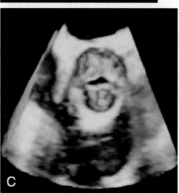

FIG. 29.3 Nonstandard parasternal long-axis view demonstrating a subaortic membrane *(arrow)*. The image is angled to show the membrane well with the result that the aortic valve (AV) is not well seen. *LA,* Left atrium. (*From Solomon SD, Wu J, Gillam L. Echocardiography. In: Mann DL, Zipes DP, Libby P, et al., eds.* Braunwald's Heart Disease: A Textbook of Cardiovascular Medicine. *10th ed. Philadelphia: Elsevier; 2015: 179–260.*)

a close inspection of the left ventricular outflow tract for evidence of subaortic obstruction that may be best seen in apical or nonstandard parasternal long-axis views. Aortic valvular regurgitation is frequently seen with subaortic membrane reflecting trauma to the valve by the subaortic stenotic jet. Supravalvular AS is a rare phenomenon consisting of a localized or diffuse narrowing of the ascending aorta distal to the sinuses of Valsalva.

VALVULAR AORTIC STENOSIS

Although the impeded cusp excursion of the bicuspid or unicuspid AV may alone result in AS, calcium deposition on a congenitally normal tricuspid AV is the most common cause of AS seen in adults. The echocardiographic appearance is one of restricted cusp excursion with irregular nodular cusp thickening (Fig. 29.4, Videos 29.10–29.12). While echocardiography can provide a semiquantitative assessment of calcium burden, computed tomography (CT) may be better suited for this purpose.

Quantitation of Aortic Stenosis Severity

Table 29.1 displays a hemodynamic classification of aortic stenotic severity with echocardiography playing a key role. For reference, a normal aortic valve area (AVA) is 3–4 cm². Application of the Bernoulli equation to continuous-wave Doppler interrogation of transvalvular flow provides accurate measures of mean and peak instantaneous gradient. Typically, the simplified form of the equation ($\Delta P = 4 V^2$) may be used, but when the left ventricular outflow tract velocity exceeds 1 meter per second, the expanded version, $\Delta P = 4 (V_2^2 - V_1^2)$ where V_2 is the transaortic velocity and V_1 is left ventricular outflow tract (LVOT) velocity, should be employed.

Recognizing the importance of recording Doppler signals parallel to flow, aortic gradients are best recorded using the apical five- or three-chamber, suprasternal notch and right parasternal windows with the highest velocities most commonly achieved using the right parasternal view (Fig. 29.5). The smaller footprint provided by the nonimaging Pedoff probe makes it essential for the optimal assessment of patients with AS. When transesophageal echo is used, velocities are recorded using the deep transgastric views. Contrast may be helpful in enhancing Doppler spectra (Fig. 29.6). It should be noted that while echocardiographically derived mean gradients are identical to those obtained invasively, the echo peak instantaneous gradient is typically higher than the peak-to-peak gradient calculated in the catheterization lab. The latter is the arithmetic difference between peak left ventricular and aortic pressures (Fig. 29.7).

While gradients alone provide a reasonable assessment of aortic stenotic severity when transaortic flow is normal, they may underestimate severity in the setting of low flow states and overestimate severity when flow is elevated (e.g., high-output states such as those caused by sepsis and anemia). For this

FIG. 29.4 Systolic TEE images of valvular aortic stenosis (tricuspid valve). (A) 2D long axis. There is minimal opening of the valve. (B) Short axis. (C) 3D. The latter two views better demonstrate the distribution of the calcium. (*From Solomon SD, Wu J, Gillam L. Echocardiography. In: Mann DL, Zipes DP, Libby P, et al., eds.* Braunwald's Heart Disease: A Textbook of Cardiovascular Medicine. *10th ed. Philadelphia: Elsevier; 2015: 179–260.*)

TABLE 29.1 Grading of Aortic Stenosis Severity

	MILD	MODERATE	SEVERE
Mean gradient mm Hg	<20	20–39	≥40
Aortic valve area cm²	>1.5	1.1–1.5	≤1.0
Peak gradient mm Hg	<36	36–63	≥64

reason, it is important to determine AVA. While direct planimetry of TEE images may be used for this purpose, TTE planimetry is not sufficiently accurate. The most common approach, therefore, is by application of the continuity equation. As shown in Fig. 29.8, AVA is calculated as AVA = (CSA $_{LVOT}$ × VTI$_{LVOT}$)/VTI$_{AV}$, where velocity time integral (VTI) represents the VTI or area under the spectral Doppler curve, and CSA represents cross-sectional area. Less desirable, is the simplified version AVA = (CSA $_{LVOT}$ × V$_{LVOT}$)/V$_{AV}$ where V represents peak velocity. The cross-sectional area of the left ventricular outflow tract is typically calculated assuming circular geometry using the formula CSA = π(D/2)², where D is the systolic left ventricular outflow tract diameter measured in the parasternal or TEE equivalent long-axis view. According to the American Society of Echocardiography (ASE) convention,[3]

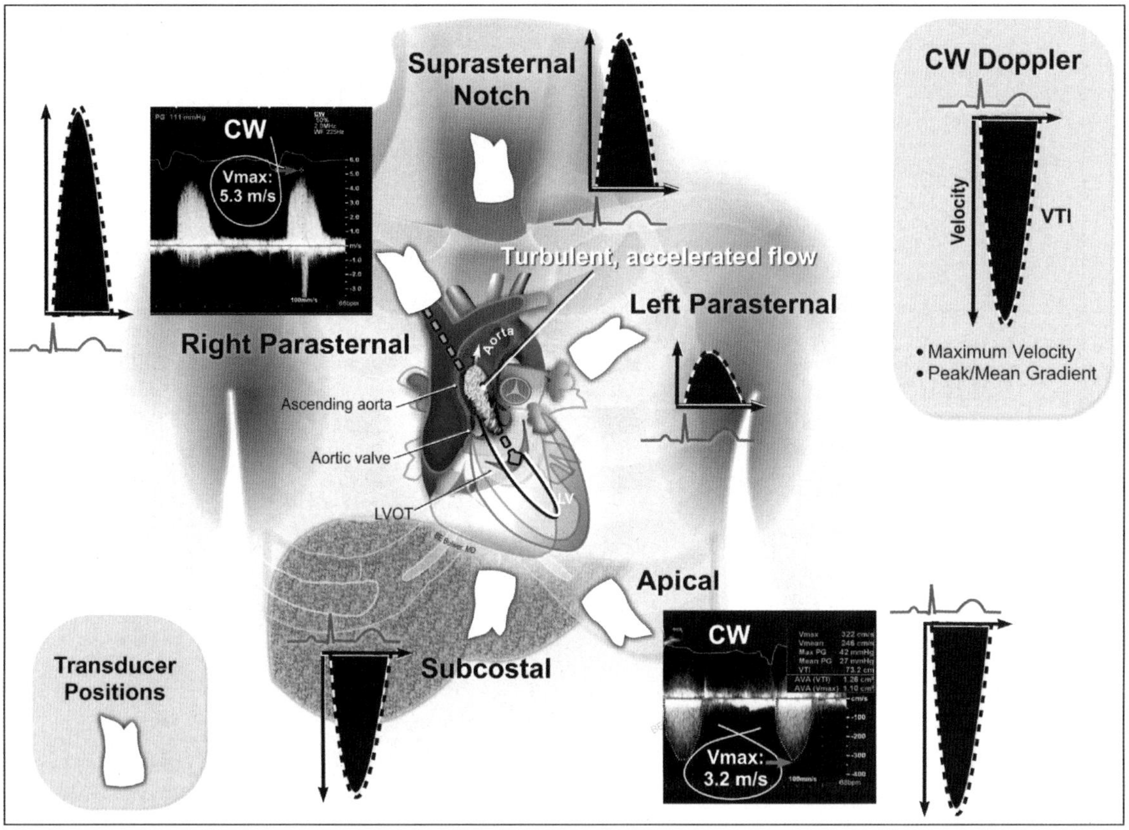

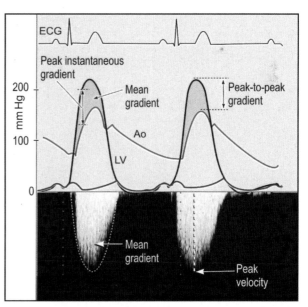

FIG. 29.5 Schematic showing continuous-wave (CW) spectra recorded from different windows in the setting of aortic stenosis. The maximal gradients are typically recorded from the right parasternal window. *LVOT,* Left ventricular outflow tract; *VTI,* velocity time integral. *(Courtesy of Bernard E. Bulwer, MD, FASE.)*

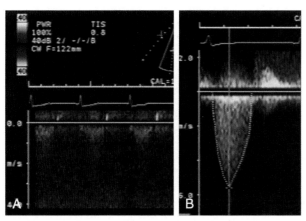

FIG. 29.6 Baseline unenhanced Doppler spectra (A) in this patient with valvular aortic stenosis are indistinct. Following administration of a contrast agent (B) the continuous-wave (CW) spectra are clearly defined. *(From Solomon SD, Wu J, Gillam L. Echocardiography. In: Mann DL, Zipes DP, Libby P, et al., eds.* Braunwald's Heart Disease: A Textbook of Cardiovascular Medicine. *10th ed. Philadelphia: Elsevier; 2015:179–260.)*

FIG. 29.7 Doppler methods provide peak instantaneous and mean gradients. The peak instantaneous gradient is typically higher than the peak-to-peak gradient calculated from invasively measured peak left ventricle (LV) and aortic pressures, although mean gradients measured with both techniques are identical. *(Courtesy of Bernard E. Bulwer, MD, FASE; From Solomon SD, Wu J, Gillam L. Echocardiography. In: Mann DL, Zipes DP, Libby P, et al., eds.* Braunwald's Heart Disease: A Textbook of Cardiovascular Medicine. *10th ed. Philadelphia: Elsevier; 2015:179–260.)*

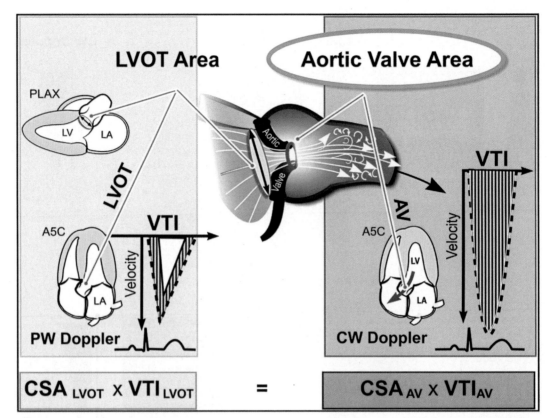

FIG. 29.8 Continuity equation approach to calculating aortic valve area. The aortic valve cross-sectional area (CSA_{AV}) is calculated as ($CSA_{LVOT} \times VTI_{LVOT}$)/$VTI_{AV}$). The left ventricular outflow tract (LVOT) cross-sectional area is calculated as Π $(D/2)^2$, where D is the LVOT diameter. The LVOT velocity time integral (VTI) should be measured from the modal rather than the maximal velocity. *CW,* Continuous wave; *LA,* left atrium; *LV,* left ventricle; *PW,* pulsed-wave Doppler. (*Courtesy of Bernard E. Bulwer, MD, FASE; From Solomon SD, Wu J, Gillam L. Echocardiography. In: Mann DL, Zipes DP, Libby P, et al., eds.* Braunwald's Heart Disease: A Textbook of Cardiovascular Medicine. *10th ed. Philadelphia: Elsevier; 2015:179–260.*)

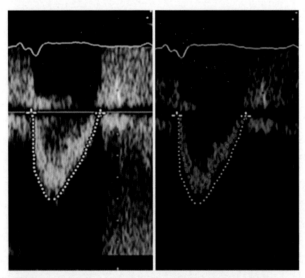

FIG. 29.9 Doppler spectra demonstrating the error that may be introduced if the maximal *(white dotted line)* rather than the modal *(red dotted line)* velocity is measured. The modal velocity (the most commonly occurring velocity) corresponds to the darkest portion of the Doppler spectrum. (*From Solomon SD, Wu J, Gillam L. Echocardiography. In: Mann DL, Zipes DP, Libby P, et al., eds.* Braunwald's Heart Disease: A Textbook of Cardiovascular Medicine. *10th ed. Philadelphia: Elsevier; 2015:179–260.*)

the diameter is measured just proximal to the aortic annulus. It should be noted that since the LVOT velocity incorporated into the calculation is the modal velocity and displayed as the densest part of the pulsed Doppler envelope, the VTI should not be traced using the outer edge of the spectrum that represents the maximal and not modal velocities at each time point (Fig. 29.9). Optimal sample volume placement is in the left ventricular outflow tract immediately proximal to the site of subvalvular flow acceleration, typically 1–2 mm proximal to the valve using the apical five- or three-chamber (TTE) or deep transgastric (TEE) views.

The advent of transcatheter AV implantation/replacement (TAVI/TAVR) has emphasized that the left ventricular outflow tract and aortic annulus are not always circular and may acquire an ovoid or irregular shape in patients with AS. In these cases, calculating the LVOT cross-sectional area and the subsequent AVA based on a single diameter will not be accurate. 3D techniques that permit direct planimetry of the LVOT and annulus solve this problem and are important tools for sizing prior to TAVI/TAVR (see also Chapter 32). However, in most situations, AVA calculations based on the concept of the circularity of the LVOT will appropriately categorize the severity of the stenosis. Nonetheless, there may be instances where a suboptimal window or the presence of calcium in the outflow tract precludes a reliable measurement of the LVOT diameter. In such instances, the dimensionless index defined as the VTI_{LVOT}/VTI_{AV} may be helpful. Values ≤0.25 indicate severe AS.

Additional Measures of Aortic Stenosis Severity

While pressure recovery is best recognized as a concern for prosthetic valves, it may also play a role in patients who have small ascending aortas. To correct for pressure recovery, the energy loss index (ELI) may be an alternative to AVA. It is calculated as follows:

(AVA × AA diam) ÷ (AA–AVA) where AA diam = ascending aortic diameter. A body surface area (BSA)-corrected ELI less than 0.5 cm^2/m^2 is considered severe AS.

Recently, the recognition of the important interplay between AS and systemic blood pressure has resulted in the introduction of valvuloarterial impedance (Z_{VA})

Z_{VA} = (SBP+Peak AV gradient)/Stroke volume indexed BSA where SBP = systolic blood pressure. This provides a measure of the total pressure load experienced by the left ventricle. Values greater than 5 mm Hg/mL per m^2 are indicative of severe obstruction.[2]

Less commonly used measures of severity are the LV % stroke work loss = (mean AV gradient/ [mean AV gradient + SBP]) *100 and AV resistance = (mean AV gradient/mean volume flow) * 1333. However, each of these is flow dependent, and there are limited outcomes data to support their clinical relevance.

Body Surface Area Correction for Aortic Valve Area

BSA-corrected AVA may be used to assess AVA in patients who are large or small. While this approach likely has merit for patients who are normal weight for height, recognizing that a valve that may be adequate for a petite woman may be inadequate for a 7-foot man, its utility in the obese has been questioned and the concept of correction for lean body size has been proposed.

Low Gradient Severe Aortic Stenosis

In the setting of reduced stroke volume due to left ventricular systolic dysfunction, the calculated effective orifice area may be small despite low gradients, and it becomes important to determine whether the valve obstruction is fixed (severe AS) or whether the valve is intrinsically capable of opening more fully (pseudo-severe AS).[4,5] Dobutamine stress echocardiography is routinely used in this setting typically with close physician supervision and a less aggressive dosing protocol (starting at 2.5–5 micrograms/kg per minute with 5 micrograms/kg per minute increments up to 20 micrograms/kg per minute), and typically longer stages than is used for testing for ischemia. With true severe AS, dobutamine augmented left ventricular systolic function will typically result in increased transvalvular gradients and a fixed effective orifice area, whereas with pseudo-severe AS, the valve area will increase with gradients that are relatively unchanged. The test will be uninterpretable if there is no augmentation of ventricular function (no contractile reserve).

Effective orifice area may also be severely reduced despite low gradients when ejection fraction (EF) is within the normal range but stroke volume is impaired (<35 mL/m²), so-called low gradient preserved EF (≥50%) severe AS. These patients are classically women with small concentrically hypertrophied ventricles in whom filling is inadequate. However, there are other causes of reduced forward stroke volume despite normal EF. These include mitral regurgitation, scenarios in which preload is reduced, such as mitral stenosis, atrial fibrillation with poorly controlled ventricular response,

pericardial constriction and restrictive physiology, as well as hypertension in which afterload is increased. In each of these, severe AS may be present despite low gradients. Low-gradient, normal stroke volume (SV), preserved EF severe AS is a more controversial condition in which error in the measurement of the LVOT and systemic hypertension must be excluded.

SUBVALVULAR OR SUPRAVALVULAR AORTIC STENOSIS

Continuous-wave Doppler echocardiographic assessment of peak and mean gradients is the cornerstone of the evaluation of patients with left ventricular outflow tract obstruction below or above the valve. However, by readily demonstrating the site of flow acceleration, color Doppler may provide a clue that obstruction is not at the level of the valve, prompting the more detailed imaging evaluation that is necessary to clarify the pathophysiology. In some patients, evaluation is complicated by the presence of obstruction at multiple levels, and due to the tradeoff between range resolution and the ability to accurately measure high velocities inherent in the pulsed wave Nyquist limit, it may be impossible to accurately delineate the gradients created at each level of obstruction.

AORTIC REGURGITATION

AR may occur in the setting of abnormalities of the valve cusps or with normal cusps whose coaptation is altered by enlargement of the annulus and/or sinuses or, rarely, by prolapse of an aortic dissection flap through the valve (Fig. 29.10, Videos 29.13–29.16). Echocardiographic imaging (transthoracic and transesophageal) will establish a causative diagnosis and typically demonstrates left ventricular end-diastolic enlargement if the regurgitation is hemodynamically significant. High-frequency fluttering of the anterior mitral leaflet caused by the impact of the regurgitant jet may be evident on

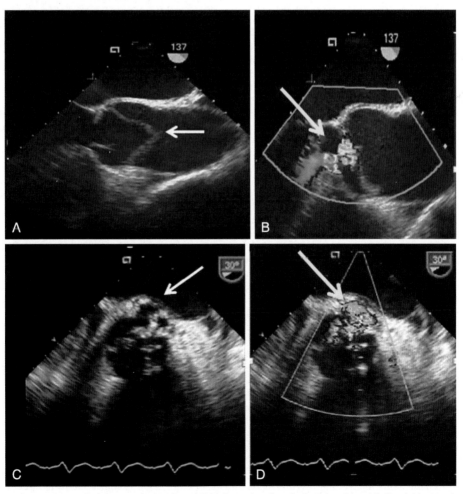

FIG. 29.10 TEE images illustrating two causes of aortic regurgitation. (A and B), In the setting of aortic dissection, the mobile flap *(white arrow)* may interfere with aortic valve closure causing aortic regurgitation *(yellow arrow)*. (C and D), Aortic valve endocarditis and root abscess *(white arrow)* may also cause aortic regurgitation.

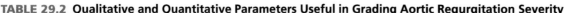

TABLE 29.2 Qualitative and Quantitative Parameters Useful in Grading Aortic Regurgitation Severity

	MILD	MODERATE	SEVERE
Structural Parameters			
LV size	Normal[a]	Normal or dilated	Usually dilated[b]
Aortic leaflets	Normal or abnormal	Normal or abnormal	Abnormal/flail, or wide coaptation defect
Doppler Parameters			
Jet width in LVOT–Color Flow[c]	Small in central jets	Intermediate	Large in central jets; variable in eccentric jets
Jet density–CW	Incomplete or faint	Dense	Dense
Jet deceleration rate–CW (PHT, ms)[d]	Slow > 500	Medium 500–200	Steep < 200
Diastolic flow reversal in descending aorta–PW	Brief, early diastolic reversal	Intermediate	Prominent holodiastolic reversal
Quantitative Parameters[e]			
VC width, cm[c]	<0.3	0.3–0.60	> 0.6
Jet width/LVOT width, %[c]	<25	25–45 46–64	≥65
Jet CSA/LVOT CSA, %[c]	<5	5–20 21–59	≥60
R Vol, ml/beat	<30	30–44 45–59	≥60
RF, %	<30	30–39 40–49	≥50
EROA, cm²	<0.10	0.10–0.19 0.20–0.29	≥0.30

[a]Unless there are other reasons for LV dilation. Normal 2D measurements: LV minor axis ≤ 2.8 cm/m², LV end-diastolic volume ≤ 82 mL/m².
[b]Exception: would be acute AR, in which chambers have not had time to dilate.
[c]At a Nyquist limit of 50–60 cm/s.
[d]PHT is shortened with increasing LV diastolic pressure and vasodilator therapy, and may be lengthened in chronic adaptation to severe AR.
[e]Quantitative parameters can subclassify the moderate regurgitation group into mild-to-moderate and moderate-to-severe regurgitation as shown.
AR, Aortic regurgitation; *CSA,* cross-sectional area; *CW,* continuous-wave Doppler; *EROA,* effective regurgitant orifice area; *LA,* left atrium; *LV,* left ventricle; *LVOT,* left ventricular outflow tract; *PHT,* pressure half-time; *PW,* pulsed-wave Doppler; *R Vol,* regurgitant volume; *RF,* regurgitant fraction; *VC,* vena contracta.
From Zoghbi WA, Adams D, Bonow R, et al. Recommendations for the noninvasive evaluation of native valvular regurgitation. J Am Soc Echocardiogr. 2017;30(4):303–371.

M-mode and, in cases of severe regurgitation, the mitral valve may close prematurely before ventricular systole, reflecting a rise in left ventricular pressure to exceed left atrial pressure before ventricular contraction.

The diagnosis of AR is most easily made when a diastolic color Doppler jet is seen in the left ventricular outflow tract. Small transient jets can be normal variants. The American Society of Echocardiography and European Association of Cardiovascular Imaging (formerly Echocardiography) recommend an integrated approach to the determination of the severity of AR[6,7] (Table 29.2) with elements including evidence of left ventricular enlargement, color jet dimensions, spectral Doppler signal intensity, pressure half time, vena contracta, and diastolic flow reversal in the descending thoracic or abdominal aorta. Regurgitant volume (RV) and regurgitant fraction can be calculated using a continuity-based approach, and RV and effective regurgitant orifice area (EROA) may be calculated using the proximal isovelocity surface area (PISA) approach.

Color jet dimensions should be assessed with Nyquist settings of 50–60 cm/s. The best dimensional predictors of angiographic severity are jet area indexed to the left ventricular short- axis area (parasternal short-axis view), and the jet diameter indexed to left ventricular outflow tract diameter immediately proximal to the valve (parasternal long-axis view). Recommended cutoffs for indexed jet area are <5% = mild, 5%–20% = mild to moderate, 21%–59% = moderate to severe, and ≥ 60% = severe, and the recommended cutoffs for the for indexed jet diameter are <25% = mild, 25%–45% = mild to moderate, 46%–64% = moderate to severe, and ≥ 65% = severe. The jet length is not a reliable index of severity.

While color jet-based assessment of severity is easy, it has many limitations, including setting dependency (particularly Nyquist limit, transmit power and gain), blood pressure (BP) and LV pressure dependence, and jet eccentricity that is prone to result in over- or underestimation if a jet is directed obliquely across the left ventricular outflow tract rather than originating from a central circular regurgitant orifice and projecting straight down into the left ventricle. This approach is also unable to handle multiple jets. Most important, the color jet is not a direct representation of the RV. For these reasons, the European Guidelines[7] state that "the color flow area of the regurgitant jet is not recommended to quantify the severity of aortic regurgitation," although jet based measurements remain in the ASE Guidelines.

The pressure half time, which reflects the rate at which aortic and left ventricular pressures equalize, is most reliable in the setting of acute regurgitation with care taken to ensure that the early diastolic velocity is accurately

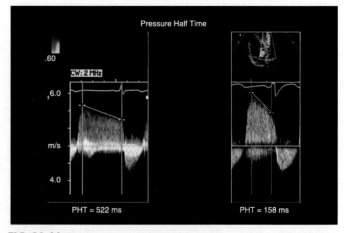

FIG. 29.11 Methods of quantitating aortic regurgitation. PHT (pressure half time) >500 ms suggests mild aortic regurgitation (AR), 200–500 ms suggests moderate AR and <200 ms suggests severe AR. *(Modified from Solomon SD, Wu J, Gillam L. Echocardiography. In: Mann DL, Zipes DP, Libby P, et al., eds.* Braunwald's Heart Disease: A Textbook of Cardiovascular Medicine. *10th ed. Philadelphia: Elsevier; 2015:179–260.)*

captured, typically at least 4 mps (Fig. 29.11). Recommended cutoffs (in ms) are >500 = mild, 200–500 = moderate, <200 = severe. However, the pressure half time is affected by systemic vascular resistance and ventricular compliance and is an insensitive method for detecting chronic severe AR.[8]

Holodiastolic flow reversal in the descending thoracic aorta, as detected with the pulsed Doppler sample volume placed near the origin of the left subclavian artery, has been reported to be a marker of at least moderate regurgitation (Fig. 29.12). The European Guidelines[7] recommend specifically that the end-diastolic velocity be at least 20 cm/s, while reversal of comparable duration as measured in the abdominal aorta generally reflects severe regurgitation. However, it should be noted that with reduced aortic compliance, there may be flow reversal in the thoracic aorta in the absence of AR, a consideration in elderly patients. Additional concerns relate to the challenges of obtaining analyzable Doppler signals and the impact of wall filters.

The vena contracta is the waist (smallest diameter) of the aortic regurgitant flow jet and is measured at the level of the valve measured in zoom mode with a parasternal long-axis or TEE equivalent

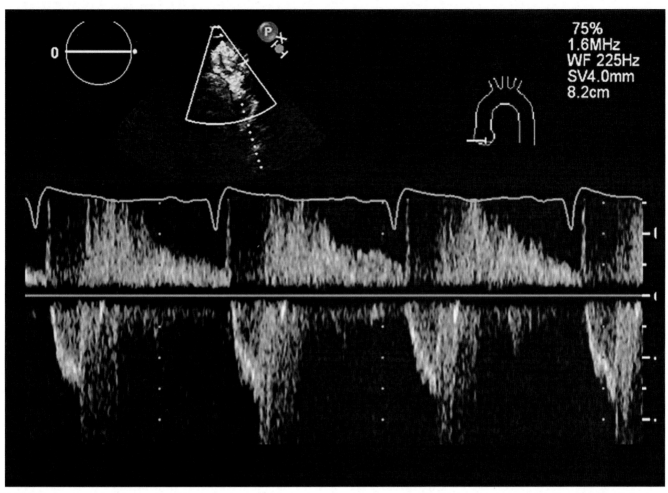

FIG. 29.12 Pulsed-wave Doppler recording with sample volume placed in the descending thoracic aorta just distal to the subclavian artery. This shows holodiastolic flow reversal with an end-diastolic velocity >20 cm/s. Holodiastolic flow reversal in the descending thoracic aorta as is shown here is typically associated with a least moderate aortic regurgitation.

view (Fig. 29.13). Recommended cutoffs (in cm) are <0.3 cm= mild, 0.3–0.6 = moderate, and >0.6 = severe. Major limitations include the spatial resolution of the measurement particularly with less-than-severe regurgitation, setting dependence (similar to jet dimensions), noncircularity of the regurgitant orifice, and inability to handle multiple jets.

While the PISA approach that is widely used to assess the severity of mitral and tricuspid regurgitation has been used to calculate EROA and RV for AR, it may be challenging to accurately measure the PISA radius when only mild regurgitation is present, particularly with TTE. An additional consideration is the angle subtending the cusps, as it has been shown that whenever this is greater than 220 degrees, the PISA calculation will be invalid (Fig. 29.14).[9] Recommended cutoffs are as follows for RV: (cc) <30 = mild, 30–44 = mild to moderate, 45–59 = moderate to severe, ≥ 60 = severe. In addition, the recommended cutoffs for EROA (cm²) are as follows: <0.10= mild, .10–.19 = mild to moderate, .20–.29 = moderate to severe, ≥ .30 = severe.[9]

The quantitative Doppler approach that calculates RV by comparing flow through the left ventricular outflow tract with that across a competent nonstenotic valve is most robust when image quality permits the use of the pulmonic valve as the reference normal flow, thereby avoiding the errors inherent when the geometrically complex mitral valve is used as the reference. The continuity equation is used to calculate transaortic and transpulmonic stroke volumes by multiplying the LVOT and right ventricular outflow tract (RVOT) VTIs by the corresponding cross-sectional areas. These are calculated assuming circular geometry and by measuring the LVOT and RVOT diameter at the level of the annulus. LVOT SV minus RVOT SV = RV and RV/LVOT stroke volume = regurgitant fraction (which is typically expressed as a percentage). Recommended cutoffs for RV (mL) are <30 = mild, 30–44 = mild to moderate, 45–59 = moderate to severe, ≥ 60 = severe, and the recommended cutoffs for regurgitant fraction (%) are <30 = mild, 30–39 = mild to moderate, 40–49 = moderate to severe, ≥ 50 = severe.

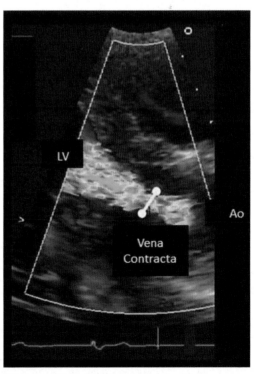

FIG. 29.13 Parasternal long-axis echocardiogram showing the measurement of the vena contracta, the narrowest portion of the aortic regurgitant jet. This is just downstream from the anatomic regurgitant orifice and is the same conceptually as the effective orifice area that is calculated by proximal isovelocity surface area. *Ao,* Aorta; *LV,* left ventricle.

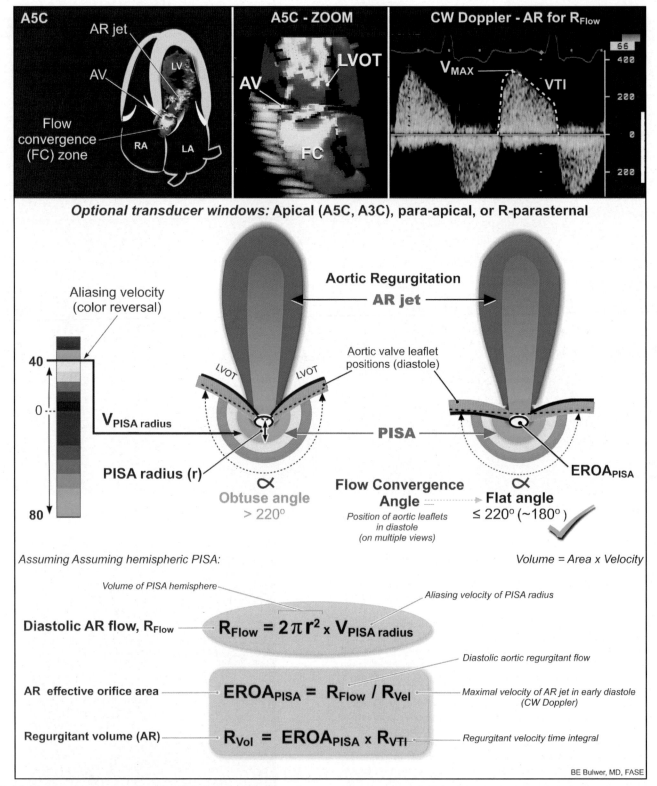

FIG. 29.14 Proximal isovelocity surface area (PISA) approach to calculating effective regurgitant orifice area (EROA) and regurgitant volume in aortic regurgitation. *AR,* Aortic regurgitation; *AV,* aortic valve; *CW,* continuous wave; *LA,* left atrium; *LVOT,* left ventricular outflow tract; *RA,* right atrium; *VTI,* velocity time integral. *(Courtesy of Bernard E. Bulwer, MD, FASE; Data from Tribouilloy CM, Enriquez-Sarano M, Fett SL, Bailey KR, Seward JB, Tajik AJ. Application of the proximal flow convergence method to calculate the effective regurgitant orifice area in aortic regurgitation. J Am Coll Cardiol. 1998;32[4]:1032–1039.)*

3D echocardiography has also been reported to be helpful in quantitating AR providing a means of direct planimetry of the effective regurgitant orifice.[10] However, the spatial resolution of this approach, particularly with TTE, limits its application in most cases of less than severe regurgitation.

Acute Versus Chronic Aortic Regurgitation

In the setting of sudden severe AR due to, for example, aortic dissection or cusp perforation due to endocarditis, the echocardiographic appearance may differ from that in chronic AR. The rapid equalization of pressures between the aorta and a left ventricle that has not had time to dilate and increase its compliance results in premature (i.e., diastolic) closure of the mitral valve. Additionally, jets may be brief and, if the patient is in extremis, of lower velocity and therefore with less mosaic flow than is typical of chronic AR. In the setting of sudden, severe AR, the murmur of AR may be difficult to hear, and peripheral manifestations including wide pulse pressure and its related findings may be absent. Thus, the clinician and echocardiographer must be alert to the diagnosis.

Suggested Reading

Baumgartner, H., Hung, J., Bermejo, J., et al. (2009). Echocardiographic assessment of valve stenosis: EAE/ASE recommendations for clinical practice. *Journal of the American Society of Echocardiography, 22,* 1–23.

Lancellotti, P., Tribouilloy, C., Hagendorff, A., et al. (2010). European Association of Echocardiography recommendations for the assessment of valvular regurgitation. Part 1: aortic and pulmonary regurgitation (native valve disease). *European Heart Journal Cardiovascular Imaging, 11,* 223–244.

Pibarot, P., & Clavel, M. A. (2015). Management of paradoxical low-flow, low-gradient aortic stenosis: need for an integrated approach, including assessment of symptoms, hypertension, and stenosis severity. *Journal of the American College of Cardiology, 65*(1), 67–71.

Pibarot, P., & Dumesnil, J. G. (2012). Low-flow, low-gradient aortic stenosis with normal and depressed left ventricular ejection fraction. *Journal of the American College of Cardiology, 60,* 1845–1853.

Zoghbi, W.A., Adams, D., Bonow, R., et al. (2017). Recommendations for noninvasive evaluation of native valve regurgitation. *Journal of the American Socieety of Echocardiography, 30,* 303–371.

A complete reference list can be found online at ExpertConsult.com.

Tricuspid and Pulmonic Valve Disease

Judy R. Mangion, Linda D. Gillam

INTRODUCTION

Echocardiography plays a unique role in the assessment of the tricuspid and pulmonic valves. However, their evaluation is often suboptimal because typical imaging protocols may overlook the views that best display pulmonic and tricuspid anatomy and function. Recent advances in percutaneous valve procedures for pulmonic and tricuspid disease have created a demand for detailed images and precise echocardiographic measurements of both the tricuspid and pulmonic valves. At the same time, advances in three-dimensional (3D) echocardiography have expanded the tools that are available.

Although the tricuspid and pulmonic valves are structurally similar to the mitral and aortic valves, they rarely undergo the chronic degenerative changes that affect their left-sided counterparts. Moreover, they are less likely to be affected directly by acquired diseases, such as rheumatic disease, endocarditis, and other inflammatory processes. This is generally attributed to the relative protection afforded by the lower right-sided pressures. Congenital abnormalities, such as Ebstein anomaly and pulmonary stenosis, are often encountered in the adult, and when the accompanying physiologic disturbance is mild, these conditions may have gone undetected in childhood. The most common form of tricuspid dysfunction is functional (i.e., when leaflet architecture is normal, but right ventricular [RV] dysfunction and remodeling prevent normal valve closure). This condition accounts for most surgical procedures performed on the tricuspid valve. RV abnormalities may be primary or secondary to pulmonary hypertension and/or left-sided abnormalities. Functional tricuspid regurgitation may also occur due to annular dilatation without ventricular abnormalities, such as that which may occur with atrial fibrillation. Myxomatous disease of the tricuspid valve and tricuspid valve prolapse may be seen in association with mitral valve myxomatous disease and prolapse, although the diagnostic criteria for tricuspid prolapse have not been clearly established. Spontaneous tricuspid flail is virtually unheard of. Although tricuspid valve endocarditis is often seen in patients with a history of intravenous drug abuse, pulmonic valve endocarditis occurs rarely, although it is possible that it is underreported. This chapter will review the echocardiographic features of these and other disorders that most commonly affect the tricuspid and pulmonic valves, and illustrate the two-dimensional (2D) and 3D echocardiographic views that can be used to image these valves most effectively. The reader is also referred to Chapter 40 for additional discussion of right-sided endocarditis.

NORMAL TRICUSPID VALVE ANATOMY

The tricuspid valve is anatomically complex, with anterior, posterior, and septal leaflets extending from the tricuspid annulus to chords and papillary muscles. The tricuspid valve annulus is normally larger than that of the mitral valve, and it is more apically positioned. The anterior leaflet is largest, with an attachment that extends from the infundibulum to the inferoposterior wall of the right ventricle. The posterior leaflet is the smallest, extending along the diaphragmatic surface of the right ventricle, and the septal leaflet attaches to the muscular and membranous interventricular septum with an irregular array of chordae. The papillary muscles that attach the RV myocardium to the tricuspid valve leaflets are variable in number, size, and position (Fig. 30.1).

TWO-DIMENSIONAL ECHO VIEWS FOR ASSESSING THE TRICUSPID VALVE

The standard 2D echocardiographic views for imaging the tricuspid valve are shown in Fig. 30.2A–E and Videos 30.1–30.5 and in composite Fig. 30.3. The initial view recorded is typically the RV inflow tract. When obtained properly, this view displays the diaphragmatic and anterior walls of the RV, and the anterior and posterior leaflets of the tricuspid valve. This is a key view for visualizing the posterior leaflet. A nonstandard but common variant of this view is recognizable by the visualization of the interventricular septum and adjacent left ventricle (LV) cavity. This view displays the anterior and septal leaflets. In the apical four-chamber view, the anterior and septal leaflets of the tricuspid valve are typically visualized. A similar view may be obtained from the transthoracic subcostal four-chamber window and from the midesophageal four-chamber transesophageal view. The subcostal short-axis view at the level of the great vessels displays the anterior and septal leaflets. A similar view may be obtained from the parasternal short-axis view. The short-axis transesophageal echocardiographic transgastric view allows visualization of all three tricuspid leaflets simultaneously. In some patients, it may be possible to obtain a comparable view using the parasternal short-axis view, particularly if the RV is dilated.

While these descriptions apply to the standard application of these views, slight changes in transducer angulation may bring different leaflets into view, as has been elucidated with 3D-derived 2D imaging. Thus, when the transducer is angulated posteriorly from the standard four-chamber view, the posterior rather than the anterior leaflet can be seen opposing the septal leaflet, and, in the parasternal short-axis view, superior and inferior angulation permits imaging of all three leaflets.[1,2]

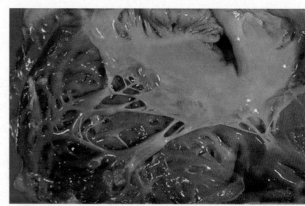

FIG. 30.1 Autopsy specimen of a normal tricuspid valve. The tricuspid valve is composed of an anterior leaflet, posterior leaflet, and septal leaflet. The anterior leaflet is the largest and the posterior leaflet is the smallest. There are a variable number of papillary muscles of different sizes and positions.

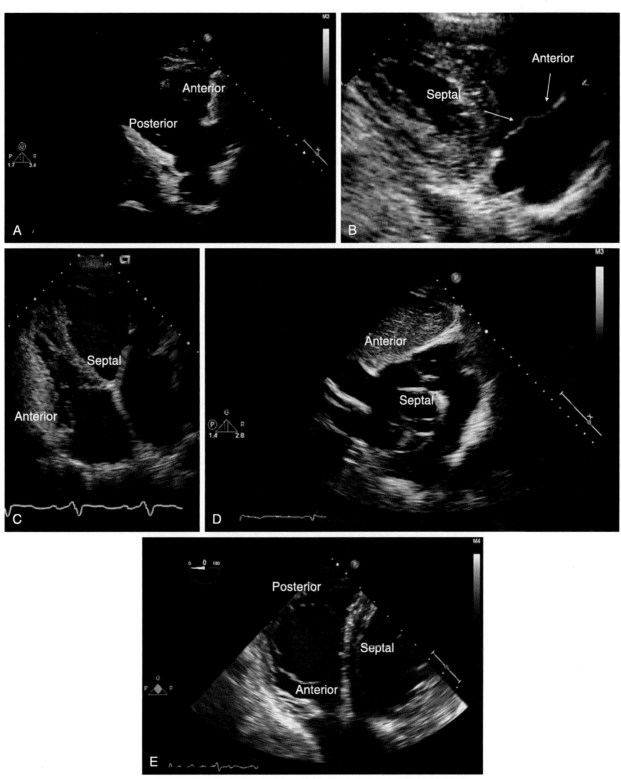

FIG. 30.2 The standard 2D echocardiographic views for imaging the tricuspid valve (A) Right ventricular inflow tract view. When obtained properly, this view displays the diaphragmatic and anterior walls of the right ventricle (RV) and the anterior and posterior leaflets of the tricuspid valve. This is a key view for visualizing the posterior leaflet. (B) A nonstandard but common variant of this view is recognizable by the visualization of the interventricular septum and adjacent left ventricle cavity. This view displays the anterior and septal leaflets (arrows). (C) This apical four-chamber view demonstrates the anterior and septal leaflets. A similar view may be obtained from the subcostal window and from the midesophageal four-chamber transesophageal echocardiographic view. (D) Subcostal short-axis view at the level of the great vessels is shown. This view displays the anterior and septal leaflets. A similar view may be obtained parasternally. (E) The short-axis transesophageal echocardiographic transgastric view is the only view that shows all leaflets simultaneously. It may be possible to obtain a comparable view using the parasternal short-axis view, particularly if the RV is dilated.

Tricuspid Valve Anatomy and Views

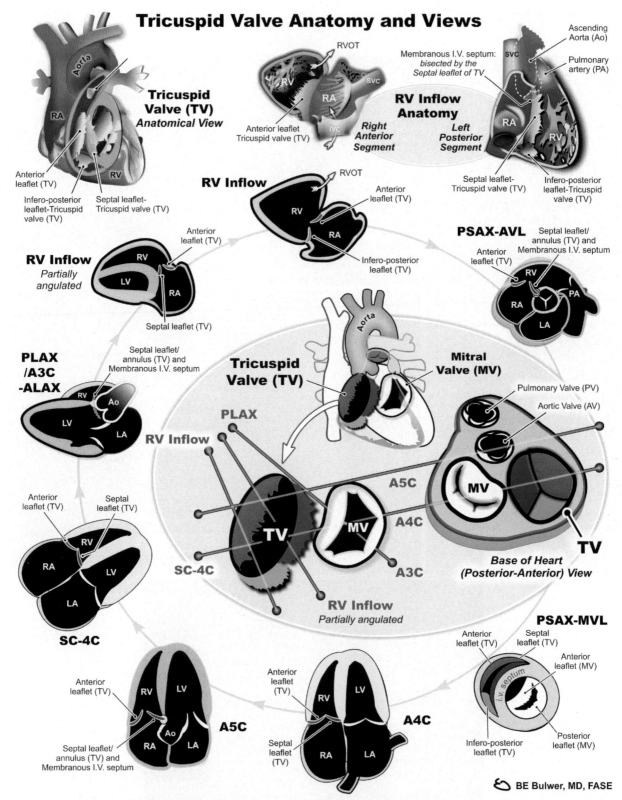

FIG. 30.3 Composite showing the key views of the tricuspid valve. *IVC,* Inferior vena cava; *RA,* right atrium; *RV,* right ventricle; *RVOT,* right ventricular outflow tract; *SVC,* superior vena cava. *(Courtesy of Bernard E. Bulwer, MD, FASE.)*

THREE-DIMENSIONAL ECHO OF THE TRICUSPID VALVE

To acquire optimal transthoracic 3D echo images of the tricuspid valve, images are best obtained from the apical four-chamber view and/or the parasternal RV inflow view, with and without color (Fig. 30.4 and Video 30.6).[3] The protocol for acquiring transesophageal echo images of the tricuspid valve involves 0- to 30-degree midesophageal four-chamber zoomed acquisitions both with and without color, as well as 40-degree transgastric views with ante-flexion with and without color. A 3D echo of the tricuspid valve has demonstrated that the tricuspid valve is saddle shaped, becoming more planar and circular with functional tricuspid insufficiency.[4,5]

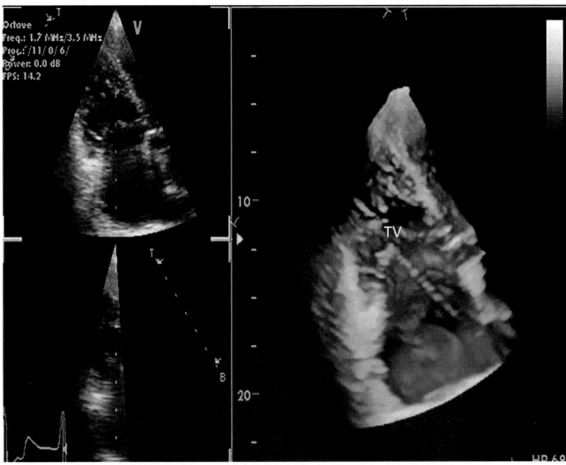

FIG. 30.4 The 3D volumes acquired using an apical window can be cropped and rotated to provide an en-face view of the valve as seen in Video 30.6. *TV,* Tricuspid valve.

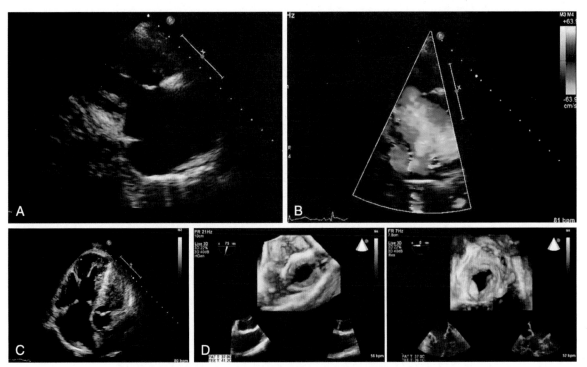

FIG. 30.5 Right ventricular inflow tract views (A and B) demonstrate the typical features of carcinoid heart disease. The leaflets are thickened, retracted, and immobilized, creating a large regurgitant orifice. As a result, there is unrestricted tricuspid regurgitation, and the color regurgitant jet may appear relatively monochromic. In the apical five-chamber view of the same patient (C) the classic "drum stick" appearance of the leaflets is evident. The valvopathy occurs when serotonin and its metabolite 5-hydroxytryptophan secreted by carcinoid tumors causes an inflammatory reaction in the valves. Because the active metabolite is inactivated in the lungs, left-sided involvement occurs only when there is an intracardiac shunt or pulmonary metastases. (D) The 3D image of the pulmonic valve *(left panel)* and tricuspid valve *(right panel)* shows en-face views of the affected valves.

ABNORMALITIES OF THE TRICUSPID VALVE

Carcinoid Valve Disease

The typical echocardiographic features of carcinoid heart disease (Fig. 30.5A–D and Videos 30.7–30.10) include tricuspid leaflets that are thickened, retracted, and immobilized, creating a large regurgitant orifice and the classic "drum stick" appearance. As a result, there is unrestricted tricuspid regurgitation, and the color Doppler regurgitant jet may appear relatively monochromic. Under these conditions, the regurgitant jet could be laminar and of relatively low velocity because of the almost complete equalization of pressures between the right atrium and right ventricle. This can lead to underestimation of the severity of tricuspid regurgitation. Similarly, estimation of pulmonary artery (PA) systolic pressure from the tricuspid regurgitation jet velocity will be inaccurate in this situation. A 3D transesophageal echo of the tricuspid valve allows high resolution and detailed visualization of the three thickened and retracted tricuspid leaflets from the right atrial or surgeon's perspective (see Fig. 30.5D, *right panel*). The valvopathy of carcinoid disease occurs when both serotonin and its metabolite 5-hydroxytryptophan are secreted by the carcinoid tumor causing an inflammatory reaction in the valves. Because the active metabolite is inactivated in the lungs, left-sided involvement occurs only when there is an intracardiac shunt or pulmonary metastases. Carcinoid heart disease is discussed in greater detail in Chapter 41, and additional images are provided there.

Rheumatic Valve Disease

Rheumatic tricuspid involvement occurs in approximately 11% of patients with rheumatic mitral valve disease. A pathognomonic echocardiographic finding in rheumatic tricuspid valve disease is diastolic leaflet doming, which is best visualized in the apical four-chamber transthoracic echocardiography (TTE) and midesophageal four-chamber transesophageal echocardiography (TEE) views (Fig. 30.6A–C and Videos 30.11–30.13). This occurs because the belly of the leaflet may remain mobile as the tip is restricted. Rheumatic tricuspid disease is generally accompanied by rheumatic mitral disease. It may be distinguished from carcinoid disease (where mitral involvement is rare) by the presence of commissural fusion and chordal thickening, whereas carcinoid is primarily a disease of the leaflets. In diastole, color flow Doppler may demonstrate proximal flow convergence, which is a marker of stenosis. Spectral Doppler in the four-chamber views can be used to derive transvalvular tricuspid gradients. In general, the severity of tricuspid stenosis is best assessed by Doppler-derived mean gradients, noting that normal mean tricuspid gradients are under 3 mm Hg.[6] Methods for calculating valve area, including the pressure half-time method, have not been validated for tricuspid stenosis. Mixed involvement with stenosis and regurgitation may occur.

Tricuspid Valve Endocarditis

Tricuspid endocarditis is typically a disease of intravenous drug abusers or the immunocompromised, although it may also occur due to contiguous spread

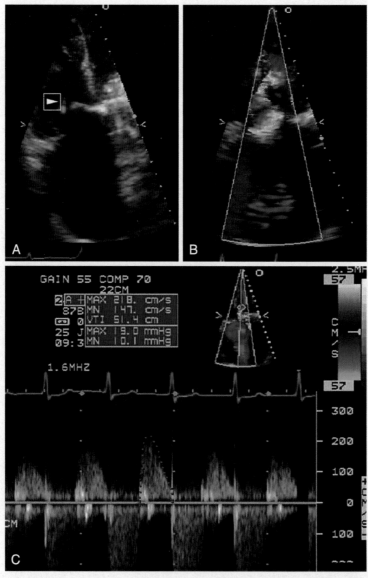

FIG. 30.6 (A) An apical four-chamber view demonstrates rheumatic tricuspid disease. A pathognomonic finding is diastolic leaflet doming *(arrowhead)* seen involving the septal leaflet. This occurs because the belly of the leaflet may remain mobile as the tip is restricted. (B) In this diastolic frame, color flow demonstrates proximal flow convergence, a marker of stenosis. This patient also had moderate to severe tricuspid regurgitation. (C) Spectral Doppler can be used to derive transvalvular gradients.

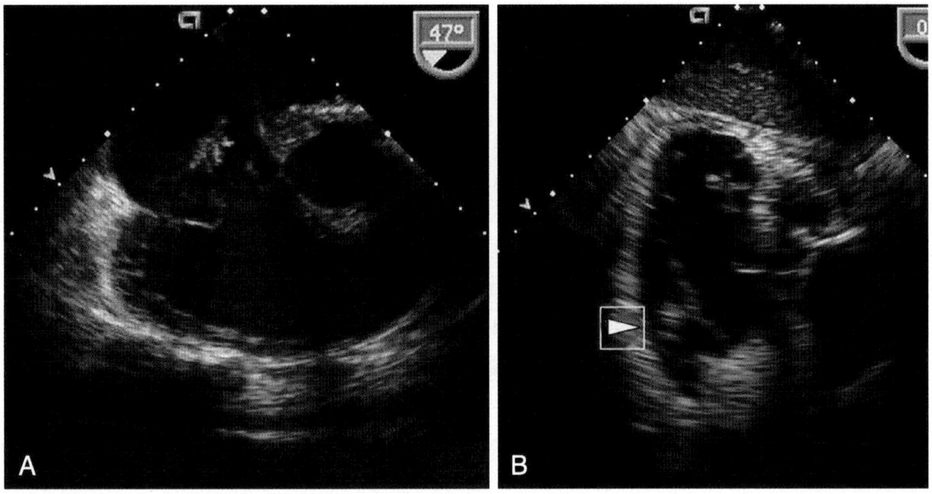

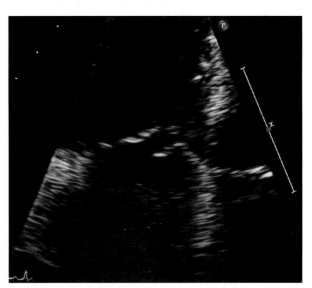

FIG. 30.7 Tricuspid valve endocarditis. Transesophageal midesophageal (A) and transgastric- (B) echocardiograms demonstrate a large irregular vegetation (B, *arrowhead*) attached to the anterior leaflet of the tricuspid valve. The chordal attachments have been disrupted, and there is severe tricuspid regurgitation.

from an aortic root abscess. In approximately 50% of primary cases, the causative organism is *Staphylococcus aureus*. *S. aureus* endocarditis may be very aggressive, significantly destroying valves within hours, and causing septic emboli to the lungs if not appropriately treated. Thus the echocardiographic appearance of valves affected by this organism can change quickly. Although TTE is often sufficient to establish the diagnosis of endocarditis in these cases, TEE offers incremental value in diagnosing disruption of the tricuspid leaflets and chordal structures, and in diagnosing annular abscess. Fig. 30.7 and Videos 30.14 and 30.15 demonstrate a large irregular vegetation attached to the anterior leaflet of the tricuspid valve. In this case, the chordal attachments have been disrupted, and there is severe tricuspid insufficiency.

Flail Tricuspid Leaflet

Flail tricuspid leaflets may be caused by trauma (e.g., acceleration-deceleration injury) or endocarditis, and it is a recognized complication of RV biopsy. Fig. 30.8 and Video 30.16 demonstrate an apical four-chamber transthoracic view of a flail tricuspid septal leaflet, which is associated with chaotic motion and resultant mal-coaptation of the leaflet. The color Doppler regurgitant jets in these cases are typically very eccentric. Other causes of iatrogenic injury to the tricuspid valve are pacer and/or defibrillator wires. Spontaneous chordal rupture or RV papillary muscle rupture is extremely rare.

Functional Tricuspid Regurgitation

Functional tricuspid regurgitation is the most common abnormality of the tricuspid valve and may be encountered as a consequence of either primary (myopathy, infarction) or secondary (pulmonary parenchymal or vascular disease, left-sided heart disease) RV dysfunction, or be due to dilation of the annulus with intact RV function, typically in the context of atrial fibrillation. The pathophysiology is likely analogous to that reported for the mitral valve with an imbalance between closure and tethering forces. Factors promoting tethering include annular dilation and geometric remodeling of the RV. Impaired RV systolic function (whether primary or secondary) reduces closure forces. The normal tricuspid valve closure pattern is best appreciated in the apical four-chamber view. The septal and anterior leaflets close in a normal linear or horizontal closure pattern in systole (Fig. 30.9A and Video 30.17). This is in contrast to the apically tethered tricuspid valve closure pattern, which is typical of functional tricuspid regurgitation (Fig. 30.9B and Video 30.18). In extreme cases, there is complete failure of leaflet coaptation with a visible regurgitant orifice and severe regurgitation occurs (Fig. 30.9C and Video 30.19).

Ebstein Anomaly of the Tricuspid Valve

Ebstein anomaly is the most common congenital anomaly of the tricuspid valve, and is associated with apical displacement (Fig. 30.10A–B and Videos 30.20 and 30.21) of the septal, posterior, and (less commonly) the anterior leaflets. As is the case here, septal tissue

FIG. 30.8 The apical four-chamber view shows a flail septal leaflet, in this case caused by trauma (acceleration-deceleration injury).

may be immobilized by an arcade-like attachment along the interventricular septum. In this case, the septal leaflet becomes mobile only at the midventricular level. The anterior leaflet is large and sail-like. Tricuspid regurgitation and interatrial shunts are common. The apically displaced origin of the tricuspid regurgitant jet is often appreciated. Although severe cases present with cyanosis in infancy due to elevated right atrial pressures and right-to-left shunting, patients with milder forms may remain asymptomatic until late adulthood.

Tricuspid Atresia

In patients with tricuspid atresia, the tricuspid valve is absent (Fig. 30.11, *arrow*), and the RV is hypoplastic. There is an associated large atrial septal defect, which directs systemic venous return to the left side of the heart. In these patients, the RV outflow tract is also small, and the pulmonary valve is abnormal. A Waterston shunt is performed to connect the ascending aorta to the main PA.

ECHO DOPPLER ASSESSMENT OF TRICUSPID REGURGITATION SEVERITY

As for valve regurgitation involving other native valves, the American Society of Echocardiography recommends an integrated approach to assessing the severity of tricuspid regurgitation as summarized in Table 30.1.[7] The European Society of Cardiovascular Imaging (formerly Echocardiography)

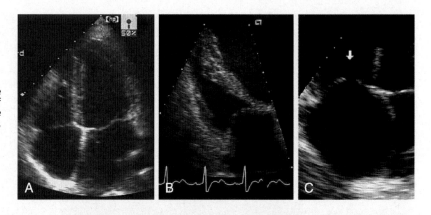

FIG. 30.9 The apical four-chamber view shows a normal closure pattern (A) and the apically tethered pattern (B), which is typical of functional tricuspid regurgitation. In extreme cases, there is complete failure of leaflet coaptation with a visible regurgitant orifice (C, *arrow*), and severe regurgitation occurs.

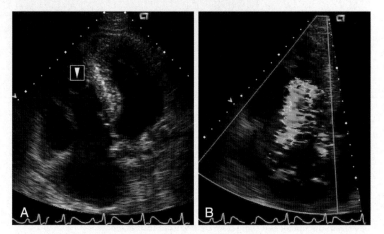

FIG. 30.10 **An apical four-chamber view of Ebstein anomaly.** This most common congenital anomaly of the tricuspid valve is associated with apical displacement (A, *arrow*) of the septal, posterior, and (less commonly) the anterior leaflets. As is the case here, septal tissue may be immobilized by an arcade-like attachment along the interventricular septum. In this case, the septal leaflet becomes mobile only at the midventricular level. The anterior leaflet is large and sail-like. Tricuspid regurgitation and interatrial shunts are common. The apically displaced origin of the tricuspid regurgitant jet is shown (B).

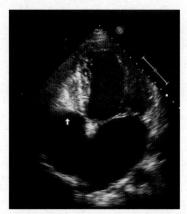

FIG. 30.11 **A four-chamber view demonstrates tricuspid atresia.** The tricuspid valve is absent *(arrow)*, and the right ventricle (RV) is hypoplastic. There is a large atrial septal defect, which directs systemic venous return to the left side of the heart. Not shown are a small RV outflow tract and an abnormal pulmonary valve. A Waterston shunt (also not shown) connects the ascending aorta to the main pulmonary artery.

recommends a similar approach.[8] The methods used to assess the severity of tricuspid regurgitation mirror those used to assess the severity of mitral regurgitation with flow reversal into the hepatic veins being analogous to pulmonary venous flow reversal. The reader is referred to Chapter 28 for a detailed discussion of these approaches. However, validation of echo approaches to assessing tricuspid regurgitation has been limited.

ROLE OF ECHOCARDIOGRAPHY IN PERCUTANEOUS TRICUSPID VALVE REPLACEMENT

Recent advances in 3D echocardiography and the development of percutaneous valve replacement procedures in the cardiac catheterization lab/hybrid operating room (OR) have created a demand for knowledge and precise echocardiographic measurements of the tricuspid valve. Although native percutaneous tricuspid valve replacements have not yet been approved, tricuspid valve-in-valve procedures have been performed with success and rely heavily on accurate 3D measurements of the prosthetic tricuspid valve annulus. Videos 30.22–30.27 are from an illustrative case. A 77-year-old male with a history of cardiac transplant presented with worsening right heart failure and renal failure. The patient had a history of a bioprosthetic tricuspid valve replacement, and initial 2D transthoracic imaging revealed a degenerated #31 Carpentier Edwards tricuspid prosthesis with pannus formation and moderate to severe tricuspid insufficiency. The patient was not deemed to be an open surgical candidate, and was referred for a determination of whether a #26 Sapien percutaneous valve could be successfully placed within his tricuspid valve. TEE with 3D reconstruction was requested to determine if the pannus had sufficiently reduced the tricuspid annular diameter so the smaller #26 Edwards-Sapien valve would seat adequately. A 2D TEE confirmed the presence of moderate to severe prosthetic tricuspid insufficiency with significant pannus. The mean transtricuspid gradient was markedly elevated at 8 mm Hg. Full-volume multibeat 3D imaging of the tricuspid prosthesis from the midesophageal four-chamber view was performed with reconstruction to visualize the tricuspid valve from the right atrial perspective. The patient was deemed to be a suitable candidate for percutaneous valve-in-valve replacement, and the patient underwent this procedure successfully without complication. Postprocedure 2D and 3D TTE confirmed the #26 Sapien valve to be in a stable position within the tricuspid bioprosthesis. There were no paravalvular leaks and the mean transtricuspid gradient measured 5 mm Hg at a heart rate (HR) of 81 bpm. There was mild valvular tricuspid insufficiency. The patient's condition was clinically improved.

A number of approaches to catheter-based intervention for tricuspid regurgitation are under investigation with echocardiography clearly identified as playing a pivotal role in patient selection and procedural guidance.[9]

ABNORMALITIES OF THE PULMONIC VALVE

Although the pulmonic valve has three cusps (right, left, and anterior), it is rare to see all three in a single, short 2D echocardiographic image.

TABLE 30.1 Echocardiographic and Doppler Parameters Used in the Evaluation of Pulmonary Regurgitation Severity: Utility, Advantages, and Limitations

PARAMETER	UTILITY/ADVANTAGES	DISADVANTAGES
RV size	RV enlargement sensitive for chronic significant PR. Normal size virtually excludes significant PR	Enlargement seen in other conditions.
Paradoxical septal motion (volume overload pattern)	Simple sign of severe PR	Not specific for PR
Jet length–color flow	Simple	Poor correlation with severity of PR
Vena contracta width	Simple quantitative method that works well for other valves	More difficult to perform; requires good images of pulmonary valve; lacks published validation
Jet deceleration rate–CW	Simple	Steep deceleration not specific for severe PR
Flow quantitation–PW	Quantitates regurgitant flow and fraction	Subject to significant errors due to difficulties of measurement of pulmonic annulus and a dynamic RVOT; not well validated

CW, Continuous wave; *PR,* pulmonic regurgitation; *PW,* pulsed wave; *RV,* right ventricle; *RVOT,* right ventricular outflow tract.
From Zoghbi WA, Enriquez-Sarano M, Foster E, et al. Recommendations for evaluation of the severity of native valvular regurgitation with two-dimensional and Doppler echocardiography. J Am Soc Echocardiogr. *2003;16(7):777-802.*

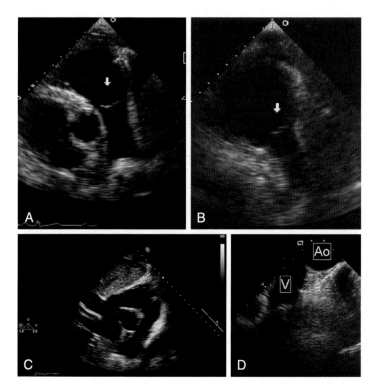

FIG. 30.12 Although the pulmonic valve has three cusps *(right, left, and anterior),* it is rare to see all three in a single, short 2D echocardiographic image. Long-axis images of the valve *(arrow)* may be obtained transthoracically using basal parasternal (A), steeply anteriorly angulated apical (B) with the valve indicated *(arrow),* and subcostal (C) windows. Comparable views may be obtained with transesophageal echocardiography (TEE). TEE offers a unique view of the valve using a high esophageal window rotated slightly from that used to image the aortic arch (D), (E) provides a schematic for the variations of the images that can be obtained from basal short-axis views. *Ao,* Aorta; *L,* left; *LV,* left ventricle; *N,* non; *PA,* pulmonary artery; *PV,* pulmonary valve; *R,* right; *RPA,* right pulmonary artery; *RV,* right ventricle; *RVOT,* right ventricular outflow tract; *V,* valve. *(Illustration courtesy of Bernard E. Bulwer, MD, FASE.)*

Long-axis images of the valve may be obtained transthoracically (Fig. 30.12A–C and Videos 30.28–30.30), using basal parasternal, steeply anteriorly angulated apical and subcostal windows. Comparable views may be obtained with TEE. TEE offers a unique view of the valve using a high esophageal window rotated slightly from that used to image the aortic arch (Fig. 30.12D and Video 30.31). Midesophageal and deep transgastric views of the pulmonic valve also can be obtained. Fig. 30.12E provides a schematic for the variations of the images that can be obtained from basal short-axis transthoracic views and the orientation of the three cusps.

The most common congenital pulmonic valve abnormality is pulmonic stenosis due to a bicuspid pulmonic valve. Acquired pulmonic valve disease is rare and includes carcinoid, endocarditis, and iatrogenic disruption of the valve because of balloon or surgical valvuloplasty.

THREE-DIMENSIONAL ECHO OF THE PULMONIC VALVE

To acquire optimal transthoracic 3D echo images of the pulmonic valve, images are best obtained from the parasternal RV outflow tract view with and without color. The protocol for acquiring transesophageal echo images of the pulmonic valve[3] involves 90-degree basal-esophageal acquisitions both with and without color, as well as 120-degree midesophageal long-axis views with and without color (Fig. 30.13A and B and Video 30.32). Whereas 2D imaging allows visualization of only two cusps simultaneously, 3D imaging of the pulmonic valve allows all three leaflets of the pulmonic valve to be evaluated concurrently. With 3D imaging of the pulmonic valve, cusp numbers can be accurately evaluated, as can involvement with carcinoid disease (see Fig. 30.5D), endocarditis, as well as supravalvular, valvular, and subvalvular measurements. Kelly et al.[10] performed live 3D TTE and full-volume 3D TTE to assess the feasibility of visualizing pulmonic valve morphology in 200 consecutive patients. 3D images were acquired from the long- and short-axis parasternal and apical four-chamber views with final volumes evaluated off line to obtain a short-axis view of the pulmonic valve. Pulmonic valve morphology could be obtained in 63% and 23% of patients using live 3D and full-volume 3D techniques, respectively. Thus, 3D echocardiography can distinguish between tricuspid, bicuspid, and unicuspid leaflet morphology in the majority of cases. 3D color methods can also quantify pulmonic regurgitation directly through direct measurement of the effective regurgitant orifice area.

Echo Anatomy of the Pulmonary Valve

Anatomical View

Aorta
SVC
Pulmonary Artery
RA
IVC
TV
RV
Pulmonary Valve (PV)
RVOT
LV

RV Outflow View

RV
RVOT
PV
PA
LV
PA

Short-Axis Anatomy
(Aortic Valve Level)

RVOT
Pulmonary Valve (PV)
Main pulmonary artery (trunk)
R
N
L
RA
Left atrial appendage
Aortic valve
LA
BE Bulwer MD

PSAX-AVL

PV
RVOT
PA
RA
LA

PSAX-PAB

PV
RVOT
RA
Ao
PA
LPA
RPA

BE Bulwer, MD, FASE

Anterior leaflet
Right
Left

Base of Heart

PV
Cardiac base
Mitral
Aortic
Tricuspid

Right

E Pulmonary Artery Bifurcation (PAB)

C6 - C7 disc
R. lung
L. lung

left pulmonary artery (LPA)
pulmonary carina
main pulmonary artery
left atrial appendage
Pulmonary valve

Ao
RA
RVOT
RV infundibulum
Left
Anterior

PAB
Aorta
RV

FIG. 30.12, cont'd

PULMONIC VALVE ENDOCARDITIS

Pulmonic valve endocarditis is rare, but may accompany tricuspid valve endocarditis or occur in the setting of congenital heart disease involving the pulmonic valve and/or PA. Fig. 30.14 and Video 30.33 demonstrate a parasternal right ventricular outflow tract (RVOT) image of a pulmonic valve with vegetation. In this case, the organism was *S. aureus*.

CONGENITAL VALVULAR PULMONIC STENOSIS

The most common congenital abnormality is valvular stenosis on the basis of developmental abnormalities that mimic those of a bicuspid aortic valve. In congenital valvular pulmonic stenosis, the imaging hallmark is systolic doming of the valve (Fig. 30.15 and Video 30.34). In real time, the valve has a jump-rope appearance because the restricted tip projects into the PA, while the belly of the cusp is mobile. Color Doppler demonstrates turbulent flow, and spectral Doppler can be used to measure transvalvular gradients. In such patients, it is important to remember that RV systolic pressure (as estimated from the tricuspid regurgitant jet) will not equal PA systolic pressure. Instead, RV systolic pressure (RVSP) = PA systolic pressure + transvalvular gradient. Failure to recognize pulmonic stenosis may result in the misdiagnosis of pulmonary hypertension. Pulmonic stenosis is most reliably quantitated with mean and peak gradients, although the continuity equation provides a means of calculating valve area.[6]

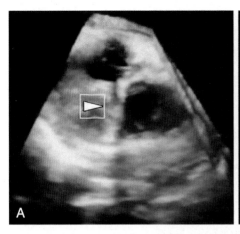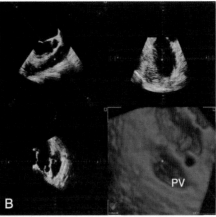

FIG. 30.13 (A) 3D echocardiographic views of the pulmonic valve *(arrowhead)* derived from a midesophageal window. A systolic frame showing all three cusps is shown. (B) Mode of acquisition of the volume and rendering to display the pulmonic valve. *PV*, Pulmonary valve.

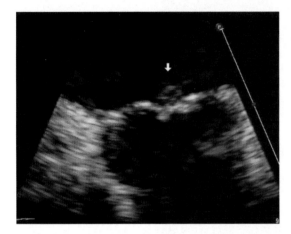

FIG. 30.14 The parasternal image demonstrates a pulmonic valve vegetation *(arrow)*.

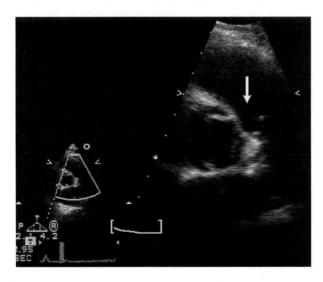

FIG. 30.15 The parasternal systolic image of congenital valvular pulmonic stenosis. The imaging hallmark is systolic doming of the valve *(arrow)*.

PULMONIC STENOSIS S/P VALVULOPLASTY

Patients with severe pulmonic valve stenosis may undergo therapeutic balloon valvuloplasty. Fig. 30.16A–C and Video 30.35 demonstrate a parasternal short-axis view of a congenitally stenotic pulmonic valve following valvuloplasty. The visualized cusp is thickened. In some cases, irregularly mobile fragments may be seen. Color flow mapping shows unrestricted regurgitation. When PA pressure is normal, the flow may not have the typical mosaic pattern of high-velocity jets, and the severity of the regurgitation may be underestimated.[7] Spectral Doppler in this case shows a laminar regurgitant signal.

CARCINOID INVOLVEMENT OF THE PULMONIC VALVE

Since traditional 2D echo does not allow for en-face simultaneous visualization of all three pulmonic leaflets, the presence and extent of carcinoid involvement of the pulmonic valve often cannot be accurately assessed with 2D methods alone. Fig. 30.5D *(left panel)* and Video 30.36 are from a 60-year-old male with a history of carcinoid syndrome who presented with severe tricuspid insufficiency and a question of severe pulmonic insufficiency on transthoracic echo. Since his overall survival rate was considered reasonable, it was recommended that he undergo surgical valve replacement to preserve his ventricular function. A 3D TEE was performed to determine

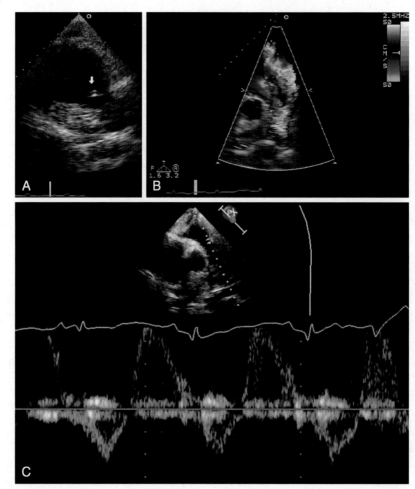

FIG. 30.16 **Post-valvotomy pulmonic valve with unrestricted pulmonic regurgitation.** (A) A parasternal short-axis view of a congenitally stenotic pulmonic valve following valvuloplasty is depicted. Visualized cusp is thickened *(arrow)*. In some cases, irregular mobile fragments may be seen. (B) Color flow mapping shows unrestricted regurgitation. When pulmonary artery pressure is normal, the flow may not have the typical mosaic pattern of high-velocity jets, and the severity of the regurgitation may be underestimated. (C) Spectral Doppler shows a laminar regurgitant signal.

the extent of carcinoid involvement of the pulmonic valve, since this was not adequately visualized by 2D methods. The 3D imaging of the pulmonic valve from the pulmonary perspective confirmed that the valve was severely thickened and retracted with carcinoid involvement and severe wide-open pulmonic insufficiency. The 3D imaging of the tricuspid valve from the right atrial perspective also confirmed severe carcinoid involvement of the tricuspid valve with unrestricted tricuspid insufficiency (see Fig. 30.5D, *right panel*). These findings were confirmed at surgery, and the patient underwent successful biprosthetic tricuspid and pulmonic valve replacement.

ECHO DOPPLER ASSESSMENT OF PULMONIC REGURGITATION SEVERITY

Although the American Society of Echocardiography recommends an integrated approach to assessing the severity of pulmonic regurgitation as summarized in Table 30.1,[7] and the European Society of Cardiovascular Imaging (formerly Echocardiography) recommends a similar approach,[8] the evidence base for assessing pulmonary regurgitation is very limited. In general, pulmonic regurgitation is most commonly quantitated on the basis of jet dimensions, with the caveat that there may be little turbulence in the setting of severe regurgitation with normal pulmonary pressure, and the possibility that its severity may be underestimated. Laminar regurgitant flow is a clue to severe regurgitation as illustrated in Fig. 30.16A–C and Videos 30.35 and 30.37.

SUMMARY

In the past, pulmonic and tricuspid valve disease did not receive the same attention as diseases of the aortic and mitral valves, just as

knowledge of diseases of the RV has historically lagged behind that of diseases of the LV. Newer and less invasive therapeutic options for treating tricuspid and pulmonic valve disease, including percutaneous valve replacement, balloon valvuloplasty, valve-in-valve replacement procedures, and, in the near future, percutaneous right-sided valve repair procedures, have increased the demand for more accurate and precise echocardiographic assessment of the anatomy and physiology of the right-sided valves. The 3D echocardiography complements traditional 2D approaches in providing this information.

Suggested Reading

Baumgartner, H., Hung, J., Bermejo, J., et al. (2009). Echocardiographic assessment of valve stenosis: EAE/ASE recommendations for clinical practice (abstr). *Journal of the American Society of Echocardiography, 22,* 1–23.

Guyer, D. E., Gillam, L. D., Foale, R. A., et al. (2008). Comparison of the echocardiographic and hemodynamic diagnosis of rheumatic tricuspid stenosis. *Journal of the American College of Cardiology, 3,* 1135–1144.

Lancellotti, P., Moura, L., Pierard, L. A., et al. (2010). European Association of Echocardiography recommendations for the assessment of valvular regurgitation. Part 2: mitral and tricuspid regurgitation (native valve disease). *European Journal of Echocardiography, 11,* 307–332.

Lang, R. M., Badano, L. P., Tsang, W., et al. (2012). EAE/ASE recommendations for image acquisition and display using three-dimensional echocardiography. *Journal of the American Society of Echocardiography, 25,* 3–46.

Mangion, J. R., & Ghosh, N. (2013). Three dimensional echocardiography to evaluate valvular disease: the value of an added dimension. In N. C. Nanda (Ed.), *Comprehensive textbook of echocardiography.* New Delhi: Jaypee Brothers Publishers.

Waller, A. H., Chatzisisis, Y. S., Moslehi, J. J., Chen, F. Y., & Mangion, J. R. (2014). Real-time three dimensional transesophageal echocardiography enables preoperative pulmonary valvulopathy assessment. *European Heart Journal Cardiovascular Imaging, 6,* 713.

Zoghbi, W. A., Enriquez-Sarano, M., Foster, E., et al. (2003). Recommendations for evaluation of the severity of native valvular regurgitation with two-dimensional and Doppler echocardiography. *Journal of the American Society of Echocardiography, 16,* 777–802.

A complete reference list can be found online at ExpertConsult.com.

31 Prosthetic Valves

Linda D. Gillam, Konstantinos Koulogiannis, Leo Marcoff

INTRODUCTION

Echocardiography is an essential tool in the evaluation and management of patients with prosthetic valves. Its use requires an understanding of valve design, normal prosthetic appearance and function, imaging artifacts introduced by valve elements, and the spectrum of valve dysfunction. This chapter will cover these topics with a focus on aortic and mitral prostheses since these are the most commonly implanted valves and those for which the largest evidence base exists. A valuable reference is the current joint document of the American Society of Echocardiography (ASE), European Association of Cardiovascular Imaging (EACVI; formerly European Association of Echocardiography), and other professional societies.[1] The reader is directed to Chapter 40 (Echocardiography in Infective Endocarditis) for a discussion of prosthetic valve endocarditis and to sections in the chapters on native valves (Chapters 28–30), which deal with the echocardiographic quantitation of valve stenosis and regurgitation, since similar approaches are used, with exceptions that are noted in this chapter. The unique considerations for echocardiography in transcatheter valves are covered in greater detail in Chapter 32 and the appropriate use of echocardiography in prosthetic valves is covered in Chapter 47.

While all echo modalities are used in the evaluation of prosthetic valves, there should be a low threshold for transesophageal echocardiography (TEE) in virtually all cases of known or suspected prosthetic valve abnormality. Also helpful are three-dimensional (3D) techniques, particularly in the setting of valve stenosis or dehiscence with paravalvular regurgitation.

NORMAL APPEARANCE AND FUNCTION

The most commonly encountered mechanical prostheses are bileaflet or single tilting-disc valves, although ball and cage valves, which are no longer implanted, may be seen as well (Fig. 31.1). The majority of bioprosthetic valves are stented porcine or bovine pericardial valves, although freestyle (stentless) xenografts, cadaveric homograft, autograft (Ross procedure), transcatheter and sutureless surgical valves, which represent a hybrid between conventional stented and transcatheter bioprostheses, are also available (Fig. 31.2). Prosthetic annular rings are also commonly used in mitral and tricuspid repair. The sewing rings of all valves, as well as the leaflets/discs of mechanical valves, may cause acoustic shadowing that limits imaging and Doppler assessment. Additionally, the material of the ball-in-cage valves transmits sound more slowly than human tissue with the result that the ball appears much larger than its actual size when imaged echocardiographically.

In general, the range of problems that can involve prosthetic valves includes pathologic stenosis and/or regurgitation and other instances where the appearance is abnormal, although function remains within normal limits. It is very helpful to know the valve type and size. At the time of implantation, patients are given wallet cards that include this information and, at the time of scheduling for echocardiographic evaluation, patients should be told to bring these cards. An alternative source of information is the operative note, which may be available in the patient's medical record. The operative note will also provide details about any deviations from standard surgical techniques, such as atypical positioning of the valve and the use of surgical glue that may translate into an atypical baseline echocardiographic appearance. It is also very helpful to have access to the intraprocedural transesophageal echocardiogram.

A core concept for prosthetic valves is that valve replacement is not curative. Thus, even normal prostheses are variably stenotic with the degree of stenosis inversely related to valve size. Additionally, trivial degrees of valvular regurgitation are normal findings[1] and, while not normal, trivial paravalvular regurgitation is not uncommon. Intraventricular micro-cavitations are often seen in the presence of mechanical valves. These findings underscore the importance of a baseline echocardiographic evaluation, which is critically important to establish gradients and the degree of regurgitation, if any, at a time when the valve is presumably normal. Typically, the baseline transthoracic echo is performed before patients are discharged or within the first 4–8 weeks post-discharge. The latter is important if the post-discharge echo is technically difficult due to residual intrathoracic air and/or the inability of the patient to move without discomfort.

Table A.15 in Appendix A provides normal echocardiographic values for the most commonly implanted valves. A rule of thumb, which is helpful when the valve size is unknown, is that for commonly sized prostheses with physiologic heart rates (HRs) and stroke volumes, the peak transaortic velocity should be less than 3 mps and the mean transmitral gradient should be ≤5 mm Hg.

Fig. 31.1 and corresponding Videos 31.1–31.6 show the most common mechanical prostheses and their transesophageal echocardiographic counterparts. All echocardiograms show valves in the mitral position. Note should be made of the reverberation artifacts caused by the mobile disc elements for the bileaflet and tilting-disc valves, as well as the acoustic shadowing caused by the sewing rings of all valves. In the case of tilting-disc valves, such an artifact also emanates from the disc pivot point. A different type of artifact is associated with ball-in-cage valves. This arises because echocardiography assumes that ultrasound waves will encounter only biologic tissue and move at a constant speed. However, sound moves through the ball of a ball-in-cage valve more slowly than it does through tissue and, thus, the trailing edge of the ball is represented as if the ball were much larger than it actually is. While ball-in-cage valves are no longer implanted, given their durability it is not unusual to encounter such valves in the echocardiography lab. Videos 31.4–31.6 demonstrate physiologic degrees of regurgitation for these valves. Note that for the bileaflet valve there are multiple jets around the perimeter as well as centrally. With a single tilting-disc valve there are also perimeter jets but the central jet is larger. Very little if any regurgitation is seen with a normally functioning ball-in-cage valve.

Fig. 31.2 shows the most commonly encountered bioprosthetic valves and their echocardiographic appearance. In these examples, all prostheses have been implanted into the aortic position. Stented bioprostheses, of which one example is provided, are the most common bioprosthetic valves. However, transcatheter aortic valves, either balloon-expandable or self-expanding, as shown here, are increasingly encountered, and are discussed in detail in Chapter 32. Note that with the balloon expandable aortic prosthesis, the support is provided by a metal frame rather than by three stents. For the balloon-expandable valve, the frame is shorter than that for the self-expanding valve, but for both there is a variable offset between the lower end of the frame and the position of the cusps. This is best appreciated in the Videos 31.7–31.9. Since valvular or paravalvular regurgitation is not invariable in bioprostheses, although still relatively common in transcatheter valves, no representative color images are provided. Similarly, since the echocardiographic appearance of stentless heterograft prostheses as well as homografts (cadaveric aortic valves) or autografts (pulmonic valve transplanted to the aortic position during the Ross procedure) is typically no different from that of the native valve, no figures are provided.

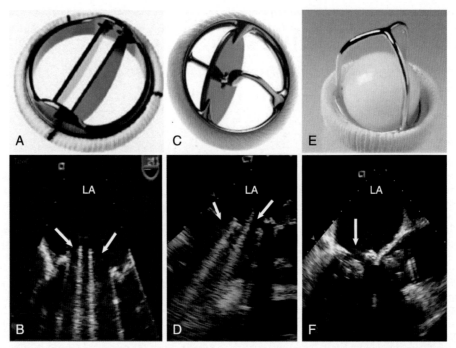

FIG. 31.1 Mechanical prostheses and their transesophageal echocardiography appearance when implanted in the mitral position. (A and B) Bileaflet (St. Jude) valve. *Arrows* indicate discs in the open position. (C and D) Medtronic-Hall tilting-disc valve. *Right arrow* indicates disc in the open position, *left arrow* indicates reverberation from the central pivot. (E and F) Starr Edwards ball and cage valve. *Arrow* points to the valve in the open position. *LA,* Left atrium. (*From Solomon SD, Wu J, Gillam L. Echocardiography. In: Mann DL, Zipes DP, Libby P, et al., eds.* Braunwald's Heart Disease: A Textbook of Cardiovascular Medicine. *10th ed. Philadelphia: Elsevier; 2015:179-260.*)

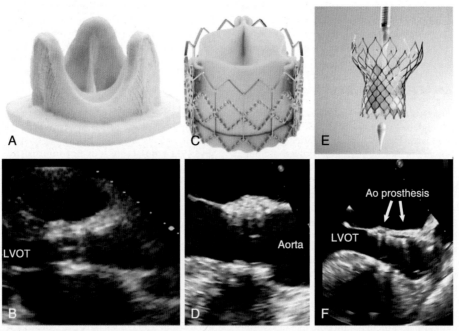

FIG. 31.2 Bioprostheses and their echocardiographic long-axis appearance when implanted in the aortic position. (A and B) Heterograft stented bioprosthesis transthoracic echocardiography (TTE). (C and D) Sapien balloon expandable bioprosthesis, transesophageal echocardiography (TEE). (E and F) CoreValve self-expanding bioprosthesis, transesophageal echocardiography (TEE). *Ao,* Aortic; *LVOT,* left ventricular outflow tract. (*From Solomon SD, Wu J, Gillam L. Echocardiography. In: Mann DL, Zipes DP, Libby P, et al., eds.* Braunwald's Heart Disease: A Textbook of Cardiovascular Medicine. *10th ed. Philadelphia: Elsevier; 2015:179-260.*)

PROSTHETIC VALVE STENOSIS

The echocardiographic tools used to identify and quantitate prosthetic valve stenosis are similar to those used for native valves. They include mean and peak gradients, and valve area calculated by the continuity equation, which is most widely used for aortic prostheses and termed the effective orifice area (EOA). While the pressure half-time can be calculated for mitral prostheses, it cannot be extrapolated to an absolute valve area, but rather can be used per se for longitudinal monitoring. The Doppler velocity index (DVI) is the prosthetic valve equivalent of the dimensionless index.

Note should be made of the impact of cardiac output and HR on prosthetic gradients, particularly for valves in the mitral position, with

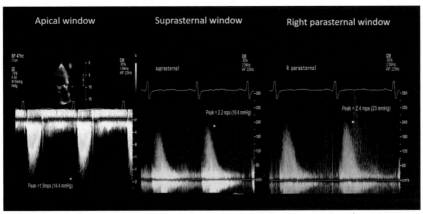

FIG. 31.3 Continuous-wave spectra recorded from the apical, suprasternal, and right parasternal windows in a patient with a normally functioning bioprosthesis. Note that the highest velocities are recorded from the right parasternal window, which is also frequently the case for native valves. Note too that the suprasternal and right parasternal spectra have been recorded using a nonimaging (Pedoff) transducer.

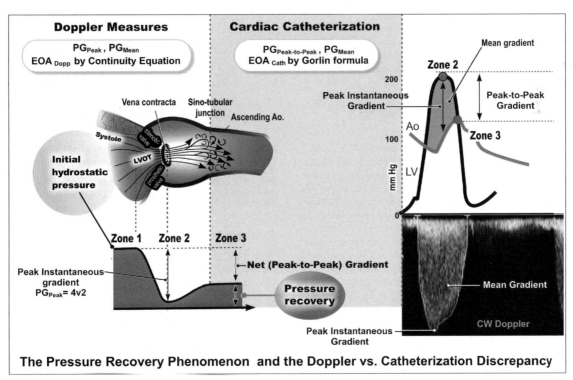

FIG. 31.4 **Schematic illustrating the concept of pressure recovery.** By recording the peak instantaneous gradient, which occurs just distal to the vena contracta, Doppler will record higher gradients than those that are recorded by catheterization, which reflect the impact of pressure recovery. This is a particular concern in the setting of small mechanical prostheses when the aorta is also small. See text for details. *Ao,* Aorta; *CW,* continuous wave; *EOA,* effective orifice area; *LV,* left ventricle; *LVOT,* left ventricular outflow tract; *PG,* pressure gradient. *(Courtesy of Bernard E. Bulwer, MD, FASE.)*

gradients being higher when stroke volume and/or HR is/are increased. The corollary of this observation is that echocardiographic reports should always make note of the HR at the time of hemodynamic evaluation.

Gradients

For native valves, it is very important to note the angle dependence of Doppler as it is used to capture velocities from which gradients are derived. Fig. 31.3 shows aortic prosthetic gradients recorded from the apical, suprasternal, and right parasternal windows demonstrating that, as is common for native valves, the gradients are typically higher when recorded from the right parasternal window.

To interpret gradients, it is important to have normal reference values, which are valve type and size specific. Table A.15 in Appendix A reproduces the values provided in the ASE–EACVI recommendations.[1]

Note that these are derived from echocardiographic rather than in vitro flow tank values, thus adjusting for pressure recovery—a concept that is discussed below. Another useful reference will be the implantation values recorded either intraoperatively or on the first postoperative transthoracic study.

Pressure Recovery

The concept of pressure recovery is not unique to prosthetic valves, although, most commonly, it is a clinical consideration in the setting of small mechanical aortic prostheses. When blood encounters an area of narrowing, pressure energy is converted to kinetic energy with the result that the pressure at the vena contracta or effective orifice will be at its lowest (Fig. 31.4), and the pressure gradient recorded at this site will be highest. Distal to the obstruction, kinetic energy can be either dispersed as thermal energy or recovered as pressure energy so that the pressure recorded distal to the obstruction will be higher, and the pressure gradient lower than that recorded at the effective orifice. Pressure recovery is more prominent when the aortic root and ascending aorta are small. Based, in part, on in vitro studies, a small aortic root is one with a diameter of ≤3 cm at the sinotubular junction, and a small prosthesis is ≤19 mm. The pressure recovery explains the discrepancy between peak instantaneous gradients measured by echocardiography and catheterization, as echocardiography measures gradients at the vena contracta, while catheterization measures the gradient distally after pressure has recovered.[2,3] It is also a consideration in the differential diagnosis of high Doppler-measured prosthetic gradients in small mechanical prostheses. Of course, there is also a fundamental difference between the peak instantaneous gradient measured by echo and the peak-to-peak gradient, which is more commonly measured invasively.

A related concept is that of the relative gradients measured across the central and lateral orifices in bileaflet mechanical prosthesis. It is recognized that the gradients across the central orifice will be higher than those across the lateral orifices, and that a continuous-wave (CW) spectrum optimized to capture the highest velocity will indeed capture that across the central orifice. For aortic prostheses, even with TEE, it is rarely possible to selectively interrogate central and lateral orifices, although this may be possible with TEE evaluation of mitral valves. Pressures measured distal to the valve will reflect a mixing of the central and lateral jets with the result that the pressure gradient will be lower than that calculated at the vena contracta. The differences are most dramatic in small valves.[4]

Valve Area and Other Measures of Valve Stenosis

Applying the continuity equation in a manner analogous to that used in native aortic valve stenosis can provide the EOA for aortic prostheses. As with native aortic stenosis, it is critical that left ventricular outflow tract sampling be proximal to the site of flow acceleration, and in the case of transcatheter or sutureless valves, that it be proximal to the inlet of the metal frame, since, in these valves, there is flow acceleration at the inlet to the metal frame as well as at the level of the cusps with both elements contributing to the total obstruction provided by the valve.[5] While the continuity equation approach to calculating EOA has been proposed for mitral prostheses, it has not been extensively validated. It has been suggested that it is best suited for mitral bioprostheses and tilting-disc mechanical prostheses, as it is limited in bileaflet valves by the tendency of Doppler to record the higher central orifice rather than lateral orifice flows. Normal valve- and size-specific values for EOA are provided in Table A.15 in Appendix A. The pressure half-time should not be used to calculate EOA in the setting of mitral prostheses, although the absolute value of the pressure half-time in milliseconds can be used for longitudinal follow-up in individual patients with progressive lengthening suggesting the development of prosthetic stenosis.

Given the challenges of measuring the left ventricular outflow tract diameter and calculating the cross-sectional area, the DVI has been proposed as an alternative measure of the degree of valve obstruction. Conceptually, this is the same as the dimensionless index for native aortic stenosis and is calculated as the ratio of the peak velocity in the left ventricular outflow tract to the peak velocity of the aortic valvular jet. A DVI less than 0.25 is considered to be highly suggestive of significant aortic valve obstruction.

The DVI calculated for the mitral valve is done somewhat differently and reflects the ratio of the velocity time integral (VTI) proximal to the mitral prosthesis to the VTI in the left ventricular outflow tract. For this index, a ratio greater than 2.5 is highly suggestive of significant mitral valve prosthetic obstruction.

For aortic prostheses, an additional semiquantitative measure of stenosis is the acceleration time of transvalvular flow, as measured by CW Doppler, with a rounded jet envelope being more suggestive of significant intrinsic dysfunction than one with a sharp upstroke. The acceleration time is calculated from the time of onset of flow to the peak velocity, and a value greater than 100 ms is suggestive of intrinsic prosthetic dysfunction.

EOA, Effective orifice area; *PPM*, patient prosthesis mismatch; *TEE*, transesophageal echocardiography.

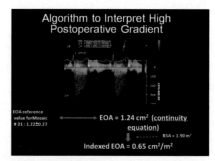

FIG. 31.5 Application of the algorithm for the diagnosis of patient prosthesis mismatch. In this case, the calculated effective orifice area (EOA) is within the reported range for a normal 21 mm Mosaic bioprosthesis. The indexed EOA is 0.65 cm²/m² consistent with patient prosthesis mismatch. Despite the calculation, the absence of functional or anatomic abnormalities of the valve should be confirmed with transesophageal echocardiography.

Patient-Prosthesis Mismatch

With prosthetic valves there are scenarios where the gradients are high but the valve has a normal appearance and a normal-for-valve type and size calculated EOA. In this case, patient prosthesis mismatch (PPM) must be considered.[6,7] Simply put, this is a scenario where the valve is too small for the patient, which is a situation that can arise when native valve geometry, typically excessive calcium, limits the size of the valve that can be implanted. In the setting of PPM, typically there will be persistence of abnormally high postoperative gradients, although PPM is defined on the basis of body surface area–indexed EOA in units of cm²/m².

For valves in the aortic position, an acceptable indexed EOA is greater than 0.85 cm²/m². Values of 0.66–0.85 cm²/m² are considered to reflect moderate PPM, and values of ≤0.65 cm²/m² are considered to reflect severe PPM. This physiology is less commonly encountered with mitral prostheses, but definitions have been proposed as follows: mild or no PPM-indexed EOA greater than 1.2 cm²/m²; moderate PPM-indexed EOA 0.9–1.2 cm²/m²; and severe PPM-indexed EOA less than 0.9 cm²/m².

The prevalence and consequences of PPM have been debated. For aortic PPM, it has been reported that there is less improvement in postoperative functional class, an increased incidence of late cardiac events, and less regression of left ventricular hypertrophy. Studies have suggested a major impact on perioperative mortality, particularly if left ventricular dysfunction is present and there is a moderate impact on late mortality; that is, after 7 years. The impact of mitral PPM has been less clearly established.

An algorithm has been proposed for the interpretation of high gradients in valve prostheses as shown in Box 31.1 and an application of the algorithm is shown in Fig. 31.5. In summary, calculated EOA is compared with reference values for the same type and size of prosthesis, and if the EOA is within the normal range for the valve as published, an indexed EOA should be calculated. Depending on the value,

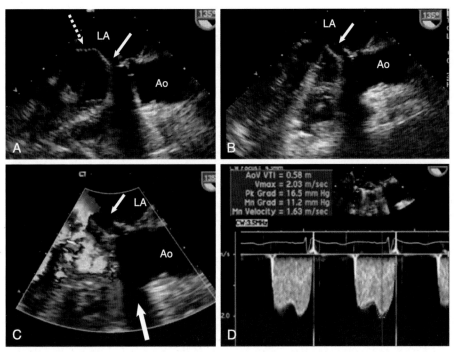

FIG. 31.6 **Transesophageal echo showing a bileaflet mechanical mitral prosthesis in which one disc is immobilized due to thrombus.** (A) The systolic frame shows that neither disc *(arrows)* closes completely. (B) While the left disc opens fully, the right disc is immobile. (C) Color flow Doppler demonstrates high velocity flow through a single orifice. The large white arrow indicates acoustic shadowing due to the mitral sewing ring. (D) Doppler demonstrates an elevated transmitral gradient (11.2 mm Hg at a heart rate of 65 bpm). *Ao,* Aorta; *LA,* left atrium. *(From Solomon SD, Wu J, Gillam L. Echocardiography. In: Mann DL, Zipes DP, Libby P, et al., eds.* Braunwald's Heart Disease: A Textbook of Cardiovascular Medicine. *10th ed. Philadelphia: Elsevier; 2015:179-260.)*

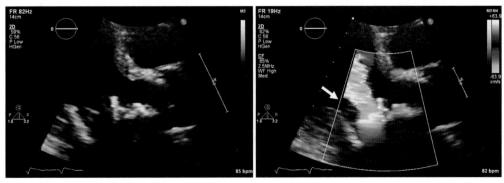

FIG. 31.7 **Apical three-chamber view of a patient with mitral prosthetic valve thrombosis.** Although it was difficult to detect impaired cusp motion or the associated valve thrombus, color Doppler showed that there was color paucity *(arrow)* highlighting the reduced leaflet excursion.

a diagnosis of PPM can be confirmed or excluded. However, it should be emphasized that because of the potential for error in the calculations, and uncertainty regarding the role of indexing, particularly in obese patients, PPM should be a diagnosis of exclusion, one made after TEE and/or fluoroscopy have been performed to definitively exclude intrinsic valve dysfunction.

Given the significance of PPM and the risks of reoperation for this condition, it has been emphasized that preoperative evaluation may reduce its occurrence. An awareness of the optimal EOA for each prosthesis allows the surgeon to determine whether the valve that has been chosen is appropriately sized. If PPM is predicted, aortic root enlargement may permit the placement of a larger valve or an alternative prosthesis with lower gradients. In some patients, an atypical position (e.g., supraannular) may permit the placement of a larger valve.[8]

Causes of Prosthetic Valve Stenosis

Despite the occurrence of PPM and pressure recovery, there are clearly instances where high gradients reflect intrinsic valve dysfunction, which is true prosthetic valve stenosis. Causes include valve degeneration, and

impeded movement of bioprosthetic leaflets or mechanical valve discs due to endocarditis (see Fig. 40.11 and Video 40.12), thrombus, pannus, or other less common causes.

Fig. 31.6 and Videos 31.10 and 31.11 demonstrate a case in which intrinsic dysfunction was suspected in the presence of high transmitral gradients in a patient with a bileaflet mechanical prosthesis who had been noncompliant with anticoagulation. TEE shows the absence of motion of one of the bileaflet valve discs, confirmed pathologically to be due to thrombus. In this case, because the disc is immobilized in the closed position, valve stenosis is the result. Had it been stuck in an open position, mitral regurgitation would have been the outcome.

Until recently, valve thrombosis was thought to be uncommon in bioprostheses, but the scrutiny of transcatheter aortic valves has brought to light its occurrence in bioprostheses as well. Since it may be difficult to see thrombi with transthoracic echocardiography (TTE) a recent study has highlighted color paucity (Fig. 31.7)—the absence of a transvalvular color signal filling the valve orifice—as a marker of valve thrombosis, and a finding that should trigger TEE. A TEE example of valve thrombus from a different patient is shown in Fig. 31.8 and Video 31.12.

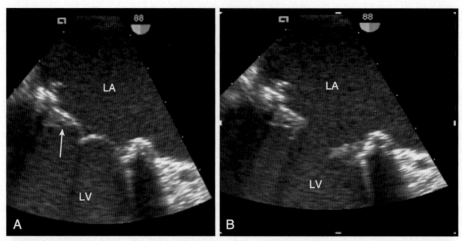

FIG. 31.8 Transesophageal echocardiographic appearance of thrombus *(arrow)* **in a mitral bioprosthesis.** (A) Systole. (B) Diastole. Note that the thrombus has immobilized the base of the left-sided cusp creating a hinge point midway along the cusp and an narrow orifice. *LA*, Left atrium; *LV*, left ventricle.

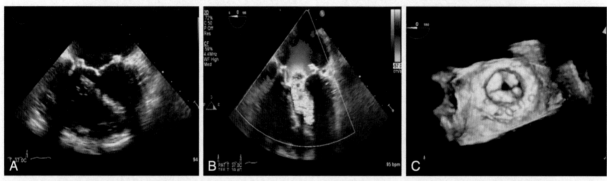

FIG. 31.9 Transesophageal echocardiography demonstrating a degenerated bioprosthesis. (A) Diastolic frame showing grossly restricted cusp motion. (B) Color Doppler demonstrates turbulent transmitral flow and an easily identifiable PISA shell. (C) 3D transesophageal echocardiography view of the prosthesis form a left atrial perspective. The mitral orifice is greatly restricted. (*From Solomon SD, Wu J, Gillam L. Echocardiography. In: Mann DL, Zipes DP, Libby P, et al., eds.* Braunwald's Heart Disease: A Textbook of Cardiovascular Medicine. *10th ed. Philadelphia: Elsevier; 2015:179-260.*)

Pannus formation, which represents fibrous ingrowth into the valve orifice, may be difficult to differentiate from thrombus on the basis of its echocardiographic appearance alone. Pannus tends to be a more chronic phenomenon, and is unrelated to anticoagulation status. The echotexture of thrombus is described as being softer, and the thrombi may be larger, more irregular, and extend beyond the sewing ring. That said, a trial of anticoagulation and/or surgical inspection may be required to differentiate between these two causes of valve stenosis.

Valve degeneration is a phenomenon that may occur somewhat unpredictably in bioprostheses, although it is more likely to occur 10 years or more after valve implantation. Occasionally the tissue of bioprosthetic valves may be rejected by the patient's immune system. An example of premature bioprosthetic degeneration of a mitral prosthesis with critical prosthetic stenosis is shown in Fig. 31.9 and Videos 31.13–31.15.

PROSTHETIC VALVE REGURGITATION

Some degree of valve regurgitation is common in mechanical valves, which has previously been described. In addition, trivial degrees of paravalvular regurgitation may be noted at the time of valve implantation but, with endothelialization, will typically disappear or not progress. However, pathologic regurgitation may occur in the setting of valve degeneration, valve dehiscence, endocarditis in which vegetations impede valve closure or cause perforations, and other etiologies of interference with valve closure in which valve stenosis and regurgitation may coexist.

The concepts of paravalvular regurgitation and valve dehiscence are related in that both reflect separation of the valve sewing ring from the

tissue to which it was attached. Regardless of the degree of separation, there will be paravalvular regurgitation (Fig. 31.10 and Videos 31.16–31.18). However, when the separation is extensive (≥ 40% of the sewing ring) the valve will rock excessively (Video 31.19; see also Videos 40.9 and 40.13 in Chapter 40). The causes of paravalvular regurgitation include infection, excessive calcification at the time of valve implantation, or abnormally friable tissue. Paravalvular regurgitation is a relatively common occurrence in transcatheter valve implantation as discussed in Chapter 32. TEE—ideally with 3D—is essential to evaluate paravalvular regurgitation as TTE may fail to identify or greatly underestimate the paravalvular leak.

The ASE/EACVI recommendations[1] provide guidance in the quantitation of valvular and paravalvular regurgitation (Tables 31.1 and 31.2). The elements are largely concordant with those for the evaluation of native valve regurgitation. For paravalvular regurgitation, it has been suggested that if less than 10% of the sewing ring is involved, the regurgitation is mild; 10%–20%, suggests moderate regurgitation; and greater than 20%, suggests severe regurgitation. However, the evidence base for this recommendation is limited.

PROSTHETIC VALVE ENDOCARDITIS

This topic is discussed in Chapter 40 (Echocardiography in Infective Endocarditis) with the following figures illustrating infection of prosthetic valves: Figs. 40.8, 40.9, 40.11, and Videos 40.8–40.10, 40.12, and 40.13.

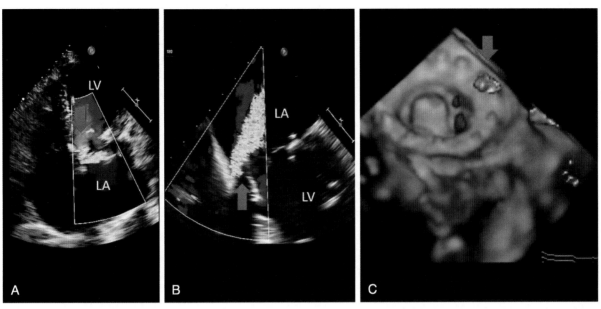

FIG. 31.10 Paravalvular regurgitation. (A) 2D apical 4 chamber TTE, (B) 2D TEE, and (C) 3D TEE, showing a paravalvular leak originating along the ventricular aspect of a mitral bioprosthesis. The spatial extent of the area of dehiscence is best appreciated with 3D where the regurgitant orifice can be planimetered to guide sizing of transcatheter closure devices. *Red arrows* point to the areas of dehiscence. *LA,* Left atrium; *LV,* left ventricle.

TABLE 31.1 Echocardiographic and Doppler Criteria for Severity of Prosthetic Mitral Regurgitation Using Findings From Transthoracic Echocardiography and Transesophageal Echocardiography

PARAMETER	MILD	MODERATE	SEVERE
Structural Parameters			
LV size	Normal[a]	Normal or dilated	Usually dilated[b]
Prosthetic valve[c]	Usually normal	Abnormal[d]	Abnormal[d]
Doppler Parameters			
Color flow jet area[c,e]	Small, central jet (usually <4 cm² or <20% of LA area)	Variable	Large central jet (usually >8 cm² or >40% of LA area) or variable size wall-impinging jet swirling in left atrium
Flow convergence[f]	None or minimal	Intermediate	Large
Jet density: CW Doppler[c]	Incomplete or faint	Dense	Dense
Jet contour: CW Doppler[c]	Parabolic	Usually parabolic	Early peaking, triangular
Pulmonary venous flow[c]	Systolic dominance[g]	Systolic blunting[g]	Systolic flow reversal[h]
Quantitative Parameters[i]			
VC width (cm)[c]	<0.3	0.3–0.59	≥0.6
R vol (mL/beat)	<30	30–59	≥60
RF (%)	<30	30–49	>50
EROA (cm²)	<0.20	0.20–0.49	≥0.50

[a]LV size applied only to chronic lesions.
[b]In the absence of other etiologies of LV enlargement and acute MR.
[c]Parameter may be best evaluated or obtained with TEE, particularly in mechanical valves.
[d]Abnormal mechanical valves, for example, immobile occluder (valvular regurgitation), dehiscence or rocking (paravalvular regurgitation); abnormal biologic valves, for example, leaflet thickening or prolapse (valvular), dehiscence or rocking (paravalvular regurgitation).
[e]At a Nyquist limit of 50–60 cm/s.
[f]Minimal and large flow convergence defined as a flow convergence radius <0.4 and ≥0.9 cm for central jets, respectively, with a baseline shift at a Nyquist limit of 40 cm/s; cutoffs for eccentric jets may be higher.
[g]Unless other reasons for systolic blunting (e.g., atrial fibrillation, elevated LA pressure).
[h]Pulmonary venous systolic flow reversal is specific but not sensitive for severe MR.
[i]These quantitative parameters are less well validated than in native MR.
CW, Continuous wave; *EROA,* effective regurgitant orifice area; *LA,* left atrium; *LV,* left ventricle; *MR,* mitral regurgitation; *RF,* regurgitant fraction; *R vol,* regurgitant volume; *VC,* vena contracta.
From Zoghbi WA, Chambers JB, Dumesnil JG, et al. Recommendations for evaluation of prosthetic valves with echocardiography and Doppler ultrasound: a report from the American Society of Echocardiography's Guidelines and Standards Committee and the Task Force on Prosthetic Valves, Developed in Conjunction With the American College of Cardiology Cardiovascular Imaging Committee, Cardiac Imaging Committee of the American Heart Association, the European Association of Echocardiography, a registered branch of the European Society of Cardiology, the Japanese Society of Echocardiography and the Canadian Society of Echocardiography, Endorsed by the American College of Cardiology Foundation, American Heart Association, European Association of Echocardiography, a registered branch of the European Society of Cardiology, the Japanese Society of Echocardiography, and Canadian Society of Echocardiography. J Am Soc Echocardiogr. 2009;22(9):975-1014.

V

VALVULAR HEART DISEASE

TABLE 31.2 Parameters for Evaluation of the Severity of Prosthetic Aortic Valve Regurgitation

PARAMETER	MILD	MODERATE	SEVERE
Valve Structure and Motion			
Mechanical or bioprosthetic	Usually normal	Abnormal[a]	Abnormal[a]
Structural Parameters			
LV size	Normal[b]	Normal or mildly dilated[b]	Dilated[b]
Doppler Parameters (Qualitative or Semiquantitative)			
Jet width in central jets (% LVO diameter): color[c]	Narrow (≤25%)	Intermediate (26%–64%)	Large (≥65%)
Jet density: CW Doppler	Incomplete or faint	Dense	Dense
Jet deceleration rate (PHT, ms): CW Doppler[d]	Slow (>500)	Variable (200–500)	Steep (<200)
LVO flow versus pulmonary flow: PW Doppler	Slightly increased	Intermediate	Greatly increased
Diastolic flow reversal in the descending aorta: PW Doppler	Absent or brief early diastolic	Intermediate	Prominent, holodiastolic
Doppler Parameters (Quantitative)			
Regurgitant volume (mL/beat)	<30	30–59	>60
Regurgitant fraction (%)	<30	30–50	>50

[a]Abnormal mechanical valves, for example, immobile occluder (valvular regurgitation), dehiscence or rocking (paravalvular regurgitation); abnormal biologic valves, for example, leaflet thickening or prolapse (valvular), dehiscence or rocking (paravalvular regurgitation).
[b]Applies to chronic, late postoperative aortic regurgitation in the absence of other etiologies.
[c]Parameter applicable to central jets and is less accurate in eccentric jets; Nyquist limit of 50–60 cm/s.
[d]Influenced by LV compliance.
CW, Continuous wave; *LV*, left ventricle; *LVO*, left ventricular outflow; *PHT*, pressure half-time; *PW*, pulsed wave.
From Zoghbi WA, Chambers JB, Dumesnil JG, et al. Recommendations for evaluation of prosthetic valves with echocardiography and Doppler ultrasound: a report from the American Society of Echocardiography's Guidelines and Standards Committee and the Task Force on Prosthetic Valves, Developed in Conjunction With the American College of Cardiology Cardiovascular Imaging Committee, Cardiac Imaging Committee of the American Heart Association, the European Association of Echocardiography, a registered branch of the European Society of Cardiology, the Japanese Society of Echocardiography and the Canadian Society of Echocardiography, Endorsed by the American College of Cardiology Foundation, American Heart Association, European Association of Echocardiography, a registered branch of the European Society of Cardiology, the Japanese Society of Echocardiography, and Canadian Society of Echocardiography. J Am Soc Echocardiogr. 2009;22(9):975-1014.

Suggested Reading

Baumgartner, H., Stefenelli, T., Niederberger, J., et al. (1999). "Overestimation" of catheter gradients by Doppler ultrasound in patients with aortic stenosis: a predictable manifestation of pressure recovery. *Journal of the American College of Cardiology, 33,* 1655–1661.

Pibarot, P., & Dumesnil, J. G. (2000). Hemodynamic and clinical impact of prosthesis-patient mismatch in the aortic valve position and its prevention. *Journal of the American College of Cardiology, 36,* 1131–1141.

Pibarot, P., & Dumesnil, J. G. (2012). Valve prosthesis-patient mismatch, 1978 to 2011: from original concept to compelling evidence. *Journal of the American College of Cardiology, 60,* 1136–1139.

Shames, S., Koczo, A., Hahn, R., Jin, Z., Picard, M. H., & Gillam, L. D. (2012). Flow characteristics of the SAPIEN aortic valve: the importance of recognizing in-stent flow acceleration for the echocardiographic assessment of valve function. *Journal of the American Society of Echocardiography, 25,* 603–609.

Zoghbi, W. A., Chambers, J. B., Dumesnil, J. G., et al. (2009). Recommendations for evaluation of prosthetic valves with echocardiography and Doppler ultrasound: a report from the American Society of Echocardiography's Guidelines and Standards Committee and the Task Force on Prosthetic Valves, Developed in Conjunction With the American College of Cardiology Cardiovascular Imaging Committee, Cardiac Imaging Committee of the American Heart Association, the European Association of Echocardiography, a registered branch of the European Society of Cardiology, the Japanese Society of Echocardiography and the Canadian Society of Echocardiography, Endorsed by the American College of Cardiology Foundation, American Heart Association, European Association of Echocardiography, a registered branch of the European Society of Cardiology, the Japanese Society of Echocardiography, and Canadian Society of Echocardiography. *Journal of the American Society of Echocardiography, 22,* 975–1014.

A complete reference list can be found online at ExpertConsult.com.

32 Echocardiography in Percutaneous Valvular Intervention

Rebecca T. Hahn

INTRODUCTION

Since the development and implantation of the first transcatheter pulmonic[1,2] and aortic[3,4] valves, there has been a rapid acceptance of transcatheter valve implantation as a solution to high-risk or inoperable patients with severe, symptomatic valve disease. Randomized trials have since supported the use of transcatheter aortic valve replacement (TAVR) for severe symptomatic aortic stenosis in these patient populations[5–8] with evidence of efficacy and safety in the intermediate surgical risk population as well.[9] These therapies have subsequently had an impact on the acceptance of percutaneous transcatheter therapies for multiple valvular heart disease pathologies. Transcatheter mitral valve repair devices have received the CE mark in Europe;[10,11] however, the MitraClip remains the only commercially available device in the United States[12] where transcatheter mitral valve replacements (TMVRs) are currently under investigation.[13–19] Transcatheter tricuspid devices have been tested in animal models[20–23] with some in their early feasibility stages in humans.[24,25] In addition, transcatheter treatment of surgical valve failure with valve-in-valve (VIV) techniques has become widely accepted.[26–30]

The preprocedural assessment of valvular heart disease severity utilizes echocardiography as the primary diagnostic imaging mode. However, this chapter will focus on the echocardiographic intraprocedural evaluation of valvular morphology and function, guidance of the transcatheter device implantation, and the postimplantation assessment for percutaneous valvular interventions.

TRANSCATHETER AORTIC VALVE REPLACEMENT

TAVR has become an accepted alternative to surgical intervention in patients with severe, symptomatic aortic stenosis who are inoperable or at high risk for surgical valve replacement.[6,7,31,32] Numerous consensus papers and guidelines suggest that echocardiography is important in the preprocedural, intraprocedural, and postprocedural evaluation of patients undergoing TAVR.[33–36] As TAVR has become more routine, some centers have advocated the use of moderate sedation rather than general anesthesia for the procedure,[37,38] limiting, but not eliminating, the ability to perform intraprocedural transesophageal echocardiography (TEE).[39]

Transthoracic echocardiography (TTE) during TAVR faces multiple challenges due to both methodologic and patient-specific issues.[40] Parasternal windows require direct placement of the probe within the fluoroscopic imaging plane with high exposure to radiation. The supine position and avoidance of the sterile field may prohibit proper transducer placement. The usual ultrasound interference rules still apply, such as chest wall deformities, emphysema, obesity, etc. Intraprocedural TTE can rule out the causes of acute hemodynamic compromise, such as pericardial effusions, underfilled or dysfunctional ventricles, and severe valvular regurgitation. However, the assessment of paravalvular regurgitation (PVR) remains challenging unless the imaging windows are ideal. Advantages and disadvantages of TTE and TEE for intraprocedural guidance during TAVR are summarized in Table 32.1. In general, the risk-benefit analysis would favor TEE imaging in patients at low risk for either general anesthesia or monitored anesthetic care. In fact, studies have suggested that using TEE imaging during TAVR may reduce mortality.[41] The final challenge to TTE imaging is the need for immediate and accurate

interpretation of the images typically requiring the presence of a physician echocardiographer in a TAVR suite. If TTE images are acquired by such physicians, they need to have proper training and experience in performing TTEs.[40] The following section will concentrate on intraprocedural TEE imaging for TAVR.[42–44]

Preimplantation Assessment

Prior to implantation of the valve, TEE is used to assess the entire "landing zone" of the transcatheter heart valve (THV) (Box 32.1). This landing zone may differ depending on the type of valve implanted (Fig. 32.1). The current commercially available balloon-expandable valve (SAPIEN 3) is short in height when fully deployed (15.5–22.5 mm depending on valve size), and the inflow (ventricular) edge is ideally positioned 1–2 mm below the level of the aortic annulus to allow the fabric skirt around the outside of the proximal portion of the valve to seal the annulus and prevent PVR. The current commercially available self-expanding THV (Evolut R) is much longer (~50 mm), with the outflow end (aortic) within the ascending aorta, and the inflow end ideally positioned 2–5 mm below the annulus. Other valve designs used commercially in Europe are currently in trials in the United States.[45,46]

Despite higher rates of PVR with the self-expanding valve,[47,48] clinical outcomes acutely, and at 1 year, do not differ significantly between the two valves.[48–50] Often, the sizing of the annulus as well as the calcium location and burden, may help to determine the ideal type of THV to implant.[51] However, as more valve types are available, other factors (i.e., bicuspid morphology, preexisting pacemaker, ease of deployment) may also influence the decision-making process.

The most important measurement currently used for THV sizing is the "annulus," which is a virtual plane at the level of the hinge-point (lowest attachment site) of the three cusps.[52] Because the annulus is often asymmetric and oval with annular diameters largest in the coronal plane and shortest in the sagittal plane, three-dimensional (3D) imaging is required.[53–55] Although, typically, multislice computed tomography (MSCT) is used for assessing average diameter, the perimeter or area of the annulus[56] may also be used. The 3D TEE has also been validated[57–59] and may be as accurate as MSCT for these measurements.[60,61]

It is important to understand the relationship between perimeter sizing and area sizing for TAVR and how this relates to the percent oversizing.[62] The percent oversizing is defined as ((THV nominal measurement/native annular measurement) −1) × 100. For a circular orifice, the percent area oversizing is two times the perimeter oversizing. However, in the setting of an oval annulus, area oversizing will be less than two times the perimeter oversizing. The current balloon-expandable valve uses area oversizing, whereas the current self-expanding valve uses perimeter oversizing. All current devices use systolic measurements, which tend to be the largest measurement during the cardiac cycle, with the lowest risk of undersizing the valve.[63] Advantages of the 3D TEE technique for preprocedural imaging include real-time imaging of the hinge-points of the cusps, and elimination of hand-tracing errors of direct planimetry. Nonetheless, 3D TEE techniques are still limited by ultrasound physics that create blooming and side-lobe artifacts as well as acoustic dropout. In addition, these techniques require expertise and practice. Advances in software packages are currently being developed and should automate many of the steps currently required to obtain 3D-derived measurements, and reduce interobserver variability of echocardiographic measurement of the aortic annulus. Two techniques have been used in

TABLE 32.1 Strengths and Weaknesses of Transthoracic Echocardiography Versus Transesophageal Echocardiography Imaging

PARAMETER	TTE	TEE
Sedation during TAVR	• None required (sedation for procedure only)	• General anesthesia, monitored anesthetic care or conscious sedation
Imaging advantages	• Standard windows for assessing ventricular and valvular structure and function	• Higher resolution with high frame rates for 2D and 3D imaging • Continuous imaging throughout procedure, irrespective of access route • Preprocedural imaging may avoid complications (i.e., paravalvular regurgitation, annular/aortic rupture, coronary occlusion) • Immediate intraprocedural diagnosis of complications
Imaging disadvantages	• Image quality dependent on patient factors (i.e., chest morphology, lung hyperinflation, suboptimal patient positioning) • Procedural delay during image acquisition (to minimize radiation exposure to imager) • Noncontinuous imaging during procedure • Low resolution with low frame rates for 2D and 3D imaging • Limited imaging windows for non-transfemoral access routes	• Special windows required for assessing ventricular and valvular structure and function • Image quality dependent on patient factors (i.e., calcific acoustic shadowing, cardiac position relative to esophagus and stomach) • Probe interference with fluoroscopic imaging (minimized by articulation of probe)
Other advantages	• Early recovery and discharge	• Need for postprocedure monitoring (Note: may not be different than for TTE)
Other disadvantages	• Possible higher radiation exposure to imager • Interference with sterile field	• Trauma to oropharynx, esophagus, or stomach

TAVR, Transcatheter aortic valve replacement; *TEE,* transesophageal echocardiography; *TTE,* transthoracic echocardiography.

the literature: direct planimetry of the short-axis (SAX) plane,[64] and indirect planimetry.[59] The steps for direct planimetry are outlined in Fig. 32.2. The steps for indirect planimetry are outlined in Fig. 32.3.

The aortic valve morphology has important implications for procedural success. The extent and distribution of calcium can impact procedural success and has been associated with excessive THV motion during deployment,[65] and PVR.[66–69] Bulky calcium increases the risk of calcific nodule displacement into the coronary ostia, annular rupture, root perforation, aortic wall hematoma, and aortic dissection (Fig. 32.4).[70–73] At this time, bicuspid aortic valve morphology is a relative contra-indication to TAVR. However, two reports of TAVR in a series of bicuspid aortic valve patients have shown that, compared to matched trileaflet aortic valve patients, there was no difference in acute procedural success, valve hemodynamics, or short-term survival.[74,75] Numerous case reports of THV

BOX 32.1 Preprocedural Structural and Functional Echocardiographic Imaging for Transcatheter Aortic Valve Replacement

Aortic Valve and Root
• Aortic valve morphology
  • Number of cusps (unicuspid, bicuspid, tricuspid)
  • Degree and location of calcium
  • Presence of commissural fusion
  • Planimetered valve area
• Annular dimensions
  • Minimum and maximum diameters
  • Perimeter
  • Area
• Aortic valve hemodynamics
  • Aortic valve peak velocity, peak and mean gradients, and calculated valve area
  • Dimensionless index
  • Stroke volume and stroke volume index
  • Impedance
• Left ventricular outflow tract
  • Extent and distribution of calcium
  • Presence of sigmoid septum and dynamic narrowing
• Aortic root dimensions and calcification
  • Sinus of Valsalva diameter and area
  • Sinotubular junction diameter, area, and calcification
  • Location of coronary ostia and risk of obstruction

Mitral Valve
• Severity of mitral regurgitation
• Presence of mitral stenosis
• Severity of ectopic calcification of the anterior leaflet

Left Ventricular Size and Function
  • Wall motion assessment
  • Exclude intracardiac thrombus
• Left ventricular mass
  • Hypertrophy and septal morphology
• Assessments of function
  • Ejection fraction
  • Strain and torsion
  • Diastolic function

Right Heart
• Right ventricular size and function
• Tricuspid valve morphology and function
• Estimate of pulmonary artery pressures

Adapted from Hahn RT, Little SH, Monaghan MJ, et al. Recommendations for comprehensive intraprocedural echocardiographic imaging during TAVR. *JACC Cardiovasc Imaging.* 2015;8(3):261–287.

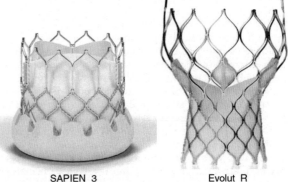

SAPIEN 3   Evolut R

FIG. 32.1 Commercially available transcatheter heart valve. In the United States, current commercially available transcatheter aortic valves are the balloon-expandable SAPIEN 3 and the self-expanding Evolut R. In the European Union, a larger array of valves have received the CE mark and are available for implantation. (*Courtesy of Edwards Lifesciences LLC, Irvine, CA; and Medtronic, Minneapolis, MN.*)

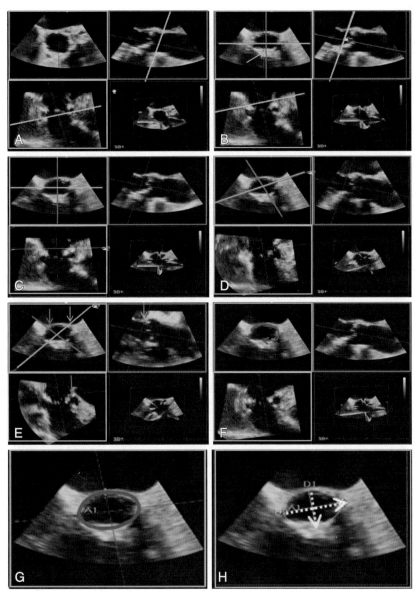

FIG. 32.2 Method of direct planimetry of the aortic annulus. The short-axis (SAX) or transverse view of the annulus is positioned in the green plane by aligning this plane in both the red (sagittal) and blue (coronal) long-axis (LAX) planes (A). The annulus is then confirmed by positioning the orthogonal LAX planes in the plane of each of the three hinge points of the leaflets. First, the right coronary cusp (B, *green arrow*) is imaged in the red plane by rotating this plane in the SAX view and the caudal/cranial position of the green plane adjusted to the level of the hinge point (C). Second, the orthogonal LAX planes are rotated from the SAX plane (D) to align with the left coronary cusp (*blue arrow*, D) and noncoronary cusp (*red arrow*); the caudal/cranial position of the SAX plane is again adjusted to align with the hinge points of these cusps. From the SAX view (F) the directly planimetered of the annulus is performed on the red plane (G) with coronal (H, *white arrow*) and sagittal dimensions (*yellow arrow*) determined for ellipticity. In this case, this results in an area of 531 mm² and circumference of 82 mm. If a balloon-expandable valve was being used, a #26 mm SAPIEN 3 valve would be appropriate.

implantations in patients with congenitally abnormal aortic valves[76–78] have limited the use of TAVR in this population because of reports of significant AR or suboptimal flow characteristics.[79,80] In the setting of stenosis and limited leaflet motion, a trileaflet valve can be determined by color flow Doppler (CFD) in all three commissures (Fig. 32.5A and Video 32.1) compared to a bicuspid valve with color Doppler in a single long commissure extending to the sinutubular junction (see Fig. 32.5B and Video 32.2).

Aortic root morphology is also important in preprocedural planning. The diastolic sinus of Valsalva diameter and height, the diastolic diameter of the sinutubular junction, and the systolic left main coronary artery ostium position may influence the size of THV selected as well as determine valve placement. The location of the coronary ostia is of primary importance since occlusion can lead to catastrophic left ventricular dysfunction. Complications associated with right coronary artery occlusion are significantly less frequent than with left coronary artery occlusion. A meta-analysis of 18 studies showed that coronary obstruction occurred

from displacement of the calcified left coronary cusp (and not typically from the stented THV) and the factors associated with coronary obstruction following TAVR include: female sex, small aortic root diameter (mean diameter = 27.8 ± 2.8 mm), and low-lying coronary artery (mean height = 10.3 ± 1.6 mm).[81] Although MSCT is often used for these measurements,[82,83] 3D TEE imaging compares favorably and allows rapid acquisition of the coronal plane for measurement of the systolic annulus-to-left main distance as well as the length of the left coronary cusp during the procedure (Fig. 32.6).[84]

INTRAPROCEDURAL IMAGING

For most of the procedure, four key standard imaging views are used for basic procedural guidance and postprocedural assessment (Fig. 32.7):
1. Midesophageal SAX view of the left ventricular outflow tract (LVOT), aortic valve, and aortic root with and left main coronary (multiplane angle of 30–60 degrees)

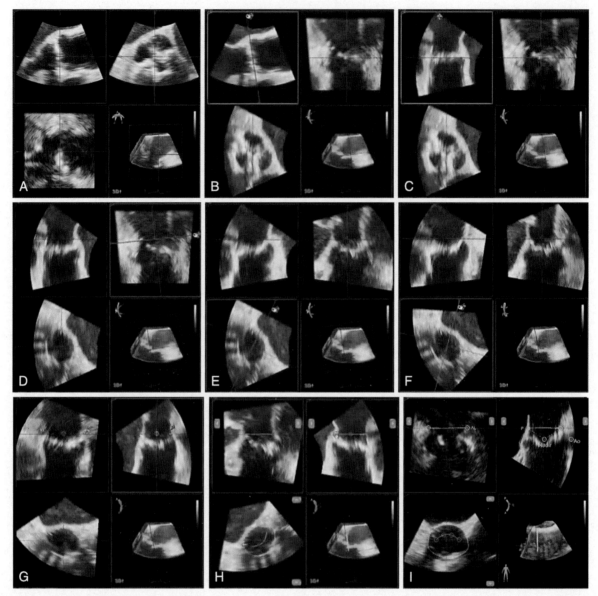

FIG. 32.3 Method of indirect planimetry of the aortic annulus. For the same patient as in Fig. 32.2, the indirect method of assessing the aortic annulus does not require direct planimetry of the annular short-axis (SAX), but rather uses points on the annulus chosen from the orthogonal long-axis (LAX) views, utilizing the program for the mitral valve annulus. A user-defined and nonsliced volume (A) is used to align the blue plane at the level of the annulus (B). The program automatically reorients the two LAX views as the green and the red planes with blue plane as the SAX view (C). Using the LAX views, the hinge points of the three aortic cusps are identified. First, the right coronary cusp (D, *green arrow*) is imaged in the green plane by rotating this plane in the SAX. Second, the orthogonal LAX planes are rotated from the SAX plane (E) to align with the left coronary cusp (*green arrow*) and noncoronary cusp (*red arrow*); fine adjustments are made (caudal/cranial position or rotation) on the blue plane within each LAX view to obtain the actual SAX (blue-plane) view. The annulus is then indirectly planimetered by finding sequential points on the two LAX views (G and H), resulting in an area of 597 mm^2 and a circumference of 88 mm (I). A #29 SAPIEN 3 valve would be appropriate, which is a size larger than predicted by the direct planimetry.

2. Midesophageal long axis (LVOT; multiplane angle of ~120–150 degrees)
3. Deep transgastric apical five-chamber view (multiplane angle 0–30 degrees) to image the aortic valve in long axis for hemodynamic assessment of the aortic valve (Video 32.3)
4. Transgastric (shallower than deep transgastric) long-axis view of the LVOT and aortic valve (multiplane angle 120–150 degrees) for hemodynamic assessment of the aortic valve (Video 32.4)

For intraprocedural imaging, a 3D-capable TEE machine is strongly recommended, but not required; simultaneous biplane imaging and live, narrow volume 3D may be the most useful modalities with rapid image acquisition and, in general, higher volume rates compared to other 3D modalities. If a preprocedural TEE was not performed, then a comprehensive TEE protocol is completed[85] with attention to the above measurements of the "landing zone."

Multiple reviews have recently been published describing the importance of imaging throughout the TAVR procedure.[42,86–88] A summary

of important imaging recommendations is listed in Table 32.2. A few caveats of imaging are discussed below.

Wire and Cannulation Position

Occasionally, the position of wires and cannulae must be confirmed. Following any wire placement into the heart, perforation and accumulation of pericardial effusion should be excluded. The right ventricular pacing wire tip is ideally in the right ventricular apex (Fig. 32.8A and Video 32.5). The position of the retrograde stiff wire within the left ventricle (LV) can also easily be assessed by echocardiography (see Fig. 32.8B and Video 32.6) with the curve of the J-wire ideally positioned at the apex of the ventricle. The transapical TAVR approach requires additional imaging. Because of the small apical window generated by the limited thoracotomy, imaging of the left ventricular apex from a midesophageal view is useful to ensure optimal location of the apical puncture (see Fig. 32.8C).

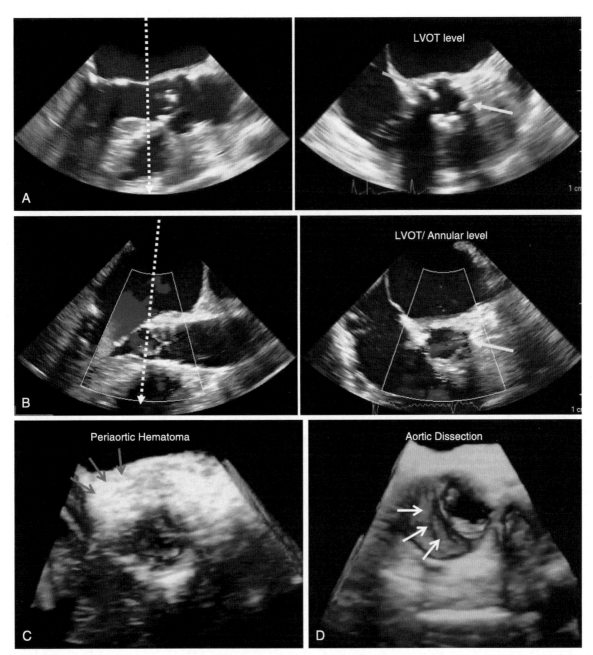

FIG. 32.4 Imaging during transcatheter aortic valve replacement. (A) Shows a simultaneous multiplane imaged of severe calcium within the left ventricular outflow tract (LVOT; *blue and yellow arrows*). (B) The same patient following transcatheter aortic valve replacement shows an annular rupture in short-axis *(yellow arrow)*. Bulky calcium increases the risk of calcific nodule displacement and root perforation resulting in peri-aortic hematoma (C, *red arrows*) or intimal disruption and aortic dissection (D, *white arrows*).

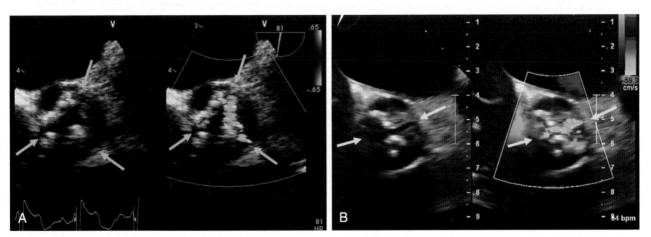

FIG. 32.5 Determining aortic valve morphology by color Doppler. These simultaneous multiplane images show how color Doppler can be used to distinguish a trileaflet valve (A) from a bicuspid valve (B). On two-dimensional (2D) imaging in systole, only two commissures are clearly imaged in (A) *(yellow and blue arrows)*; however, the associated color Doppler image shows flow in all three commissures *(blue arrows)*. In (B), only two commissures *(yellow arrows)* are seen on both 2D and color Doppler imaging.

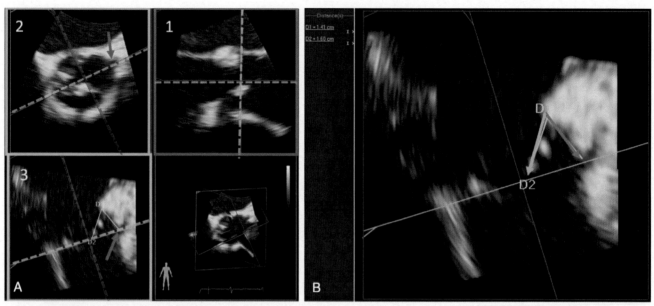

FIG. 32.6 Use of three-dimensional volumes to assess risk of coronary occlusion. (A) Using multiplanar reconstruction, the long axis (LAX) of the aorta is in the red plane *(1)*, the short-axis (SAX) image of the aortic root at the level of the left main coronary artery is imaged in the green plane *(2)*. From this SAX view, the blue plane is then rotated to bisect the left main coronary artery *(red arrow)*, which then comes into the LAX blue plane *(3, red arrow)*. (B) A zoom view of the blue panel showing the measurement of the height of the left main coronary *(red arrow)* and length of the left coronary cusp *(green arrow)*.

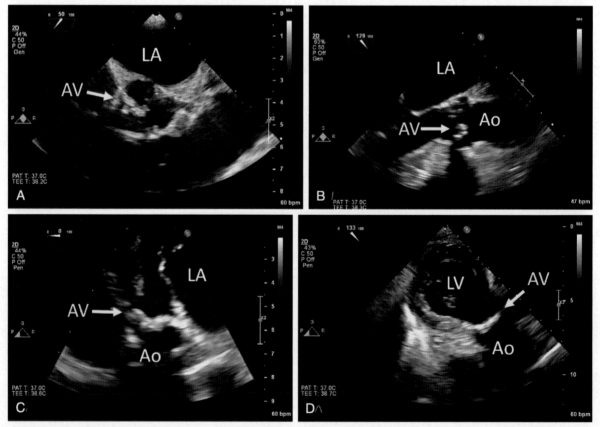

FIG. 32.7 Four key standard imaging views of the aortic valve. (A) The midesophageal short-axis (SAX) view of the aortic valve (multiplane angle of 30–60 degrees). From this view, slight retroflexion will image the left ventricular outflow tract (LVOT) and slight ante-flexion will image the left main coronary artery. (B) The midesophageal long-axis (LAX) view (multiplane angle of approximately 120–150 degrees). (C) The deep transgastric apical five-chamber view (multiplane angle 0–30 degrees) which aligns transaortic flow with the Doppler beam and allows hemodynamic assessment of the aortic valve. (D) A shallower transgastric LAX view of the LVOT and aortic valve (multiplane angle 120–150 degrees), which aligns transaortic flows that may be more anteriorly directed. *Ao,* Aorta; *AV,* aortic valve; *LA,* left atrium; *LV,* left ventricle.

TABLE 32.2 Summary of Intraprocedural Imaging Recommendations for Transcatheter Aortic Valve Replacement

PROCEDURAL STEP	IMAGING RECOMMENDATIONS
Pacing wire position	1. Confirm position in the right ventricle 2. Exclude perforation and pericardial effusion (pre- and postprocedure)
Stiff wire position	1. Imaging of wire: ensure stable position in the ventricle without entanglement in mitral apparatus/worsening mitral regurgitation 2. Exclude perforation and pericardial effusion
Balloon aortic valvuloplasty (BAV)	1. Image during and immediately following BAV for aortic leaflet motion and aortic regurgitation 2. Image the coronary arteries (particularly the left main) for obstruction by the calcified leaflets 3. Image the location of the displaced calcified leaflets for possible deformation of the aortic wall or risk for annular rupture

Positioning of transcatheter valve	1. Balloon-expandable valve:
	  a. SAPIEN XT: inflow (or proximal or ventricular) edge of the THV should be 5–6 mm below the annulus. Optimal final position is ~2 mm below the annulus and covers the native leaflets
	  b. SAPIEN 3: outflow (or distal or aortic) edge of the THV should cover the native leaflets while being below the sinotubular junction. Optimal final position covers the native leaflets
	2. Self-expanding valve:
	  a. CoreValve Classic: Edge of the proximal stent (posterior typically) should be 4–5 mm below the annulus. Optimal position is <10 mm below the annulus to avoid conduction disturbance
	  b. Evolut R: Edge of the proximal stent should be 2–5 mm below the annulus

Transapical cannulation	1. Confirm location of the transapical puncture site by imaging the apex (either from midesophageal views or transgastric views). Optimal position will avoid the right ventricle, and be angulated away from the interventricular septum

Postdeployment	1. Assess stent positioning, shape and leaflet motion; perform comprehensive hemodynamic measurements including effective orifice area
	  a. New LVOT diameter can be the outer-to-outer stent diameter at the inflow edge if well-positioned, or inner-to-inner stent diameter at the level of the leaflets if THV is too low
	  b. Match the velocity-time-integral for the location of the LVOT diameter measurement
	2. Assess paravalvular regurgitation relying on short-axis images of the LVOT just apical to the inflow edge of the THV to confirm jet reaches the ventricle (and gastric views for confirmation)
	3. Assess coronary artery patency and ventricular function; confirm ventricular size and function are similar to baseline or improved
	4. Assess mitral valve morphology and function
	5. Assess tricuspid regurgitation velocities and estimate pulmonary artery pressures
	6. Exclude perforation and pericardial effusion

LVOT, Left ventricular outflow tract; *THV*, transcatheter heart valve.
Adapted from Hahn RT, Little SH, Monaghan MJ, et al. Recommendations for comprehensive intraprocedural echocardiographic imaging during TAVR. JACC Cardiovasc Imaging. 2015;8(3):261–287.

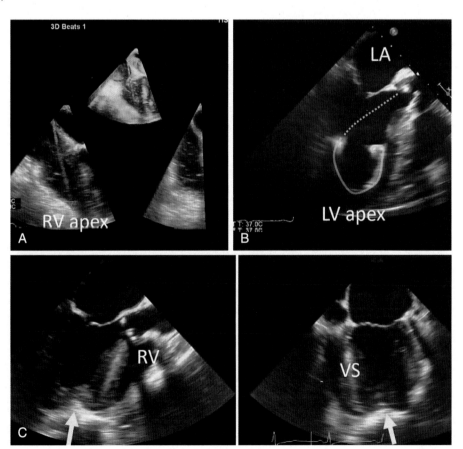

FIG. 32.8 Wire positioning and apical puncture site. The right ventricular pacing wire tip is ideally in the right ventricular (RV) apex (A, *red arrow*). The position of the retrograde stiff wire should be imaged with the curve of the J-wire ideally at the left ventricular (LV) apex of the ventricle (B, *blue line*). The intended transapical transcatheter aortic valve replacement apical puncture site is imaged by locating the surgeon's finger (C, *yellow arrows*) to ensure the site is clear of the RV and the ventricular septum (VS). *LA*, Left atrium.

Balloon Aortic Valvuloplasty

Balloon aortic valvuloplasty (BAV) prior to TAVR is used to increase cusp excursion and to ensure adequate cardiac output during THV positioning. Although some studies have suggested preimplant BAV is not required for the implantation of some valve types,[89] other THV types require BAV.[46] A recent study has suggested that BAV prior to implantation of a balloon-expandable valve[90] may reduce cerebral ischemic lesions. BAV can be used diagnostically for both the confirmation of annular sizing, and the prediction of calcium displacement (into the aorta, left main coronary or annular/subannular region) during final THV deployment.[91–93] Therefore, imaging during and following BAV is important to assess the functional results of the dilatation and possible adverse events.

Ventricular and Baseline Valvular Function

A qualitative assessment of mitral regurgitation (MR), tricuspid regurgitation, and biventricular function should be made prior to implantation. Changes in the severity of MR may indicate mechanical compromise of the mitral apparatus from stiff wires, the THV, left ventricular dysfunction (particularly following pacing), systolic anterior motion following the abrupt reduction in afterload that occurs with valve deployment, increases in blood pressure, or severe aortic regurgitation (AR). An acute reduction in left ventricular or right ventricular function may be a clue to coronary artery compromise during the procedure. Quantitation of right ventricular stroke volume is attempted in order to aid in the final assessment of AR.[94] Deep gastric views of the aortic valve are crucial, allowing accurate Doppler calculation of effective orifice area by continuity equation and assessment of the presence, location, and severity of AR.

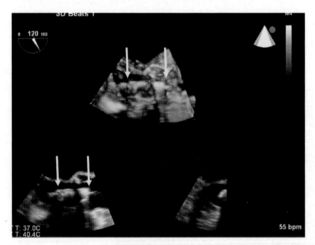

FIG. 32.9 Imaging the balloon-expandable valve. The long-axis view (top and lower left) is used to optimize imaging of the crimped stented valve (between yellow arrows) and supporting balloon catheter.

Transcatheter Valve Positioning

It is critically important to precisely position the THV in order to prevent complications, such as embolization, coronary obstruction, PVR, and pacemaker implantation. Although fluoroscopy plays a central role,[65] TEE, with its wide field of view, allows continuous imaging of not just the landing zone, but also of the ventricles and the mitral valve. TEE imaging can be used to confirm the THV location as well as the displacement of calcium during valve positioning, and may minimize the use of fluoroscopy and contrast.

For the third-generation balloon-expandable valve, precise positioning can be accomplished since the cell design of the stented valve results in foreshortening of the valve at the inflow portion of the valve with a stable position of the outflow portion of the valve throughout deployment. Thus echocardiographic positioning should focus on the long-axis view, optimizing the imaging of the entire stented valve and the supporting balloon catheter. In order to do this, small adjustments in image angulation or probe rotation should be used (Fig. 32.9 and Video 32.7). This distal (i.e., aortic or outflow) edge of the THV stent should cover the native leaflets but remain below the sinotubular junction during the pacing run. Although simultaneous multiplane imaging is not required, it can be useful on occasion to image the orthogonal SAX, focusing on previously identified high-risk regions. For instance, bulky calcified leaflets may threaten the aorta (Fig. 32.10A) or coronary ostia (see Fig. 32.10B), and early identification may help avoid a catastrophic complication.

For the second-generation, repositionable self-expanding valve, deployment is driven by fluoroscopic imaging. However, on occasion, simultaneous TEE imaging may diagnose an impingement of the mitral valve with resulting significant MR (Fig. 32.11A) or malpositioning that is poorly imaged by noncoaxial fluoroscopic views (see Fig. 32.11B).

POSTIMPLANTATION ASSESSMENT

A comprehensive evaluation of chamber and valvular morphology and function should be performed after TAVR. Table 32.3 summarizes the parameters that should be assessed. For hemodynamic evaluation of valve function, deep gastric views are imperative to align transaortic flow with the Doppler insonation beam (Fig. 32.12).

Paravalvular Regurgitation

Multiple studies have shown a higher incidence of PVR in the TAVR population compared to the surgical aortic valve replacement population, with moderate or severe PVR seen in 0%–24% of TAVR patients.[73,95–104] Studies also suggest that AR is an important predictor of mortality.[100,105–107] The varying incidence of this complication, as well as the differences in prognostic significance for various grades of PVR, are likely attributed not only to differences in imaging modalities, but also to the absence of a unified grading scheme.[94] A rapid assessment of PVR following TAVR is essential since this post-TAVR complication can be treated intraprocedurally with balloon dilatation, VIV salvage, or paravalvular

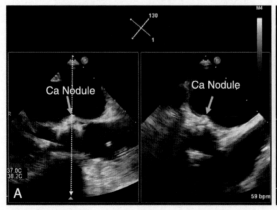
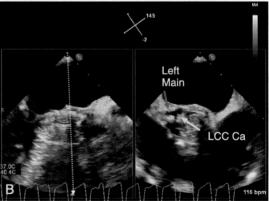

FIG. 32.10 Simultaneous multiplane imaging during deployment. Simultaneous multiplane imaging may be helpful for imaging high-risk regions during deployment. Bulky calcium (Ca) nodules may threaten the aorta (A, blue arrow) and when imaged, may warrant a slower balloon inflation. During balloon aortic valvuloplasty, when bulky calcium of the left coronary cusp (LCC) threatens to occlude the left main coronary ostia (B, red arrow), protecting the coronary artery may be warranted.

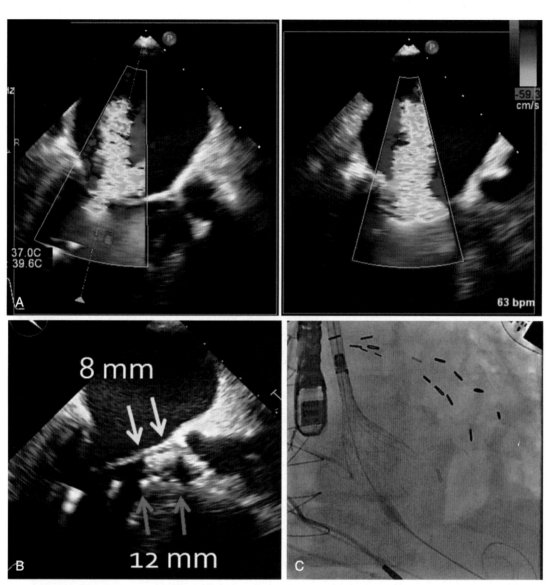

FIG. 32.11 Impingement of the mitral valve. Echocardiographic imaging during deployment of the self-expanding valve diagnosed impingement of the mitral valve with resulting significant mitral regurgitation (A) due to low positioning of the valve (B) (the THV distance below the annulus posteriorly *[yellow arrows]* and anteriorly *[red arrows]*), which was poorly imaged by a non-co-axial fluoroscopic view (C).

TABLE 32.3 Comprehensive Echocardiographic Assessment Following Transcatheter Aortic Valve Replacement

	CHAMBER	TRANSCATHETER VALVE
Structure	• Left ventricular dimensions and volume (systolic and diastolic), wall thickness, mass • Right ventricular dimensions (diastolic), wall thickness, function • Left atrial volume (biplane preferred over single plane) • Right atrial volume	• Position in relation to the annulus • Stability/motion of the transcatheter valve • Expansion/shape and regions of separation from the annulus • Leaflet appearance including leaflet thickness, calcification, or abnormal echodensities • Aortic annulus and root morphology and size
Function	• Ejection fraction • Global longitudinal strain	• Leaflet motion including an assessment of opening as well as closure
Hemodynamics	• Left ventricular stroke volume, stroke volume indexed to body surface area • Cardiac output and cardiac index • Left atrial filling pressure • Right atrial filling pressure • Pulmonary artery pressure	• Peak transaortic velocity • Peak and mean transaortic gradient • Aortic valve area • Regurgitant severity and location
Other	• Other concomitant valve disease • Left ventricular outflow tract obstruction	• Impingement or compromise of adjacent anatomic structures

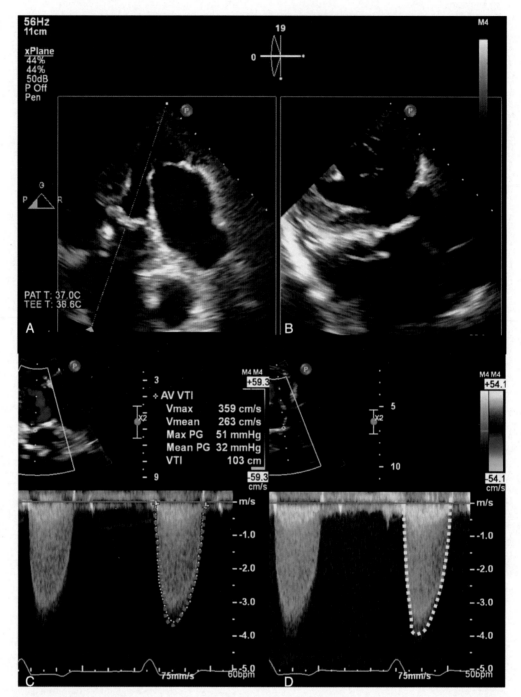

FIG. 32.12 Transgastric views of the aortic valve. For accurate hemodynamic evaluation of valve function, transgastric views are imperative to align transaortic flow with the Doppler insonation beam. In the simultaneous multiplane image shown, the 0- to 30-degree (A) Doppler is shown in C with peak velocity of 3.6 m/s. The orthogonal view (B), which aligns a more anteriorly directed transaortic jet results in a spectral profile with peak velocity of 4.0 m/s (D).

device implantation.[43,44] Although multiple modalities can be used to confirm severity, echocardiography remains a major modality that can determine location (central or paravalvular) and, thus, the need for and type of further intervention. Fortunately, with the newer iterations and types of THVs, this problem may become less significant.[45,108,109]

Because of multiple grading schemes used for grading AR using both numerical scales[110] and simple categories,[111] a more granular 5-class grading scheme has been suggested[94]: 0 = none or trace; 1 = mild; 2 = mild-to-moderate; 3 = moderate; 4 = moderate-to-severe; and 5 = severe. These five classes of grading can easily be collapsed into the 3-class scheme recommended by the American Society of Echocardiography (ASE)—European Association of Cardiovascular Imaging (EACVI) guidelines[111–113] as follows: mild in a 3-class scheme = class 1 plus class 2 of a 5-class scheme; moderate in a 3-class scheme = class 3 plus class 4 of a 5-class scheme;

and severe in a 3-class scheme = class 5 in a 5-class scheme. Unlike early reports of mortality associated with mild AR following TAVR,[114] more recent studies utilizing this grading scheme have shown that mild and mild-moderate regurgitation do not affect the outcome.[108]

There are a number of caveats to assessing PVR severity by echocardiography. First, while suboptimal stent shape and position may support Doppler findings of PVR, they lack sensitivity and specificity, particularly since valve design typically allows for a range of acceptable THV positions and shapes. Second, the use of ventricular size and remodeling as a clue to the severity of AR may not apply to this population with preexisting aortic stenosis and significant left ventricular hypertrophy. Third, the patient population of those preexisting severe, symptomatic aortic stenosis, as well as the atypical and irregular nature of the PVR jets, may limit the accuracy of qualitative, semiquantitative, and quantitative parameters

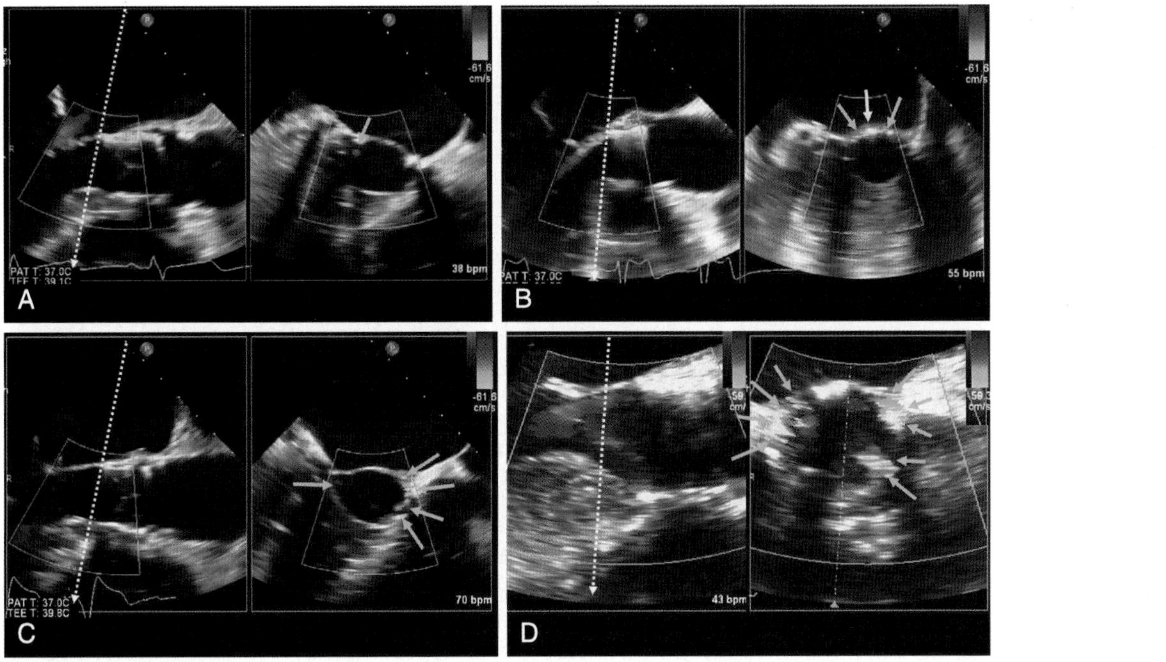

FIG. 32.13 Examples of grades of paravalvular regurgitation. The *blue arrows* point to paravalvular regurgitation (PVR) seen in the orthogonal short-axis views. (A) A trivial jet. (B) Mild PVR in the setting of focal calcium (*yellow arrow*) in the left ventricular outflow tract. (C) A moderate jet (<30% of the circumference). (D) Severe PVR with multiple jets with net circumferential extent of >30%.

used for native or surgical valve disease, and thus change the approach to grading severity. Also, there are imaging limitations that are similar to those encountered with surgical prostheses[111] with acoustic shadowing of the far field (anterior paravalvular region for TEE and posterior paravalvular region for TTE) requiring an extensive search for jets by the use of multiple imaging windows (parasternal, apical, and subcostal for TTE, midesophageal, transgastric, and deep transgastric for TEE) as well as subtle angulation/translation of the transducer within each window.

Note that reduced compliance of both the ventricle and aorta will influence pressure halftime, making this particular parameter less useful. Similar issues exist for flow reversal in the aorta, which can occur in the setting of aortic noncompliance and hypertension,[115,116] although true holodiastolic reversal may still be useful. Recent modeling has confirmed the limitation of using pressure halftime as a measure of regurgitant severity in this patient population, with shorter pressure halftime with both reduced LV and aortic compliance independent of aortic regurgitant severity.[117]

Although THV shape and position may be clues to PVR severity, CFD imaging is the primary method of assessment. CFD imaging of PVR relies heavily on a multiwindow, multilevel approach, first documenting that the suspected PVR jet actually extends beyond the skirt into the LVOT. It is important to scan from distal (aortic) to proximal (ventricular) ends of the THV to identify jet locations and direction. The use of simultaneous multiplane imaging allows a rapid assessment of multiple SAX levels, using the long-axis image as the guide. Central prosthetic AR jets will occur at the level of leaflet coaptation, whereas PVR will be seen at the proximal (ventricular) edge of the THV. For grading severity of PVR, the imaging plane, which visualizes the smallest jet area or width, representative of the vena contracta of the jet, must be assessed. Although this region is typically near the proximal region of the THV stent, ensuring that the visualized jet reaches the ventricle (and is not sealed by the THV skirt) requires visualization of the sub-THV region as well. Multiple imaging planes are used to assess the entire circumference at the level of the vena contracta(e). Imaging of color flow around the THV within the sinuses of Valsalva should not be mistaken for PVR, since the THV skirt at the lowest inflow (ventricular) edge of the stented valve may prevent flow in the sinuses from reaching the ventricle.

Decisions about acute intraprocedural treatment (postdilatation, VIV salvage or paravalvular leak closure device) are typically made by assessment of color Doppler imaging from multiple views. Although quantitation is not typically performed, a qualitative assessment of jet location(s), number,

and direction, as well as vena contracta(e) diameter or area, will allow a rapid decision to be made. Fig. 32.13 shows examples of various grades of PVR, with greater than mild regurgitation an indication for postdilatation in the absence of high-risk features. The high-risk features include bulky calcium that may occlude the left main or injure the aorta or aortic annulus, and hemodynamic issues that may be affected by a second pacing run. In addition, in the presence of severe calcification of the LVOT, the effectiveness of a postdilatation is reduced, and some paravalvular jets may be more appropriately treated with a closure device (Fig. 32.14A). Severe central regurgitation typically arises from malpositioning of the valve and can be treated with a second transcatheter valve (see Fig. 32.14B).

Other complications of TAVR have been extensively reviewed for both the balloon-expandable and self-expanding valves.[43,44] A summary of the types of complications that can be imaged are listed in Table 32.4.

TRANSCATHETER MITRAL VALVE REPAIR

The MitraClip device (Abbott Vascular Structural Heart, Menlo Park, California) was designed after the surgical edge-to-edge repair[118] was first introduced in the early 1990s as a method to rapidly treat complex mitral valve disease[118] and has gained widespread acceptance.[119–124] The MitraClip system uses a tri-axial catheter system with an implantable clip. The tapered and steerable guide catheter (GC) is delivered across the posterior-superior region of the interatrial septum with a tapered dilator. The distal end of the GC is easily imaged on both fluoroscopy and echocardiography. The Clip Delivery System (CDS) with the MitraClip attached to its distal end, is introduced through the GC. This CDS uses two dials that permit medial-lateral and anteroposterior steering. The MitraClip device (Fig. 32.15) is a 4-mm-wide metal implant (the current device is cobalt/chromium) with two polyester-covered arms that open to about 2 cm (7–8 mm on either side of a center post). Attached to the center post, and opposite the two arms, are two "grippers" that secure the leaflets as they are "captured" during closure of the arms. Once in position on the ventricular side of the mitral leaflets, each leaflet is independently secured between an arm and a gripper, and the two arms close in synchrony for leaflet capture. If one leaflet is not captured, both arms must be opened for recapture. The procedure is performed with the patient under general anesthesia, with the use of fluoroscopy and TEE and, on occasion, TTE guidance.

TEE is integral to the successful implantation of the MitraClip device: guiding catheter insertion, clip delivery, and positioning, the grasping of leaflet tissue, and the determining of procedural success.[125,126] The 3D TEE

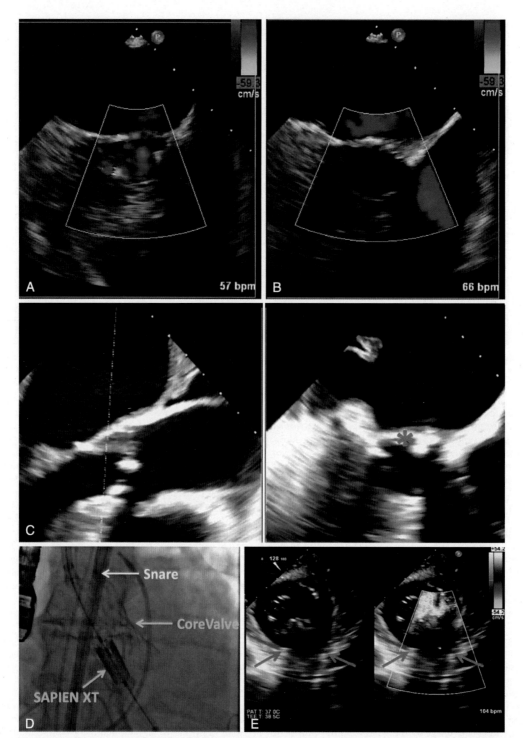

FIG. 32.14 Intraprocedural management of significant paravalvular regurgitation. Three methods of managing significant paravalvular regurgitation (PVR) include postdilatation, closure device, or valve-in-valve (VIV). (A) The baseline short-axis view following transcatheter aortic valve replacement (TAVR). (B) The same patient following a postdilatation with trivial residual PVR. (C) A simultaneous biplane image of a patient whose significant left ventricular outflow tract calcium was high risk for annular rupture. A vascular plug was placed at the location of the *red asterisk* following TAVR. (D) The fluoroscopic image of a patient who required a VIV procedure for severe PVR following a CoreValve *(orange arrow)*. The valve was snared *(yellow arrow)* and then secured in a more aortic position using a balloon expandable valve *(blue arrow)*. (E) is a transgastric color-compare image with no residual aortic regurgitation following the balloon-expandable valve implantation *(red arrows)*.

may further improve procedural success and shorten procedure time.[126–128] Compared to 2D TEE, 3D TEE has been reported to be advantageous in 9 of 11 steps of the percutaneous mitral repair procedure, including: optimizing the transseptal puncture site, guiding the CDS, precise positioning of the CDS simultaneously in anterior–posterior and lateral-medial directions, determining valvular regurgitation jet position, adjusting and visualizing the clip position relative to the valvular orifice, and assessing the remaining regurgitant jets.[128] Following MitraClip, the assessment of residual regurgitation also can be assessed by 3D color Doppler.[129] A greater

than 50% reduction in regurgitant volume using the product of vena contracta areas defined by direct planimetry of real-time 3D color Doppler and velocity time integral using continuous-wave Doppler, has been reported to be associated with greater left atrial and ventricular remodeling.

PREPROCEDURAL IMAGING

Understanding the anatomy of the mitral valve, ventricles, and atria is key to a successful MitraClip procedure. The important elements of

TABLE 32.4 Complications of Transcatheter Aortic Valve Replacement

COMPLICATION	TRANSESOPHAGEAL ECHO ASSESSMENT
Hemodynamic Instability	
Severe transvalvular or paravalvular aortic regurgitation	• Assess location of regurgitation (central vs. paravalvular) • Assess position of the transcatheter valve • Assess severity of aortic regurgitation
Severe mitral regurgitation	• Evaluate severity of mitral regurgitation and anatomy of the mitral apparatus: look for valvular perforation, ruptured chordae, tethering of the leaflets
Pericardial effusion	• Assess for tamponade physiology and possible etiology (i.e., chamber perforation, aortic dissection)
Ventricular dysfunction	• Evaluate for regional or global wall motion abnormalities of the LV or RV • Identify the coronary ostium; use color flow Doppler to assess blood flow
Aortic rupture or dissection	• Examine the aortic root/ascending aorta for peri-aortic hematoma, aortic dissection, or rupture • Assess for pericardial effusion/tamponade
Major bleeding	• Assess ventricular size and function (wall collapse due to hypovolemia)
Other Procedural Complications	
Balloon aortic valvuloplasty complication	• Assess severity of aortic regurgitation • Examine the aortic root/ascending aorta for peri-aortic hematoma, aortic dissection, or rupture • Identify the left main ostium; use color flow Doppler to assess blood flow
Mal-positioning of the transcatheter heart valve	• Too high or too low within the annulus with resulting hemodynamic instability: rapid deployment of a second valve can be performed • Embolization of the valve (into the LV or into the aorta) may require surgical intervention
Fistula	• Ventricular septal defect • Aorto-cameral fistula (typically into the right ventricular outflow tract or right atrium)

LV, Left ventricle; *RV*, right ventricle.
From Hahn RT, Little SH, Monaghan MJ, et al. Recommendations for comprehensive intraprocedural echocardiographic imaging during TAVR. JACC Cardiovasc Imaging. 2015;8(3):261–287.

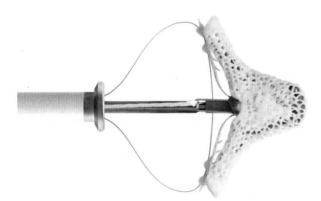

FIG. 32.15 MitraClip device. The MitraClip device is a 4-mm-wide metal (current device is cobalt/chromium) implant with two polyester-covered arms that open to about 2 cm (7–8 mm on either side of a center post). (Courtesy of Abbott, Abbott Park, IL.)

BOX 32.2 Preprocedural Assessment for the MitraClip Procedure

Mitral Valve Assessment
• Morphology/etiology (primary or secondary mitral regurgitation)
• Severity and location of mitral regurgitation: both qualitative and quantitative assessment essential
• Mitral valve area by planimetry
• Peak and mean transmitral gradient
• Assessment of the grasping region

Left Ventricular Size and Function
• Left ventricular volumes (diastolic and systolic)
• Assessments of function
    • Ejection fraction
    • Strain and torsion

Atrial Morphology
• Left atrial size/length of the interatrial septum
• Exclude congenital atrial septal defect
• Exclude left atrial thrombus
• Interatrial septum morphology and ideal site of transseptal puncture

Right Heart
• Right ventricular size and function
• Tricuspid valve morphology and function
• Estimate of pulmonary artery pressures

the preprocedural assessment for the MitraClip procedure are listed in Box 32.2. For the initial investigational MitraClip trials, degenerative (or primary) as well as functional (or secondary) mitral regurgitant etiologies were included. The key anatomic inclusion criteria for entry into the randomized trials[120,130] included a regurgitant jet origin associated with the A2 to P2 segments of the mitral valve and, for patients with functional MR, a coaptation length of at least 2 mm and a coaptation depth of no more than 11 mm; and for patients with leaflet flail, a flail gap less than 10 mm and a flail width less than 15 mm.[12] In addition, the mitral valve area by planimetry should be greater than 4.0 cm², and the leaflet length at the grasping site should be greater than 7 mm and relatively free of thickening or calcium. With additional experience with the device and the adoption of 3D TEE guidance, there are a number of other anatomic abnormalities of the mitral valve that can be successfully treated with this device.[88]

INTRAPROCEDURAL GUIDANCE

3D echocardiography has dramatically changed the accuracy of catheter and clip positioning for this procedure, allowing operators to place clips in both typical[131] and atypical positions.[122,124] 2D imaging, frequently derived from 3D simultaneous multiplane imaging, as well as user-defined 3D rendering of the mitral valve (from en-face, surgically correct views), are the primary imaging modalities for this procedure. Coregistration of TEE and fluoroscopic images may further enhance the ease and accuracy of the procedure.[132] A summary of the intraprocedural imaging steps is shown in Table 32.5.

The majority of procedural guidance utilizes four key standard TEE views (Fig. 32.16):
1. Midesophageal bicaval view (multiplane angle of ~60–90 degrees) at the base of the heart is typically used to perform transseptal catheterization and image GC, and initial CDS position and clip introduction. Using simultaneous multiplane imaging may allow measurement of the height of the puncture above the annular plane, depending on patient anatomy.
2. Midesophageal commissural view (multiplane angle of ~60 degrees) is used for medial-lateral and axial adjustments of the system. This view must be centered on the A2 scallop; simultaneous multiplane

TABLE 32.5 Summary of Intraprocedural Imaging Recommendations for MitraClip

PROCEDURAL STEP	IMAGING RECOMMENDATIONS

Transseptal puncture	1. Locate the position and direction of transseptal catheter puncture
	  a. Optimal height is ~3.5–4.0 cm above the mitral annular plane
	  b. Optimal position is the superior, posterior quadrant of the fossa ovalis
	2. Avoid punctures too anterior/superior (adjacent to the aorta)
	3. Avoid punctures too posterior/superior (into the right pulmonary vein and oblique sinus)

Advancing the guide catheter and clip delivery system	1. Position the MitraClip guiding catheter so that the tip (double-echodensity) is across the interatrial septum 2. Continuously image the guide catheter as the delivery catheter system (with clip) is introduced into the left atrium. The catheter should avoid contact with lateral structures in the left atrium. 3. Guide the manipulation of the steering mechanisms to position the clip above the A2–P2 scallops (or primary regurgitant jet)

Positioning and orienting the MitraClip	1. Based on the preprocedural anatomic imaging (TEE) of the mitral valve, the clip is positioned over the regurgitant orifice
	2. The clip arms are partially opened to determine orientation and position
	3. Guide the orientation/rotation of the clip arms to be perpendicular to the leaflets at the site of the regurgitant orifice
	  a. Note: although typically the clip is perpendicular to the commissures, maximum reduction in regurgitant volume may require an off-axis orientation of the clip
	  b. Use color Doppler to confirm positioning above the regurgitant jet
	4. Check the trajectory of the clip when crossing the annular plane (typically with a closed clip)

Grasping the mitral leaflets	1. Follow the open clip across the mitral orifice into the left ventricle 2. Once the clip arms are opened within the left ventricle, document the orientation of the clip adjusting the clip and guide if needed 3. Continuously image the two clip arms as the interventionalist withdraws the clip (toward the leaflets) and grasps both anterior and posterior leaflets with the device grippers 4. Verify capture of both leaflets prior to full closure of the clip using multiplane 2D imaging or real-time 3D imaging a. Release and recapture may be necessary if confirmation of capture cannot be made 5. With incremental closure of the clip verify mitral regurgitation reduction

Prerelease assessment	1. Assess MitraClip positioning and stability
	2. Assess residual mitral regurgitation
	  a. Qualitative grading (including vena contracta of regurgitant jet, systolic reversal of flow in pulmonary veins)
	  b. Quantitative grading of regurgitant volume, regurgitant orifice area and regurgitant fraction (using 3D color Doppler or other quantitative methods)
	3. Assess mitral valve area
	  a. Peak and mean transmitral gradients
	  b. Planimetered area of new orifice(s)

Postdeployment assessment	1. Assess final MitraClip positioning and stability
	2. Assess residual mitral regurgitation
	  a. Qualitative grading (including systolic reversal of flow in pulmonary veins)
	  b. Quantitative grading of regurgitant volume, regurgitant orifice area, and regurgitant fraction
	3. Assess final mitral valve area
	  a. Peak and mean transmitral gradients
	  b. Planimetered area of new orifice(s)
	4. Assess need for another MitraClip
	  a. If a second clip is needed, the steps above are repeated with the exception of crossing the annular plane with a closed clip
	5. Assess ventricular function; confirm ventricular size and function are similar to baseline or improved.
	6. Assess interatrial septum: size and direction of shunt
	7. Assess tricuspid regurgitation velocities and estimate pulmonary artery pressures
	8. Exclude perforation and pericardial effusion

TEE, Transesophageal echocardiography.

orthogonal view should be the long-axis view. The midesophageal probe position is also ideal for Doppler assessment of regurgitation and transmitral gradients.

3. Midesophageal long axis (LVOT; multiplane angle of ~120–150 degrees) is used for anterior–posterior system adjustments and imaging of leaflet capture.

4. 3D volume of the mitral valve (from any midesophageal view) is used for alignment of the clip arms perpendicular to the line of coaptation, and positioning of the clip at the site of regurgitation. This modality is also used to directly planimeter the mitral valve orifice as well as the color Doppler regurgitant vena contracta(e) at baseline and following device placement.

Because of 3D TEE, transgastric SAX views are rarely utilized, although deep gastric views may still be useful for quantifying forward stroke volume (across the LVOT), which may significantly increase following a successful MitraClip, and assessing the severity of the interatrial shunt (Qp/Qs) following removal of the transseptal catheters.

Prior to the procedure, a Heart Team discussion should consider the location of the regurgitation, the anatomy of the leaflets in and around

this region, the ideal location for the transseptal puncture, the proposed number of clips, and the criteria for terminating the procedure. A full baseline TEE should be performed, paying particular attention to:

1. Qualitative parameters of regurgitant severity (i.e., reversal of flow in the pulmonary veins)

2. Quantification of mitral regurgitation (effective regurgitation orifice area and regurgitation volume) with particular attention to the 3D quantification

3. Mitral valve area by planimetry; pressure halftime and continuity equations are inaccurate in the setting of severe mitral regurgitation. Early studies showed that the mitral valve area is reduced by 40%–50% with a single clip.[133]

4. Peak and mean transmitral gradients.

Transseptal Puncture

The transseptal puncture is typically guided equally by fluoroscopy and echocardiography. The position of this puncture is ideally in the superior/posterior fossa ovalis, and some caveats are worth noting

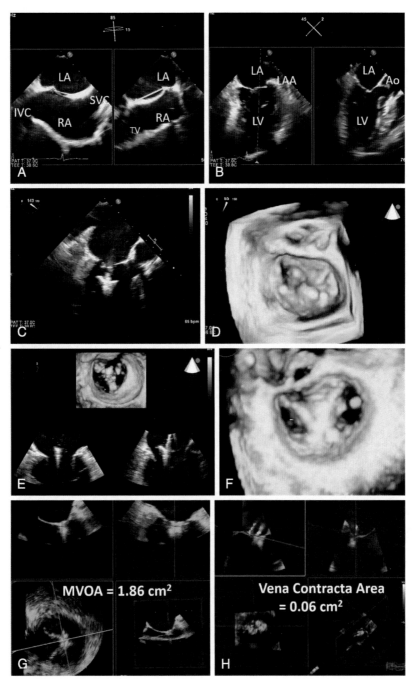

FIG. 32.16 MitraClip procedural guidance. The majority of procedural guidance utilizes four key standard transesophageal echocardiography views: midesophageal bicaval view (multiplane angle of ~60–90 degrees) (A) is typically used to perform the transseptal puncture. Using simultaneous multiplane imaging may allow measurement of the height of the puncture above the annular plane *(yellow arrow)* depending on patient anatomy. The midesophageal commissural view (multiplane angle of ~60 degrees) is used for medial-lateral and axial adjustments of the MitraClip (B), and the simultaneous multiplane orthogonal view should be the long-axis view, which is used for anterior–posterior adjustments. A single-plane midesophageal left ventricular outflow tract view (C, multiplane angle of ~120–150 degrees) may be used for leaflet capture (C) because of the greater resolution. Three-dimensional volumes of the mitral valve (from any midesophageal view) are used for imaging native anatomy and preprocedural planning (D), alignment of the clip arms perpendicular to the line of coaptation or jet, and the positioning of the clip at the site of regurgitation (E). A user-defined volume at the end of the study (F) is also used to directly planimeter the mitral valve orifice (G) and a 3D color Doppler regurgitant vena contracta (H). *Ao,* Aorta; *IVC,* inferior vena cava; *LA,* left atrium; *LAA,* left atrial appendage; *LV,* left ventricle; *MVOA,* mitral valve orifice area; *RA,* right atrium; *SVC,* superior vena cava; *TV,* tricuspid valve.

(Fig. 32.17). First, the typical transseptal puncture in the anterior/superior portion of the fossa ovalis or crossing a patent foramen ovale should be avoided. Being too anterior or creating an anterior trajectory by the "flap" of the primum septum will make positioning of the clip at the line of coaptation more difficult, and will create an angle of the clip arms that may reduce the chances of adequate bileaflet capture. Second, the CDS requires enough (but not too much) height above leaflet coaptation, ideally 4 cm. This means that for functional MR, where the coaptation of the leaflets is apical to the annulus, the

transseptal puncture may be lower in relation to the annulus. For degenerative mitral regurgitation in the setting of a flail or myxomatous valve, where coaptation is within the left atrium, a transseptal puncture may need to be higher relative to the annulus. Finally, small left atria, which can be seen with acute degenerative regurgitation, may limit the height that can be achieved, and care should be taken to avoid puncturing near the inflow of the right pulmonary veins. In this region there is no interatrial septum, but rather, pericardial reflection and the oblique sinus around the base of the veins that abut

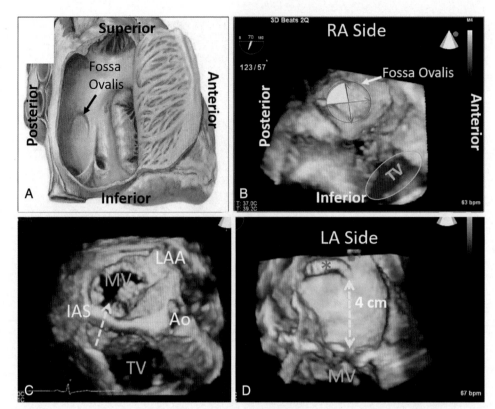

FIG. 32.17 Transseptal puncture. The position of the transseptal puncture is ideally in the superior, posterior fossa ovalis. (A) A drawing of the right atrial (RA) side of the interatrial septum (IAS) with the fossa ovalis near the center. (B) A 3D volume also from the RA side with the superior, posterior quadrant (*yellow triangle*) marked. (C) Looking from the roof of the atria down on the mitral valve (MV) and tricuspid valve (TV), the IAS is well imaged with the ideal posterior puncture site (*yellow dashed arrow*). (D) A 3D volume of the left atrial side of the IAS with a guide catheter (*red ** **) in the correct superior position, 4 cm above the mitral annulus. *Ao*, Aorta; *LA*, left atrium; *LAA*, left atrial appendage.

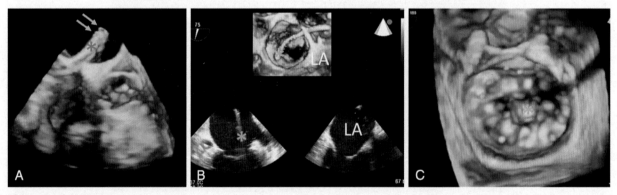

FIG. 32.18 Positioning the MitraClip. The steerable guide catheter (*red ** **) is positioned with the tip 1–2 cm across the interatrial septum (A). The tip of the guide catheter is easily imaged on both fluoroscopy and echocardiography as a double ring (*blue arrows*). The Clip Delivery System (CDS) is introduced into the guide catheter, and the MitraClip (*green ** **) is advanced into the left atrium (B), making sure to image the adjacent atrial structures to avoid injury and perforation. Using en-face 3D surgical views of the mitral valve (C) the CDS (*blue ** **) is positioned above the coaptation line of the leaflets and approximately at the location of the regurgitant jet. *LA*, Left atrium.

the dome of the right atrium. If perforation of the right atrium/right pulmonary vein is not recognized prior to introduction of the large guide delivery catheter, a significant pericardial effusion may result, which sometimes may require surgical correction.

Advancing the Guide Catheter and Clip Delivery System

After transseptal puncture, the steerable GC is positioned with the tip 1–2 cm across the interatrial septum (Fig. 32.18A). The tip of the GC is easily imaged on both fluoroscopy and echocardiography as a double ring. The CDS is introduced into the GC, and the MitraClip device is advanced into the left atrium, making sure to image the adjacent atrial structures to avoid injury and perforation (see Fig. 32.18B). Using en-face 3D surgical

views of the mitral valve, the CDS is positioned above the coaptation line of the leaflets and approximately at the location of the regurgitant jet (see Fig. 32.18C).

Positioning and Orienting the MitraClip

The clip arms are open, and using echocardiographic and fluoroscopic guidance, the clip is steered and reoriented until centered and axially aligned over the origin of the regurgitant jet (Fig. 32.19A and B). This may require frequent interchanging of 2D and 3D views (with and without color Doppler). Given the steering capabilities of the CDS, atypical clip orientations and positions may be achieved, allowing for treatment of a wide variety of anatomies with this device. Determining the trajectory of the device in both the medial-lateral and anteroposterior dimensions

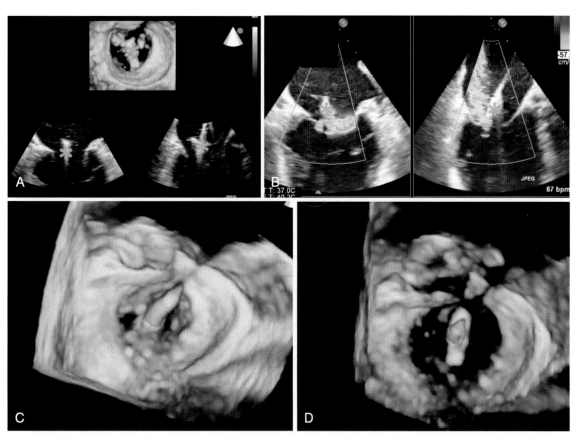

FIG. 32.19 **Orienting the MitraClip.** The clip arms are open (A) and using echocardiographic and fluoroscopic guidance, the clip *(green asterisk)* is steered and reoriented until centered, and axially aligned over the origin of the regurgitant jet (B). The clip arms are then reopened and the clip advanced into the left ventricle (LV) below the mitral leaflets; reducing the gain (C) will eliminate the thin mitral leaflets to reveal the orientation of the clip arms below the leaflets. *LA,* Left atrium.

is typically performed from a simultaneous biplane image of the commissural and LAX views, with a closed clip. For the first clip, the two arms are then re-opened, and the clip is advanced into the LV below the mitral leaflets (see Fig. 32.19C and Videos 32.8 and 32.9).

Grasping the Mitral Leaflets

Clip advancement across the mitral annulus is continuously imaged to avoid contact with lateral structures, particularly the chordal apparatus. The position and rotation of the clip is confirmed since advancing the clip into the LV frequently changes the orientation. To image leaflet grasp, the LAX view, which images symmetric open "V"-shaped clip arms, is acquired (Fig. 32.20A). This may require small adjustments in rotation of the probe and multiplane angles. If multiplane imaging is not of sufficient resolution (lateral, axis, or temporal), then simple 2D (single-plane) images can be used. From this view, the clip is retracted until both leaflets are grasped and then closed to capture the mitral leaflets. Leaflet insertion into the clip and MR reduction are assessed by the use of 2D and Doppler echocardiography (see Fig. 32.20B). Confirmation of leaflet grasp must be made from multiple views in addition to the grasping LAX view (see Fig. 32.20C). Simultaneous multiplane imaging from the commissural view allows orthogonal imaging to either side of the 4-mm-wide clip and ensures enough leaflet length has been captured to assure clip stability (see Fig. 32.20D). If necessary, the clip can be reopened and the leaflets released and then repositioned. If the clip must be withdrawn into the left atrium, the arms may be inverted in the ventricle, providing a smooth device profile for retraction to prevent entangling the chordae tendineae. Importantly, echocardiography can frequently image chordal entanglement, and this should be relayed to the interventionalist to avoid chordal rupture.

Prerelease Assessment

Prior to clip release, echocardiography must be used to quantify residual regurgitation and planimeter the double orifice (usually by 3D methods;

see Fig. 32.16G and H), and assess the mean gradient. Importantly, the mean gradient across either orifice should be the same, reflecting the flow across summed orifice area. On-axis imaging (flow parallel to the insonation beam) is essential for an accurate assessment of gradient, with off-axis Doppler imaging the most common reason for a difference in mean gradients across the two orifices. Typically, the densest spectral profile with the highest gradient is the most accurate. If the planimetered valve area is less than 2.0 cm^2, and/or the mean gradient under physiologic conditions is greater than 6 mm Hg, an individualized decision of whether to reposition or remove the clip should be made. Small or inactive patients may tolerate smaller valve areas or higher resting gradients. After adequate reduction of MR has been achieved and confirmed under hemodynamic challenge, the clip is deployed, and the CDS and GC are withdrawn. If a second MitraClip is required, the same procedures are repeated, except the clip is advanced into the LV in the closed position. As a general rule, inverting and withdrawing a second clip is discouraged because of the significant risk of native valve apparatus injury.

Post-MitraClip Assessment

After clip release, echocardiography must confirm the stability of the device, and quantify the procedural results: residual regurgitation, orifice area, and mean gradients. Quantifying the orifice area is typically performed by planimetry of the double orifice. Although deep gastric views were used in the past, 3D quantitation improves the accuracy of the measurement and is now the standard. In addition, qualitative assessment of regurgitation also should be performed (i.e., pulmonary vein systolic reversal). Documentation of the following is also essential: change in ventricular size/function, the presence of a new or change in pericardial effusion, and the size of the residual interatrial shunt following catheter removal. The latter assessment may be important for predicting outcomes, since some studies suggest that a residual atrial septal defect, occurring in approximately 50% of cases, is associated with worse outcomes.[134]

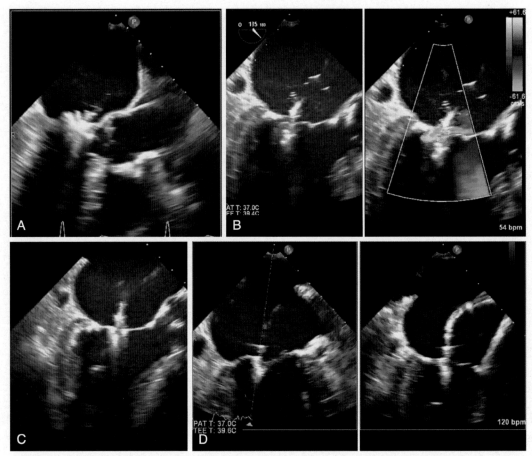

FIG. 32.20 **Leaflet grasp.** The long-axis (LAX) view is used to image leaflet grasp with the "v"-shaped clip arms clearly imaged (A). To improve frame rates, a single-plane 2D image (B) can be used. Leaflet insertion into the clip and mitral regurgitation reduction are assessed by the use of 2D and Doppler echocardiography. Confirmation of leaflet grasp must be made from multiple views in addition to the grasping LAX view (C). Simultaneous multiplane imaging from the commissural view, allows orthogonal imaging to either side of the 4-mm-wide clip, and ensures enough leaflet length has been captured to assure clip stability (D).

Quantitative assessment of postclip residual MR is significantly more difficult with echocardiography, compared to native valve disease, with multiple eccentric jets, flow acceleration from the reduced valve area, and artifact from the clips. Cardiovascular magnetic resonance (CMR) imaging can accurately and reproducibly quantify left and right ventricular volumes, which, in combination with phase-contrast flow imaging, can quantify mitral regurgitant fraction.[135] Although the proximal isovelocity surface area method should be avoided because of flow interference by the MitraClip, calculating relative stroke volumes using 2D LV biplane volumes and LVOT stroke volume has been reported to allow an assessment of regurgitant volume and regurgitant fraction.[135] These same authors also quantified the transmitral stroke volume by standard methods as recommended by the ASE.[136] Although there was significant variability in these measurements, regurgitant fractions by Doppler quantification had substantially improved reproducibility over expert readers' subjective assessment, which underlines the importance of quantitative metrics over-and-above visual qualitative analysis.

OTHER TRANSCATHETER MITRAL VALVE REPAIR DEVICES AND TRANSCATHETER MITRAL VALVE REPLACEMENT

A number of other transcatheter mitral valve repair devices have been or are now being evaluated for a CE mark in Europe. These include the CARILLON Mitral Contour System (Cardiac Dimensions, Inc., Kirkland, Washington), the Cardioband System (Valtech Cardio Ltd., Or Yehuda, Israel), Mitralign Percutaneous Annuloplasty System (Mitralign, Tewksbury, Massachusetts), NeoChord System (NeoChord, Inc., Eden Prairie, Minnesota), and the Arto System (MVRx, Inc., Belmont, California). All these devices have specific imaging needs, but share the use of TEE as the primary imaging modality. Imaging protocols are also under development.

Although implantation of the aortic transcatheter device into native calcific, degenerative, mitral stenosis has been reported,[137] valve-specific TMVR has been proposed as a viable solution to significant mitral regurgitation in high-risk patients.[17,19,138,139] Although preprocedural imaging with computed tomography gives precise information about mitral valve, annular, and subannular anatomy, intraprocedural imaging with primarily TEE and occasionally intracardiac echocardiography (ICE) has significant advantages of continuous, uninterrupted imaging of high quality and reproducibility. The intraprocedural echocardiographic protocols for these devices are currently being developed and cannot be discussed in detail at this time. However, a few considerations may give the imager some perspective on this developing field.

The basic anatomy of the transmitral devices is similar; a stented frame holds the bioprosthetic leaflets, with an atrial stabilizer and an anchoring mechanism. Some anchoring mechanisms use the native annulus, others the native leaflets, and still others, a left ventricular apical tethering device. The access for the majority of devices is currently transapical; however, transfemoral venous approaches are being investigated, and this solution will likely be the access of choice in the future.

TMVR devices require proper sizing of the mitral annulus as well as a detailed characterization of the landing zone, including the morphology of the leaflets; adjacent basal left atrium and annulus; subannular and subvalvular apparatus; and the surrounding ventricle (particularly the LVOT). Although the dynamic nature of the annulus changes with the valve and ventricular pathology, annular dimensions should be assessed at multiple time points throughout the cardiac cycle (e.g., end systole and end diastole). Excessive mitral annular calcification or subvalvular calcification that could interfere with proper seating and sealing of the device may be contraindicated for TMVR. Specific devices designed for implantation into severe degenerative mitral annular calcification are also under development.

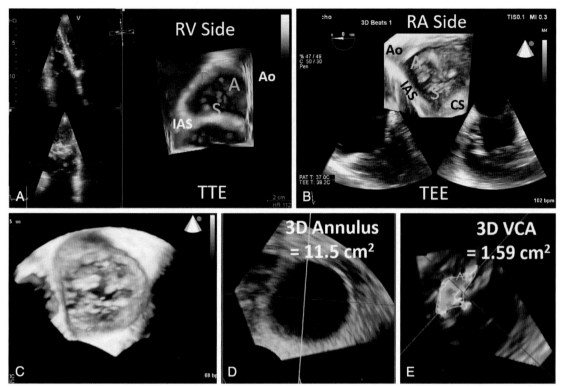

FIG. 32.21 Three-dimensional tricuspid valve imaging. Imaging of the tricuspid valve can be performed on transthoracic imaging (TTE) in A, with the right ventricular (RV) side of the leaflets oriented with the septal leaflet (*blue S*) in the far field and the anterior leaflet (*green A*) to the right and posterior leaflet (*red P*) to the left. (B) Transesophageal (TEE) imaging of the tricuspid valve is ideal for imaging the tricuspid valve from the right atrial (RA) side. Using the three-dimensional (3D) user-defined TEE volume (C), the annular area (D), and 3D color Doppler planimetry (E) of the vena contract area (VCA) can help quantify the tricuspid valve complex. *Ao,* Aorta; *CS,* coronary sinus; *IAS,* interatrial septum.

One of the major concerns of TMVR is LVOT obstruction. In contrast to surgical bioprosthetic mitral valves, the native leaflets are intact following TMVR. Thus, the anterior leaflet has the potential to create either a dynamic or fixed obstruction of the LVOT. In addition, if the THV stent struts are covered by synthetic material,[16,17,19] the device itself may protrude into the LV cavity and encroach upon the LVOT. Finally, the relative angle of the LVOT and mitral annulus, as well as the size and dynamism of the septal myocardium, will influence the development of LVOT obstruction. In this context, LVOT obstruction actually refers to creation of a small-sized neo-LVOT rather than obstruction of the native LVOT.[140]

Thus, intraprocedural imaging for TMVR will likely involve a number of steps:
1. Preprocedural confirming of "landing zone" morphology (including LVOT)
2. Guiding access (transapical or transseptal; Note: direct atrial access may also be an option)
3. Guiding positioning of the valve within the annulus (particularly for noncircular designs)
4. Ensuring the anchoring device is functioning properly
5. Ensuring the absence of interaction with adjacent cardiac structures
6. Imaging of deployment
7. Assessing postdeployment valve function and/or complications.

TRICUSPID REPAIR DEVICES

Given the advanced echocardiographic imaging techniques, which allow for consistent and accurate real-time imaging of the tricuspid valve, transcatheter solutions to tricuspid regurgitation are now possible. As with mitral repair devices, TEE will likely play an integral role in the use of tricuspid devices. While the development of wide-angle intracardiac echocardiographic probes may increase the utility of this technology,[141] TEE permits imaging with higher frequencies for improved spatial resolution, a larger number of windows for a more comprehensive evaluation of the tricuspid valve apparatus, and consistent acquisition of these images. The new ASE guideline for performing a comprehensive TEE examination[85]

and the guideline for 3D imaging[142] describe image acquisition and standard display specific to the tricuspid valve. The 3D TEE in particular has significantly improved the accuracy of imaging as well as the identification of the tricuspid leaflets and associated anatomic components of the tricuspid valve complex, and already has been shown to be integral to tricuspid valve interventions (Fig. 32.21 and Videos 32.10 and 32.11).[24]

Patients with severe tricuspid regurgitation experience symptoms of chronic right-sided heart failure (peripheral edema, ascites, and orthopnea) with congestive hepatopathy. Thus, treatment of the upstream effect of severe TR may be a reasonable approach to reducing symptoms, although the effect on outcomes is unclear. Lauten et al.[25,143] succeeded in placing two custom-made transcatheter valves into the superior vena cava (SVC) and inferior vena cava (IVC), reducing short-term symptoms while improving liver function.

The surgical edge-to-edge repair of the tricuspid valve has been used with mixed success.[144] For the mitral valve, imaging is likely to play an important role for the placement of a MitraClip device on the tricuspid valve. The only published use of the MitraClip for tricuspid regurgitation has been in a patient with congenitally corrected transposition of the great arteries (thus on a left-sided atrioventricular valve).[145] However, multiple unpublished cases of this technique (personal communication have been successfully performed in non-congenitally abnormal tricuspid valves via both the transjugular and the transfemoral approaches. There are numerous advantages to the use of this system; operators are familiar with the manipulation of this device; both functional and degenerative etiologies of tricuspid regurgitation may be successfully addressed; the clip may be positioned anywhere along the lines of coaptation; and significant re-configuring of the current device is probably not required. This solution should be studied in a formal registry or trial.

Numerous studies have shown that in functional TR the tricuspid annulus dilates in the septo-to-lateral direction. Knowing this pathoanatomy, investigators of The TriCinch System (4TECH Cardio, Galway, Ireland) have developed a tethering device that cinches the anteroposterior dimension of the annulus in order to improve coaptation. The Percutaneous Treatment of Tricuspid Valve Regurgitation with the TriCinch System (PREVENT) trial is currently enrolling.

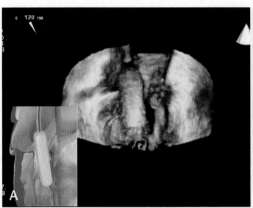
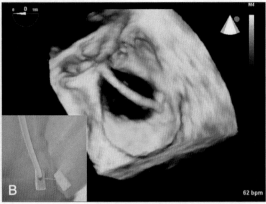

FIG. 32.22 Transcatheter tricuspid valve devices. The FORMA spacer device (A) is a foam-filled device that sits across tricuspid annulus and allows the leaflets to close against the surface, reducing the regurgitant orifice. The Trialign system places two pledgeted sutures within the tricuspid valve annulus and plicates the annulus (B), effectively bringing the anterior and septal leaflets together and bicuspidizing the tricuspid valve.

The Forma Spacer (Edwards Lifesciences, Irvine, California) device uses a simple approach to tricuspid regurgitation by placing a tubular-shaped foam-filled spacer in the center of the regurgitant orifice, forming a surface against which the leaflet tips coapt. This device is implanted from a left subclavian vein approach, introducing an anchor, which is attached to a foam-filled spacer device. The anchor is positioned within the right ventricular wall at the apex, ensuring the stability of the device, and the attached spacer is positioned within the central coaptation of the leaflets (Fig. 32.22A). The procedure is guided by TEE. A number of devices have been implanted on a compassionate use basis; however, no published results are available. The Early Feasibility Study of the Edwards Tricuspid Transcatheter Repair System is underway.

The Titralign system (Mitralign Inc.), has completed its CE mark trial in Europe and recently reported their first-in-human implantation of their device on the tricuspid annulus.[24] The Tiralign system places pledgeted sutures within the tricuspid valve annulus by means of a transjugular venous approach, aiming to bicuspidize the tricuspid valve by annular reduction adjacent to the posterior leaflet (see Fig. 32.22B). Their early compassionate use data have not been published; however, the data presented at TCT 2015 showed a 40%–50% reduction in regurgitant orifice and a greater than 50% reduction in annular area with a single pair of cinched pledgets. Early Feasibility of the Mitralign Percutaneous TriCuspid Valve Annuloplasty System (PTVAS) in patients with Chronic Functional Tricuspid Regurgitation (SCOUT) trial has enrolled its initial 15 patients with positive results recently reported but not yet published.

Numerous investigators have studied transcatheter tricuspid valve replacement in animal models.20–23 Although early in development, this technology appears feasible and may become another transcatheter tool to treat tricuspid valve regurgitation. Similar to the mitral side, issues of valve anchoring and interference with subvalvular apparatus must be solved. Although outflow tract obstruction, which is an issue for the mitral valve replacement technology, is unlikely to be an issue with the discontinuity of the inflow and outflow tracts on the right side, the proximity of the vena cavae and the angulation of the annulus will be new challenges for transcatheter tricuspid valve replacement. Assessment of the valve using MSCT and echocardiography is likely warranted with intraprocedural TEE guidance.

ECHOCARDIOGRAPHY IN TRANSCATHETER VALVE-IN-SURGICAL-VALVE PROCEDURES

Reoperation for bioprosthetic valve dysfunction is associated with an operative mortality of 5%–11%,[146–149] which increases to 15% with concomitant coronary artery disease.[150] Numerous investigators have reported the feasibility of THV implantation into failed surgical heart valves (SHVs; the VIV procedure).[26,27,151–153] A recent report from the Valve-in-Valve International Data (VIVID) Registry included data on 459 patients from 55 participating sites undergoing VIV with either a balloon-expandable or self-expanding prosthesis between 2007 and 2013.[27] The reported 30-day mortality of 7.6% (higher for stenotic valves than regurgitant valves) suggests this procedure may be an acceptable alternative to surgical reoperation for degenerated bioprosthetic valves.

Recent reviews for the use of multimodality imaging in VIV therapy have been published.[30,154,155] Similar to TAVR, the success of this procedure hinges on accurate sizing and our understanding of true internal diameter (TD) of the stent diameter (SD)—neither of which is equivalent to the labeled valve size. For VIV therapy, there are essentially three types of valves: porcine leaflets mounted inside the stent frame in which the TD is 2 mm smaller than the SD, pericardial leaflets mounted inside the stent frame in which the TD is 1 mm smaller than the SD, and pericardial leaflets mounted outside the stent frame in which the TD equals the SD. To choose the correct THV valve size, a general rule is to oversize TD for an aortic VIV by 1 mm, and for a mitral VIV by 2–3 mm. Both computed tomography and TEE have been used to confirm the TD of the SHV.[156–158] Confirmation of aortic or mitral prosthetic TD by echocardiography is typically performed using 3D TEE (Fig. 32.23A).[157–159] User-defined or zoom 3D volumes are acquired during a single cardiac cycle as multi-beat acquisitions may introduce splice artifacts. With multiplanar reconstruction, on-axis SAXs of the sewing ring are acquired to measure the sewing ring TD. Care is taken to avoid the measurement of acoustic "blooming" by reducing gain and measuring only the densest border. LVOT obstruction following mitral VIV procedure is a specific complication of this procedure.[155] Because the bioprosthetic leaflets form the equivalent of a "covered stent" once a THV is deployed in the prosthesis, the relationship of the SHV to the LV outflow tract is of significant concern. The risk of outflow obstruction can be accurately estimated by MSCT; however, 3D echocardiography can also be considered (see Fig. 32.23B).

INTRAPROCEDURAL IMAGING

The positioning of the THV in the aortic position will depend on the type of surgical valve and its implantation location (annular or supraannular), as well as the landing zone characteristics (i.e., sewing ring appearance, aortic root size/height, sinotubular junction, and coronary ostia location). Bapat et al. have demonstrated that the narrowest portion of the SHV is at the level of the sewing ring. In many cases, this can be identified fluoroscopically and used as a reference point during the VIV procedure.[160] However, this is not feasible when the sewing ring is radiolucent and, in these cases, echocardiographic imaging may prove particularly useful.[161] For the second-generation balloon-expandable valve (SAPIEN XT), the final position of the THV should be ~1–2 mm below the surgical sewing ring, and the position on echocardiography during pacing should be approximately ~4–5 mm below the ventricular edge of the SHV sewing ring. Because the SAPIEN 3 valve shortens from the ventricular end only, and the final length of the valve is dependent on the degree of deployment (shorter when fully deployed), the final position of this valve is less predictable. For the positioning of the second-generation self-expanding valve (EVOLUT R), the lowest edge of the THV (posterior typically)

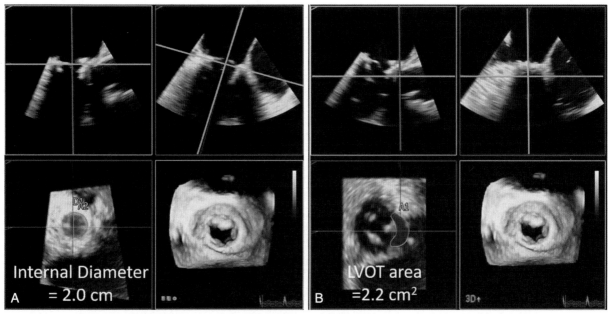

FIG. 32.23 **Valve-in-bioprosthetic valve imaging.** In A, the multiplanar reconstruction of the 3D transesophageal echocardiography image measures an internal diameter of a bioprosthetic valve of 2.0 cm and a 23 mm SAPIEN 3 valve would be appropriate. The risk of left ventricular outflow tract (LVOT) obstruction can also be estimated (B), and, in this case, is low with an estimated LVOT area of 2.2 cm².

should be at most 4–6 mm below the lowest edge of the imaged sewing ring, and often can be much higher. This will ensure that the lowest edges of the THV skirt cover the lowest edge of the prosthetic sewing ring and that the functioning THV valve remains supraannular.

For aortic VIV, malpositioning of the THV increases the risk of complications.[162] High implantation of either the balloon-expandable or self-expanding THV risks THV embolization or coronary obstruction. Low VIV implantation of the balloon-expandable valve can result in AR or prosthetic leaflet overhang, which affects valve hemodynamics. The latter complication may be a risk only in taller SHVs (i.e., Mitroflow and Trifecta) and less likely with the longer SAPIEN 3 valve. Low implantation of the self-expanding valve may result in mitral leaflet impingement or loss of the supraannular position (and thus maximum opening) of the THV leaflets. Coronary obstruction may be related to the relative location of the artery to the surgical stent posts and to the bioprosthetic leaflets. There is a higher risk of obstruction with supraannular valves, low-lying coronary arteries, narrow sinuses and sinotubular junction, bulky prosthetic leaflets, and lack of a stent frame (i.e., homograft or stentless valve).[27]

For VIV in the mitral valve position, either a transapical or transseptal approach can be attempted. The current self-expanding valve is too tall for the mitral position and balloon-expandable or other lower profile valves can be used. If a transapical approach is used, confirming the cannulation site position as described in the TAVR section is essential to the safety of the procedure, allowing the surgeon to avoid right ventricular perforation, ventricular septal disruption, or papillary muscle transection. If a transseptal approach is used, then the techniques described in the MitraClip section apply. Because the SAPIEN 3 valve shortens from the atrial side during deployment, the center marker of the crimped valve is positioned at, or just ventricular to, the top of the sewing ring on fluoroscopy; by echocardiography, the ventricular side of the crimped valve should be just ventricular to the bioprosthetic valve (Fig. 32.24A). The atrial edge of the valve may protrude well into the left atrium; however, with deployment it will protrude approximately 2 mm above the sewing ring of the failed valve (see Fig. 32.24B). Oversizing the TD by 2–3 mm should result in a conical-shaped THV, which should prevent early and late migration; if this is not seen on either fluoroscopy or echo, then a postdilatation may be warranted.

Following the VIV implantation, intraprocedural echocardiography is used to assess procedural results: transcatheter valve position and stability, leaflet excursion, gradients, and valve area (see Fig. 32.24C and D).

Complications of the procedure should always be excluded: the presence and severity of intra- and intervalvular regurgitation, a change in ventricular size and function, and a change in pericardial effusion. Small intervalvular jets between the SHV and THV are not uncommon and may resolve over time. Patients with more than mild intervalvular regurgitation should be considered for a second balloon dilatation. Location-specific concerns must be carefully evaluated: coronary obstruction for aortic VIV and LVOT obstruction for mitral VIV. However, the incidence of various complications for the VIV procedure differs from native valve TAVR (Table 32.6).

Prosthetic Paravalvular Regurgitation Treatment

PVR occurs in 2%–10% of aortic prosthetic valves and 7%–17% of mitral prosthetic valves.[163] Whereas most of these patients are asymptomatic, 1%–3% of patients may present with heart failure, hemolysis, or both. In symptomatic patients with severe PVR, the risk of adverse outcome with repeat surgery is up to 16%,[164,165] which increases with each reoperation.[165] A number of studies have shown that percutaneous closure of PVR is not only possible using a number of different devices,[166–170] but can treat both heart failure and hemolysis.[171–174] Clinical success is determined by the procedural success and the presenting symptom(s). Improvement in heart failure symptoms is typically limited to patients with mild or no residual regurgitation following closure.[173] However, patients with hemolytic anemia often fail to improve despite successful closure.[175] Persistent or worsening hemolysis may be due to the typical off-label use of devices used to close these leaks, which are woven from a larger-caliber nitinol mesh and fail to conform to the irregular shapes of the paravalvular defects and create small, high-velocity jets between the nitinol mesh. More recently, the Amplatzer vascular plug (AVP II and IV) devices have been used. These have a smaller profile and conform to the shape of the defect allowing them to fit better into the small, irregular paravalvular defects, resulting in reduced para-device leak.

PROCEDURAL APPROACH

The choice of access site is determined in part by the location of the surgical valve and related paravalvular leak. Periaortic leaks typically can be approached via a retrograde aortic approach. Transcatheter closure of mitral PVR can be achieved from a retrograde or antegrade approach.

The retrograde method for the mitral prostheses can be performed from a femoral arterial approach (and thus across the aortic valve into

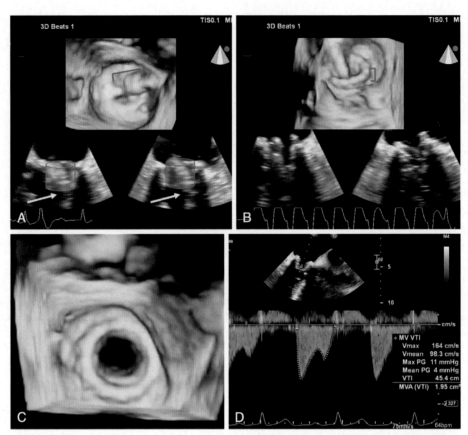

FIG. 32.24 Mitral valve-in-valve positioning. On transesophageal echocardiography, the ventricular side of the crimped valve should be just ventricular to the bioprosthetic valve (A, *yellow arrows*). The atrial edge of the valve may protrude well into the left atrium *(red bracket)*. With deployment, the transcatheter valve will protrude approximately 2 mm above the sewing ring of the failed valve (B). Following the valve-in-valve implantation, transcatheter valve position and stability, leaflet excursion, gradients, and valve area (C and D) should be assessed.

TABLE 32.6 Adverse Events Reported With Aortic Valve-In-Valve Procedures

RISK PROFILE	ADVERSE EVENT
Lower risk than in native TAVR	Significant peri-valvular leak
	Tamponade
	Annular rupture
	Aortic dissection
	Conduction defect
Higher risk than in native TAVR	Device malposition
	Ostial coronary occlusion
	Elevated postprocedural gradients

TAVR, Transcatheter aortic valve replacement.
Adapted from Dvir D, Barbanti M, Tan J, Webb JG. Transcatheter aortic valve-in-valve implantation for patients with degenerative surgical bioprosthetic valves. Curr Probl Cardiol. 2014;39(1):7–27.

the ventricle), or a direct transapical approach; the latter may be ideal for patients requiring multiple devices since multiple wires can be introduced simultaneously through the apex, either by direct puncture or with a small surgical apical window. The transapical approach for mitral paravalvular leak closure has been shown to reduce procedural and fluoroscopy time.[176]

The antegrade method requires a transseptal puncture and 3D transesophageal guidance may be helpful in identifying the optimal location for the puncture. The steerable GC (i.e., Agilis) has made the antegrade approach highly feasible for any para-mitral paravalvular defect.

INTRAPROCEDURAL IMAGING

Standard transesophageal imaging views for the aortic and mitral valves should be used throughout preinterventional imaging and procedural guidance.[85] Much of the preprocedural assessment of paravalvular leaks

are performed by 3D imaging.[142] The standardization of acquisition and display, emphasize creating an anatomic view of the mitral valve[142] that places the aortic valve anterior (or at 12 o'clock) with the left atrial appendage identifying the medial sewing ring (9 o'clock), and the inter-atrial septum the medial sewing ring (3 o'clock). More recently, fusion imaging has been used and may improve communication and reduce procedure time, particularly in paravalvular closure procedures (Fig. 32.25A).[177]

Preprocedural planning by the Heart Team for transcatheter closure of PVR requires a determination of: (a) the number and location of defects; (b) the shape and exact size of each defect; and (c) the distance and orientation of the defect to the sewing ring or prosthesis. This assessment requires extensive 2D and 3D transesophageal imaging.[87,172,178] The shape and size of the defect determine the choice of device. Long, crescent-shaped leaks often require multiple closure devices. Para-aortic leaks tend to be smaller than para-mitral leaks, and simultaneous or sequential closure devices are rarely necessary.

Echocardiographic imaging for aortic prostheses can be limited by acoustic shadowing of the anterior sewing ring. Thus off-axis imaging (deep esophageal or transgastric views) may be necessary (see Fig. 32.25B) and, occasionally, transthoracic imaging may be better than transesophageal imaging. Defects in the posterior sewing ring are easily imaged on TEE. Alternatively, ICE can be used, but the experience with this imaging modality during paravalvular leak closure is more limited. The recommended 3D orientation of the valve places the left sinus of the Valsalva anterior and to the right with the right sinus of Valsalva directly posterior (6 o'clock).

The location of the defect may influence the success of the procedure. Anterolateral para-mitral defects close to the left atrial appendage frequently have a serpiginous superior-to-inferior orientation because of massive left atrial dilation, with the inferior (or left ventricular origin) of the defect located closer to the valve prosthesis. This orientation of the defect may result in a 90-degree rotation of the device after deployment,

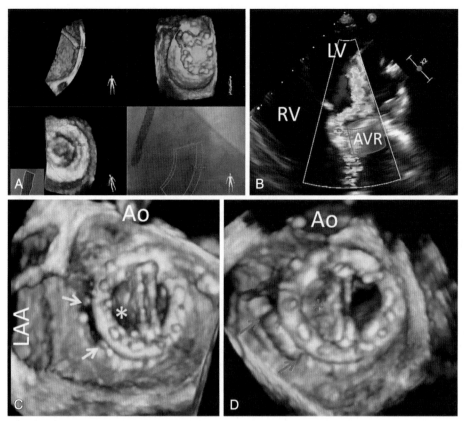

FIG. 32.25 Imaging for transcatheter paravalvular regurgitation closure. Fusion imaging for paravalvular regurgitation (A) can place a fiduciary point on an echocardiographic image *(red dot)*, and this same point is then coregistered on the fluoroscopic image. Paravalvular imaging of aortic valve prostheses can be limited by acoustic shadowing of the anterior sewing ring. (B) This shows a large paravalvular jet imaged only from deep transgastric views. This anterolateral paravalvular mitral defect close to the left atrial appendage (LAA; C, *between yellow arrows*) has a superior-to-inferior orientation. Of note, the mechanical disc near the defect opens normally *(yellow *)*. After deployment of an AVP II device (D, *between red arrows*), there was a 90-degree rotation of the device resulting in the obstruction of the mechanical occluder *(red *)*. *Ao,* Aorta; *AVR,* aortic valve replacement; *LV,* left ventricle; *RV,* right ventricle.

resulting in protrusion of the device across the prosthetic orifice and obstruction of the mechanical occluder or biologic leaflet (see Fig. 32.25C and D).[179] This complication may be recognized on fluoroscopy as well. Once deployed in a suboptimal position (or if embolized), removal of the device can be accomplished with a snare or a long, flexible bioptome, thus avoiding the need for open retrieval.

Following device deployment, a full assessment of prosthetic valve function should be performed. This includes (but is not limited to): 2D and 3D imaging of the prosthesis to assess function; continuous-wave Doppler across the prosthetic orifice for assessment of peak/mean gradients; 2D and 3D color Doppler assessment of residual PVR; Doppler assessment of the effect of device placement on flow in the pulmonary veins as well as pulmonary artery pressures, and residual transseptal defect.

CONCLUSION

Echocardiography is an essential imaging tool for structural heart disease interventions. This imaging modality is ideal for preprocedural planning, intraprocedural guidance, and postprocedural assessment of every transcatheter intervention.

Suggested Reading

Altiok, E., Becker, M., Hamada, S., et al. (2011). Optimized guidance of percutaneous edge-to edge repair of the mitral valve using real-time 3-D transesophageal echocardiography. *Clinical Research in Cardiology, 100,* 675–681.

Baumgartner, H., Hung, J., Bermejo, J., et al. (2009). Echocardiographic assessment of valve stenosis: EAE/ ASE recommendations for clinical practice. *Journal of the American Society of Echocardiography, 22,* 1–23 [quiz 101-102].

Bloomfield, G. S., Gillam, L. D., Hahn, R. T., et al. (2012). A practical guide to multimodality imaging of transcatheter aortic valve replacement. *JACC Cardiovascular Imaging, 5,* 441–455.

Hahn, R. T., Abraham, T., Adams, M. S., et al. (2013). Guidelines for performing a comprehensive transesophageal echocardiographic examination: recommendations from the American Society of Echocardiography and the Society of Cardiovascular Anesthesiologists. *Journal of the American Society of Echocardiography, 26,* 921–964.

Hahn, R. T., Gillam, L. D., & Little, S. H. (2015). Echocardiographic imaging of procedural complications during self-expandable transcatheter aortic valve replacement. *JACC Cardiovascular Imaging, 8,* 319–336.

Hahn, R. T., Kodali, S., Tuzcu, E. M., et al. (2015). Echocardiographic imaging of procedural complications during balloon-expandable transcatheter aortic valve replacement. *JACC Cardiovascular Imaging, 8,* 288–318.

Hahn, R. T., Little, S. H., Monaghan, M. J., et al. (2015). Recommendations for comprehensive intraprocedural echocardiographic imaging during TAVR. *JACC Cardiovascular Imaging, 8,* 261–287.

Tzikas, A., Schultz, C. J., Piazza, N., et al. (2011). Assessment of the aortic annulus by multislice computed tomography, contrast aortography, and trans-thoracic echocardiography in patients referred for transcatheter aortic valve implantation. *Catheterization and Cardiovascular Interventions, 77,* 868–875.

A complete reference list can be found online at ExpertConsult.com.

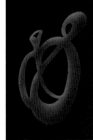

DISEASES OF THE PERICARDIUM AND GREAT VESSELS

33 Pericardial Disease

Sheila M. Hegde

INTRODUCTION

The pericardium is a thin-walled structure composed of two layers, a serous visceral layer (epicardium) and a fibrous parietal layer, both of which surround and protect the heart. Between these layers, up to 50 mL of pericardial fluid normally cushion the heart while the pericardium serves as a barrier to inflammation and infection.[1-3]

Limited epidemiologic data are available for the incidence and prevalence of pericardial disease. Marked variability exists depending on the clinical setting, whether in a developed or developing country and according to the availability of subspecialty care. The etiology of pericardial disease may be attributed to infection, autoimmune, postmyocardial infarction, malignant, metabolic, traumatic, drug-related, congenital, or iatrogenic causes.[4]

Transthoracic echocardiography is the first-line noninvasive test of choice in patients with suspected pericardial disease. The pericardium is typically seen as a bright, linear structure surrounding the heart due to its interface with lung tissue.[3] Although the pericardium can be assessed with M-mode, two-dimensional (2D), or three-dimensional echocardiography, 2D echocardiography is most frequently used for assessing pericardial effusions and their hemodynamic significance and also serves as the most cost-effective imaging modality.[4]

This chapter reviews the echocardiographic evaluation of the pericardium in various pericardial syndromes: pericardial effusion, pericarditis, pericardial constriction, and other pericardial disorders.

PERICARDIAL FLUID

Fluid Characteristics

Pericardial fluid is the serous fluid secreted by the serous layer of the pericardium and is typically echo free by ultrasound. Effusions are often not distributed uniformly in the pericardial space. Hemorrhagic pericardial fluid may serve as a marker of disease (e.g., malignancy) or trauma (e.g., ventricular rupture, coronary artery trauma). Hemopericardium may appear echo free at its onset because echo-free fluid is the same density as the intracardiac blood pool; however, with time the fluid may increase in echodensity, consistent with organizing thrombus. Purulent fluid is consistent with an infectious etiology and associated with elevated fluid protein levels. Such an exudative fluid may also demonstrate stranding or adhesions, consistent with an inflammatory and more complicated disease process. Purulent pericarditis should be managed aggressively with urgent pericardiocentesis, and these effusions are often loculated. Chylous fluid is consistent with trauma or infiltration of the thoracic duct; computed tomography (CT) with and without contrast can aid in the diagnosis.

Effusion Size

The end-diastolic distance of echo-free space between the visceral and parietal pericardium defines the size of a pericardial effusion: trivial (seen only in systole), small (<10 mm), moderate (10–20 mm), large (>20 mm), or very large (>25 mm) (Fig. 33.1 and Videos 33.1 and 33.2). Descriptions of effusions should include the size and location of the measurements made. Although there is not a strict correlation between linear dimensions and volume, one may very roughly expect a fluid volume of ≤250 mL from the small effusions, 250–500 mL from the moderate effusions, and greater than 500 mL from pericardiocentesis of large circumferential effusions. Loculated effusions that may occur in the postsurgical setting or secondary to inflammatory disease may not be visible on standard transthoracic echocardiography, and a transesophageal echocardiogram may be necessary.

Distinguishing Features

The position of the descending thoracic aorta relative to the fluid collection is often key to distinguishing a left pleural effusion from a pericardial effusion. Because the visceral pericardium remains closely apposed to the heart muscle itself, fluid anterior to the descending thoracic aorta is more likely to be pericardial, whereas fluid posterior the aorta is more likely to be pleural (Fig. 33.2 and Video 33.3). The descending thoracic aorta can often be identified in apical four-chamber views as well (see Fig. 13.5) and used in exactly the same way as a landmark to distinguish pericardial from left pleural effusions.

Epicardial fat sits between the visceral pericardium and the myocardium. Variable amounts can be found over the right ventricle (RV) and the atrioventricular and interventricular grooves.[1] This is often seen as isolated echo-free space anterior to the RV. Increasing the gain settings will show increased texture or brightness relative to the myocardium, which is consistent with epicardial fat. In addition, epicardial fat will move together with the myocardium.

ACUTE PERICARDITIS

Acute pericarditis most commonly presents with chest pain that is characterized as sharp, substernal, and pleuritic, with an improvement in symptoms by sitting up and leaning forward. Diagnostic criteria include the presence of two of the following: characteristic chest pain, pericardial rub, widespread ST segment-elevation or PR segment depression on electrocardiogram (ECG), and a new or worsening pericardial effusion.[1,5]

In the absence of a pericardial rub and ECG changes, imaging of the heart is necessary to make the fourth diagnostic criteria. Although the chest x-ray is likely the first imaging study obtained in a patient with chest pain, the cardiothoracic ratio is often normal in acute pericarditis; the ratio generally only increases once a pericardial effusion is greater than 200–300 mL.[4,6]

Transthoracic echocardiography will demonstrate the presence of even small pericardial effusions and allow for characterization of the fluid density and size of the effusion. Pericardial effusions may be present without

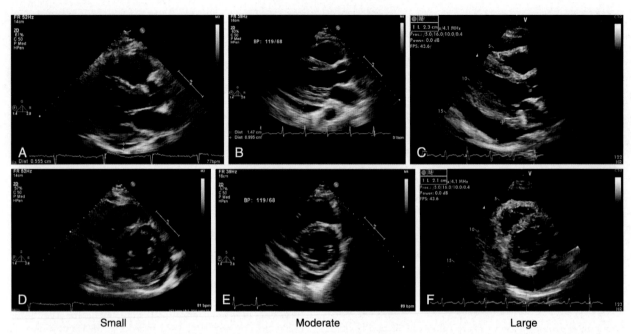

Small   Moderate   Large

FIG. 33.1 Pericardial effusion. (A and D) Parasternal long- and short-axis views demonstrating a small (<10–20), circumferential pericardial effusion. (B and E) Parasternal long- and short-axis views demonstrating a moderate (10–20 mm), circumferential pericardial effusion. (C and F) Parasternal long and short-axis views demonstrating a large (>20 mm), circumferential pericardial effusion.

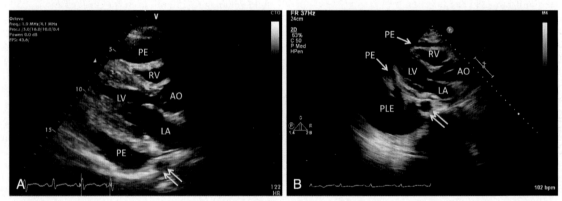

FIG. 33.2 Distinguishing pericardial and pleural effusions. (A) Parasternal long-axis view demonstrating a large, circumferential pericardial effusion (PE), seen at the same level as the descending thoracic aorta *(double arrows)*. (B) Parasternal long-axis view demonstrating a small, circumferential pericardial effusion *(single arrows)*, seen anterior to the descending thoracic aorta *(double arrows)*. A pleural effusion (PLE) is also present and seen posterior to the descending thoracic aorta. *Ao,* Aorta; *LA,* left atrium; *LV,* left ventricle; *RV,* right ventricle.

or with tamponade physiology (seen in up to 3% of patients).[1] In some cases, the pericardium may appear bright. The echocardiogram may also appear normal with normal left ventricular function and a trace to small pericardial effusion. Echo imaging may also be helpful in excluding wall motion abnormalities in the setting of myocardial infarction although up to 5% of patients may exhibit wall motion abnormalities with pericarditis, due to concomitant inflammation of the myocardium.[1] Concurrent myopericarditis may present with new focal or global left ventricular dysfunction and elevated cardiac biomarkers.

Several major and minor high-risk features have been associated with an increased risk of subsequent complications from acute pericarditis. Major risk factors include high fever, large pericardial effusion, subacute course, cardiac tamponade, and no response to 7 days of nonsteroidal antiinflammatory drugs (NSAIDs).[5] Minor risk factors include oral anticoagulant therapy, trauma, immunosuppression, and concomitant myocarditis (myopericarditis).[1,5]

RECURRENT PERICARDITIS

Recurrent pericarditis occurs in 15%–30% of patients after the initial diagnosis.[1] The diagnosis of recurrent pericarditis is made after a 6-week symptom-free interval following the first episode of pericarditis. A patient must also meet the same two of four diagnostic criteria for acute pericarditis.

Echocardiography may demonstrate the presence of a pericardial effusion. Complications such as cardiac tamponade and constriction are less common in recurrent pericarditis.[7] Additional findings may include a septal bounce and other signs of constrictive pericarditis (see later). Cardiac CT may be helpful in assessing pericardial thickness, and delayed gadolinium enhancement with cardiac magnetic resonance imaging (MRI) may be helpful in demonstrating inflammation of the pericardium.

PERICARDIAL TAMPONADE

The hemodynamic response to a pericardial effusion is most closely related to the speed with which the fluid accumulates, the distensibility of the pericardium, and the filling pressures and compliance of the cardiac chambers rather than the size or total volume.[5] Pericardial tamponade describes the state in which excessive pericardial fluid with elevated intrapericardial pressures limits cardiac filling. As the amount of pericardial fluid increases, pericardial pressure rises, which results in a compensatory rise in pulmonary and systemic venous pressures to maintain cardiac output.[1] Eventually, the compensatory mechanisms fail and preload can no longer support cardiac filling.

Two-dimensional echocardiography will often demonstrate a large pericardial effusion in tamponade. Irrespective of the size of the effusion, the most worrisome signs include the presence of dilated hepatic veins

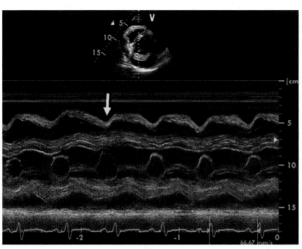

FIG. 33.3 M-mode of pericardial tamponade. Note the right ventricle (RV) outflow tract collapsing *(arrow)* in diastole (when the mitral valve is open), as well as the reciprocal variation in RV and left ventricle sizes over time with respiration (ventricular interdependence).

TABLE 33.1 Comparison of Findings in Pericardial Constriction and Tamponade

	PERICARDIAL CONSTRICTION	TAMPONADE
Two-Dimensional Echo Findings		
Pericardial space	± Effusion	Effusion
Inferior vena cava	Dilated, diminished collapse	Dilated, diminished collapse
Septal position	Ventricular interdependence (Septal shift, varies with respiration)	Ventricular interdependence (Septal shift, varies with respiration)
Echo Doppler Findings		
Respiratory variation in E wave (mitral)	>25%	>25%
Respiratory variation in E wave (tricuspid)	>40%	>40%
Hepatic vein flow	Diastolic reversal	Diastolic reversal
M-mode Findings		
Septal position	Ventricular interdependence (Septal shift, varies with respiration)	Ventricular interdependence (Septal shift, varies with respiration)
	Septal bounce	
	Left ventricle posterior wall flattening	
Clinical Findings		
Jugular venous pressure	Elevated	Elevated
Pulsus paradoxus	Uncommon	Common
Kussmaul sign	Present	Absent
Cardiac Catheterization Findings		
Y descent	Exaggerated (Prominent early diastolic filling)	Blunted (Prominent systolic filling)

Data from Klein AL, Abbara S, Agler DA, et al. American Society of Echocardiography clinical recommendations for multimodality cardiovascular imaging of patients with pericardial disease. J Am Soc Echocardiogr. 2013;26(9):965–1012.

and a dilated inferior vena cava (see Fig. 13.4), which together represent the presence of elevated systemic venous pressures. These findings together with a small left ventricle (LV) suggest the presence of a reduction in stroke volume and cardiac output. Additional findings of elevated intrapericardial pressure include early diastolic collapse of the RV and inversion of the right atrium for greater than one-third of the cardiac cycle (see Fig. 13.6 and Videos 13.9 through 13.11). Collapse of the atria occurs near the peak of the R wave, whereas collapse of the ventricles occurs at the end of the T wave in early diastole. Due to thin wall of the right atrium, collapse of the chamber may be seen in patients without tamponade; however, if the duration of RA inversion is greater than one-third of the cardiac cycle, this finding has been described to be 100% sensitive and specific for cardiac tamponade.[1] The severity of tamponade increases with the duration of chamber collapse. The right-sided chambers are most susceptible to compression due to its lower filling pressures. Examples are shown and discussed in Chapter 13.

M-mode echocardiography is particularly well suited to demonstrate changes in chamber dimensions, right-sided chamber collapse, and interventricular dependence in relation to respiratory variation, in part due to the increase in temporal resolution with this technique (Fig. 33.3; see also Fig. 13.6). These patients are often tachycardic, so an M-mode cursor through the chamber or wall of interest can aid in the judgment of duration and timing of chamber collapse. As fluid accumulates in the pericardial space, intrapericardial pressure rises and hemodynamics mimic constrictive physiology. With inspiration, increased filling to the RV results in a leftward shift of the ventricular septum and decreased filling of the LV. With expiration, increased filling to the LV results in a reciprocal rightward shift of the ventricular septum and decreased filling of the RV. This relationship can be appreciated on M-mode and 2D echocardiography.

Doppler echocardiographic findings include exaggerated respiratory variation in mitral (>25%) and tricuspid (>40%) inflow velocities due to the ventricular interdependence that develops as intrapericardial pressure rises (as in Fig. 13.7). The respiratory changes are highest on the first beats of inspiration and expiration.[1] The consensus for calculation is (expiration-inspiration)/expiration for both mitral and tricuspid inflow.[1] Respiratory variation can also be demonstrated in LV outflow tract and RV outflow tract flows. In addition, hepatic vein velocities will be reduced, reflecting the reduction in cardiac filling. As the degree of tamponade increases, blunting or reversal of diastolic flow in expiration may be appreciated in the hepatic veins.[1]

Special consideration should be given to patients with history of elevated right-sided chamber pressures prior to the development of the pericardial effusion. In this setting, right-sided chamber collapse may occur later in the development of tamponade physiology because it will take an even greater intrapericardial pressure to collapse the right-sided chambers in diastole. Similarly, low intracardiac pressures, such as in

hypovolemia, may result in earlier collapse of right-sided chambers. In those with loculated pericardial effusions, attention should be given to the left-sided chambers and any cardiac chambers adjacent to the effusion (see Videos 13.13 and 13.14).

Pericardial constriction and tamponade share many similar characteristics, including echocardiographic findings (Table 33.1). Aside from the presence of a pericardial effusion, clinical characteristics seen at the bedside and hemodynamics in the cardiac catheterization lab can help distinguish the two diagnoses.

PERICARDIAL CONSTRICTION

Pericardial constriction describes the impaired cardiac filling that occurs due to a thickened, scarred, and/or calcified pericardium. Constriction can occur as result of any long-standing pericardial inflammatory process, and the likelihood of progression is related to the etiology; constrictive pericarditis is more frequently seen as a result of bacterial pericarditis and relatively less common as a result of viral or idiopathic acute pericarditis.[8] In developing countries and immunosuppressed patients, the etiology is most commonly secondary to tuberculosis, whereas in developed areas, the most common etiologies are idiopathic, cardiac surgery, pericarditis, and mediastinal radiation.[1,9]

Two-dimensional echocardiography may show pericardial thickening and calcification (Fig. 33.4). Although pericardial thickness cannot be reliably measured by transthoracic echocardiography, measurements by transesophageal echocardiography have been shown to be reproducible in

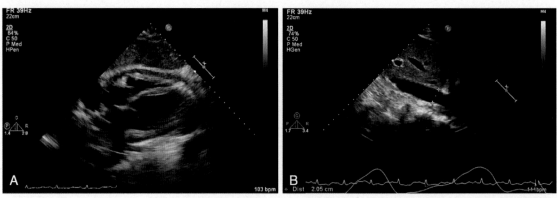

FIG. 33.4 Pericardial constriction. (A) Subcostal view demonstrating a thickened pericardium with echo-dense material in the pericardial space. (B) Subcostal view demonstrating a dilated inferior vena cava.

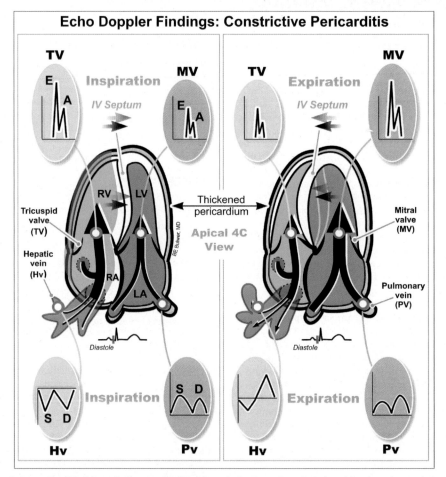

FIG. 33.5 Schematic of constrictive pericarditis. Schematic demonstrating hemodynamic changes and ventricular interdependence in constrictive pericarditis during inspiration and expiration. The overall cardiac volume is relatively fixed due to a noncompliant pericardium. With inspiration, the increased filling to the right-sided chambers results in decreased filling of the left ventricle (LV). The ventricular septum shifts to the left and the tricuspid inflow E velocity and hepatic vein diastolic forward flow velocity increase. With expiration, diastolic filling of the LV increases, which results in a rightward shift of the ventricular septum and decreased filling of the RV. The tricuspid inflow E velocity and hepatic vein diastolic forward flow velocity decrease; the hepatic vein Doppler also may demonstrate diastolic flow reversal. *A wave,* Late diastolic filling; *D,* pulmonary vein diastolic wave; *E wave,* early diastolic filling; *IV,* intraventricular; *LA,* left atrium; *RA,* right atrium; *RV,* right ventricle; *S,* pulmonary vein systolic wave. (*Courtesy of Bernard E. Bulwer, MD, FASE; Adapted from Solomon SD, Wu J, Gillam L. Echocardiography. In: Mann DL, Zipes DP, Libby P, et al., eds.* Braunwald's Heart Disease: A Textbook of Cardiovascular Medicine. *10th ed. Philadelphia: Elsevier; 2015:179–260.*)

comparison to CT.[10] Exaggerated ventricular interdependence may also be apparent by the presence of a characteristic diastolic septal bounce, as well as an associated respiratory variation in the position of the interventricular septum (similar to tamponade).

In constrictive pericarditis the overall cardiac volume is relatively fixed due to the noncompliant pericardium and minimal respiratory changes in intrapericardial pressure. The rigid pericardium also causes dissociation of intrathoracic and intracardiac pressures. As a result, diastolic filling of both ventricles exhibits reciprocal changes with respiration due to the ventricular interdependence (Fig. 33.5 and Video 33.4). With inspiration, there is

rapid early diastolic filling of the right heart, which abruptly halts when the cardiac volume constrained by the rigid pericardium is reached. The increased filling to the right-sided chambers results in shifting of the interventricular septum to the left; simultaneously, due to the thick pericardium surrounding the left heart but not the thorax, there is less of a pressure gradient driving flow between the pulmonary veins and the left atrium, which further exacerbates the decreased filling of the LV. The ventricular septum shifts to the left and the tricuspid inflow E velocity and hepatic vein diastolic forward flow velocity increase. With expiration, diastolic filling of the LV increases, which results in a rightward shift of the ventricular septum

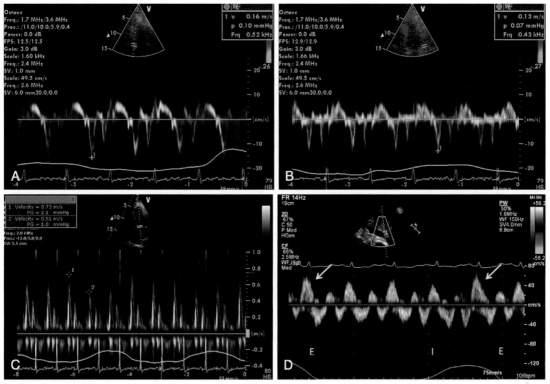

FIG. 33.6 **Doppler findings in pericardial constriction.** (A) Preserved medial mitral annular early diastolic velocity (>8 cm/s). (B) Preserved lateral mitral annular early dia-stolic velocity (>8 cm/s). (C) Exaggerated respiratory variation in the mitral inflow (>25%). (D) Pulsed-wave Doppler of the hepatic veins demonstrating exaggerated diastolic flow reversal in expiration. *E,* Expiration; *I,* inspiration.

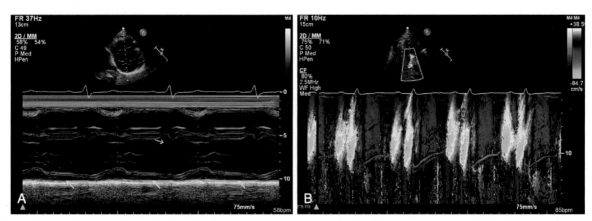

FIG. 33.7 **M-mode (two-dimensional and color Doppler) in pericardial constriction.** (A) M-mode of parasternal short axis at the papillary muscle level demonstrating abnormal septal motion *(white arrows)* and flattening of the left ventricle posterior wall in diastole *(yellow arrows).* (B) Color M-mode of the apical four-chamber view demon-strating a brisk mitral flow propagation velocity (Vp) consistent with normal myocardial relaxation.

and decreased filling of the RV. The tricuspid inflow E velocity and hepatic vein diastolic forward flow velocity decrease; the hepatic vein Doppler also may demonstrate diastolic flow reversal. The inferior vena cava is typically dilated with reduced collapse during respiration (see Fig. 33.4 and Video 33.5). Similar to tamponade, Doppler echocardiography will demonstrate a restricted filling pattern of the mitral valve inflow profile, with greater than 25% respiratory variation in the mitral inflow velocity and greater than 40% respiratory variation in the tricuspid inflow velocity.[1]

Additional findings of constriction include a preserved early diastolic mitral annular tissue Doppler velocity (E′ velocity >8 cm/s), which has been associated with an 89% sensitivity and 100% specificity for dis-tinguishing constriction from restriction (Fig. 33.6).[11] The high and/or preserved E′ tissue velocities may be more pronounced at the medial annulus. The presence of "annulus reversus," which is described as a higher medial E′ velocity compared with the lateral E′ velocity, has been associated with constrictive pericarditis and thought to be due to tether-ing of the pericardium impairing lateral mitral annular motion.[12] Recent work suggests the presence of a similar relationship between septal and

lateral wall motion with a more attenuated regional longitudinal systolic strain in the LV anterolateral wall compared with the septal wall, which may be more robust than the tissue Doppler velocity ratios in distinguish-ing constriction from restriction.[13] In addition, other research has shown a more attenuated LV basal longitudinal strain in restriction and a more attenuated circumferential strain in constriction.[14]

Using color M-mode flow analysis, the presence of rapid diastolic flow propagation (Vp > 55 cm/s) to the apex has been associated with a 74% sensitivity and 91% specificity for distinguishing patients with constriction from restrictive cardiomyopathy (Fig. 33.7B).[11] 2D M-mode echocardiography is useful because of its superior temporal resolution. It may demonstrate (1) abnormal diastolic septal bounce, or "notching" as the septum fleetingly shifts left, then right in early diastole (as the right, then left atrioventricular valves open) and then again in late diastole with (right, then left) atrial contraction; (2) a relatively gradual septal shift to the left with inspiration; and (3) flattening of the LV posterior wall in diastole (see Fig. 33.7A and Video 33.6), which can be seen by both M-mode and 2D imaging. Because the impact of respiration is integral

TABLE 33.2 Comparison of Echocardiographic Findings in Pericardial Constriction and Restrictive Cardiomyopathy

	PERICARDIAL CONSTRICTION	RESTRICTIVE CARDIOMYOPATHY
Two-Dimensional Findings		
Pericardium	± Thickening/calcification	Normal
Inferior vena cava	Dilated, diminished collapse	Dilated, diminished collapse
Septal position	Ventricular interdependence (Septal shift, varies with respiration)	Normal
Atrial size	± Enlarged	Enlarged
M-mode Findings		
Septal position	Ventricular interdependence (Septal shift, varies with respiration)	Normal
Color M-mode mitral valve Vp	Increased (>55 cm/s)	Reduced
Doppler Findings		
Mitral valve inflow pattern	Restrictive	Restrictive
Deceleration time	Short	Short
Respiratory variation in E wave (mitral)	>25%	Normal
Respiratory variation in E wave (tricuspid)	>40%	Normal
Mitral annulus early diastolic velocity (E′)	Normal	Reduced
Pulmonary hypertension	Uncommon	Common

Data from Klein AL, Abbara S, Agler DA, et al. American Society of Echocardiography clinical recommendations for multimodality cardiovascular imaging of patients with pericardial disease. J Am Soc Echocardiogr. 2013;26(9):965–1012.

to the assessment of pericardial disease, image acquisitions should include long (up to 10 beats or more) captures with respiratory gating, particularly for Doppler and M-mode images.

Three forms of constrictive pericarditis have been described. *Transient constrictive pericarditis* has been associated with acute pericarditis with mild pericardial effusion and resolution within several weeks of antiinflammatory treatment.[5] In the absence of signs of chronic pericarditis, management is often conservative prior to recommendation for a pericardiectomy.[5] *Effusive-constrictive pericarditis* may be characterized by the presence of a pericardial effusion, signs of constriction, or both. Noninvasive imaging by echocardiography and/or cardiac MRI can aid in the diagnosis. Echocardiography will demonstrate Doppler findings of constriction and ventricular interdependence with a septal bounce. Effusions may be large enough that a patient will exhibit concomitant signs and symptoms of tamponade; however, these may be difficult to distinguish from constrictive pericarditis (see Table 33.1). Persistently elevated right atrial pressure following pericardiocentesis suggests the presence of constrictive pericarditis.[1,9,15] Treatment involves visceral pericardiectomy because the visceral layer of the pericardium is responsible for constriction.[5] *Chronic constrictive pericarditis* is the third form of constrictive disease for which pericardiectomy is the standard therapy in those with persistent symptoms.

Distinguishing pericardial constriction from restrictive cardiomyopathy (see Chapter 24) can be challenging even after multimodality testing with echocardiography, cardiac CT, cardiac MRI, and cardiac catheterization. By Doppler echocardiography, there are a few distinct characteristics, albeit with limited specificity (24%–57%; Table 33.2).[9] Patients with pericardial constriction have marked mitral inflow respiratory variation (>25%) in contrast to minimal respiratory variation in those with

restrictive cardiomyopathy. The early diastolic mitral annular velocity (E′) is normal in patients with pericardial constriction, but E′ is typically reduced (<8 cm/s) in those with restrictive cardiomyopathy.[11,16] Rapid diastolic flow propagation is typically preserved or increased (Vp > 100 cm/s) in constriction but decreased in restriction.[1,5,11] Furthermore, conditions with exaggerated intrathoracic pressure variation, such as asthma or chronic obstructive pulmonary disease, can result in a false positive diagnosis of constrictive pericarditis due to increased respiratory variation in mitral and tricuspid inflow; superior vena cava flow will show marked respiratory variation in pulmonary disease compared to the minimal variation seen with constrictive pericarditis.[1,3,17]

OTHER PERICARDIAL DISORDERS AND ABNORMALITIES

Congenital Absence of Pericardium

Congenital absence of the pericardium is a rare finding that can occur in either complete or partial forms. More commonly, a portion of the left pericardium is absent. Congenital absence of the pericardium has been associated with bicuspid aortic valve, atrial septal defects, and bronchogenic cysts and occurs more often in males.[18–20] Absence of the pericardium is associated with a leftward shift of the heart, resulting in exaggerated cardiac motion. Partial left-sided defects carry a higher risk of compression, herniation, or strangulation of the great vessels, cardiac chambers, or coronary arteries.[1] Echocardiography will demonstrate prominent right-cardiac chambers and abnormal septal motion, which may together resemble a pattern of RV volume overload or atrial septal defect. CT or cardiac MRI can confirm the diagnosis.

Pericardial Cysts

Pericardial cysts are rare mediastinal findings characterized as cystic formations or diverticulae. In contrast to diverticulae, cysts do not communicate with the pericardial space. Cysts can present as single cysts or multiloculated cysts, and they are often found at the costophrenic angles. The overall incidence is as low as 1 in 100,000 patients, and they account for 33% of mediastinal cysts and 6% of mediastinal masses.[5] The majority are located at the right cardiophrenic angle. Pericardial cysts are often detected incidentally. Echocardiography can be used to confirm location (Fig. 33.8 and Videos 33.7 and 33.8). Contrast echocardiography can be useful in excluding an anomalous systemic vein, whereas color Doppler and pulsed Doppler at low velocities can help to ensure that there is no phasic flow in the structure. Evaluation often includes additional imaging with CT and cardiac MRI to further characterize the structure (Fig. 33.9). The differential diagnosis includes loculated pericardial effusions, pericardial fat pad, diaphragmatic hernia, benign pericardial masses, and malignant pericardial masses. No treatment is necessary in asymptomatic patients.

Pericardial Involvement in Malignancy

Primary tumors of the pericardium are very rare and may be benign (lipoma, fibroma, hemangioma, lymphangioma) or malignant (mesothelioma, angiosarcoma, fibrosarcoma). An example of pericardial mesothelioma is shown in Fig. 37.9. Lung cancer, breast cancer, melanoma, lymphoma, and leukemias are more commonly the cause of secondary malignant tumors of the pericardium (Fig. 33.10 and Video 33.9).[1,5] Malignant pericardial effusions can be of any size, often recur, and may then require creation of a pericardial window to allow drainage of the effusion into the pleural space. Increased or layering echodensities within the pericardial space, particularly if they appear as solid masses, infiltrate the myocardium, or are associated with constrictive physiology should increase suspicion for malignant involvement of the pericardium (see Chapter 37).

MULTIMODALITY IMAGING

Although echocardiography is often used as first-line imaging in pericardial disease, cardiac CT and cardiac MRI provide complementary diagnostic information (Chapter 48). Advantages to echocardiography

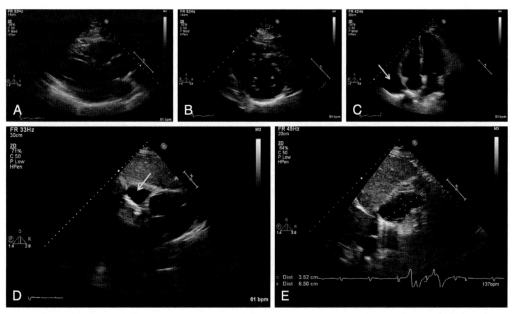

FIG. 33.8 **Pericardial cyst on echocardiography.** (A and B) Parasternal long-axis and short-axis views demonstrating no pericardial effusion and no apparent pericardial cyst on these windows. (C and D) Apical four-chamber view and off-axis subcostal view demonstrating the pericardial cyst, seen as an echo-free space *(arrows)* adjacent to the right atrium and right ventricle. (E) Off-axis subcostal view further demonstrating the pericardial cyst (measuring 3.5 × 6.5 cm).

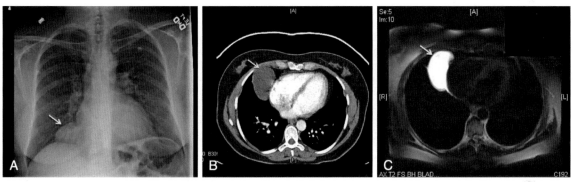

FIG. 33.9 **Pericardial cyst by radiologic modalities.** Pericardial cysts *(arrows)* are often an incidental diagnosis, most commonly diagnosed incidentally by chest x-ray (A). Cardiac CT (B) and cardiac MRI (C) provide complementary diagnostic information and can help to distinguish a pericardial cyst from a pericardial diverticulum, pericardial mass, or pericardial effusion.

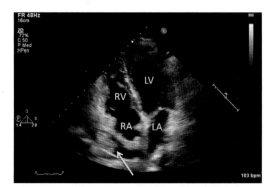

FIG. 33.10 **Pericardial mass.** Echocardiographic images from a patient with breast cancer. Apical four-chamber view demonstrating an echogenic mass *(arrow)* in the pericardial space adjacent to the right atrium, which proved to be metastatic breast cancer. *LA,* Left atrium; *LV,* left ventricle; *RA,* right atrium; *RV,* right ventricle.

include its low cost, portability, safety profile, high frame rate, and ability to correlate dynamic physiologic changes with a respirometer, whereas limitations include operator dependence, low signal-to-noise ratio of the pericardium, limited tissue characterization, limited windows, and technical limitations in image acquisition particularly in those with obesity, chronic obstructive pulmonary disease, or in a

postoperative state.[1] Consideration of patient presentation, clinical context, and availability of imaging modalities should drive the choice of testing.

CONCLUSION

Echocardiography remains the first imaging modality of choice in evaluating pericardial disease and its hemodynamic significance. The finding of a pericardial effusion demands careful interpretation of its size and clinical implications. Distinguishing between restrictive and constrictive pericarditis remains challenging given their similar hemodynamic findings. A careful history, physical examination, high index of clinical suspicion, multimodality imaging, and invasive hemodynamic assessment by cardiac catheterization may ultimately assist in making the diagnosis.

Suggested Reading

Adler, Y., Charron, P., Imazio, M., et al. (2015). 2015 ESC guidelines for the diagnosis and management of pericardial diseases: The Task Force for the Diagnosis and Management of Pericardial Diseases of the European Society of Cardiology (ESC). Endorsed by: The European Association for Cardio-Thoracic Surgery (EACTS). *European Heart Journal, 36,* 2921–2964.

Khandaker, M. H., Espinosa, R. E., Nishimura, R. A., et al. (2010). Pericardial disease: diagnosis and management. *Mayo Clinic Proceedings, 85,* 572–593.

Klein, A. L., Abbara, S., Agler, D. A., et al. (2013). American Society of Echocardiography clinical recommendations for multimodality cardiovascular imaging of patients with pericardial disease. *Journal of American Society Echocardiography, 26,* 965–1012.e15.

Little, W. C. (2006). Pericardial disease. *Circulation, 113,* 1622–1632.

A complete reference list can be found online at ExpertConsult.com.

34 Diseases of the Aorta

Eliza P. Teo, Eric M. Isselbacher

INTRODUCTION

An evaluation of the aorta is a routine part of the standard echocardiographic examination. Indeed, aortic pathology is often first discovered on an echocardiogram that was ordered for other indications.

ANATOMY, NOMENCLATURE, AND DIMENSIONS

The thoracic aorta is divided into four segments (Fig. 34.1), both because of anatomical distinctions and because they are affected differentially by conditions that affect the aorta. The aortic root is the most proximal segment, extending from the annulus of the aortic valve and extending to the sinotubular junction (STJ); and the aortic root is composed of the right, left, and noncoronary sinuses of Valsalva. The ascending thoracic aorta is tubular and extends from the STJ to the ostium of the innominate (brachiocephalic) artery. Many cardiologists and radiologists refer to the entire proximal aorta, both the root and ascending aorta, as the "aortic root." However, this is a misnomer, as only the segment below the STJ is truly the "root," and using the correct nomenclature is critical to communicate accurately and effectively regarding a given patient's aortic pathology. Both the aortic root and ascending aorta lie within the pericardial space, which means that the ascending aorta can be surrounded by pericardial fluid in the setting of an effusion; it also means that rupture of the ascending thoracic aorta can cause cardiac tamponade. The aortic arch extends from the proximal ostium of the innominate artery to just beyond the left subclavian artery at the ligamentum arteriosum. The normal aortic arch gives rise to the innominate (also known as brachiocephalic) artery, left common carotid, and left subclavian arteries. In a minority of patients, the innominate and left common carotid arteries arise as a common trunk in a conformation known as a "bovine arch." The descending thoracic aorta begins just distal to the origin of the left subclavian artery, courses distally under the pleura and just to the left of the vertebral column, and extends to the crux of the diaphragm. The abdominal aorta extends from the diaphragm to the aortic bifurcation; its proximal and distal portions are referred to as the suprarenal and infrarenal abdominal aorta, respectively.

Aortic Measurements and Dimensions

The diameter of the aorta decreases as it moves distally, and therefore each segment has a different range of normal diameters. Because the aorta is not a straight tube running from cephalad to caudal, axial imaging (computed tomography [CT] and magnetic resonance imaging [MRI]) often cuts the aorta obliquely, leading to an overestimate of its true diameter (Fig. 34.2). Even on echocardiography, the aorta can be imaged obliquely, so one must be careful to ensure that the aorta is measured along the axis perpendicular to its long axis (the axis of blood flow).

The aortic root diameter is typically measured in the parasternal long-axis (PLAX) view from the right-coronary sinus to the opposite sinus of Valsalva (usually the noncoronary sinus). It is occasionally difficult to obtain a long-axis image that shows both sinuses of Valsalva, in which case, the root may be measured more accurately in the parasternal short-axis view. However, there is not universal agreement about the optimal landmarks from which to measure the root diameter in short axis. Some experts advocate taking the diameter from the right coronary sinus to the opposite commissure (between the left- and noncoronary sinuses), whereas others advocate measuring to the more posterior of the opposite sinuses (Fig. 34.3); that latter method generally leads to a diameter measurement about 2 mm larger than the former. We prefer the sinus-to-sinus

approach, as it most closely approximates the diameter measurement made in the parasternal view, and it reflects the true maximal diameter that dictates maximal aortic wall stress according to the law of Laplace.

Measurements of the aortic root and ascending aorta are typically performed at end diastole, as this phase of the cardiac cycle demonstrates the resting aortic diameter; since the aorta is elastic, measurement at end systole can be several millimeters larger, especially in young people, as the aorta is actively distended by peak systolic pressure. In contrast, the aortic annulus is typically measured in mid-systole.

Historically, aortic root measurements had been made using M-mode echocardiography, and over several decades, multiple clinical and epidemiologic studies have used the M-mode leading-edge to leading-edge method. Multiple guidelines have reported normal limits based on this method and, consequently, the American Society of Echocardiography has also recommended using the leading-edge to leading-edge approach for measuring the aortic root.[1] However, measurements using two-dimensional images are preferred over M-mode images, as the latter may be off-axis and are subject to aortic motion during the cardiac cycle that may produce erroneous measurements. Moreover, harmonic imaging has improved the ability to visualize the blood-tissue interface, permitting more accurate inner-edge to inner-edge measurements (Fig. 34.4). It should be noted, however, that measurements made using the leading-edge to leading-edge method are approximately 2 mm larger than those made using the inner-edge to inner-edge method.[2] Regardless of the technique employed, echocardiography laboratories should use the same method consistently to allow accurate reporting of changes in aortic diameters over time. Complicating the issue further is the fact that in the interpretation of CT and MRI, many radiologists measure the aorta from outer-edge to outer-edge,[3] which results in a diameter about 1–2 mm larger than that obtained by echocardiography.

In adults, aortic dimensions are strongly correlated with age and body size. Because of the differential in body size, the aorta is on average 2 mm smaller in women compared to men;[4] and the upper limit of normal for the diameter of the aorta is defined as 2 standard deviations greater than the mean predicted diameter,[5] as shown in Table 34.1. More refined stratification by age and body surface area have been published by society consensus.[1]

For the more distal aortic segments, the upper limit of normal is approximately 3.6 cm for the aortic arch, 3.0 cm for the proximal descending thoracic aorta, and 2.0 cm for the distal descending thoracic aorta.

ECHOCARDIOGRAPHIC VIEWS

Transthoracic Echocardiography

Transthoracic echocardiography (TTE) can visualize the aortic root, proximal ascending aorta, aortic arch, and a short segment of the descending aorta. The aortic root and the proximal 4 cm of the ascending aorta are typically well seen on the PLAX view. However, positioning the transducer one rib space higher than the usual PLAX view may provide better visualization of the proximal ascending aorta. Moreover, in some patients, especially in the setting of ascending aorta dilatation, the right parasternal view (Fig. 34.5) may better image the mid and distal ascending thoracic aorta. The aortic arch and its branches are imaged from the suprasternal notch view. The proximal descending thoracic aorta can also be seen from the suprasternal notch view, but the mid-descending thoracic aorta is best imaged in short axis from the PLAX and apical four-chamber views and in long axis from the apical two-chamber view. From the subcostal view, the distal descending thoracic aorta and suprarenal abdominal aorta are usually well visualized.

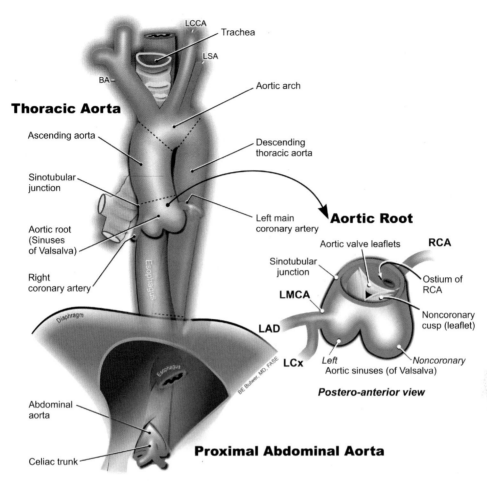

FIG. 34.1 Names and landmarks of the different segment of the aorta. *BA*, Brachiocephalic (innominate) artery; *LAD*, left anterior descending; *LCCA*, left common carotid artery; *LCx*, left circumflex; *LMCA*, left main coronary artery; *LSA*, left subclavian artery; *RCA*, right coronary artery. *(Courtesy of Bernard E. Bulwer, MD, FASE.)*

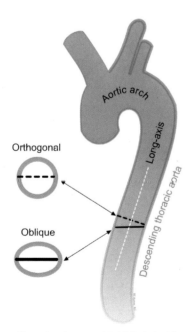

FIG. 34.2 Diagram illustrating the potential pitfall of obtaining an oblique imaging plane resulting in an ellipsoid cross section that overestimates the true diameter. This is particularly a problem when the descending aorta is tortuous. *(Courtesy of Bernard E. Bulwer, MD, FASE.)*

Transesophageal Echocardiography

The quality of TTE images of the aorta is limited by both the distance of the aorta from the transducer as well as acoustic interference by both ribs and lung. A clear advantage of transesophageal echocardiography (TEE)

is the close proximity of the esophagus to the aorta, such that the transducer is within several centimeters of the aorta and there is no acoustic interference, except for a "blind spot" where the interposition of the air-filled trachea and right main bronchus obstruct the view of the distal ascending thoracic aorta (Fig. 34.6).

From the mid-esophageal transducer position, the aortic root and proximal ascending aorta are well visualized in both short axis and long axis, typically at omniplane angles of 0–45 degrees and 90–135 degrees, respectively (Fig. 34.7A–D). Slight withdrawal of the probe then permits visualization of the mid-ascending thoracic aorta in both short and long axes, but further withdrawal of the probe leads to the blind spot, in which the airway obscures the distal ascending thoracic aorta.

The descending aorta is readily visualized from the left subclavian artery to the celiac trunk, because the esophagus is immediately adjacent to this portion of the aorta. However, the probe's proximity is sometimes a limitation in that it can be difficult to capture both side walls of the aorta within the one field of view because of the limited angle of beam (see Fig. 34.7E and F). The typical TEE exam of the descending thoracic aorta begins with imaging the most distal visible segment, followed by progressive withdrawal of the probe to image the mid- and then proximal segments.

The aortic arch is most easily visualized by slowly withdrawing the probe with the omniplane at 0 degrees after imaging the most proximal segment of the descending aorta. When the probe is withdrawn to most proximal segment of the descending aorta, the distal arch appears to the left of the screen, after which, rotating the probe clockwise and advancing slightly will reveal a long-axis view of the mid and distal arch. Following this, rotating the imaging plane to 90 degrees provides a short-axis view of the mid-arch. The ostia of the left common carotid and left subclavian arteries can usually be identified, but the proximal arch and ostium of the innominate artery are typically obscured by the blind spot and are thus not visible.

Aortic Root Diameters

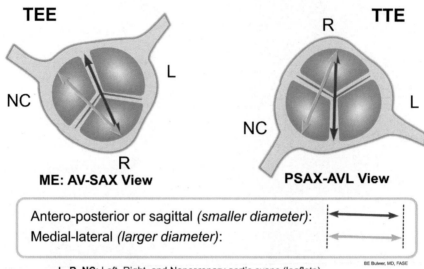

BE Bulwer, MD, FASE

L, R, NC: Left, Right, and Noncoronary aortic cusps (leaflets)
ME: AV-SAX: Mid-esophageal aortic valve short-axis
PSAX-AVL: Parasternal short-axis aortic valve level
TEE: Transesophageal echocardiography; **TTE:** Transthoracic echocardiography

FIG. 34.3 Methods of measuring the aortic root in the parasternal short-axis view. The aortic root diameter is typically about 2 mm larger when measured by the sinus-to-sinus *(blue arrow)* than by the sinus-to-commissure *(green arrow)* method. *(Courtesy of Bernard E. Bulwer, MD, FASE.)*

Aortic Diameter Measurements

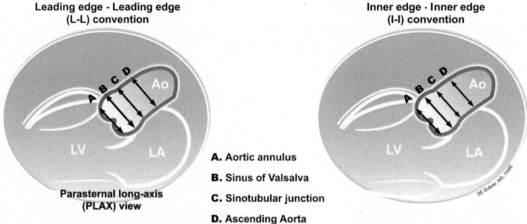

A. Aortic annulus

B. Sinus of Valsalva

C. Sinotubular junction

D. Ascending Aorta

FIG. 34.4 Transthoracic echocardiography (TTE) views of the aortic root and ascending thoracic aorta in which measurements are made at the level of the aortic annulus, sinuses of Valsalva, sinotubular junction, and ascending aorta. Measurements were performed using the leading-edge to leading-edge method on the left and inner-edge to inner-edge method on the right. *Ao*, Aorta; *LA*, left atrium; *LV*, left ventricle. *(Courtesy of Bernard E. Bulwer, MD, FASE.)*

Doppler Flows in the Aorta

To document flow profiles and velocities on TTE, Doppler interrogation is typically performed in the suprasternal or subcostal views. Normal antegrade systolic aortic flow has a brisk upstroke, with a peak velocity of approximately 1 m/s. Even in normal patients, the wave of antegrade systolic flow is typically followed by a brief and low-velocity wave of retrograde flow in early diastole (Fig. 34.8A) that is thought to result from reflection of the pressure wave by the distal arterial circulation.

Abnormal flow patterns may be seen in the setting of significant aortic valve or thoracic aortic disease. For example, holodiastolic flow reversal with an end-diastolic velocity of greater than 20 cm/s occurs in the setting of severe aortic regurgitation (see Fig. 34.8B).[6] A flow profile in the descending thoracic aorta that demonstrates a slow systolic upstroke followed by persistent antegrade diastolic flow occurs in the setting of significant coarctation of the aorta (see later discussion).

AORTIC ANEURYSMS

Thoracic aortic aneurysms are typically asymptomatic, and most produce no findings on physical exam. Consequently, the large majority of thoracic aortic aneurysms go undetected until discovered incidentally on imaging studies ordered for other indications. Aneurysms tend to involve primarily one segment of the aorta, such as the aortic root, ascending aorta, arch, or descending aorta, although some will extend from one segment into the next. Rarely, the entire thoracic aorta can be aneurysmal.

TABLE 34.1 Upper Limits of Normal for Diameters of the Aortic Root and Ascending Thoracic Aorta, Estimated From the Mean Diameter ± 2 Standard Deviations

	MEN (CM)	WOMEN (CM)	INDEXED FOR BSA (CM/M²) FOR BOTH MEN AND WOMEN
Sinus of Valsalva	4.0	3.6	2.1
Sinotubular junction	3.6	3.2	1.9
Proximal ascending aorta	3.8	3.5	2.1

BSA, Body surface area.
Adapted from Roman MJ, Devereux RB, Kramer-Fox R, O'Loughlin J. Two-dimensional echocardiographic aortic root dimensions in normal children and adults. Am J Cardiol. 1989;64(8):507–512.

The standard definition of an "aneurysm" is a vessel that is dilated to a diameter of 50% greater than an adjacent normal segment or the vessel's expected diameter for age and body size, and that definition applies well to most arteries, including the descending thoracic and abdominal aorta. However, that definition has not been used routinely for aneurysms of the aortic root and ascending thoracic aorta, because it would require that the aorta reach a diameter of close to 6.0 cm before being called an aneurysm, which makes little sense when the threshold for surgical repair is a diameter of just 5.0–5.5 cm. Consequently, most cardiologists and cardiac surgeons consider a dilated root or ascending thoracic aorta to be an "aneurysm" when it reaches a diameter of 4.5 cm or larger.

Most aortic aneurysms are *fusiform*, a shape in which the walls of the aorta bulge outward symmetrically (Fig. 34.9). Less common are *saccular* aneurysms, in which one wall of the aorta protrudes asymmetrically (Fig. 34.10). *Pseudoaneurysms* are rare, and unlike true aneurysms, they

Transthoracic Echocardiographic Views of the Aorta

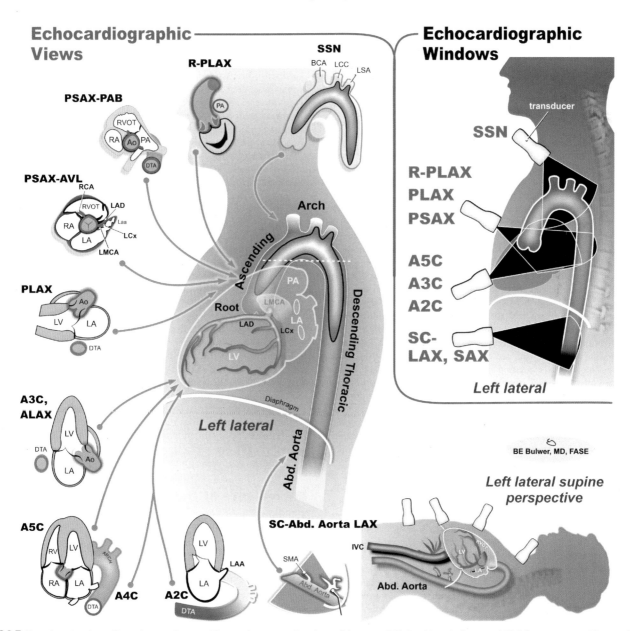

FIG. 34.5 Transthoracic echocardiography transducer positions and corresponding views of the aorta. *BCA,* Brachiocephalic artery; *LCC,* left common carotid artery; *LSA,* left subclavian artery, *SMA,* superior mesenteric artery. *(Courtesy of Bernard E. Bulwer, MD, FASE.)*

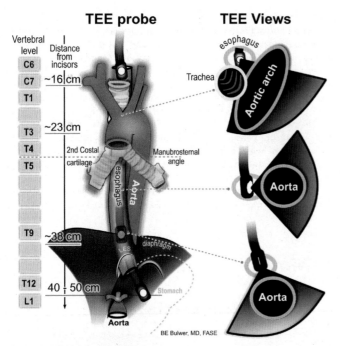

FIG. 34.6 Anatomic relationships of the esophagus, aorta, trachea, and bronchi. Interposition of the airways typically obstructs the imaging of the distal ascending aorta and proximal aortic arch. *LES,* Lower esophageal sphincter; *TEE,* transesophageal echocardiogram. *(Courtesy of Bernard E. Bulwer, MD, FASE.)*

result from a focal rupture of the aortic wall that is contained either by the remaining adventitia or by surrounding mediastinal structures. Most pseudoaneurysms arise at sites of penetrating atherosclerotic ulcers (see later Fig. 34.17), surgical anastomoses, or sites of prior surgical cannulation.

Of thoracic aortic aneurysms, those involving the aortic root or ascending aorta are most common (60%), followed by the descending aorta (40%), the aortic arch (10%), or the thoracoabdominal aorta (10%);[7] the percentages add up to greater than 100% because, although most aneurysms are localized, some extend across more than one segment, such as ascending aortic aneurysms that extend into the arch. Moreover, patients with aneurysms in one segment of the aorta may develop discrete aneurysms elsewhere in the aorta; consequently, when an aortic aneurysm is first detected, one should image the remainder of the thoracic and abdominal aorta to see that there are no unrecognized aneurysms elsewhere. However, given the limitations of echocardiographic imaging, surveillance of the entire aorta is best performed using either CT or MRI.

The most common known causes of aneurysms of the aortic root and/or ascending aorta are bicuspid aortic valve disease, familial thoracic aortic aneurysm syndrome, Marfan syndrome, and Turner syndrome. Less common connective tissue disorders, such as Loey-Dietz syndrome and Ehlers-Danlos syndrome type IV (vascular type), or systemic arteritides such as giant cell arteritis can cause aneurysms as well. However, the majority of ascending thoracic aortic aneurysms remain idiopathic. Marfan syndrome affects primarily the aortic root with relative sparing of the ascending thoracic aorta (Fig. 34.11A), but there is sometimes effacement of the STJ that produces pear-shaped aortic dilatation that is often referred to as *annuloaortic ectasia* (see Fig. 34.11B). In patients with bicuspid aortic valves, most often the ascending thoracic aorta alone is dilated (see Fig. 34.11C), less often the root alone is dilated, and in some cases, both the root and ascending aorta are dilated (see Fig. 34.11D).

Aneurysms of the aortic arch often arise from distal extension of an ascending aneurysm. When discrete aneurysms of the aortic arch do occur, they are often saccular or pseudoaneurysms. Descending thoracic aortic aneurysms often arise in the setting of chronic hypertension and atherosclerosis, and they commonly extend into the abdominal aorta (known as thoracoabdominal aortic aneurysms). Tertiary syphilis, now very rare, can cause aortitis and subsequent descending aortic aneurysms and dissections. Complex aneurysms of the distal arch and proximal descending aorta are often seen in patients with coarctation of the aorta and can even arise late after surgical repair.

Sinus of Valsalva Aneurysms

Sinus of Valsalva aneurysms can be congenital or acquired. A congenital sinus of Valsalva aneurysm is rare and can either be uniformly smooth (Video 34.1) or have a highly irregular and mobile "windsock" appearance (Fig. 34.12A). In the short-axis view, the affected sinus appears asymmetrically dilated, and ventricular septal defects (perimembranous and supracristal) can lead to acquired sinus of Valsalva defects. The aortic sinus (most commonly the right sinus) prolapses toward the septal defect in an attempt to close it; however, over time, an aneurysm forms. Aortic regurgitation commonly accompanies this due to malcoaptation of the aortic valve leaflets.

Most sinus of Valsalva aneurysms are asymptomatic and discovered incidentally on echocardiograms obtained for other indications, and some will present with aortic regurgitation. On occasion, the sinus of Valsalva aneurysm can compress a coronary artery and result in coronary insufficiency and ischemia. A sinus of Valsalva aneurysm can rupture and create a fistula into adjacent structures, but most often rupture occurs into the right atrium or right ventricle and less often into the left atrium. Color and continuous-wave Doppler imaging demonstrates continuous flow from the high-pressure aorta into the lower-pressured surrounding chambers (see Fig. 34.12B and C).

Associated Abnormalities

Aortic insufficiency (AI) frequently accompanies dilatation of the aortic root or ascending aorta. Although sometimes the AI can be due to underlying intrinsic aortic valve pathology (e.g., bicuspid aortic valve or senile degeneration of tricuspid valves), often the AI is actually secondary to the aortic dilatation itself. The aortic cusps are suspended from their commissures at the level of the STJ. When either the aortic root or ascending aorta dilates, the STJ widens and the aortic leaflets are pulled outward and become tethered. Such tethering keeps the leaflets from closing completely in diastole, resulting in a central orifice and a corresponding central jet of AI (Fig. 34.13).

Tethering of the aortic valve by the dilated aorta also reduces the cusps outward excursion in systole and produces a triangular-shaped orifice often referred to as the "triangle sign." If the echocardiographic findings suggest that the AI is secondary to incomplete aortic valve closure by a dilated aorta, then surgical repair of the aortic aneurysm with restoration of normal root geometry may well be all that is needed to restore effective leaflet cooptation and eliminate the AI, thus avoiding the need for aortic valve replacement.

In large aneurysms, especially those of the descending aorta, one may see spontaneous echo-contrast (often referred to as "smoke") swirling within the aortic lumen (Fig. 34.14A). Such spontaneous echo-contrast is due to slow flow through the dilated aortic segment. Slow flow occurs even in the setting of a normal cardiac output. Since the volume of blood flow through an aneurysm is effectively the same as flow through a normal aorta, and since blood flow = velocity × cross-sectional area, if the aneurysm diameter were twice normal, then its cross-sectional area would be four times normal; thus, the velocity of blood flow would fall to one-fourth normal. Consequently, systolic blood flow within a large aneurysm slows markedly. Furthermore, when blood stagnates against the wall of a dilated aorta, mural thrombus may form (see Fig. 34.14 and Video 34.2).

Surveillance of Thoracic Aortic Aneurysms

TTE can be used for surveillance imaging of aortic root aneurysms and is also often used for surveillance of aneurysms of the proximal-to-mid ascending thoracic aorta when the affected segments are adequately visualized. Although TEE provides better resolution of the ascending thoracic aorta, because it is a semiinvasive procedure, it is typically not preferred for surveillance imaging. Surveillance of aneurysms involving the aortic arch and descending thoracic aorta is usually undertaken with computed tomographic angiography (CTA) or magnetic resonance angiography (MRA).

When a dilated thoracic aorta is first discovered, repeat imaging is usually recommended in 6 months to confirm that the aneurysm is relatively stable rather than rapidly expanding. Assuming that there is no significant growth at 6 months, surveillance imaging can be performed

Short axis   Long axis

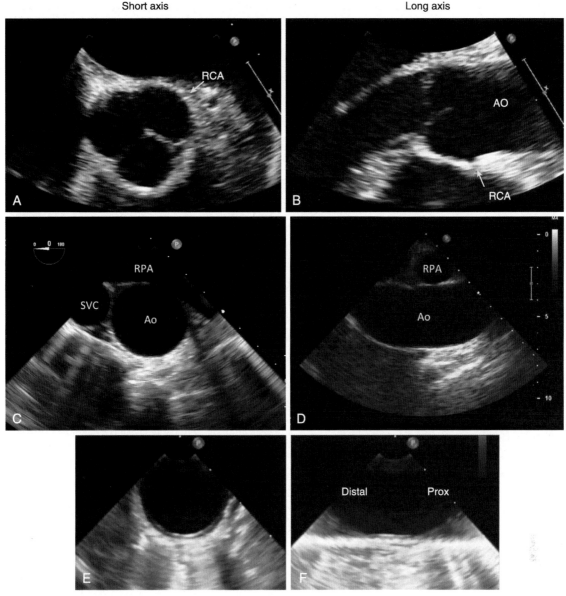

FIG. 34.7 **Transesophageal echocardiogram views of the thoracic aorta from the midesophageal transducer position. Left column are short-axis images, and the right column contains long-axis images.** (A and B) Aortic root (in diastole with closed leaflets). (C and D) Proximal ascending aorta. (E and F) Descending thoracic aorta. In the long-axis view of F, the near wall of the aorta is too close to the transducer to be well visualized. *Ao,* Aorta; *RCA,* ostium of the right coronary artery; *RPA,* right pulmonary artery; *SVC,* superior vena cava, as indicated by a *yellow arrow.*

annually thereafter. Moreover, when aortic growth is minimal over a number of years, the frequency of surveillance imaging can reasonably be decreased to every other (or even every third) year. Ideally surveillance imaging should be performed with the same technique and at the same center so that like images can be compared directly.[7]

AORTIC DISRUPTIONS (ACUTE AORTIC SYNDROMES)

Aortic dissection is a tear in the aortic intima that enables blood to force its way between the other layers of the vessel wall, forming an intimal flap that divides the aorta into a true and false lumen. Although dissection can arise in relatively normal-appearing aortas, it is associated with aortic aneurysm and shares the same risk factors, including connective tissue disorders, a personal or family history of aortic valve disease (particularly bicuspid valves), hypertension, smoking, and atherosclerosis. The acute aortic syndromes, including classical aortic dissection and its variants (below), typically present with acute severe chest or back pain and have high mortality rates (17%–26% early mortality in patients undergoing surgery). Rapid diagnosis is essential to proper management and can be

accomplished at the bedside by TEE, but more complete imaging may require CT or MRI (see Chapter 48).[8,9]

Aortic dissection is classified according to the location and extent of the dissection flap: Stanford type A involves the ascending aorta, and Stanford type B involves the descending aorta, that is from the origin of the left subclavian artery and distally. In the DeBakey classification, type I involves both ascending aorta and the arch and possibly beyond, type II involves the ascending aorta only, and type III the descending or thoracoabdominal aorta.

Echocardiography is often the first tool deployed to investigate for dissection in urgent circumstances, as it can be done by the bedside even on largely immobilized patients without the use of contrast agents. TTE allows visualization of the aortic root and proximal ascending aorta and ideally a portion of the arch, but only very limited sections of the descending thoracic and abdominal aorta. An example of a dissection flap (in a Marfan patient, postpartum) is shown in Video 34.3. Although the sensitivity is limited (70%–80% for all locations, with higher sensitivity in type A dissections), it can serve as a rapid bedside screening tool (with specificity of 63%–93%) and also allows one to look for associated AI or pericardial effusion. TEE is more invasive but allows higher-resolution images of a far greater percentage of the aorta. The sensitivity of TEE reaches 99% and specificity 89%, particularly with respect to type A dissections. TEE also has the advantage of allowing surgeons to examine the coronary ostia and great arteries and better determine the extent of the dissection flap.

Dissection tends to propagate anterograde from the proximal toward the distal aorta, and when the dissection flap enters the brachiocephalic, common carotid, or subclavian arteries, flow to the brain and arms may be compromised (see example in Video 34.4). However, retrograde extension may also occur all the way back to the sinuses, causing AI (see Video 34.5) or occlusion of coronary artery ostia (see Video 34.6). On TTE or TEE, the hallmark of aortic dissection is the presence of an independently mobile linear intimal flap, delineating a true lumen and false lumen. *Care should be taken to rule out artifacts*, such as linear reverberation in the aortic root (typically from the anterior wall of the left atrium or posterior wall of the right pulmonary artery), which can mimic a flap; this can be

assessed by M-mode echocardiography to document that the putative flap moves independently from the surrounding walls and additional orthogonal views to ensure that the putative flap respects true tissue borders. Occasionally, TEE is able to pinpoint one or more sites of communication between the lumina that may represent the entry or starting point of the dissection (Fig. 34.15F). Distinguishing true from false lumen takes on importance when it comes to determining which supplies the vessels to the brain, kidneys, limbs, and other viscera as flow off the false lumen may be reduced or obliterated by the flap or thrombosis. Furthermore, in cases such as aortography, surgery, or endovascular procedures, where one needs to cannulate the true lumen, it is crucial to distinguish which space a guidewire or catheter has entered to avoid propagating further dissection. Table 34.2 and Fig. 34.15 detail ways to differentiate the lumina on echocardiography. Importantly, size is not a distinguishing feature, and very often, the false lumen is much larger than the true lumen. The true lumen typically expands during systole, has antegrade flow during systole, and typically, flow by color Doppler will be seen to be from true to false lumen. The false lumen is more likely to contain organized thrombus, particularly in chronic dissections (see Fig. 34.15G).

Aortic dissection can also be iatrogenic rather than spontaneous in nature. Recent aortic manipulation—as occurs during cardiac catheterization, cardiac surgical bypass or placement of intraaortic balloon pumps, and intravascular stenting—puts the patient at risk. Blunt trauma is also responsible for cases of dissection, frank rupture, and even complete transection, and blunt trauma is typically from high-speed motor vehicle accidents in which there is sudden deceleration causing shear at the aortic isthmus (see Chapter 13).

There are other aortic syndromes that are considered variants of aortic dissection, and it is possible that they may coexist or evolve into one another: these include aortic intramural hematoma and penetrating aortic ulcer. TEE is clearly superior to TTE in diagnosing these entities. *Intramural hematoma* is a term that refers to blood or thrombus localized within the aortic wall medial layer without identified intimal injury. Video 34.6 shows an example in the ascending aorta. The intramural hematoma is distinguished from dissection in that there is no freely mobile intimal flap or blood flow through the intima and is distinguished from atherosclerotic plaque by its smooth contours (in long and short axes) and homogeneous swelling below the intima. It is possible that intramural hematoma represents either a precursor to aortic dissection or, alternatively, an aortic dissection with thrombosis of the false lumen and cryptic or healed intimal site of injury.

Penetrating aortic ulcer is a focal area of aortic injury that usually occurs within or at the edges of an atherosclerotic plaque, and an example is shown in Fig. 34.16 and Video 34.7. The disruption is a denuded area of intima with injury extending variably through the aortic wall layers, occasionally all the way through to the adventitia. There is occasionally associated thrombus layered on the lumenal side and/or subadventitial hematoma. Although the mechanisms by which aortic dissection,

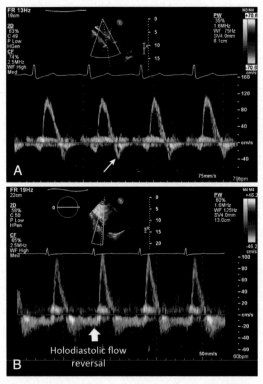

FIG. 34.8 Spectral Doppler flow profiles in the thoracoabdominal aorta from the subcostal position. (A) A normal flow profile with a rapid systolic upstroke followed by brief early-diastolic flow reversal *(arrow)*. (B) Evidence of holodiastolic flow reversal *(block arrow)* that is indicative of severe aortic regurgitation.

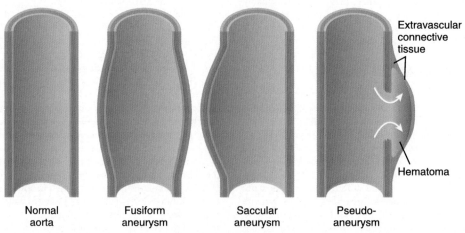

Types of aortic aneurysms

FIG. 34.9 Morphologic types of aortic aneurysms: fusiform, saccular, and pseudoaneurysms.

intramural hematoma, and penetrating aortic ulcer arise and their relationship to each other may overlap, all possess the risk for progressing to rupture; thus, the decision algorithms for pursuing medical versus surgical or endovascular surgery are similar.

A *pseudoaneurysm* of the native aorta occurs when there is a rupture through the aortic intima and media that is contained by either the remaining layer of adventitia or the surrounding mediastinal structures, resulting in a peri-aortic hematoma (see Fig. 34.9). Pseudoaneurysms can be caused by contained rupture of an aortic aneurysm or penetrating atherosclerotic ulcer, from a mycotic aneurysm or aortic paravalvular abscess, or by dehiscence of a surgical anastomosis or suture line. Pseudoaneurysms can also result from aortic transsection. They typically appear on echocardiography as a cavity adjacent to the aorta (Fig. 34.17) with little or sluggish flow by Doppler. The pseudoaneurysm cavity is

sometimes partially filled with thrombus and may pulsate a bit as blood from the aorta flows into and out of the cavity with each cardiac cycle.

PERIOPERATIVE AND POSTOPERATIVE IMAGING

To accurately and effectively interpret and communicate the findings of perioperative and postoperative echocardiographic images, it is essential that the echocardiographer be familiar with the various surgical aortic repair techniques and their appearance on imaging studies.

The most commonly performed thoracic aortic repair is replacement of an isolated aneurysm of the ascending thoracic aorta. The standard repair involves resecting the ascending aortic segment (above the STJ) and replacing it with an interposition Dacron tube graft (Fig. 34.18A). The presence of an ascending thoracic aortic graft can be difficult to

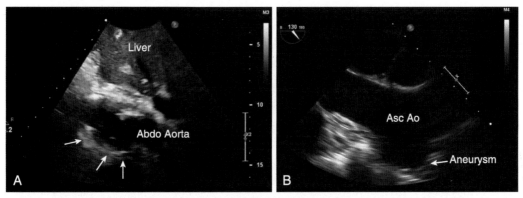

FIG. 34.10 Saccular aneurysms. (A) A subcostal transthoracic echocardiography (TTE) image showing a saccular aneurysm *(arrows)* of the suprarenal abdominal aorta. (B) A long-axis TEE view from the midesophageal position of the mid-ascending aorta demonstrating a saccular aneurysm *(arrow)* of unknown etiology.

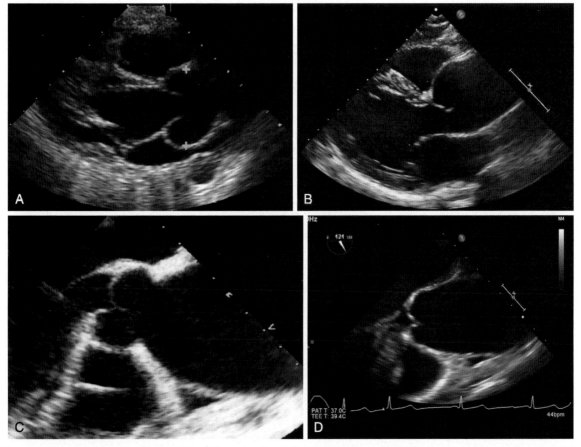

FIG. 34.11 Long-axis transesophageal echocardiogram views of the root and ascending thoracic aorta, demonstrating several aneurysm morphologies. (A) An isolated root aneurysm with sparing of the ascending thoracic aorta in a patient with Marfan syndrome. (B) A root aneurysm with effacement of the sinotubular junction (STJ) and dilatation of the proximal ascending thoracic aorta, producing pear-shaped aortic dilatation known as annuloaortic ectasia. (C) An ascending aortic aneurysm with complete sparing of the aortic root and preservation of a normal STJ. (D) Diffuse dilatation of both the root and ascending aorta.

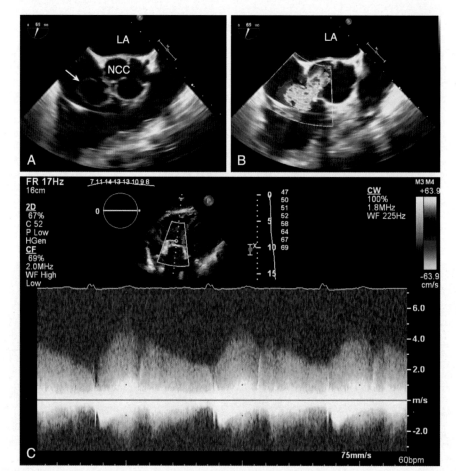

FIG. 34.12 A ruptured sinus of Valsalva aneurysm. (A) A short-axis transesophageal echocardiogram image from the midesophageal position demonstrating the aortic root with an aneurysm of the noncoronary sinus of Valsalva protruding as a windsock into the cavity of the right atrium *(arrow)*. (B) A similar image with color Doppler demonstrating brisk diastolic flow from the aortic root via the ruptured aneurysm and into the right atrium. (C) A subcostal TTE image demonstrating continuous (both systolic and diastolic) flow into the right atrium through the ruptured aneurysm. *LA,* Left atrium; *NCC,* noncoronary sinus of Valsalva.

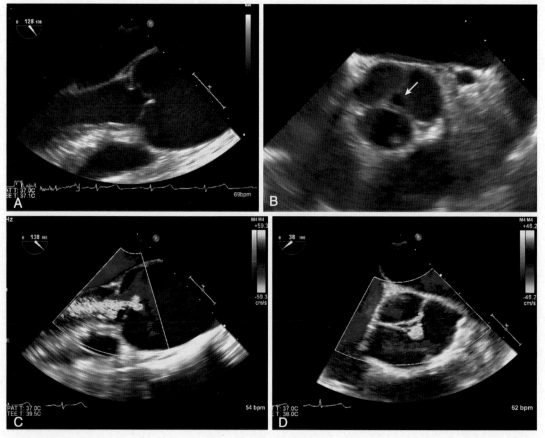

FIG. 34.13 Transesophageal echocardiogram long-axis views (on the left) and short-axis views (on the right) demonstrating aortic valve function. (A, B) 2D images showing incomplete aortic valve closure in diastole due to leaflet tethering, resulting in a diastolic orifice between the leaflets *(arrow)*. (C, D) Color Doppler images that demonstrate a centrally directed jet of moderate aortic insufficiency.

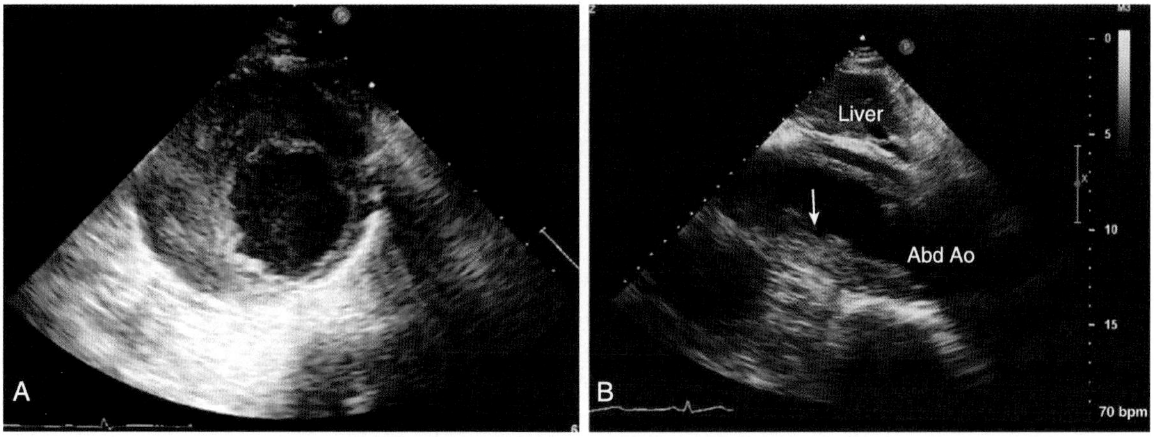

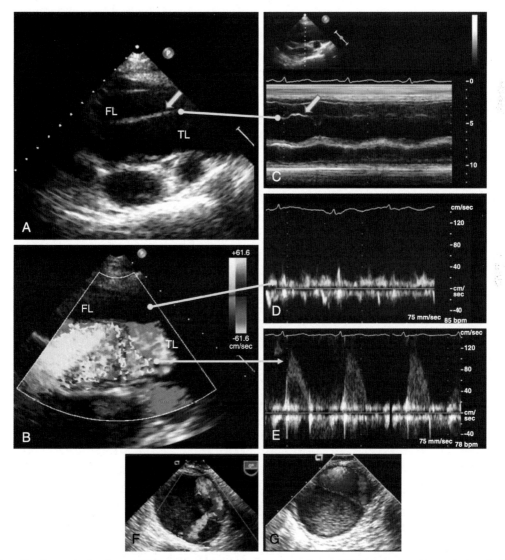

FIG. 34.14 **Consequences of the slow flow of blood through a thoracic aortic aneurysm.** (A) Transesophageal echocardiogram (TEE) image from the midesophageal position showing spontaneous echo-contrast ("smoke") within the lumen of a descending thoracic aortic aneurysm that is lined with mural thrombus. (B) TTE subcostal view showing extensive mural thrombus *(arrow)* along the posterior wall of a 5-cm thoracoabdominal aortic aneurysm.

FIG. 34.15 **Aortic dissection demonstrating true and false lumens.** (A) Transthoracic echocardiogram (TTE) high parasternal long-axis view of a type A aortic dissection. The linear dissection flap is indicated by the *arrow*. (B) TTE view at the same level with color flow Doppler illustrating brisk and turbulent color flow within the true lumen. (C) M-mode illustrating systolic pulsation of the dissection flap *(arrow)* outward from the true aortic lumen. (D) Low-velocity spectral Doppler flow without clear cyclical variation in the false lumen. (E) Systolic forward high-velocity spectral Doppler flow in the true lumen. (F) Transesophageal echocardiogram (TEE) short-axis view of the ascending aorta in a different type A dissection case demonstrating flow at an entry point into the false lumen by color Doppler. (G) TEE short-axis view of the ascending aorta showing spontaneous echocardiographic contrast in the false (larger) lumen and brisk systolic flow in the true (smaller) lumen by color Doppler. *FL,* False lumen; *TL,* true lumen. (*A–E, G from Solomon SD, Wu J, Gillam L. Echocardiography. In: Mann DL, Zipes DP, Libby P, et al., eds.* Braunwauld's Heart Disease: A Textbook of Cardiovascular Medicine. *10th ed. Philadelphia: Elsevier; 2015:234.*)

distinguish on transthoracic imaging, but is usually evident on transesophageal imaging because the graft material is ribbed, producing a beaded appearance to the aortic wall, and is more echogenic than the native aortic wall (Fig. 34.19A).

In the past, ascending thoracic aortic repair was sometimes performed using the inclusion technique, which involves insertion of an artificial tube graft that is then wrapped inside the retained diseased native aorta. This technique results in a potential space between the graft and native aorta that may, on follow-up imaging, mimic an aortic dissection or pseudoaneurysm.

The traditional surgical repair of an aneurysm aortic root involves resecting the native root as well as the aortic valve, because the valve is suspended within the root. This necessitates replacing both the aortic root and valve, which is accomplished by inserting a composite aortic graft (a single prosthesis with an artificial valve sewn onto the end of a graft), in what is known as the Bentall procedure. The two coronary arteries are then reanastomosed as tissue buttons onto the aortic root graft (see Fig. 34.18B). While this procedure is both effective and durable, it requires replacing the aortic valve in many cases in which the valve itself is not diseased. In the modern era, when patients have aortic root aneurysms

but an otherwise healthy aortic valve, the aneurysm can be replaced while sparing the valve by resuspending the native valve within the prosthetic aortic graft using a procedure known as a valve-sparing root repair, and the most common of which is called the David-procedure (see Fig. 34.18C). When performing a perioperative TEE during this procedure, following cardiopulmonary bypass, it is essential for the echocardiographer to document normal aortic valve function with little or no AI.

Aneurysms of the ascending thoracic aorta often extend into the proximal aortic arch. When repairing the ascending thoracic aorta, it is therefore ideal to remodel the dilated proximal arch as well. To accomplish this without having to perform a total aortic arch replacement, surgeons often repair the underside of the proximal arch by beveling the distal prosthetic graft; this technique is known as a hemiarch repair (see Fig. 34.18D). When the mid or distal aortic arch is also abnormal, a total aortic arch replacement is preferred. This is most often performed using a branched graft and sewing individual anastomoses to each of the arch's branch arteries (see Fig. 34.18E). When the aneurysmal disease extends beyond the arch and into the descending thoracic aorta, surgeons will often add an additional segment of graft to the distal anastomosis of the arch graft and let that segment dangle within the dilated descending aorta. Such a segment of graft is referred to as an elephant trunk and can be used at a later date either to permit the surgeon to cross clamp the proximal aortic segment during an open descending aortic repair or to serve as a proximal landing zone for a thoracic endovascular stent-graft repair. On echocardiography, an elephant trunk can mimic an aortic dissection, because the aorta appears to have an inner and an outer wall (see Fig. 34.19A) and there is a differential color Doppler flow profile on the inside and outside of the intraluminal prosthetic graft. Indeed, thrombus can even from between the native aortic wall and the elephant trunk near its proximal anastomosis, mimicking thrombus formation within a false lumen (see Fig. 34.19B). The well-defined tubular shape of elephant trunk and the ribbed texture of the prosthetic graft wall are the key findings that distinguish it from a true aortic dissection.

Aneurysms of the descending thoracic aorta can be repaired surgically. This is usually performed with an interposition aortic graft that is then wrapped by the native descending thoracic aortic tissue (see Fig. 34.18G) to protect the graft and reduce the risk of fistulae to the esophagus, trachea,

TABLE 34.2 Differentiation Between True and False Lumina

	TRUE LUMEN	FALSE LUMEN
Size	True < false	Most often: false > true lumen
Pulsation	Systolic expansion	Systolic compression
Flow direction	Systolic antegrade flow	Systolic antegrade flow reduced or absent, or retrograde flow
Communication flow	From true to false lumen in systole	
Contrast echo flow	Early and fast	Delayed and slow

From Evangelista A, Flachskampf FA, Erbel R, et al. Echocardiography in aortic diseases: EAE recommendations for clinical practice. Eur Heart J Cardiovasc Imaging. 2010;11(8):645–658.

Short axis   Long axis

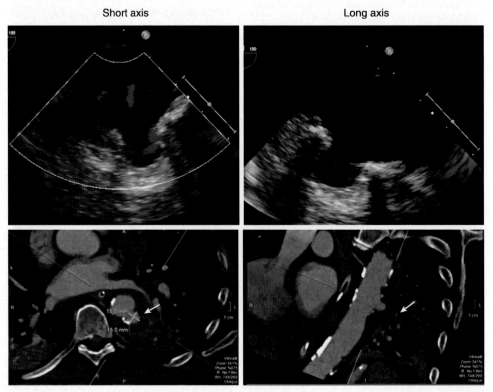

FIG. 34.16 Penetrating aortic ulcers in the descending thoracic aorta on transesophageal echocardiogram *(upper panels)* and CT angiography *(lower panels)*. The left panels illustrate short-axis or cross-sectional views, and the right panels illustrate long-axis or sagittal views of a 1.5-cm penetrating aortic ulcer *(arrows)* occurring in the region of calcified plaque in a dilated segment of the descending thoracic aorta.

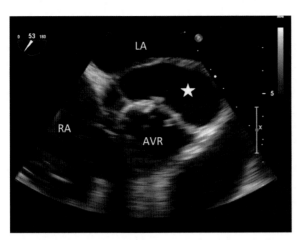

FIG. 34.17 Abscess and pseudoaneurysm. A transesophageal short-axis view of the aortic root in a patient with endocarditis of a bioprosthetic valve (AVR) with an associated aortic root abscess; the abscess has broken down and formed a large pseudoaneurysm *(star)* posterior to the root and ascending aorta that communicates with the aortic root above the sewing ring. *LA,* Left atrium; *RA,* right atrium.

or bronchus. In recent years, an increasing percentage of descending aortic aneurysms are being repaired using thoracic endovascular stent-grafting, which is commonly referred to as thoracic endovascular stent-grafting or TEVAR (see Fig. 34.18H). Sometimes endovascular surgeons will perform such stent-graft repairs under TEE guidance.

Postoperative Imaging

Following aortic valve replacement or aortic root surgery, postoperative echocardiographic imaging typically reveals soft tissue thickening of up to 10 mm around the aortic root, and the thickening may persist up to 3 months (Fig. 34.20). If one were unaware of a patient's early postoperative status, it could be difficult to differentiate such normal postoperative thickening from true peri-aortic pathology such as a peri-graft infection. However, normal postoperative thickening appears homogeneous, is not associated with other echocardiographic evidence of infection or dehiscence, and improves over time, whereas thickening due to a peri-graft infection tends to be heterogeneous in appearance and the thickening increases over time. Hence, obtaining baseline images even after uncomplicated surgery may be expedient.

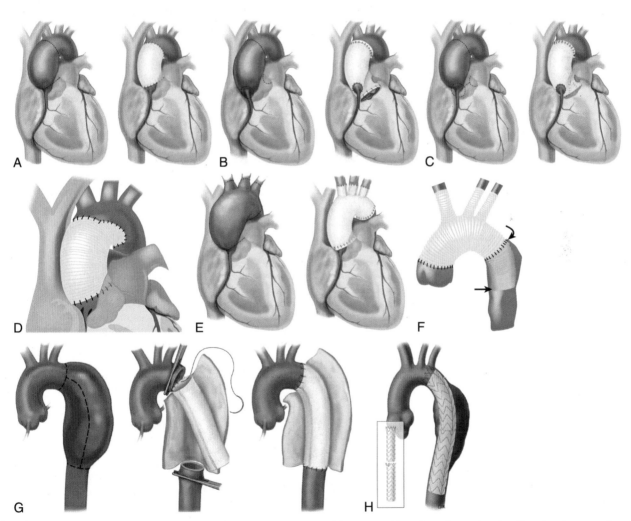

FIG. 34.18 Surgical procedures for repair of various thoracic aortic aneurysms. (A) An interposition tube graft to replace the affected aortic segment in an isolated ascending thoracic aortic aneurysm. (B) A composite aortic graft (a prosthetic aortic valve initially sewn to a Dacron tube graft before insertion) to repair a dilated aortic root and adjacent segment of the ascending aorta, with the coronary arteries reimplanted as tissue buttons. (C) Valve-sparing root repair using the David technique to replace a diseased aortic root with a tube graft but then resuspending the native aortic valve within the tube graft. (D) Ascending thoracic aortic replacement with a hemiarch repair in which a beveled distal tongue of graft material replaces a portion of the underside of the aortic arch. (E) Total arch replacement in which each of the branch vessels is anastomosed to separate branches off the arch graft. (F) Total arch repair with an elephant trunk, which is an additional segment of tube graft attached to the distal arch anastomosis *(curved arrow)* and left dangling *(straight arrow)* within the lumen of the dilated descending thoracic aorta to facilitate subsequent distal repair procedures. (G) Surgical graft replacement of a descending thoracic aortic aneurysm, in which the native aortic wall is wrapped around the graft following repair to protect the graft reduces the risk of postoperative complications. (H) Thoracic endovascular stent-graft repair of a descending thoracic aortic aneurysm using two interlocking stent-graft segments. *(A–C, E, G, H copyright Massachusetts General Hospital Thoracic Aortic Center, used with permission.)*

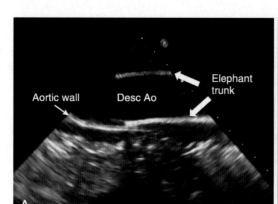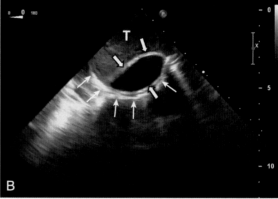

FIG. 34.19 Transesophageal echocardiogram images of the distal segments of elephant trunk grafts. (A) Long-axis view of the descending thoracic aorta with the elephant trunk graft (note its ribbed appearance) dangling within the aortic lumen, with the distal end of the graft (toward the left) free and unattached. (B) Short-axis view of the proximal descending thoracic aorta with an elephant trunk *(block arrows)* inside the lumen of the descending thoracic aorta *(narrow arrows)* with thrombus (T) having formed in the space between the two.

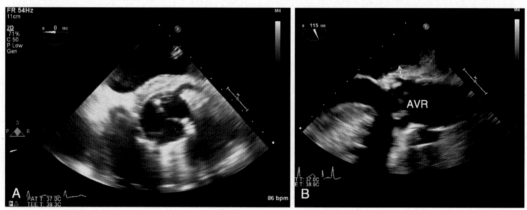

FIG. 34.20 Intraoperative short- (A) and long-axis (B) transesophageal echocardiogram images after coming off cardiopulmonary bypass following surgical aortic valve replacement with a pericardial prosthetic valve (AVR). The aortic root appears thickened up to 7 mm *(arrow)*. Thickening up to 10 mm is accepted as within the expected postoperative range.

INTRALUMINAL PATHOLOGY

Atheroma

Aortic atheromas, also known as "atheromata," result from an accumulation of lipids, macrophages, connective tissue, and calcium within the intimal layer of the aortic wall. Such collections begin as atherosclerotic plaques that line the wall of the aorta, but they can subsequently grow and bulge into the aortic lumen to form "protruding atheromas" (Fig. 34.21). Moreover, on TEE imaging, some atheromas will have mobile components that protrude even further into the lumen (see Fig. 34.21B and Video 34.8); it is believed that these mobile components represent thrombus superimposed on the underlying atherosclerotic plaque. TEE produces high-resolution images of the intimal surface of the thoracic aorta and is therefore the modality of choice to assess the location, size, severity, and mobility of aortic atheromas.

The thickness of a healthy intimal layer is normally ≤1 mm; consequently, an irregular intima with a thickness of ≥2 mm is considered to be an atheroma.[1] The presence of aortic atheromas with a thickness of greater than 4 mm is associated with increased risk of embolic events.[10] The presence of superimposed mobile components further increases the risk of embolization. A grading systems exists (Table 34.3) that classifies atheromas based on maximal thickness and the presence of mobile or ulcerated components, assigning them a grade of 1–5.[1] However, many find it easier to use a descriptive scale, ranging from mild to complex. When significant atheromas are present, the echocardiography report should comment on location, the atheroma thickness, and the presence of mobile segments.

Aortic Thrombus

Mural thrombus is a common finding in descending thoracic aortic, particularly in ectatic and aneurysmal portions, as discussed previously with aneurysms (and shown in Fig. 34.14).

Rarely, primary thrombi form in patients with seemingly normal aortas, that is, with no evidence of aneurysm, atheromatous disease, penetrating atherosclerotic ulcer, or other pathology. They appear most commonly in the proximal descending thoracic aorta,[11] but they can also arise in the ascending thoracic aorta or arch. The thrombi tend to be large (≥1 cm), pedunculated, and mobile (Fig. 34.22), and therefore quite distinct from the laminated mural thrombus commonly seen in the setting of large thoracic aortic aneurysms. Patients are most often asymptomatic until they present with symptoms or signs of peripheral embolization. The etiology of such thrombi is uncertain, and hypercoagulability workups are usually negative. Fortunately, the thrombi invariably resolve with systemic anticoagulation.

Aortic Tumors

Aortic tumors are rare and typically present with embolic or obstructive phenomena, and the tumors may be primary or secondary: Primary aortic tumors are mesenchymal in origin and include angiosarcoma, histiocytoma, intimal sarcoma, leiomyosarcoma, and undifferentiated sarcoma; secondary tumors arise either from direct invasion by neighboring cancers (Fig. 34.23) or as secondary metastases from tumors of the lung or esophagus. Intraluminal tumors appear polypoid on imaging and can mimic protruding atheromas or thrombi. Invasive tumors may encase the aorta and can affect the periaortic tissues and surrounding organs.

COARCTATION OF THE AORTA

Coarctation of the aorta is a congenital anomaly in which a short segment of the descending aorta is narrowed at the region of the ligamentum arteriosum. It is commonly associated with a bicuspid aortic valve, subaortic membrane, mitral valve abnormalities (such as parachute mitral

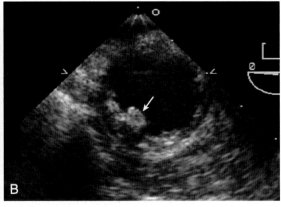

FIG. 34.21 Transesophageal echocardiogram short-axis images of the descending thoracic aorta demonstrating atheromas. (A) Atheromas up to 5 mm in thickness but without evidence of mobile elements. (B) Protruding atheromas with a superimposed mobile element *(arrow)*.

TABLE 34.3 Grades of Aortic Atheromas

GRADE	MAXIMAL ATHEROMA THICKNESS	DESCRIPTIVE SCALE
1	<2 mm	Normal
2	2–3 mm	Mild
3	>3–5 mm, no mobile or ulcerated elements	Moderate
4	>5 mm, no mobile or ulcerated elements	Severe
5	Grade 2, 3 or 4 with mobile or ulcerated elements	Complex

Modified from Goldstein SA, Evangelista A, Abbara S, et al. Multimodality imaging of diseases of the thoracic aorta in adults: from the American Society of Echocardiography and the European Association of Cardiovascular Imaging: endorsed by the Society of Cardiovascular Computed Tomography and Society for Cardiovascular Magnetic Resonance. J Am Soc Echocardiogr. 2015;28(2):119–182.

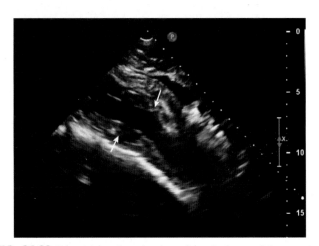

FIG. 34.23 Subcostal transthoracic echocardiography image of the suprarenal abdominal aorta demonstrating secondary tumor invasion of the aorta *(arrows)* in a patient with extensive B-cell lymphoma.

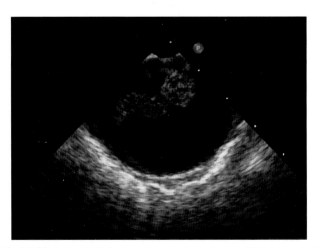

FIG. 34.22 A short-axis transesophageal echocardiogram (TEE) image of the descending thoracic aorta demonstrating a pedunculated, highly mobile, 3 cm × 1 cm mass consistent with an intraluminal thrombus. The patient had presented with acute left flank pain and was diagnosed by CTA with a splenic infarct. The patient was treated with anticoagulation and a repeat TEE several weeks later showed a normal underlying aortic wall with no evidence of residual thrombus.

valve), ventricular septal defect, and varying degrees of arch hypoplasia.[12] Unrecognized hemodynamically significant coarctation is rare in adults older than the age of 40 because the unoperated survival is 35 years of age with 75% mortality by 46 years of age.[12]

The diagnosis of coarctation of the aorta is readily made by TTE with two-dimensional (2D) and Doppler imaging. In the suprasternal view, when the aortic arch is imaged in its long axis, there is typically a discrete narrowing of the aortic lumen, with a shelf-like appearance, just distal to the origin of the left subclavian artery (Fig. 34.24A). Color

Doppler interrogation of the descending thoracic aorta demonstrates flow acceleration and turbulence at the site of coarctation (see Fig. 34.24B). Continuous-wave Doppler at the site reveals increased peak and mean gradients (see Fig. 34.24C). Pulsed-wave Doppler interrogation, performed in a stepwise fashion along the affected descending thoracic aorta, can demonstrate the level of coarctation.

Doppler flow profiles of the abdominal aorta are useful not only as supportive evidence, but also in screening for unsuspecting coarctation. A normal pulsed-Doppler profile demonstrates laminar flow with a rapid systolic upstroke and little forward flow into diastole (see Fig. 34.8A). Conversely, accompanying significant coarctation is turbulent rather than laminar flow, a delay in the systolic Doppler upstroke, and a continuation of antegrade flow into or through diastole (see Fig. 34.24D); such holodiastolic "runoff" is pathognomonic of a hemodynamically significant coarctation.

A minority of patients with severe coarctation develop sizeable collaterals as a means to physiologically bypass the aortic obstruction. In such cases, the Doppler gradients across the coarctation will likely be falsely low because of reduced volume of antegrade flow across the narrowed aortic lumen, which in turn can lead to an underestimate of the true severity of the obstruction. Abnormal flow via collaterals may be detected with color and pulsed-wave Doppler.

Some patients with thoracic aortic disease present with a long tubular narrowing of the descending aorta without a discrete obstruction, and although such narrowings can cause flow acceleration and increased peak velocities, strictly speaking, they are not considered to be true coarctations of the aorta.

When performing and interpreting echocardiograms in patients with coarctation of the aorta, measurements of the aortic root, ascending aorta, and aortic arch should be reported. The morphology of the aortic valve should be determined, and the left ventricular size, systolic function, and

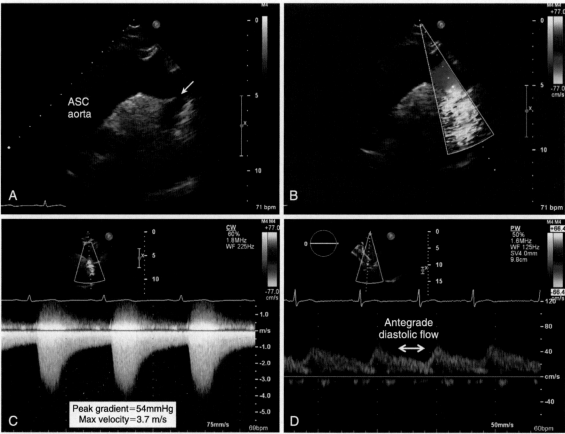

FIG. 34.24 **Transthoracic echocardiography imaging of a significant coarctation of the aorta just distal to the origin of the subclavian artery.** (A) In the suprasternal notch view, there is a visible shelf-like narrowing the aortic lumen. (B) In the same view, there is turbulence demonstrated by color Doppler at the level of the coarctation. (C) In the same view, interrogation with continuous-wave Doppler demonstrates an increased peak gradient of 54 mm Hg across the coarctation. (D) Spectral Doppler of the descending aorta from the subcostal position demonstrating a slow systolic upstroke as well as persistent antegrade diastolic flow, consistent with a hemodynamically significant coarctation.

mass should be assessed. One should also inspect for evidence of associated abnormalities, such as ventricular septal defect and parachute mitral valve. Targeted stress echocardiography to document gradients both at rest and with stress can be helpful in clinical decision making.

Patients with mild degrees of coarctation should undergo annual surveillance by TTE to monitor for changes in the gradients and aortic anatomy. Following coarctation repair, TTE is used most often for routine surveillance to detect recurrent coarctation, which is not uncommon; since it can be difficult to visualize the site of repair by 2D imaging, the use of spectral Doppler to measure gradients plays a vital role. Another potential late complication following coarctation repair is the appearance of pseudoaneurysms at the sites of surgical patch repairs or

anastomoses, and such pseudoaneurysms are better detected and defined by CTA or MRA.

Suggested Reading

Beretta, P., Patel, H. J., Gleason, T. G., et al. (2016). IRAD experience on surgical type A acute dissection patients: results and predictors of mortality. *Annals of Cardiothoracic Surgery, 5,* 346–351.

Evangelista, A., Flachskampf, F. A., Erbel, R., et al. (2010). Echocardiography in aortic diseases: EAE recommendations for clinical practice. *European Heart Journal Cardiovascular Imaging, 11,* 645–658.

Goldstein, S. A., Evangelista, A., Abbara, S., et al. (2015). Multimodality imaging of diseases of the thoracic aorta in adults: From the American Society of Echocardiography and the European Association of Cardiovascular Imaging: endorsed by the Society of Cardiovascular Computed Tomography and Society for Cardiovascular Magnetic Resonance. *Journal of the American Society of Echocardiography, 28*(2), 119–182.

A complete reference list can be found online at ExpertConsult.com

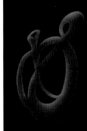

DISEASES OF THE PULMONARY ARTERY AND VEINS

35 Pulmonary Embolism

Scott D. Solomon

INTRODUCTION

Pulmonary embolism (PE) is associated with substantial morbidity and mortality, accounting for over 50,000 deaths per year in the United States. PE coexists with other cardiac and pulmonary diseases and remains a diagnosis that continues to elude clinicians. Indeed, PE has been called "the great masquerader" because the signs and symptoms of PE mimic that of other diseases. The emergence of interventional strategies that remove or dissolve thrombus, including thrombolysis and surgical or suction embolectomy, makes accurate diagnosis and risk stratification in PE essential. PE is generally a consequence of thrombi that form in the deep veins, which have the potential to migrate to the right side of the heart and lodge in the pulmonary vasculature. Thus, PE is a subset of thromboembolic disease and venous thromboembolism disease, and PEs need to be viewed as a continuum.

UTILITY OF ECHOCARDIOGRAPHY IN PULMONARY EMBOLISM

Echocardiography can be extremely helpful in the diagnosis and management of acute PE, and there are several characteristic echocardiographic features in acute PE (Box 35.1). While generally not used as the primary method to diagnose PE—a role reserved for spiral computed tomography (CT) and ventilation/perfusion scanning—echocardiography provides supportive information to complement other diagnostic tests in this disorder. Nevertheless, echocardiography can often be the first imaging test obtained in patients with acute PE, as it is commonly used as a screening test to determine the etiology of nonspecific signs and symptoms. Indeed, echocardiography can be used to distinguish PE from other causes of chest pain, shortness of breath, and hypotension, such as myocardial infarction, tamponade, and aortic dissection.

Identification of Thrombus by Echocardiography

Thrombi that result in PE generally arise from the deep venous system in the legs (Fig. 35.1), although they can form de novo in the right side of the heart. Echocardiography can visualize thrombus in the venous system anywhere from the vena cava through the proximal pulmonary arteries. All masses in the heart that might represent potential thrombi need to be distinguished from other cardiac masses, including myxomas, fibroelastomas, and other cardiac tumors (see Chapter 39). Thrombi in the pulmonary arteries (Fig. 35.2) can generally be visualized to approximately just past the bifurcation with transthoracic echocardiography (TTE), and somewhat further with transesophageal echocardiography (TEE). Thrombi from the deep venous system of the legs tend to be linear in appearance, although can dissociate and become more rounded, and can be visualized extending from the inferior vena cava (Fig. 35.3 and Video 35.1), in the right atrium (Fig. 35.4 and Video 35.2), right ventricle (RV) (Fig. 35.5 and Video 35.3), or pulmonary outflow tract (Figs. 35.6–35.8

and Videos 35.4–35.6). It is not uncommon for so-called saddle emboli to become lodged at the bifurcation (see Figs. 35.6–35.8 and Videos 35.4–35.6), and the pulmonary artery bifurcation should be carefully assessed from the short-axis views in patients with suspected PE.

Assessment of the Right Ventricle in Pulmonary Embolism

Beyond identification of thrombus in the right side of the heart, echocardiography is particular useful in assessing the effect of PE on cardiac function, particularly right ventricular function. The unique physiology of the RV (see Chapter 16) contributes to the characteristic echocardiographic findings in PE. The normal RV, generally accustomed to low pulmonary vascular resistance, and hence very low afterload, needs only to generate relatively low pressures (normal right ventricular systolic pressures are generally no higher than about 25 mm Hg; Fig. 35.9, *left panel*). In the

---

BOX 35.1 Echocardiographic Features in Pulmonary Embolism

Right ventricular dilatation
Right ventricular dysfunction (global and regional)
Normal or hyperdynamic left ventricular function
Paradoxic septal motion, interventricular septal flattening
Tricuspid regurgitation
Pulmonary artery dilatation
Attenuation of normal inspiratory collapse of inferior vena cava
Decrease in right ventricular fractional area change

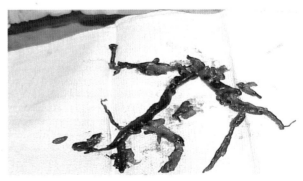

FIG. 35.1 Thrombi arising from the deep veins of the legs after extraction from pulmonary artery.

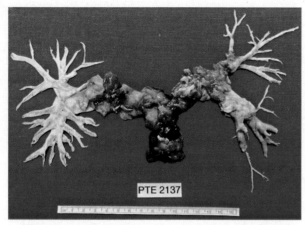

FIG. 35.2 Thrombi in pulmonary artery at autopsy. *(From Jaff MR, McMurtry MS, Archer SL, et al. Management of massive and submassive pulmonary embolism, iliofemoral deep vein thrombosis, and chronic thromboembolic pulmonary hypertension: a scientific statement from the American Heart Association. Circulation. 2011;123(16):1788–1830.)*

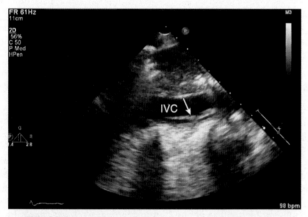

FIG. 35.3 Linear embolus *(arrow)* in the inferior vena cava (IVC).

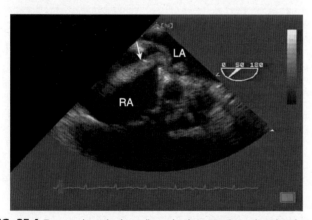

FIG. 35.4 Transesophageal echocardiography demonstrating a thrombus *(arrow)* passing through a patent foramen ovale between the right atrium (RA) and left atrium (LA) in a patient who had both a pulmonary embolism and a stroke.

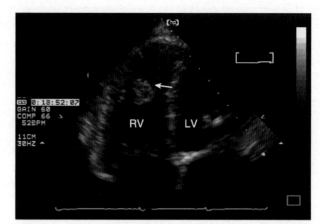

FIG. 35.5 Round thrombus *(arrow)* in the right ventricle (RV). *LV,* Left ventricle.

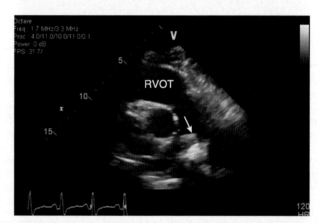

FIG. 35.6 Saddle embolus *(arrow)* in the right ventricular outflow tract (RVOT) at the bifurcation of the pulmonary arteries in a parasternal short-axis view.

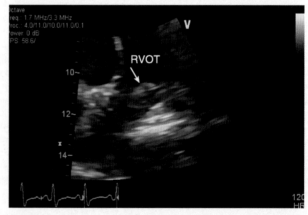

FIG. 35.7 Close-up view of pulmonary bifurcation saddle embolism *(arrow)* seen in Fig. 35.6. *RVOT,* Right ventricular outflow tract.

setting of acute PE, pulmonary vascular resistance rises abruptly and substantially, resulting in RV dilatation and, in severe cases, RV failure (see Fig. 35.9, *right panel*). The right ventricular dilatation and dysfunction that can occur in this setting can result in reduced right ventricular cardiac output, which can in turn lead to a reduction in left ventricular preload, and ultimately a reduction in cardiac output, with resultant hypotension. Hypotension can lead to reduced coronary perfusion, which can contribute to ischemia or even infarction of the RV. Moreover, increased right ventricular afterload can lead to an increase in right ventricular wall stress, which can increase RV myocardial oxygen demand. The combination of increased oxygen demand and reduced oxygen supply can lead to further RV dysfunction (Fig. 35.10).

RV dilatation is the echocardiographic hallmark of PE. This is best visualized from the apical four-chamber view where classic findings include RV diameter greater than left ventricle (LV) diameter, relatively normal LV function, with a small underfilled LV. While right ventricular diameter in the apical four-chamber view is rarely greater than 2.7 cm in normal individuals, these measures can vary widely, and a good rule of thumb is to compare right ventricular diameter to left ventricular diameter in the mid-ventricular regions and the apical four-chamber views.

Regional Right Ventricular Dysfunction: The "Mcconnell" Sign

A distinctive regional wall motion abnormality has been recognized in acute PE in which the RV mid free wall becomes dyskinetic, with relative sparing of the apex and the base. This pattern, alternatively known as the

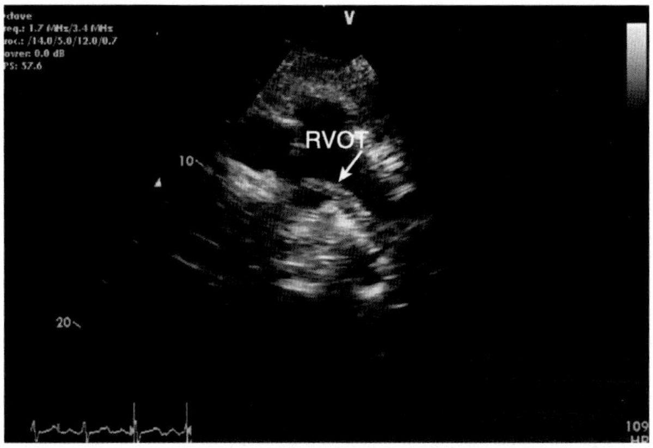

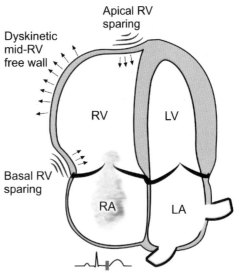

FIG. 35.8 Linear thrombus *(arrow)* at the bifurcation of the pulmonary arteries. *RVOT,* Right ventricular outflow tract.

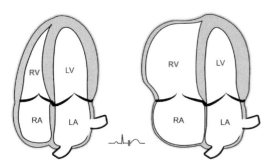

Normal Right Ventricle (RV)   Right Ventricle post pulmonary embolism

FIG. 35.9 Schematic of normal right ventricle *(left panel)* and right ventricle after pulmonary embolism *(right panel)*. Notice the severe right ventricular dilatation. *LA,* Left atrium; *LV,* left ventricle; *RA,* right atrium; *RV,* right ventricle.

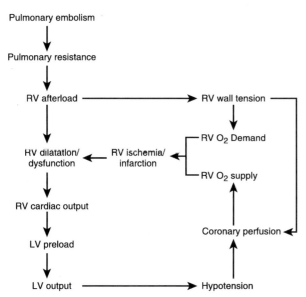

FIG. 35.10 Pathophysiology of acute pulmonary embolism. See text. *LV,* Left ventricle; *O₂,* oxygen; *RV,* right ventricle. *(Adapted from Lualdi JC, Goldhaber SZ. Right ventricular dysfunction after acute pulmonary embolism: pathophysiologic factors, detection, and therapeutic implications. Am Heart J. 1995;130(6):1276–1282.)*

right ventricular strain pattern or McConnell sign (Figs. 35.11–35.13; Videos 35.7–35.10), is visually quite characteristic and recognizable. It is highly specific for acute PE, although can be seen rarely in other conditions in which pulmonary vascular resistance increases abruptly, such as acute pneumonia or interstitial lung disease. Nevertheless, acute PE remains the predominant condition in which the "McConnell sign" is seen.

FIG. 35.11 Regional right ventricular dysfunction in acute pulmonary embolism (McConnell sign). Note dyskinesis of mid right ventricular free wall *(blue arrows)* and relative sparing of the apex and the base *(green arrows)*. *LA,* Left atrium; *LV,* left ventricle; *RA,* right atrium; *RV,* right ventricle.

The Influence of Elevated Pulmonary Pressures on Echocardiographic Features in Pulmonary Embolism

The characteristic findings of right ventricular dilatation and dysfunction in acute PE are most apparent in patients with previously normal RVs that have not been chronically exposed to high pulmonary pressures. In patients with chronic thromboembolic disease, these findings can be obscured to some extent as right ventricular hypertrophy (RVH), and will compensate for chronically elevated right ventricular afterload. Thus, both RV dilatation and RV regional dysfunction will be less apparent in patients in whom pulmonary vascular resistance has been elevated for a longer period of time. In these patients, the RV hypertrophies and pulmonary pressures will ultimately rise, and the RV may not show evidence of dilatation or dysfunction in the setting of PE. Thus, these echocardiographic findings are less likely to be useful in patients with long-standing pulmonary hypertension, chronic obstructive pulmonary disease (COPD), or chronic thromboembolic disease in which pulmonary hypertension has been long-standing.

In patients without prior history of pulmonary hypertension, pulmonary pressures are generally not elevated in acute PE, and tricuspid regurgitation (TR) velocities will be relatively normal and rarely above 3 m/s. Patients with preexisting pulmonary vascular disease, however, may have increased TR velocity consistent with elevation in pulmonary systolic pressures.

ECHOCARDIOGRAPHY IN PROGNOSIS AND MANAGEMENT OF PULMONARY EMBOLISM

Assessment of right ventricular function has become central to the management algorithms in acute PE. The presence of RV dilatation or dysfunction in acute PE has important prognostic significance, as these patients have been shown to have increased risk for short- and medium-term mortality. Patients with RV dysfunction who also have elevation in cardiac markers such as troponin or natriuretic peptides are at marked increased risk for death (Fig. 35.14). Current guidelines suggest that this high-risk group should be considered for interventional therapy such as thrombolysis, suction, or surgical embolectomy (Fig. 35.15). Current treatment algorithms now incorporate assessment of right ventricular function (Fig. 35.16). Patients with confirmed PE that is considered of intermediate risk on clinical grounds should have RV function assessed either by CT or by echocardiography, and biomarker testing performed. If there is evidence of biomarker elevation (particularly troponin elevation) *and* evidence of right ventricular dysfunction, patients are considered intermediate–high risk (although the presence of only one of these puts patients in the intermediate–low risk category). High-risk patients should be considered for reperfusion therapy.

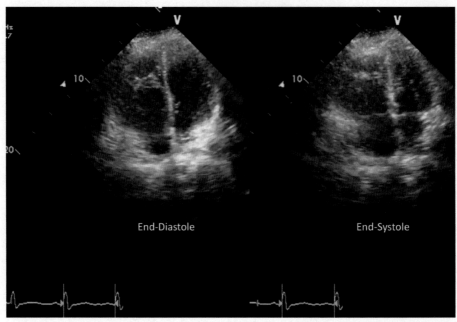

FIG. 35.12 End-diastolic and end-systolic views of a patient with "McConnell sign." Note that the right ventricle is dilated in both diastole and systole. See videos.

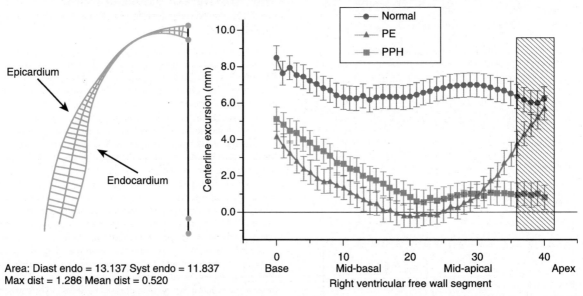

FIG. 35.13 Assessment of regional wall motion in patients with pulmonary embolism using the "centerline" method *(left panel)*. *Right panel* shows regional deformation from base to apex demonstrating relatively similar deformation throughout the right ventricular (RV) free wall in patients with normal RVs *(circles)*, and mid-RV dysfunction in patients with acute pulmonary embolism (PE; *triangles*) where basal and apical motion is spared, compared with patients with pulmonary hypertension *(squares)* who lack the apical sparing. *PPH*, Primary pulmonary hypertension. (*Right panel from McConnell MV, Solomon SD, Rayan ME, Come PC, Goldhaber SZ, Lee RT. Regional right ventricular dysfunction detected by echocardiography in acute pulmonary embolism. Am J Cardiol. 1996;78(4):469–473.*)

Echocardiography in Assessment of Response to Therapy in Pulmonary Embolism

In addition to its utility in prognosis, echocardiography can be used to assess the response to therapy in acute PE. Improvement in RV function can be seen within several days of successful treatment (such as embolectomy or thrombolysis) of PE and can be useful for determining whether additional interventional therapy is required (Videos 35.11 and 35.12).

Novel Methods to Assess Right Ventricular Function in Pulmonary Embolism

Myocardial strain imaging may have some utility in RV assessment and has been shown to be substantially abnormal in patients with acute PE (Fig. 35.17, Videos 35.13 and 35.14). In particular, strain imaging can be used to visualize the classic regional right ventricular dysfunction seen in PE. While these methods are likely not required in most clinical

circumstances, incorporation of automated assessment of the RV into echocardiographic equipment may occur in the future and may make these techniques more clinically useful.

Handheld echocardiography, performed in the emergency setting, can also be quite useful in acute PE (see Chapter 13). While handheld devices lack the power and penetration of traditional echo equipment, they are generally able to visualize right ventricular dilatation and dysfunction and distinguish PE from other acute conditions.

Transesophageal Echocardiography in Pulmonary Embolism

TEE can visualize thrombus further in the pulmonary vasculature than can TTE, and can be useful in the identification of relatively proximal pulmonary emboli, thrombi in the RV or right atrium, or inferior vena cava. However, TEE is rarely used as a primary diagnostic modality in PE.

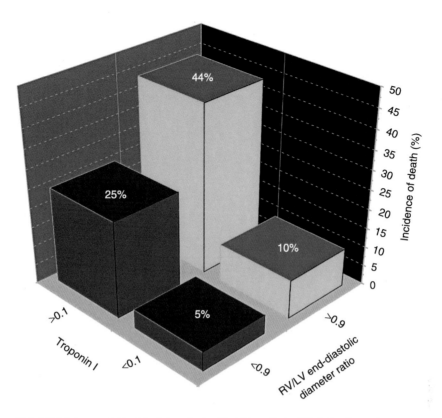

FIG. 35.14 Increased risk of death in patients with right ventricular (RV) dysfunction and elevation in troponin. *LV*, Left ventricle. (*From Scridon T, Scridon C, Skali H, Alvarez A, Goldhaber SZ, Solomon SD. Prognostic significance of troponin elevation and right ventricular enlargement in acute pulmonary embolism. Am J Cardiol. 2005;96(2):303–305.*)

Classification of patients with acute PE based on early mortality risk					
Early mortality risk		**Risk parameters and scores**			
		Shock or hypotension	PESI class III-V or sPESI >I[a]	Signs of RV dysfunction on an imaging test[b]	Cardiac laboratory biomarkers[c]
High		+	(+)[d]	+	(+)[d]
Intermediate	Intermediate-high	−	+	Both positive	
	Intermediate-low	−	+	Either one (or none) positive[e]	
Low		−	−	Assessment optional; if assessed, both negative[e]	

[a]PESI Class III to V indicates moderate to very high 30-day mortality risk; sPESI ≥ 1 point(s) indicate high 30-day mortality risk.

[b]Echocardiographic criteria of RV dysfunction include RV dilation and/or an increased end-diastolic RV–LV diameter ratio (in most studies, the reported threshold value was 0.9 or 1.0); hypokinesia of the free RV wall; increased velocity of the tricuspid regurgitation jet; or combinations of the above. On computed tomographic (CT) angiography (4-chamber views of the heart), RV dysfunction is defined as an increased end-diastolic RV/LV (left ventricular) diameter ratio (with a threshold of 0.9 or 1.0).

[c]Markers of myocardial injury (e.g. elevated cardiac troponin I or -T concentrations in plasma), or of heart failure as a result of (right) ventricular dysfunction (elevated natriuretic peptide concentrations in plasma).

[d]Neither calculation of the PESI (or sPESI) nor laboratory testing are considered necessary in patients with hypotension or shock.

[e]Patients in the PESI Class I–II, or with sPESI of 0, and elevated cardiac biomarkers or signs of RV dysfunction on imaging tests, are also to be classified into the intermediate-low-risk category. This might apply to situations in which imaging or biomarker results become available before calculation of the clinical severity index.

PE, Pulmonary embolism; *PESI*, pulmonary embolism severity index; *RV*, right ventricular; *sPESI*, simplified pulmonary embolism severity index.

FIG. 35.15 Risk stratification for acute pulmonary embolism based on 2014 European Society of Cardiology (ESC) guidelines. (*From Konstantinides SV, Torbicki A, Agnelli G, et al. 2014 ESC Guidelines on the diagnosis and management of acute pulmonary embolism. Eur Heart J. 2014;35(45):3033–3080.*)

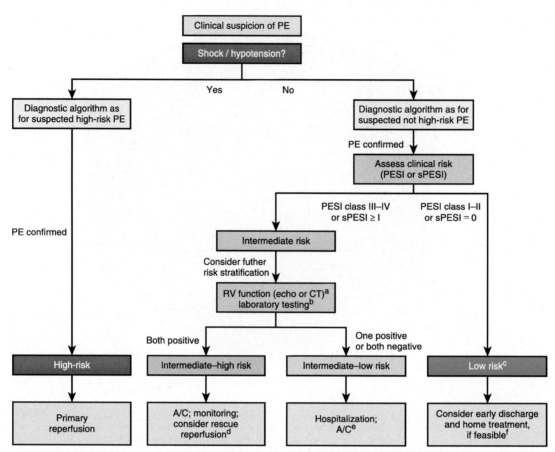

FIG. 35.16 European Society of Cardiology (ESC) algorithm for risk stratification in acute pulmonary embolism. See Fig. 35.15 for notations. *A/C*, Anticoagulation; *CT*, computed tomography; *PE*, pulmonary embolism; *PESI*, pulmonary embolism severity index; *RV*, right ventricular; *sPESI*, simplified pulmonary embolism severity index. (*From Konstantinides SV, Torbicki A, Agnelli G, et al. 2014 ESC guidelines on the diagnosis and management of acute pulmonary embolism. Eur Heart J. 2014;35(45): 3033–3080.*)

[a]If echocardiography has already been performed during diagnostic work-up for PE and detected RV dysfunction, or if the CT already performed for diagnostic work-up has shown RV enlargement (RV/LV) ratio >0.9, a cardiac troponin test should be performed except for cases in which primary reperfusion is not a therapeutic option (e.g., due to severe comorbidity or limited life expectancy of the patient).

[b]Markers of myocardial injury (e.g., elevated cardiac troponin I or T concentrations in plasma), or of heart failure as a result of (right) ventricular dysfunction (elevated natriuretic peptide concentrations in plasma). If a laboratory test for a cardiac biomarker has already been performed during initial diagnostic work-up (e.g., in the chest pain unit) and was positive, then an echocardiogram should be considered to assess RV function, or RV size should be (re)assessed on CT.

[c]Patients in the PESI Class I–II, or with sPESI of 0, and elevated cardiac biomarkers or signs of RV dysfunction on imaging tests, are also to be classified into the intermediate–low risk category. This might apply to situations in which imaging or biomarker results become available before calculation of the clinical severity index. These patients are probably not candidates for home treatment.

[d]Thrombolysis, if (and as soon as) clinical signs of hemodynamic decompensation appear; surgical pulmonary embolectomy or percutaneous catheter-directed treatment may be considered as alternative options to systemic thrombolysis, particularly if the bleeding risk is high.

[e]Monitoring should be considered for patients with confirmed PE and a positive troponin test, even if there is no evidence of RV dysfunction on echocardiography or CT.

[f]The simplified version of the PESI has not been validated in prospective home treatment trials; inclusion criteria other than the PESI were used in two single-armed (nonrandomized) management studies.

Because TEEs require patients to receive conscious sedation or to be intubated, most consider the technique of limited utility in patients with acute shortness of breath who are not intubated. Moreover, TEE is no better than TTE in assessment of the RV under most conditions, and because TEE can only visualize thrombus in the proximal pulmonary arteries, the overall sensitivity and specificity for diagnosis of PE will be quite low.

DISTINGUISHING PULMONARY EMBOLISM FROM PULMONARY HYPERTENSION

The echocardiographic features of PE display both similarities and differences to those seen in pulmonary hypertension (see Chapter 36). Patients with pulmonary hypertension typically demonstrate RVH and dilatation, elevated tricuspid regurgitant velocities consistent with elevated pulmonary systolic pressure, dilatation of the pulmonary artery, and bowing of the interventricular septum (IVS) toward the left side of the heart throughout the cardiac cycle due to right-sided pressures that can approach left-sided pressures (Table 35.1). While regional right ventricular dysfunction can be seen in pulmonary hypertension, there is generally a lack of apical sparing typically seen in PE (Figs. 35.18 and 35.19; Videos 35.15 and 35.16). In acute PE where there was no prior elevation in pulmonary pressures, features of right ventricular dilatation and failure predominate but without bowing of the IVS throughout the cardiac cycle and without elevated tricuspid regurgitant velocities. Nevertheless, in those patients with prior elevation of pulmonary pressures, such as those

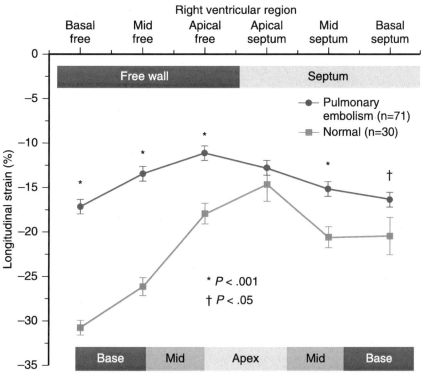

FIG. 35.17 Right ventricular strain in acute pulmonary embolism. (*From Platz E, Hassanein AH, Shah A, Goldhaber SZ, Solomon SD. Regional right ventricular strain pattern in patients with acute pulmonary embolism. Echocardiography. 2012;29(4):464–470.*)

TABLE 35.1 Comparison of Echocardiographic Findings in Pulmonary Embolism and Pulmonary Hypertension

PULMONARY EMBOLISM	PULMONARY HYPERTENSION
No RVH (unless chronic)	RVH
Normal TR velocity	Increased TR velocity
Flattening of IVS, diastole only	Flattening of IVS diastole and possibly systole
Regional RV dysfunction—sparing of apex	RV dysfunction—apex included

IVS, Interventricular septum; *RV*, right ventricle; *RVH*, right ventricular hypertrophy; *TR*, tricuspid regurgitation.

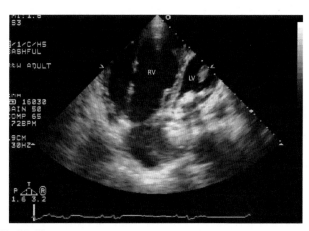

FIG. 35.19 Right ventricular dilatation in pulmonary hypertension (apical four-chamber view). Note marked enlargement of right ventricle and small left ventricle.

with chronic thromboembolic disease, the echocardiographic findings in PE can become more similar to those seen in pulmonary hypertension. Indeed, the right ventricular dysfunction seen in acute PE can be obscured in those patients with chronic elevation in pulmonary pressures and RVH.

Suggested Reading

Goldhaber, S. Z. (1998). Clinical overview of venous thromboembolism. *Vascular Medical*, 3(1), 35–40.
Goldhaber, S. Z. (2002). Echocardiography in the management of pulmonary embolism. *Annals of Internal Medicine*, 136(9), 691–700.
McConnell, M. V., Solomon, S. D., Rayan, M. E., Come, P. C., Goldhaber, S. Z., & Lee, R. T. (1996). Regional right ventricular dysfunction detected by echocardiography in acute pulmonary embolism. *The American Journal of Cardiology*, 78(4), 469–473.
Nass, N., McConnell, M. V., Goldhaber, S. Z., Chyu, S., & Solomon, S. D. (1999). Recovery of regional right ventricular function after thrombolysis for pulmonary embolism. *The American Journal of Cardiology*, 83(5), 804–806, A10.

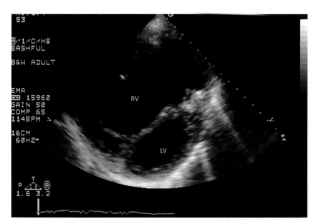

FIG. 35.18 Right ventricular dilatation in pulmonary hypertension (short axis view). Note marked enlargement of right ventricle and small left ventricle.

36 Pulmonary Hypertension

André La Gerche, Leah Wright

INTRODUCTION

The echocardiographic assessment of pulmonary hypertension (PH) must include an appreciation of the interaction between the load imposed on the ventricle by the increased resistance of the pulmonary arteries and the contractile force of the right ventricle (RV). It is a combination of these two factors that determines the right ventricular and pulmonary artery pressures (Fig. 36.1). Thus, the first principle is that an echocardiographic assessment must include assessment of both the pulmonary arterial load and the RV function.

The second principle is that the interaction between pulmonary vascular load and cardiac performance is not constant but rather is marked by differing phases as PH progresses. In early disease, RV contractility increases to compensate for the increase in pulmonary vascular resistance (PVR). This phase is marked by increased pulmonary artery pressures, maintained cardiac output, and few or no symptoms. Then there is a stage where the RV contractility is no longer able to compensate for the increase in PVR; the cardiac output starts to fall and progressive symptoms develop. At first, these occur only during exertion, so measures appear reasonably compensated when measured at rest. Finally, there is a completely decompensated phase in which reduction in RV function is so significant that cardiac output falls even under resting conditions. This results in a fall in pulmonary artery pressures despite the continued increase in PVR (Fig. 36.2).

Thus, the echocardiographic assessment that follows will describe measures that assess pulmonary vascular load, measures of RV function, and some measures that attempt to quantify RV/pulmonary arterial coupling; that is, the degree to which the RV is compensating for the increase in load.

ASSESSMENT OF RIGHT VENTRICLE AFTERLOAD/PULMONARY VASCULAR FUNCTION

Pulmonary Artery Systolic Pressure

Pulmonary artery systolic pressure (PASP) can be reliably estimated from a continuous-wave Doppler assessment of the tricuspid regurgitation (TR) jet (Fig. 36.3; Bernoulli equation; $4 \times$ TR velocity^2 = max pressure gradient) and has been validated in numerous studies.[1-3] As Doppler intercept angle affects the measurement, multiple acoustic windows should be interrogated. Saline or contrast enhancement also should be available (Fig. 36.4) to increase the intensity of the regurgitant signal and the sensitivity of results.

The regurgitant velocity represents the pressure gradient between the RV and right atrium. Thus, it measures RV systolic pressure (RVSP) minus the right atrial pressure (RAP). To use this clinically, an estimate of RAP can be made (see below) and then RVSP = $4 \times$ TR velocity^2 + RAP. The RVSP is equivalent to PASP, except when there is a significant gradient across the right ventricular outflow tract (RVOT) or pulmonary valve. Thus, in pulmonary stenosis, the systolic gradient would need to be considered when estimating PASP.

The other setting in which the Bernoulli equation needs to be used with caution is in severe TR. The early equalization of pressures between the RV and RA can result in considerable underestimation of PASP.

Diastolic Pulmonary Artery Pressure

Diastolic pulmonary artery pressure (dPAP) is calculated from a measurement of the peak velocity of pulmonary regurgitation (PR) at the end of diastole. This usually occurs simultaneously with the Q wave of

the electrocardiogram (ECG) and after a small "notch" that reflects atrial contraction (Fig. 36.5).

$$dPAP = 4(V_{PR}end - diastole)^2 + RAP$$

Mean Pulmonary Artery Pressure

Mean pulmonary artery pressure (mPAP) can be calculated using a number of methods:

1. The Chemla formula that is derived from linear regression of the reasonably consistent relationship between PASP and mPAP. Thus, PASP can be measured from the maximal tricuspid regurgitant velocity, as depicted in Fig. 36.3, and then mPAP is calculated using the formula: mPAP = 0.61*PASP + 2 mm Hg.[4]
2. An average of all instantaneous pressure estimates, which is obtained by tracing the maximal instantaneous velocities across the TR regurgitant signal and averaged. The RAP pressure estimate is again added (Fig. 36.6).[5]
3. Deriving PASP and dPAP using the methodologies stated above and incorporating these values into the formula: mPAP = ⅓ PASP + ⅔ dPAP.

The Right Atrium and Right Atrial Pressure

The *right atrial size* is traced from the RV apical view. The transducer should be rotated to ensure that the RA is as elongated as possible. This may require a different acquisition from that used to measure the left atrium. Recent guidelines have proposed the area–length measurement, with body surface area (BSA)–indexed values of 25 ± 7 mL/m^2 and 21 ± 6 mL/m^2 representing the average upper limit of normal measures for males and females, respectively.[6]

RAP is typically estimated based on dimensions of the inferior vena cava (IVC). IVC measurements are made from the subcostal view, 1–2 cm from the junction of the right atrium (from a long-axis view). The maximum dimension can be measured from M-mode or 2D. IVC distensibility is calculated in response to respiratory measures that alter intrathoracic pressure;[7] 50% collapsibility provides optimal sensitivity and specificity for detecting RAP greater or less than 10 mm Hg, but RAP is often underestimated when values exceed 12 mm Hg. Values are as follows (Fig. 36.7):

- IVC <2.1 cm and collapsible >50%, RAP~ 3 mm Hg.
- IVC >2.1 cm and collapsible >50% or IVC < 2.1 cm and collapsible ≤ 50%, RAP~ 8 mm Hg.
- IVC >2.1 cm and collapsible <50%, RAP~ 15 mm Hg.

Velocity-time integrals (VTIs) of the hepatic veins (or superior vena cava) provide an indication of elevated RAP. Hepatic vein systolic filling fraction (VTI systolic/VTI systolic + VTI diastolic) can provide semiquantitative assessment of RAP, with a measurement of <55% predicting RAP >8 mm Hg with good sensitivity and specificity.[7] This technique offers advantages over IVC measurements in patients with falsely elevated IVC diameters (athletes, large BSA, and mechanically ventilated patients).

OTHER MEASURES OF RIGHT VENTRICLE AFTERLOAD

Pulmonary Arterial Acceleration Time

Pulmonary arterial acceleration time (PAT) is calculated via pulsed-wave Doppler, at the level of the pulmonary valve leaflets. Acceleration time is measured along the modal velocity from the baseline to peak (Fig. 36.8). This method is less reliable than other methods of assessing PASP and

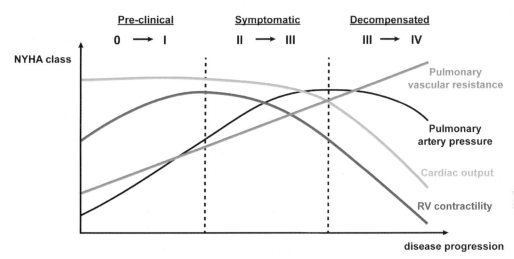

FIG. 36.1 The relationship between pulmonary artery pressures, right ventricular (RV) function and vascular load. Pulmonary artery pressures are determined by both the ability of the RV pump to generate pressure and by the load against which this pump must push. The RV afterload is determined by pulmonary vascular factors (resistance, compliance, and impedance) and by left atrial pressures. (*From La Gerche A, Claessen G, Van De Bruaene A. Right ventricular structure and function during exercise. In: Gaine SP, Naeije R, Peacock AJ, eds.* The Right Heart. *London: Springer; 2014: 83–98.*)

FIG. 36.2 The progression of measures of disease severity in pulmonary hypertension. As the disease progresses (increase in pulmonary vascular disease), there is an initial compensated phase in which right ventricle (RV) contractility increases to meet the increase in resistance, and maintains cardiac output. Symptoms start to develop when the RV exhausts its contractile reserve and can no longer compensate for the increases in pulmonary artery pressures during exercise. Finally, RV function declines to the extent that it can no longer maintain cardiac output at rest against the increased afterload. *NYHA,* New York Heart Association (classification of heart failure symptoms).

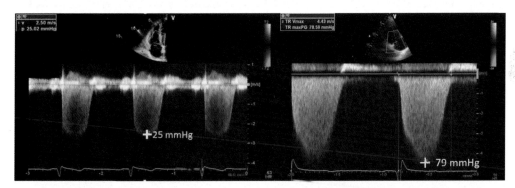

FIG. 36.3 Estimations of normal and severely elevated pulmonary artery systolic pressures (PASP) are estimated with the Bernoulli equation (PASP = 4 × TR velocity^2). *TR,* Tricuspid regurgitation.

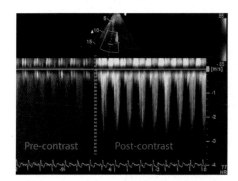

FIG. 36.4 Contrast enhancement. Injection of agitated contrast (saline or colloid) is very effective at increasing the intensity of the Doppler regurgitant signal. The *pink dotted line* indicates the agitated contrast entering the right ventricle (RV), enhancing the signal and enabling the PASP to be estimated.

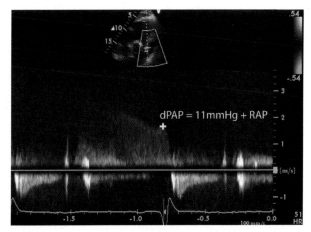

FIG. 36.5 Estimation of diastolic pulmonary artery pressure (dPAP). Estimated from the peak pulmonary regurgitant velocity at end diastole with the addition of right atrial pressure.

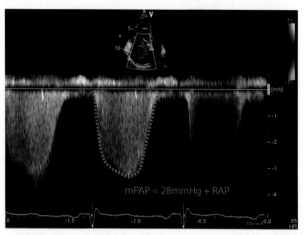

FIG. 36.6 Estimation of mean pulmonary artery pressure (mPAP). The tricuspid regurgitation time-velocity integral can be traced to determine the mean RV-RA gradient to which an estimate of RAP is added. *RA,* Right atrium; *RAP,* right atrial pressure; *RV,* right ventricle.

is heart-rate dependent. It should not be applied when the heart rate is outside the range of 60–100 bpm. PAT <100 ms has been proposed to indicate a PASP >38 mm Hg (normal PAT is >120 ms)

Notching of the Right Ventricular Outflow Tract Signal

A qualitative measure of pulmonary arterial hypertension (PAH) is "notching" of the RVOT signal (see Fig. 36.8), although its absence cannot "rule-out" PH. This can give us insight into the underlying physiology of the PH. In large artery stiffness, an early notch relates to a restricted vascular bed, whereas a late notch could imply secondary PH due to left heart disease.

Echocardiographic Estimates of Pulmonary Vascular Resistance

PVR is calculated as the pressure gradient across the pulmonary vasculature (mPAP—left atrial pressure [LAP]) divided by cardiac output. Each of these factors can be estimated by echocardiography. In the absence of shunts, cardiac output can be measured using the left ventricle (LV) or RV as these should be equal. However, often the VTI of the RV outflow tract is used (Fig. 36.9). Abbas et al. estimated PVR as PASP/RVOT$_{VTI}$,

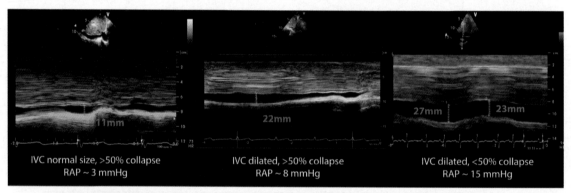

FIG. 36.7 Estimation of right atrial pressure (RAP). See text for details. *IVC,* Inferior vena cava.

IVC normal size, >50% collapse
RAP ~ 3 mmHg

IVC dilated, >50% collapse
RAP ~ 8 mmHg

IVC dilated, <50% collapse
RAP ~ 15 mmHg

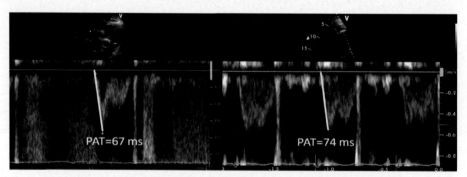

FIG. 36.8 Two patients with short pulmonary acceleration time (PAT) and notching of flow consistent with pulmonary hypertension.

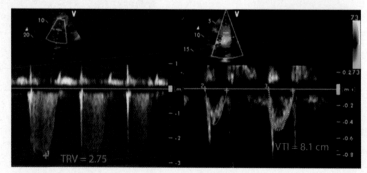

FIG. 36.9 Measures used to estimate pulmonary vascular resistance. *Left panel* shows the peak tricuspid regurgitation jet velocity (TRV = 2.75 mps), while the *right panel* shows the right ventricular outflow tract velocity-time integral (VTI) measured from pulsed Doppler spectra (8.1 cm).

but a very significant limitation of this formula was that the heart rate was ignored,[8] which is a problem when one considers that heart rate represents the most important means of augmenting cardiac output. Thus, Haddad et al. improved this formula with the addition of heart rate (PVR = PASP/[HR × TVI$_{RVOT}$]) so that the calculation more closely approximates the pulmonary pressure gradient divided by cardiac output.[9]

The other big limitation in applying these formulas to estimate PVR is that LAP is ignored. In situations in which LAP is elevated, these formulas will grossly overestimate PVR.

Defining Pre- Versus Postcapillary Pulmonary Hypertension

Echocardiography can be used to aid with the differentiation of precapillary (PAH) versus postcapillary PH. The current clinical standard requires right heart catheterization and the estimation of LAP by means of the pulmonary artery occlusion pressure (PAOP), which is otherwise known as the pulmonary capillary wedge pressure (PWCP), with values >15 mm Hg suggesting that PH is consistent with a diagnosis of raised LAPs due to left heart disease. There have been a number of attempts to develop a noninvasive estimate of LAP to assist in identifying those patients with precapillary (Class I PAH) or postcapillary (Class II PH due to left heart disease) causes of raised pulmonary pressures.[10] This is a critical distinction because pulmonary vasodilators have demonstrated efficacy in pre- but not postcapillary causes of PH. However, it is controversial as to whether echocardiographic surrogates have a role in clinical decision making. Given the significance of the outcomes, current recommendations would be that patients with elevated estimates of PASP on echocardiography should undergo right heart catheterization both to confirm the result and to assess the contribution from left heart disease.

Despite this, noninvasive estimates of PCWP have been proposed from measures of pulsed-wave mitral inflow, and tissue Doppler of the mitral septal annulus,[11] using the formula:

$$PCWP = 1.24 * E/e' + 1.9$$

where

E = mitral inflow E wave and
e' = septal annular e wave as measured by Doppler tissue imaging (DTI).

A disadvantage of this is that in severe PH, the septal motion of the mitral annulus is restricted due to tethering of the RV.[12] Despite this, some recent indices that combine TR velocities and E/e' estimates of LAP have shown promising results in the differentiation of pre- and postcapillary PH.[13]

RIGHT VENTRICULAR STRUCTURE AND FUNCTION

Right Ventricular Wall Thickness

A 2D (Fig. 36.10A) or M-mode (Fig. 36.10B) measurement of the right ventricular free wall is traditionally performed from the subcostal view, zoomed to maximize spatial resolution. The inner edge to inner edge method should be used, taking care to exclude trabeculae and papillary muscles. This measurement is subjective to tangential cuts, and measurement from a single view of the RV free wall may not be representative of the heterogeneity of the RV structure.

Tricuspid Annular Plane Systolic Excursion

Tricuspid annular plane systolic excursion (TAPSE) is measured as the displacement of the lateral tricuspid annulus toward the apex during systole. It is predicated on the argument that longitudinal RV function is the dominant means by which the RV generates stroke volume, although this may not necessarily track with disease progression in PH, as it has been demonstrated that function becomes progressively more dependent on radial function.[14]

• TAPSE is measured by aligning an M-mode cursor parallel with the RV free wall as it meets the tricuspid annulus from the RV apical four-chamber view (Fig. 36.11). Values <17 mm are abnormal. This measure is easy to perform, is very widely available, and has strong associations with the outcome in PH.

However, specific to patients with PH is the fact that an imbalance between left and right ventricular contractility means that the apex of the heart is often pulled toward the LV during systole. As a result, the tricuspid annulus is pulled along in unison, even in the absence of actual shortening or deformation of the RV. This artefactual overestimation of TAPSE due to "apical rocking" can be a profound confounder and is a good reason why strain measures (see below) of the RV are preferable in patients with PH.[15]

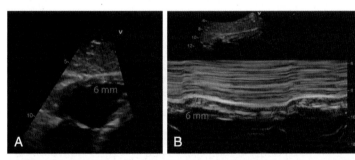

FIG. 36.10 Measuring right ventricle wall thickness. Performed in a subcostal acquisition using 2D (A) or M-mode (B) echocardiography.

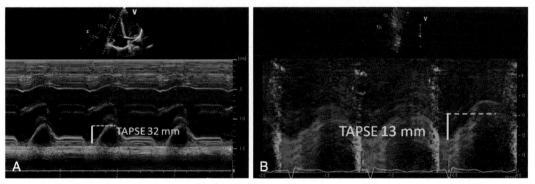

FIG. 36.11 Tricuspid annular plane systolic excursion (TAPSE). A patient with normal tricuspid excursion (A) compared with a patient with pulmonary hypertension and reduced tricuspid motion (B). Tissue Doppler overlay is used to highlight the direction of motion in the latter example.

Right Ventricular Eccentricity Index/Inter Ventricular Septal Shift

"D-shaped" flattening of the interventricular septum during systole (pressure overload) and diastole (volume overload) provides a qualitative assessment of load excess. A quantitative assessment of this principle is also possible. From the parasternal short-axis view (level of the papillary muscles), two left ventricular axis measurements are made; one parallel (anteroposterior diameter) and one perpendicular (septo-lateral diameter) to the inter ventricular septum (Fig. 36.12).[16] The eccentricity index is calculated as anteroposterior diameter/septo-lateral diameter, with a ratio >1.1 in systole, which suggests a pressure

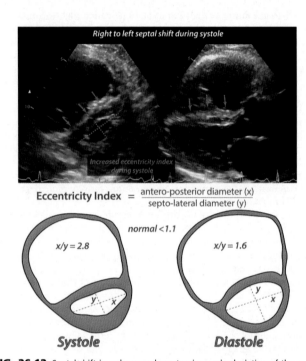

FIG. 36.12 Septal shift in pulmonary hypertension and calculation of the eccentricity index. *Arrows* identify the interventricular septum in the parasternal short-axis *(left)* and long-axis *(right)* views. Note the D-shaped contour in the short-axis view.

excess in the RV. The separation between volume and pressure overload is rarely absolute. Part of the reason for this is physiological because volume loading is an early compensatory mechanism in PH (an attempt to get "free" stroke volume through greater reliance on the Starling preload stretch-recoil).

Right Ventricular Area Assessment

The RV end-diastolic and end-systolic areas (RVEDA and RVESA) can be manually traced from an apical four-chamber view optimized to focus on the RV. The RV apex can be densely trabeculated; thus, adequate care should be taken when tracing myocardial borders. The ultrasound probe should be carefully rotated so that the maximal RV area is visualized. Given the variable crescent shaped anatomy of the RV, it is critical that care is taken to maximize the RV area (Fig. 36.13). RV fractional area change (FAC) is calculated according to the formula:

$$RV\ FAC = 100 \times (RVEDA - RVESA)/RVEDA$$

RV FAC <35% is indicative of reduced RV function (Fig. 36.14).

Three-Dimensional Volume Assessment

Although technically challenging, three-dimensional (3D) right ventricular volume assessment can give further insight into changes in RV chamber size, and has improved accuracy (compared to two-dimensional [2D] echocardiography) when measured against cardiac magnetic resonance imaging.[17] Acquisition can be improved when the probe is positioned very laterally, with breath holds to capture a full volume acquisition. A number of proprietors now have packages specifically designed to measure RV 3D volumes and ejection fraction (Fig. 36.15), which has decreased postprocessing time.

Doppler Tissue Imagings' cm/s

A pulsed-wave Doppler region of interest (ROI) is aligned with the tricuspid annulus, to measure the peak systolic velocity (Fig. 36.16A). This is an easy measure to perform, although it is important to align the motion of free wall displacement with the angle of the ultrasound beam. A value of <9.5 cm/s indicates RV dysfunction.

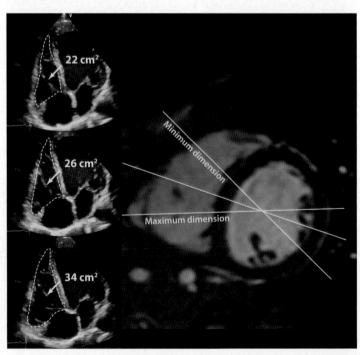

FIG. 36.13 Standardizing right ventricle (RV) area acquisitions. The ultrasound probe should be rotated so that the maximal area is obtained. Marked differences in RV areas can result if this is not carefully performed.

Iso-Volumetric Acceleration

This measure, as opposed to the right ventricular annular systolic velocity, utilizes the isovolumetric contraction time (IVCT) spike on the basal free wall DTI tracing.[18] The isovolumetric peak velocity is divided by the time over which this presystolic spike develops (see Fig. 36.16B). This measure is relatively load independent and, thus, may be one of few measures in which estimates of PASP do not need to be considered in interpreting values. A normal value of >1.1 m/s^2 has been suggested. A significant issue with this measure is that the reproducibility is questionable given the limited dynamic range of the measure compared against the considerable margin for measurement error.

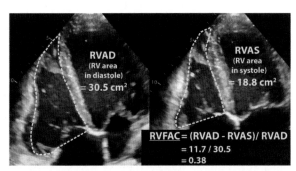

FIG. 36.14 Measurement of right ventricle (RV) fractional area change (FAC). In this case, the FAC is 0.38 × 100 = 38%.

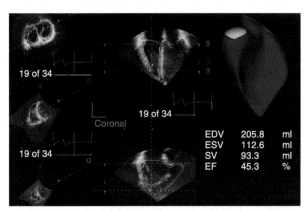

FIG. 36.15 A three-dimensional (3D) volume quantification of right ventricle (RV) function. Commercially available software is used to orientate a 3D dataset in multiple planes on which the endocardial contour is traced. The endocardial contours are then interpolated for the remainder of the cavity, and temporal propagation enables volume estimation throughout the cardiac cycle. This promising technique minimizes approximation, and more directly incorporates the complexity of geometry. The major disadvantage is that it can be difficult to acquire the full volume of the RV, particularly including the apex and outflow tract in the one data set. This is a concern with the enlarged right ventricles, which are frequent in patients with pulmonary hypertension. *EDV,* End-diastolic volume; *EF,* ejection fraction; *ESV,* end-systolic volume; *SV,* stroke volume.

Right Ventricular E/e′

Estimation of RV filling pressures can be performed through methods similar to those used for the LV. A pulsed-wave Doppler of the tricuspid inflow is acquired, with the peak E wave divided by the lateral DTI e′ of the RV free wall. This provides a modest correlation with RAP, although there is limited data on the range of normal values.[6]

Strain/Strain Rate

Longitudinal deformation of the right ventricular myocardium can be measured with speckle tracking. This is performed from the RV apical four-chamber focused view, with the ROI set to track the RV free wall (Fig. 36.17A). Mean RV strain values of –28% are higher than for the LV (normal range –20% to –39% with more negative values representing better function).[7] There is also a normal deformation gradient with slightly higher strain values moving from the base to the apex, although a degree of individual variation and disease-specific patterns exist.[19] As with the LV, care needs to be taken not to include pericardium or trabeculae within the ROI. Pulmonary pressure should be taken into account as this value is load dependent. It is also possible to quantify strain and strain rate from color-coded Doppler tissue acquisitions, although this technique has become less popular due to the considerable time required for analysis (see Fig. 36.17C and D). An ROI is placed within the myocardium and needs to be tracked throughout the cardiac cycle. The advantage of this technique is the high temporal resolution, which is most suitable for resolving events of short duration—particularly peak values of strain rate (see Fig. 36.17D).

Studies have shown links between RV strain and outcomes, with this measurement now available on systems from a wide variety of ultrasound vendors. Although intervendor differences are decreasing, sequential follow-up should be performed on the same vendor systems. Additional normative data are still needed.

The strain rate reflects the rate of deformation per time unit. Therefore, it is based on local tissue deformation, and not translational movement. As stated previously, it can be measured with DTI (benefit of higher frame rates), with three sample volumes placed at the basal, mid, and apical RV free wall segments (see Fig. 36.17D). There are fewer data concerning the link between strain rate and outcomes in patients with pulmonary artery hypertension.

TIMING MEASUREMENTS

Right Ventricular Isovolumetric Relaxation Time Measurement

The isovolumetric relaxation time (IVRT) is measured via a DTI trace of the lateral tricuspid annulus. This is a simple measurement of RV function. In healthy subjects, RV IVRT should not be appreciable (see Fig. 36.16A), but it increases in length with increasing pulmonary arterial pressures and/or RV dysfunction (see Fig. 36.16B). It can serve as an excellent qualitative screening test for the presence of uncoupling between RV function and the pulmonary vascular load.

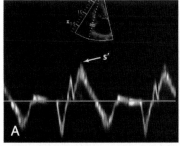
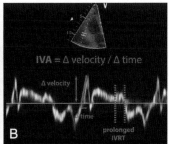

FIG. 36.16 Doppler tissue annular velocities comparing a normal subject and a patient with pulmonary hypertension. Pulse-wave Doppler velocity of the lateral tricuspid annulus in a healthy subject demonstrating normal systolic velocity and an absence of an isovolumetric relaxation time (A). In comparison, the patient with pulmonary hypertension has reduced systolic velocities and a prolonged isovolumetric relaxation time (B). Isovolumetric acceleration is calculated as velocity/time of the presystolic contractile spike. *IVA,* Iso-volumetric acceleration.

Myocardial Performance Index or Tei Index

Reflecting a combination of systolic and diastolic function, the myocardial performance index (MPI) can be measured from either tissue Doppler or a combination of Doppler flow measures. The latter involves two steps. First, tricuspid regurgitant time (TRT) is measured from the continuous-wave Doppler trace of the TR jet. Second, a pulsed-wave Doppler of the RV outflow tract flow is used to measure the RV ejection time (RVET; Fig. 36.18A). From this, the sum of IVCT and IVRT is calculated as (TRT–RVET) and thus $MPI_{FLOW} = TRT–RVET /RVET$ (<0.43 Normal).[6] The DTI approach involves using the pulsed-wave DTI (PW DTI) sample acquired from the RV basal segment (see Fig. 36.18B).

$$MPI_{TISSUE} = \frac{(IVRT + IVCT)}{ET\ (\ <0.54\ Normal)}$$

Note the difference in normal values for MPI according to the method used reflecting the fact that the time in which flow can be measured through the pulmonary valve exceeds the time period in which myocardial contraction occurs (due to flow inertia).

Importance of Considering Right-Sided Ventricular-Arterial Interactions

As discussed at the outset of this chapter, RV function is exquisitely dependent upon load, in large part because the range of load is greater than that commonly experienced for the LV. In PH, the afterload can be fourfold greater than normal values, or even more. Having now presented the methods for evaluating RV afterload in PH (i.e., the estimation of pulmonary arterial pressures and resistance) and the methods for assessing RV function, it is important to recognize that these measures need to be considered together in order to fully appreciate the burden of disease in PH. As illustrated in Fig. 36.2, measures of RV function, pulmonary artery pressure estimates, and cardiac output can determine whether the patient is in a compensated or decompensated phase of disease, and this may be important to determine treatment.

Although RV contractility and function are often used as synonyms, they are quite different. RV contractility refers to the intrinsic contractile ability of the RV *independent* of loading conditions. This would be valuable to be able to quantify, as it would enable us to know whether the RV has the ability to recover some function if the PVR could improve. Loss of RV contractility progresses with disease severity (see Fig. 36.2). There are two ways to estimate RV contractility using echocardiography:

1. *Load independent measures.* All cardiac measures have some load dependence, but some are *relatively* independent of pulmonary artery pressures. The two measures that have been demonstrated to be least affected are RV isovolumetric acceleration and RV systolic strain rate. However, both of these measures can be challenging to use, and their reproducibility is far from perfect.
2. *Composite measures.* The gold standard measure of contractility uses a combination of pressure and volume (i.e., load and function) and this approach can be utilized using echocardiography. Ratios can be used that express function relative to pulmonary artery pressures. For example, the ratio of TAPSE to PASP has been used to define RV performance in patients with PH complicating left-sided heart failure.[20] Similarly, the ratio of RVESA to PASP (termed the RV end-systolic pressure area relationship or RV ESPAR) has been validated against invasive measures of RV contractility.[3] The MPI (see Figs. 36.18A and B) also incorporates measures of both function and load, and more closely represents RV contractility than do geometric, volume, or strain measures when used in isolation.

Echocardiographic Measures as Prognostic Markers in Pulmonary Hypertension

The current methods used for predicting the risk of disease progression and death in PAH are nonspecific. The 2015 European Guidelines for the management of PAH provide a prognostic guide in which nine measures (comprising clinical, invasive hemodynamic, biochemical and imaging) can be each stratified into mild, intermediate, and high risk.[10] However, patients frequently present with imaging, biochemical markers, and hemodynamic measures of severity that are discordant. Most current evidence is derived from the Registry to Evaluate Early and Long-Term Pulmonary Arterial Hypertension Disease Management (REVEAL) registry of PAH patients[21] that included only basic echocardiographic measures.

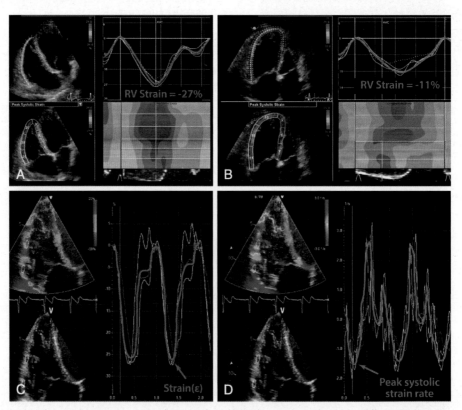

FIG. 36.17 Strain rate imaging in pulmonary hypertension. A two-dimensional speckle tracking strain can be used to differentiate between normal right ventricle (RV) free wall strain (A) and reduced strain in a patient with pulmonary hypertension (B). Alternatively, color Doppler tissue imaging can be used to derive strain (C) and strain rate (D).

There is great potential for improving current prognostic tools using evidence from a number of well-performed studies that demonstrate the importance of RV function on PAH outcomes,[22,23] and arguments that RV quantification could serve as the most useful surrogate endpoint in PAH trials.[24] Overall, markers of RV function appear to do better at predicting survival than echocardiographic measures of hemodynamics. RV function markers that have been associated with survival include TAPSE, FAC, MPI, and RV free wall strain. RV free wall thickness also has prognostic value.[25] The most consistent markers of prognosis appear to be right atrial area and the presence of pericardial effusion.

Right Ventricular Assessment During Exercise

There is evolving interest in the assessment of the RV during exercise as a means of assessing pulmonary vascular function and RV contractile reserve. Although the concept of exercise-induced PH is not endorsed by international guidelines regarding the diagnosis of PH, there is relatively robust evidence relating measures obtained during exercise to outcomes in patients with PH.[26,27] When compared with direct invasive gold standards, pulmonary artery pressure estimates derived from tricuspid valve regurgitation velocities are reliable at rest and during exercise. Similarly, quantitative measures of RV function, such as RV FAC, are relatively accurate at rest and during exercise when compared with the cardiovascular magnetic resonance(CMR)–derived RV ejection fraction.[3] Assessment of the RV during exercise has the potential to enable earlier and potentially more accurate diagnosis of pathology in patients with early PH, and may assist in improved risk stratification in those with established disease. However, this remains a largely research pursuit, and further evidence of incremental clinical utility is required.

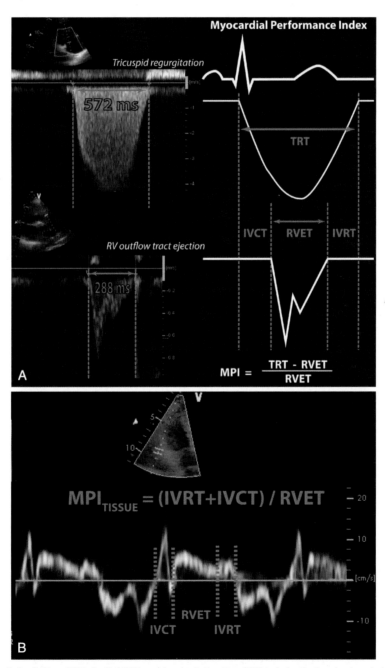

FIG. 36.18 Myocardial performance index (MPI or "Tei Index"). (A) Tricuspid regurgitation time (TRT) includes the isovolumic periods, whereas right ventricle ejection time (RVET) does not. Thus, the total isovolumic period can be deduced from subtracting RVET from TRT. Thus, the myocardial performance index, which is the ratio of isovolumic contraction time plus isovolumetric relaxation time (IVCT+IVRT)/RVET can then be expressed as a ratio of (TRT–RVET)/RVET. (B) An alternative approach uses Doppler tissue imaging (DTI) of the tricuspid valve free wall annulus to directly measure IVCT, IVRT, and RVET.

Suggested Reading

Grunig, E., & Peacock, A. J. (2015). Imaging the heart in pulmonary hypertension: an update. *European Respiratory Review*, *24*(138), 653–664.

Jurcut, R., Giusca, S., La Gerche, A., Vasile, S., Ginghina, C., & Voigt, J. U. (2010). The echocardiographic assessment of the right ventricle: what to do in 2010? *European Journal of Echocardiography*, *11*(2), 81–96.

Rudski, L. G., Lai, W. W., Afilalo, J., et al. (2010). Guidelines for the echocardiographic assessment of the right heart in adults: a report from the American Society of Echocardiography endorsed by the European Association of Echocardiography, a registered branch of the European Society of Cardiology, and the Canadian Society of Echocardiography. *Journal of the American Society of Echocardiography*, *23*(7), 685–713.

van de Veerdonk, M. C., Kind, T., Marcus, J. T., et al. (2011). Progressive right ventricular dysfunction in patients with pulmonary arterial hypertension responding to therapy. *Journal of the American College of Cardiology*, *58*(24), 2511–2519.

Wright, L. M., Dwyer, N., Celermajer, D., Kritharides, L., & Marwick, T. H. (2016). Follow-up of pulmonary hypertension with echocardiography. *JACC Cardiovascular Imaging*, *9*(6), 733–746.

A complete reference list can be found online at ExpertConsult.com.

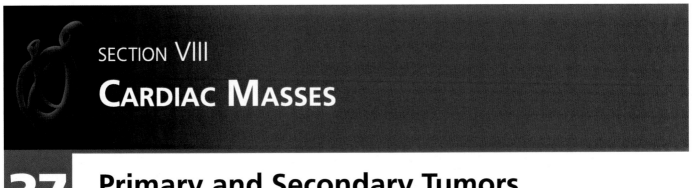

37 Primary and Secondary Tumors

Justina C. Wu

INTRODUCTION

The first demonstration of a left atrial myxoma by ultrasound occurred in Germany in 1959.[1] Since then echocardiography has evolved to become the usual initial modality for detecting a cardiac tumor. Cardiac neoplasms are found in only 1%–2% of cases in general autopsy series. For this reason, routine screening to rule out cancer in the heart is not appropriate and would undoubtedly lead to many false positives. This is generally true even in cancer patients, in whom there is higher risk (autopsy incidence reported in up to 4%–8%) of cardiac tumors. However, there are exceptional circumstances, such as familial tumor syndromes and carcinoid, in which screening may be justified. Because of the rarity of primary malignancies, the best data available originate from autopsy studies and larger specialized single-center studies, supplemented by case reports in the literature.

A fair proportion of heart tumors are clinically silent and discovered as incidental findings in the process of ancillary testing or workup prior to a surgery. In other cases, systemic embolization or pericardial involvement with hemodynamic effect may be the sentinel event that initiates a cardiac workup. Even more rarely, large masses of the heart may impede cardiac inflow or outflow, cause valvular regurgitation, and hence cause heart failure or syncope.

With knowledge of the general distribution of cardiac tumors and by taking the patient's age and comorbidities into consideration, along with the location and echocardiographic features of the mass, the clinician can make an educated guess as to the likely nature of the tumor. After the possibilities are narrowed down, one can formulate a diagnostic and therapeutic plan, which may involve further imaging with intravenous (IV) echo contrast, three-dimensional (3D) echocardiography, transesophageal echocardiography (TEE), or other modalities to better define the tumor boundaries and stage before deciding upon observation, surgery, or other treatment. Echocardiography also serves to monitor for growth, recurrence after treatment, or adverse sequelae of tumors.

TUMOR TYPES

Primary Versus Secondary Tumors

The best data for the actual frequency distribution of cardiac tumors are decades old and come from autopsy series, as summarized in Fig. 37.1.[2,3] Primary tumors of the heart (see Fig. 37.1A and B) occur in only 0.02% of autopsy series and represent only 2%–5% of all cardiac tumors. The vast majority are secondary, metastatic neoplasms (see Fig. 37.1C). Although most clinicians recognize the significance of this binary classification system, the World Health Organization (WHO) has updated and refined their classification and nomenclature in 2015 to better describe rare tumors and those with variable or unknown natural history.[4]

Primary Benign Tumors

Of the primary tumors, approximately 75% are benign, and approximately 30% of these in the general population (up to 50% in adults) are myxomas. The next most common primary tumors are lipomas (10%) and papillary fibroelastomas (8% of general population). Echocardiographic characteristics and patient demographics are often enough to distinguish these three entities. (Of note, the prevalence of tumors reported in the literature from living patients may differ slightly from incidence rates reported from autopsy series, particularly for benign tumors).

Myxoma

Cardiac myxomas are the most common type of primary cardiac tumor, particularly in adults. They are believed to arise from endocardial (mesenchymal) cells. The classic myxoma arises in the left atrium (in 75% of the cases), but 20% of cases arise in the right atrium, and the remaining 5% occur in the ventricles. It is common for the myxoma to be attached to the interatrial septum near the fossa ovalis via a stalk or pedicle, although attachments to the mitral valve have also been described.

On echocardiography, myxomas often appear as compact, gelatinous-appearing masses that can be globular, ovoid, or multilobular (Fig. 37.2 and Video 37.1). However, there exists a spectrum of morphologies. Smaller tumors are often more papillary or villous in appearance, are friable, and are more prone to embolization. In contrast, larger bulky myxomas tend to be more discrete, with a smoother surface or "cluster of grapes" appearance. These can grow large enough to fill the left atrium and are renowned for causing both mitral stenosis, with a diastolic rumble and a tumor "plop" on auscultation, as the mass prolapses into the left ventricle in diastole (Video 37.2). TEE can help determine if the myxoma extends into the pulmonary veins or vena cavae.

There is an autosomal dominant form of myxoma, which constitutes approximately 7% of cases, that tend to present earlier in life (i.e., second decade) than the sporadic myxomas. Individuals affected by this mutation in the PRKAR1A gene (which encodes a regulatory subunit of protein kinase A) or alternatively by a chromosome 2p16 mutation, tend to develop myxomas in atypical locations, even extracardiac locations, with multiple and recurrent sites.[4] The "Carney complex" is a syndrome associated with these mutations that consists of myxomas, hyperpigmented skin spots (lentiginosis), and endocrine overactivity. First-degree relatives of identified patients should be screened by echocardiography, and the patients themselves must be surveyed frequently for recurrence of myxoma.

Lipoma

Lipomas represent slightly more than 8% of benign cardiac tumors. The tumor consists of benign fat cells that are encapsulated. They can arise anywhere in the heart but have been described most frequently in the

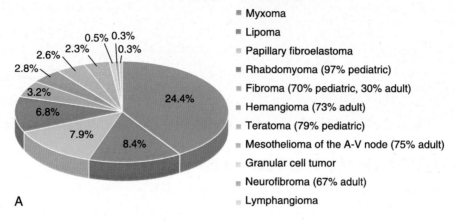

Primary Benign Tumors of the Heart

- Myxoma
- Lipoma
- Papillary fibroelastoma
- Rhabdomyoma (97% pediatric)
- Fibroma (70% pediatric, 30% adult)
- Hemangioma (73% adult)
- Teratoma (79% pediatric)
- Mesothelioma of the A-V node (75% adult)
- Granular cell tumor
- Neurofibroma (67% adult)
- Lymphangioma

A

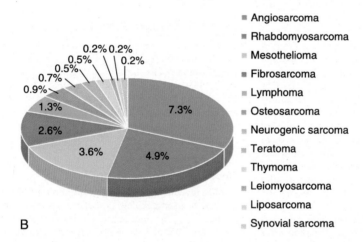

Primary Malignant Tumors of the Heart

- Angiosarcoma
- Rhabdomyosarcoma
- Mesothelioma
- Fibrosarcoma
- Lymphoma
- Osteosarcoma
- Neurogenic sarcoma
- Teratoma
- Thymoma
- Leiomyosarcoma
- Liposarcoma
- Synovial sarcoma

B

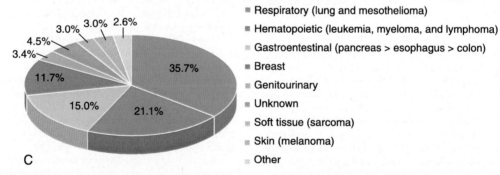

Secondary Tumors Metastatic to the Heart

- Respiratory (lung and mesothelioma)
- Hematopoietic (leukemia, myeloma, and lymphoma)
- Gastroentestinal (pancreas > esophagus > colon)
- Breast
- Genitourinary
- Unknown
- Soft tissue (sarcoma)
- Skin (melanoma)
- Other

C

FIG. 37.1 Frequency distribution of cardiac tumors, data obtained from the US autopsy series from the Armed Forces Institute of Pathology, most recently updated in 1996. Note that: (1) percentages are the percent of total primary tumors, n = 533 (408 benign and 125 malignant); (2) pericardial and bronchogenic cysts, which represent 16.7% (n = 89) of all primary cardiac masses in this autopsy series, are excluded from the above analysis; and (3) pediatric was defined as patients ≤15 years old. *(Adapted from Wu JC. Cardiac tumors and masses. In: Stergiopoulous K, Brown DL, eds.* Evidence-Based Cardiology Consult. *New York: Springer; 2014:377-390.)*

left ventricle, right atrium, and atrial septum, usually in the subepicardial or subendocardial regions. On echocardiograms, they appear as homogeneous circumscribed masses that may be hyperechoic or hypoechoic. Those in the interatrial septum need to be distinguished from lipomatous hypertrophy, which is a normal finding (see Chapter 39). Lipomas tend to grow progressively and may intrude into the pericardial space. Accordingly, they are surgically excised if the patient becomes symptomatic due to mass effect or arrhythmia. An example, along with differential diagnoses and corresponding cardiac magnetic resonance imaging (MRI), is shown in Fig. 37.3.

Papillary Fibroelastoma

Papillary fibroelastomas are the most common valvular tumor and have recently surpassed myxomas in being the most commonly excised cardiac masses.[4] They represent approximately 8% of benign cardiac tumors and most commonly develop in older adults. Most (>80%) arise on the left-sided valves, and a minority may be multivalvular. They often appear on the aortic valve, less frequently on the mitral valve; a fraction manifest at multiple valves. On echocardiogram, fibroelastomas may appear irregular, frequently threadlike or fingerlike in shape, can often branch or have flowerlike fronds, and be quite mobile. They may attach to either

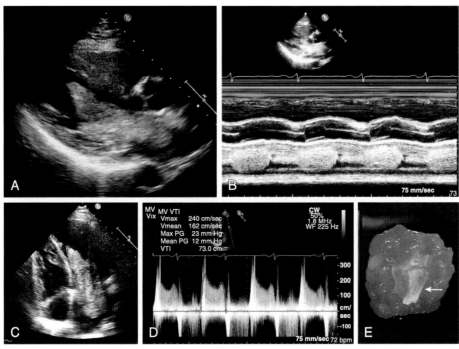

FIG. 37.2 **Left atrial myxoma.** See also corresponding Video 37.1. (A) Parasternal long-axis view. (B) M-mode view showing the mass prolapsing into the left atrium in systole. (C) Apical four-chamber view. (D) Transmitral gradients (mitral stenosis) as shown by continuous wave Doppler, with peak and mean gradients of 23 and 12 mm Hg. (E) Gross pathologic specimen of a left atrial myxoma, which appears as a clusterlike, gelatinous myxoid mass with an attached fragment *(arrow)* of atrial myocardium and interatrial septum. *(A–D modified from Wu JC. Cardiac tumors and masses. In: Stergiopoulous K, Brown DL, eds.* Evidence-Based Cardiology Consult. *New York: Springer; 2014:377-390.)*

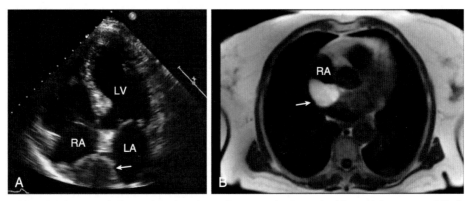

FIG. 37.3 **Lipoma.** (A) Apical four-chamber view of a lipoma *(arrow)* residing in the interatrial septum. The differential diagnoses would be lipomatous hypertrophy of the interatrial septum, myxoma, or metastatic tumor. (B) Cardiac magnetic resonance imaging (MRI) T1-weighted short-axis image at the base of the heart, showing the well-circumscribed hyperintense mass *(arrow)*, which was hypointense after fat suppression and did not enhance during or after first pass perfusion. This was consistent with cardiac lipoma, which was confirmed upon surgical excision. *LA,* Left atrium, *LV,* left ventricle, *RA,* right atrium. *(Courtesy Swathy Kolli, MD, Brigham and Women's Hospital. Adapted from Wu JC. Cardiac tumors and masses. In: Stergiopoulous K, Brown DL, eds.* Evidence-Based Cardiology Consult. *New York: Springer; 2014:377-390.)*

left ventricular outflow tract (LVOT) or aortic aspect of the aortic valve (Fig. 37.4A and Video 37.3). They tend to occur more on the atrial side of the mitral valve but have been found attached to mitral chordae or papillary muscles as well (see Fig. 37.4B and Video 37.4). Pathologically, fibroelastomas appear to be endocardial papillary growths that are larger and more exuberant forms of Lambl's (degenerative) excrescences. Studies indicate that fibroelastomas larger than 1 cm in length have greater potential to embolize and hence are often resected (with preservation of the underlying valve) for primary or secondary prevention. Interestingly, up to 30% of papillary fibroelastomas are findings discovered incidentally upon echocardiography, cardiac surgery, or autopsy.[5]

Rhabdomyomas

Rhabdomyomas are less common primary tumors, representing approximately 7% of total population, but represent the most common primary heart tumor in children. Greater than 95% of rhabdomyomas occur in

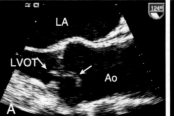

FIG. 37.4 **Papillary fibroelastomas.** (A) Aortic valve fibroelastoma on transesophageal echocardiography (TEE). Note the 1.5-cm long wormlike mobile echodensity on the aortic aspect of the valve, as well as a second short filamentous fibroelastoma on the left ventricular outflow tract (LVOT) aspect of the valve. See also corresponding Video 37.3. (B) Papillary fibroelastoma of the left ventricle (LV). This three-dimensional (3D) transthoracic echocardiogram (TTE) apical four-chamber view shows the fibroelastoma *(arrow)* attached to a mitral chorda. See also corresponding Video 37.4. *Ao,* Aorta; *RV,* left ventricle.

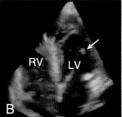

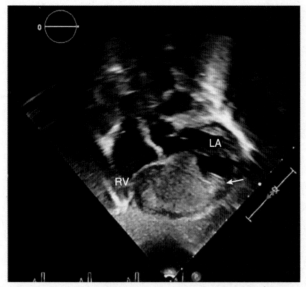

FIG. 37.5 Fibroma in child. Transthoracic pediatric echocardiogram five-chamber view showing a large 5-cm fibroma *(arrow)* arising in the distal left ventricle and exerting mass effect upon the right ventricle (RV). *LA,* Left atrium.

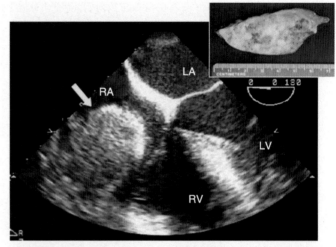

FIG. 37.6 Hemangioma. The *arrow* indicates a large mass arising from the right atrioventricular groove occupying the right atrium (RA) on this transesophageal four-chamber view. The mass was fed by the right coronary artery and also partially compressed it. It was confirmed on surgical resection *(inset)* to be a hemangioma with both cavernous and capillary (red) blood-filled areas. *LA,* Left atrium; *LV,* left ventricle; *RV,* right ventricle.

young children, often before a year of age or even detected on prenatal ultrasonography. Approximately half of all cases are associated with the genetic disorder tuberous sclerosis, but these tumors can also arise spontaneously. They appear as well-demarcated, round, homogeneously hyperechoic masses or discrete foci of thickened myocardium, most frequently located in the ventricles (80% of cases, with 15% arising in the right ventricle). They frequently occur in multiples and have not been reported to arise on cardiac valves. Rhabdomyomas carry a relatively good prognosis because they tend to regress, partially or completely, with time. For this reason, unless they cause severe obstruction, valve dysfunction, or intractable arrhythmias, they are observed expectantly.

The remaining tumors, which together make up less than 10% of primary benign cardiac tumors, include fibromas, hemangiomas, and teratomas. The fibromas and teratomas also occur predominantly in the pediatric population.[6] Fibromas are the second most common benign cardiac tumor found in children and fetuses and appear as a solid very echodense mass of fibroblasts and collagen (an example is shown in Fig. 37.5). They typically arise in the ventricular myocardium, usually the LV free wall or interventricular septum (where they may mimic hypertrophic cardiomyopathy). They are always solitary and may have calcified centers (in contrast to rhabdomyomas). Unlike rhabdomyomas, the growth of fibromas appears to be variable. Some can grow over time and cause ventricular arrhythmias (often reentrant ventricular tachycardia) or less often obstruction or valvular dysfunction, in which case surgical resection may be necessary. Others have been observed over decades and shown regression, although they may never resolve completely.[7] Of the remaining benign cardiac tumors, hemangiomas may be distinguished as being highly vascularized and hence may take up IV echocardiographic contrast (Fig. 37.6). These are rare, can be found at any age, and are mostly located in the right atrium (particularly in children) and ventricles. The natural history is variable.[8] Teratomas are usually found in the anterior mediastinum rather than intracardiac locations, particularly in the pericardium, where they may be attached to the ascending aorta and hemorrhage.[4] These tumors are distinct in that they may possess elements of all three germ cell layers, as well as hair, skin, and muscle, and the propensity for malignancy is related to the degree of differentiation.

Benign Versus Malignant

Primary Malignant Tumors

Approximately one-fourth of all primary cardiac tumors are malignant, and most are sarcomas.[9] Histologically, sarcomas can be subclassified as: angiosarcomas, sarcomas of varying lines of differentiation

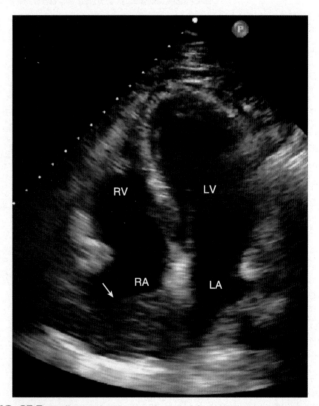

FIG. 37.7 Cardiac angiosarcoma. This apical four-chamber transthoracic view displays a right atrial (RA) mass *(arrow),* which was initially presumed to be a myxoma but subsequently on pathology found to be a high-grade angiosarcoma with spindle cell elements and transmural invasion through the right atrial wall. *LA,* Left atrium; *LV,* left ventricle; *RV,* right ventricle.

(undifferentiated, myxofibrosarcomas, sarcomas with bone matrix elements), and rhabdomyosarcoma. Angiosarcomas are the most common type in adults (Fig. 37.7). These have a predilection for the right atrium, where they may invade the vena cava and tricuspid apparatus. They often appear bulky and multilobular, are broad based, grow rapidly in an exophytic manner, and present with intracardiac obstruction. The next most common primary heart malignancy is the rhabdomyosarcoma, which can arise in any cardiac chamber and is often multifocal. With all cardiac sarcomas, those that affect the left heart tend to present more often with congestive heart failure. Mesothelioma, fibrosarcoma, and cardiac lymphoma are rarer cardiac malignancies. Regardless of the histologic type of sarcoma, the treatment options and prognosis are usually dictated largely by the tumor's anatomic location and effect on the heart. All the primary cardiac malignancies share a predilection for rapid invasive growth and metastasis with frequent extension to the pericardium, which may limit the options for complete resection. All confer a poor prognosis even with complete resection and systemic chemotherapy or radiotherapy. Unlike the benign cardiac tumors, there have been no demonstrated linkages of these malignancies with specific genetic mutations.

Secondary Tumors

As stated previously, secondary or metastatic masses are 20–40 times more likely to be found in the heart than primary tumors.[2,10] The frequency distribution of malignancies found in the heart is shown in Fig. 37.1C. More than one-third of these malignancies arise from the respiratory system (lung and mesothelioma). Approximately one-fifth (21%) originate from hematopoietic malignancies such as leukemia, lymphoma, and myeloma. Gastrointestinal and breast cancer account for much of the remaining fraction of secondary tumors. Given how relatively rare primary cardiac tumors are, if there is no obvious extracardiac malignancy seen by conventional radiologic methods (computed tomography [CT] or MRI), then positron emission tomography (PET) scanning is often undertaken to search the body for a primary source.

TUMOR LOCATIONS: SITE-SPECIFIC DIFFERENTIAL

The location in which a tumor arises within the heart is often the strongest clue to its type and origin. Certain malignancies (e.g., renal cell and bronchogenic carcinomas) have a predilection for invading the heart by specific pathways, whereas other distributions are simply observed cumulatively from the literature and experience.[6] Table 37.1 summarizes the site-specific differential diagnoses for cardiac tumors. The most common findings are presented here.

Atrial Tumors

In the left atrium the most common mass overall is not in fact a neoplasm but is the thrombus (see Chapter 38). Thrombus should be ruled out particularly in patients with atrial fibrillation, enlarged left atria or prior cardiac surgery, and mitral stenosis. MRI or CT angiography can be used to distinguish thrombus from tissue, and thrombi usually regress with adequate anticoagulation. The most common neoplasm in the left atrium is myxoma; if the mass has the prototypical location, appearance, and attaches to the interatrial septum, further diagnostic modalities are often not required and treatment may proceed directly with surgical resection. Another primary tumor that may involve the atria is the lipoma. In smokers, bronchogenic carcinomas, which invade the left atrium via the pulmonary veins, are a distinct possibility and chest CT may be indicated to look for the primary neoplasm. TEE or cardiac MRI may be used to assess invasion and patency of the pulmonary veins.

Right atrial tumors frequently turn out to be myxomas as well. However, secondary tumors from the kidney (renal cell carcinoma or nephroblastoma), liver (hepatocellular carcinoma), and the adrenal glands (adrenaloma) are notorious for extending up the inferior vena cava and invading the right atrium. Fig. 37.8 is an example of renal cell carcinoma. Thrombus alone or superimposed on such tumors may also extend to the right atrium. From the other direction, lung and thyroid carcinomas may grow down the superior vena cava into the right atrium. Of the rare primary malignant cardiac tumors of adulthood, angiosarcomas are known to have a predilection for the right atrium.

Ventricular Tumors

In contrast to the atrial tumors, which generally are intracavitary, ventricular masses are rare and usually arise intramurally. They are rare and seen mostly in the pediatric population. Both rhabdomyomas

TABLE 37.1 Site-Specific Differential Diagnoses for Neoplasms Detected on Echocardiography[a]

	PRIMARY	SECONDARY (METASTATIC)
Left atrium	**Myxoma** **Lipoma** *Sarcomas (undifferentiated and angiosarcomas)* **Hemangioma** **Paraganglioma** (10% malignant)	Lung (bronchogenic) carcinoma Lymphoma
Right atrium	**Myxoma** *Sarcoma (especially angiosarcoma)* **Paraganglioma** (10% malignant)	Nephroblastoma, renal cell cancer Hepatocellular carcinoma Adrenal tumors Pancreatic carcinoma
Left ventricle	**Rhabdomyoma** (often multiple) **Fibroma** **Hamartomas** **Purkinje cell tumors** (usually infants)	
Right ventricle	**Rhabdomyoma** **Fibroma**	
Valves/Annuli	**Papillary fibroelastoma** **Myxoma** **Hamartoma** **Lipomas**	
Pericardium	*Mesothelioma* *Lymphoma* **Solitary fibrous tumor** (rarely malignant) *Sarcomas (fibrosarcomas, angiosarcomas, synovial sarcomas)* **Lipoma** **Germ cell tumors:** **Teratoma** *(malignant if immature)* *Yolk sac tumor* **Paraganglioma** (10% malignant)	Lung (bronchogenic) carcinoma Breast carcinoma Lymphoma/leukemia GI cancer Melanoma Liposarcoma
Anterior mediastinum		Lymphoma Thymoma and thymic carcinoma Thyroid carcinoma Teratoma

[a]For primary cardiac tumors, **bold text** is used for benign tumors, and *italic text* for malignant tumors. Some tumors have uncertain or variable biologic behavior (e.g., paragangliomas and teratomas), or very few cases described.

(the most common pediatric cardiac tumor) and fibromas tend to occur predominantly in the left ventricle, although the latter may also arise in the interventricular septum. Taking into perspective the rarity of ventricular tumors, noncancerous masses such as papillary muscles, thrombi, and degenerative or traumatic changes need to be excluded first.

Valvular Tumors

Tumors involving the valves frequently turn out to be papillary fibroelastomas in older individuals, although myxomas involving the mitral valve can occur in younger patients. Because these tumors are often smaller, more amorphous, and very mobile, real-time imaging by TEE can often visualize them better than the cardiac MRI or CT. Pragmatically, it may also be prudent to exclude endocarditis, either infectious or marantic in etiology, when valvular masses are seen in the context of a concomitant fever.

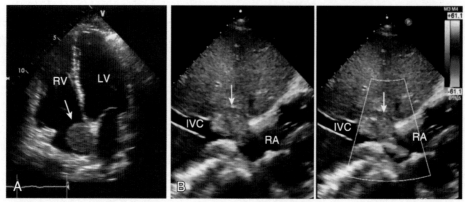

FIG. 37.8 Renal cell carcinoma. (A) This carcinoma *(arrow)* appears as a mobile mass that is invading the right atrium from the IVC. The mass was composed of carcinoma but also much tumor-associated thrombus. (B) Renal cell carcinoma at the IVC/RA junction, causing partial obstruction of flow. This was subsequently stented as a palliative measure. (See also Video 37.5). *IVC,* Inferior vena cava; *LV,* left ventricle; *RA,* right atrium; *RV,* right ventricle.

Pericardial Tumors

The most frequent causes of malignant pericardial disease are due to dissemination from lung, lymphoma/leukemia, and breast cancer, presumably due to their high overall prevalence in the general population. Direct extension of tumor from adjacent lung, pleura (mesothelioma), or mediastinum (such as in lymphoma) is also not uncommon. Of all the malignancies, melanoma has the highest predilection to metastasize to the pericardium. Autopsy studies have shown that melanoma causes cardiac involvement in 38%–50% of cases, yet only 2% of patients become symptomatic. Tumor involvement may appear as simple as an echolucent pericardial effusion, which upon pericardiocentesis turns out to contain malignant cells. However, aggressive solid tumors may invade the pericardial parietal surface, become partially space occupying or even completely infiltrate the pericardium as a solid mass. They may also invade further to the visceral pericardial surface and enter the myocardium (Fig. 37.9).

CLINICAL PRESENTATION OF TUMORS

Neoplasms involving the heart may come to a patient or clinician's attention in many ways and can affect not only the structure and function of the heart but also other organ systems. Knowing the classic or common patterns of tumor presentation can tune the sonographer into examining the relevant portions of the heart more astutely.

The myxoma is notorious for producing a constellation of systemic and constitutional symptoms, including fever, fatigue, malaise, arthralgias, and weight loss. However, the presence of these symptoms plus systemic embolization, particularly with a new murmur of mitral valve obstruction (i.e., a diastolic rumble of stenosis or tumor "plop") or regurgitation, is the classic presentation of left atrial myxoma.

Larger tumors may exert a mass effect on heart chambers. This can occur via extrinsic compression, such as a mediastinal tumor impinging upon the heart. The right ventricular (RV) outflow tract may be susceptible to anterior mediastinal tumors and metastatic masses that compress the area around the pulmonary artery (Fig. 37.10A). Intracavitary lesions may grow large enough to intrinsically obstruct atrial or ventricular inflow and outflow (Fig. 37.10B). Obstruction of the superior vena cava will cause facial, neck, and upper extremity swelling and potentially dyspnea and cough. Lung adenocarcinoma, lymphoma, and metastatic mediastinal tumors account for greater than 90% of cases.[11] The clinical sequelae to RV or LV outflow obstruction is syncope.

Smaller tumors, if located intramyocardially, can lead to reentrant circuits and tachyarrhythmias, or heart block if the AV conducting system is invaded. More widespread involvement of myocardium by primary or malignant tumors can cause focal wall motion abnormalities, restrictive physiology, and congestive heart failure.

Involvement of the valves by tumors can obviously lead to stenosis and/or regurgitation. However, systemic embolization of tumor bits or

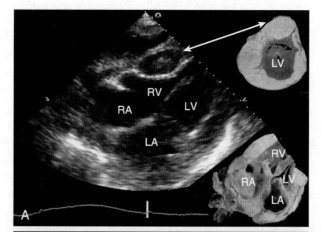

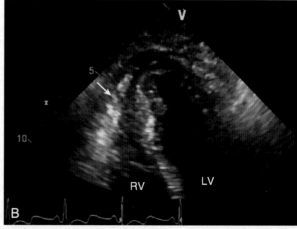

FIG. 37.9 (A) Invasion of pericardium and myocardium by pericardial mesothelioma. This subcostal four-chamber view illustrates severe thickening and inhomogeneous echodensity of the pericardium circumferentially around the heart, causing constriction. The insets show similarly oriented gross heart specimen *(lower right)* and apical short-axis section *(upper right),* with the thick light-hued mesothelioma encasing the heart. (B) Lung carcinoma invading the right ventricle (RV) apex as a solid mass. There was also an associated malignant pericardial effusion (not shown). *LA,* Left atrium; *LV,* left ventricle; *RA,* right atrium.

tumor-associated thrombus may be the first sign of a cardiac neoplasm. This is frequently a presenting symptom and feared complication of papillary fibroelastomas. "Showering" of emboli to more than one organ, including the brain, kidneys, spleen, extremities, and even the coronary arteries should always cause one to suspect a cardiac source and is a strong

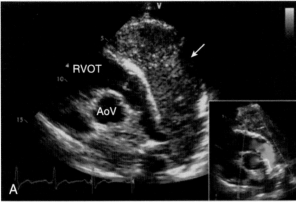
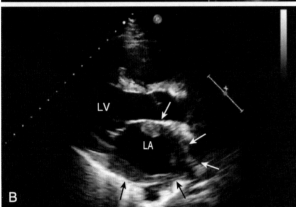

indication for echocardiography. Tumors that are more likely to embolize are those associated with the aortic valve or left atrium, those with increased mobility, and those with friable elements.[5,12,13] Right-sided masses can obviously cause pulmonary emboli, but may also be the source of paradoxical (systemic) emboli if there is a patent foramen ovale which allows interatrial communication.

Lastly, malignancies can directly invade the pericardium or alternatively seed them with metastases (via hematogenous or lymphangitic routes). In these cases, cardiac tamponade, constriction, or both physiologies can ensue (see Fig. 37.9).

Suggested Reading

Bruce, C. J. (2011). Cardiac tumours: diagnosis and management. *Heart, 97*, 151–160.
Burke, A., & Tavora, F. (2016). The 2015 WHO classification of tumors of the heart and pericardium. *Journal of Thoracic Oncology, 11*, 441–452.
Guimaraes, M. D., Bitencourt, A. G., Marchiori, E., Chojniak, R., Gross, J. L., & Kundra, V. (2014). Imaging acute complications in cancer patients: what should be evaluated in the emergency setting? *Cancer Imaging, 29*, 14–18.

A complete reference list can be found online at ExpertConsult.com.

FIG. 37.10 **Space-occupying presentations of tumors: lymphoma.** (A) Lymphoma presenting as an anterior mediastinal mass *(arrow)* impinging upon the pulmonary artery and insinuating between the aorta and pulmonary artery, causing flow acceleration in the supravalvular region (inset color Doppler) in this parasternal short-axis view at the base of the heart. (B) Non-Hodgkin B-cell lymphoma *(arrows)* infiltrating the left atrium circumferentially and invading into the pulmonary veins, in parasternal long-axis window. *AoV,* Aortic valve; *LA,* left atrium; *LV,* left ventricle; *RVOT,* right ventricular outflow tract.

38 Identification of Intracardiac Thrombus

Jordan B. Strom, Warren J. Manning

INTRODUCTION

Intracardiac thrombi represent a subset of cardiac sources of embolism, are common in a variety of cardiac disease states, and account for 15%–20% of the 500,000 annual strokes in the United States. In addition, they are important sources of systemic emboli to other vascular beds.[1] Thrombi may exist in all cardiac chambers and can either originate from an extracardiac source with migration to the heart (i.e., clot-in-transit) or arise de novo in the cardiac chambers (i.e., left atrial appendage [LAA] thrombi). In the following, we will review the appearance and differential diagnosis of thrombus and other sources of emboli and the echocardiographic methods of detecting thrombi.

INTRACARDIAC SOURCES OF EMBOLI

Similar to venous thromboembolism, arterial and intracardiac thrombi likely arise from disturbances in flow and vessel characteristics, described by Virchow triad in which there are alterations in blood flow (i.e., stasis), endothelial damage, and inherited or acquired variations in prothrombotic blood constituents.[2] Intracardiac sources of embolism may be divided into thrombotic and nonthrombotic etiologies.

Left Ventricle

Thrombus in the left ventricle (LV) typically is as a result of myocardial infarction (MI) and subsequent local akinesis/aneurysm with stasis and exposure of prothrombotic collagen to the blood pool. As a result, thrombus almost invariably occurs in areas of hypokinesis, akinesis, or dyskinesis of the underlying LV wall segments, most commonly in the setting of an apical aneurysm. It may also occur in the setting of underlying non-ischemic cardiomyopathy with reduced global ejection fraction; specific cardiomyopathies (e.g., noncompaction, Chagas, and Loeffler endocarditis) appear more predisposed to thrombus formation, presumably due to local stasis and hypercoagulability. Echocardiography is useful in detecting LV thrombi directly, as well as identifying risk factors for thrombus formation, including wall motion abnormalities and spontaneous echo contrast (SEC). There are caveats: visualization of the endocardial border and therefore clear resolution of thrombus from surrounding trabeculae may be difficult in patients with poor acoustic windows, without the use of echocardiographic contrast. Transesophageal echocardiography (TEE), despite its high resolution, may foreshorten the ventricular apex, and thus transthoracic echocardiography (TTE) is actually preferred for the identification of apical thrombi. Occasionally, even with appropriate contrast opacification, other imaging modalities such as computed tomography (CT) and cardiac magnetic resonance imaging (CMR) may be required to identify thrombus with higher fidelity.[3]

Left Atrium

The LAA represents the most common location for atrial thrombus formation. Ninety percent of thrombi occur in the setting of atrial fibrillation of atrial flutter as a result of disorganized and ineffective contraction of the LAA causing local stasis (Fig. 38.1 and Video 38.1).[4] When the LAA ejection velocity, measured using pulsed-wave Doppler 1 cm into the mouth of the appendage, is less than 0.4 m/s, there is an increased risk of thrombus formation (Fig. 38.2).[5] Rheumatic mitral stenosis may also contribute to left atrial (LA) enlargement, stasis, and an increased risk for LA thrombus formation and thromboembolism despite sinus rhythm.

The incidence of LA thrombus with mitral stenosis in sinus rhythm is estimated to be 2.4%–13.5%, with risk factors including age greater than 44 years, LA inferosuperior dimension greater than 6.9 cm, mean mitral gradient greater than 18 mm Hg, and dense SEC.[6] Some consider TEE warranted if any of the aforementioned risk factors are present; the absence of SEC on TEE is highly predictive of thrombus absence.[6] In contrast to the stasis and predisposition to thrombus formation seen in mitral stenosis, significant mitral regurgitation has been associated with a lower incidence of thrombus formation and thromboembolization in individuals with rheumatic mitral valvular disease.[7] Owing to the complex three-dimensional anatomy of the LAA with its one to four lobes, trabeculation, and interindividual variability in morphology, distinguishing thrombus from normal anatomical structures by TEE can be difficult, especially in patients with SEC (Fig. 38.3).

Right Ventricle/Right Atrium

Although the same disease processes involved in formation of LV thrombi occur in the right ventricle (RV), the prevalence and specific predictors of RV thrombi have not been identified to date. Certain cardiomyopathies predominantly involving the RV, most notably arrhythmogenic right ventricular cardiomyopathy (ARVC), have been noted in case series to be associated with RV thrombi and may identify a group at risk of RV thrombus formation.[8] Loeffler endocarditis (also called endomyocardial fibroelastosis) is often associated with both right and left ventricular restrictive physiology and thrombi, typically mural and involving the apices of the heart (see Chapter 24). In theory, one would presume that there is a higher risk for thrombus formation for mechanical prostheses in the tricuspid position due to the lower ventricular pressures in the RV versus LV, but supportive data are limited. With the increasing use of right-sided intracardiac devices such as pacemaker and defibrillator leads, whose artificial surfaces are predisposed to thrombus formation, RV thrombi are likely to be of greater importance in the future (Fig. 38.4 and Video 38.2). Venous thromboembolism that is visualized in the right atrium (RA) or RV, so called clot-in-transit, is high risk for subsequent pulmonary embolism and may appear "sausage-like" in shape on echocardiography, representing a cast of the originating lower extremity vein (Fig. 38.5 and Video 38.3; see also Fig. 35.1 and Video 35.2). The RA appendage (RAA) is broad based compared with the LA and can be a source of pulmonary embolism in setting of atrial fibrillation or atrial flutter.

Prosthetic Valves

With their thrombogenic artificial surfaces, mechanical valve prostheses are common sources of intracardiac embolism, particularly in the tricuspid and mitral positions where chamber pressures are lower and there may be areas of stagnation. Subtherapeutic anticoagulation is a major risk factor. Because thrombus on echocardiography may appear similar to pannus or vegetation, both of which may also affect prosthetic valves, the clinical history (in particular the acuity of onset of symptoms, and any history of lapse in anticoagulant therapy), laboratory data including the international normalized ratio (INR), and echocardiographic characteristics such as mobility are all paramount to proper identification of prostheses-associated intracardiac masses (see Chapter 31). Although the risk of thrombus and embolization is higher in mechanical valves, thromboembolism may occur with bioprosthetic valves as well, particularly in the first several months after implantation. Due to shadowing and reverberations from the carbon/titanium valve occluders or supporting rings, identification

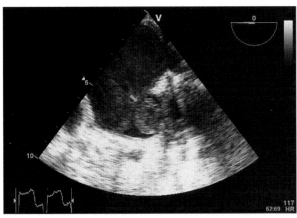

FIG. 38.1 Transesophageal echocardiography of the left atrial appendage shows a round 2 × 1 cm structure with the echodensity and location consistent with thrombus *(arrow)*. Note the overlying spontaneous echo contrast. See corresponding Video 38.1.

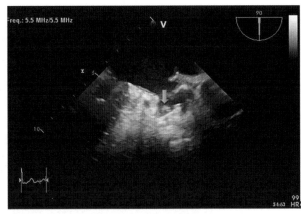

FIG. 38.3 Transesophageal echocardiogram two-chamber image of the left atrial appendage, showing a multilobulated left atrial appendage with at least four lobes visualized in this particular scan plane. A small thrombus is also seen *(arrow)*.

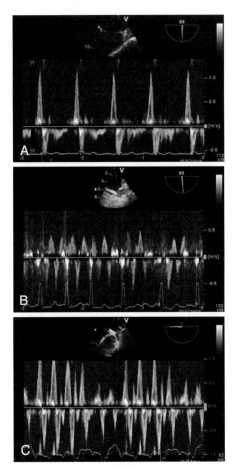

FIG. 38.2 Pulsed-wave Doppler at the entrance to the left atrial appendage during transesophageal echocardiography displaying (A) normal amplitude, regular contraction consistent with normal sinus rhythm, (B) variably reduced and disorganized contraction velocities in the setting of underlying atrial fibrillation, and (C) higher amplitude and more organized contraction velocities consistent with atrial flutter, compared with that of atrial fibrillation above.

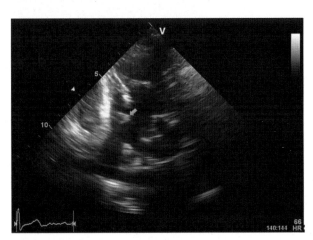

FIG. 38.4 Transthoracic echocardiogram, parasternal short-axis view at the base of the heart, demonstrating a pacemaker wire extending into the right ventricle with a rectangular thrombus *(arrow)* attached to its tip. See corresponding Video 38.2.

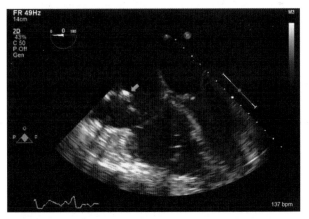

FIG. 38.5 Transesophageal 4-chamber view showing an echogenic thrombus *(arrow)* prolapsing through a stretched tricuspid valve annulus, so-called, clot-in-transit. Note that the right ventricle (RV) appears dilated in the setting of a preexisting pulmonary embolism and RV pressure overload. See corresponding Video 38.3.

Interatrial and Interventricular Septum

of prosthetic valve thrombi usually requires TEE for mitral and tricuspid valve prostheses or a combination of TTE and TEE for aortic and pulmonic prostheses. In some cases, no discrete thrombus is visualized but is suggested by an increase in transvalvular velocities, diminished valve clicks, and clinical deterioration (Fig. 38.6). Furthermore, thrombi may be very small and obscured by prosthetic material. Thus, in the absence of other risk factors for cardiac thromboembolism, a prosthetic valve should be considered to be the likely source of embolism in most cases.

Paradoxical embolism of a venous thrombus or mass to the systemic arterial bed (see Video 35.2) may occur in the setting of an intracardiac septal defect, either at the atrial or ventricular level, with intermittent or continuous right-to-left flow. Similarly, although a patent foramen ovale (PFO) is present in 25%–30% of the population at autopsy, it is noted with higher prevalence in younger adults with stroke.[9] Particularly in association with an atrial septal aneurysm, it may predispose to a higher risk of

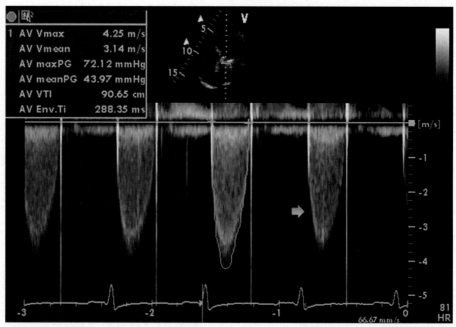

1 AV Vmax	4.25 m/s
AV Vmean	3.14 m/s
AV maxPG	72.12 mmHg
AV meanPG	43.97 mmHg
AV VTI	90.65 cm
AV Env.Ti	288.35 ms

FIG. 38.6 Continuous-wave Doppler through the aortic valve in a patient with a bileaflet mechanical aortic valve prosthesis demonstrates a diminished opening valve click *(arrow)* and higher transvalvular velocities than expected for this type of prosthesis. This is suggestive of prosthetic valve obstruction.

paradoxical embolism in patients less than 55 years old. However, current data are conflicting on the benefit of PFO closure to reduce this risk, in part due to the overall low rate of recurrence of stroke in those populations without other identified sources of embolus (i.e., cryptogenic stroke).

Nonthrombotic Causes of Embolism

Nonthrombotic masses may also embolize to the systemic arterial bed and are an important consideration on the differential diagnosis of systemic embolization. Primary intracardiac tumors most commonly myxomas and fibroelastomas, infectious or noninfectious vegetations, and complex arterial atheromas (>4 mm thick or mobile) can all embolize (see Chapters 37 and 39). In addition, intracardiac structures such as mitral annular calcification with overlying thrombus may be a rare source of embolism.

PREVALENCE OF AND RISK FACTORS FOR LEFT VENTRICULAR AND ATRIAL THROMBI

Prior MI represents the greatest risk for LV thrombus formation, with the likelihood of thrombus formation related to infarct size and location. Patients with large anterior MIs with anteroapical aneurysms are particularly at risk. Using LV ejection fraction as a surrogate for infarct size post-MI, in the Gruppo Italiano per lo Studio della Sopravvivenza nell'infarto Miocardico (GISSI-3) database, individuals with an left ventricular ejection fraction (LVEF) ≤40% had a higher incidence of LV thrombus (17.8% in the setting of anterior MI, 5.4% at other sites) compared with those with a higher LVEF (9.6% in anterior MI, 1.8% at other sites).[10,11] Although those with an LVEF less than 20% are at highest risk of LV thrombus formation, Doppler echocardiography can be used to identify abnormal spatial flow patterns, predictive of LV thrombus formation.[12] Specifically, persistence of abnormal flow patterns noted at 24 hours post MI, defined as (1) delay between onset of blood motion at the mitral valve and apical level (best demonstrated by high pulse repetition frequency Doppler), (2) a continuous positive Doppler shift near the lateral wall, or (3) continuous negative Doppler shift during the cardiac cycle near the interventricular septum, identified individuals who developed LV thrombus at 3 months. The abnormal Doppler flow patterns are thought to reflect larger ring-type vortices or smaller local apical rotating flow patterns engendered by areas of dysfunctional ventricle.

Most thrombi develop within a median of 5–6 days after MI, with one series suggesting an incidence of 27% at less than 24 hours, 75% by 1

week, and 96% by 2 weeks.[13] In the era of reperfusion, estimates of prevalence appear to have decreased to 4%–17% incidence in several small series of individuals undergoing reperfusion therapy (with either fibrinolysis or percutaneous coronary intervention [PCI]), compared with the 40% incidence noted previously.[14] In a meta-analysis of six trials and 390 patients with prior anterior MI and LV thrombus, fibrinolysis reduced the odds of LV thrombus formation by 0.48 (95% CI 0.29–0.79), likely by reducing infarct size and accelerating endogenous fibrinolysis.[15] The prevalence of LV thrombus after primary PCI for ST elevation myocardial infarction (STEMI) is similar to that seen with fibrinolysis. In one study of 163 patients, TTE performed within 3–5 days after MI had a prevalence of 10.4% thrombus in anterior MI and 4.3% overall.[10] In another study of 1059 patients receiving primary PCI, risk factors for LV thrombus included reduced LVEF, anterior MI, and use of glycoprotein IIb/IIIa inhibitors. It is likely that the prevalence of LV thrombus after MI has been underestimated as the aforementioned studies did not use echocardiographic contrast, used TTE instead of CMR, which have shown higher rates of detection of LV thrombi, and excluded those with severe heart failure.[16]

The prevalence for LV and LA thrombus may vary according to comorbid and genetic risk, as well as medication compliance. For example, although LAA thrombi are more common in those with atrial fibrillation, this risk varies according to presence and adequacy of anticoagulation and comorbid conditions known to predispose to LV and LA thrombi (e.g., heparin-induced thrombocytopenia and polycythemia vera). Furthermore, prothrombotic tendencies that show a strong familial inheritance but are not yet been localized to single mutations may account for the increased risk of thrombus formation in individuals in whom no etiology for thrombus formation has been identified. In addition, specific disease states, in particular the cardiomyopathies associated with diminished LV systolic function, are associated with a higher LV thrombus risk. In noncompaction cardiomyopathy, developmental failure of compaction of the spongiform myocardium contributes to diminished LV systolic function and large intramyocardial recesses in continuity with the LV chamber. Resulting stasis and thrombus formation are more common (Fig. 38.7; see also Videos 22.5 and 22.6). Thus individuals with noncompaction cardiomyopathy may be at higher risk for systemic embolization. Certain cardiomyopathies associated with apical akinesis or aneurysm (i.e., Chagas disease, hypertrophic cardiomyopathy with apical aneurysm, and Takotsubo cardiomyopathy) are associated with a risk of thrombus formation and embolization (see Chapter 22).[17–19] Furthermore, cardiomyopathies in which there is disturbance of the

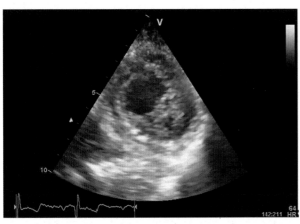

FIG. 38.7 Transthoracic echocardiogram parasternal short-axis view at the apex in a patient with noncompaction cardiomyopathy showing prominent trabeculations (*arrow*) and intramyocardial recesses that predispose to thrombus formation.

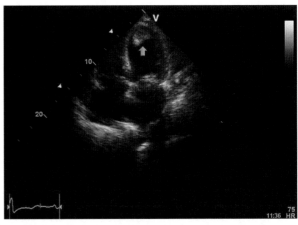

FIG. 38.8 Transthoracic echocardiogram apical four-chamber view demonstrating a large apical thrombus (*arrow*). Note the highly reflective surface and protrusion into the left ventricular cavity suggesting recent formation. See corresponding Video 38.4.

blood-endocardium barrier (e.g., Loeffler endocarditis, hypereosinophilic syndromes, and ARVC) are also at risk.[8,20]

Other imaging modalities may be more sensitive than TTE for identification of thrombus and should be considered if further imaging will change the overall treatment plan. In one study, late gadolinium enhancement CMR identified thrombi in 21% of 57 patients with prior MI or ischemic cardiomyopathy versus only 8.8% identified by TTE with the nonvisualized thrombi primarily located at the LV apex.[21] Another retrospective study of 160 patients with remote MI and confirmed LV thrombus at surgery or autopsy, the sensitivity of LV thrombus with CMR was 88%, versus 23% with TTE and 40% with TEE.[16] CT angiography has evolved to become a useful modality, particularly for visualizing abnormalities in aortic mechanical prostheses, which can be difficult to visualize on both TTE and TEE due to acoustic shadowing (see Chapter 48).

ECHOCARDIOGRAPHIC APPEARANCE

The echocardiographic appearance of LV thrombus may be difficult to distinguish from other cardiac masses, and the diagnosis of thrombus may depend on the absence of characteristics of other masses. Furthermore, no consensus exists currently on which measurements or characteristics should be used to describe or categorize thrombi. For example, although thrombi are often described according to their major and minor axis lengths, it is unclear whether using the major axis length alone or the area or volume of a thrombus is more relevant to clinical outcomes. Similarly, while thrombus mobility is associated with increased risk of embolization, no consensus exists on what degree of mobility confers an impact on patient outcomes. Furthermore, LV thrombus appearance is variable and is impacted by age of the thrombus. New thrombus is often highly mobile, with a reflective surface, protruding into the LV cavity (Fig. 38.8 and Video 38.4; see also Fig. 20.2 and Video 20.3). Older thrombi resemble the tissue characteristics of the liver, have a smooth, often concave, surface, and tend to be less mobile (Fig. 38.9; see also Fig. 20.2 and Video 20.4). Furthermore, pedunculated (as opposed to mural) and multiple LV thrombi are at higher risk of systemic embolization even with anticoagulation.[22] Additional independent risk factors included a history of cardiac arrest (pretreatment), a dilated LV, prior cerebrovascular accident, and female gender. These high-risk groups may warrant more aggressive therapy and close follow-up with serial echocardiography.

Several intracardiac masses may have similar echocardiographic appearances to thrombus (see Chapter 39). Normal structures may be confused with thrombus. For example, the "warfarin ridge," a ridge of tissue separating the LAA from the left upper pulmonary vein, is named for its predilection to be confused with thrombi requiring anticoagulation. It may be nodular or linear in appearance and may even undulate with cardiac motion (Fig. 38.10; see also Video 49.7). The location of the warfarin ridge distinguishes it from thrombus. Similarly, prominent LAA trabeculations known as "false tendons" may be confused for thrombi, although typically are the same echotexture as the underlying myocardium and attach to the adjacent myocardium. Other normal

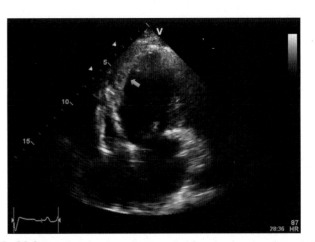

FIG. 38.9 Transthoracic echocardiogram apical four-chamber view demonstrating a mural thrombus (*arrow*), adherent to the septal wall and apex. Note the firm echotexture similar to that of the liver and concave appearance suggesting its chronicity.

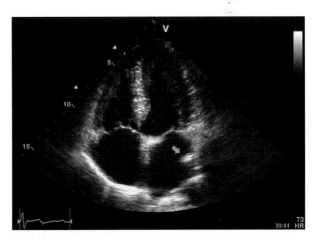

FIG. 38.10 Transthoracic echocardiogram apical four-chamber view demonstrating a prominent "warfarin ridge" (*arrow*), separating the left atrial appendage (above) from the left upper pulmonary vein (below). This normal structure is sometimes confused for thrombus.

structures commonly confused with thrombus include the eustachian valve (Fig. 38.11) and a fenestrated eustachian valve known as a Chiari network, typically located in the RA (see also Fig. 29.1 and Video 49.1). An aneurysmal atrial septum, defined as a combined total excursion of the interatrial septum of ≥15 mm may be confused for thrombus, is commonly associated with PFO, and is an independent risk factor for

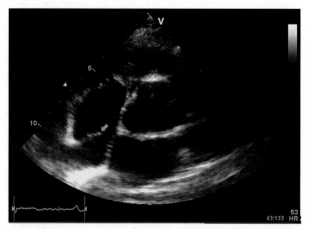

FIG. 38.11 Transthoracic echocardiogram parasternal short-axis view at the level of the aortic valve showing a prominent eustachian valve *(arrow)*, a normal embryologic structure often confused for thrombus.

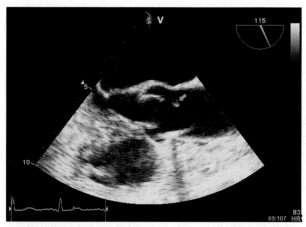

FIG. 38.13 Zoomed transesophageal echocardiogram of the aortic valve image demonstrating a filamentous structure attached to the downstream side of the non-coronary aortic valve cusp consistent with a Lambl excrescence *(arrow)*.

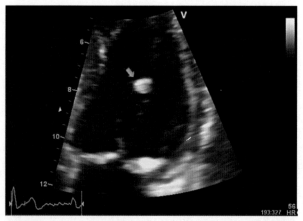

FIG. 38.12 Zoomed image of a transthoracic echocardiogram four-chamber view demonstrating a round papillary fibroelastoma *(arrow)* attached to the chordal structures. Note the downstream location relative to the mitral valve.

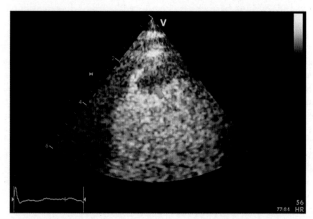

FIG. 38.14 Zoomed image of a transthoracic echocardiography apical four-chamber view focused on the apex using a myocardial contrast agent to opacify the left ventricle chamber. The filling defect seen is an apical thrombus *(arrow)* and demonstrates how intravenous echocardiographic contrast can be used to identify apical thrombi with greater accuracy and confidence. See corresponding Video 38.7.

paradoxical embolism (Video 38.5).[23] Thrombus may form within the "pouch" of the aneurysm and embolize through the PFO, as well as embolize from the venous system through an associated PFO.

Other masses with similar appearance to thrombus include tumors (see Chapter 37) and vegetations (see Chapter 40). Cardiac myxomas account for 27% of primary cardiac tumors and can either be single or multiple.[24] They typically arise from the interatrial septum (although can arise from other locations) with a pedunculated stalk, irregular borders, and occasional areas of calcification. Papillary fibroelastomas are common pedunculated cardiac tumors usually located on downstream surface of the aortic and mitral valves, often appearing speckled with echolucent edges, and may be associated with systemic embolization, especially when greater than 1 cm in length (Fig. 38.12; see also Videos 47.3 and 47.4). Mobile filamentous fibrin strands, referred to as Lambl excrescences, similar in histology to papillary fibroelastomas, can be seen on native or prosthetic valves with increased prevalence in those with recent cerebral ischemia (Fig. 38.13).[25] Lipomatous hypertrophy of the interatrial septum is clearly distinguished from thrombus by its location and typical "barbell" appearance, sparing the fossa ovalis region (see Fig. 49.1C). Malignant cardiac tumors are most commonly metastatic and unlike thrombi may cross tissue planes and show prominent pericardial involvement. Vegetations are seen as irregular, mobile oscillating masses, typically on the upstream surface of the valve, and may be infectious or noninfectious. Infectious vegetations are typically associated with other evidence of systemic infection including bacteremia, fever, constitutional symptoms, and leukocytosis, although may not reliably be distinguished from thrombus in their absence, even though valvular disruption and pathologic regurgitation may suggest an underlying infection. Noninfectious vegetations may include from microscopic aggregates of platelets or large

platelet thrombi and are most commonly seen in those with advanced malignancy, severe burns, or systemic inflammatory diseases (i.e., systemic lupus erythematosus, rheumatoid arthritis).

Both thrombus and pannus may contribute to prosthetic valve obstruction and clinical symptoms and may be difficult to distinguish. As thrombus but not pannus may be treated with fibrinolysis; this distinction is clinically important. In one surgical series of 23 patients with valvular obstruction undergoing valve reoperation, predictors of thrombus (versus pannus) included shorter duration of time from valve insertion to malfunction, shorter duration of symptoms (<1 month), inadequate anticoagulation, mass size (2.8 cm vs. 1.2 cm with pannus), and ultrasound videointensity relative to the prosthetic valve of less than 0.7.[26] Pannus was more common in the aortic position. Larger thrombi were more common in the mitral and tricuspid position, often protruding into the respective atria.

SEC is thought to represent erythrocyte aggregation in the setting of low shear stress states.[27] Its presence and appearance are dependent on gain settings and it may be seen in the LA, LAA, or LV (Video 38.6). It may be associated with an underlying thrombus or predispose to thrombus formation because it is found in 80% of those with atrial fibrillation and a LAA thrombus.[28] The presence of SEC increases the embolic rate in individuals with atrial fibrillation from 3% to 12% per year.[29]

The use of echocardiographic contrast improves the detection and diagnosis of LV thrombus. In published series the sensitivity of TTE for detection of LV thrombus has ranged from 50% to 95%. Although in one study, TTE was noted to be 95% sensitive and 86% specific for LV thrombus, in another series of 78 patients with known LV thrombus at autopsy or surgery, the positive predictive value was only 86% and declined to

29% if the initial study was equivocal.[30] In individuals with poor image quality, intravenous (IV) contrast agents can improve the sensitivity and specificity of LV thrombus detection. With contrast, the LV thrombus appears as a filling defect separated distinctly from the myocardium (Fig. 38.14 and Video 38.7). In one study, LV contrast doubled the sensitivity (61% vs. 33%) and improved the accuracy (92% vs. 82%) for detection of LV thrombi, particularly in those with low LVEF, but may still miss small mural thrombi detected by late gadolinium enhancement CMR.[31]

RISK FACTORS FOR EMBOLIZATION

The risk of embolization of LV thrombus has been estimated at 10%–15%. In a meta-analysis of 856 patients with a prior anterior MI, LV thrombus was associated an increased odds ratio of 5.5 (95% CI 3.0–9.8) for an embolic event with most events occurring within the first 3–4 months.[15,32] TTE risk factors for thromboembolism include thrombus mobility and protrusion with embolization occurring in 58% of patients with free thrombus mobility compared with 3% without.[33] Similarly, 58% of those with thrombus protrusion into the LV cavity had subsequent embolic events compared with only 4% without protrusion.[33] For prosthetic valves, there are little data from controlled trials, but in general obstructive thrombi are associated with a high risk of adverse events with any treatment (surgery, anticoagulation, or fibrinolysis), and smaller (<5 mm) nonobstructive thrombi appear to have a lower risk of stroke or valve obstruction.

CHOICE OF INITIAL TEST

TTE plays a crucial role in the identification of cardiac source of embolism and may be used to identify or exclude LV thrombi, as well as to evaluate for risk factors for thrombus formation. Although hand-held point-of-care ultrasound is being used with increasing frequency for clinical management decisions, the sensitivity and specificity of point-of-care ultrasound for detection of intracardiac thrombi has not been established and use at this time for this purpose is not recommended. Given the ease and noninvasive nature of examination, minimal risk, and widespread availability, TTE should be used as the initial test of choice for the majority of patients with a suspected cardiac source of embolism. As mentioned previously, TTE is superior to TEE for visualization of the LV apex and detection of apical thrombi due to foreshortening of the apical segments on TEE. It may also be more accurate to rule out prosthetic stenosis, because the angle of insonation from apical windows is also more likely to be colinear with transvalvular blood flow particularly for the aortic valve. For those individuals with atrial fibrillation for whom there is a strong suspicion of LA/LAA thrombus, TEE is reasonable as the initial test of choice if the detection of thrombus would impact clinical management decisions. TEE has a sensitivity of 100% and specificity of 99% for the detection of LAA thrombus as compared with direct visualization at the time of surgery, in contrast to a sensitivity and specificity of 39% and 65%, respectively, for TTE.[34] For detection of LV thrombus, late gadolinium-enhancement CMR has been associated with a 3-fold higher diagnostic accuracy than TTE, attributable to a markedly higher sensitivity of CMR of 88% versus 23%.[16] Late gadolinium-enhancement CMR is more sensitive than TTE for detection of chronic LV thrombus from ischemic cardiomyopathy.[16] Cardiac CT is also useful for detection of LV thrombi with a sensitivity and specificity of 80% and 100%, respectively, and overall accuracy of 87%.[35] In this latter study, CMR was more sensitive than CT (93% vs. 80%) but had an overall similar accuracy (88%). As mentioned previously, the use of echocardiographic contrast improves sensitivity for detection of LV thrombus. In addition, echocardiographic contrast may opacify structures with prominent vascularity, improving the detection of tumor versus thrombus (see Chapter 12). Where TTE visualization is suboptimal or inconclusive, cardiac CT and CMR may represent important alternative means of diagnosis.

TEE may be more useful in certain groups of individuals as the initial test of choice. For patients younger than 45 years without known cardiovascular disease, for individuals with a high pretest probability of a cardiac embolic source for whom a negative TTE would likely be falsely negative, for patients with suspected aortic dissection, or for those with mechanical prosthetic valves, TEE is a reasonable first test given the

higher overall superior sensitivity versus TTE. Other imaging modalities may also be useful for detection of LAA thrombus, including cardiac CT and CMR. Dual enhanced cardiac CT with prospective gating was noted in one study of 83 patients with stroke to have a sensitivity and specificity of 96% and 100%, respectively, relative to TEE for detection of LAA thrombus.[36] In patients with atrial fibrillation presenting for pulmonary vein isolation who underwent both CMR and TEE, long inversion time late gadolinium-enhancement CMR had a sensitivity, specificity, and accuracy of 100%, 99.2%, and 99.2%, respectively, for LAA thrombus as compared with TEE.[37] Thus CMR represents a reasonable first test for detection of LAA thrombus in selected individuals but is limited by cost and availability. Similarly, intracardiac echocardiography (ICE) has shown comparable if not improved detection for LAA thrombus in several small series of individuals undergoing ablation of atrial arrhythmias.[38,39]

ROLE OF FOLLOW-UP IMAGING

TTE may be useful in serial evaluations to document LV thrombus resolution and monitor for improvement in LVEF and wall motion abnormalities. LV thrombus resolution has been noted in a 47% of patients at 6 months and 1 year and 76% at 2 years by serial TTE evaluation.[40–42] Absence of apical dyskinesis at 6 weeks after infarction is currently the only known predictor of LV thrombus resolution. Therapy with warfarin is *not* actually associated with thrombus resolution but is associated with lower rates of embolization.[11,42] Given the moderately invasive nature of TEE, routine serial TEE evaluation for resolution of LAA thrombus is not generally recommended, although CT and CMR may provide an adequate noninvasive means of serial monitoring of LAA thrombus in the future. For those with new onset nonvalvular atrial fibrillation, data suggest thrombus resolution of 80% after 4–6 weeks of warfarin (target INR 2–3).[43] Serial follow-up imaging for intracardiac thrombus should only be obtained if the results are likely to change management (i.e., allow for safe electrical cardioversion).

PREVENTION OF THROMBOEMBOLISM

Prevention of thromboembolism is the primary goal of detection and treatment of intracardiac thrombi. Although a comprehensive discussion of anticoagulation prevention and treatment is beyond the scope of this chapter, prevention of thromboembolism may be broadly categorized into prevention of thrombus formation and prevention of thromboembolism after thrombus identification. Crucial to the former strategy is early reperfusion and treatment with parenteral anticoagulants at the time of MI. As smaller infarct sizes have been associated with lower prevalence of LV thrombus, early use of fibrinolysis or PCI is of vital importance. Furthermore, the early administration of heparin (within 48 hours after MI) has been found in some but not all studies to decrease thrombus formation.[15] Therapy with warfarin has been shown to prevent thrombus embolization with a approximately 86% reduction in the odds of embolization compared with placebo in a meta-analysis of 270 patients with anterior MI.[15] Dual antiplatelet therapy and the group of non-vitamin K oral anticoagulant (NOAC) agents (direct thrombin and factor Xa inhibitors) have not been studied for their impact on left ventricular thrombus resolution.

Approaches to stroke prevention in patients with atrial fibrillation encompasses a topic far broader than the scope of this chapter, but mainstays of therapy include warfarin, NOACs, antiplatelet therapy, and IV unfractionated heparin or low-molecular-weight heparin with the choice of one or more agents weighted after consideration of the patient's risks, benefits, cardiac condition, and other comorbidities. In patients with atrial fibrillation or at risk for recurrent atrial fibrillation who are undergoing open heart (usually valvular or coronary artery bypass grafting) surgery, it is not uncommon for the surgeons to ligate or completely remove the LAA. This is usually done as part of a surgical Maze procedure, in which a number of linear transmural lesions are made within the left and RA, with either surgical incision or now more commonly with a radiofrequency/cryothermal ablation device, to form scar tissue that disrupts any potential reentrant circuits. This can also be done via minimally invasive approach using a microwave probe to create long continuous lesions around the pulmonary veins and isolate them electrically. For patients not undergoing cardiac surgery who have a contraindication to anticoagulation, more recent developments are percutaneous devices such as the Watchman device and Amplatzer cardiac plugs, which occlude the mouth of the appendage. For the Watchman device,[44] TEE is imperative prior to the procedure to rule out LAA thrombus and to measure the appendage itself in multiple onmiplane views, so that the appropriate device size may be selected. For this device the length of the appendage needs to be greater than the width of the appendage neck to deliver the device. For both of the occlusion devices, CT angiography to determine morphology of the LAA is also required. TEE is also used intraprocedurally to guide implantation and document lack of residual flow around the device, and post implant at prespecified intervals to monitor leakage and inform whether additional antithrombotic therapy is still required (Video 38.8). The Lariat system[45] is a percutaneous device currently used "off-label" in the United States for ligation of the LAA: it uses two magnet-tipped guidewires and a balloon catheter placed within the appendage to place an epicardial lasso around the LAA, with subsequent tightening to snare the neck of the appendage shut (Video 38.9). TEE is required to guide placement of the balloon catheter within the appendage, ensure that the coronary sinus is not snared, and to document closure of the appendage. Postprocedurally, even in appendages that are surgically ligated, it may be possible to see residual flow entering and exiting the LAA even years after the procedure; if present, such leakage in theory argue that the LAA still has some potential for harboring cardiac sources of emboli. There are many other percutaneous systems and approaches being tested and in the pipeline as well.

CONCLUSIONS

Intracardiac thrombi represent an importance source of morbidity and mortality in cardiovascular diseases and a common source of embolism to the systemic arterial bed. Both TTE and TEE play a crucial role in the identification and serial monitoring of intracardiac thrombi, as well as other cardiac masses that must be distinguished from thrombi. With improvements in three-dimensional echocardiography, strain imaging, and echocardiographic contrast, it is likely that novel techniques may be further applied toward the detection, risk stratification, and evaluation of intracardiac masses, with the adjunctive use of other noninvasive imaging modalities such as cardiac CT and CMR.

Suggested Reading

Collins, L. J., Silverman, D. I., Douglas, P. S., & Manning, W. J. (1995). Cardioversion of nonrheumatic atrial fibrillation: Reduced thromboembolic complications with 4 weeks of precardioversion anticoagulation are related to atrial thrombus resolution. *Circulation, 92*(2), 160–163.
Kitkungvan, D., Nabi, F., Ghosn, M. G., et al. (2015). Detection of left atrial and left atrial appendage thrombus by cardiovascular magnetic resonance in patients referred for pulmonary vein isolation. *JACC: Cardiovascular Imaging, 9*(7), 809–818.
Saric, M., Armour, A. C., Arnaout, M. S., et al. (2016). Guidelines for the use of echocardiography in the evaluation of a cardiac source of embolism. *Journal of the American Society of Echocardiography, 29*(1), 1–42.
Silvestry, F. E., Cohen, M. S., Armsby, L. B., et al. (2015). Guidelines for the echocardiographic assessment of atrial septal defect and patent foramen ovale: From the American Society of Echocardiography and Society for Cardiac Angiography and Interventions. *Journal of the American Society of Echocardiography, 28*(8), 910–958.
Weinsaft, J. W., Kim, H. W., Crowley, A. L., et al. (2011). Left ventricular thrombus detection by routine echocardiography: Insights into performance characteristics using delayed enhancement CMR. *JACC: Cardiovascular Imaging, 4*(7), 702–712.

A complete reference list can be found online at ExpertConsult.com

Other Cardiac Masses

Justina C. Wu

INTRODUCTION

Among cardiac masses, the three most common types are tumors, thrombi, and vegetation.[1] However, there are a variety of other structures that can be misinterpreted as cardiac tumors. These include normal anatomic structures or variants of the heart, abnormal structures, and echo artifacts.

With the abundance of echocardiograms being performed today, it is inevitable that variants of normal structure, echo artifacts, degenerative or acquired lesions, and noncancerous masses will be detected. The sonographer and cardiologist must be able to recognize this possibility and try to distinguish between the following entities, which can be called pseudo-neoplasms. This may require additional ultrasound transducer angles and techniques, or the adjunctive use of cardiac computed tomography (CT) or magnetic resonance imaging (MRI). Potential pseudo-neoplasms and their causes are summarized in Table 39.1. Differentiating between true masses and false pathology is obviously particularly important if one is performing echocardiography to rule out cardiac sources of embolus or flow obstruction.

Thrombi and vegetations are discussed fully in separate chapters (Chapters 38 and 40). Thrombi should be suspected if the mass is noted in akinetic or dyskinetic areas of the ventricle, or in the left atrial appendage. Fibrin collections (which are essentially small thrombi) can also occur on pacemaker and automated internal cardiac defibrillator (AICD) wires, as well as indwelling catheter tips, and may not necessarily imply

that removal is clinically necessary. Vegetations typically occur on valves that are predisposed to infection (e.g., myxomatous, bicuspid, or calcified valves) and are usually associated with some degree of regurgitation. It should be noted that chronic or old healed vegetations can remain almost indefinitely, but tend to become smaller and more echobright with time.[2]

VARIANTS OF NORMAL STRUCTURE

In the right atrium (RA), remnants of normal embryonic structures (from incomplete resorption of the right sinus venosus valve) can remain and may be mistaken for pathology (Fig. 39.1).[3] The eustachian valve is a caudal remnant that can be prominent and elongated, but will always be anchored to the RA-inferior vena cava (IVC) junction. A Chiari network is an extension of the eustachian valve, which is reported to be found in 2%–15% of normal hearts. It appears as a reticulated network of filaments with a characteristic oscillating or whiplike motion within the right atrium (Video 39.1). This can be seen on short-axis windows of the base of the heart, right ventricle (RV) inflow views, and apical four-chamber windows; the network may be attached to one or all of: the eustachian valve, the interatrial septum, and the upper atrium. Although they are normal structures, the eustachian valve and Chiari network can become nidi for vegetations in the presence of intravenous (IV) drug use, infected lines, or pacemaker/AICD wires.[4] They may also become associated with thrombus in rare cases.[5] In

TABLE 39.1 Site-Specific Differential Diagnoses for Nonneoplastic Cardiac Masses

	NON-NEOPLASTIC MASSES	NORMAL OR VARIANT STRUCTURES	ECHO ARTIFACT
Left atrium	Thrombus Endocardial blood cyst	Left upper pulmonary vein (LUPV) limbus (a.k.a. "Coumadin ridge") Lipomatous hypertrophy of the interatrial septum Interatrial septal aneurysm External compression: from hernia, thoracic aorta, esophageal bezoar, scoliosis (vertebrae), pericardial thrombus (postcardiac surgery) Atrial suture anastomosis postheart transplant Inverted LA appendage (postoperative) LA appendage pectinate muscles and trabeculations	Reverberation artifact from LUPV limbus
Right atrium	Thrombus (deep venous or in situ) or fibrin cast (if prior indwelling catheter/wire) Vegetation (on pacemaker/AICD wires) Lipomatous hypertrophy of the interatrial septum	Eustachian valve Chiari network Crista terminalis External compression: from pectus excavatum, liver/elevated hemidiaphragm	—
Left ventricle	Thrombus Apical hypertrophic cardiomyopathy Hydatid cyst (*Echinococcus*)	Calcified or multilobed papillary muscles Redundant or severed mitral chordae Trabeculations	Near-field clutter
Right ventricle	Thromboemboli	Redundant tricuspid chordae Tricuspid papillary muscle Moderator band	
Valves	Lambl excrescences Caseous mitral annular calcification Vegetation Marantic endocarditis Abscess or aneurysm Blood cyst Rheumatoid nodule	Nodules of Arantius Myxomatous/degenerative changes Pannus, loose suture, bioglue or pledgets around prosthetic valves	
Pericardium	Pericardial or bronchogenic cyst Rheumatoid nodule Thrombus Hydatid cyst (*Echinococcus*)	Epicardial or mediastinal fat Pectus excavatum Atelectatic lung or fibrin within pleural/peritoneal spaces Vascular pseudoaneurysm	

AICD, Automated internal cardiac defibrillator; *LA,* left atrium.

certain invasive procedures, such as patent foramen ovale (PFO) closures or MitraClip placement, both can also interfere with the manipulation of catheters and entrap devices (see Fig. 39.1B).

In the left atrium, on both transthoracic and transesophageal echocardiography (TEE), the left upper pulmonary vein (LUPV) limbus (i.e., the fold between the LUPV and left atrial appendage), can appear prominent and has frequently been mistaken for a mass or thrombus (see Fig. 39.1D). However, its typical position and continuity with the appendage and atrial wall should help distinguish it, along with the lack of any associated spontaneous echo contrast. Reverberation artifact from the LUPV limbus is also frequently confused with thrombus (see Video 39.9), thus giving this tissue fold the informal moniker of "the Coumadin ridge."[6] Lipomatous hypertrophy is a focal echogenic thickening of the epicardial fat surrounding the interatrial septum that develops frequently in elderly or obese patients, and can be exacerbated by steroid use. It is caused an expansion (hyperplasia) of normal fat cells, which are contained within the epicardial recesses between the atria.[7] This encroaches upon (but spares) the fossa ovalis, producing a characteristic dumbbell-shaped mass on echocardiography (see Fig. 39.1C). It is distinguished from lipoma and other neoplasms by both its characteristic location and its lack of a discrete capsule. Although lipomatous hypertrophy may become impressively large (>2 cm), no treatment is required unless there are associated atrial arrhythmias or caval obstruction.

In the left ventricle (LV), prominent or accessory papillary muscles may be mistaken for neoplasm or thrombus (Fig. 39.2 and Videos 39.2–39.4). Multiple imaging planes and sweeping the transducer to demonstrate the structure's attachment to the LV myocardium, the relationship with mitral chordae, and the systolic contractility will help distinguish these. In some cases, IV echo contrast (to both delineate and assess for vascularization) and/or cardiac MRI may be required to definitively distinguish between these masses and malignancy or thrombus. Other LV structures such as prominent apical trabeculations or false tendons (as in Fig. 39.4A and Video 39.5) may be mistaken for thrombi. In the RV, the moderator band and tricuspid papillary muscles may mimic neoplasms.

Similar to lipomatous hypertrophy, other pericardial fat pads may be mistaken for tumors. Most are located in a typical location anteriorly, near the right atrial/right ventricular junction or at the RV apex.[8] Pericardial cysts are a rare benign congenital anomaly, which is theorized to arise from failure of fusion of one of the mesenchymal lacunae that forms the pericardial sac during embryogenesis. They may be found incidentally on chest x-ray or ultrasound, as they usually do not cause symptoms. On echocardiography, they appear as echolucent, simply rimmed structures, typically at the right costophrenic angle. A small number of cases have been associated with hemodynamic effect from compression of the right heart, chronic cough, chest pain, and dyspnea. There are also case reports of spontaneous or traumatic hemorrhage into the pericardial cysts and subsequent tamponade.[9] The differential for pericardial cysts includes inflammatory cysts and loculated pericardial effusions. Although echocardiography is an excellent modality for follow-up or guiding aspiration of the cyst (if indicated), it may miss pericardial cysts that are in atypical locations. Congenital cysts can arise elsewhere in the heart: blood cysts (so-called because they contain venous blood and hence appear as echolucent, thin-walled structures) are very rare, benign, endothelial malformations that usually arise on the atrioventricular valves.[10]

DEGENERATIVE/ACQUIRED MASSES

Elderly patients as well as those with renal failure are prone to developing prominent degenerative and calcific changes. Caseous mitral annular calcification is a variant of this process in which inner foci of the calcified portions undergo an atypical liquefaction necrosis. The calcified mass may enlarge, distort the annulus, and bulge into the myocardium or chambers to the extent that it actually resembles an abscess or tumor (Fig. 39.3).[11] The absence of associated fever, bacteremia, and stability of the lesion over time should make endocarditis a less likely diagnosis. In ambiguous cases, cardiac CT is an extremely helpful modality for distinguishing this from an abscess. Cardiac MRI may also be useful, but can be limited due to the presence of surrounding calcium. Most of these masses

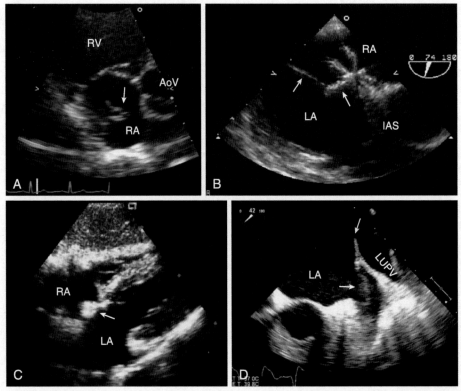

FIG. 39.1 Normal structures and anatomic variants. (**A**) A Chiari network *(arrow)*, extending from the right atrial-caval junction into the right atrium (RA) on this parasternal short-axis window. (See also corresponding Video 39.1.) (**B**) Eustachian valve *(yellow arrow)*, seen entangled in and tethering the anterior right atrial corner *(white arrow)* of a Cardioseal septal occluder, which impedes it from apposing properly to the interatrial septum (IAS) in this transesophageal echocardiography (TEE) image. (**C**) Lipomatous hypertrophy of the interatrial septum, with the characteristic dumbbell shape *(arrow)*. (**D**) TEE view of the left atrium and left atrial appendage, illustrating the fold, or limbus *(yellow arrow)* between the left upper pulmonary vein (LUPV) and left atrial appendage (see also corresponding Video 39.9). Note the reverberation artifact *(white arrow)* below it, which mimics a thrombus floating within the appendage. *AoV,* Aortic valve; *LA,* left atrium; *RV,* right ventricle.

are conventionally thought to be stable and benign. However, they can cause complications of mitral regurgitation or stenosis, systemic embolization of microfragments or associated thrombi, and atrioventricular block. Cases of spontaneous resolution or even recurrence after surgical excision have also been reported.

POSTSURGICAL MASSES

In patients with older mechanical or biologic valve prostheses, fibrotic and inflammatory scar tissue known as "pannus" can proliferate and grow inward

from the periphery of the prosthesis, as well as outward toward the adjacent chambers. This may cause stenosis (from obstruction of the valve orifice or impedance of disc motion at the hinges), regurgitation (by preventing leaflet coaptation or discs from closing flush with the surgical ring), and often both problems concomitantly within the involved valve (see Chapter 31). Formation of pannus is usually more common on aortic prostheses than mitral prostheses.[12] TEE is usually required for better evaluation of the type and physiologic impact of the perivalvular mass: although neither size nor mobility of the mass can reliably distinguish between pannus and thrombus; pannus tends to be more echobright than thrombus. Masses that are close

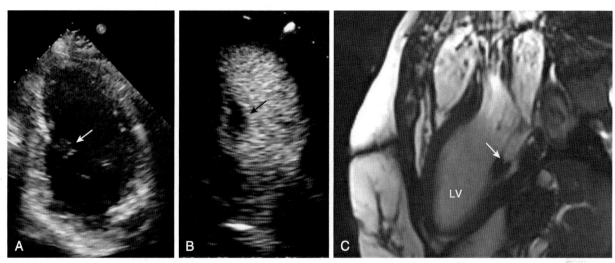

FIG. 39.2 Bilobed papillary muscle *(arrows)* **in the left ventricle.** (**A**) A small, mobile mass was initially detected on this apical two-chamber transthoracic view of the left ventricle (LV), which appeared associated with the inferior wall and mitral chordae. (**B**) The same two-chamber view, with intravenous echocardiographic contrast after flash destruction of microbubbles to assess for neovascularization of the mass. This study was negative for perfusion of the mass. (**C**) Cardiac magnetic resonance imaging demonstrates that the mass was in fact a bilobed posterolateral papillary muscle, with the more prominent head connecting via a chorda to the anterior mitral leaflet. (See also corresponding Videos 39.2–39.4.)

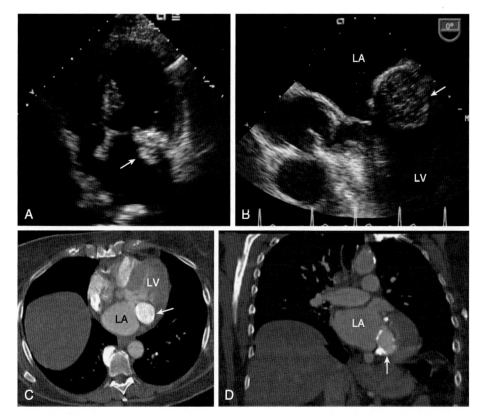

FIG. 39.3 Caseous mitral annular calcification. (**A**) Apical four-chamber view showing a rounded 3.5 cm heterogeneously echogenic mass at the mitral annulus protruding into the left heart chambers. (**B**) Transesophageal echocardiography four-chamber view. Note the acoustic shadowing due to the calcification on the atrial surface of the mass. Cardiac computed tomographic scans are shown in (**C**) short-axis and (**D**) coronal view. *Arrows* in all panels indicate the caseous mitral annular calcification. *LA,* Left atrium; *LV,* left ventricle. (*Modified from Wu JC. Cardiac tumors and masses. In: Stergiopoulous K, Brown DL, eds.* Evidence-Based Cardiology Consult. *New York: Springer; 2014:377–390.*)

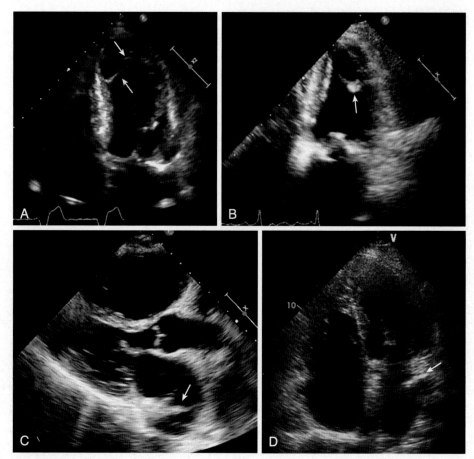

FIG. 39.4 Cardiomyopathic and postsurgical changes. (A) This apical four-chamber view illustrates three findings that are not uncommon in the left ventricle, particularly if the ejection fraction is low: apical trabeculations *(white arrow)*, a false tendon *(yellow arrow)*, and slight spontaneous echo contrast are seen in the left ventricle (best appreciated in accompanying Video 39.5). **(B)** A severed and much thickened chorda in a patient after mitral valve replacement with a bioprosthesis. The surgeon resected the anterior leaflet and chordae, but was able to leave the posterior leaflet and chords intact. (See corresponding Video 39.6.). **(C** and **D)** Parasternal long and apical four-chamber windows of hearts following transplant via bi-atrial anastomoses. A circumferential bulky ridge of echobright tissue *(arrows)* is noted where the recipient atria and donor heart are sutured together.

to the ultrasound intensity of the most highly echogenic part of mechanical prostheses are very likely to be pannus. In cases where there is limited visibility on echocardiogram due to acoustic shadowing from the prosthesis, a parallel finding (increased radiodensity) on cardiac CT can be a valuable adjunctive tool.[13] Of note, the best distinguishing predictor is not echo based, but clinical: patients who are under-anticoagulated are far more likely to have thrombus. Furthermore, in one surgical series of obstructed mechanical valves, half of all cases found to have pannus also had associated thrombus.[14]

During mitral valve replacements, surgeons attempt to preserve as much of the mitral chordal apparatus as possible, since the continuity between the papillary muscles and the annulus helps preserve LV contractility. This can be accomplished by resecting a triangular or quadrangular wedge of redundant tissue, leaving the chordae attached to the remaining leaflet. However, if the chordae are already damaged or must be sacrificed, the severed remnants can appear as elongated string-like mobile echodensities still attached to the left ventricular wall. In patients with rheumatic disease, these chordae can be quite thickened and less mobile (see Fig. 39.4B and Video 39.6). If chordae are already ruptured, the surgeon may also create new Gore-tex chordae to resuspend the papillary muscles, which can be visualized on echocardiogram as very thin echobright filaments that tighten during systole and loosen with each diastole.

Patients who have had cardiac transplants using bi-atrial anastomoses (i.e., the standard Shumway-Lower technique, which has been used for three decades) often have prominent plication of tissue at the anastamotic line, where the newly transplanted heart needs to be sewn to the caps of the enlarged recipient atria. These can be misinterpreted on both transthoracic and TEE as thrombi, but careful inspection will reveal circumferential fixed tissue thickening and echodensity at the expected suture line, which can create an hour-glass appearance of the left atrium in four-chamber views (see Fig. 39.4C and D). Currently, there is an increasing trend for cardiac transplants to be performed via bicaval anastomoses or total heart transplant (with

pulmonary venous anastomoses), where there is only left atrial or no recipient atrial tissue remaining. The bicaval technique in particular appears to improve the atrial geometry and lessen the risk for atrial fibrillation and postoperative tricuspid regurgitation, and is associated with slightly better survival.[15,16]

EXTRACARDIAC STRUCTURES

There are extracardiac structures that can impinge or distort the appearance of the heart, but should be distinguished from actual neoplasms (Fig. 39.5 and Video 39.7). These include esophageal hernias, thoracic aortic aneurysms, and extracardiac or pericardial thrombi (which may indent the posterior left atrial wall) and vertebral bodies (which can indent the left atrium in apical windows). A simple front-line technique to illustrate the esophageal hernia is to have the patient drink an oral echo contrast agent (carbonated soda) during the echo exam.[17] The influx of bubbles into the gastrointestinal (GI) lumen is usually easily visible on imaging (Video 39.8). Deformity from an anterior structure, such as the sternum in pectus excavatum deformity (Fig. 39.6), has the distinctive effect of indenting the right atrium and ventricle, and confirmation should be obvious from physical exam or a lateral x-ray.

ULTRASOUND ARTIFACTS

Last, there are echocardiographic artifacts that can falsely produce the appearance of a mass or thrombus (see Chapter 7). Of these, the most common are near-field artifacts, which can mimic LV apical thrombi in apical windows (see Fig. 7.10 and Videos 7.5 and 7.6). These are caused by high-amplitude oscillations of the piezoelectric crystals of the transducer, and can be eliminated by harmonic imaging or by using a different frequency transducer. Even with harmonics, occasionally the presence of echo artifact can still fool inexperienced observers and confound the ability to definitively exclude a real clot in the area. IV echocardiographic

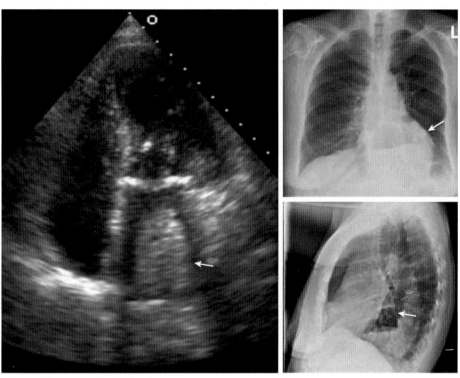

FIG. 39.5 Extracardiac impingement producing pseudomasses. An echogenic mass *(arrow)* appears to be "free-floating" within the left atrial cavity on this apical four-chamber view. No attachments to the left atrial wall or any structure could be demonstrated on echocardiogram. However, the right panels show posterioranterior (PA) *(upper panel)* and lateral *(lower panel)* chest X rays confirming that the patient in fact had a large esophageal hernia *(arrows)*, seen as a fluid-filled stomach bubble above the diaphragm pushing posteriorly upon the left atrium. (See Videos 39.7 and 39.8; oral echo contrast within the gastrointestinal [GI] lumen).

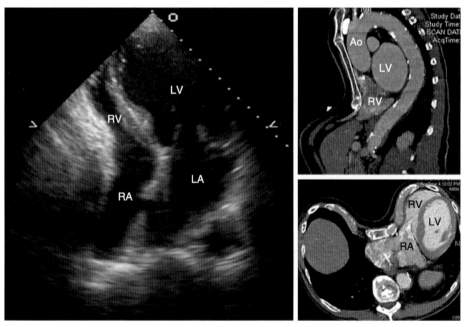

FIG. 39.6 Pectus excavatum. The sternum is bowed inward, indenting the right heart on apical four-chamber windows *(left panel)*. The right panels are a cardiac-gated computed tomographic study *(upper panel* = axial, and *lower panel* = sagittal section), illustrating how the severe pectus deformity has displaced the entire heart leftward and indented the right atrium and ventricle. *Ao,* Aorta; *LA,* left atrium; *LV,* left ventricle; *RA,* right atrium; *RV,* right ventricle.

contrast or zooming in on the apex with color Doppler at a low Nyquist limit are two techniques that are useful; if "fill in" of the LV apex occurs and the trabeculations are noted to be in continuity with the rest of the LV apex, then thrombus is unlikely. Adjusting near-field gains and varying the transducer frequency may also eliminate this artifact. Reverberation and side-lobe artifacts may also fool the observer with apparent pseudomasses, but should be distinguishable by imaging the involved structure from orthogonal aspects and different windows to remove the reflecting interface. Fig. 39.1D and Video 39.9 are a TEE view of the left atrial appendage, which demonstrates how the LUPV limbus (which can itself

be mistaken for a mass) casts a reverberation artifact onto the left atrial appendage that is often mistaken for a thrombus.

Suggested Reading

Elgendy, I. Y., & Conti, C. R. (2013). Caseous calcification of the mitral annulus: a review. *Clinical Cardiology, 36,* E27–E31.

Peters, P. J., & Reinhardt, S. (2006). The echocardiographic evaluation of intracardiac masses: a review. *Journal of the American Society of Echocardiography, 19,* 230–240.

Silbiger, J. J., Bazaz, R., & Trost, B. (2010). Lipomatous hypertrophy of the interatrial septum revisited. *Journal of the American Society of Echocardiography, 23,* 789–790.

A complete reference list can be found online at ExpertConsult.com.

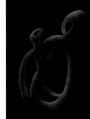

SECTION IX

SYSTEMIC DISEASES INVOLVING THE HEART

40 Echocardiography in Infective Endocarditis

Linda D. Gillam, Leo Marcoff, Konstantinos Koulogiannis

INTRODUCTION

Infective endocarditis (IE) is a serious infection of the heart that, despite advances in diagnosis and treatment, is associated with in-hospital and 1-year mortalities of approximately 20% and 40%, respectively. IE is also associated with major morbidity with embolic events (stroke in 17% of patients, non-neurologic embolus in 23%, heart failure (32%), abscess (14%), and the need for surgery (48%) being relatively common events. With an overall incidence of 3–10 per 100,000 patient years, in the United States alone there are over 50,000 cases per year, the majority of which affect the left side of the heart.[1–3] Risk factors for endocarditis include the presence of a valve prosthesis or other implanted device, intravenous drug abuse, diabetes, and immunosuppression.

Echocardiography is integral to the diagnosis and management of this condition because it can identify vegetations and complications associated with spreading infection, assess the severity of concomitant valve dysfunction, and document the impact of the disease on ventricular function and cardiovascular hemodynamics including pulmonary artery pressure. This chapter focuses on the role of echocardiography in IE with an emphasis on native and prosthetic valves. It discusses the imaging features of vegetations and complications of endocarditis including embolus, abscess, perforation, and other forms of valvular disruption, and in the case of prosthetic valves, variable degrees of dehiscence. It also covers the prognostic role of echocardiography, particularly in the prediction of embolic risk, and emphasize the important role that echocardiography plays during follow-up of treatment, and for intraprocedural guidance during surgical intervention. Where specific recommendations for the use of echocardiography are provided, they are consistent with the current American College of Cardiology/American Heart Association (ACC/AHA) Guidelines for the Management of Patients with Valvular Heart Disease,[1] (with the 2017 update including no changes related to echocardiography) European Society of Cardiology (ESC) Guidelines for the Management of Infective Endocarditis,[2] ESC Recommendations for the Practice of Echocardiography in Infective Endocarditis,[4] the AHA Scientific Statement on Infective Endocarditis,[3] and ACCF/ASE/AHA/ASNC/HFSA/HRS/SCAI/SCCM/SCCT/SCMR 2011 Appropriate Use Criteria for Echocardiography.[5]

Although a full discussion of the etiology, pathophysiology, natural history, and optimal approaches to management such as surgical decision making is beyond the scope of this chapter, the reader is referred to the ACC/AHA[1] and ESC[2] Guidelines and AHA Scientific Statement[3] for this information. It is worth noting that echocardiography has served as a research tool in many of the studies that form the basis for these documents. Additionally, the echocardiographic assessment of the hemodynamic severity of valve lesions caused by IE and associated changes in cardiac function are critical to clinical decision making in IE, and the reader is referred to Chapters 8–10 and 28–31 for a more detailed discussion of the tools that are used to make these assessments.

DIAGNOSIS

Indications for Transthoracic Echocardiography and Transesophageal Echocardiography

Echocardiography is essential for the diagnosis of IE (Table 40.1). Endocarditis may be suspected in a wide variety of situations, most commonly with otherwise unexplained fever lasting at least 48 hours, bacteremia, a new regurgitant heart murmur, new conduction disturbance, and/or embolic events. Although 90% of cases of IE are associated with bacteremia, 10% have culture-negative endocarditis, which may reflect the presence of difficult-to-culture organisms such as the HACEK (*Haemophilus, Aggregatibacter, Cardiobacterium hominis, Eikenella corrodens,* and *Kingella*) species or the institution of antibiotic therapy before blood cultures are drawn. Although the clinical presentation is most typically subacute, valvular disruption and associated sudden severe valvular regurgitation may be associated with acute heart failure or shock.

The diagnosis of endocarditis is typically based on the Modified Duke criteria (Tables 40.2 and 40.3).[6] In these criteria, echocardiographic evidence of endocarditis, as defined by the presence of vegetation, abscess, or new dehiscence of a prosthetic valve, is one of the major criteria; new valvular regurgitation, which can also be identified by echocardiography, is a second major criterion.

New valvular regurgitation may be on the basis of cusp/leaflet perforation, chordal rupture, or altered cusp/leaflet coaptation caused by bulky vegetations. Valve stenosis is a less common complication but may occur with prosthetic valve IE in which a bulky vegetation obstructs the orifice or a strategically placed smaller vegetation impedes mechanical disk motion. Note that it may be difficult to distinguish superimposed vegetation when there is a flail segment due to chordal rupture. Although transthoracic echocardiography (TTE) is typically the initial study (Class I in ACC/AHA and ESC Guidelines; see Table 40.1), there should be a low threshold for transesophageal echocardiography (TEE). Indeed, as listed in Table 40.1, there are number of scenarios for which TEE has Class I, IIA, and IIB indications for diagnosis. The IIB indication (TEE may be considered) for nosocomial *Staphylococcus aureus* bacteremia with a portal of entry from a known extracardiac source exists because IE has been reported to occur in approximately 30% of patients with *S. aureus* bacteremia particularly in patients with osteomyelitis, prolonged bacteremia, or hemodialysis catheters.[1] The European recommendations[4] (see Table 40.1) offer expanded recommendations for TEE including its use in patients with a high clinical suspicion of infectious endocarditis but a normal TTE and suggest that TEE should be considered in the majority of adult patients with suspected IE even when the TTE is positive. TEE should not be performed in patients with a negative TTE of excellent quality when there is a low clinical suspicion of IE.

TABLE 40.1 Role of Echocardiography in Infective Endocarditis

	2014 ACC/AHA GUIDELINES			2015 ESC GUIDELINES			2011 ASE APPROPRIATE USE CRITERIA	
	Should Be Performed (Class I)	Reasonable to Perform (Class IIa)	May Be Considered (Class IIb)	Recommended/Indicated (Class I)	Should Be Considered (Class IIa)	May Be Considered (Class IIb)	Appropriate	Rarely Appropriate
TTE	• To identify vegetations, characterize the hemodynamic severity of valvular lesions, assess ventricular function and pulmonary pressures, and detect complications (LOE: B)			• As the first-line imaging modality in suspected IE. (LOE: B) • At completion of antibiotic therapy for evaluation of cardiac and valve morphology and function (LOE: C)			• Initial evaluation of suspected IE with positive blood cultures or a new murmur • Reevaluation of IE at high risk for progression or complication or with a change in clinical status or cardiac exam	• Transient fever without evidence of bacteremia or a new murmur • Transient bacteremia with a pathogen not typically associated with IE and/or a documented non-endovascular source of infection • Routine surveillance of uncomplicated IE when no change in management is contemplated
TEE	• When TTE is non-diagnostic, when complications are suspected, or when intracardiac device is present (LOE: B)	• In patients with Staphylococcal aureus (S. aureus) bacteremia without a known source (LOE: B) • In patients with prosthetic valve and persistent fever without bacteremia or a new murmur (LOE: B)	• In patients with nosocomial S. aureus bacteremia with a known portal of entry from an extracardiac source (LOE: B)	• Clinical suspicion of IE and a negative or nondiagnostic TTE. (LOE: B) Clinical suspicion of IE, when a prosthetic valve or an intracardiac device is present. (LOE: B) • Suspected cardiac device-related IE to evaluate lead-related endocarditis and heart valve infection (LOE: C)	• Suspected IE, even in cases with positive TTE, except in isolated right-sided native valve IE with good-quality TTE with unequivocal findings (LOE: C)		• Reevaluation of prior TEE finding for interval change (e.g., resolution of vegetation after antibiotic therapy) when a change in therapy is anticipated • To diagnose IE with a moderate or high pretest probability (e.g., staph bacteremia, fungemia, prosthetic heart valve, or intracardiac device)	• To diagnose IE with a low pretest probability (e.g., transient fever, known alternative source of infection, or negative blood cultures/atypical pathogen for endocarditis) • Surveillance of prior TEE finding for interval change (e.g., resolution of vegetation after antibiotic therapy) when no change in therapy is anticipated

	2014 ACC/AHA GUIDELINES			2015 ESC GUIDELINES			2011 ASE APPROPRIATE USE CRITERIA	
	Should Be Performed (Class I)	Reasonable to Perform (Class IIa)	May Be Considered (Class IIb)	Recommended/Indicated (Class I)	Should Be Considered (Class IIa)	May Be Considered (Class IIb)	Appropriate	Rarely Appropriate
TTE and/or TEE	• Change in clinical signs or symptoms (e.g., new murmur, embolism, persistent fever, HF, abscess, or atrioventricular heart block) and in patients at high risk of complications (e.g., extensive infected tissue/large vegetation on initial echocardiogram or staphylococcal, enterococcal, fungal infections) (LOE: B)			• Within 5–7 days in case of initially negative examination when clinical suspicion of IE remains high (LOE: C) • As soon as a new complication of IE is suspected (new murmur, embolism, persisting fever, HF, abscess, atrioventricular block) (LOE: B)	• S. aureus bacteremia. (LOE: B) • During follow-up of uncomplicated IE, to detect new silent complications and monitor vegetation size. The timing and mode (TTE or TEE) of repeat examination depend on the initial findings, type of microorganism, and initial response to therapy. (LOE: B)			
Intraoperative TEE	• Patients undergoing valve surgery for IE (LOE: B)			• All cases of IE requiring surgery (LOE: B)				
Intracardiac echo						• Suspected cardiac device-related IE, positive blood cultures and negative TTE and TEE results (LOE: C)		

ACC, American College of Cardiology; AHA, American Heart Association; ESC, European Society of Cardiology; HF, heart failure; IE, infective endocarditis; LOE, level of evidence; TEE, transesophageal echocardiogram; TTE, transthoracic echocardiogram.

Data from Nishimura RA, Otto CM, Bonow RO, et al. 2014 AHA/ACC guideline for the management of patients with valvular heart disease: executive summary: a report of the American College of Cardiology/American Heart Association Task Force on Practice Guidelines. J Am Coll Cardiol. 2014;63(22):2438-2488; Habib G, Badano L, Tribouilloy C, et al. Recommendations for the practice of echocardiography in infective endocarditis. Eur J Echocardiogr. 2010;11(2):202-219; and Douglas PS, Garcia MJ, Haines DE, et al. 2011 appropriate use criteria for echocardiography. J Am Coll Cardiol. 2011;57(9):1126-1166.

TABLE 40.2 Modified Duke Criteria for Diagnosis of Infective Endocarditis

DEFINITE IE	POSSIBLE IE	REJECTED IE
Presence of ANY of the following: Pathologic criteria 1. Microorganisms demonstrated by culture or histologic examination of a vegetation, a vegetation that has embolized, or an intracardiac abscess specimen; or 2. Pathologic lesions; vegetation or intracardiac abscess confirmed by histologic examination showing active endocarditis Clinical criteria[b] 1. 2 major; or 2. 1 major and 3 minor; or 3. 5 minor criteria	1. 1 major and 1 minor[a]; or 2. 3 minor criteria[a]	1. Firm alternate diagnosis explaining evidence of IE; or 2. Resolution of IE syndrome with antibiotic therapy for ≤4 days; or 3. No pathologic evidence of IE at surgery or autopsy, with antibiotic therapy for ≤4 days; or 4. Does not meet criteria for possible IE as above.

IE, Infective endocarditis.
[a]Modification from the original Duke criteria.
[b]See Table 40.3 for definitions of major and minor criteria.
Adapted from Li JS, Sexton DJ, Mick N, et al. Proposed modifications to the Duke criteria for the diagnosis of infective endocarditis. Clin Infect Dis. *2000;30(4):633-638.*

TABLE 40.3 Definition of Terms Used in the Modified Duke Criteria for Diagnosis of Infective Endocarditis

MAJOR CRITERIA	MINOR CRITERIA

Blood culture positive for IE
• Typical microorganisms consistent with IE from two separate blood cultures:
  • Viridans streptococci, *Streptococcus gallolyticus* (formerly *S. bovis*), including nutritional variant strains (*Granulicatella spp.* and *Abiotrophia defectiva*), HACEK group, *Staphylococcus aureus*; or community-acquired enterococci, in the absence of a primary focus; or
• Microorganisms consistent with IE from persistently positive blood cultures, defined as follows:
  • At least two positive cultures of blood samples drawn 12 h apart; or
  • All of three or a majority of ≥4 separate cultures of blood (with first and last sample drawn at least 1 h apart)
• Single positive blood culture for *Coxiella burnetii* or antiphase I IgG antibody titer >1: 800[a]
	Predisposition, predisposing heart condition, or injection drug use

Evidence of endocardial involvement	Fever, temperature >38°C (100.4°F)
Echocardiogram positive for IE, defined as follows: • Oscillating intracardiac mass on valve or supporting structures, in the path of regurgitant jets, or on implanted material in the absence of an alternative anatomic explanation; or • Abscess; or • New partial dehiscence of prosthetic valve Note: TEE is recommended in patients with prosthetic valves, rated at least "possible IE" by clinical criteria, or complicated IE (paravalvular abscess); TTE is first test in other patients.[a]	Vascular phenomena, major arterial emboli, septic pulmonary infarcts, mycotic aneurysm, intracranial hemorrhage, conjunctival hemorrhages, and Janeway lesions
New valvular regurgitation (worsening or changing of pre-existing murmur not sufficient)	Immunologic phenomena: glomerulonephritis, Osler's nodes, Roth's spots, and rheumatoid factor
	Microbiological evidence: positive blood cultures that do not meet major criteria; or serologic evidence of active infection with organism consistent with IE
	Echocardiographic minor criteria eliminated[a]

HACEK, Haemophilus, Aggregatibacter, Cardiobacterium hominis, Eikenella corrodens, and *Kingella; IE*, infective endocarditis; *TEE*, transesophageal echocardiogram; *TTE*, transthoracic echocardiogram.
[a]Modification from the original Duke criteria.
Adapted from Li JS, Sexton DJ, Mick N, et al. Proposed modifications to the Duke criteria for the diagnosis of infective endocarditis. Clin Infect Dis. *2000;30(4):633-638.*

TTE has a reported sensitivity of 62%–82% and a specificity of 91%–100% for native valve endocarditis[4] and is most likely to detect vegetations larger than 3 mm in size. For prosthetic valve endocarditis, the sensitivity is only 36%–69%.[4] TEE with spatial resolution of 1–2 mm has a reported sensitivity of 87%–100% and specificity of 91%–100% for native valve endocarditis. Notably, although the sensitivity of TEE for prosthetic valve endocarditis is significantly higher than that of TTE, it is still somewhat lower than that for native valve endocarditis, but can increase with follow-up studies when the initial study is negative but the clinical suspicion of IE is high. TEE has a specificity of over 90% for prosthetic valve endocarditis.

As discussed later, there are a number of reasons for which echocardiography, even TEE, may be negative in cases of IE. Therefore, if the clinical suspicion of endocarditis remains high, it is reasonable to repeat echocardiography, typically after 7–10 days. A similar approach is reasonable in cases of suspected abscess, but a shorter interval between initial and subsequent echoes is probably warranted because there can be dramatic changes in the appearance of an abscess over the course of even several hours. Additional indications for repeat echocardiographic evaluation include a clinical change in a patient with established endocarditis and surveillance without clinical change in patients at high risk for complications based on the extent of infection or organism (*Staphylococcus, Enterococcus* or fungus [AHA/ACC Class I]). Conversely, there is no indication for TEE or follow-up TTE when the initial transthoracic echo is of high quality and there is a low clinical suspicion of endocarditis.

VEGETATIONS

Vegetations are identified by the presence of echogenic masses of variable size that typically have oscillating motion independent of the surface to which they are attached (Fig. 40.1 and Videos 40.1 and 40.2). Their echotexture is typically similar to that of the myocardium although they can become more echodense during the course of treatment (Fig. 40.2 and Video 40.3). They have irregular shapes and may prolapse from one chamber to the other during the cardiac cycle. By far the most common location for vegetations is on the cardiac valves, either native or prosthetic, but they may also be encountered on indwelling foreign bodies such as pacer/automated implantable cardioverter defibrillator (AICD) leads and central lines. Rarely, vegetations are encountered on the endocardial surface of the ventricles or aorta at sites impacted by jet lesions (for example, on the right ventricular side of a restrictive ventricular septal defect [VSD]).

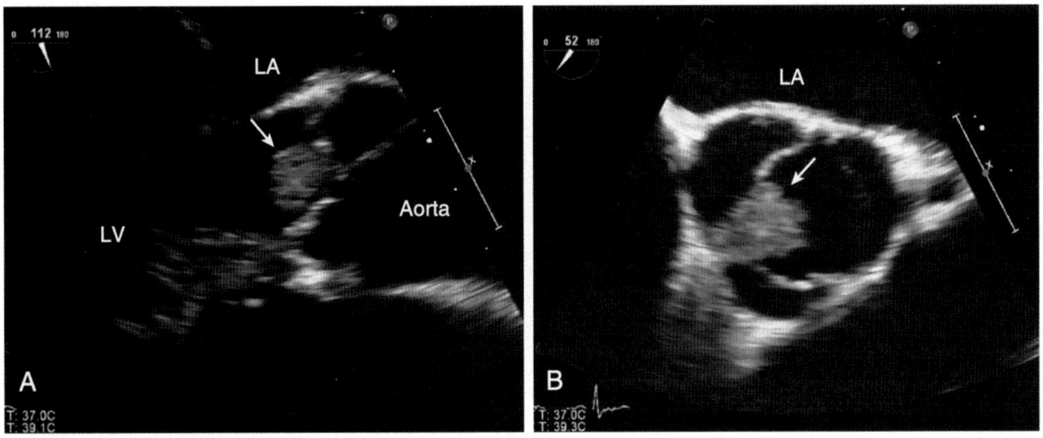

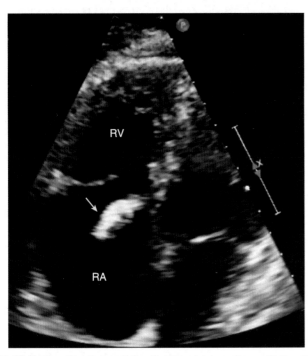

FIG. 40.1 Aortic valve vegetation. Transesophageal echocardiogram. Midesophageal aortic valve long-axis (A) and short-axis (B) views showing a large vegetation *(arrow)* on the left ventricular aspect of the aortic valve. *LA,* Left atrium; *LV,* left ventricle.

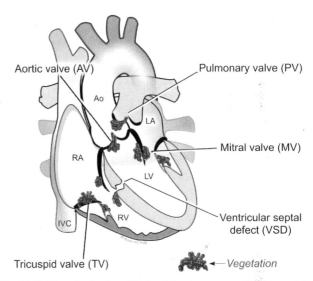

FIG. 40.2 Tricuspid valve vegetation. Transthoracic echocardiogram. Right ventricular modified apical four-chamber view. A vegetation *(yellow arrow)* is seen on the right atrial aspect of the tricuspid valve septal leaflet. *RA,* Right atrium; *RV,* right ventricle.

FIG. 40.3 Schematic drawing of the heart showing common sites for vegetations. *Ao,* Aorta; *LA,* left atrium; *LV,* left ventricle; *RA,* right atrium; *RV,* right ventricle. *(Courtesy of Bernard E. Bulwer, MD, FASE.)*

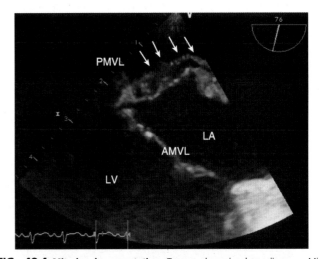

FIG. 40.4 Mitral valve vegetation. Transesophageal echocardiogram. Midesophageal mitral valve view showing large posterior leaflet vegetation *(arrows).* The location and the length of the vegetation pose an increased risk for embolization. Note the echolucency within the vegetation. *AMVL,* Anterior mitral valve leaflet; *LA,* left atrium; *LV,* left ventricle; *PMVL,* posterior mitral valve leaflet.

Vegetations are typically seen on the low-pressure aspect of valves or shunts (Fig. 40.3) and usually at the site of endothelial damage, which may be the result of preexisting structural disease. With endothelial damage, blood-borne organisms can adhere to associated platelet and fibrin aggregates. Thus, vegetations are more common on the ventricular surface of the aortic valve, particularly in the presence of aortic regurgitation, and on the atrial surface of the mitral and tricuspid valves, particularly in the presence of mitral or tricuspid regurgitation. Pulmonic valve endocarditis is a very rare entity but in the absence of data, it would be predicted that pulmonic endocarditis would have a predilection for the right ventricular aspect of the valve. The presence of a mass that might be confused with vegetation on the high-pressure aspect of the valve favors an etiology other than vegetation. However, these rules are by no means definitive, and it should be noted that the ventricular surface of the anterior mitral leaflet may be infected when in the path of an aortic regurgitant jet and chordal involvement of both the mitral and tricuspid valves may also occur.

Although the echotexture of vegetations is frequently homogeneous, inhomogeneity with areas of echolucency may also occur, particularly if vegetations are very large (Fig. 40.4). When IE is suspected, nonstandard views are essential, and when involvement of the mitral and tricuspid valves is suspected, it is imperative to get multiple views so that each of the scallops and leaflets is visualized (see Chapters 28 and 30 for a description of the views needed to image all six mitral scallops and three tricuspid leaflets). With prosthetic valves, particularly mechanical prostheses, vegetations may be smaller and more difficult to detect because of shadowing from prosthetic elements. Additionally, mechanical prosthetic valves are more likely to have early perivalvular spread with abscess, pseudoaneurysms, and dehiscence, than bioprostheses in which infection is more likely to involve the cusps.

Echocardiography should address the number, size, shape, location, mobility, and echogenicity of vegetations, because many of these features have prognostic value as discussed later. Although not widely used, a scoring system has been proposed with mobility broken down by grade, with grade 1 being fixed, grade 2 a fixed base but a free edge, grade 3 pedunculated, and grade 4 prolapsing.[7] Increased echogenicity suggests a degree of organization or chronicity (see Fig. 40.2 and Video 40.3).

Reasons for which echocardiography, even TEE, may be unable to detect vegetations, include situations in which vegetations are very small, atypically located, sessile, or obscured by calcification. Thus, repeat echocardiography is warranted in cases where the clinical suspicion is high.

Although the diagnosis of vegetation may be strongly suspected based on its echocardiographic appearance, it is important that the echocardiographic findings be interpreted in clinical context. The differential diagnosis for vegetation includes thrombus, neoplasm such as fibroelastoma (see Fig. 37.4 in Chapter 37), mobile calcific elements, aortic valve Lambl excrescences, Libman-Sacks (noninfective) endocarditis, or benign degenerative strands. Less commonly, prosthetic valve suture may be confused with vegetation, as can the variable valve thickening of myxomatous mitral disease or the normal right atrial variants of the eustachian valve or Chiari network. As a rule of thumb, masses with an echotexture similar to that of calcium or the pericardium are unlikely to be vegetations, as are linear strand-like masses that have a narrow attachment to the valve.

It is impossible to identify the infecting organism based on the echocardiographic appearance of vegetations, although fungal vegetations do tend to be large.

COMPLICATIONS OF ENDOCARDITIS

Complications of endocarditis include those due to the local extension of the infective process and distal complications related to embolus or secondary seeding of distal sites by endocarditis-associated bacteremia.

Abscess, Pseudoaneurysm, and Fistula

Perivalvular abscesses occur due to contiguous spread of infection and are most commonly encountered in the setting of aortic valve or prosthetic valve endocarditis. Involvement of the conduction system may cause atrioventricular conduction disturbances, which may be clinical clues to aortic root or, less commonly, mitral or tricuspid abscess formation.

The echocardiographic appearance of an abscess is one of initial thickening, which typically acquires variable degrees of echolucency with progression (Fig. 40.5, Videos 40.4 and 40.5). Septation and loculation are common. Transthoracic echo has a reported sensitivity of approximately 50% for the detection of abscesses with a sensitivity of up to 90%. For TEE, the sensitivity is 60%–90% with specificity of approximately 90%. For both TTE and TEE, nonstandard views are important and TTE and TEE should be viewed as complementary techniques. For example, TTE may be superior to TEE in identifying anterior aortic root abscesses in the setting of aortic prostheses due to acoustic shadowing by the prosthesis in standard midesophageal TEE views. It is imperative that abscess formation detected or suspected on TTE be followed by TEE for better delineation. The most common location for an abscess is in the vicinity of aortic-mitral intervalvular fibrosa at the junction of the aortic annulus and anterior mitral leaflet. However, abscesses can extend circumferentially and involve any location in the aortic annulus. Mitral annular abscesses are less common in the absence of a prosthetic valve, although mitral annular calcification may be secondarily infected.

It should be noted that the appearance of the aortic root following aortic root repair or homograft/allograft aortic valve replacement may mimic the thickening associated with an abscess, particularly if surgical glue has been used. This underscores the importance of intraoperative postprocedural TEE and subsequent baseline TTE for any valve surgery or root reconstructive procedure.

When the abscess ruptures into the adjacent blood pool, there may be to and fro or unidirectional flow with **pseudoaneurysm** formation (Figs. 40.6 and 40.7, Videos 40.6 and 40.7). The diagnosis is established with color flow Doppler. In the case of aortic root abscesses, secondary rupture into the left ventricle may also occur with resultant severe regurgitation. If the abscess is extensive it may extend toward the right atrium, right ventricle, or left atrial appendage (Fig. 40.8, Video 40.8). It may also be associated with infection of adjacent structures, particularly the septal leaflet of the tricuspid valve, which is closely positioned relative to the aortic root. It is essential to use nonstandard images and extend the examination to adjacent structures if one is to capture the full extent of the infectious process.

An abscess may also progress to **fistula** formation (Fig. 40.9, Videos 40.9 and 40.10) with the abscess creating a communication between the aorta and the atrium or ventricle, or between the cardiac chambers. Fistulae may be in direct communication or have a more serpiginous course, and depending on the size and location of the communication, be associated with catastrophic hemodynamic compromise. Color flow mapping may provide the first echocardiographic clue that a fistula exists and help map out its course.

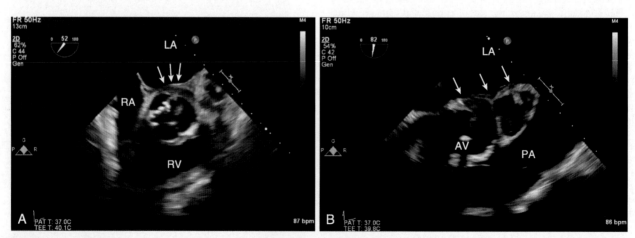

FIG. 40.5 Aortic root abscess. Transesophageal echocardiogram. (A) Midesophageal aortic valve short-axis view shows thickening and echolucency of the aortic root *(arrows)* in the region of the left and the noncoronary sinuses of Valsalva. (B) Modified midesophageal aortic valve long-axis view showing extension of the aortic root abscess into the ascending aorta *(arrows)*. *AV,* Aortic valve; *LA,* left atrium; *PA,* pulmonary artery; *RA,* right atrium; *RV,* right ventricle.

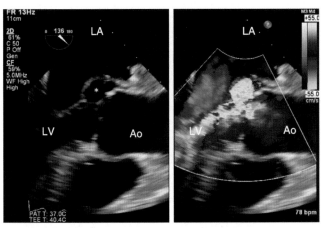

FIG. 40.6 Aortic root abscess with pseudoaneurysm formation. Transesophageal echocardiogram. Midesophageal aortic valve long-axis view in color-compare mode showing simultaneous 2D *(left)* and 2D with color Doppler interrogation *(right)* of the aortic valve and root in diastole. There is an abscess cavity *(asterisk)* involving the intervalvular fibrosa. Color flow Doppler demonstrates turbulent diastolic flow through a small perforation in the wall of the sinus into the cavity (pseudoaneurysm) and out to the left ventricle (LV). *Ao,* Aorta; *LA,* left atrium.

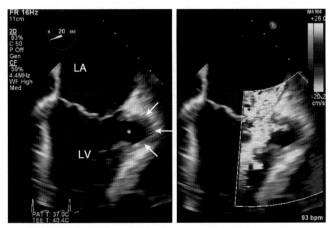

FIG. 40.7 Mitral valve endocarditis: perivalvular myocardial abscess. Transesophageal echocardiogram. Midesophageal four-chamber view in color-compare mode showing simultaneous 2D *(left)* and 2D with color Doppler interrogation *(right)* of the mitral valve and the adjacent basal anterolateral myocardial abscess *(asterisk)*. Note the advancing echolucent front *(arrows)* of the abscess toward the pericardium. Color Doppler interrogation shows flow within the abscess cavity. Note that the Nyquist limit had to be lowered significantly to reveal the low-velocity flow within the cavity. *LA,* Left atrium; *LV,* left ventricle.

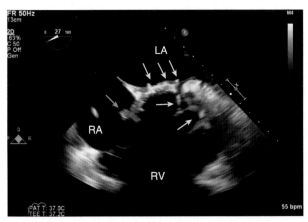

FIG. 40.8 Aortic root abscess with extension into right atrium. Transesophageal echocardiogram. Midesophageal aortic valve short-axis view demonstrating an aortic bioprosthesis enveloped by a large aortic root abscess *(yellow arrows)*. Abscess extension into the right atrium (RA) is demonstrated by the presence of a vegetative mass on the RA surface of the aortic abscess *(green arrow)*. *LA,* Left atrium; *RV,* right ventricle.

Mechanical Disruption of the Valve Apparatus: Perforation and Dehiscence

Cusp/leaflet perforation may complicate IE and may be present even when there is no clear-cut nearby vegetation. Involvement may start with a small outpouching of the affected cusp or leaflet with progressive aneurysm formation before full perforation occurs (Fig. 40.10, Video 40.11). Note that mitral perforation can occur in the setting of aortic valve endocarditis as an outcome of seeding of the anterior leaflet where it is traumatized by a bacteria-laden aortic regurgitant jet. Because echo dropout may false positively create the appearance of a perforation, color confirmation of associated valve regurgitation is essential to establish the diagnosis of perforation.

When the mitral subvalvular apparatus is involved, infection can also result in chordal or rarely papillary muscle rupture, the appearance of which may be difficult to distinguish from spontaneous chordal rupture or postinfarction papillary muscle rupture. However, the context in which this occurs usually makes a diagnosis obvious.

Each of these complications is typically associated with significant regurgitation while, as previously noted, valve stenosis complicating IE is unusual and limited to prosthetic valves (Fig. 40.11, Video 40.12).

Prosthetic valve dehiscence and paravalvular regurgitation can occur with perivalvular infection that undermines the seating of the prosthesis. As infection spreads, there may be evidence of echo dropout and progressive regurgitation; the latter is required to confirm that the area of dropout is not an artifact. Three-dimensional echocardiography is particularly helpful in delineating the extent of valve dehiscence particularly for mitral valves. When extreme, valve dehiscence is associated with valve rocking and the risk of valve embolization (see Videos 40.9 and 40.13). Note that in some instances mitral prostheses are implanted onto the basal leaflets when there is excessive annular calcification and that, for these valves, some degree of rocking would typically be the case. This is another argument for the importance of a baseline postoperative study.

RIGHT-SIDED ENDOCARDITIS

Right-sided endocarditis is most typically encountered in intravenous drug abusers or alcoholics with tricuspid valve involvement accounting for the vast majority of cases (see Fig. 40.2, Video 40.3). The tricuspid valve may also be secondarily seeded due to extension of aortic valve or right-sided device endocarditis. In general, TTE performs well in the assessment of the tricuspid valve as long as care is taken to ensure that all three leaflets are adequately seen. This requires parasternal, apical, and subcostal views as discussed in detail in Chapter 30. Tricuspid vegetations can be extremely large with size greater than 2 cm identified as being a predictor of IE-related mortality. Pulmonic valve endocarditis is rare (see also Chapter 30) but perhaps underappreciated due to the challenges of imaging this valve.

Although infection may also involve the eustachian valve or Chiari network, typically in the setting of pacing lead or indwelling line infection, it may be challenging to distinguish vegetation from the normal appearance of these structures or from superimposed thrombus.

NONVALVULAR ENDOCARDITIS

Device-Related Infective Endocarditis

In addition to prosthetic valves, all implantable cardiac devices including pacemakers, cardioverter defibrillators, and devices used in structural heart interventions are vulnerable to infection during generalized bacteremia. In addition, local pacemaker pocket infections may extend along implanted leads to involve the heart as well. The ability of echocardiography to detect infection in segments of the superior vena cava (SVC) remote from the heart is limited, but adjacent segments and the leads within the heart can be evaluated adequately with TEE. TTE plays a limited role in this setting. The appearance of lead-related vegetation may be indistinguishable from that of thrombus (Video 40.14), emphasizing the importance of interpreting imaging findings in clinical context.

Lead and pacing device removal is essential in the setting of infection and is typically performed percutaneously, but it has been suggested that when vegetations greater than 25 mm in size are present, surgery may be

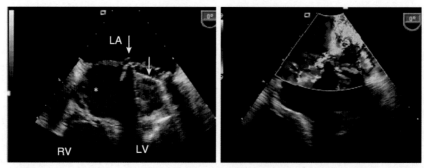

FIG. 40.9 Intervalvular fibrosa abscess with fistula into the left atrium. Transesophageal echocardiogram. Midesophageal modified four-chamber view demonstrating an abscess of the intervalvular fibrosa *(asterisk)* complicating mechanical mitral prosthetic endocarditis. There is a fistula between the abscess and the left atrium *(white arrow)*. Mitral prosthesis, *yellow arrow*. Color Doppler *(right panel)* confirms the communication. *LA*, Left atrium; *LV*, left ventricle; *RV*, right ventricle.

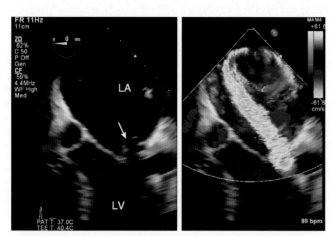

FIG. 40.10 Mitral valve endocarditis: leaflet perforation. Transesophageal echocardiogram. Midesophageal five-chamber view in color-compare mode showing simultaneous 2D *(left)* and 2D with color Doppler interrogation *(right)* of the mitral valve in systole. There is perforation in the posterior mitral leaflet *(arrow)* resulting in a characteristically turbulent and narrow jet of mitral regurgitation *(right panel)*. *LA*, Left atrium; *LV*, left ventricle.

the preferred approach. In the case of right-sided devices, it is important to determine whether there is a patent foramen ovalis, because this provides a window for infection to spread to the left side of the heart and for systemic embolus.

Infection of Cardiac Shunts

Atrial septal defects pose very low risk of infection while VSDs or patent ducti (PDAs) are at greater risk. As with valvular endocarditis, shunt infection is typically on the low-pressure side (see Fig. 40.3)

PURULENT PERICARDITIS

Purulent pericarditis is a rare complication of endocarditis that is most likely to occur in the setting of a mitral or tricuspid annular abscess, although cases attributable to myocardial abscesses, myocarditis, or pseudoaneurysm of the proximal aorta have also been reported. As with other more common causes of pericardial effusion, echocardiography is helpful in identifying the presence and hemodynamic consequences of such fluid collections. Purulent pericardial effusions may have a less echo-free appearance than typical transudative effusions with strand-like echodensities suspended within the fluid (Fig. 40.12).

ECHOCARDIOGRAPHIC PREDICTORS OF OUTCOMES

Embolism

Clinically evident embolic events occur in 20%–40% of patients with IE;[8] they are more common within the first days after the initiation of antibiotic treatment and then diminish. They are rare events after the completion of a successful course of antibiotics. With left-sided IE, the most common sites of clinically detected embolus are the brain and spleen, although coronary artery embolus may occur particularly if IE involves the aortic valve (Fig. 40.13). Although pulmonary embolism is predictably most common in the setting of right-sided endocarditis, right-sided lesions may occasionally be associated with emboli in the systemic circulation if there is a coexistent patent foramen. It is estimated that roughly one-fifth of embolic events are clinically silent.

The major predictor of embolic risk is vegetation size with reports that vegetations greater than 10 mm in any dimension as sized by 2D TEE pose high risk with even higher risk assigned to those greater than 15 mm (see Figs. 40.4 and 40.14). Highly mobile vegetations, particularly those on the anterior mitral leaflet, are also associated with increased embolic risk (Video 40.15), as are vegetations that increase in size during antibiotic treatment. Although the data are inconsistent, it has also been reported that decreasing vegetation size during treatment is a risk factor. Increased echogenicity suggests a degree of organization, and echodense vegetations are reported to be unlikely to embolize.

Echocardiographic assessment should therefore include the number, size, shape, location, mobility, and echogenicity of vegetations. Although not widely used, a scoring system for mobility has been proposed with the following elements:[7] grade 1, fixed; grade 2, fixed base but free edge; grade 3, pedunculated; grade 4, prolapsing. Note, however, that the ability of echocardiography to predict an embolic event in an individual patient is limited.

Overall Prognosis

Echocardiographic findings reported to be associated with worse prognosis are perhaps intuitive given an understanding of the natural history of the disease. They include evidence of perivalvular extension, severe valve dysfunction, reduced left ventricular systolic function and/or elevated filling pressures, pulmonary artery hypertension, and very large vegetations.

SURGERY FOR ENDOCARDITIS

Echocardiographic Indicators for Surgery

In general, evidence has pointed to the advantages of early versus delayed surgery in endocarditis with early surgery, defined as during initial hospitalization and before completion of a full therapeutic course of antibiotics, performed in almost 50% of IE cases. Indications are provided in Table 40.4 and include heart failure, embolic events on therapy, and evidence of extension characterized by an abscess, pseudoaneurysm, fistula, or complete heart block. For prosthetic valves, surgery is also indicated when there is recurrent bacteremia after a course of antibiotic therapy with subsequent negative blood cultures when there is no other identifiable source of infection. For a detailed discussion of the indications for surgery, the reader is referred to the relevant guidelines of the ESC[2] and ACC/AHA.[1]

FIG. 40.11 Pulmonic bioprosthetic endocarditis and stenosis. Upper esophageal aortic arch long-axis view. The pulmonic valve can be well visualized from the upper esophageal position. There is extensive endocarditis *(arrow)* of the pulmonic bioprosthesis (A) with color Doppler (B) and spectral Doppler (C) evidence of severe stenosis. Pulmonic bioprosthesis peak gradient = 111 mm Hg. *PA,* Pulmonary artery; *RVOT,* right ventricular outflow tract.

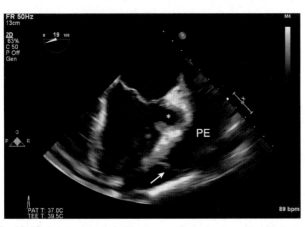

FIG. 40.12 Purulent pericarditis. Transesophageal echocardiogram from the same patient as in Fig. 40.7. Note the abscess cavity *(asterisk)* and the echolucent advancing front of the abscess toward the pericardium. There is a large, likely loculated pericardial effusion with stranding *(arrow)*. *PE,* Pericardial effusion.

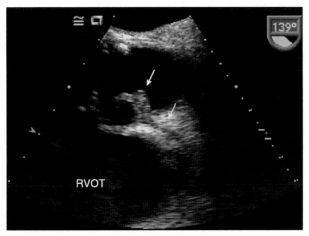

FIG. 40.13 Embolic coronary occlusion. Transesophageal echocardiogram. Midesophageal long-axis view of the proximal aorta showing a plug-like occlusion of the right coronary artery *(yellow arrow)* by a vegetation *(white arrow)* that embolized as a complication of aortic prosthetic endocarditis. *RVOT,* Right ventricular outflow tract.

Intraoperative Transesophageal Echocardiography

A detailed preprocedural intraoperative TEE is essential even if there has been a recent preoperative TEE. Because of the potential for IE to spread aggressively, there may have been an important interval change, even if a TEE has been performed even hours before surgery. It is particularly important to recognize when there has been spread to contiguous structures not previously involved; for example, the tricuspid valve in aortic valve endocarditis. It has been reported that a preprocedural intraoperative TEE can change the surgical plan in 11% of cases. In addition, once the surgical intervention has been completed, it is important to carry out a thorough reevaluation. It is not uncommon that in complex repairs there is residual valvular or paravalvular regurgitation and, if significant, this should prompt surgical revision. Patients with endocarditis are at increased risk of recurrent endocarditis and recognition of such is contingent on understanding the baseline appearance of the valves. Because repair frequently involves nonstandard valve replacement, there may be areas of thickening that could easily be confused with an early or recurrent root abscess. Finally, intraprocedural TEE provides a sense of baseline postoperative function of the left and right ventricles. Having access to 3D echocardiography can be very helpful because it can provide a better understanding of the location and spatial extent of the infective process. This is particularly true for mitral valve endocarditis (see Fig. 40.14 and Video 40.15).

Frequency of Echocardiography

Given the heterogeneity in the presentation and clinical course of infectious endocarditis, there are no hard and fast rules as to the frequency of follow-up.

The most recent ACCF Appropriate Use Criteria for echocardiography, also endorsed by the American Society of Echocardiography (see Table 40.1),[5] designate reevaluation of IE at high risk for progression or complication and/or with a change in clinical status on cardiac exam as being an appropriate use of echocardiography. Routine surveillance of uncomplicated native or prosthetic valve IE when no change in management is contemplated is considered inappropriate. This might be the case in patients with comorbidities or other circumstances that might make them ineligible for surgery regardless of echocardiographic findings. Other scenarios in which echocardiography is inappropriate are noted in Table 40.1. The European guidelines recommend a baseline transthoracic echo predischarge and/or following the completion of a full course of antimicrobial therapy with serial examinations at 1, 3, 6, and 12 months thereafter.[4] Follow-up TEE should be limited to those in whom there is new or persistent valve dysfunction or clinical suspicion of recurrent infection. Note that vegetations may not disappear even with bacteriologic cure although they may become more echodense and smaller.

Role of 3D Echocardiography

As 3D echocardiography has become more widely available and has improved its spatial and temporal resolution, an expanding role is emerging in the setting of IE. That said, the resolution may still be inadequate for the identification of small oscillating vegetations and the identification of small pathologic jets. However, 3D echocardiography is ideally

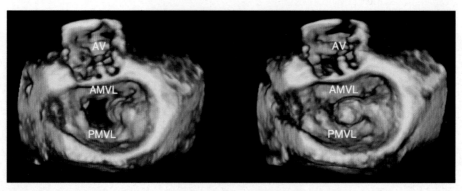

FIG. 40.14 Mitral valve endocarditis: large mobile vegetation. Three-dimensional transesophageal echocardiogram showing the mitral valve in diastole *(left)* and systole *(right)* in the "surgeon's view" with the aortic valve at the top. There is a large mobile vegetation attached by a broad stalk just above the medial commissure of the mitral valve. *AV,* Aortic valve; *AMVL,* anterior mitral valve leaflet; *PMVL,* posterior mitral valve leaflet.

TABLE 40.4 Current Indications for and Timing of Surgery in Infective Endocarditis

2014 ACC/AHA GUIDELINES			2015 ESC GUIDELINES		
Should Be Performed (Class I)	**Reasonable to Perform (Class IIa)**	**May Be Considered (Class IIb)**	**Recommended/ Indicated (Class I)**	**Should Be Considered (Class IIa)**	**May Be Considered (Class IIb)**
• Early surgery[a] for IE with valve dysfunction resulting in symptoms of HF (LOE: B) • Early surgery for left-sided IE caused by *Staphylococcus aureus*, fungal, or other highly resistant organisms (LOE: B) • Early surgery for IE complicated by heart block, annular or aortic abscess, or destructive penetrating lesions (LOE: B) • Early surgery for evidence of persistent infection as manifested by persistent bacteremia or fevers lasting longer than 5–7 days after onset of appropriate antimicrobial therapy (LOE: B) • Surgery for PVE and relapsing infection (defined as recurrence of bacteremia after a complete course of appropriate antibiotics and subsequently negative blood cultures) without other identifiable source for portal of infection (LOE: C) • Complete removal of pacemaker or defibrillator systems, including all leads and the generator, is indicated as part of the early management plan in patients with IE with documented infection of the device or leads (LOE: B)	• Complete removal of pacemaker or defibrillator systems, including all leads and the generator in patients with valvular IE caused by *S. aureus* or fungi, even without evidence of device or lead infection (LOE: B) • Complete removal of pacemaker or defibrillator systems, including all leads and the generator in patients undergoing valve surgery for valvular IE (LOE: C) • Early surgery for patients with IE who present with recurrent emboli and persistent vegetations despite appropriate antibiotic therapy (LOE: B)	• Early surgery for patients with NVE who exhibit mobile vegetations greater than 10 mm in length (with or without clinical evidence of embolic phenomenon) (LOE: B)	• Emergency[b] surgery for aortic or mitral NVE or PVE with severe acute regurgitation, obstruction or fistula causing refractory pulmonary edema or cardiogenic shock (LOE: B) • Urgent[c] surgery for aortic or mitral NVE or PVE with severe regurgitation or obstruction causing symptoms of HF or echocardiographic signs of poor hemodynamic tolerance (LOE: B) • Urgent surgery for locally uncontrolled infection (abscess, false aneurysm, fistula, enlarging vegetation) (LOE: B) • Urgent/elective[d] surgery for infection caused by fungi or multiresistant organisms (LOE: C) • Urgent surgery for aortic or mitral NVE or PVE with persistent vegetations >10 mm after one or more embolic episode(s) despite appropriate antibiotic therapy (LOE: B)	• Urgent surgery for persistent positive blood cultures despite appropriate antibiotic therapy and adequate control of septic metastatic foci (LOE: B) • Urgent/elective surgery for PVE caused by staphylococci or non-HACEK Gram-negative bacteria (LOE: C) • Urgent surgery for aortic or mitral NVE with vegetations >10 mm, associated with severe valve stenosis or regurgitation, and low operative risk (LOE: B) • Urgent surgery for aortic or mitral NVE or PVE with isolated very large vegetations (>30 mm) (LOE: B) • Complete hardware removal should be considered on the basis of occult infection without another apparent source of infection (LOE: C) • RIGHT-SIDED IE: Surgical treatment should be considered in the following scenarios: • Microorganisms difficult to eradicate (e.g., persistent fungi) or bacteremia for 7 days (e.g., *S. aureus, Pseudomonas aeruginosa*) despite adequate antimicrobial therapy or • Persistent tricuspid valve vegetations >20 mm after recurrent pulmonary emboli with or without concomitant right heart failure or • Right HF secondary to severe tricuspid regurgitation with poor response to diuretic therapy (LOE: C)	• Urgent surgery for aortic or mitral NVE or PVE with isolated large vegetations (>15 mm) and no other indication for surgery[e] (LOE: C) • In patients with NVE or PVE and an intracardiac device with no evidence of associated device infection, complete hardware extraction may be considered (LOE: C)

ACC, American College of Cardiology; *AHA,* American Heart Association; *ESC,* European Society of Cardiology; *HACEK,* Haemophilus, Aggregatibacter, Cardiobacterium hominis, Eikenella corrodens, and Kingella; *HF,* heart failure; *IE,* infective endocarditis; *LOE,* level of evidence; *NVE,* native valve endocarditis; *PVE,* prosthetic valve endocarditis.
[a]Early surgery is one taking place during initial hospitalization before completion of a full therapeutic course of antibiotics.
[b]Emergency surgery: surgery performed within 24 hours.
[c]Urgent surgery: within a few days; elective surgery: after at least 1–2 weeks of antibiotic therapy.
[d]Elective surgery: after at least 1–2 weeks of antibiotic therapy.
[e]Surgery may be preferred if a procedure preserving the native valve is feasible.
Data from Nishimura RA, Otto CM, Bonow RO, et al. 2014 AHA/ACC guideline for the management of patients with valvular heart disease: executive summary: a report of the American College of Cardiology/American Heart Association Task Force on Practice Guidelines. J Am Coll Cardiol. 2014;63(22):2438-2488; and Habib G, Badano L, Tribouilloy C, et al. Recommendations for the practice of echocardiography in infective endocarditis. Eur J Echocardiogr. 2010;11(2):202-219.

suited to characterize perivalvular abscesses and the spatial extent of large vegetations. It has been suggested that 3D is better able to size valve vegetations and that it generally provides measurements that are larger than those obtained by transthoracic echo. A single study has suggested that vegetations larger than 20 mm as sized by 3D TEE pose a greater risk of embolic events.[9] However, this cutoff has not yet been widely adopted or incorporated into current guidelines.

Suggested Reading

Baddour, L. M., Wilson, W. R., Bayer, A. S., et al. (2015). Infective endocarditis in adults: Diagnosis, antimicrobial therapy, and management of complications. *Circulation, 132*(15), 1435–1486.

Douglas, P. S., Garcia, M. J., Haines, D. E., et al. (2011). ACCF/ASE/AHA/ASNC/HFSA/HRS/SCAI/SCCM/SCCT/SCMR 2011 Appropriate Use Criteria for Echocardiography. A Report of the American College of Cardiology Foundation Appropriate Use Criteria Task Force, American Society of Echocardiography, American Heart Association, American Society of Nuclear Cardiology, Heart Failure Society of America, Heart Rhythm Society, Society for Cardiovascular Angiography and Interventions, Society of Critical Care Medicine, Society of Cardiovascular Computed Tomography, and Society for Cardiovascular Magnetic Resonance Endorsed by the American College of Chest Physicians. *Journal of the American Society of Echocardiography, 57*(9), 1126–1166.

Habib, G., Badano, L., Tribouilloy, C., et al. (2010). Recommendations for the practice of echocardiography in infective endocarditis. *European Journal of Echocardiography, 11*(2), 202–219.

Habib, G., Lancellotti, P., Antunes, M. J., et al. (2015). 2015 ESC guidelines for the management of infective endocarditis. *European Heart Journal, 36*(44), 3075–3128.

Nishimura, R. A., Otto, C. M., Bonow, R. O., et al. (2014). 2014 AHA/ACC guideline for the management of patients with valvular heart disease: A report of the American College of Cardiology/American Heart Association Task Force on Practice Guidelines. *Journal of the American College of Cardiology, 63*(22), e57–e185.

A complete reference list can be found online at ExpertConsult.com

41 Other Systemic Diseases and the Heart

Linda D. Gillam, Lillian Aldaia, Konstantinos Koulogiannis

INTRODUCTION

While echocardiography is, of course, critical in the evaluation of primary diseases of the heart, it is an equally important tool in identifying and monitoring the cardiovascular sequelae of systemic diseases and their treatment. Many of these are discussed in variable detail in prior chapters including those on dilated cardiomyopathies (see Chapter 22), Restrictive Cardiomyopathies (see Chapter 24), Mitral Valve Disease (see Chapter 28), Diseases of the Aorta (see Chapter 34), and Malignant Diseases (see Chapter 42). This chapter focuses on those not previously covered or those conditions with manifestations that are not limited to a single cardiac structure.

SARCOIDOSIS

Sarcoidosis is a granulomatous disease of uncertain etiology that primarily affects the lungs and lymphatic system. It has an annual incidence of 5–40 cases per 100,000 in the United States and Europe, with blacks at threefold greater risk. Cardiac involvement occurs in 25%–40% of patients overall. The hallmark of sarcoidosis is the development and accumulation of noncaseating granulomas composed of organized collections of macrophages and epithelioid cells surrounded by lymphocytes. Over time, granulomas and associated edema progress to fibrosis, thinning, and scar. Cardiac granulomas and scar occur most commonly in the basal interventricular septum and free wall of the left ventricle (particularly the basal inferior wall). Less common sites of myocardial involvement are the papillary muscles, atrial walls, and right ventricle. Involvement of the valves, pericardium, conduction system, and, rarely, the coronary arteries also occurs. Involvement tends to be patchy and, because of this, the diagnostic yield of myocardial biopsy is only 20%.

Cardiac involvement may be manifest as regional wall motion abnormalities, aneurysms (often atypically located), dilated cardiomyopathy, conduction abnormalities, arrhythmias, valvular regurgitation, pericardial effusion and rarely as acute coronary syndromes due to coronary vasculitis.

Two-dimensional transthoracic echocardiography is typically the first screening tool in the evaluation of cardiac sarcoidosis although note should be made of the important roles played by nuclear cardiology and cardiac magnetic resonance in patients with known or suspected sarcoid.[1] Echocardiographic features of cardiac sarcoidosis include abnormal septal thickness (may be increased initially and then progress to thinning), left ventricular (LV) systolic dysfunction, and segmental wall motion abnormalities in a noncoronary distribution. Ventricular aneurysms in atypical locations, right ventricular (RV) dysfunction, valvular abnormalities, and pericardial effusion may also be seen.[2]

The most common echocardiographic presentation of sarcoid is localized thinning of the basal interventricular septum (Fig. 41.1, Video 41.1). This otherwise unusual pattern should raise the possibility of sarcoidosis. Ventricular aneurysms, most commonly of the basal inferior wall, may be more discrete than is typical of those caused by coronary disease (Fig. 41.2, Video 41.2). These aneurysms may not correspond to typical coronary artery distributions and instead be due to the presence of granulomas within the myocardium. When there is segmental dysfunction, abnormal wall motion is most commonly seen in the anterior and apical LV segments. Impaired global longitudinal strain rate may also be seen in patients with cardiac sarcoidosis, often before the disease is evident clinically.[3]

One of the earliest signs of sarcoid involvement in the heart is diastolic dysfunction, including lower mitral annular tissue velocities of the septal wall. A restrictive pattern is unusual. Valvular dysfunction is also seen in patients with sarcoid due to either granulomatous deposition within the valve leaflets or secondary to ventricular dysfunction or pulmonary hypertension. Mitral and tricuspid regurgitation are the most common abnormalities with transesophageal echocardiography (TEE) playing an important role in understanding the pathophysiology. Pulmonary hypertension and secondary RV dysfunction can result from sarcoid lung involvement and be detected on echocardiographic evaluation. Direct involvement of the right ventricle by granuloma deposition can lead to regional or global RV systolic dysfunction.

Echocardiographic abnormalities may occur in the absence of extracardiac evidence of disease, symptoms, or ECG abnormalities. Conversely, the absence of echocardiographic findings does not exclude the diagnosis of cardiac sarcoid (negative predictive value of only 32%).[4] Fig. 41.3 provides a composite reference for the cardiac findings with cardiac sarcoid.

HYPEREOSINOPHILIC SYNDROME (LOEFFLER ENDOCARDITIS)

Hypereosinophilic syndrome (HES) refers to a family of disorders that share blood eosinophil counts of $>1.5 \times 10^9$/L and have directly attributable organ damage, frequently the heart. The hypereosinophilia may be idiopathic or due to leukemia, chronic parasitic infections, allergies, granulomatous disease, hypersensitivity, or neoplastic disorders. There is overlap with Churg-Strauss syndrome and endomyocardial fibrosis.

There are three phases of the cardiac involvement of HES: an acute inflammatory and necrotic state, followed by thrombotic and then fibrotic stages. Either or both ventricles of the heart may be affected and show endocardial thickening of the inflow regions and ventricular apices (Fig. 41.4, Video 41.3). There is also regional thickening of the basal inferior segment of the left ventricle that may impair the movement of the posterior leaflet of the mitral valve and cause significant mitral regurgitation, a mechanism that can be delineated by TEE. The apex may be filled with thrombus contributing to the appearance of Merlon sign, hypercontractility of the base with dysfunction of the apex. Contrast perfusion imaging may be helpful in separating thrombus from muscle in instances where there might be confusion between HES and apical hypertrophic cardiomyopathy. The atria are generally dilated, and there may be additional features of diastolic dysfunction and restrictive myopathy in later stages as well as pericardial effusion.[5]

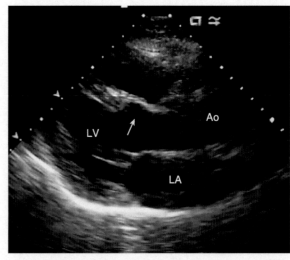

FIG. 41.1 Cardiac sarcoidosis. Transthoracic echocardiogram. Parasternal long-axis view. Thinning of the basal interventricular septum *(arrow)*. *Ao,* Aorta; *LA,* left atrium; *LV,* left ventricle.

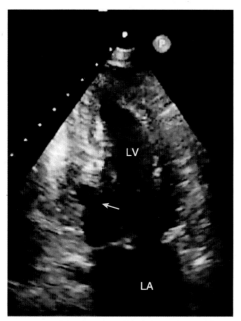

FIG. 41.2 Cardiac sarcoidosis. Transthoracic echocardiogram. Apical two-chamber view. There is a ventricular aneurysm of the basal inferior wall *(arrow)*. *LA*, Left atrium; *LV*, left ventricle.

THYROID DISEASE

The main mechanism by which thyroid disease affects the cardiovascular system is perturbation of the amount of thyroid hormone present in the circulation. Both hypothyroidism and hyperthyroidism have long been known to produce changes in the cardiovascular system by causing changes in cardiac contractility, myocardial oxygen consumption, and cardiac output. In addition, both hyperthyroidism and hypothyroidism are known to affect the electrical system of the heart and predispose afflicted individuals to atrial fibrillation and ventricular arrhythmias. Because hyperthyroidism is known to be associated with pulmonary hypertension, LV dysfunction, and mitral valve prolapse, echocardiographic evaluation of the heart in patients with hyperthyroidism should address right heart function and estimation of pulmonary artery systolic pressure, LV systolic function, and mitral valve structure and function. More sophisticated tools such as strain and Doppler tissue imaging are important to assess diastolic function and identify subclinical systolic dysfunction.

Hypothyroidism is associated with decreased cardiac contractility and cardiac output, altered diastolic function, and heart failure. Echocardiographic evaluation of the patient with hypothyroidism should focus on LV systolic and diastolic function, again taking advantage of strain and Doppler tissue imaging indices.[6] Pericardial effusion may also be present and may cause tamponade. Lipid levels are typically elevated in patients with hypothyroidism, and these patients may also exhibit accelerated atherosclerosis. Therefore, stress echocardiography in this subset of patients may be helpful in evaluating pain syndromes.

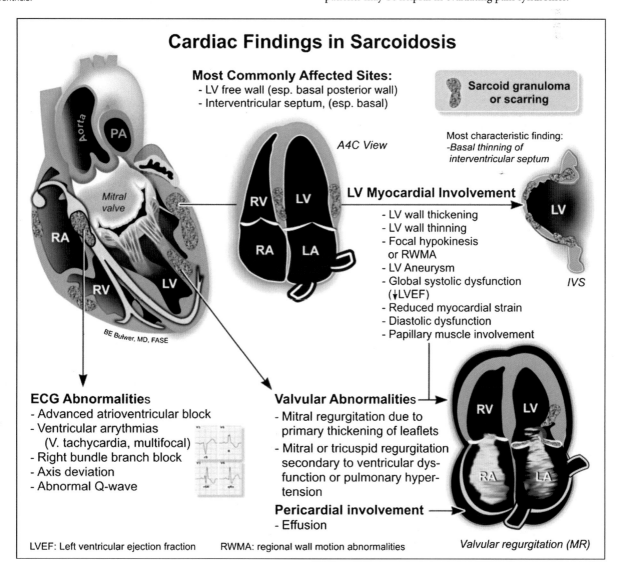

FIG. 41.3 Cardiac involvement in sarcoid. *A4C,* Apical four-chamber; *LA,* left atrium; *LV,* left ventricle; *PA,* pulmonary artery; *RA,* right atrium; *RV,* right ventricle. *(Courtesy of Bernard E. Bulwer, MD, FASE.)*

CARCINOID HEART DISEASE (SEE ALSO CHAPTER 30)

Carcinoid tumors are neuroendocrine malignancies most commonly located in the gastrointestinal tract. The most frequent locations are the appendix and terminal ileum. Rarely, they may be found in the bronchus and gonads. The presentation of the majority of patients is related to detection of the primary tumor alone, but carcinoid heart disease may be the presenting problem in 20% of patients, making this a diagnosis that can be made in the echo lab. Frequently, carcinoid heart disease is accompanied by other elements of carcinoid syndrome (secretory diarrhea, flushing, and bronchospasm).

The hallmark of carcinoid heart disease is valvular thickening and leaflet retraction due to the paraneoplastic effects of vasoactive substances secreted by the tumors. These substances include serotonin (5-hydroxytryptamine), 5-hydroxytryptophan, histamine, tachykinins, bradykinins, and prostaglandins. Pathologic changes include endocardial plaques of fibrous tissue that typically involve the tricuspid and pulmonary valves, right sided cardiac chambers, vena cavae, pulmonary artery, and coronary sinus. The tissue is most commonly deposited on the ventricular aspect of the tricuspid valve and pulmonary arterial aspect of the pulmonic valve, and the underlying architecture is not altered. Generally, only carcinoid tumors that have metastasized to the liver affect the heart and involvement is typically limited

to the right side, because the vasoactive substances are largely inactivated in the lungs. The presence of left-sided involvement, which occurs in 10% of cases, implies the presence of an intracardiac right- to-left shunt or pulmonary metastases.

On echocardiography, the most common finding is tricuspid valve leaflet and subvalvular apparatus thickening, shortening, and retraction so that the leaflets acquire a drumstick appearance. The valve leaflets cannot coapt normally with resultant tricuspid regurgitation, which is often severe (Fig. 41.5, Video 41.4). The continuous-wave Doppler profile may show a characteristic "dagger" shape, corresponding to an early peak and rapidly declining RV to right atrium (RA) pressure gradient, corresponding to rapid equalization of the RV and right atrial pressures. Because such flow will be color-coded as monochromatic, rather than the typical mosaic appearance of valve regurgitation, the severity may be underestimated by color Doppler. However, tricuspid stenosis is rare. The pulmonic valve may also be affected and appear thickened and retracted, resulting in either pulmonic regurgitation or stenosis. In addition to cusp involvement, the annulus may be constricted, but calcification of the valve is generally not seen in carcinoid heart disease.

In the presence of significant right-sided valve regurgitation, RV enlargement and diastolic flattening of the interventricular septum are common. Once established, valve abnormalities do not regress with otherwise successful medical or surgical treatment of the tumor.[7]

Carcinoid tricuspid valve disease can be distinguished from rheumatic disease by the absence of diastolic doming which occurs because the belly of the leaflet typically retains some mobility in rheumatic disease, unlike the full-length contraction and scarring seen in carcinoid. The absence of concomitant mitral disease also favors the diagnosis of sarcoid.

HEMOCHROMATOSIS

Hereditary hemochromatosis is an autosomal recessive disorder characterized by excess iron deposition in the solid organs (primarily the liver), joints, thyroid, pancreas, and heart. Although patients are generally asymptomatic in their youth, by middle age, iron levels may surpass the storage capacity of cells and end-organ damage occurs. Secondary hemochromatosis occurs secondary to iron overload due to other conditions such as certain anemias, chronic and recurrent blood transfusions, long-term hemodialysis, and chronic liver disease.

Under either circumstance, the heart can be infiltrated with iron. In the early stages, this may manifest as a restrictive myopathy with increased wall thickness, although in later stages, the appearance is indistinguishable

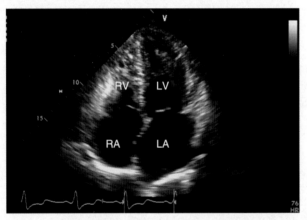

FIG. 41.4 Hypereosinophilic syndrome (Loeffler endocarditis). Transthoracic echocardiogram. Apical four-chamber view. The apices of the left ventricle (LV) and right ventricle (RV) are filled with thrombus. *LA*, Left atrium; *RA*, right atrium.

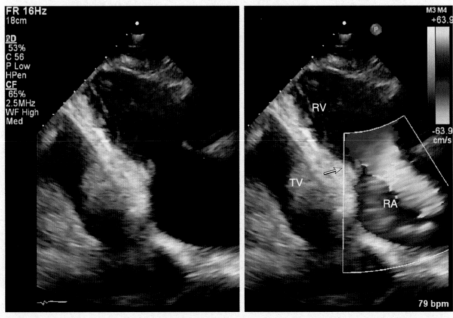

FIG. 41.5 Carcinoid heart disease. Transthoracic echocardiogram. The right ventricular inflow view is seen in diastole. The tricuspid valve leaflets and subvalvular apparatus are thickened, shortened, and retracted, leading to a "drumstick" appearance. The leaflets cannot fully coapt, and there is severe tricuspid regurgitation with laminar flow across the tricuspid valve *(arrow)*. *RA*, Right atrium; *RV*, right ventricle; *TV*, tricuspid valve.

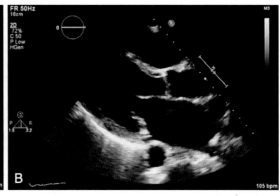

FIG. 41.6 **Late-stage hemochromatosis.** Transthoracic echocardiogram. Parasternal long-axis view. (A) Systole. (B) Diastole. In the later stages of the disease, the most common finding is a dilated cardiomyopathy. This echocardiogram is from a patient with hemochromatosis.

from that of dilated cardiomyopathies of other causes. This is by far the most common presentation of hemochromatotic heart disease (Fig. 41.6, Video 41.5).[8]

MUSCULAR DYSTROPHIES

The muscular dystrophies are a heterogeneous group of inherited disorders of the skeletal muscle system and are generally characterized by progressive wasting of the skeletal muscles. The four most common types of muscular dystrophies that are known to affect the cardiovascular system are dystrophin-associated disease (Duchenne and Becker muscular dystrophy), Emery-Dreifuss muscular dystrophy, limb-girdle muscular dystrophy, and myotonic dystrophy. Duchenne and Becker muscular dystrophies are associated with dilated cardiomyopathy and ventricular arrhythmias. Emery-Dreifuss muscular dystrophy is associated with dilated cardiomyopathy and atrioventricular conduction abnormalities. Limb-girdle muscular dystrophy is associated with dilated cardiomyopathy, RV and LV fatty infiltration, and conduction abnormalities. Cardiac involvement may be the only sign of disease in heterozygotes. In patients with myotonic dystrophy, dilated cardiomyopathy and conduction disturbances are also seen.

LYSOSOMAL STORAGE DISEASES

Glycogen Storage Diseases

Glycogen storage diseases (GSDs), of which there are 22 types, are conditions caused by autosomal or X-linked recessive mutations that result in specific enzyme deficiencies that render muscles unable to use glycogen as an energy substrate. Only three types (IIa also known as Pompe disease), III, and IXd are associated with myocardial dysfunction due to glycogen accumulation; while in type IIb, there is increased myocardial glycogen but function remains intact.[9] Cardiac manifestations include massive left and RV hypertrophy with "tumor like" enlargement of the papillary muscles.[10] Congestive heart failure can be seen in Pompe disease. Type IIb GSD is X-linked and associated with increased wall thickness but preserved function.

Fabry Disease

Fabry disease is an X-linked recessive condition that results in a deficiency of alpha-galactosidase A causing an accumulation of glycosphingolipids in endothelial lysosomes of the heart, skin, kidney, nervous system, and cornea. Within the heart, there is diffuse involvement of the myocardium, coronary artery endothelium, and cardiac heart valves (most significantly, the mitral valve). On echocardiographic evaluation, findings include increased LV wall thickness that may be asymmetric and mimic hypertrophic cardiomyopathy (including causing LV outflow tract obstruction) and aortic root dilation (Fig. 41.7, Video 41.6).[10] Abnormalities of both systolic and diastolic function have been reported, and strain and strain rate imaging may be particularly important in identifying early stages of the disease.[11] While a binary sign (echo-bright

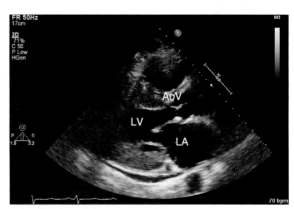

FIG. 41.7 **Fabry disease.** Transthoracic echocardiogram. Parasternal long-axis view. There is increased left ventricular wall thickness. *AoV*, Aortic valve; *LA*, left atrium; *LV*, left ventricle.

endocardium with an adjacent hyporeflective subendocardial layer that discriminates it from the myocardial midwall at end-diastole) has been reported to be a distinguishing feature of Fabry (Fig. 41.8),[12] others have argued that the sensitivity (35%), in particular, and specificity (79%) are too low to make this clinically helpful.[10,13]

Mucopolysaccharidoses

The mucopolysaccharidoses are composed of a family of diseases in which the lysosomal enzymes needed to break down glycosaminoglycans are deficient or ineffective. They include Hurler, Scheie, Hunter, Sanfilippo, Morquio, Maroteaux-Lamy, Sly, and Natowicz syndromes. These disorders are autosomal recessive, with the exception of Hunter syndrome, which is X-linked recessive. All these disorders share various cardiac manifestations including valvular thickening, regurgitation and stenosis, endomyocardial infiltration, myocardial fibrosis, left and RV hypertrophy, stenosis of the coronary arteries, and arterial hypertension. Dilated cardiomyopathy is also seen, but this is less frequent. In addition, there are no echocardiographic features that are unique to these conditions.

Sphingolipidoses

The most common of the sphingolipidoses that affect the cardiovascular system is Gaucher disease (beta-glucocerebrosidase deficiency). Gaucher disease is a heritable (autosomal recessive) deficiency of beta-glucocerebrosidase, which causes cerebrosides to accumulate in the spleen, liver, bone marrow, lymph nodes, brain, and heart. Cardiac manifestations include increased wall thickness with septal predominance and a stiffened ventricle with reduced chamber compliance. Regional wall motion abnormalities involving the apex can occur as can LV dilatation, pericardial effusion (rare), and sclerotic, calcified left-sided valves. Secondary elevation of pulmonary artery (PA) systolic pressure may also occur.[10]

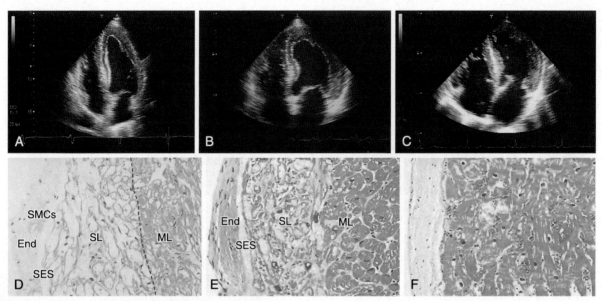

FIG. 41.8 Fabry disease. Two-dimensional echocardiography in four-chamber apical view and left ventricular endomyocardial biopsy from two patients with Fabry disease cardiomyopathy (A, D and B, E, respectively) and a patient with hypertrophic cardiomyopathy (C, F). Comparison of the three echocardiographic frames reveals the presence of a binary appearance of left ventricular endocardial border in the two Fabry patients (A, B). This echocardiographic finding shows the glycosphingolipids compartmentalization involving a thickened endocardium (End) with enlarged and engulfed smooth muscle cells (SMC), a subendocardial empty space (SES), and a prominent involvement of subendocardial myocardial layer (SL), while the middle layer (ML) appears partially spared (D, E). The echocardiographic pattern is absent in hypertrophic cardiomyopathy (C), despite a similar thickening of the endocardium (F). (*From Pieroni M, Chimenti C, De Cobelli F, et al. Fabry's disease cardiomyopathy: echocardiographic detection of endomyocardial glycosphingolipid compartmentalization.* J Am Coll Cardiol. *2006;47[8]:1663–1671.*)

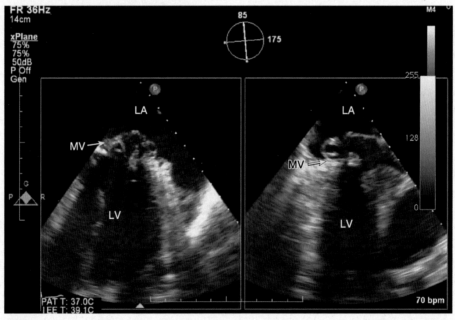

FIG. 41.9 Ehler-Danlos syndrome. Transesophageal echocardiogram, midesophageal commissural, and long-axis views. There is florid mitral valve prolapse *(arrow)*. *LA*, Left atrium; *LV*, left ventricle; *MV*, mitral valve.

CONNECTIVE TISSUE DISORDERS

Ehlers-Danlos Syndrome

Ehlers-Danlos syndrome (EDS) is an inherited connective tissue disorder. The main features include skin hyperextensibility, abnormal wound healing, and joint hypermobility. Cardiac manifestations are uncommon in classic EDS; however, mitral valve prolapse and tricuspid valve prolapse are known to occur. In severe cases of classic EDS, there may be dilatation of the aortic root and spontaneous rupture of the large arteries. A cardiac valvular form of EDS is an autosomal recessive disorder that results in the absence of a protein in type I collagen. Florid mitral valve prolapse and concomitant mitral regurgitation may be encountered in this condition (Fig. 41.9, Video 41.7) as can similar findings of the tricuspid valve (Video 41.8).

Marfan Syndrome

Marfan syndrome is an autosomal dominant inherited disease that affects the ocular, skeletal, and cardiovascular systems. Cardiac manifestations include dilatation of the aorta (Fig. 41.10, Video 41.9) with predisposition for aortic dissection and rupture, mitral and tricuspid valve prolapse, and enlargement of the proximal pulmonary artery.

MARANTIC ENDOCARDITIS

Marantic endocarditis refers to non-bacterial thrombotic endocarditis and covers a spectrum of lesions ranging from small platelet aggregations to large vegetations in the absence of bacteremia. It is rare, and it is often associated with hypercoagulable states, advanced malignancy, disseminated

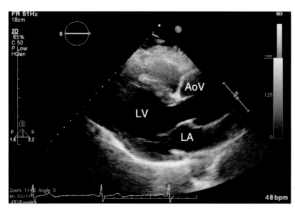

FIG. 41.10 Marfan syndrome. Transthoracic echocardiogram. Parasternal long-axis view. The aortic root is severely dilated. *AoV,* Aortic valve; *LA,* left atrium; *LV,* left ventricle.

intravascular coagulation, uremia, burns, systemic lupus erythematosus, valvular heart disease, and the presence of intracardiac catheters. It also occurs at the valve closure contact line on the atrial surfaces of the mitral and tricuspid valves (Video 41.10), and on the ventricular surfaces of the aortic and pulmonic valves. Marantic vegetations may serve as a nidus for bacterial superinfection, and marantic endocarditis is typically a diagnosis of exclusion based on clinical presentation with imaging features that mimic those of infective endocarditis (see Chapter 40).

DIABETES, HYPERTENSION, AND OBESITY

Diabetes, hypertension, and obesity are associated with diastolic dysfunction and heart failure with normal ejection fraction. Although patients with diabetes mellitus often have concomitant renal dysfunction, hypertension, and coronary artery disease, there are direct effects of hyperglycemia on the heart including myocyte hypertrophy, fibrosis, and coronary artery disease, especially of the microvasculature.

Hypertensive patients are also at increased risk for diastolic dysfunction, as chronic high blood pressure is a stimulus for remodeling. In hypertensive heart disease, there is LV hypertrophy, increasing ventricular stiffness and impaired relaxation, which leads to diastolic dysfunction. These patients often have elevated resting filling pressures and will respond with a greater-than-expected increase in filling pressures in the setting of coronary ischemia.

For obese patients, the increased weight increases the work of the heart and adipose tissue is metabolically active, producing substances linked to chronic inflammation. Obesity aggravates the challenges of appropriate body size-adjustment of measures of cardiac structure and function with there being no consensus as to whether lean body mass rather than total body mass provides the preferred approach.

For each of these conditions, echocardiographic techniques including Doppler tissue imaging and speckle tracking echocardiography at rest and with stress have been shown to identify abnormalities at an earlier stage than conventional resting imaging and spectral Doppler. For a more comprehensive discussion of echocardiographic findings in these conditions, the reader is referred to reviews and guidelines on these topics.[14–16]

Suggested Reading

Alizad, A., & Seward, J. B. (2000). Echocardiographic features of genetic diseases: Part 2. Storage disease. *Journal of the American Society of Echocardiography, 13*(2), 164–170.

Blankstein, R., & Waller, A. H. (2016). Evaluation of known or suspected cardiac sarcoidosis. *Circulation: Cardiovascular Imaging, 9*(3), e000867.

Click, R. L., Olson, L. J., Edwards, W. D., et al. (1994). Echocardiography and systemic diseases. *Journal of the American Society of Echocardiography, 7*(2), 201–216.

Connolly, H. M., & Pellikka, P. A. (2006). Carcinoid heart disease. *Current Cardiology Reports, 8*(2), 96–101.

Cuspidi, C., Rescaldani, M. F., Sala, C. F., & Grassi, G. (2014). Left-ventricular hypertrophy and obesity: A systematic review and meta-analysis of echocardiographic studies. *Journal of Hypertension, 32*(1), 16–25.

Mankad, R., Bonnichsen, C., & Mankad, S. (2016). Hypereosinophilic syndrome: Cardiac diagnosis and management. *Heart, 102*(2), 100–106.

Marwick, T. H., Gillebert, T. C., Aurigemma, G., et al. (2015). Recommendations on the use of echocardiography in adult hypertension: A report from the European Association of Cardiovascular Imaging (EACVI) and the American Society of Echocardiography (ASE). *Journal of the American Society of Echocardiography, 28*(7), 727–754.

Wang, Y., & Marwick, T. H. (2016). Update on echocardiographic assessment in diabetes mellitus. *Current Cardiology Reports, 18*(9), 1–6.

A complete reference list can be found online at ExpertConsult.com.

42 Echocardiography in Malignant Disease

Sarah Cuddy, John D. Groarke

INTRODUCTION

Approximately two out of every five people will be diagnosed with cancer at some point during their lifetime. Significant improvements in cancer care have improved 5-year survival for all cancer sites from 49% in 1980 to 67% currently, such that there are over 14 million people living with cancer in the United States today.[1] Multiple factors contribute to an increasing prevalence of clinically significant cardiotoxicity during or after cancer treatments (Box 42.1). Echocardiography is the mainstay of cardiac assessment before, during, and after cancer treatments. This chapter reviews increasing applications of standard and advanced echocardiographic techniques in patients along the entire cancer survivorship continuum that now account for a significant proportion of the referrals for echocardiography.

BASELINE ASSESSMENT PRIOR TO INITIATION OF CANCER TREATMENTS

Echocardiography should ideally be performed for baseline evaluation of cardiac function prior to initiation of potentially cardiotoxic cancer treatments; however, this often does not occur routinely in clinical practice. At the very least, the authors advocate that pretreatment echocardiography should be strongly considered in the context of any baseline characteristics outlined in Box 42.2. Furthermore, echocardiography should be part of a more comprehensive baseline cardiovascular (CV) assessment that includes history, physical examination, and electrocardiography. This baseline assessment provides an opportunity to modify proposed cancer treatment protocols if necessary, to optimize pretreatment CV comorbidities, and to identify "higher risk" patients who may warrant closer CV surveillance during cancer treatment, in the hope of minimizing risk of cardiotoxicity.

DURING CANCER TREATMENT

Echocardiography is indicated for patients who develop symptoms and/or signs of cardiac disease during cancer treatment. Echocardiographic surveillance in the absence of clinical symptoms and signs is recommended for certain therapies with significant cardiotoxic potential, such as anthracyclines and trastuzumab. In addition, empiric surveillance using echocardiography is often used for "higher risk" patients with predisposing risk factors for cardiotoxicity undergoing cancer treatment. The primary focus of echocardiographic assessment is to detect cancer

therapeutics-related cardiac dysfunction (CTRCD). CTRCD can complicate many cancer therapies and is defined as a decrease in left ventricular ejection fraction (LVEF) of greater than 10%, to a value of less than 53%.[2] CTRCD can be either symptomatic or asymptomatic and can be further categorized based on reversibility as either of the following:
1. Reversible CTRCD: LVEF recovery to within 5% of baseline
2. Partially reversible CTRCD: LVEF recovery by ≥10% but remains greater than 5% below baseline
3. Irreversible CTRCD: LVEF recovery less than 10% and remains greater than 5% below baseline.

The diagnosis of CTRCD should be confirmed by reassessment of LVEF 2–3 weeks after initial detection.[3]

Serial Assessment of Left Ventricular Ejection Fraction

The modified biplane Simpson technique is the method of choice for two-dimensional (2D) echocardiographic assessment of LVEF and left ventricular (LV) volumes. However, this technique is limited by test-retest, and inter- and intraobserver variability, such that changes over time may indicate random measurement or reporting variability rather than true clinically meaningful findings.[4] Indeed, it has been reported that 11% is the smallest change in LVEF that can be recognized with 95% confidence by 2D echocardiographic techniques,[5] which is higher than the difference to be detected based on the definition of CTRCD. Sequential quantification of LVEF and LV volumes in patients undergoing cancer treatments is the exact scenario that calls for better reproducibility due to implications for clinical chemotherapeutic decisions. There are ways to improve reproducibility: contrast echocardiography and 3D echocardiography can reduce temporal and acquisition-related variability in serial LVEF quantification. For a given patient, serial LVEF measurements should be performed using the same technique throughout follow-up, and ideally with the same observer and equipment, to ensure meaningful comparisons.

Contrast Echocardiography

LV opacification with an intravenous contrast agent should be employed when ≥2 contiguous LV segments are not seen on non-contrast 2D

BOX 42.1 Factors Associated With Increasing Prevalence of Cardiovascular Toxicities Associated With Cancer Treatments

- Increasing survivorship
- Increasing age and cardiovascular comorbidities of cancer patients
- Increasing range of targeted cancer drugs with potential for cardiovascular toxicity
- Increasing use of combinations of cancer agents and adjuvant thoracic irradiation
- Increasing duration of treatment (e.g., maintenance treatment with BCR-ABL tyrosine kinase inhibitors in chronic myeloid leukemia)
- Increasing treatment of patients with recurrent or second malignancies with prior exposure to cancer treatments

---

BOX 42.2 Baseline Characteristics That Should Prompt Consideration for Transthoracic Echocardiogram Prior to Initiation of Cancer Treatments

- Preexisting cardiovascular disease (e.g., ischemic heart disease, valvular heart disease, cardiomyopathies)
- Risk factors for cardiovascular disease (e.g., hypertension, diabetes mellitus)
- History of left ventricular dysfunction
- Signs or symptoms of heart failure
- Older patients (>65 years of age)
- Planned treatment with anthracyclines
- Planned treatment with trastuzumab
- Planned treatment with any cancer therapy with higher risk of incident cardiac dysfunction
- Planned surgery as part of cancer treatment that is not considered low risk with respect to morbidity
- Patients with recurrent or second cancers and history of prior chemotherapy exposure and/or thoracic irradiation

echocardiographic apical images.[6] Cancer patients are particularly predisposed to suboptimal echocardiographic windows that warrant consideration for contrast usage as a result of prior surgery (e.g., left mastectomy and breast reconstruction, left thoracotomies). Two-dimensional echocardiographic evaluation of LV volumes and LVEF is more accurate and reproducible when a contrast agent is used.[7] Its use should be consistent at each study time point throughout the surveillance period.

Three-Dimensional Echocardiography

Where available, 3D-echocardiography is the preferred technique for longitudinal assessment of LV function in patients undergoing treatment for cancer.[2] Noncontrast 3D-echocardiography demonstrated significantly lower temporal variability, test-retest variability, and observer variability in a study comparing 2D and 3D techniques with and without contrast administration for serial evaluation of LVEF and LV volumes in patients undergoing chemotherapy over 1 year of follow-up.[5] This is in keeping with a meta-analysis of studies performed in noncancer populations comparing echocardiography and cardiac magnetic resonance imaging (CMR), which demonstrated that 3D-echocardiography is more accurate for LV volumes and LVEF than traditional 2D methods.[8] However, widespread clinical application of 3D-echocardiography in oncology patients is limited by availability, operator experience, cost, and dependence on good 2D echocardiographic-image quality. As the technology becomes more widely available, a 3D-volumetric approach for quantification of LV function will be increasingly used in longitudinal assessment of patients with cancer. At this time, contrast agents are not recommended in conjunction with 3D-echocardiography in the serial assessment of patients with cancer.[2]

Other Imaging Modalities

Echocardiography has emerged as the modality of choice for serial assessment of oncology patients in clinical practice due to widespread availability, relatively competitive cost, absence of radiation exposure, and opportunity to assess cardiac structures other than the LV. If echocardiographic assessment is inadequate for reasons such as poor windows, nuclear multiple gated acquisition (MUGA) scans or CMR may be considered. MUGA scans are well suited for serial assessment of LVEF due to high reproducibility and low variability and were extensively used for this indication in the 1980s and 1990s. However, limitations of radiation exposure and failure to provide any meaningful data beyond LVEF underlie the recent transition to echocardiography in most patients. CMR offers very accurate and reproducible quantification of biventricular function and is particularly suited to evaluate cardiac tumors and pericardial disease. Gadolinium-based imaging techniques are helpful in detection and quantification of myocardial fibrosis that can be a feature of CTRCD. Cost and availability issues, in addition to contraindications to CMR (e.g., pacemakers/defibrillators), limit widespread application of this modality in serial assessment. Nevertheless, it remains a very useful adjunct to echocardiography in select oncology patients. It is important that there is consistent application of the same modality for surveillance for cardiotoxicity in the same patient to facilitate meaningful inter-study comparisons.

Left Ventricular Ejection Fraction Surveillance Schedules

Although the risk associated with specific cancer treatments varies, CTRCD is linked to a large number of traditional cytostatics (e.g., anthracyclines) and newer targeted anticancer drugs that include monoclonal antibodies (e.g., trastuzumab), protein kinase inhibitors (e.g., tyrosine kinase inhibitors), and proteasome inhibitors (e.g., carfilzomib).[9] The 2013 American College of Cardiology Foundation/American Heart Association Guideline for the Management of Heart Failure recognizes this risk of heart failure (HF) by categorizing patients without structural heart disease or symptoms of HF who receive cancer therapies with cardiotoxic potential as having stage A HF and recommend careful optimization of other modifiable risk factors that may lead to or contribute to HF.[10] Although guidelines for cardiovascular surveillance of patients treated with trastuzumab and anthracyclines are available, similar guidelines for surveillance of patients receiving newer cancer therapies are lacking.

Anthracyclines

Anthracyclines are highly effective chemotherapies used in the treatment of many solid and hematological malignancies. Cardinale et al. reported an overall incidence of 9% of cardiotoxicity (defined as a decrease in LVEF by >10% from baseline and absolute LVEF <50%) in a prospective study that performed periodic echocardiography in 2625 patients receiving anthracyclines.[11] A dose-response relationship between cumulative anthracycline exposure and risk of cardiomyopathy is well recognized.[12] Baseline assessment of LVEF should be performed in all patients prior to anthracycline exposure and repeated at any time if signs or symptoms of heart failure develop during or after treatment. For asymptomatic patients, the European Society for Medical Oncology (ESMO) Clinical Practice Guidelines propose repeating LVEF assessment at 6 months after conclusion of anthracycline treatment, annually for 2–3 years thereafter, and then at 3- to 5-year intervals for life.[13] Patients considered at higher risk, such as those exposed to a high cumulative dose of anthracycline (e.g., >300 mg/m² of doxorubicin or equivalent) may require more frequent monitoring. Indeed, an expert consensus statement from the American Society of Echocardiography and the European Association of Cardiovascular Imaging advocates for an evaluation of LVEF before each additional cycle of anthracycline once the dose exceeds 240 mg/m².[2] The Children's Oncology Group Long-Term Follow-up Guidelines recommend lifelong serial echocardiographic screening for survivors of childhood cancers every 1–5 years based on age at treatment, cumulative anthracycline exposure, and whether the heart was irradiated.[14] Given that over 90% of cases of cardiotoxicity occur within the first year of anthracycline treatment, focusing LVEF screening to this higher-risk period could significantly increase yield, as well as physician and patient adherence.[15]

The clinical benefits, yield, and cost effectiveness of LVEF surveillance schedules for detection of asymptomatic LV dysfunction in patients exposed to cardiotoxic cancer therapies are uncertain. Rationalizing lifelong surveillance schedules used in childhood cancer survivors exposed to anthracyclines may be necessary to improve cost effectiveness.[16,17]

Trastuzumab

Trastuzumab (Herceptin) is a humanized monoclonal antibody directed against the Human Epidermal Growth Factor Receptor 2 (HER2) receptor that is overexpressed in approximately 15% of breast cancers. Use of trastuzumab in HER2 positive breast cancer is associated with significant reduction in cancer recurrence and improvement in survival. However, trastuzumab is well recognized to cause cardiotoxicity. The addition of trastuzumab to chemotherapy regimens is associated with HF in 1.7%–4.1% and LV dysfunction in 7.1%–18.6%, although the incidence is likely higher in clinical practice.[18] Risk factors associated with trastuzumab cardiotoxicity include adjuvant chemotherapy (particularly anthracyclines), advancing age, and CV comorbidities.[19]

Serial evaluation of LVEF is recommended for patients receiving trastuzumab every 3 months during therapy[2,13,20] or at any time in the event of clinical signs or symptoms of HF. An algorithm for the continuation and discontinuation of trastuzumab based on LVEF assessment is presented in Fig. 42.1. Although the role of HF treatment in trastuzumab-induced LV dysfunction has not yet been established,[21] patients are treated according to international guidelines for HF management.[10] In clinical practice, an angiotensin-converting enzyme (ACE) inhibitor is often introduced with the aim of preventing further deterioration in LVEF or development of clinical HF when LVEF is between 40% and 50%.[20]

Left Ventricular Diastolic Function

Left ventricular diastolic dysfunction is common in patients with cancer before, during, and after treatment. The American Society of Echocardiography and the European Association of Cardiovascular Imaging conclude that despite suggestions that alterations in LV diastolic function (as evaluated by Doppler indices of mitral inflow and e′ velocity of the mitral annulus) precede overt reductions in LVEF, these indices are not useful for prediction of later CTRCD based on available evidence.[2] The therapeutic implications of alterations in echocardiographic measures of LV diastolic function have not been determined, and there is no evidence that cancer treatments should be modified based on these findings. In addition, it is important to remember that loading conditions can fluctuate in the context of volume contraction due to cancer treatment-associated gastrointestinal side effects and volume expansion due to intravenous administration of cancer drugs. These fluctuations in loading conditions may underlie changes in E and

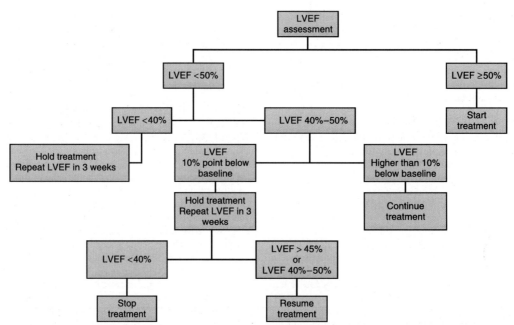

FIG. 42.1 Algorithm for management of trastuzumab based on serial left ventricular ejection fraction (LVEF) assessments. (*From Curugliano G, Cardinale D, Suter T, et al. Cardiovascular toxicity induced by chemotherapy, targeted agents and radiotherapy: ESMO Clinical Practice Guidelines. Ann Oncol. 2012;23[suppl 7]:vii155-166.*)

e′ velocities in oncology patients rather than true alterations in LV diastolic function. Nonetheless, a conventional assessment of LV diastolic function as outlined in Chapter 15 is often included in the echocardiographic protocol for oncology patients.

Early Detection of Subclinical Left Ventricular Dysfunction Using Myocardial Strain Imaging

Overt reductions in LVEF may be a relatively late marker of cardiotoxicity. Detection of early subclinical markers of LV injury may offer the potential to intervene at an earlier time point where likelihood of full recovery is higher. This is a growing body of literature to support the use of myocardial deformation parameters in detection of early myocardial injury and in prediction of subsequent decrease in LVEF.[22] Myocardial deformation or strain can be measured using Doppler tissue imaging or two-dimensional strain rate echocardiography (SRE), as described in Chapter 6. The role of various indices of myocardial strain (longitudinal, radial, and circumferential strain, strain rate, twist) have been evaluated in the detection of early myocardial changes in patients receiving chemotherapy, and global longitudinal strain (GLS) has emerged as the most optimal parameter of deformation for early detection of subclinical LV dysfunction and prediction of subsequent LVEF reductions.[2,3]

A relative reduction in GLS of less than 8% from baseline during cancer treatment does not appear to be clinically meaningful, whereas a relative percentage reduction of greater than 15% from baseline is very likely to have clinical significance.[2,3] Changes in loading conditions will influence GLS values, and the abnormal GLS value should be confirmed by a repeat study performed after 2–3 weeks. Given intervendor variability in strain measurement, the same machine and software version should be employed in serial evaluation of patients for meaningful interstudy comparisons. Based on available evidence at present, GLS-based evidence of subclinical myocardial dysfunction alone is not sufficient reason to introduce cardioprotective therapies or to modify cancer treatments.[3]

Other

Right Ventricular Function

Right ventricular (RV) abnormalities in oncology patients may be a consequence of preexisting disease, cardiotoxicity of cancer treatments, or direct tumor involvement. The frequency of RV involvement in cases of CTRCD is uncertain. Echocardiography protocols for oncology patients should include qualitative and quantitative measures of RV size and function as

> **BOX 42.3 Echocardiographic Features of Radiation-Induced Valvular Heart Disease**
>
> - Left-sided valve disease (i.e., mitral and aortic valves) is much more common than right sided valve disease
> - Calcification of aortic root and aortic valve annulus
> - Calcification of aortic leaflets
> - Calcification of the aortic-mitral intervalvular fibrosa
> - Calcification of the mitral valve annulus and mitral leaflets with sparing of the mitral valve tips and commissures (in contrast to rheumatic mitral valve disease, which is characterized by commissural fusion and involvement of the leaflet tips)

discussed in Chapter 16, in addition to specific comments on any signs of RV overload that may accompany elevations in pulmonary artery pressures.

Valvular Assessment

While anticancer drugs do not directly affect heart valves, radiation-induced valve disease is well recognized. Risk of clinically significant valvular disease increases with time from chest radiation. Refinement of modern-day radiation treatment protocols has reduced incidental radiation exposure to the heart and risk of subsequent valve disease compared to traditional protocols. Echocardiographic features of radiation-induced valvular disease are summarized in Box 42.3. In the aortic and mitral positions, early thickening and calcification are the usual result. In addition, Fig. 42.2 and corresponding Videos 42.1 and 42.2 show an example of radiation-induced mitral stenosis. Early calcification of the aortic valve as well is not uncommon, as shown in Video 42.3. In contrast, although the tricuspid valve may become thickened and retracted due to radiation, the result is usually tricuspid regurgitation (Fig. 42.3 and Video 42.4) with ensuing right heart failure. Grading severity of valvular disease should follow international guidelines and are described in Chapters 28–30.

Other causes of valvular disease in oncology patients include preexisting valvular disease or valvular dysfunction secondary to CTRCD. In addition, patients undergoing treatment for malignancy are predisposed to infective endocarditis due to risk factors such as indwelling vascular catheters and immunosuppression. Finally, cancer itself can have direct effects on the heart valves, as in the case of carcinoid heart disease discussed in Chapter 30. Carcinoid valvular disease predominantly affects right sided valves and is most commonly associated with hepatic metastases, which allow humoral tumor

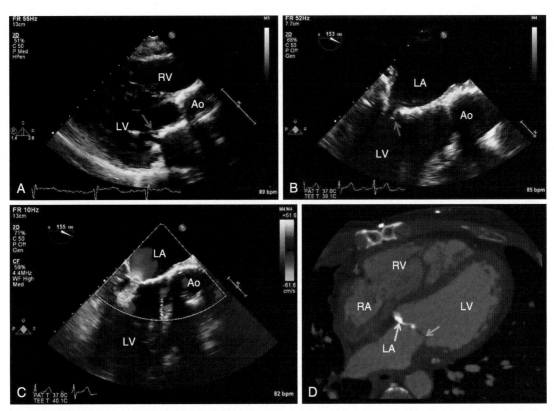

FIG. 42.2 Radiation-induced mitral stenosis in a 59-year-old male survivor of Hodgkin lymphoma who presented with progressive dyspnea on exertion 19 years following mantle radiation. (A) Parasternal long-axis view from a transthoracic echocardiogram demonstrated thickening of the mitral valve annulus and mitral leaflets with relative sparing of the leaflet tips *(arrow)*. (B) Midesophageal long-axis view from a transesophageal echocardiogram performed in the same patient confirmed thickening of the mitral valve leaflets with relative sparing of the leaflet tips *(arrow)*. (C) Midesophageal long-axis view from B with color Doppler demonstrated flow convergence on the left atrial side of the mitral valve due to radiation-induced mitral stenosis. (D) Four-chamber view from a gated thoracic computed tomography performed on the same patient demonstrated calcification of the anterior mitral valve leaflet *(yellow arrow)* with sparing of the leaflet tips *(green arrow)*. Ao, Aortic root; LA, left atrium; LV, left ventricle; RA, right atrium; RV, right ventricle.

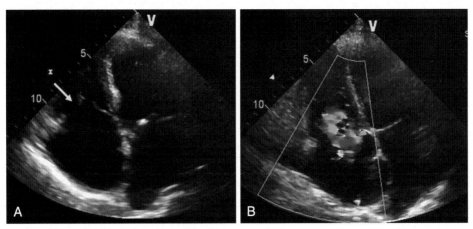

FIG. 42.3 Radiation-induced tricuspid valvulopathy in a 79-year-old female who received radiation and lumpectomy for breast cancer at age 50. (A) There is thickening and retraction of the tricuspid valve *(arrow)* with incomplete closure, with ensuing right atrium and right ventricle (RV) dilatation and hypokinesis. (B) Severe tricuspid regurgitation into a markedly dilated right atrium is shown by color Doppler. The jet is relatively low velocity but very broad, due to a wide-open orifice and diminished RV contractile function.

products to reach the right side of the heart evading inactivation by first-pass metabolism in the liver. Otherwise, vasoactive substances can also bypass hepatic inactivation via gonadal venous drainage from carcinoid tumor in the gonads and lymphatic drainage from retroperitoneal lymph node metastases via the thoracic duct. Left-sided valves are involved in carcinoid heart disease in less than 10% due to inactivation of humoral substances within the pulmonary circulation.[23] Carcinoid involvement of left-sided valves should prompt evaluation for a right-to-left shunt but can also occur in the setting of a primary bronchial carcinoid or very poorly controlled carcinoid disease.

Pericardial Disease

Pericardial disease is common in cancer patients and can occur as a consequence of metastatic disease or as a complication of cancer therapies including radiation therapy (RT). Cancer drugs that are associated

with pericarditis and/or pericardial effusions are outlined in Box 42.4. Whereas acute pericarditis that complicated chest radiation prior to the 1970s rarely occurs today due to lower radiation doses and modern techniques, 7%–20% of patients will develop constrictive pericarditis ≥10 years after thoracic radiation.[24] Survivors of Hodgkin lymphoma treated with mantle radiation are at particularly high risk of late pericardial complications. Transthoracic echocardiography (TTE) is the method of choice for assessment of suspected pericardial disease in cancer patients, and should follow standard practice outlined in Chapter 33.

Pulmonary Arterial Hypertension

Pulmonary arterial hypertension (PAH) is a rare but serious complication of certain cancer therapies. For example, reversible PAH is a recognized complication of dasatinib, a BCR-ABL tyrosine kinase inhibitor used in

---

BOX 42.4 Cancer Drugs Associated with Pericarditis and/or Pericardial Effusions

- Anthracyclines
- Cyclophosphamide
- Cytarabine
- Imatinib and dasatinib (pericardial and pleural effusions)
- Interferon-alpha
- Busulfan
- Methotrexate
- 5-fluorouracil
- Docetaxel

Data from Plana JC, Galderisi M, Barac A, et al. Expert consensus for multimodality imaging evaluation of adult patients during and after cancer therapy: a report from the American Society of Echocardiography and the European Association of Cardiovascular Imaging. *J Am Soc Echocardiogr.* 2014;27(9):911-939.

---

the treatment of chronic myelogenous leukemia. In addition, alkylating agents including cyclophosphamide have been linked to development of pulmonary veno-occlusive disease.[25] Echocardiographic assessment of pulmonary artery systolic pressure should be considered in all patients during treatment with cancer agents known to cause PAH if symptoms of dyspnea, fatigue, or angina develop, or every 3–6 months in asymptomatic patients.[3]

Cardiac Masses

Echocardiographic assessment of primary and secondary cardiac masses in oncology patients is discussed in Chapter 37.

Stress Echocardiography

In addition to the standard indications outlined in Chapter 27, stress echocardiography may be helpful in patients with intermediate or high probability for coronary artery disease who will receive cancer treatment regimens that may provoke ischemia (e.g., fluoropyrimidines). In addition, stress-induced reductions in contractile reserve as a marker of subclinical LV dysfunction and as a predictor of subsequent overt reductions in LVEF in patients exposed to cancer treatments with cardiotoxic potential is a focus of clinical research.[26,27]

Chest radiation is known to cause vascular injury and accelerate arteriosclerosis.[28,29] Hence, tests for inducible ischemia such as stress echocardiography should be considered for patients with prior thoracic irradiation who develop anginal symptoms or who manifest new regional wall motion abnormalities on resting TTE or new ECG abnormalities. Furthermore, it is reasonable to consider noninvasive stress imaging to screen for obstructive coronary artery disease in *asymptomatic* patients following anterior or left chest irradiation with high-risk criteria (e.g., high cumulative radiation dose [>30 Gray], and age <50 years at time of RT), with repeated stress testing every 5 years thereafter if first exam is unremarkable.[27]

AFTER TREATMENT: SURVIVORSHIP

Survivors of Thoracic Radiation Therapy

RT is used as adjuvant therapy in the management of many malignancies. Radiation-induced heart disease (RIHD) can manifest as pericardial disease, cardiomyopathy, coronary artery disease, conduction system disease, or valvular heart disease. Thoracic RT can also result in medium and large vessel vasculopathy, for example, porcelain aorta. Presentation can be delayed, with an estimated aggregate incidence of RIHD of 10%–30% by 5–10 years after thoracic irradiation.[30] Risk factors for RIHD include higher radiation dose, minimal or no cardiac shielding at time of RT, younger age at irradiation, increasing interval from time of RT, preexisting CV risk factors, and concomitant chemotherapy.[24] New cardiopulmonary symptoms or clinical signs should prompt TTE to evaluate for RIHD. Furthermore, asymptomatic patients should undergo screening echocardiography 10 years after thoracic irradiation and every 5 years thereafter; patients with a history of anterior or left-sided irradiation and ≥1 risk factor for RIHD may warrant earlier initiation of screening at 5 years following exposure.[24,27]

Thoracic irradiation can cause constrictive pericarditis and/or restrictive cardiomyopathy; echocardiography assessment of these disease processes is discussed in Chapters 24 and 33.

Survivors of Childhood Malignancies

Advances in cancer care have significantly improved survival in childhood cancers. CV complications are recognized as a leading cause of morbidity and mortality in long-term survivors of childhood cancers. Survivors with a history of exposure to anthracyclines or chest radiation are at risk of developing congestive heart failure and often transition through asymptomatic cardiomyopathy before signs and symptoms of HF manifest. Screening of asymptomatic survivors of childhood cancers to detect "silent" cardiomyopathy is recommended in certain scenarios in the hope that early intervention prevents/delays progression. The International Late Effects of Childhood Cancer Guideline Harmonization Group recommends echocardiography as the primary cardiomyopathy surveillance modality for assessment of LV systolic function.[12] This Group risk stratifies survivors into three groups based on radiation and anthracycline exposure and provides risk-specific guidance on cardiomyopathy surveillance as follows:

1. High-risk group: Patients are considered high risk for cardiomyopathy if exposure history includes high-dose (≥250 mg/m²) anthracycline, high-dose (≥35 Gy) chest radiation, or moderate-high dose (≥100 mg/m²) anthracycline in addition to moderate-high dose (≥15 Gy) chest radiation. Cardiomyopathy surveillance *is recommended* for this group to begin no later than 2 years after completion of cancer treatments, repeated at 5 years after diagnosis, and every 5 years thereafter.
2. Moderate-risk group: This group includes patients exposed to more than 100 and less than 250 mg/m² anthracycline in whom cardiomyopathy surveillance *is reasonable*, and patients treated with ≥15 and less than 35 Gy chest radiation in whom surveillance *may be reasonable.* The suggested frequency of surveillance is similar to the schedule described above for the high-risk group.
3. Low-risk group: Patients treated with low dose (<100 mg/m²) anthracycline are considered low risk, and cardiomyopathy surveillance *may be reasonable.* The Group provides no recommendation for surveillance in survivors treated with low-dose (<15 Gy) chest radiation.

Cardiomyopathy surveillance *is reasonable* prior to pregnancy or in the first trimester for all female survivors with a history of anthracycline or chest radiation exposure. In addition to heart failure, survivors of childhood cancer demonstrate a greater than fourfold relative risk of valvular dysfunction;[31] radiation-induced valvular disease is discussed earlier.

FUTURE DIRECTIONS

The ability of echocardiographic markers of subclinical LV dysfunction to predict subsequent overt and prognistically significant cardiotoxicity in oncology patients needs to be examined in large multicenter studies. Similarly, the utility of these sensitive echocardiographic measures in directing decisions on cardioprotective treatments and modifications in oncology treatment regimens requires study. The role of cardiac biomarkers in detection and prediction of cardiotoxicity in patients exposed to cancer treatments is an area of much interest. Elevated troponins in patients receiving cancer therapies with cardiotoxic potential may be a sensitive and early marker of cardiotoxicity. The challenge is to distinguish clinically insignificant and transient subclinical cardiotoxicity that may manifest during cancer treatment from functionally and prognostically relevant cardiotoxicity that warrants intervention. There is a need to establish how best to integrate echocardiographic and biomarker data to predict subsequent CTRCD, and treatment algorithms to direct therapeutic decisions based on these data need to be developed. These surveillance strategies and associated treatment algorithms will need to be treatment specific to reflect differing cardiotoxic potentials of anticancer drugs. Moreover, surveillance strategies for established and emerging cardiotoxic cancer treatments need to consider cost efficiency and pretest probability of cardiotoxicity based on individual risk assessment. Such future directions should aim to achieve maximal oncologic benefit of cancer treatments with minimal cardiotoxicity.

CONCLUSION

Standard and advanced echocardiographic techniques are central to assessment of and surveillance for cardiotoxicity in oncology patients. Echocardiographers will increasingly encounter patients referred for cardio-oncological indications given the rising prevalence of cardiotoxicity among a growing population of patients with cancer undergoing active treatment and cancer survivors. There is a need for clinical research to guide refinement and expansion of consensus guidelines for more optimal application of echocardiography in the oncology population.

Suggested Reading

Curigliano, G., Cardinale, D., Suter, T., et al. (2012). Cardiovascular toxicity induced by chemotherapy, targeted agents and radiotherapy: ESMO Clinical Practice Guidelines. *Annals of Oncology, 23*(Suppl. 7), vii155–166.

Groarke, J. D., Nguyen, P. L., Nohria, A., Ferrari, R., Cheng, S., & Moslehi, J. (2014). Cardiovascular complications of radiation therapy for thoracic malignancies: the role for non-invasive imaging for detection of cardiovascular disease. *European Heart Journal, 35*(10), 612–623.

Lancellotti, P., Nkomo, V. T., Badano, L. P., et al. (2013). Expert consensus for multi-modality imaging evaluation of cardiovascular complications of radiotherapy in adults: a report from the European Association of Cardiovascular Imaging and the American Society of Echocardiography. *European Heart Journal - Cardiovascular Imaging, 14*(8), 721–740.

Plana, J. C., Galderisi, M., Barac, A., et al. (2014). Expert consensus for multimodality imaging evaluation of adult patients during and after cancer therapy: a report from the American Society of Echocardiography and the European Association of Cardiovascular Imaging. *Journal of the American Society of Echocardiography, 27*(9), 911–939.

Zamorano, J. L., Lancellotti, P., Rodriguez Muñoz, D., et al. (2016). 2016 ESC Position Paper on cancer treatments and cardiovascular toxicity developed under the auspices of the ESC Committee for Practice Guidelines: The Task Force for cancer treatments and cardiovascular toxicity of the European Society of Cardiology (ESC). *European Heart Journal, 37*(36), 2768–2801.

A complete reference list can be found online at ExpertConsult.com.

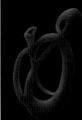
43 Atrial Septal Defect

Keri Shafer, M. Elizabeth Brickner

INTRODUCTION

Atrial septal defects (ASDs) occur in 0.1% of the population and represent the largest group of congenital defects in the adult population. Echocardiographic evaluation of ASDs should include characterization of the defect, evaluation for additional associated lesions, and description of the physiologic effect of the ASD. Here we characterize a standardized approach as well as highlight some common pitfalls.

ANATOMY/EMBRYOLOGY

Atrial septation occurs early in embryologic formation and is nearly complete by 2 months' gestation. Embryologic formation of the atrial septum is a complex series of changes but is simplified here. Septation occurs with the formation of two membranes. The first membrane that occurs on the left atrium (LA) side is called the septum primum, and the second membrane is the septum secundum. Initially, these membranes function to allow for continuous inferior vena cava (IVC)-LA flow in utero (via the foramen ovale).[1,2] After birth, the membranes fuse (in the majority of patients) to form the fossa ovalis.

PATENT FORAMEN OVALE

In most patients, the foramen ovale closes by the second month of life. In adulthood, persistence of a patent foramen ovale (PFO) is a variant existing in 20%–25% of the general population.[3] Although the clinical importance of PFO is unclear, there are some specific circumstances when diagnosis is important. Examples include patients with right atrial hypertension (e.g., pulmonary hypertension), pre-cardiopulmonary bypass, in anticipation of procedures that require interatrial access (such as left atrial ablation), and in patients with recurrent embolic events. On transthoracic echocardiogram (TTE), diagnosis can be made with either color Doppler or agitated saline contrast.
1. Color Doppler: On TTE, the interatrial septum is best imaged in the apical four-chamber view, subcostal four-chamber, and the parasternal short-axis view at the aortic valve level. However, because of the frequently poor color Doppler signal in the subcostal four-chamber position in adults, this image can have low sensitivity, particularly in the setting of abdominal obesity. Color flow typically has a tunnel-like appearance. On transesophageal imaging, the atrial septum is best imaged in the bicaval view. Typically, a clockwise rotation of the probe, which scans the septum and fossa ovalis from left to right, is needed to detect and identify the exact location of the PFO. In both TTE and transesophageal echocardiography (TEE), a low Nyquist limit with a high frame rate is required to detect the low velocity, intermittent flow of a PFO. Video 43.1 shows an example on TTE. (A TEE example is shown in Chapter 17, Fig. 17.8, and Video 17.2.)
2. Agitated saline contrast: using the same views for color Doppler, saline contrast can be used to determine the presence of an interatrial connections. Imaging should begin prior to the opacification of the right

atrium (RA). PFO flow typically occurs 3–5 beats after right ventricle (RV) opacification. In contrast, ASD flow is even faster, almost instantaneous (Video 43.2). In contrast, extracardiac shunting occurs after five beats. In patients with very low right atrial pressure, additional maneuvers such as Valsalva are requisite to increase the RA pressure enough to force right to left flow of the saline contrast across the septum.

CLINICAL PRESENTATION OF ATRIAL LEVEL DEFECTS

Unrepaired atrial level defects presenting in adulthood can be found incidentally, as many patients are asymptomatic. If symptomatic, the most common complaints include dyspnea, fatigue, palpitations, and chest pain.[4] Clinical findings suggestive of an unrepaired atrial level defect include a pulmonary flow murmur and fixed split S2. On electrocardiogram (ECG) patients often have right bundle branch block.

ATRIAL SEPTAL DEFECTS

Defects in the atrial septum are the most common type of adult congenital heart disease, but there are actually only two types of defects of the true atrial septum: secundum and primum (Fig. 43.1). Secundum ASDs occur as a result of a deficiency in septum primum and occur near the center of the atrial septum. In contrast, primum ASDs result from incomplete endocardial cushion formation. For this reason, primum ASDs are often associated with other lesions that result from incomplete endocardial cushion formation such as inlet ventricular septal defects and cleft atrioventricular (AV) valves.

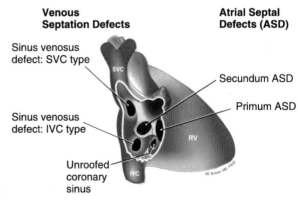

FIG. 43.1 Atrial level defects fall into two categories: atrial septal defects and venous septation defects. *IVC*, Inferior vena cava; *RV*, right ventricle; *SVC*, superior vena cava. *(Courtesy of Bernard E. Bulwer, MD, FASE; Adapted from Solomon D, Wu J, Gillam L. Echocardiography. In: Mann DL, Zipes DP, Libby P, et al., eds. Braunwald's Heart Disease: A Textbook of Cardiovascular Medicine. 10th ed. Philadelphia: Elsevier; 2015:179–260.)*

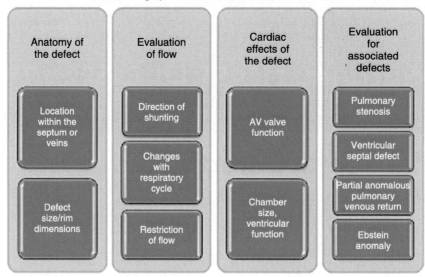

Echocardiographic assessment of atrial level defects

FIG. 43.2 Standardized approach to echo evaluation.

VENOUS SEPTATION DEFECTS

While venous septation defects are physiologically similar to ASDs, they are anatomically distinct. Understanding of this anatomic distinction is critical to appropriate image acquisition and interpretation. Defects can occur at the insertion of the superior vena cava (SVC) or the IVC and the edge of the atrial septum. Typically, there is also incomplete septation of the associated right pulmonary vein. Coronary sinus defects occur as the coronary sinus passes behind the LA a defect ("unroofing") in this wall can occur, causing a communication between the LA and coronary sinus and flow from right to left at the atrial level.

IMAGING APPROACH

The approach to imaging of atrial level shunting focuses on anatomic characterization and evaluation of physiologic effects (Fig. 43.2). Additionally, complete imaging of the rims of the secundum ASD is particularly important, as it is currently the only type of ASD that is a candidate for percutaneous closure.

1. Anatomy of the defect: The initial approach is to describe the location and dimensions of the defect. Detailed description of secundum defects are particularly important due to the potential for percutaneous closure. TEE is needed for complete evaluation of the secundum ASD rims, and three-dimensional (3D) imaging can be very useful to reconstruct the entire defect.
   a. Secundum: Visualization of each "rim" of tissue in reference to its associated structure. Typically, the rims are identified as the aortic, tricuspid, superior, posterior, and inferior (Fig. 43.3). For adequate device position, each rim should measure at least 0.5 cm. Often the anterior, or retro-aortic rim, is the smallest as shown in Fig. 43.4.
2. Evaluation of flow: Similar to PFOs, ASDs and venous defects are typically first diagnosed with color Doppler. Flow is best visualized with low Nyquist and high frame rates. Additionally, the direction of flow should be evaluated typically with color flow Doppler, but pulsed wave Doppler is also used. Direction of flow can change typically due to either:
   a. Change in ventricular compliance: In most cases, flow is typically left to right owing to the very compliant nature of the RA and RV. Compliance can change due to ventricular scar formation (e.g., due to volume loading), and shunt direction can change.
   b. Change in pulmonary vascular resistance (pulmonary hypertension): if the patient develops pulmonary hypertension due to increasing pulmonary vascular resistance, atrial level shunting can shift from right to left (Eisenmenger syndrome).

c. In rare situations, right-to-left shunting can occur due to anatomic factors (e.g., a prominent eustachian valve can direct IVC flow preferentially across the ASD) or mechanical distortion of the atrial septum (e.g., after pneumonectomy, ascending aortic aneurysm) or in the setting of pericardial effusion or constriction. In these settings, pulmonary pressures are not necessarily elevated. Changes can even occur transiently with body position, causing a "platypnea-orthodeoxia" syndrome in which a patient desaturates when going from recumbent to upright position.

3. Cardiac effects of the defect: As shunts are typically left to right, the RA and RV typically dilate. Characterization of right atrial dilation as well as right ventricular dilation and function are useful in determination of the physiologic effects of the defect. When there is persistent flow and development of pulmonary hypertension or right sided chamber dilation, tricuspid regurgitation can develop.

4. Evaluation for associated defects: Most commonly, secundum ASDs are associated with pulmonary stenosis, ventricular septal defects, partial anomalous pulmonary veins, and Ebstein anomaly. Primum ASDs are often seen together with other endocardial cushion defects such as inlet ventricular septal defect, cleft mitral valve, and cleft tricuspid valve. In addition, evaluation for additional ASDs is done by interrogating the entire septum. Other septation defects can be present, including venous septation defects (Table 43.1).

ATRIAL LEVEL SHUNTING CLOSURE

The ACC/AHA guidelines recommend that closure should be considered in patients with the following[5]:
- Right atrial and right ventricular enlargement regardless of symptoms (Class I, LOE B)
- Paradoxical embolism (Class IIa, LOE C)
- Documented platypnea-orthodeoxia (Class IIa, LOE B)

Closure is not recommended in patients who have severe, irreversible pulmonary hypertension. Some devices require that the defect has greater than 0.5 cm rims (recommendations regarding the required retroaortic rim dimension is variable).

IMAGING DURING PERCUTANEOUS CLOSURE

Periprocedural TEE is often used during the device closure for secundum ASDs. This TEE should evaluate for the following:
1. Sufficient rims to seat the device (discussed above).
2. Evaluation of size and number of secundum defect(s): Patients may have multiple defects or a fenestrated atrial septum, which will affect the decision regarding size of device as well as appropriateness of percutaneous closure. Video 43.3 shows an example of multiple defects.

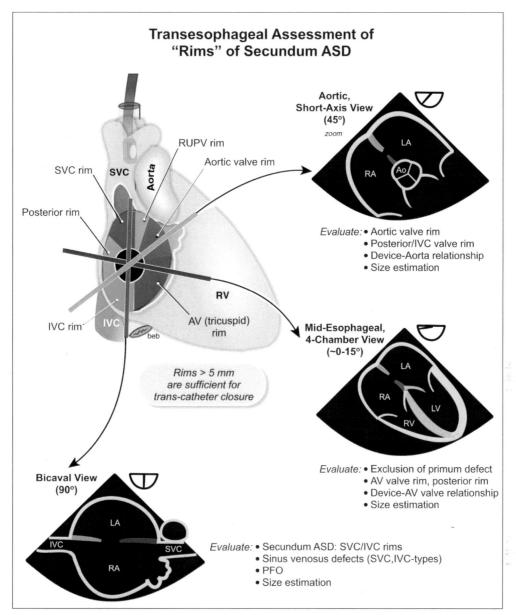

FIG. 43.3 Transesophageal approach to the evaluation of secundum atrial septal defects. *ASD,* Atrial septal defect; *IVC,* inferior vena cava; *LA,* left atrium; *LV,* left ventricle; *PFO,* patent foramen ovale; *RA,* right atrium; *RUPV,* right upper pulmonary vein; *RV,* right ventricle; *SVC,* superior vena cava. (*Courtesy of Bernard E. Bulwer, MD, FASE; Data from Silvestry FE, Cohen MS, Armsby LB, et al. Guidelines for the echocardiographic assessment of atrial septal defect and patent foramen ovale: from the American Society of Echocardiography and Society for Cardiac Angiography and Interventions.J Am Soc Echocardiogr. 2015,28[8].910–958.*)

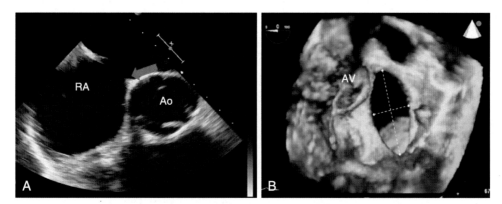

FIG. 43.4 Transesophageal imaging of a secundum atrial septal defect (ASD). (A) Midesophageal transesophageal echocardiography (TEE) image at ~45 degrees demonstrates a deficient retroaortic rim *(red arrow).* (B) 3D TEE view demonstrating all rims as viewed from the left atrial aspect. Note that use of 3D TEE can avoid underestimation of ASD diameters due to 2D imaging alone, although balloon-sizing is also used to measure the size of the balloon-stretched defect. *Ao,* Aortic valve; *AV,* aortic valve; *RA,* right atrium. (*B, Modified from Solomon D, Wu J, Gillam L. Echocardiography. In: Mann DL, Zipes DP, Libby P, et al., eds. Braunwald's Heart Disease: A Textbook of Cardiovascular Medicine. 10th ed. Philadelphia: Elsevier, 2015:179–260.*)

TABLE 43.1 Transthoracic Imaging Approach to Atrial Level Defects

TYPE OF DEFECT	DESCRIPTION	TYPICAL TTE IMAGING VIEW	ADDITIONAL VIEWS	ASSOCIATED DEFECTS
Secundum ASD	Defect of ostium primum, near central portion of septum secundum, potentially closed percutaneously	• Apical 4-chamber • Subcostal 4-chamber[a]	• Parasternal short axis at aortic valve level (useful for visualizing aortic rims) • Subcostal long axis (similar to bicaval view)	• Ventricular septal defect • Pulmonary stenosis • Ebstein anomaly • Partial anomalous pulmonary vein return/connection
Primum ASD	Defect of the superior portion of the endocardial cushion	• Apical 4-chamber • Subcostal 4-chamber[a]	• Parasternal long axis, sweep	• Inlet VSD • Cleft mitral valve • Cleft tricuspid valve • LV outflow tract obstruction ("gooseneck deformity")
Sinus venosus defect (superior)	Absence of the SVC septation	Limited	• Apical 4-chamber superiorly angled • Right parasternal long axis	• Partial anomalous venous return
Sinus venosus defect (inferior)	Absence of the IVC septation	Limited	• Apical 4-chamber inferiorly angled • Right parasternal long axis, inferior	Partial anomalous venous return
Coronary sinus defect	Absence of coronary sinus–left atrium septation	Limited	• Apical 4-chamber inferiorly angled • Parasternal short axis at the level of the mitral valve, posteriorly angled	

[a]Subcostal imaging views may be inadequate if abdominal obesity is present.
ASD, Atrial septal defect; *IVC,* inferior vena cava; *LV,* left ventricle; *SVC,* superior vena cava; *TTE,* transthoracic echocardiography; *VSD,* ventricular septal defect.

3. Evaluation for associated defects: secundum ASDs can be associated with anomalous pulmonary veins, ventricular septal defects, and pulmonary stenosis (as well as other defects if not done on preprocedure imaging). These should be identified before closure is undertaken.

4. During closure:
   a. A guidewire is passed across the defect and usually "parked" in a left pulmonary vein for use as a rail. Care should be taken to make sure it does not enter the left atrial appendage, which is very thin-walled.
   b. Sizing balloon: A sizing balloon filled with contrast medium is used to cross and measure the balloon-stretched diameter of the defect. This confirms that the patient will tolerate closure but also that an appropriate-sized device is selected. This is achieved by measuring the waist of the balloon on both echocardiography and fluoroscopy. Evaluation for color flow around the balloon can be performed to confirm that the defect is completely occluded by the balloon.
   c. Seating of the device: After the device is placed and before release from the delivery catheter, imaging should confirm that the device is appropriately seated with occluders on either side of the interatrial septum. It should not impinge on surrounding structures (i.e., obstruct caval inflow or indenting the aortic root). After complete release of the device, color Doppler and agitated saline contrast can be utilized to assess for significant residual interatrial shunting.

5. Two different devices used for percutaneous secundum ASD closure are seen in Fig. 43.5, with slightly different double-disc designs. An ASD is shown in Video 43.4 (preclosure) and postclosure (Video 43.5) with an Amplatzer device. An implanted Helex device is shown in Video 43.6.

Imaging post percutaneous device closure should be performed to evaluate for device erosion or embolization. Device erosion is rare (~0.2%) but has been reported both into the walls of the atria causing hemopericardium as well as into the aorta, both being life threatening events.

ADDITIONAL TECHNIQUES AND PITFALLS

Clues To Undiagnosed Atrial Level Shunting

1. High pulmonary artery flow (all atrial level defects) (Fig. 43.6 and Video 43.7)
2. Isolated RV/RA dilation (all atrial level defects)

3. Mitral and tricuspid valves are not offset (primum ASD) (Fig. 43.7)

These should prompt the use of IV saline contrast to rule out ASD. If the #1 and/or #2 are found but there is no evidence of a primum or secundum ASD, the patient may have a sinus venosus or coronary sinus defect. While these defects are usually easier to see by transesophageal echo (Fig. 43.8 and Video 43.8) or cross-sectional imaging, attempts can be made on transthoracic imaging.

Evaluation for sinus venosus defect: This defect can be superior or inferior in origin and occurs because of unroofing of the pulmonary vein as it goes behind the vena cava. Superior sinus venosus defects can be evaluated by a right parasternal plane placing color Doppler near the insertion of the SVC (Fig. 43.9). If anteriorly directed flow is seen, this suggests a sinus venosus defect. Both superior and inferior sinus venosus defects can be evaluated in the subcostal view at the insertion of the vena cavae (Fig. 43.10).

Common Mistakes in Diagnosis

1. IVC flow: many physiologic states are associated with prominent IVC flow. However, this is sometimes mistaken for ASD flow. Typically, the correct diagnosis can be made with additional imaging views, absence of RA and RV dilation, and agitated saline contrast

2. Missing atypical defects: sinus venosus and coronary sinus defects in particular are commonly missed, as they are not typically seen on standard imaging. In the presence of the clues mentioned, additional TTE views (see Table 43.1) can be obtained to further investigate. However, additional imaging (TEE or cardiac magnetic resonance imaging [MRI]) are often required to confirm the diagnosis.

3. Miscalculation of Qp:Qs: Due to the difficulty in estimating pulmonary outflow Doppler and right ventricular outflow tract diameter, estimations of shunt ratios are typically inaccurate in atrial level defects. Often, cardiac catheterization or cardiac MRI is required to adequately assess shunting.

4. Low frame rate and high Nyquist limits: Atrial level flow typically has a low velocity and may not occur throughout the cardiac cycle. Particularly in those with limited acoustic windows, atrial level shunting requires careful and dedicated imaging.

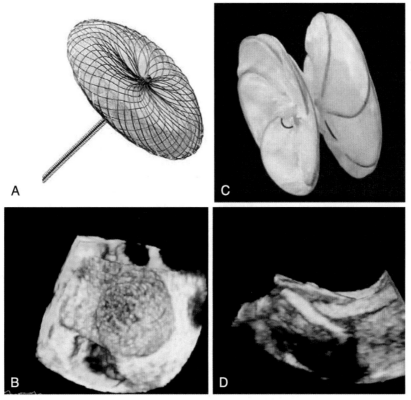

FIG. 43.5 Atrial septal defect closure devices. (A) Amplatzer septal occluder, which is a double umbrella–type device. (B) 3D transesophageal echocardiography (TEE) view of the Amplatzer device seated across the interatrial septum. (C) Gore-Helex occluder device. (D) 3D-TEE view of the Helex device with the interatrial septum sandwiched within. (*A, AMPLATZER and St. Jude Medical are trademarks of St. Jude Medical, LLC or its related companies. Reproduced with permission of St. Jude Medical, ©2017. All rights reserved; C, Courtesy of Gore Medical, Flagstaff, AZ.*)

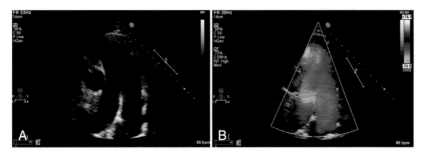

FIG. 43.6 Parasternal short-axis view, dilated pulmonary arteries due to high-flow atrial shunt. (A) 2D image, and (B) with color Doppler.

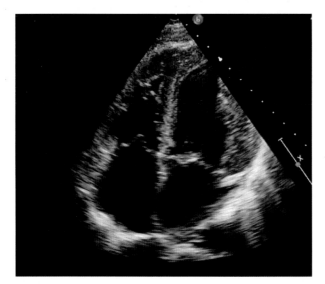

FIG. 43.7 Repaired primum atrial septal defect. Note that the mitral and tricuspid valves are at the same level, that is, not offset with the tricuspid valve closer to the apex as normal, in this apical four-chamber view.

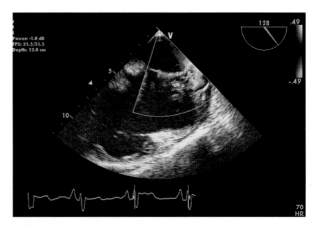

FIG. 43.8 Transesophageal image at ~120 degrees showing flow through a superior sinus venosus defect.

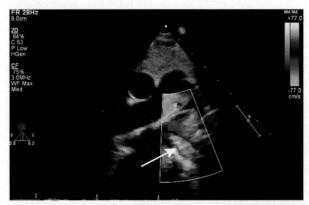

FIG. 43.9 Right parasternal long-axis image of sinus venosus defect. Note the superiorly directed *(red)* flow of the right upper pulmonary vein into the superior vena cava through the sinus venosus defect *(arrow)*.

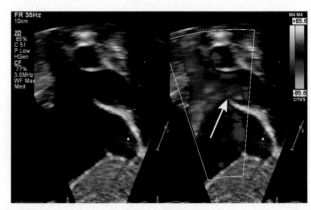

FIG. 43.10 Subcostal image (pediatric convention) of sinus venosus defect. Note the superior vena cava flow *(red)* into both the left and right atria through the defect *(arrow)*.

Suggested Reading

Geva, T., Martins, J. D., & Wald, R. M. (2014). Atrial septal defects. *Lancet, 383,* 1921–1932.

Lai, W. W., Mertens, L. L., Cohen, M. S., & Geva, T. (Eds.). (2016). *Echocardiography in Pediatric and Congenital Heart Disease: From Fetus to Adult* (2nd ed.). Hoboken, NJ: Wiley-Blackwell.

Roberson, D. A., & Cui, V. W. (2014). Three-dimensional transesophageal echocardiography of atrial septal defect device closure. *Current Cardiology Reports, 16,* 453.

Silvestry, F. E., Cohen, M. S., Armsby, L. B., et al. (2015). Guidelines for the echocardiographic assessment of atrial septal defect and patent foramen ovale: from the American Society of Echocardiography and Society for Cardiac Angiography and Interventions. *Journal of the American Society of Echocardiography, 28,* 910–958.

A complete reference list can be found online at ExpertConsult.com.

44 Ventricular Septal Defect

Keri Shafer, M. Elizabeth Brickner

INTRODUCTION

Ventricular septal defects (VSDs) represent the most common type of congenital heart disease in childhood (~40%). As a significant proportion of VSDs spontaneously close in childhood (predominantly muscular defects), the prevalence in adulthood decreases and is closer to 25%.[1,2]

ADULT PRESENTATION

Most commonly, VSDs are diagnosed in childhood. Often, large VSDs are diagnosed due to recurrent infections or evidence of over-circulation, while small VSDs often present with loud murmurs. If small VSDs are diagnosed in adulthood, they can present with a murmur, the development of endocarditis, or valve damage related to the flow through the VSD. Large unrepaired VSDs can present in adulthood with evidence of pulmonary hypertension and reversal of the shunt (Eisenmenger syndrome). Additionally, increases in left ventricle (LV) systolic and diastolic pressures with aging can increase the degree of left-to-right (L–R) shunting. Common associated findings at the time of presentation include double-chambered right ventricle, subaortic stenosis, aortic prolapse, and arrhythmias. Additionally, adults can develop VSDs as a result of large myocardial infarctions (see Chapter 19). When evaluating VSDs by echocardiography, evaluation of ventricular size and function, valve function, estimate of pulmonary pressures, and exclusion of associated defects must be performed.

TYPES/LOCATIONS OF VENTRICULAR SEPTAL DEFECTS

Based on the embryologic origins of the ventricular septum, VSDs can be categorized based on their location and structure, as shown in Fig. 44.1.

Perimembranous Ventricular Septal Defects

Defects of the membranous septum are the second most common type of defect in childhood but represent a larger portion of defects in adulthood as they are much less likely to spontaneously close.[3] Membranous VSDs often occur in the setting of other types of congenital heart disease. They are often detectable in the parasternal long axis but may require slightly off-axis imaging to visualize the entire jet (Fig. 44.2 and Video 44.1). Based on their size and extension (VSDs may extend into the inlet, trabecular, or outlet septum), they can be associated with either aortic or tricuspid valve dysfunction, which is typically related to leaflet prolapse and regurgitation (Video 44.2). If the defect is more significantly associated with the right ventricular outflow tract with anterior malalignment of the infundibular septum, it is called a conoventricular defect and is seen in tetralogy of Fallot. Thus, careful evaluation of valve function should be included in the echocardiographic exam of a VSD. Other imaging views to evaluate membranous VSDs include the parasternal short axis at the aortic valve level and the apical five-chamber view.

Muscular/Trabecular Ventricular Septal Defects

VSDs occurring solely in the muscular/trabecular septum constitute up to 20% of all VSDs. These can spontaneously close in infancy/childhood, but if persistently patent they can be closed percutaneously. Evaluation should include further characterization of location within the muscular septum (anterior, mid, apical, or posterior) as well as a

meticulous search for multiple defects. At times, small jets of flow within the trabecula will occur that are not complete defects (i.e., no true shunt). Demonstration of flow through the septum is imperative and may require off-axis imaging or sweeping loop (Fig. 44.3 and Video 44.3). When imaging these defects, it is important to inspect each portion of the ventricular septum with a narrow color Doppler box to prevent missing small defects with bidirectional shunting. Screening for muscular VSDs can be done in the apical four-chamber view as well as the short-axis view at each level (vs. sweeping loops through the septum at each view).

Outlet Ventricular Septal Defects

The pulmonary artery connects to the heart via a ring of muscle (conus) that partially forms the outlet portion of the ventricular septum, which extends to the membranous septum. Due to the location, several different names for these defects have been given, including subpulmonic, doubly committed subarterial, conal, and supracristal. Slight changes in the location of the VSD in relationship to the great arteries can change the physiology of the defect. For example, if the defect is predominantly associated with the aorta, prolapse of the aortic valve can occur resulting in regurgitation and progressive valvular damage. Aortic valve damage can occur with both outlet and membranous defects.[4] Outlet VSDs can be seen on the parasternal long axis when angled towards the outflow tracts, and in the short-axis view with the color Doppler sector focused on the conal septum (Fig. 44.4).

Inlet Ventricular Septal Defects

Inlet defects occur as a result of deficiency in the ventricular septum between the inlet/atrioventricular valves (mitral and tricuspid), also called atrioventricular canal VSD. These defects can be diagnosed on transthoracic imaging at the level of the inlet valves, typically in the apical four-chamber view. Inlet VSDs constitute approximately 5% of all VSDs.[5] The majority of the time they are associated with other defects with similar embryologic origin (endocardial cushion), such as cleft mitral valve, cleft tricuspid valve, and primum atrial septal defect (ASD). Collectively, this pattern is called an atrioventricular septal defect (AVSD) or endocardial cushion defect (shown in Fig. 44.5).

Diagnostic Clues to Inlet Ventricular Septal Defect or Atrioventricular Septal Defect

- The atrioventricular (AV) valves lie at the same level (rather than slight apical displacement of the tricuspid valve), when viewed in apical windows.
- Associated syndromes: A number of genetic defects have been associated with inlet VSDs, most notably trisomy 21 (Down syndrome), in which it is the most common congenital heart abnormality. Other associated syndromes include CHARGE, VATER, Noonan, and Holt-Oram.[5,6]
- Unusual left ventricular outflow tract (LVOT) shape: Because of the shorter inlet septum in AVSD patients, an elongated and narrowed left ventricular outflow tract can occur (gooseneck deformity) occasionally with LVOT obstruction.
- Postsurgical repair: Echogenic material will be seen in both the inlet septum and the medial portions of the mitral or tricuspid valve at the site of VSD and cleft valve repair.
- Best imaged in the apical four-chamber view, but can be visualized in the subcostal long-axis view.

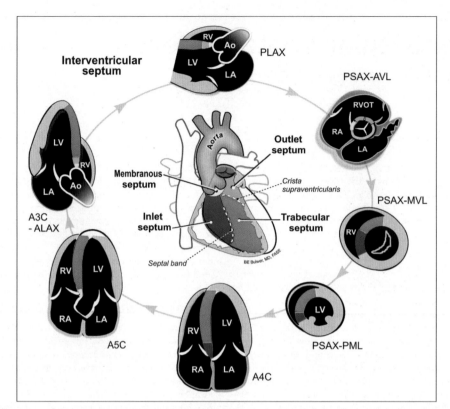

FIG. 44.1 The ventricular septum can be separated into four sections primarily based on embryologic origins. The portions of the septum imaged with each echocardiographic plane are shown. *ALAX*, Apical long-axis; *Ao*, aorta; *LA*, left atrium; *AVL*, aortic valve level; *LV*, left ventricle; *MVL*, mitral valve level; *PLAX*, parasternal long-axis; *PSAX*, parasternal short-axis; *PVL*, papillary muscle level; *RA*, right atrium; *RV*, right ventricle. (*Modified from Bulwer BE, Rivero JM, eds.* Echocardiography Pocket Guide: The Transthoracic Examination. *Burlington, MA: Jones & Bartlett Learning, 2011;2013:142.*)

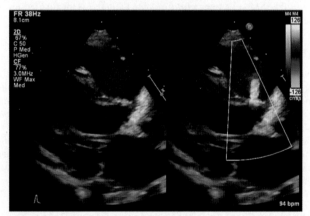

FIG. 44.2 Small perimembranous ventricular septal defect with left-to-right flow on parasternal long-axis window.

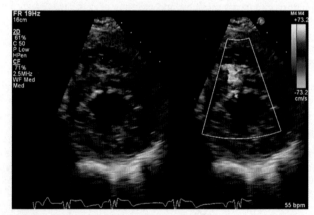

FIG. 44.3 A restrictive, serpiginous ventricular septal defect is shown in the parasternal short axis at the mid-ventricular level with turbulent left-to-right flow.

Transthoracic imaging   Transesophageal imaging

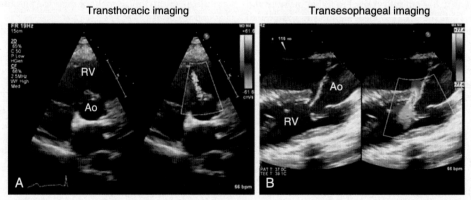

FIG. 44.4 A small outlet ventricular septal defect with left-to-right flow is shown in both transthoracic imaging (A) and transesophageal (B) imaging. *Ao*, Aorta; *RV*, right ventricle.

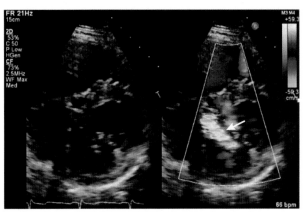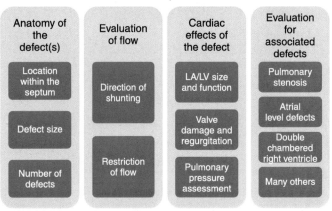

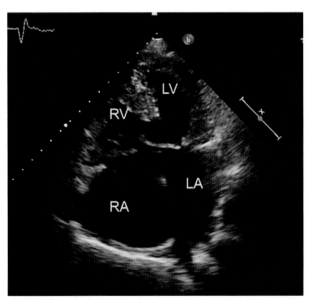

FIG. 44.5 An unrepaired atrioventricular septal defect is shown from the apical four-chamber view. Note that the patient has an inlet ventricular septal defect, primum atrial septal defect, and AV valves at the same level. *ALAX*, Apical long-axis; *AV*, atrioventricular; *AVL*, aortic valve level; *LA*, left atrium; *LV*, left ventricle; *MVL*, mitral valve level; *PLAX*, parasternal long-axis; *PSAX*, parasternal short-axis; *PVL*, papillary muscle level; *RA*, right atrium; *RV*, right ventricle. (See Fig. 43.1 and Table 43.1.)

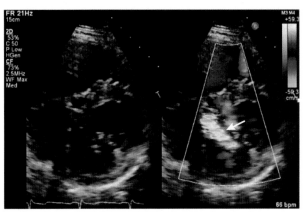

FIG. 44.6 Cleft mitral valve, parasternal short-axis image of cleft mitral valve. *Arrow* denotes flow through the anterior leaflet of the cleft mitral valve.

- The abnormal morphology of the AV valves can be visualized in the short-axis view at the level of the mitral and tricuspid valves (Fig. 44.6). Partial AV canal defects will be associated with cleft mitral valve, and in complete canal defects there is often a common AV valve.

BASIC IMAGING APPROACH TO VENTRICULAR SEPTAL DEFECTS

As with atrial septal defects, the imaging approach to VSDs should define the anatomic location and the physiologic effects of the defect. The ventricular septum is a curved structure and cannot be visualized completely in any one plane; thus, imaging must be performed in multiple planes. VSDs are sometimes easier to visualize on the LV surface of the septum (smooth septal surface), rather than the trabeculated surface of the right ventricle (RV). In addition to defining the VSD, evaluation should be made for associated defects. A systematic assessment of VSDs is as follows (Fig. 44.7):

1. Description of flow: VSDs in adults are typically first diagnosed by color Doppler given the difficulty in visualization of small VSDs with 2D imaging alone. Small VSDs typically have high velocity flow in systole, thus Nyquist limits can remain at the usual 60 cm/s. However, given that flow does not occur throughout the cardiac cycle, high frame rates (>20 Hz) are critical for diagnosis. Additionally, the direction of flow should be evaluated with both color and pulsed or

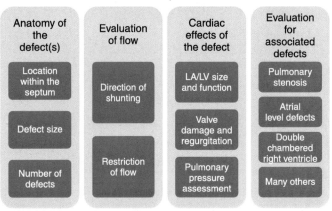

FIG. 44.7 An echocardiographic approach to assessing ventricular septal defects. *LA*, left atrium; *LV*, left ventricle.

continuous-wave Doppler. Direction of flow can change typically due to either:
   a. Change in ventricular compliance: In most cases, flow is typically L–R owing to the very compliant nature of the RV. Compliance in both ventricles may change with age.
   b. Change in vascular resistance: If the patient develops pulmonary hypertension due to increasing pulmonary vascular resistance, ventricular level shunting can decrease and may eventually reverse (R–L).
2. Size/restriction:
   a. Size can be categorized in relation to the aortic diameter: small (<25% aortic diameter), moderate (25%–75%), or large (>75%).[7]
   b. Restriction: Restrictive defects have a pressure gradient between the ventricles where LV pressure is higher than RV pressure. Small defects are typically restrictive with minimal flow volume. If there is no significant pressure difference between the ventricles (as may be seen with a large VSD), the defect is considered "nonrestrictive." Although there is no established standard for categorizing restrictive, at least 20–40 mm Hg pressure gradient would be considered restrictive.[7] Assessment of left atrium (LA) and LV size is an important indicator of the hemodynamic significance of the shunt.
3. Location and number of defects:
   a. The location nomenclature highlighted in Fig. 44.1 limits the defects to four general regions of the ventricular septum: membranous, outlet, inlet, and muscular (as discussed above). It is recommended that the laboratory adopt a standard terminology to be used across providers.
   b. VSDs can be single or multiple. Particularly in the case of trabecular/muscular defects or post-myocardial infarction (MI) VSDs, a complete interrogation of the entire ventricular septum is imperative.
4. Effects on other cardiac structures:
   a. LV/LA size: in patients with significant shunting, LA and LV dimensions can increase. Evidence of significant LV dilation is among the criteria for consideration for VSD closure.
   b. Valve regurgitation: Depending on the location of flow across the VSD as well as the potential Venturi effect, surrounding valves may be damaged as a result of high-velocity VSD flow. Careful initial and serial valve evaluation is critical in echocardiographic evaluation.
      1) Aortic cusp prolapse with resulting aortic regurgitation may occur with either perimembranous defects or conal (outlet) defects due to inadequate support of the aortic valve leaflets.
      2) Tricuspid leaflet prolapse: With perimembranous defects, the defect may be closed or decreases in size by adhesion of a portion of the tricuspid septal leaflet to the margins of the septal defect. As this septal leaflet tissue bulges out into the RV, it is often

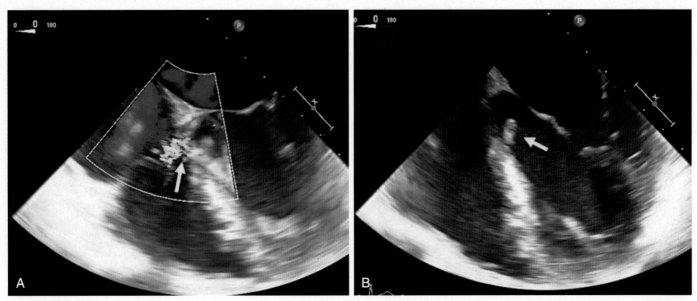

FIG. 44.8 Membranous ventricular septal defect with vegetation. Transesophageal echocardiography four-chamber view showing a membranous ventricular septal defect (VSD) with left-to-right flow (A, *arrow*), and a vegetation (B, *arrow*) discovered on the left ventricle side at the periphery. This patient also had mild aortic insufficiency that likely contributed to turbulence on the left ventricular outflow tract (LVOT) aspect of the VSD.

called a "ventricular septal aneurysm." Distortion of the septal leaflet or tissue or displacement of the anterior leaflet by the VSD jet can result in tricuspid regurgitation (see Video 44.2).

c. Development of pulmonary hypertension: Shunts with a significant increase in pulmonary blood flow may be associated with the remodeling of pulmonary vasculature, an increase in pulmonary vascular resistance, and, thus, an increase in pulmonary pressure. Evaluation for pulmonary hypertension is an important part of the evaluation of patients with a VSD. In some cases, severe pulmonary hypertension with shunt reversal (Eisenmenger syndrome) may occur. VSDs are the most common congenital heart defect associated with Eisenmenger syndrome.

5. Associated lesions:
   a. VSDs are associated with additional lesions up to 50% of the time. Most commonly associated lesions include:
      1) Atrial septal defects (~10%–15%)
      2) Pulmonary stenosis (~15%)
      3) Double-chambered right ventricle (~10%).

6. Endocarditis risk: In part due to turbulent flow and endothelial injury, there is an increased risk for endocarditis in unrepaired VSDs. Depending on the location of the VSD and the direction of the VSD jet, vegetations may occur on adjacent cardiac valve leaflets, on the ventricular endocardial surface where the jet strikes, or on a prior surgical patch. Careful evaluation of valves and any prosthetic material is compulsory for all initial VSD echoes, and in any patient with clinical concern for infection (see example in Fig. 44.8).

7. Qp:Qs: Echocardiographic evaluation of cardiac output can be difficult to do reliably. Evaluation of the LV and RV outflow velocity time integral can be used to estimate the relative flow (stroke volume) in the LV versus the RV and to estimate the approximate Qp:Qs. However, given the difficulties with reproducibility and reliability, echo assessment of the shunt fraction should be considered an approximation at best.

8. Pulmonary hypertension assessment: An estimation of RV systolic pressure (RVSP) is important in determining whether or not pulmonary hypertension is present. Typically, the tricuspid regurgitant jet is used to estimate RVSP. However, if the VSD jet enters the RV near the tricuspid valve (as it does in perimembranous defects), the tricuspid regurgitation (TR) jet is often contaminated by the VSD jet making assessment of RVSP inaccurate. If the Doppler cursor can be aligned through the VSD jet in a relatively perpendicular orientation, the LV to RV pressure gradient can be assessed from the peak velocity of the VSD jet, and this measurement can be used to determine whether or not significant pulmonary hypertension is present.

RVSP = Systolic BP − 4 (peak interventricular pressure gradient in m/s)^2

As a caveat, if the VSD is serpiginous or tortuous in its course through the septum, the LV–RV gradient measured across the VSD may be inaccurate.

UNIQUE VENTRICULAR SEPTAL DEFECT PHYSIOLOGY

Double-Chambered Right Ventricle

A commonly missed defect in adult echocardiography is the double-chambered RV. A double-chambered RV occurs when progressive focal hypertrophy of the RV at the border between the inlet and outlet portion of the RV results in subpulmonary stenosis. This creates an intracavitary gradient within the RV. The outlet portion of the RV typically has low pressure while the inlet portion of the RV has high pressure, with a significant gradient between the two portions. The mechanism is unclear, but hypothesized to be hypertrophy of the crista supraventricularis (an RV internal muscular ridge) due to flow across the VSD jet; the resulting increased pulmonary blood flow may be at least partially related (Fig. 44.9 and Video 44.4).[8]

Eisenmenger Syndrome

In patients with long-standing VSD with high L–R flow, remodeling of the pulmonary vasculature can occur, resulting in pulmonary hypertension with increased pulmonary vascular resistance (PVR) and reversal of the VSD flow. As PVR increases, flow across the VSD decreases and eventually reverses. At these lower flow rates, the velocities across the VSD are markedly decreased and eventually reverse in this setting; the flow no longer appears "turbulent" and often requires a lower Nyquist limit and a high frame rate for diagnosis and evaluation. Additionally, interrogation with pulse Doppler can be helpful in determining the flow direction. In these patients, significant pulmonary hypertension occurs, resulting in right ventricular hypertrophy in response to the elevated pulmonary pressures (Video 44.5). TR and RV systolic dysfunction may occur in later stages of the disease. Echocardiographic evaluation in these patients mirrors the assessment in patients with other types of pulmonary hypertension, and focuses on the size and function of the RV and tricuspid valve.

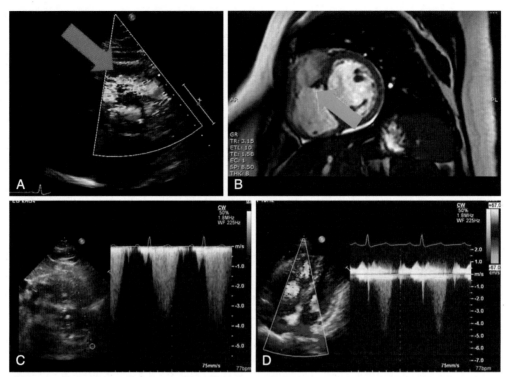

FIG. 44.9 Double-chambered right ventricle (RV). (A) Color Doppler evidence of the double-chambered ventricle with flow turbulence starting well below the level of the pulmonic valve *(red arrow)*, on parasternal short-axis window. (B) Cardiovascular magnetic resonance image for the same patient, which demonstrates the discrete subpulmonic stenosis *(green arrow)*. (C) Continuous-wave (CW) Doppler across the right ventricular outflow tract (RVOT) and pulmonic valve, showing a high late systolic-peaking gradient of infundibular stenosis. Note the atrial systolic antegrade flow due to right atrium (RA) "kick" with very high RA pressures, which are capable of opening the pulmonic valve. (D) CW Doppler revealing the intracavitary pressure gradient within the RV, with high pressure at the RV apex. See also Video 44.4.

Suggested Reading

Hadeed, K., Hascoet, S., Amadieu, R., et al. (2016). Assessment of ventricular septal defect size and morphology by three-dimensional transthoracic echocardiography. *Journal of the American Society of Echocardiography, 29,* 777–785.

Lai, W. W., Mertens, L. L., Cohen, M. S., & Geva, T. (Eds.). (2016). *Echocardiography in Pediatric and Congenital Heart Disease: From Fetus to Adult* (2nd ed.). Hoboken, NJ: Wiley-Blackwell.

Menting, M. E., Cuypers, J. A., Opić, P., et al. (2015). The unnatural history of the ventricular septal defect: outcome up to 40 years after surgical closure. *Journal of the American College of Cardiology, 65,* 1941–1951.

A complete reference list can be found online at ExpertConsult.com.

45 Other Common Congenital Defects in Adults

Keri Shafer, M. Elizabeth Brickner

INTRODUCTION

Due to improvements in surgical techniques and medical therapies in recent years, there has been an increase in survival to adulthood in those with complex congenital heart disease.[1] While complex congenital heart disease requires a careful and individualized approach, there are some fundamental assessments that should occur based on anatomic diagnosis.

SEGMENTAL ANATOMY

In patients with complex congenital heart disease, it is important to first assess the segmental anatomy of the heart. A systematic approach, which evaluates each level of blood flow—from the inferior vena cava (IVC) to the descending aorta—can be useful. Heart position is often best assessed with a subcostal sweep evaluating the location of the cardiac organ and the direction of the ventricular apex. This approach determines levocardia (leftward apex) from mesocardia (midline apex) from dextrocardia (rightward apex) (Video 45.1). A careful evaluation of the systemic venous flow, atrial position, atrioventricular valves, ventricular morphology, pulmonary venous return, great vessel location, aortic arch, and descending aorta anatomy should follow. A brief review of the more common congenital heart lesions is presented here. A review of atrial septal defect (ASD) and ventricular septal defects (VSDs) is in Chapters 43 and 44. The full scope of complex congenital heart disease is addressed in the congenital echocardiography references listed at the end of this chapter.

PATENT DUCTUS ARTERIOSUS

The ductus arteriosus is a connection of the descending aorta and pulmonary arteries that functions to deliver oxygenated blood from the placenta to the pulmonary arteries in the fetal circulation. In the vast majority of newborns, the ductus closes by 1 month of age. However, a persistently patent ductus arteriosus (PDA) can occur (estimated at approximately 3/10,000 live births). With the rapid decline of pulmonary vascular resistance after birth, flow across the PDA is directed "left to right" from the aorta to the pulmonary arteries. If the PDA persists into adulthood, it results in overcirculation of blood through the pulmonary arteries, the pulmonary veins, the left atrium (LA), and the left ventricle (LV).

In an adult with a PDA, the findings include:
1. Dilated LA and LV without other etiology
2. Persistent flow across the PDA, which, on echocardiography, is best visualized in the parasternal short-axis image at the base of the heart or suprasternal notch imaging of the descending aorta
3. Right ventricle (RV) hypertension and pulmonary hypertension (as a result of Eisenmenger syndrome)

Diagnosis of a PDA is often made in the parasternal short-axis view with color Doppler evaluation. Imaging should focus on the pulmonary artery bifurcation (Fig. 45.1 and Video 45.2). Flow from a PDA originates near the origin of the left pulmonary artery with continuous flow into the pulmonary artery shown by color Doppler. Usually, the color flow jet is visible, but visualization of the actual ductus is often difficult in adults. Suprasternal imaging of the aortic arch may be used with color Doppler with the imaging plane angulated towards the left pulmonary artery (Video 45.3). Flow from the aorta to the pulmonary artery through the ductus can be visualized in this view.

Continuous-wave Doppler interrogation of the flow through a PDA with left-to-right shunting will demonstrate continuous flow

from the aorta to the pulmonary artery. Flow velocity will vary between systole and diastole, with the higher flow velocities in systole, reflecting the larger pressure gradient. An estimation of the pressure gradient across the ductus can be helpful to determine whether pulmonary hypertension is present. Measurement of the peak velocity during systole (at or just after the R wave on electrocardiogram) reflects the pressure difference between aortic and pulmonary artery systolic pressure. Low velocity flow across a PDA suggests pulmonary hypertension.

TETRALOGY OF FALLOT

Tetralogy of Fallot (TOF) represents one of the largest groups of adults with complex congenital heart disease.[2] Initial palliative surgeries were performed in the 1940s, with ultimate repairs being accomplished by the mid-1950s.[3] As a result, there is a growing cohort of adults with repaired TOF with improving survival but a risk for morbidity.[4]

Imaging Approach to the Adult With Repaired Tetralogy of Fallot

1. Understanding of baseline anatomy:
   a. Unrepaired: Although uncommon in adulthood, patients can present with TOF without repair. Diagnosis is made by defining the VSD (often termed the conoventricular VSD), overriding aorta, right ventricular outflow tract (RVOT) obstruction, and RV hypertrophy (Fig. 45.2).
   b. Initial surgical shunting: Most patients have had palliative shunting that may have included aortopulmonary shunts or subclavian to pulmonary artery shunts. Prior shunt sites can become stenotic or aneurysmal, thus specific evaluation is needed.
   c. Repair type: While the majority of adult patients had a transannular patch (Fig. 45.3), RVOT patches or RV-pulmonary artery (PA) conduits (Fig. 45.4) have also been used.
   d. Pulmonary artery anatomy: Significant hypoplasia or pulmonary artery atresia can occur, resulting in significantly abnormal PA development and function
   e. Aortic arch sidedness: Approximately 10% to 25% of TOF patients have right aortic arches.
2. Evaluation of right atrium (RA) and RV: RA and RV size should be near normal in a patient with a good repair and no residual or recurrent lesions. A dilated RV suggests the presence of significant pulmonary regurgitation, tricuspid regurgitation (TR), or both. A hypertrophied RV suggests the presence of residual or recurrent RV outflow obstruction. Residual dilation and hypertrophy also can be secondary to significant delay in repair.
3. Repair integrity/results:
   a. Ventricular septal patch: Evaluation for residual defects or aneurysm. Color Doppler interrogation should be performed in multiple views with the color box encompassing the patch. Most residual defects occur at the margin of the patch.
   b. RVOT/pulmonary valve function: By using two-dimensional (2D) imaging, color and spectral Doppler evaluation for obstruction should be performed at the level of the infundibulum, pulmonary valve, main or branch PAs. Some patients will have a valved RV-to-PA conduit or pulmonary homograft. The origin of

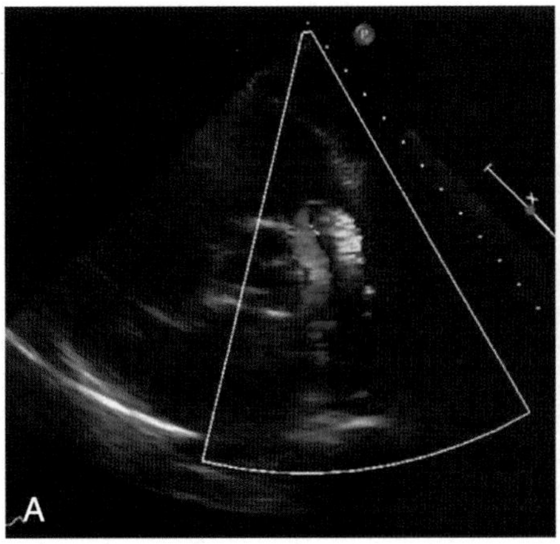

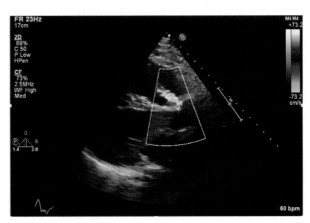

FIG. 45.1 Parasternal long axis with anteriorly directed color flow *(red)* of a patent ductus arteriosus on parasternal short-axis view of the bifurcation (A), and suprasternal window (B). See also Videos 45.2 and 45.3.

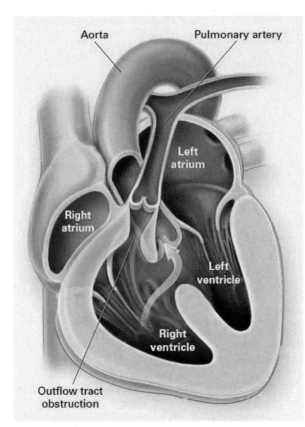

FIG. 45.2 Diagram of the native anatomy of tetralogy of Fallot. *(From Brickner ME, Hillis LD, Lange RA: Congenital heart disease in adults. Second of two parts. N Engl J Med. 2000;342(5):334–342. Copyright © 2000 Massachusetts Medical Society. Reprinted with permission.)*

RV-to-PA conduits may require off-axis imaging to identify the origin of the conduit and to appropriately align the Doppler cursor to interrogate the valve/conduit (see Fig. 45.4).
4. Left ventricular systolic and diastolic function
5. Aortic root dilation: The aortic root is frequently dilated in patients with TOF, and can be associated with aortic valve regurgitation. Aortic regurgitant jets are frequently angled towards the VSD patch, and it is important to visualize/assess the jet origin.

Key Imaging Views

In addition to the standard adult protocol, TOF imaging should include:
1. Evaluation for residual VSD-parasternal long-axis view
2. Pulmonary valve function and evaluation for pulmonary artery stenoses with pulsed Doppler along the RVOT to branch PAs, continuous

FIG. 45.3 Parasternal long axis of a patient with repaired tetralogy of Fallot. Note the small patch margin defect with left-to-right flow.

Doppler across the RVOT for pulmonary regurgitation and stenosis evaluation (parasternal short axis, long axis).
  a. For patients with a history of significant pulmonary stenosis or pulmonary atresia, extended views can be performed in the parasternal short-axis orientation. By shifting the imaging probe slightly towards the diaphragm and angling superiorly, the branch pulmonary arteries may come into view. Additionally, anastomotic sites of the RV-PA conduit should be imaged.

TRANSPOSITION OF THE GREAT ARTERIES

Transposition of the great arteries (TGA) has two predominant types. The most common type is often referred to as D-loop TGA. The less common form is called physiologically or congenitally corrected transposition (also known as L-loop TGA). Embryologically, as the heart is forming, the heart tube makes a rightward loop (i.e., a D-loop). In patients with D-Loop TGA, their ventricles are in the typical location. If the heart loops incorrectly, it has an L-loop and the ventricles have an inverted relationship.

In D-loop TGA, the great arteries are transposed so the aorta is located anterior and rightward to the pulmonary artery. The aorta is associated with the RV and the pulmonary artery to the LV. As this circulation is not physiologically sustainable, an initial palliative procedure must be done to increase arterial and venous mixing until the ultimate repair is completed (e.g., balloon atrial septostomy). Based on era and location of birth, the final procedure to restore systemic venous blood circulation to the pulmonary artery and pulmonary venous blood to the aorta was either an atrial switch or an arterial switch (Fig. 45.5).
1. Atrial switch: Fundamentally, in this procedure, systemic venous blood is re-routed (baffled) directly to the LV to ultimately go to the pulmonary artery. The pulmonary venous blood is then baffled to the

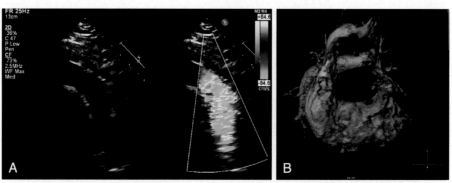

FIG. 45.4 Right ventricle–pulmonary atresia (RV-PA) conduit for tetralogy of Fallot. (A) RV-PA conduit shown in the parasternal long axis angled superiorly. The *right image* shows turbulent flow in the conduit. (B) The same conduit as in (A) shown on cardiac magnetic resonance imaging in three-dimensional reconstruction.

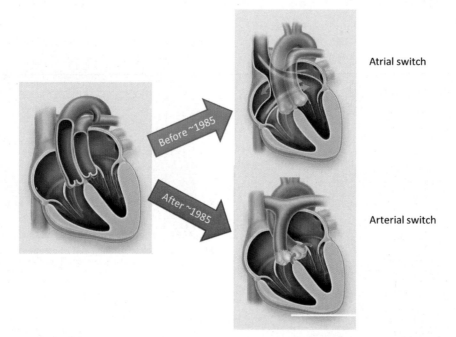

FIG. 45.5 Diagram of the transposition of the great arteries with surgical options. Prior to about 1985, most institutions performed the atrial switch procedure. After that date, most institutions performed the arterial switch. (*Modified from Brickner ME, Hillis LD, Lange RA. Congenital heart disease in adults. Second of two parts. N Engl J Med. 2000;342(5):334–342. Copyright © 2000 Massachusetts Medical Society. Reprinted with permission.*)

RV and on to the aorta. At least one patch is made in the coronal plane to septate the atria anterior-to-posterior rather than right-to-left.

a. Imaging approach:

i. The ventricles: The ventricles in the atrial switch patients can be best visualized in the apical four-chamber and the parasternal short-axis view. In the apical four-chamber view, the RV appears enlarged and hypertrophied while the LV (subpulmonary ventricle) appears small. In short-axis views, the anterior RV (which generates systemic pressure) flattens the posteriorly positioned LV (which pumps to the pulmonary artery). Assessment of the systemic RV (both systolic and diastolic function) and the systemic AV valve (tricuspid valve) is important, since a significant number of these patients develop heart failure with systemic (RV) ventricular dysfunction and TR.

ii. Systemic and pulmonary venous baffles: superior vena cava (SVC) and IVC blood are redirected to the mitral valve and subpulmonic LV. Pulmonary vein flow is directed around the systemic venous baffle to the tricuspid valve and the systemic RV. In the apical four-chamber view, a portion of the baffle system can be easily seen in the LA, bisecting the LA. The portion of the LA closest to the mitral valve receives inflow from the SVC and IVC limbs. Pulmonary venous return to the posterior portion of the atrium flows across the pulmonary venous channel (where the atrial septum has been resected) into the RA. Flow across the pulmonary vein channel should be low velocity (unobstructed). The areas of baffle anastomosis and along the contour of the baffle can become stenosed, aneurysmal, and/or develop leaks. Thus careful evaluation of the baffle with both 2D imaging, low Nyquist/high-frame-rate color Doppler and pulsed-wave Doppler is important (Fig. 45.6). Screening for baffle leaks can be done with agitated saline contrast (Fig. 45.7A shows a normal baffle, and Fig. 45.7B shows a baffle leak). See also Video 45.4.

iii. The great arteries are situated side by side, with the aorta arising anteriorly from the RV (Video 45.5). Non-standard imaging planes are usually required to visualize the aorta and the aortic valve.

iv. Common errors: Failure to recognize transposition can lead to an incorrect diagnosis of pulmonary hypertension, based on the enlarged RV, the septal flattening, and the incorrect use of the TR jet to estimate pulmonary pressure. In evaluation of transposition patients, the great vessels are commonly mislabeled. It is imperative to know that in the patient s/p atrial switch, the aorta remains the anterior vessel, and the pulmonary artery is posteriorly situated.

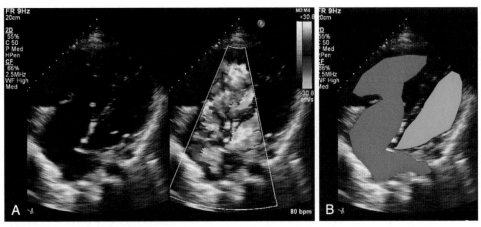

FIG. 45.6 Atrial switch baffle. (A) Apical four-chamber view of the atrial switch baffle in D-loop transposition of the great arteries. (B) Blue blood is shown coming across the systemic venous baffle and red blood from the pulmonary venous baffle.

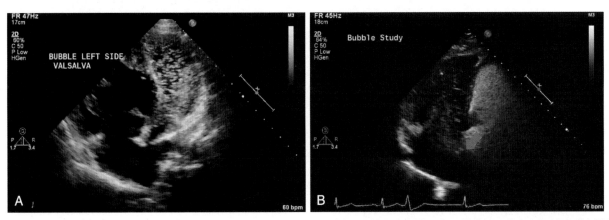

FIG. 45.7 Agitated saline contrast to evaluate atrial switch baffles in D-loop transposition of the great arteries. (A) An intact and normally functioning baffle. (B) The site of the baffle leak is indicated with a *red arrow*.

2. Arterial switch: This represents a near anatomic correction of the transposed vessels. The aorta and pulmonary arteries are transected above the level of the valve and are switched. The pulmonary arteries are usually brought forward in front of the aorta (LeCompte maneuver). The coronary arteries are transferred posteriorly via coronary buttons. In comparison to the atrial switch procedure, the postarterial switch operation (ASO) great vessel location looks closer to normal. The great arteries are still aligned in parallel, and the PA bifurcation is usually anterior to the aorta (LeCompte maneuver). Thus, in the traditional parasternal short-axis view, the branch pulmonary arteries are not well-visualized.

   b. Imaging of arterial switch:

      i. Evaluation of biventricular size and function: Early surgeries had variable success with coronary artery button transfer. At times, patients had a compromise of coronary flow, which can result in permanent regional wall motion abnormalities due to infarction.

      ii. Evaluation of anastomotic sites: Patients are at risk for supra-pulmonary stenosis and supra-aortic stenosis at the site of anastomosis. Additionally, aortic dilation can be seen (Fig. 45.8)

      iii. Branch pulmonary artery flow: Due to the LeCompte maneuver, the branch pulmonary arteries can become stretched across the aorta causing branch pulmonary stenosis (Fig. 45.9)

COARCTATION

Coarctation is a narrowing of the aorta just at or past the left subclavian artery (otherwise known as the aortic isthmus). In the top five most frequent defects, coarctation can be missed in childhood, as it may not immediately manifest with hypertension or murmur. It can be diagnosed in adolescence or adulthood in the evaluation of secondary causes of hypertension. Coarctation is associated with other defects. Up to 50% of patients have bicuspid aortic valves but may also have ventricular septal defects or additional left sided obstructive lesions such as subaortic

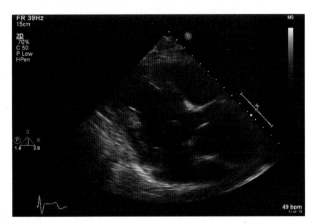

FIG. 45.8 After the arterial switch procedure for the D-transposition of the great arteries, a dilated neo-aortic root is common.

stenosis or supramitral ring. If the patient has serial left sided outflow tract obstruction, it is termed Shone's complex. Additionally, in significantly narrowed coarctation, collateral vessels can be seen (Fig. 45.10), which occur to increase flow to the descending aorta in the setting of significant obstruction across the coarctation.

Imaging approach: A similar imaging approach is used for both native (unrepaired) coarctation and repaired coarctation.

   a. Suprasternal notch imaging to visualize location of coarctation (difficult in some adults)

      i. 2D imaging is performed to assess the location of narrowing, and the aortic arch and isthmus dimensions. Color Doppler assesses for turbulent flow, location of obstruction, and collateral vessels (Fig. 45.11 and Video 45.6).

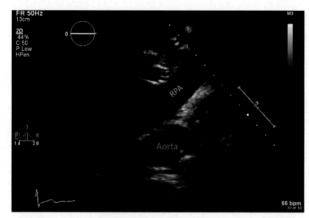

FIG. 45.9 Arterial switch for D-transposition of the great arteries. Due to the LeCompte maneuver, the right pulmonary artery is seen anterior to the aorta. Structures are shown in the parasternal short axis.

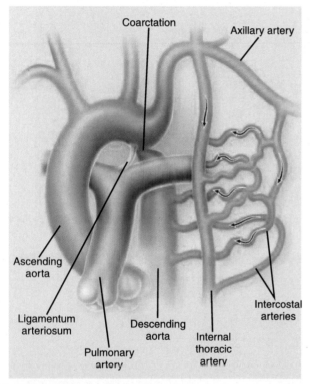

FIG. 45.10 Diagram of coarctation of the aorta. Due to the significant stenosis, accessory arteries can dilate to collateralize the descending aorta. (*From Brickner ME, Hillis LD, Lange RA: Congenital heart disease in adults. First of two parts. N Engl J Med. 2000;342(4):256–263. Copyright © 2000 Massachusetts Medical Society. Reprinted with permission.*)

   ii. Gradient/velocity assessment: When assessing for peak gradients, it is important to ensure that the angle of interrogation is aimed directly and collinearly down the narrowest region of the coarctation to prevent underestimation of the obstruction. Of note, in long areas of stenosis or with extensive collaterals, continuous-wave assessment may be inaccurate as an indicator of stenoses severity in part due to decreased flow across the coarctation and tortuosity.

b. Abdominal aorta: Pulsed-wave (PW) Doppler assessment is used for screening for coarctation as the waveform has a signature appearance and can be performed in nearly all adult patients. Coarctation results in PW tracing with blunted, late peak systolic flow and diastolic forward flow (Fig. 45.12).

c. Postoperative patients: The sonographer should evaluate for re-coarctation, aneurysm formation at the repair site, and associated aortopathy in other areas of the aorta.

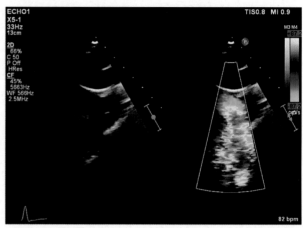

FIG. 45.11 Aortic coarctation. Suprasternal notch imaging shows the region of stenosis best depicted with color Doppler flow acceleration and turbulence (see Video 45.6).

FONTAN

When patients have incompletely developed or malformed ventricles, biventricular repair is often not possible. Commonly, these patients with single ventricle physiology are palliated with the Fontan procedure. Underlying cardiac anatomy can vary widely (e.g., tricuspid atresia, hypoplastic left or right heart, double inlet LV), and often, several palliative shunts have been performed prior to the Fontan completion. The Fontan circulation is one in which systemic venous flow is directed to the pulmonary arteries without an intervening pump (i.e., ventricle) to promote forward flow, and is created to separate systemic venous (deoxygenated) and pulmonary venous (oxygenated) flows. For forward flow to occur, there must be serially lower resistances that result in a systemic venous pressure and pulmonary artery pressure that are higher than the LA pressure. Flow through the Fontan circuit is low velocity, biphasic, and minimally, if at all, pulsatile. The single ventricle provides the driving force for the entire circulation. This is a palliative procedure, which, unfortunately, in the long term, eventually leads to ventricular dysfunction, arrhythmias, and other complications.

Imaging approach:

1. Ventricular and valve function: It is critical to recognize that there is only one functional ventricle (which may be LV or RV in morphology, with a hypoplastic RV or LV). Based on the underlying ventricular anatomy, there may be one or two atrioventricular valves, for which quantification of regurgitation and stenosis is helpful.

2. Aortic valve: Blood has been surgically routed to exclusively go to the aorta. The origin of the aorta from the ventricle is variable, depending on the underlying defect. The pulmonary artery (if present) is usually oversewn, with all pulmonary blood flow coming directly from the SVC and IVC. Imaging assessment should focus on both definition of the aortic dimensions and valve function. Further evaluation should be performed to determine if a pulmonary artery stump is present to evaluate for flow into the stump and to screen for thrombi.

3. Fontan baffle assessment: Although the ultimate physiologic circulation is similar across the patients, there are multiple anatomic variants of the Fontan procedure. In a Glenn shunt, SVC blood is channeled directly to the pulmonary artery. A direct connection of the RA to the pulmonary artery (i.e., atriopulmonary connection) was used in the past and often resulted in massive dilatation of the RA. Other versions of the Fontan have resulted in more efficient blood flow through the Fontan circuit and potentially fewer arrhythmias. In addition to a Glenn shunt, patients may either have: a lateral tunnel Fontan is a conduit within the RA directing IVC blood flow to the pulmonary artery; an extracardiac Fontan is a conduit adjacent to the atrium directing IVC blood flow to the pulmonary artery. Flow through the Fontan to the LA depends on a compliant left atrium and left ventricle with low atrial pressure. Any condition that results in increased ventricular diastolic or atrial pressure will decrease the efficiency of the Fontan circulation and decrease flow. Imaging should focus on the anastomotic sites for stenosis or leak. Additionally, color Doppler flow

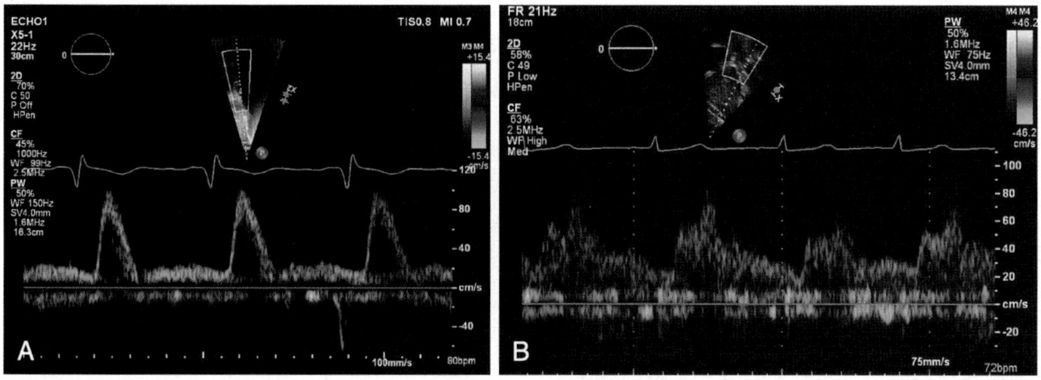

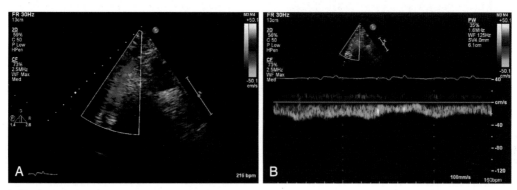

FIG. 45.12 Pulsed-wave Doppler of the abdominal aorta in (A) normal state, and (B) coarctation, in which there is delayed upstroke and diastolic forward flow suggesting coarctation.

FIG. 45.13 Fontan baffle. (A) Suprasternal imaging of Fontan baffle showing no turbulence of the superior vena cava as it drains into the right pulmonary arter (RPA) (see corresponding Video 45.7). (B) Pulsed-wave Doppler with sample volume placed within the Fontan shows low velocity flow, which is suggestive of no significant Fontan obstruction.

should assess for turbulence or concern for thrombus. The Fontan is best assessed in the subcostal views as well as the suprasternal notch (Fig. 45.13 and Videos 45.7 and 45.8). However, full assessment of the Fontan circulation requires cross-sectional imaging (e.g., MRI or CT).

EBSTEIN ANOMALY

Ebstein anomaly is a rare condition, but depending on the severity of valvular dysfunction, it can be diagnosed in adulthood. The tricuspid valve has the appearance of apical displacement as a result of incomplete delamination of the septal, and sometimes inferior/posterior, leaflets. The hinge point of these leaflets are displaced, resulting in malcoaptation of the valve and atrialization of a portion of the RV. Ebstein anomaly displacement of the valve has been defined as greater than 0.8 mm/m^2.[5] The RV is divided into an "atrialized portion" and the functional contractile RV (Fig. 45.14). However, the RV is typically also dysfunctional. Ebstein anomaly is often associated with patent foramen ovale (PFO) or ASD, which can have bidirectional or right-to-left shunting, depending on the compliance of the RV. Ebstein anomaly is also associated with accessory conduction pathways leading to Wolff-Parkinson-White syndrome. Additionally, patients may also have abnormal left ventricular myocardium with a non-compaction-like appearance. Cases in which the tricuspid valve is not actually apically displaced, but the tricuspid valve leaflets are malformed, are termed *tricuspid valve dysplasia*.

Imaging assessment of Ebstein anomaly and dysplastic tricuspid valves includes an assessment to determine:

- Relative size of atrialized RV and functional RV, which correlates with the severity of apical displacement of the tricuspid valve (Fig. 45.15 and Video 45.9)
- Function of the residual or "functional" RV
- Degree of tricuspid regurgitation. This is often difficult to fully assess given the need for off-axis imaging to fully view the displaced coaptation plane. TR may be "wide open" and thus appear to be a smooth and low-velocity flow

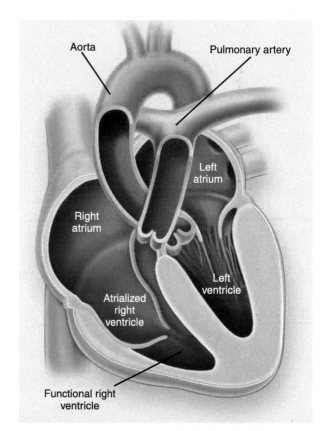

FIG. 45.14 Ebstein anomaly. Diagram depicting the apically displaced tricuspid valve. (*From Brickner ME, Hillis LD, Lange RA: Congenital heart disease in adults. Second of two parts. N Engl J Med. 2000;342(5):334–342. Copyright © 2000 Massachusetts Medical Society. Reprinted with permission.*)

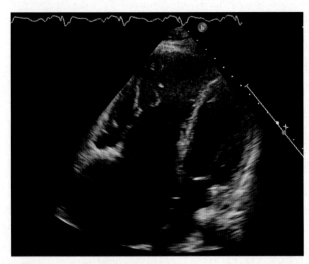

FIG. 45.15 Severe Ebstein anomaly. Apical four-chamber view of the apically displaced tricuspid valve and atrialized right ventricle.

- Characterization of the tricuspid valve attachments and annular displacement. This is often needed prior to surgical repair and may be best assessed by three-dimensional (3D) imaging
- Degree of atrial level shunting by using both color Doppler and agitated saline
- Left ventricular function.

Suggested Reading

Brickner, M. E., Hillis, L. D., & Lange, R. A. (2000). Congenital heart disease in adults. First of two parts. *New England Journal of Medicine, 342*, 256–263.

Brickner, M. E., Hillis, L. D., & Lange, R. A. (2000). Congenital heart disease in adults. Second of two parts. *New England Journal of Medicine, 342*, 334–342.

Cohen, M. S., Eidem, B. W., Cetta, F., et al. (2016). Multimodality imaging guidelines of patients with transposition of the great arteries: a report from the American Society of Echocardiography Developed in Collaboration with the Society for Cardiovascular Magnetic Resonance and the Society of Cardiovascular Computed Tomography. *Journal of the American Society of Echocardiography, 29,* 571–621.

Lai, W. W., Mertens, L. L., Cohen, M. S., & Geva, T. (Eds.). (2016). *Echocardiography in pediatric and congenital heart disease: from fetus to adult* (2nd ed.). Hoboken, NJ: Wiley-Blackwell.

Valente, A. M., Cook, S., Festa, P., et al. (2014). Multimodality imaging guidelines for patients with repaired tetralogy of Fallot: a report from the American Society of Echocardiography Developed in Collaboration with the Society for Cardiovascular Magnetic Resonance and the Society for Pediatric Radiology. *Journal of the American Society of Echocardiography, 27,* 111–141.

A complete reference list can be found online at ExpertConsult.com.

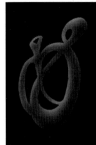

46 Handheld Echocardiography

Faraz Pathan, Jagat Narula, Thomas H. Marwick

INTRODUCTION

Although Moore's law of increasing computing capabilities (including processing power and memory) has propelled the development of all imaging modalities, its most tangible manifestation has been in the field of ultrasonography. Unrestrained by the physical limitations (gantry size and power requirements) of the other modalities, echocardiography machines have evolved from large, cumbersome pieces of equipment to handheld echocardiography (HHE) devices that are the size of a mobile phone (Fig. 46.1).[1]

Three aspects of miniaturization have been particularly important for HHE. The display interface has benefited tremendously from technological evolution—cathode ray tube monitors have been replaced by lightweight, high-resolution liquid crystal display (LCD) screens. Developments in microprocessors have led to a shift in the balance between hardware and software so that it is closer to the transducer, usurping some of the functionalities previously performed by the scanner (Fig. 46.2).[2] Likewise, there has been a progressive drop in the size of digital beamforming components from 1 μm to 100 nm. Freeing the handheld device from the ECG leads through fixed time acquisitions or more complex tracking iterations using mitral annular movement of speckle tracking has led to increased portability and reduced size.

The inextricable connection between energy transmitted by a system and the information gained has led powerful, high-end systems to hold an advantage over their battery-dependent counterparts. These power-to-performance issues have benefited from greater efficiency of systems and greater integration, although the limitations imposed by their size continue to leave HHE at one end of the spectrum of ultrasound devices.

CURRENT HANDHELD DEVICES

A modern HHE device is characteristically lightweight, portable, and can fit into a coat pocket—in contrast to previous miniaturized models. These devices provide B mode grayscale imaging and in some cases color Doppler. Unlike their fully functional mobile (but non-HHE) counterparts, which are essentially complete echocardiographic devices, most HHE devices do not provide spectral Doppler. They also have smaller screens and a display that is lower in resolution than standard echocardiographic devices (Fig. 46.3). Their various properties are described in Table 46.1. It is important to remember that comparison with standard echocardiography is only reasonable if these devices are touted as a replacement for echocardiography rather than an extension of the physical examination.

The limitations of HHE are related to the imaging modes, processing, display, and ability to do measurements. None of the devices have continuous-wave Doppler, and only one has pulsed-wave Doppler capability. Because Doppler wave-form analysis is a cornerstone in the severity assessment of valvular and diastolic heart disease, this represents an important (and potentially avoidable) limitation. The high-resolution display of high-end devices provides high-fidelity images that are difficult to reproduce on HHE devices. Finally, post-acquisition analysis and measurements are a key component of analysis. Although three devices enable measurement of distances and area, volumetric assessments are not possible. Adjustment of imaging parameters such as zoom, changing focal point, narrowing sector width to improve frame rate, changing mechanical index for contrast studies, harmonic imaging, changing dynamic range or grayscale maps, and changing frequency are all currently unavailable on such devices. Future iterations may overcome some if not all of these limitations, but currently there is a clear difference between a standard echocardiogram and HHE equipment.

THE LEARNING CURVE

The acquisition of information from the traditional physical examination is less reliable than in former times. HHE is a potential replacement for bedside diagnosis, but ultrasonography has not been as well taught and is currently restricted to certain physicians, surgeons, and sonographers. The relative cost, portability, and applicability of HHE devices make them ideal for more widespread dissemination. However, for those unfamiliar with echocardiography, there needs to be a learning process and assessment of competence. The recommended training requirements for performance and reporting of echocardiography are summarized in Table 46.2.

Clearly Level 2– and 3–trained individuals will readily adapt to HHE; both American Society of Echocardiography (ASE) and European Association of Echocardiography (EAE) recommend that experienced cardiologists and sonographers should be able to use handheld devices.[3] Miniaturization of technology has outpaced training and accreditation guidelines, and ultrasonography has moved from the field of radiologists and subspecialty physicians to residents and general physicians. The ASE advises additional training for Level 1–trained individuals and EAE recommends additional training for cardiologists not fully conversant with echocardiography.[3,4] The American College of Emergency Physicians (ACEP) has addressed the role of focused cardiac ultrasound (FCU) in the emergency department and provided guidelines on the acquisition and interpretation of ultrasound images on a range of diagnostic possibilities.[5] At an earlier stage in training, HHE can also be used as teaching aide to visualize anatomy and physiology at the bedside.[6] Wittich demonstrated that 79% of medical students could produce a satisfactory parasternal long axis (PLAX) image within 3 weeks of didactic and practical sessions.[7] It seems feasible to use HHE to acquire images and interpret basic cardiac function early during medical school.

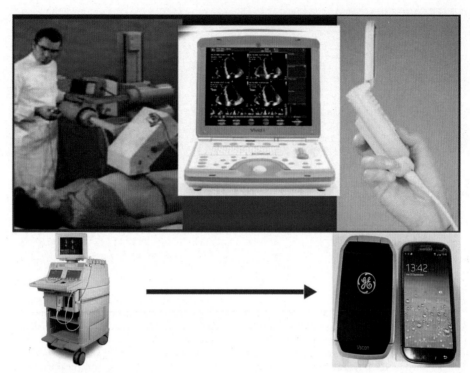

FIG. 46.1 Progressive reduction in the size of ultrasound devices. The original devices were large and of limited mobility. Echocardiograms became more mobile, eventually being transferred to equipment about the size of a laptop. Handheld devices represent the fruits of ongoing miniaturization, and are analogous in size to a smartphone. (*Modified from Marwick TH. The future of echocardiography.* Eur J Echocardiogr. *2009;10(5):594–601.*)

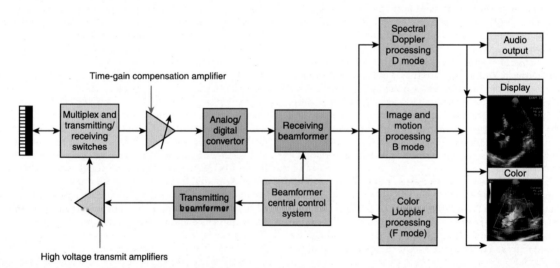

FIG. 46.2 Changes in the balance between hardware and software. The *blue boxes* indicate system functionality that has been transferred to software or microprocessors. The *yellow boxes* show steps performed by digital application-specific integrated circuits. The receive (RX) beamforming component has also been incorporated into software applications, and the remainder of the boxes contain analog signal processing units that have been incorporated into the probe itself, thereby reducing volume required on the display end. (*Modified from Thomenius KE. Miniaturization of ultrasound scanners.* Ultrasound Clin. *2009;4(3):385–389.*)

There have been multiple previous comparisons of HHE and physical examination—a recent example is summarized in Table 46.3.[8] There is clear incremental value of HHE over the traditional physical examination; the area under the receiver operating characteristic (ROC) curve was 1.97 for physical examination, 2.42 for ECG and physical examination, and 6.23 for HHE-based echocardiography.[9]

Handheld ultrasonography can be applied to any organ system, although for the purposes of this chapter it will refer solely to the examination of the cardiovascular system. FCU is a specific adaptation—involving HHE—that provides a "Focused examination of the cardiovascular system performed by a physician using an ultrasound as an adjunct to the physical examination to recognise specific ultrasonic signals that represent a narrow list of potential diagnosis in specific clinical settings." This

must be differentiated from limited transthoracic echocardiography, which refers to a reduced number of images performed on a standard and thus a high-end machine by an echocardiographer with appropriate qualifications and interpreted by a cardiologist with the necessary level of experience. The training recommendations on FCU by the ASE comprise three educational components—a didactic component (ultrasound physics, basic cardiac anatomy and views), practical training (image acquisition and correction of technique by experienced echocardiographers), and image interpretation. Recent literature has demonstrated that electronic modules were equivalent to didactic teaching, but there is no substitute for "hands-on" sonographer-based training,[10] or the use of a training log to track the number of successful echocardiographic interrogations for specific cardiac pathologic conditions.[11] There is considerable

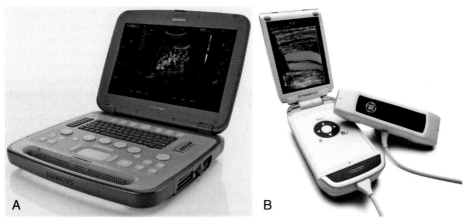

FIG. 46.3 Currently available "handheld" devices. The technical capabilities of the (A) AcusonP10 (Siemens, Mountain View, California), and (B) Vscan (GE Medical Systems, Milwaukee, Wisconsin) are listed in Table 46.1. (*[A] Courtesy Siemens; B, Courtesy GE Healthcare.*)

TABLE 46.1 Properties of Current Handheld Echocardiography Equipment

	MOBIUS™ SP1	VSCAN V1.2	ACUSON P10™	SIGNOSRT
Company	MobiSante	GE Healthcare	Siemens	Signostics
Weight (g)	330	390	725	392
Display Size (Inches)	4.1	3.5	3.7 (Diagonal)	4.5 (height)
Imaging options	Gray scale	Grayscale Color Doppler	Grayscale	Gray scale M-mode PW Doppler
Transducer Frequency (MHz)	3.5–5.0 (and 7.5) Mechanical Single element	1.7–3.8 Phased Array	2–4 Phased array	3.0–5.0
Interface with PC	USB synch	Micro SD card	Software	Micro SD card
Battery Capacity (minutes)	60	90	100	120

PW, Pulsed-wave Doppler.
Data from company product information statements.

TABLE 46.2 Training Duration and Levels of Echocardiographic Expertise

LEVEL	DURATION OF TRAINING (M)	CUMULATIVE DURATION OF TRAINING (M)	MINIMAL NO. OF TTE EXAMS PERFORMED	MINIMAL NO. OF TTE EXAMS INTERPRETED
1	3	3	75	150
2	3	6	150	300
3	6	12	300	750

TTE, Transthoracic echocardiography.

TABLE 46.3 Comparison of Handheld Echocardiography and Physical Examination

ECHOCARDIOGRAM FINDINGS	HHE % CORRECT	PE % CORRECT	INCREMENTAL %	P
Normal LV function	89	58	31	<0.0001
Abnormal LV function	96	35	61	<0.0001
Normal RV function	94	57	37	<0.0001
Abnormal RV function	68	21	47	0
Pulmonary hypertension absent	92	89	3.1	0.36
Pulmonary hypertension present	53	42	10	0.33
Valve disease, mild or absent	94	91	3.5	0.23
Valve disease, moderate or severe	71	31	39	0.00
Miscellaneous findings absent	77	64	13	0.02
Miscellaneous findings present	47	3	44	<0.0001

HHE, Handheld echocardiography; *PE*, physical examination.

variation in the duration of training programs depending on the level of experience of operators, opportunity to scan, time, and resources.[12–15] The length of the learning curve is variable. General practitioners with 8 hours of supervised training using HHE were able to assess left ventricle (LV) function with a sensitivity of 83% and a specificity of 78%.[16] A regression model based on more than 230 HHE examinations performed and interpreted by 30 residents and audited against cardiologists' measurements suggested improvements every 10 scans and that 30 scans would result in a minimal overall difference. It must be noted that with all R^2 values of less than 0.2, the fit and predictive value of the model was limited.[17]

VALIDATION OF HANDHELD DEVICES

Table 46.4 summarizes the literature reporting sensitivity, specificity, or agreement between HHE and standard echocardiography.[8,9,15,18–39] Reported levels of sensitivity, specificity, agreement, and weighted Kappa values, depend on multiple factors including technology used (availability of color Doppler, ability to make measurements), skill level of the operator and interpreter (echocardiographer/cardiologist vs. internist/general resident) and the exact target. Categorical evaluations (presence vs. absence of pathology) are likely to be more robust than quantitative evaluations (e.g., severity of a valvular lesion). The variability in Table 46.4 also reflects that in addition to the progressive development of HHE, there has been an evolution of standard echocardiography over time, with a shifting paradigm toward quantitative analysis using tools such as strain, 3D volumetric analysis, and a focus on quantitative assessment of Doppler waveforms. The variation in agreement despite evolution of handheld technology does not necessarily represent a decline in diagnostic ability; rather, it is testament to the evolution of high-end echocardiography.

A consensus statement published by the ASE found that the use of HHE for assessment of LV enlargement (6 studies), LV hypertrophy (8), LV systolic function (19), left atrium (LA) enlargement (9), right ventricle (RV) enlargement (3), RV systolic function (6), pericardial effusion (11), and inferior vena cava (IVC) size (2) have all been well validated.[40] Similarly, recent literature has attempted to categorize accuracy of HHE as excellent (Sn ≥ 90%, Sp ≥ 95%) including studies by nonexperts, good (Sn ≥ 90%, Sp ≥ 95%) by experts, fair (Sn ≈ 80%, Sp≈ 80%), and variable. Using this categorization, HHE for detection of pericardial effusion was considered to have excellent accuracy. Good accuracy was demonstrated for LV size, LV systolic function, regional wall motion abnormalities (RWMA), ultrasound lung comets, pleural effusion, and abdominal aortic aneurysm (AAA) detection. The accuracy was deemed fair for LA size and assessment of the presence and severity of aortic and mitral valve disease. The accuracy of HHE for RV and IVC assessment was considered to be quite variable.[41]

SUGGESTED PROTOCOL

HHE may be used for a targeted assessment, for example, IVC diameter, a limited examination (apical views only), or a more comprehensive assessment. Any protocol recommendations need to balance the comprehensiveness of an examination with expediency.

Clearly the clinical context will determine the best approach and duration of echocardiography. In an emergent setting such as cardiac arrest, HHE can be used to guide resuscitation. Images can be acquired in the 5- to 10-second window during pulse check or between defibrillations, with the aim to exclude potential causes, including hypovolemic shock (small cavity with contact of ventricular walls), saddle pulmonary embolism (dilated, dysfunctional RV, systolic flattening of septum), cardiogenic shock (markedly reduced ejection fraction [EF]), or pericardial tamponade.[42] The detection of a significant pericardial effusion can be achieved easily and rapidly as shown in Fig. 46.4.

TABLE 46.4 Comparison of Handheld Echocardiography With Standard Echocardiography

AUTHOR	YEAR	DEVICE	OPERATOR	CONCORDANCE WITH SE (AG, K, R)	ACCURACY (AC, SN, SP)	COMMENTS
Fukuda	2009	Acuson P10	Sonographer	r 0.87–0.98	(RWMA) Sn 88%, Sp 95%	Valves not assessed (no color Doppler)
Galderisi	2010	Vscan	Experts/Trainee	k 0.84	Sn 97%, Sp 84%	Calcification k 1.00 (AS not reported)
Andersen	2011	Vscan	Cardiologists	r 0.62–1.00	Sn 63%–100%, Sp 68%–100%	Moderate correlation with AS (r 0.62), poor specificity for LA size (Sp 68%)
Gianstefani	2011	Vscan	Sonographers	Ag 79%, k 0.47	X	No k or Ag data for valvular disease, reported good concordance
Giusca	2011	AcusonP10	Cardiology trainees	k 0.56–0.81	Sn 56%–71%, Sp 90%–100%	No color Doppler
Lafitte	2011	Vscan	Expert physician	k 0.64–0.91	x	Moderate agreement with aortic root size (k 0.64)
Liebo	2011	Vscan	Fellow/Physician	x	Ac (0.58–0.91)	Lowest accuracy for IVC size (0.54)
Prinz	2011	Vscan	Cardiologists	k 0.21–1.00	x	Severity AS (k 0.21), qualitative valve disease (k 0.9 any regurgitation), (K 1.0 any AS/calcification)
Razi	2011	Vscan	Residents	Ag LVSD 86%–98%	EF < 40% Sn 94%, Sp 94%	LV function study
Reant	2011	Vscan	Residents	k 0.86–0.90	x	LV function, MR and PE assessment
Amiel	2012	Vscan	Sonographers	k 0.75	x	LV function study
Biais	2012	Vscan	Experienced physician	k 0.70–0.90	Sn 77%–94%, Sp 96%–100%	Good agreement for severe RV dilatation (k 0.87)
Kimura	2012	AcusonP10	Sonographer	x	x	EPSS Ac 82%, Sn 47%, Sp 98%, LA Ac 64%, Sn 79%, Sp 52%
Mjolstad	2012	Vscan	Cardiologist/Internist	Overall ≥0.85	Sn/Sp ≥89% (valvular)	LV sz/fn (Sn/ Sp 97%/ 99%) LA r 0.65,IVC r 0.68

TABLE 46.4 Comparison of Handheld Echocardiography With Standard Echocardiography—cont'd

AUTHOR	YEAR	DEVICE	OPERATOR	CONCORDANCE WITH SE (AG, K, R)	ACCURACY (AC, SN, SP)	COMMENTS
Prinz	2012	Vscan	Sonographer	r 0.60–1.0	x	LV Fn r >0.6, valvular regurgitation k 0.10–0.90
Abe	2013	Vscan	Sonographer	AS score k 0.85	Mod-Sev AS Sn 84%, Sp 90%	AS study
Kitada	2013	Vscan	Expert physician	Ag 90%	X	Cost-effectiveness study
Mjolstad	2013	Vscan	Residents	r 0.44–0.86	Sn 40%–92%, Sp 81%–94%	Poor sensitivity for Rv functional assessment
Testuz	2013	Vscan	Cardiologists	k 0.46–0.90	X	RV size and LV size k 0.46, K 0.59 (function and valvular k ≥0.60)
Beaton	2014	Vscan	Pediatric cardiologist	X	Sn 90%, Sp 93% for RHD	Modified assessment of RHD
Cullen	2014	Vscan	Sonographers	k 0.49–0.91	X	LVH, atrial size, PE k ≤0.55, valvular and fn ≥0.61
Khan	2014	Vscan	Cardiology fellows	Ag 90%–97%	Sn 79%–96%, Sp 92%–99%	Cost-effectiveness study/good overall agreement
Mehta	2014	Vscan	Cardiology fellows	% correct- 82%	x	LV fn (89% N, 96% Abn), RV fn (N 94%, abn 68%), overall valve (absent/mild 94%, mod-sev 71%)
Riley	2014	Vscan	Cardiologists	k 0.82	Sn 75%	Pediatric patients
Di Bello	2015	Vscan	Cardiologists	k 0.82, Ag 94%	Sn 94%, Sp 88%	Comparison to physical examination. Incremental area under ROC curve.

Abn, Abnormal; *Ac,* accuracy; *Ag,* agreement; *AS,* aortic stenosis; *EF,* ejection fraction; *EPSS,* E point systolic separation; *Fn,* function, *IVC,* inferior vena cava; *K,* kappa/weighted kappa; *LA,* left atrium; *LV,* left ventricle; *LVH,* left ventricular hypertrophy; *LVSD,* left ventricular systolic dysfunction; *MR,* mitral regurgitation; *N,* normal; *r,* correlation coefficient; *ROC,* receiver operating characteristic; *RHD,* rheumatic heart disease; *RV,* right ventricle; *RWMA,* regional wall motion abnormalities; *Sn,* sensitivity; *Sp,* specificity.

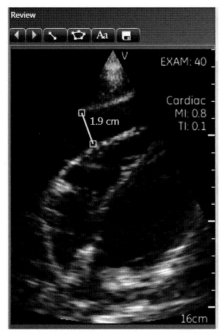

FIG. 46.4 Use of handheld echocardiography to identify pericardial effusion. In this subcostal view, the effusion can be recognized as loculated and moderate in size.

The international consensus has recommended a systematic approach of obtaining multiple views in a protocoled manner. HHE does not require the execution of all views used on standard echocardiography. The suggested views for an FCU examination include subcostal long axis, subcostal IVC, parasternal long axis, parasternal short axis, and apical four chamber.[43] Clearly these recommendations should be seen as the minimum necessary number of views and have been designed to limit duration of the examination in time-sensitive scenarios. When appropriate, we also recommend the acquisition of apical two- and three-chamber views. In a time-limited examination, there is a need to employ whichever views are necessary to answer the clinical question, informed by the insight that all may not be possible with HHE (Fig. 46.5). If the device is equipped with color, then this should be employed in each view as well.

Documentation of results is also necessary. The ASE has recommended that in addition to identification data and results, limitations of the study and recommendations for additional studies should be reported.[5] A suggested template is shown in Fig. 46.6.[8]

QUANTITATIVE ASSESSMENT WITH HANDHELD ECHOCARDIOGRAPHY

The size of a regurgitant jet by color Doppler and its temporal resolution are influenced by transducer frequency, settings such as gain, output power, Nyquist limit, and depth of the sector. HHE devices do not have the ability to significantly change these settings. The predominant strength of handheld echocardiography lies in its immediate ability to facilitate bedside decisions based on "eye-balling" chamber size, function, and severity of valvular lesions. However, a semiquantitative approach can also be implemented depending on the features available on a device.[44]

Visual estimation and template matching have been the predominant manner with which to evaluate EF.[19,20,24,25,35,45–47] However, semiquantitative approaches including linear measurements (Fig. 46.7), with the Teichholz or Quinones formula to calculate EF, or mitral annular systolic plane excursion (mitral annular plane systolic excursion [MAPSE]; normal MAPSE is greater than 11 mm for women and greater than 13 mm for men) can be employed.[16,37] In the future, models incorporating speckle tracking technology, initialized and constrained by a deformable model may offer an automated approach to assessment of the severity of LV dysfunction with HHE.[48] The assessment of volume status may be assisted by evaluation of IVC size, and pulmonary congestion may be identified by the detection of "lung comets" caused by fluid in the

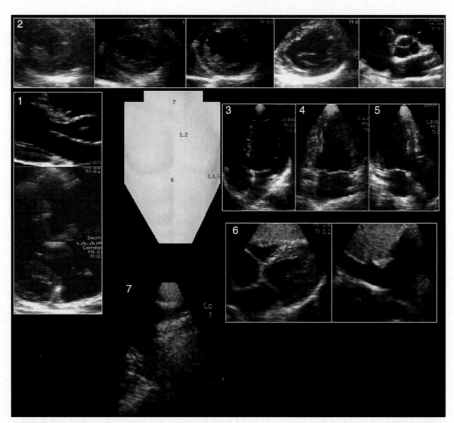

FIG. 46.5 Suggested views for handheld echocardiography. (1 and 2) Parasternal long axis view (PLAX) and parasternal short-axis view (PSAX) (including modified views of pulmonary, tricuspid valve, and short-axis sweep for LV function and regional wall motion assessment. (3, 4, and 5) Apical views 2ch, 3ch, 4ch as illustrated and 5ch for AR, AS assessment. (6) Subcostal long-axis and IVC views 7) aortic arch view.

Study Number		Date		
Subject Name		Age	Sex	
BMI		Medical Record #:		
Primary indication for standard echocardiogram				

Findings:

Normal cardiac examination:	Yes	No		
Mitral stenosis:	None	Mild	Moderate	Severe
Mitral regurgitation:	None	Mild	Moderate	Severe
Mitral valve prolapse:	Yes	No		
Aortic stenosis:	None	Mild	Moderate	Severe
Aortic regurgitation:	None	Mild	Moderate	Severe
Ascending aortic dilatation:	Yes	No		
Pulmonic stenosis:	None	Mild		
Pulmonic regurgitation:	None	Mild	Moderate	Severe
Tricuspid stenosis:	None	Mild	Moderate	Severe
Tricuspid regurgitation:	None	Mild	Moderate	Severe
Pulmonary hypertension:	Yes	No	Moderate	Severe
Atrial septal defect:	Yes	No		
Ventricular septal defect:	Yes	No		
Hypertrophic cardiomyopathy:	Yes	No		
LV hypertrophy:	Yes	No		
LV dilatation:	Yes	No		
LV function:	Normal	Reduced (LV ejection fraction <40%)		
RV dilatation:	Yes	No		
RV function:	Normal	Reduced (tricuspid annular systolic excursion <1.5 cm)		
Estimated right atrial pressure:	Normal	Elevated		
Pericardial effusion:	Yes	No		
Other congenital heart disease:				

FIG. 46.6 Proposed handheld echocardiography report. In addition to a description of all valves and chambers, the report should include commentary about particular limitations and guidance for additional testing. (*From Mehta M, Jacobson T, Peters D, et al. Handheld ultrasound versus physical examination in patients referred for transthoracic echocardiography for a suspected cardiac condition. JACC Cardiovasc Imag. 2014;7(10):983–990.*)

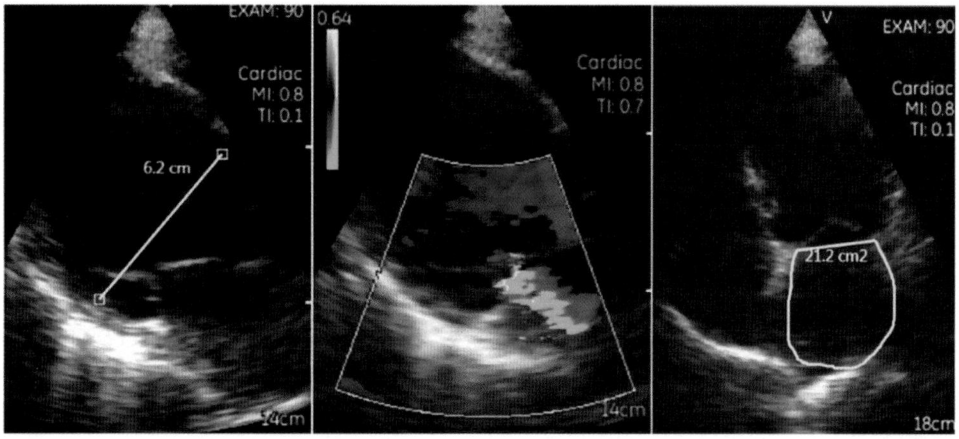

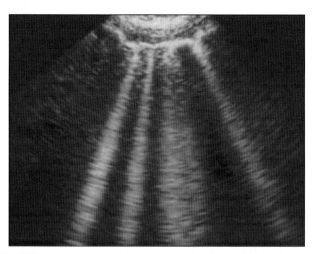

FIG. 46.7 Approach to the patient with left ventricle (LV) dysfunction. Multiple views should include measurement of LV size, recognition of mitral regurgitation and its severity, and measurement of left atrium enlargement.

FIG. 46.8 Lung ultrasound for evidence of pulmonary congestion. This "comet tail" phenomenon is thought to be a consequence of fluid in the pulmonary septa.

interlobular septa (Fig. 46.8). The use of IVC collapsibility and lung comets facilitate differentiation of cardiogenic from pulmonary causes of dyspnea.[49]

As a means to facilitate more accurate determination of valvular heart disease, Beaton et al. have modified the classification of pathological valvular lesions by the World Heart Federation (WHF) (Table 46.5).[36] HHE-acquired examples of mitral regurgitation (MR) (see Fig. 46.7) and aortic regurgitation (Fig. 46.9) can be assessed using this methodology. The importance of nonstandard views is demonstrated in a patient with carcinoid syndrome with moderate pulmonary and severe tricuspid regurgitation (Fig. 46.10).

The current generation of handheld devices cannot determine valvular stenosis, diastolic dysfunction, and pulmonary pressures with a satisfactory degree of accuracy. Stenotic lesions present a unique challenge for HHE, because continuous-wave (CW)-derived mean and peak gradients and valve areas cannot be calculated. A unique strategy has been developed to assess the significance of aortic stenosis, in addition to assessing the degree of calcification. The mobility of each cusp is scored as 0, 1, 2 with increments based on degree of restriction. A score of 3 or more has a sensitivity of 84% and a specificity of 90% for moderate to severe aortic stenosis and has demonstrated incremental diagnostic value over and above physical examination for assessment of aortic valve pathology (Fig. 46.11).[33]

The use of HHE for assessment of pulmonary stenosis and pulmonary hypertension are compromised by the absence of CW Doppler. Certain morphological features can indicate the presence of increased RV afterload, including increased RV wall thickness and systolic flattening of the interventricular septum.

TABLE 46.5 Modification of World Heart Federation Criteria to Recognize Significant Mitral Regurgitation and Aortic Regurgitation

CRITERIA	PATHOLOGIC MR	PATHOLOGIC AR
2012 WHF criteria	Seen in 2 views	Seen in 2 views
	In at least 1 view jet length >2 cm	In at least 1 view, jet length >1 cm
	Velocity >3 m/sec for one complete envelope	Velocity >3 m/s in early diastole
	Pansystolic jet in at least 1 envelope	Pansystolic jet in at least 1 envelope
Modified criteria		
	Seen in 2 views	Seen in 2 views
	In at least 1 view jet length >2 cm	In at least 1 view, jet length >1 cm
	Pansystolic jet (by color Doppler)	Pansystolic jet (by color Doppler)

AR, Aortic regurgitation; *MR,* Mitral regurgitation; *WHF,* World Heart Federation.

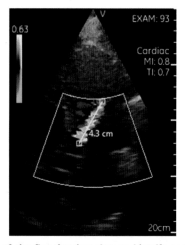

FIG. 46.9 Use of the five-chamber view to identify aortic regurgitation (AR). Quantification of AR severity remains challenging even on full echocardiography machines and the recognition of significant AR at handheld echocardiography is best followed up with a full echocardiogram.

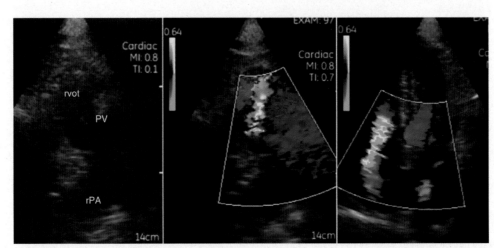

FIG. 46.10 Assessment of right-sided heart valves using handheld echocardiography, leading to diagnosis of carcinoid syndrome. The use of modified parasternal long axis view (PLAX) *(left, center panels)* confirms the presence of moderate pulmonary regurgitation (PR). Severe tricuspid regurgitation (TR) can be recognized in the modified A4C view.

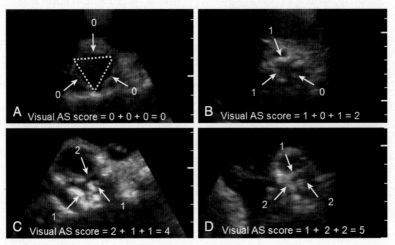

FIG. 46.11 **Semiquantitative analysis of aortic stenosis.** The mobility of each cusp is scored as 0, 1, 2 with increments based on degree of restriction. A score of 3 or more has a sensitivity of 84% and a specificity of 90% for moderate-to-severe aortic stenosis and has demonstrated incremental diagnostic value over and above physical examination for assessment of aortic valve pathology. *(From Abe Y, Ito M, Tanaka C, et al. A novel and simple method using pocket-sized echocardiography to screen for aortic stenosis. J Am Soc Echocardiogr. 2013;26(6):589–596.)*

SPECIFIC ROLES FOR HANDHELD ECHOCARDIOGRAPHY

The ASE consensus document has identified three appropriate settings for use of HHE[40]:

1. The need for clinical evaluation is emergent or urgent, echocardiography is not immediately available, and where the findings from HHE-facilitated physical examination would allow more rapid triage and directed clinical management
2. When echocardiography is not practical (e.g., frequent serial exams to follow up an ultrasound finding)
3. In underserved or remote populations where standard platforms are unavailable (e.g., rural and remote applications, or for screening athletes away from a medical facility)

HANDHELD ECHOCARDIOGRAPHY AS A SCREENING TOOL

The screening of asymptomatic populations implies an initial risk-evaluation process,[50] and requires certain specifications to be fulfilled. The findings should be identifiable with HHE, somewhat prevalent, associated with morbidity, and easily missed on physical examination. The findings need to translate into a therapeutic response (e.g., LV dysfunction in asymptomatic patients). Populations that have been subject to HHE screening protocols include hypertensive patients

screened for presence of left ventricular hypertrophy (LVH), rheumatic heart disease screening in rural or remote settings, athletes, patients at risk of asymptomatic LV dysfunction, and valvular heart disease in the elderly.

Preparticipation cardiovascular screening is the practice of systematically evaluating large, general populations of athletes before participation in sports with the purpose of identifying abnormalities where exertion could provoke disease progression or cardiac death. The American Heart Association (AHA) guidelines recommend a history and physical examination, whereas the European guidelines additionally recommend a 12-lead ECG.[51,52] HHE echocardiography is not currently in preparticipation guidelines, but may prove to be an inexpensive way of adding incremental diagnostic information.[53,54]

LV dysfunction is a precursor to heart failure, but the ideal screening modality is unclear. The prevalence of asymptomatic left ventricular systolic dysfunction (LVSD) ranges from 2% to 8% in adults and up to 20% in selected high-risk population groups.[55] HHE is a feasible and accurate test for detection of asymptomatic impairment of EF,[46,56] but the detection of more subtle indices of LV systolic and diastolic dysfunction remain problematic.

There is tremendous potential for HHE in rural and remote communities, where the scarcity of resources and funds often necessitate an inexpensive approach. Beaton evaluated the modified WHF criteria for evaluating rheumatic heart disease in Uganda using HHE and found good sensitivity and specificity compared to standard echocardiography (79% and 87% respectively).[36,57] In addition to the portability and cost benefits, the rapid transmission of data enables remote, expert consultation.[58] HHE has been used to evaluate 1023 studies that were uploaded from rural and remote regions of India to a cloud server enabling reading by expert physicians.[59]

COST AND WORKFLOW ISSUES

The use of echocardiography has steadily increased, reflecting the population burden of cardiovascular disease. The development of appropriate use criteria has been a response to curb the cost burden and inappropriate use that has paralleled the growth of echocardiography.[60] HHE has been proposed as a modality that may reduce complete echocardiograms, improve work flow, and have cost benefits as well. Further routine utilization of HHE in the outpatient and inpatient settings may reduce the need for standard echocardiograms and thereby reduce cost.[34,38,61] The workflow in an echocardiography lab can be improved upon by triaging echocardiography requests and providing a less cumbersome alternative to periprocedural assistance. Similarly, multiple repeat assessment for LV function, fluid status, or pericardial effusion size evaluation can be assessed with HHE. There are also fewer quantifiable benefits to earlier confirmation or exclusion of a provisional diagnosis enabling streamlined care. A comparison of physical examination and HHE-guided decision making yielded a higher diagnostic yield and cost saving per person using the HHE approach.[8]

FUTURE DEVELOPMENTS

Miniaturization and integration have heralded the smartphone revolution. An HHE device already connects to and relies on powerful and ubiquitous commercial smartphone devices for processing. The use of HHE in the education of medical students and junior doctors will position such a smartphone device as a useful addition to the physical examination.

The growth of HHE will be facilitated by adding functionality to handheld devices—particularly spectral Doppler. The key is to maintain simplicity while improving diagnostic yield and functionality. Thus, automated assessment of dimension and function—now a feature of high-end scanners—could be implemented on these devices.[62] This would enable HHE to be a rapid bedside diagnostic tool with a built-in safety threshold for inexperienced users.

A large amount of literature is dedicated to comparing SE to physical examination and HHE. Further evaluation is mandated to assess its role as an alternative to standard echocardiography in specific situations. This may require future randomized controlled trials.

Finally, a regulatory framework needs to be established around the documentation, storage, and transfer of data that preserves patient confidentiality. Issues regarding reimbursement and legal liabilities need to be discussed in appropriate forums. Indeed, the primary costs will reflect logistical issues including storage, preservation, and security of information rather than the time taken for echocardiography. Inherent in the regulatory framework and legal requirements is accreditation and validation of devices, which is likely to become a challenge as more devices enter the market.

Suggested Reading

Beaton, A., Lu, J. C., Aliku, T., et al. (2015). The utility of handheld echocardiography for early rheumatic heart disease diagnosis: a field study. *European Heart Journal Cardiovascular Imaging, 16*(5), 475–482.

Mehta, M., Jacobson, T., Peters, D., et al. (2014). Handheld ultrasound versus physical examination in patients referred for transthoracic echocardiography for a suspected cardiac condition. *JACC Cardiovascular Imaging, 7*(10), 983–990.

Mirabel, M., Celermajer, D., Beraud, A. S., et al. (2015). Pocket-sized focused cardiac ultrasound: strengths and limitations. *Archives of Cardiovascular Diseases, 108*(3), 197–205.

Spencer, K. T., Kimura, B. J., Korcarz, C. E., et al. (2013). Focused cardiac ultrasound: recommendations from the American Society of Echocardiography. *Journal of the American Society of Echocardiography, 26*(6), 567–581.

Thomenius, K. E. (2009). Miniaturization of ultrasound scanners. *Ultrasound Clinics, 4*(3), 385–389.

A complete reference list can be found online at ExpertConsult.com.

Appropriate Use of Echocardiography

Rory B. Weiner

INTRODUCTION

Echocardiography is an important tool in the diagnosis and management of cardiovascular disease. The detailed cardiac structural and functional information that echocardiography provides, coupled with its portability and lack of ionizing radiation, has established this imaging modality as a critical tool in the care of patients with known or suspected cardiovascular disease. However, there has been concern in recent years regarding the rapid growth of echocardiography utilization, which was estimated at 6%–8% per year in the early 2000s.[1,2] Although the widespread use of echocardiography has been in keeping with the overall growth in cardiac imaging services,[2] geographic variation[3] and concerns regarding appropriate use[4] have helped stimulate a drive for improved utilization of clinical echocardiography services.

DEVELOPMENT OF APPROPRIATE USE CRITERIA

The American College of Cardiology Foundation (ACCF), along with other subspecialty societies, developed Appropriate Use Criteria (AUC)[5] in an effort to promote more effective utilization of diagnostic testing and procedures in cardiovascular medicine, and echocardiography has been a focus of the AUC. The AUC were developed primarily out of concern regarding an increase in the use of noninvasive cardiac imaging services and Medicare spending between 1995 and 2006, and the ACCF published its first AUC document in 2005.[5] AUC are distinct from clinical practice guidelines, as guidelines are intended to inform clinicians when a diagnostic test or procedure should or should not be performed. In contrast, AUC delineate clinical scenarios in which ordering a test or procedure may be considered appropriate or less appropriate.

Initial AUC for transthoracic (TTE) and transesophageal (TEE) echocardiography were published in 2007[4] and stress echocardiography (SE) AUC were released in 2008.[6] The AUC are based on a number of common clinical scenarios in which echocardiography is most often used. Revised and updated AUC covering adult TTE, TEE, and SE were published in 2011;[7] however, this document does not address the use of perioperative TEE. AUC for initial outpatient pediatric echocardiography were published in 2014.[8] The 2011 revised AUC for adult echocardiography incorporated data and recommendations provided by interval clinical data and standards documents published after the release of the initial AUC in 2007 and 2008. Additionally, the revised AUC clarified areas in which omissions or lack of clarity existed in the original criteria. The approach for the revised 2011 AUC for adult echocardiography was to create five broad types of clinical scenarios regarding the possible use of echocardiography: (1) for initial diagnosis; (2) to guide therapy or management, regardless of symptom status; (3) to evaluate a change in clinical status or cardiac exam; (4) for early follow-up without change in clinical status; and (5) for late follow-up without change in clinical status. Certain specific clinical scenarios were addressed with additional focused indications. The evaluation of heart failure provides an example of the main types of clinical scenarios found in the AUC for TTE (Fig. 47.1).

The scenarios are rated by a panel with a broad array of expertise (i.e., including not only echocardiographers) to evaluate the "appropriateness" of echocardiography in each situation. AUC ratings are created by applying the validated, prospectively based modified RAND (Research and Development) appropriateness method.[9] Briefly, this process involves: (1) the development of a list of clinical indications, assumptions, and definitions by a writing group; (2) a review of indications and feedback from a review panel; and (3) two rounds of indication ratings by a rating panel (first round, no interaction among panel members; second round, panel interaction) and determination of a composite appropriate use score (Fig. 47.2).

An appropriate imaging study is defined as "one in which the expected incremental information, combined with clinical judgment, exceeds the expected negative consequences by a sufficiently wide margin for a specific indication that the procedure is generally considered acceptable care and a reasonable approach for the indication."[5] Ratings are made on a scale of 1–9, in which a score of 9 indicates highly appropriate use of testing. Using the iterative modified Delphi exercise process described previously, a final rating score is established for each indication, and grouped as A, a score of 7–9, indicating an appropriate test for the specific indication (the test *is* generally acceptable and *is* a reasonable approach for the indication); U, a score of 4–6, indicating uncertainty for the specific indication (the test *may* be generally acceptable and *may* be a reasonable approach for the indication); and I, a score of 1–3, indicating an inappropriate test for that indication (the test *is not* generally acceptable and *is not* a reasonable approach for the indication).[5]

The AUC methodology has subsequently evolved over time.[10] Importantly, the terminology used to describe the three appropriateness categories has changed. As mentioned previously, studies for specific clinical indications were initially divided into appropriate, uncertain, or inappropriate categories. The revised terminology specifies "appropriate care," "may be appropriate care," and "rarely appropriate care." It is therefore more explicitly recognized that a rarely appropriate study may be correct for a specific patient at a specific time; therefore, the goal for rarely appropriate studies is not necessarily zero.

APPLICATION OF APPROPRIATE USE CRITERIA

One of the first uses of the AUC for echocardiography was to characterize practice patterns and determine appropriateness rates in clinical practice. A number of studies evaluated the 2007 AUC for TTE in various practice settings, including academic medical centers,[11–13] Veterans Affairs (VA) hospitals,[14] and community settings.[15,16] Several common themes emerged, namely that 10%–15% of TTEs could not be classified by the AUC; however, of those classified, the majority (~90%) were deemed appropriate. The influence of practice location was noted, as the rate of

Evaluation of Heart Failure with TTE	Score
Initial evaluation of known or suspected HF (systolic or diastolic)	A (9)
Re-evaluation of known HF with a change in clinical status *without* a clear precipitating factor	A (8)
Re-evaluation of known HF with a change in clinical status *with* a clear precipitating factor	U (4)
Re-evaluation of known HF to guide therapy	A (9)
Routine surveillance (<1 yr) when there is no change in clinical status or cardiac exam	I (2)
Routine surveillance (≥1 yr) when there is no change in clinical status or cardiac exam	U (6)

FIG. 47.1 Appropriate use criteria for transthoracic echocardiography for the evaluation of heart failure. Clinical indications are typically organized around basic types of clinical scenarios (for initial diagnosis, to guide therapy or management, to evaluate change in clinical status or physical examination, and for early or late follow-up without change in clinical status). *A,* Appropriate; *I,* inappropriate (rarely appropriate); *HF,* heart failure; *TTE,* transthoracic echocardiography; *U,* uncertain (may be appropriate). (*Adapted from Douglas PS, Garcia MJ, Haines DE, et al. ACCF/ASE/AHA/ASNC/HFSA/HRS/ SCAI/SCCM/SCCT/SCMR 2011 appropriate use criteria for echocardiography.* J Am Coll Cardiol. *2011;57(9):1126–1166.*)

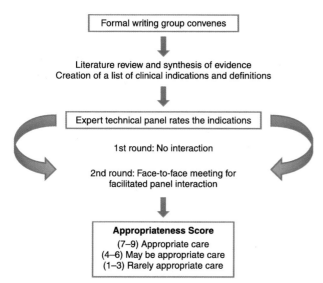

FIG. 47.2 The RAND method with modified Delphi process for developing Appropriate Use Criteria. The clinical indications developed by the writing group are circulated for external review prior to rating by the technical panel. The expert technical panel rating the indications is a diverse group, not just echocardiographers, with a broad array of expertise in various cardiac imaging modalities and clinical care. (*Modified from Patel MR, Spertus JA, Brindis RG, et al. ACCF proposed method for evaluating the appropriateness of cardiovascular imaging. J Am Coll Cardiol. 2005;46(8):1606–1613.*)

inappropriate studies was higher in the outpatient (vs. inpatient) environment. Subsequent studies at academic medical centers utilizing the 2011 AUC showed that the updated AUC were able to classify the vast majority of TTEs and filled virtually all of the gaps in the initial AUC.[17,18] Another finding was that with the improved classification of TTEs with the 2011 AUC, it appeared that the appropriate rate of TTEs was not as high as initially thought (e.g., previously unclassified studies were more likely to be categorized as rarely appropriate).[18] This indicated that there may be more opportunities for practice improvement and improved utilization than initially realized. Studies of TEE utilization in general show higher appropriate rates,[17,19] possibly due to the more invasive nature of the procedure and the associated case review and need for informed consent. Studies of SE show lower appropriate rates,[20] which is consistent with studies of other forms of stress testing.[21] Furthermore, recent analyses indicate that AUC have relevance beyond the United States, with a recent study in the United Kingdom reporting similar rarely appropriate rates for TTE.[22]

In addition to characterizing the percentage of appropriate and rarely appropriate studies, the analyses of practice patterns identified a relatively small number of specific indications that constituted the most common rarely appropriate indications, which varied based on practice setting (outpatient vs. inpatient) (Box 47.1). In the outpatient setting, the most common rarely appropriate TTEs are mainly "surveillance" studies, referring to repeat studies in patients with known cardiovascular disease, but no change in clinical status or physical examination.[17,18] In this context, if echocardiograms are ordered prior to prespecified time intervals (e.g., within 3 years in the case of mild valvular disease, and no change in clinical status or examination) they are classified as rarely appropriate.

Moving beyond a description of ordering patterns in clinical practice, educational intervention studies have been designed, which incorporate AUC into the process of educating ordering clinicians. The aim of such studies is to reduce the number of rarely appropriate TTEs. The first study was conducted on the inpatient medical service of an academic medical center.[23] In this time-series analysis, an educational intervention consisting of a didactic lecture, a pocket card applying the AUC to common clinical scenarios, and twice-monthly feedback emails of ordering behavior resulted in a significant reduction in inappropriate TTEs, and a significant increase in appropriate TTEs. This study was limited by the fact that it was conducted in the inpatient environment and lacked a randomized study design. A subsequent randomized controlled study attempted to address these limitations by utilizing a similar AUC-based educational intervention in an outpatient cardiology environment.[24] This study was limited to physicians-in-training, with a study population consisting of

BOX 47.1 Common Rarely Appropriate Indications for Transthoracic Echocardiography in Outpatient and Inpatient Settings

Outpatient
- Routine surveillance (<3 year) of mild valvular stenosis without change in clinical status or cardiac examination
- Routine reevaluation for surveillance of known ascending aortic dilation or history of aortic dissection without change in clinical status or cardiac examination, and findings will not change management or therapy
- Routine evaluation of systemic hypertension without symptoms or signs of hypertensive heart disease
- Evaluation of left ventricular function with previous ventricular function evaluation showing normal function in patients without change in clinical status or cardiac examination
- Routine perioperative evaluation of ventricular function with no symptoms or signs of cardiovascular disease

Inpatient
- Transient fever without evidence of bacteremia or a new murmur
- Transient bacteremia with a pathogen not typically associated with infective endocarditis and/or a documented nonendovascular source of infection
- Lightheadedness/presyncope without other signs/symptoms of cardiac disease
- Suspected pulmonary embolism in order to establish diagnosis

cardiovascular medicine fellows. Nonetheless, the proportion of rarely appropriate TTEs was significantly lower in the intervention group than in the control group, and the proportion of appropriate TTEs ordered by the intervention group was significantly higher. These studies indicate that it is feasible to teach clinicians about appropriate use, and that providing feedback about ordering behavior may improve utilization. Additionally, it appears that knowledge of local practice patterns and "targeting" the educational intervention toward the most common rarely appropriate indications for TTE may aid in creating a successful intervention.

Despite the encouraging results of the educational intervention studies aimed at TTE ordering, it should be emphasized that attempts to utilize AUC to improve utilization of other cardiovascular imaging modalities (e.g., single-photon emission computed tomography [SPECT]) have been met with limited success (Table 47.1).[25] Similarly, a study of SE showed that educating the ordering providers failed to reduce the rate of rarely appropriate studies.[26] Attempting to explain the variability in the effectiveness of educational interventions, it is important to note that the "successful" TTE studies used active feedback as a component of the intervention, whereas the SPECT and SE studies did not. The importance and role of feedback in AUC-based educational efforts is supported by the results of another study of TTE and SPECT in a large multisite cardiovascular practice over a wide geographic area.[27] Another component of an education-based quality improvement initiative that may enhance success in improving utilization is the threat of loss of reimbursement, as documented in a study of coronary computed tomographic angiography (CTA).[28] It therefore appears that AUC-based interventions that focus on feedback and financial implications may be most effective. The available literature also suggest that it may be more difficult to improve the utilization of stress testing (SPECT or SE) compared to resting examinations (TTE or CTA).[29]

Other unanswered questions remain regarding the use of AUC as a tool to improve patient selection for cardiac imaging. One is with respect to the sustainability of the AUC-based intervention to improve utilization. The CTA study with financial ramifications[28] showed sustained benefit at 6 months. However, the inpatient echocardiography study[23] appeared to lose its benefit after cessation of the educational intervention,[30] and the outpatient study[24] did not provide this type of follow-up data. Another issue with respect to the TTE studies is that they focused on physicians-in-training at an academic medical center. Testing this

TABLE 47.1 Appropriate Use Criteria-Based Educational Intervention Studies in Cardiovascular Imaging

FIRST AUTHOR	IMAGING MODALITY	RANDOMIZED TRIAL (Y/N)	DECREASE IN RARELY APPROPRIATE (Y/N)	PRE- VERSUS POST-RARELY APPROPRIATE (%)	FEEDBACK UTILIZED (Y/N)
Bhatia[23]	TTE	N	Y	13 vs. 5	Y
Bhatia[24]	TTE	Y	Y	13 vs. 34[a]	Y
Gibbons[25]	SPECT	N	N	14.4 vs. 11.7	N
Willens[26]	SE	N	N	31.5 vs. 32.4	N
Johnson[27]	TTE	N	Y	18.5 vs. 6.9	Y
	SPECT		Y	20.5 vs. 11.1	Y
Chinnaiyan[28]	CTA	N	Y	14.6 vs. 5.8	Y

CTA, Coronary computed tomographic angiography; *SPECT,* single photon emission computed tomography; *TTE,* transthoracic echocardiography.
[a]% rarely appropriate in the intervention versus control groups.

type of AUC-based educational intervention in attending physicians—and even in physician extenders—in various academic and community practice settings is necessary, and is an area of active research.[31]

Recent data indicate that the rate at which echocardiography is performed is no longer increasing, but has begun to decrease.[32] The United States General Accounting Office reported in 2008 that Medicare spending on cardiac imaging services more than doubled from 2000 to 2006, while a subsequent Medicare Payment Advisory Commission report to Congress noted that the annual rate of growth in the number of echocardiograms provided per Medicare beneficiary was only 2.6% between 2005 and 2009, and decreased by 0.8% per year between 2009 and 2010.[33] The explanation for this finding is not clear, and multiple factors may be at play. It is possible that the AUC for echocardiography played a role in improved patient selection and improved utilization. A meta-analysis suggests that since the release of AUC, rates of appropriate TTE have increased, but SE and TEE have not seen the same improvement in appropriate rates.[29] This may be due to the initial high rate of appropriate TEEs and the finding that it has been more challenging to improve utilization of stress testing. Other educational programs have also been championed during this time period, including the American Board of Internal Medicine's Choosing Wisely campaign, which has been directed at patients and providers.[34]

FUTURE DIRECTIONS FOR APPROPRIATE USE CRITERIA

The optimal approach to incorporate AUC into patient selection remains to be determined, and it should be emphasized that clinical judgment remains important and is not to be replaced by criteria. Several other remaining issues persist when contemplating incorporating AUC into the clinical care of patients. First, one must consider the documented variation in inter-rater reliability when using AUC to classify cardiac imaging studies[35] and the need to better standardize the process of AUC classification. Second, further investigation into assessing the clinical impact of appropriate versus rarely appropriate studies is needed, as there are conflicting data on this subject. In one study, new and important TTE abnormalities were more frequently found in appropriate studies compared with rarely appropriate studies in both academic and community practice settings,[15] although the rate of new findings in the rarely appropriate category is not zero. A separate study at an academic medical center documented a high rate of appropriate TTEs; however, it reported that less than one-third of TTEs resulted in an active change in clinical care.[36] This study fails to account for the fact that continuation of current care may be an important impact of an echocardiogram, and highlights difficulties in determining the clinical impact of appropriate versus rarely appropriate studies. Furthermore, a recent study examined the AUC as a prognostic tool in patients with valvular heart disease undergoing SE.[37] In this study, the 12-month event-free survival was significantly reduced in patients with appropriate (or uncertain) studies compared to patients with rarely appropriate studies. This suggests that in certain patient populations, appropriateness designations of echocardiograms may help differentiate patients with high and low risks of cardiac events. This finding requires validation in other patient populations and with other echocardiographic modalities beyond SE.

Tracking the appropriateness of echocardiograms is also an important issue, and is now a requirement for Intersocietal Accreditation Commission (IAC) accreditation.[38] The development of automated tools may facilitate real-time tracking of appropriateness. In one study, an electronic application was shown to allow for rapid and accurate implementation of the AUC for TTE at the point of service.[39] There was excellent agreement between the electronic classification and investigator-determined classification, and the mean time required for electronic classification was 55 seconds. Incorporation of AUC-based decision support at the time of order entry warrants study as an approach to improve patient selection for echocardiography. In a prospective multi-center study, which included various imaging modalities for assessment of coronary artery disease (including SE), a point-of-order AUC-based decision support tool enabled rapid determination of test appropriateness, and was associated with improved utilization.[40] The optimal use of AUC in decision support, and whether or not a "hard stop" should be in place for rarely appropriate studies, has not been clearly defined and warrants further study. A related issue is how AUC-based determinations correlate with other metrics to determine the appropriateness of echocardiography. In an SE study, AUC designations were compared to pre-authorization determinations, based on radiology benefit managers' pre-certification guidelines, and there were a large number of appropriate and uncertain studies that would not have received pre-authorization.[41] Whether AUC should be considered the "gold standard" is debatable, although this study calls for the need for greater consistency in the methods used to determine the appropriateness of echocardiograms. A potential framework for how AUC may be incorporated into clinical care to help improve patient selection for echocardiography is provided in Fig. 47.3. Adherence to AUC and the subsequent impact on clinical outcomes, although difficult to study, is a critical area in need of further investigation.

Much of the focus of AUC in echocardiography is on overutilization, or inappropriate utilization, of this imaging modality. However, AUC have also helped to identify an often forgotten issue, namely that of underutilization. In one study, an analysis of hospitalized patients on a medical service who were discharged without being referred for an echocardiogram showed that in nearly 16% of patients a TTE would have been appropriate.[42] Although provocative, AUC are not practice guidelines, meaning that even if a study is appropriate it does not mean that it should necessarily be performed (e.g., not having what would be considered an appropriate study may be acceptable in certain situations). To further investigate underutilization, a more recent analysis of patients with at least moderate valvular dysfunction showed that only 59% underwent follow-up echocardiography within the time period recommended by practice guidelines.[43] This indicates that the issue of underutilization is real, and AUC may help characterize practice patterns in an effort to identify groups of patients who may not be receiving desired or necessary follow-up imaging.

The focus of this chapter is the appropriate use of echocardiography. It must be recognized that clinical echocardiograms are performed in the context of other existing and complimentary imaging modalities, such as SPECT, CTA, and cardiac magnetic resonance imaging. As such, the most recent AUC publications focus on specific disease conditions, such

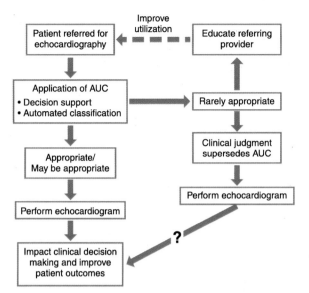

FIG. 47.3 Appropriate selection of patients for echocardiography. A possible approach for application of Appropriate Use Criteria *(AUC)* to help improve patient selection and minimize rarely appropriate echocardiograms. Adherence to AUC and the subsequent impact on clinical outcomes needs further investigation.

as stable ischemic heart disease[44] and heart failure,[45] and describe the appropriate use of various imaging modalities in parallel for each clinical situation. Future AUC will most likely be developed and integrated into clinical care in a multimodality fashion, as opposed to each individual imaging test in isolation.

A final consideration is the integration of AUC in the larger context of quality improvement in echocardiography. The mandate for continuous quality improvement initiatives in echocardiography dates back to the 1990s.[46] There are many key components of echocardiography laboratory quality, including the laboratory structure (physical laboratory, equipment, sonographers, and physicians) and the imaging process (patient selection, image acquisition, image interpretation, results communication, and the incorporation of results into care).[47] AUC fall mainly in the patient selection area of the imaging process. In order to achieve overall quality in echocardiography, AUC must be utilized in conjunction with other laboratory processes that promote quality, such as efforts to reduce intra- and inter-reader variability in image interpretation,[48] improving access to care, and strategic planning for new reimbursement models.[49]

Suggested Reading

Douglas, P., Iskandrian, A. E., Krumholz, H. M., et al. (2006). Achieving quality in cardiovascular imaging: proceedings from the American College of Cardiology-Duke University Medical Center Think Tank on Quality in Cardiovascular Imaging. *Journal of the American College of Cardiology, 48*(10), 2141–2151.

Douglas, P. S., Garcia, M. J., Haines, D. E., et al. (2011). ACCF/ASE/AHA/ASNC/HFSA/HRS/ SCAI/ SCCM/SCCT/SCMR 2011 appropriate use criteria for echocardiography. *Journal of the American College of Cardiology, 57*(9), 1126–1166.

Douglas, P. S., & Picard, M. H. (2013). Healthcare reform for imagers: finding a way forward now. *JACC Cardiovascular Imaging, 6*(3), 385–391.

Hendel, R. C., Patel, M. R., Allen, J. M., et al. (2013). Appropriate use of cardiovascular technology: 2013 ACCF appropriate use criteria methodology update: a report of the American College of Cardiology Foundation appropriate use criteria task force. *Journal of the American College of Cardiology, 61*(12), 1305–1317.

Wiener, D. H. (2014). Achieving high-value cardiac imaging: challenges and opportunities. *Journal of the American Society of Echocardiography, 27*(1), 1–7.

A complete reference list can be found online at ExpertConsult.com.

48 Echocardiography in the Context of Other Cardiac Imaging Modalities

Stephen J. Horgan, Seth Uretsky

INTRODUCTION

Despite advances in imaging technology over the past 20 years, echocardiography has maintained its central role in cardiovascular medicine. Although some of this relates to the fact that echocardiographic technology is also progressing steadily, the primary reason is by virtue of the unique advantages of echocardiography including portability, rapid availability, safety, and excellent temporal resolution. As a result, echocardiography is generally the first tool implemented for the evaluation of a wide variety of clinical indications. Its superior temporal resolution permits better assessment of small or thin mobile structures as well as the physiologic and hemodynamic consequences of disease. Although echocardiography is effectively a real-time imaging modality regarding temporal resolution, cardiac magnetic resonance (CMR) imaging comes in second place, with nuclear imaging and coronary computed tomographic angiography (CCTA) lagging further behind (Table 48.1). On the other hand, the spatial resolution of CCTA and CMR is superior compared with echocardiography. Although spatial resolution is improved with positron emission tomography (PET) compared with single-photon emission computed tomography (SPECT), this imaging characteristic is the Achilles heel of nuclear imaging. Along with ionizing radiation, these properties of the four main imaging modalities are invariably taken into account when considering further evaluation with noninvasive cardiac imaging techniques. Careful consideration should also be given to the cost effectiveness of a diagnostic pathway.

It is rare for a patient to undergo a CMR, CCTA, SPECT, or PET without first having an echocardiogram. Multimodality imaging and echocardiography have a complementary or synergistic relationship. It is always extremely useful to review the prior imaging of a patient when considering the next best test or when protocoling and subsequently analyzing the new study. To address the role of multimodality imaging in the context of echocardiography, seven main topics are discussed as outlined in Fig. 48.1.

CHAMBER QUANTIFICATION: VOLUMES AND FUNCTION

Echocardiography is the mainstay, although not the gold standard, for evaluating chamber size and function through linear measurement, and volume quantification. End-diastolic and end-systolic dimensions and volumes are the most commonly used parameters to describe left ventricular cavity size and function. Volumes derived from linear measurements are confined to the assumption that the left ventricle (LV) is a fixed geometric shape, such as a prolate ellipsoid. As a result, the Recommendations for Cardiac Chamber Quantification by Echocardiography in Adults outline that the Teichholz and Quinone methods for calculating LV volumes are no longer recommended for clinical use.[1] The recommended method for two-dimensional echocardiographic (2DE) volume calculation is the biplane method of disks summation or modified Simpson's rule. Volume is generated by taking an average of the apical four- and two-chamber views, and the measurements are standardized by indexing to body surface area. Foreshortening of the ventricle and wall motion abnormalities can cause erroneous results. Poor endocardial definition is improved by administration of contrast agents. Although contrast-enhanced images provide larger volumes than unenhanced images, these measurements are closer to those found with cardiac magnetic resonance imaging (MRI).[2]

Three-dimensional echocardiographic (3DE) volume measurement is accurate and reproducible and eliminates the error introduced by geometric assumptions in 2DE.[3] It should also be remembered that volume measurements from different imaging modalities should not be used interchangeably. For instance, CT can overestimate and echocardiography underestimate right ventricular (RV) volume when compared with the gold standard CMR.[4] Although accurate and comparable to CMR, 3D-transthoracic echocardiography (TTE) and 3D-transesophageal echocardiography (TEE) tend to underestimate volume and function.[5]

Accurate estimation of LV systolic function is of particular importance in patients under consideration for an implantable cardioverter defibrillator or resynchronization therapy, for those whose profession is dependent on a certain cutoff for LV ejection fraction (LVEF), and in patients undergoing chemotherapy with cardiotoxic agents. Deformation imaging by echocardiography using strain or two-dimensional (2D) speckle tracking permits accurate assessment of global and regional LV systolic function. Strain analysis increases the sensitivity for detecting subclinical myocardial dysfunction in cardiomyopathies before there is an overt drop in LVEF. Multimodality imaging is required when there is some doubt as to the exact LVEF. In this setting, multigated acquisition (MUGA) nuclear imaging or CMR are usually performed and are considered to be the most accurate and reproducible methods for the assessment of LV systolic function. Retrospectively gated CCTA also provides a very accurate evaluation of LVEF but is generally reserved for other indications.

Assessment of RV size and function is challenging due to the complex geometry of the RV chamber. On TTE, RV size is often estimated by visual assessment or "eyeballing." Various surrogates are used to assess size and function, each with their own limitations. 3DE allows volumetric assessment and complements 2D measurements. Although 3DE is accurate, it is time consuming and tends to underestimate volumes compared with CMR. Few laboratories measure RV size and function by 3DE. CMR is the gold standard for the assessment of RV size and function. The usefulness of the echocardiographic "eyeball" method to estimate RV size and systolic function in patients with right heart disease is limited when compared with CMR, specifically with regard to interobserver variability between echocardiographers.[6] Cardiac CT provides accurate and reproducible RV volume measurements when compared with CMR and, like 3DE, is an alternative for patients who have a contraindication to CMR.[7]

The "overloading" effect of chronic regurgitant valve lesions, as well as intracardiac and extracardiac shunts, is best measured by the degree of ventricular dilatation. The accurate assessment of the severity of mitral regurgitation (MR) and aortic insufficiency (AI) by echocardiography is difficult when the lesions are in the moderate to severe range. Although the vena contracta, effective regurgitant orifice area, and flow reversal (pulmonary vein in MR and holodiastolic flow reversal in the aorta in AI) are all useful measures of the severity of valvular dysfunction, regurgitant volume, regurgitant fraction, and LV dilatation are key when determining the need for surgical or transcatheter intervention. Echocardiography is an excellent tool for assessing and monitoring valvular heart disease and carries a class 1B indication for AI and MR. CMR is indicated in patients with moderate or severe AI (stages B, C, and D) and suboptimal echo images for the assessment of LV systolic and diastolic volumes, function, and measurement of AI severity.[8] Like echo, CMR has a class 1B recommendation for the evaluation of AI and is a useful screening tool for associated aortopathies. Aortic magnetic resonance angiography (MRA) or CTA is also indicated in patients with a bicuspid AV when morphology of the aortic sinuses, sinotubular junction, and thoracic aorta cannot be assessed accurately or fully by echo (class 1C). Serial assessment of size and morphology can be achieved with any one of the three modalities (class 1C). CMR is also indicated in patients with chronic primary MR to assess LV and RV volumes, function, and MR severity when these issues are not satisfactorily addressed by TTE (class 1B). There is also evidence to suggest that CMR should be considered when MR severity as assessed by TTE is influencing important clinical decisions, such as the decision to undergo mitral valve surgery (Figs. 48.2 and 48.3; Videos 48.1–48.4).[9] TEE is indicated for the evaluation of chronic primary MR in whom noninvasive imaging provides nondiagnostic information about the severity of MR, mechanism of MR, and/or status of LV function (class 1C).

Unexpected chamber dilatation raises the question of a cardiovascular shunt and is often a finding noticed on TTE. The right atrium and right ventricle are usually dilated when there is a significant shunt proximal to the tricuspid valve, whereas a shunt distal to the tricuspid valve results in LV dilatation (e.g., ventricular septal defect or patent ductus arteriosus). There are other clues on TTE as to the presence of a shunt; for instance,

RV function is usually preserved, and there are increased velocities across the pulmonary valve in shunts proximal to the tricuspid valve. TEE can be performed to localize and define morphology of the shunt. Qp:Qs can also be evaluated during TEE and is defined as $(CSA^{RVOT} \times VTI^{RVOT})/(CSA^{LVOT} \times VTI^{LVOT})$. A patent foramen ovale is best picked up on echocardiography compared with other imaging modalities. Although echocardiography and angiography have traditionally been the primary tools used for the evaluation of cardiac shunts, CCTA and particularly CMR are proving to be very useful in this setting.

CCTA is an excellent modality for demonstrating structural heart disease including septal defects, anomalous pulmonary venous return, and arterial and venous anatomy but is limited in terms of functional analysis. Volumetric analysis can be performed with CT but is hampered by the presence of regurgitant valve lesions and higher doses of radiation with the necessity for retrospective gating. CMR has emerged as an accurate noninvasive alternative for characterization of anatomy and assessment of function. Precise shunt quantification is achieved with CMR using both volumetric cine imaging and phase-contrast cine imaging (see Fig. 48.3; see Videos 48.3–48.5). Phase contrast techniques derive contrast between flowing blood and stationary tissue by manipulating the phase of the

TABLE 48.1 Comparison of Mainstream Noninvasive Cardiovascular Imaging Modalities

	TRANSTHORACIC ECHOCARDIOGRAPHY	TRANSESOPHAGEAL ECHOCARDIOGRAPHY	COMPUTED TOMOGRAPHY	MAGNETIC RESONANCE	SPECT AND PET
Availability	Readily available Portable/bedside if required	Available in most centers but operator dependent	Cardiac CTA only available in centers of expertise	CMR only available in centers of expertise	SPECT usually available PET only available in centers of expertise
Cost	Low	Low to intermediate	Intermediate	High	Intermediate to high
Safety	Safe	Procedural complications are relatively rare	Ionizing radiation (1–14 mSv) Iodinated contrast usually C/I if eGFR <30 mls/min	No radiation Gadolinium based contrast C/I if eGFR <30 mls/min C/I if patient has a device, for example, PPMs[a], ICDs[a], LVADs	Ionizing radiation (3–21 mSv)
Arrhythmia	Impairs quality of 3D imaging (stitch artifact)	Impairs quality of 3D imaging (stitch artifact)	Impairs gating resulting in suboptimal images	Impairs gating resulting in suboptimal images	Impairs gated images
Patient-related factors limiting image quality	Limited windows Narrow field of view Limited by obesity, COPD, and postoperative setting	Esophageal pathology Sedation usually required	Hemodynamically stable only Poor breath-holder	Hemodynamically stable only Claustrophobia Poor breath-holder	Hemodynamically stable only
Temporal resolution	Almost real-time Long loop acquisitions possible	Almost real-time Long loop acquisitions possible	160–200 ms Retrospective acquisition required for full cardiac cycle	30–50 ms with SSFP	8–16 frames per cardiac cycle
Spatial resolution	Dependent on US frequency and depth	Better than transthoracic (increased US frequency possible)	0.5 mm with later generation CT scanners	5–8 mm 0.9–1.2 mm when ECG and respiratory gated (3D acquisition)	9–10 mm A-SPECT or 4–5 mm D-SPECT 4–5 mm PET
Myocardial perfusion imaging	Contrast echo with microbubbles— promising but not FDA approved	Not applicable	Fair—not yet mainstream. Improves diagnostic accuracy of CT	Good	Excellent PET > SPECT
Pericardial assessment	Best modality for evaluating hemodynamic effect	Reasonable for anatomic assessment	Excellent for anatomy (including calcification)	Excellent for both anatomy and hemodynamic effect	Not applicable
Tissue characterization	Limited Contrast enhanced	Limited	Good Hounsfield unit	Excellent	Good Molecular imaging techniques for scar, inflammation, etc.
Extracardiac structures	Limited	Limited	Excellent	Excellent	Limited unless performed with CT attenuation correction

CMR, Cardiac magnetic resonance imaging; CTA, computed tomographic angiogram; C/I, contraindicated; COPD, chronic obstructive pulmonary disease; eGFR, estimated glomerular filtration rate; ECG, electrocardiogram; FDA, Food and Drug Administration; ICD, implantable cardioverter defibrillator; LVAD, left ventricular assist device; PET, positron emission tomography; PPM, permanent pacemaker; SPECT, single-photon emission computed tomography; SSFP, steady-state free precession.
[a]Note is made of MRI-safe PPMs and the fact that some centers perform CMR on patients with ICDs.

magnetization. This method provides accurate measurements of volumes and velocities in the absence of significant turbulence and is the most accurate of the noninvasive modalities.

MORPHOLOGY

LV mass is a prognostically important parameter and should be reported in imaging studies where possible, particularly in patients with hypertension. There are different methods to measure LV mass on TTE, including M-mode and 2DE linear equations, and other 2D-based formulae, such as the truncated ellipsoid and the area-length method. For the linear method, mass is calculated using the unidimensional Devereux formula indexed to body surface area and relies on a normally shaped LV. 3DE has an advantage over 2DE in that potential errors from geometric assumptions are removed. In fact, the estimation of LV mass by 3DE has similar accuracy to the gold standard CMR.[10] Although generally not performed, LV mass may also be assessed by CT with reasonable accuracy.[11] Estimation of mass is less accurate with nuclear techniques.

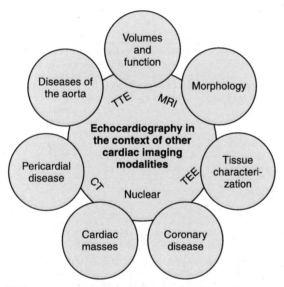

FIG. 48.1 **Chapter outline.** Seven main topics are discussed when addressing echocardiography in the context of other imaging modalities. *CMR,* Cardiac magnetic resonance imaging; *CT,* computed tomography; *TTE,* transthoracic echocardiogram; *TEE,* transesophageal echocardiography.

Abnormal morphology in the setting of congenital or acquired heart disease is usually identified on TTE initially. Pattern recognition allows the experienced sonographer and reader to infer a likely cause or differential diagnosis. Dilated chambers as described previously provide a hint as to the abnormality, but it is anatomic imaging in the form of 3D volumes that permits precise localization of the defect or altered anatomy. Volumetric imaging in 3DE, CCTA, and CMR permits multiplanar reconstruction of congenital abnormalities. Indeed, multimodality imaging is paramount in terms of diagnosis, decision to intervene, and suitability for different therapies, as well as monitoring and follow-up. Congenital heart disease (CHD) is something that adult cardiologists are now seeing more often as infants born with CHD survive into adulthood and require lifelong follow-up and care. Although echocardiography is routinely used in all patients, complementary multimodality imaging is frequently required particularly in postsurgical patients or those with complex CHD. Three-dimensional volume sets with both CT and CMR allow comprehensive assessment of cardiac anatomy, the aorta, pulmonary arteries, and venous return. Quantification of ventricular volumes and function can be achieved with 3DE, CT, and CMR, as discussed. Although CT has superior spatial resolution, CMR has the benefit of complex flow measurements for shunt evaluation.

Anomalies of the coronary arteries are rare, with an incidence of 0.2%–1%.[12] Patients presenting with symptoms resulting from coronary artery anomalies are usually younger and can present with symptoms relating to episodic myocardial ischemia such as chest pain, syncope, ventricular arrhythmia, or sudden cardiac death. In patients with suspected anomalous coronary arteries, echocardiography may establish the diagnosis, but the predictive value remains controversial.[13] Pediatric cardiologists are better versed in looking for anomalous origins of the coronary arteries by TTE compared with adult cardiologists. A particular strength of CCTA is the depiction of coronary artery anatomy including the ostia and course of the coronary vessels (refer to Fig. 48.12, later). The appropriate use criteria ascribe a score of 9 to CCTA for the evaluation of anomalous coronary arteries.[14] CMR is also useful in delineating the proximal course of the coronary arteries and is often considered in younger patients when avoidance of ionizing radiation is preferred.

Another instance in which an initial evaluation with echocardiography leads to further multimodality imaging is acquired abnormal chamber morphology. Examples include excessive hypertrophy/hypertrophic cardiomyopathy, dilated and restrictive cardiomyopathies of uncertain etiology, LV noncompaction, endomyocardial fibrosis, and occasionally Takotsubo cardiomyopathy (Fig. 48.4; Videos 48.6–48.9) to name but a few. CMR is usually recommended when a new diagnosis is made or suggested by TTE. As well as excellent anatomic imaging, CMR offers

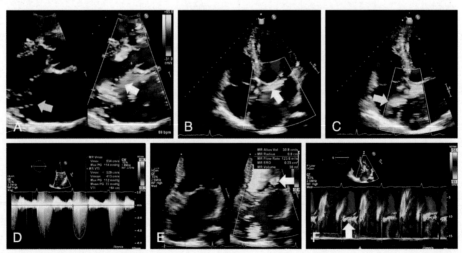

FIG. 48.2 **Mitral regurgitation in the presence of an ASD (TTE).** A 58-year-old male presented with dyspnea and was found to have a systolic murmur. TTE revealed significant mitral regurgitation and an ASD. Accurate echocardiographic quantification was challenging due to the dual pathology and the patient was referred for CMR (see Fig. 48.3). A flail P2 scallop is demonstrated in A (TTE PSLA, see Video 48.1) indicated by the *green arrow.* An eccentric anteriorly directed jet of mitral regurgitation is demonstrated in A (see Video 48.1) and B (TTE A4Ch) indicated by the *white arrow.* Color M-mode is consistent with holosystolic mitral regurgitation (*white arrow,* F). The mitral regurgitant volume using the PISA formula was 38 mL (D and E, PISA radius indicated by the *white arrow*). Systolic flow across the ASD is seen in C (TTE A4Ch, see Video 48.2) indicated by the *orange arrow.* CMR images are shown in Fig. 48.2B. *A4Ch,* Apical four-chamber view; *ASD,* atrial septal defect; *CMR,* cardiac magnetic resonance imaging; *PISA,* proximal isovelocity surface area; *PSLA,* parasternal long axis; *TTE,* transthoracic echocardiogram.

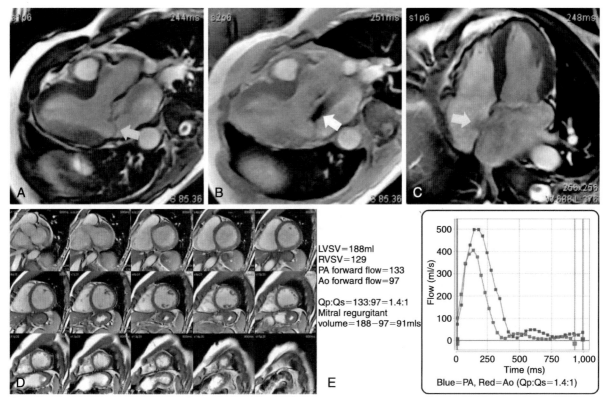

LVSV=188ml
RVSV=129
PA forward flow=133
Ao forward flow=97

Qp:Qs=133:97=1.4:1
Mitral regurgitant
volume=188−97=91mls

Blue=PA, Red=Ao (Qp:Qs=1.4:1)

FIG. 48.3 Mitral regurgitation in the presence of an ASD (CMR). CMR findings for the patient with mitral regurgitation and an ASD described in Fig. 48.2 are shown. The flail P2 scallop is clearly seen in panel A (3Ch SSFP, see Video 48.3) indicated by the *green arrow*. The eccentric anteriorly directed jet of mitral regurgitation is demonstrated in B (3Ch FSPGR) indicated by the *white arrow*. Systolic flow across the ASD is seen in C (4Ch SSFP, see Video 48.4) and indicated by the *orange arrow*. Left and right ventricular end diastolic and end systolic volumes were obtained by tracing the endocardium of every slice on the CMR short-axis stack (D, SSFP and see Video 48.5) providing LVSV and RVSV. Pulmonary artery and aorta forward flow volumes were also assessed using phase contrast sequences (flow curves shown in E). Qp:Qs was 1.4:1 and mitral regurgitant volume was 91 mL. This case illustrates how mitral regurgitant volumes can be underestimated on TTE when a significant ASD is present and the utility of CMR in such cases. *4Ch*, Four-chamber view; *3Ch*, three-chamber view; *ASD*, atrial septal defect; *CMR*, cardiac magnetic resonance imaging; *FSPGR*, fast spoiled gradient echo; *LVSV*, left ventricular stroke volume; *PISA*, proximal isovelocity surface area; *RVSV*, right ventricular stroke volume; *SSFP*, steady-state free precession imaging; *TTE*, transthoracic echocardiogram.

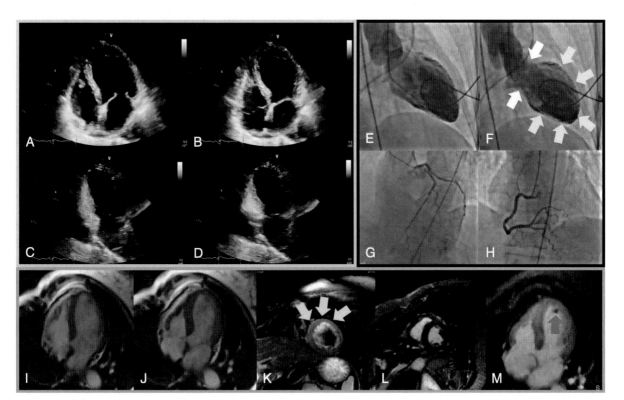

FIG. 48.4 Takotsubo cardiomyopathy. A 67-year-old female patient presented with chest pain and dyspnea triggered by exercise. ECG showed repolarization abnormalities and troponin was mildly elevated. TTE images are shown in A to D *(orange border)*, left heart catheterization in E to H *(black border)* and CMR images in I to M *(gray border)*. TTE on presentation demonstrated akinesis of all mid and apical segments with hyperdynamic basal function (A4Ch and A2Ch views in A and C are diastole and B and D are systole, see Video 48.6). Left heart catheterization reveals the classical "octopus pot" appearance in systole (F, *orange arrows:* akinesis of all mid and apical segments, *white arrows:* hyperdynamic basal function). There was nonobstructive coronary disease (G and H showing left and right coronary arteries respectively). CMR was performed to rule out myocarditis. 4 and 2Ch SSFP demonstrate the previously mentioned wall motion abnormalities (I and J, see Video 48.7). Fat-suppressed T2-weighted imaging suggests inflammation in the mid *(green arrows)* and apical segments (K). There was no hyperenhancement on late gadolinium enhancement imaging consistent with the absence of infarction or infiltration and a finding consistent with a diagnosis of Takotsubo cardiomyopathy (L). An apical thrombus *(red arrow)* was discovered on post gadolinium long TI time sequences (M). Repeat TTE on admission day 5 demonstrated complete recovery of left ventricular systolic function (see Video 48.8). The apical thrombus persists and is identified using contrast-enhanced TTE (see Video 48.9). *A4Ch*, Apical four-chamber view; *A2Ch*, apical two-chamber view; *CMR*, cardiac magnetic resonance imaging; *SSFP*, steady-state free precession imaging; *TTE*, transthoracic echocardiogram.

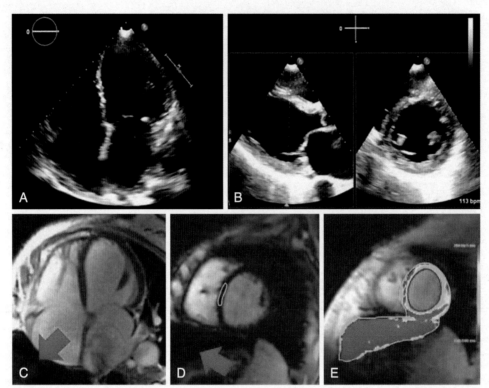

FIG. 48.5 Iron overload cardiomyopathy. Representative TTE (A and B) and CMR (C, D, and E) images from a 70-year-old female with severe nonischemic dilated cardiomyopathy are shown. The LV is LV with severely depressed LV systolic function (A and B are A4Ch, PSLA, PSSA views respectively, see Video 48.10). CMR was performed and revealed increased iron accumulation in the myocardium confirmed by T2* analysis. The liver appears unusually dark on SSFP sequences (C, *red arrow*), which can be suggestive of an iron overload state. A T2* map was acquired and a region of interest drawn around the myocardium in the septum (D, short axis of the LV). Subsequent analysis (E) revealed strongly positive T2* values with a mean of 5 ms, normal is greater than 20 ms. *A4Ch,* Apical four-chamber view; *CMR,* cardiac magnetic resonance imaging; *LV,* left ventricle; *PSLA,* parasternal long axis; *PSSA,* parasternal short axis; *SSFP,* steady-state free precession imaging; *TTE,* transthoracic echocardiogram.

the additional benefit of tissue characterization, which may be pathognomonic in certain cardiomyopathies. After the diagnosis has been made by complementary imaging techniques, surveillance and follow-up are usually accomplished with TTE.

TISSUE CHARACTERIZATION

Characterization of myocardial tissue provides virtual in vivo histology in patients with cardiomyopathy and unexplained increased LV mass. There are a variety of potential causes of excessive mass beyond hypertension and aortic stenosis, which may have important implications in terms of treatment and prognosis. Further evaluation should be considered when the degree of LV hypertrophy or wall thickening is out of keeping with clinical picture. Options for the evaluation of myocardial tissue characterization by TTE are limited and include measures of tissue reflection (a surrogate for tissue density) and dynamic changes as a result of alterations in myocardial ultrastructure.[15] Ultrasonic scatter from small reflectors also known as integrated backscatter is the only available echo tool to evaluate tissue density. Collagen within the tissue results in scatter and attenuation and is the primary determinant; however, feasibility with this method is limited. On the other hand, tissue characterization is a major strength of CMR and to less extent cardiac PET.

Inflammation, infarction, and infiltration are demonstrated on CMR primarily with late gadolinium enhancement (LGE) but also with other specialized sequences permitting characterization of pathologic tissue without the need for contrast. Long T2 relaxation times of water-specific contrast results in high signal intensity of edematous tissue. Harnessing this property in combination with black blood imaging allows detection of acute myocyte swelling and interstitial fluid accumulation.[16] This technique is used to identify acute inflammation in myocarditis, acute myocardial infarction, stress cardiomyopathy (Takotsubo), and transplant rejection and will be somewhat refined with the advent of T2 mapping. On the other hand, T1-weighted sequences result in a high signal intensity of fatty tissue. These sequences are useful in the assessment of the pericardium as epicardial, and pericardial fat layers provide

an excellent contrast for margins of the visceral and parietal pericardium respectively. Fatty infiltration in the context of arrhythmogenic RV cardiomyopathy or cardiac tumors is also identified with this technique. Iron accumulation in the myocardium is evaluated by CMR in the form of a unique myocardial T2 star map (Fig. 48.5 and Video 48.10). This method has been validated with in vivo histology and allows direct detection and quantification of myocardial iron in vivo.[17] There are three ways in which myocardium can be characterized with gadolinium contrast agents. As the contrast is administered, rest or stress myocardial first pass perfusion is observed with dynamic imaging. Early gadolinium enhancement occurs within 1–3 minutes of injection and LGE is observed 5–20 minutes post administration. Gadolinium is a heavy metal that accumulates in expanded extracellular space and when present LGE represents inflammation (edema), fibrosis, or infiltration. The pattern of enhancement is crucial, with LGE extending from the endocardium across the myocardium (subendocardial LGE) usually indicating varying degrees of myocardial infarction. The specificity of the LGE pattern in ischemic cardiomyopathy has been confirmed in numerous studies in which coronary angiography and CMR were performed in patients with systolic dysfunction of unknown etiology.[18] Mid-wall or subepicardial LGE is found in myocarditis as well as various cardiomyopathies. The segmental location, distribution (focal or patchy) and extent of LGE often holds a clue as to the underlying pathologic process.[19] Occasionally extensive systemic amyloidosis involving the heart results in a classical dilemma where the myocardium cannot be adequately "nulled" due to altered gadolinium kinetics relating to sequestration of gadolinium by other organs infiltrated with amyloid plaques (Figs. 48.6 and 48.7; Videos 48.11–48.13). T1 mapping will further differentiate the underlying cause of various cardiomyopathies as well as permit earlier detection of myocardial interstitial fibrosis.

Molecular imaging of inflammation, scar, and hibernating myocardium is also achieved with nuclear imaging. In terms of PET, myocardial metabolism is manipulated to image either viable/hibernating myocardium or inflammation including granulomatous inflammation and infection. In the case of inflammation, the patient is prescribed a

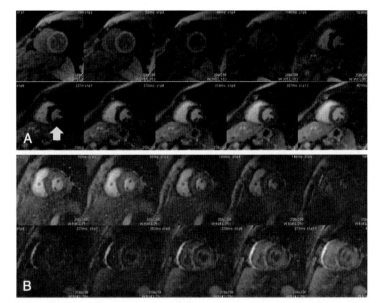

FIG. 48.6 Altered gadolinium kinetics in cardiac amyloidosis. A is a row or map of 10 consecutive T1-weighted inversion times (TI) times in a normal patient 8 minutes post gadolinium administration. The sixth image in this sequence *(orange arrow)* is the appropriate TI time as the myocardium is adequately nulled and the blood pool is bright. This sequence is run to choose the correct TI time for myocardial delayed enhancement imaging. B is the same sequence in the patient in Fig. 48.5A performed 5 minutes after gadolinium administration. An appropriate TI time cannot be chosen due to the altered kinetics of gadolinium by extensive systemic and cardiac amyloidosis.

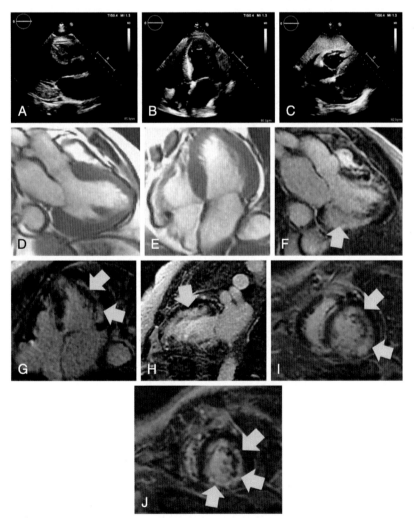

FIG. 48.7 Cardiac amyloidosis. A to J are TTE and CMR images demonstrating the features of cardiac amyloidosis in a 70-year-old male who was originally diagnosed with heart failure with preserved ejection fraction. The TTE PSLA and A4Ch views (A and B, see Video 48.11) show severe concentric LV hypertrophy with preserved LV systolic function. There is biatrial enlargement and a pericardial effusion. RV hypertrophy as well as thickening of the interatrial septum are appreciated on the subcostal view (C, see Video 48.12). CMR SSFP sequences show similar findings (D and E are 3 and 4Ch views respectively, see Video 48.13). F to J are myocardial delayed enhancement gradient echo sequences demonstrating diffuse subendocardial *(green arrows)* late gadolinium enhancement consistent with extensive cardiac amyloidosis (F, G, and H are 3, 4, and 2Ch views respectively and I and J are SA views). *A4Ch,* Apical four-chamber view; *CMR,* cardiac magnetic resonance imaging; *LV,* left ventricle; *PSLA,* parasternal long axis; *RV,* right ventricle; *SA,* short axis; *SSFP,* steady-state free precession imaging; *TTE,* transthoracic echocardiogram.

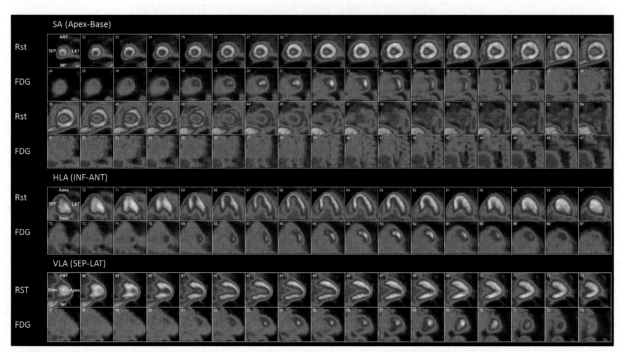

FIG. 48.8 Cardiac sarcoidosis. A 45-year-old man with nonischemic cardiomyopathy and recurrent ventricular tachycardia underwent a cardiac PET sarcoid study. SA, HLA and VLA views are shown with rest perfusion images in the *top row* (Rst) and metabolism or FDG images in the *second row* (FDG). The images demonstrate avid FDG uptake in the lateral wall with normal perfusion suggesting active inflammation in this territory without scar formation. These findings are highly suggestive of cardiac sarcoidosis. *ANT,* Anterior; *FDG,* F18-fluorodeoxyglucose; *HLA,* horizontal long axis; *INF,* inferior; *LAT,* lateral; *PET,* positron emission tomography; *Rst,* rest; *SA,* short axis; *SEP,* septal; *VLA,* vertical long axis.

high-fat high-protein diet with no carbohydrate for 12–16 hours. This dietary modification manipulates the energy source for normal cardiomyocytes, resulting in almost exclusive fatty acid metabolism. F18-fluorodeoxyglucose (FDG) is subsequently administered, and PET images are acquired 45–60 minutes later. In a well-prepared patient, FDG avidity is demonstrated in regions of inflammation resulting from ingestion of FDG by macrophages and neutrophils (Fig. 48.8). This technique is used in the diagnosis and therapeutic monitoring of cardiac sarcoidosis and in patients with possible intracardiac infections such as device infections or prosthetic valve endocarditis. The other way in which myocardial metabolism is manipulated is by administration of a glucose load with subsequent delivery of intravenous insulin to drive glucose as well as FDG into ischemic or hibernating cardiomyocytes. The predominant metabolism of normal cardiomyocytes is fatty acid metabolism (ratio 80:20 fatty acid to glucose). However, hibernating myocardium uses almost exclusively glycolysis. Rest perfusion is performed during a PET viability protocol when a resting severe defect represents either scar or hibernating myocardium. The presence of FDG avidity within the severe resting perfusion defect is termed a perfusion:metabolism mismatch and suggests hibernating myocardium or viability. Other molecular techniques used to characterize myocardial tissue include SPECT with technetium 99–labeled pyrophosphate, which can differentiate transthyretin (TTR) amyloid from other forms of cardiac amyloidosis such as AL amyloid.

The utility of CT in terms of characterizing myocardial tissue pathology is under investigation and is limited by higher radiation doses (for instance, precontrast and postcontrast imaging). On the other hand, CT is extremely good at identifying calcification and thinned or scarred myocardium. The Hounsfield scale is used when evaluating cardiac masses and pericardial disease and differentiates fat, water, air, blood products, and calcium with reasonable accuracy.

CORONARY DISEASE

A sound knowledge of the advantages and disadvantages of the different imaging modalities in the evaluation of coronary artery disease (CAD) is imperative. With various imaging tools at our disposal (Figs. 48.9–48.12), we are capable of evaluating the presence and impact of coronary stenosis with various forms of stress testing, demonstrate the anatomy of the coronary arteries including plaque morphology, assess viability of

infarcted myocardium, and observe for sequelae of ischemic heart disease (IHD).

Standard exercise stress testing without imaging has a class IA recommendation in patients with an intermediate pretest probability for IHD, an interpretable electrocardiogram (ECG), and at least moderate physical functioning or no disabling comorbidity.[20] Although standard exercise stress testing provides excellent prognostic information, its diagnostic accuracy is modest at best as evidenced by a sensitivity and specificity of 73%–90% and 50%–74%, respectively.[21] Exercise stress testing with TTE or nuclear myocardial perfusion imaging (MPI) is recommended for patients with intermediate to high pretest probability who have an uninterpretable ECG and at least moderate physical functioning or no disabling comorbidity (class IB recommendation) (see Figs. 48.9 and 48.10; Videos 48.14 and 48.15). CMR with pharmacologic stress is also an option in such patients (class IIa) (see Fig. 48.11; Video 48.16). When the same group of patients have an interpretable ECG, stress testing with TTE and nuclear MPI is considered reasonable (class IIa). CCTA is assigned a class IIb indication in this particular group of patients. In the same group of patients who are incapable of at least moderate physical functioning or have a disabling comorbidity, pharmacologic stress with TTE or nuclear MPI is recommended (class IB). When the pretest probability is low in these patients, pharmacologic TTE is reasonable (class IIa). CCTA gains a class IIa recommendation when pretest probability is low to intermediate and is also reasonable for patients with an intermediate pretest probability who have continued symptoms with prior normal test findings, inconclusive results from prior stress testing, or are unable to undergo nuclear MPI or TTE. Coronary calcium score receives a class IIb recommendation for patients with a low to intermediate pretest probability of obstructive IHD. In summary, the cardiologist or internist has many options to choose from and there may not be one particular optimal test. The preferred imaging modality for the evaluation of CAD varies from center to center and often relates to quality and the availability of the imaging tools. Additional information acquired with PET coronary flow reserve and perfusion with CMR in terms of microvascular disease should also be considered when making a selection. Fractional flow reserve by CCTA improves specificity and is likely to become an additional clinical tool in the CT armamentarium.[22]

In terms of coronary artery anatomic imaging, echocardiography can determine the origin of the coronary arteries to some degree but, like

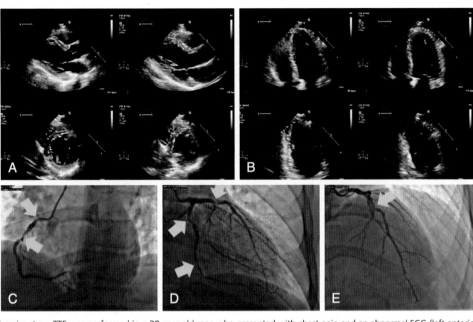

FIG. 48.9 Stress echo. Exercise stress TTE was performed in a 39-year-old man who presented with chest pain and an abnormal ECG (left anterior fascicular block). He exercised for 9:02 minutes, reaching 10 Mets and 88% target heart rate. The stress test was stopped due to shortness of breath and 1 mm of ST depression in the precordial leads. There is resting inferolateral hypokinesis and the LVEF at rest was 55% (A and B, best appreciated in Videos 48.14 and 48.15). There was stress-induced severe hypokinesia of the mid to distal anterolateral and inferolateral walls and ventricular apex with a mildly depressed LVEF of 45% (A and B, best appreciated in Videos 48.14 and 48.15). LHC revealed triple vessel CAD with moderate stenosis in the RCA (C, *green arrows*) and severe stenoses in the LAD and LCx (D and E, *green arrows*). *CAD,* Coronary artery disease; *ECG,* electrocardiogram; *LAD,* left anterior descending artery; *LCx,* left circumflex coronary artery; *LHC,* left heart catheterization; *LVEF,* left ventricular ejection fraction; *Mets,* metabolic equivalents; *RCA,* right coronary artery; *TTE,* transthoracic echocardiogram.

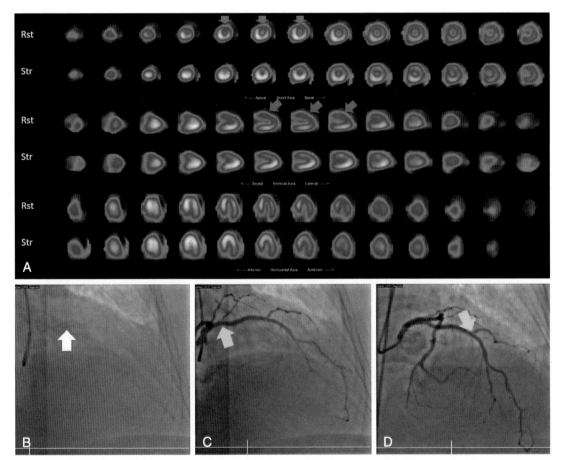

FIG. 48.10 **Nuclear stress test.** A shows an exercise SPECT perfusion scan of a 65-year-old woman who was experiencing exertional chest pain post PCI to the LAD (B, *white arrow* indicating a coronary stent precontrast injection). She exercised for 5:30 minutes, reaching 6 Mets and 78% target heart rate. The stress test was stopped due to chest pain and 2 mm of ST depression in the lateral precordial leads. The SPECT images demonstrate a reversible perfusion defect in the anterior wall (A, *red arrows; top rows:* stress perfusion; *bottom rows:* rest perfusion). LHC revealed ostial stenoses of the first (jailed) and second diagonal branches of the LAD (C and D respectively, *green arrows*). *LAD,* Left anterior descending artery; *LHC,* left heart catheterization; *PCI,* percutaneous intervention; *SPECT,* single-photon emission computed tomography.

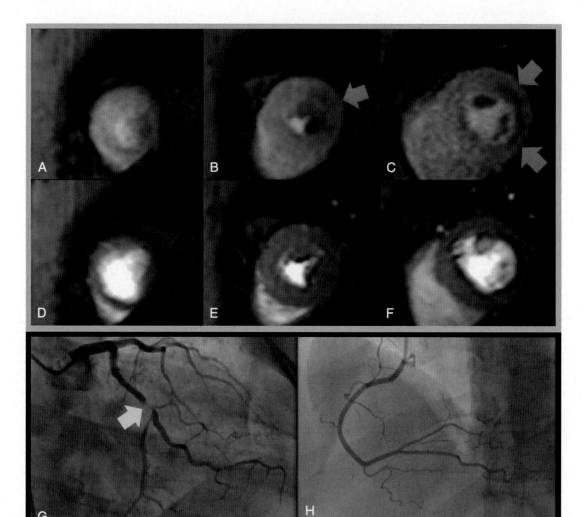

FIG. 48.11 Stress cardiac MRI. Images A to F *(gray border)* show a positive vasodilator (Regadenoson) stress CMR in a 50-year-old woman with scleroderma who presented with chest pressure and mildly elevated troponin *(top row:* stress perfusion [A to C]; *bottom row:* rest perfusion [D to F, see Video 48.16]). Stress perfusion demonstrates a severe basal and mid lateral wall perfusion defect *(red arrows)*. LHC (G is the left coronary artery, and H is the right coronary artery) revealed a severe discrete stenosis in the proximal LCx *(green arrow)*. *CMR,* Cardiac magnetic resonance imaging; *LCx,* left circumflex coronary artery; *LHC,* left heart catheterization.

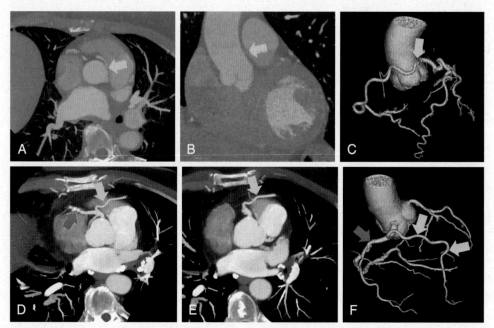

FIG. 48.12 **Coronary CT angiography.** A to F demonstrate the utility of CT coronary angiography in terms of evaluation of anomalous coronary arteries. A and B show an anomalous RCA coursing between the aorta and main pulmonary artery (interarterial course). There is an acute take-off angle (A, *green arrow*), which is slitlike in short axis (B, *green arrow*). C is a 3D reconstruction that shows the origin of the RCA adjacent to the LCA at the left coronary cusp *(green arrow)*. D and E demonstrate an anomalous LAD *(green arrow)* arising from the proximal RCA *(red arrow,* there is also calcification of the RCA) and coursing anteriorly (prepulmonic course). F is a 3D reconstruction that clearly shows the LAD arising from the RCA. *3D,* 3-dimensional; *CT,* computed tomography; *LAD,* left anterior descending artery; *RCA,* right coronary artery.

nuclear MPI, is not capable of evaluating the lumen of the vessel. CMR with MRA is useful for evaluating the proximal course of the coronary arteries, ruling out anomalies and in time may provide an alternative to CCTA for anatomic imaging of the coronaries. However, CCTA is the gold standard, with modern equipment providing a full volume of the cardiac anatomy in a single heart beat with excellent spatial resolution. The anatomy, origins, and course of the coronary arteries are laid out. The wall and lumen of the vessels are evaluated, providing an estimation of stenosis and unique information about plaque composition with certain features suggesting more high-risk lesions. Along with the indications mentioned previously, CCTA should also be considered when investigating coronary disease in new onset heart failure or intermediate/high-risk patients undergoing intermediate-risk noncardiac surgery, evaluation of bypass grafts in acute chest pain and in suspected or known coronary anomalies (see Fig. 48.124).

The utility of CMR for triaging patients presenting with chest pain in the emergency department has been demonstrated. CMR rest perfusion in conjunction with LGE in patients presenting with chest pain and nondiagnostic ECG is very accurate in detecting acute coronary syndromes (sensitivity 100% for non-ST elevation myocardial infarction, and sensitivity and specificity for ACS of 84% and 85%, respectively).[23] In troponin-positive chest pain patients, CMR is also a powerful tool in identifying a cause such as obstructive CAD missed on left heart catheterization, myocarditis, or stress cardiomyopathy.

Echocardiography is the principal test when evaluating the sequelae of IHD and myocardial infarction. Evaluation of chamber size and function, wall motion, and thinning/scar; mechanical complications such as valvular regurgitation, ventricular septal defect, and free wall rupture, and aneurysm formation are all easily assessed by TTE and can be monitored over time in the acute or chronic setting. TTE with contrast is a sensitive tool for the identification of LV thrombus. The utility of CMR in ischemic cardiomyopathy from diagnosis to sequelae and viability assessment is also well described in the literature. Precise evaluation of function, wall motion abnormalities, wall thinning, and secondary MR is achieved with CMR, as described in the previous sections. Location, size, and wall thickness of aneurysms can be accurately characterized. CMR also has a proven ability to detect or confirm the presence of thrombus. Using a long TI time post gadolinium provides excellent contrast between myocardium and avascular thrombus (see Fig. 48.4M).

Assessment of myocardial viability is a controversial area in cardiovascular imaging, and three methods currently exist to assess whether or not the muscle is still alive, including dobutamine stress echocardiography (DSE), contrast-enhanced CMR, and nuclear viability studies. In patients with inducible ischemia and hibernating myocardium, revascularization is likely to result in improvement of regional and global LV function, heart failure symptoms, and long-term prognosis.[24] DSE estimates contractile reserve but is the least sensitive of all imaging viability studies. SPECT is marginally better at identifying hibernation, but the utility of both modalities has been challenged by the STICH (Surgical Treatment for Ischemic Heart Failure) trial.[25] PET has high sensitivity and superior spatial resolution to SPECT. Regions that show a concordant reduction in both myocardial blood flow (ammonia or rubidium) and FDG uptake (perfusion:metabolism match) are considered to be irreversibly injured, whereas regions of FDG uptake that are relatively preserved or increased despite having a perfusion defect (perfusion:metabolism mismatch) are considered ischemic but viable.[26] Three parameters are used to help determine viability by CMR: end-diastolic wall thickness, low-dose dobutamine stress CMR, and LGE. An end-diastolic wall thickness of less than 5.5 or 6 mm was found to be associated with a low likelihood of functional recovery after revascularization.[27,28] Low-dose dobutamine (≤10 μg/kg per minute) stress CMR is also used to evaluate myocardial viability.[28,29] Wall thickening of greater than 2 mm during systole suggests likely functional recovery with revascularization. Extent transmurality of LGE is the gold standard technique for viability assessment by CMR. LGE with a cutoff of less than 50% transmurality of scar tissue had a high sensitivity and a high negative predictive value to predict functional recovery.[30,31] Contrast-enhanced CMR in combination with low-dose dobutamine stimulation seems to be the most accurate method, with a growing body of evidence to support it.

CARDIAC MASSES

Based upon data from 22 large autopsy series, the prevalence of primary cardiac tumors is approximately 0.02% (200 tumors per million autopsies with one in four being malignant).[32] On the other hand, metastatic tumors to the heart are 20–40 times more common. Nonneoplastic cardiac masses can also masquerade as cardiac tumors, examples of which include thrombi, pericardial cysts/tumors, and prominent anatomic structures. The number of possible causes of a cardiac mass renders diagnosis challenging. However, multimodality imaging has led to an in vivo almost histologic characterization of cardiac masses, which plays a crucial role in diagnosis and surgical planning.

Cardiac masses are often picked up incidentally on echocardiography, which remains the first line modality in the evaluation of a mass (Fig. 48.13; Videos 48.17–48.19). High temporal resolution in real-time allows excellent determination of the mobility of a mass, as well as demonstrating the presence of compromise of cardiac or valvular function. 3DE and TEE result in more accurate assessment of morphology. TEE also provides clearer imaging with higher definition, particularly when the mass arises in the atria, and is a useful tool for intraoperative guidance of percutaneous biopsy of intracardiac lesions. Tumor size is monitored safely with echocardiography. As described earlier, contrast echocardiography allows more accurate delineation of the location and size of cardiac masses. However, TTE and TEE are limited in terms of tissue characterization and in the evaluation of extracardiac structures.

The location, attachment, appearance, and mobility of a mass picked up on TTE is often suggestive of the underlying etiology. However, it is with multimodality imaging that the differential diagnosis is narrowed down further. CT is often preferred in the setting of small lesions, owing to its advantageous spatial resolution. For the same reason, CT provides superior anatomic information, along with global evaluation of cardiac and extracardiac structures. Analysis of the volumetric dataset on a 3D workstation better identifies the anatomic features of the lesion. Vascularity/enhancement, vascular invasion, and occasionally neovascular recruitment are also appreciated with CT. An added bonus is the evaluation of the coronary arteries in patients under consideration for mass resection. CCTA is typically considered in suspected valvular lesions such as papillary fibroelastoma or valvular vegetations. CT is also optimal for evaluation of calcified masses and serves as an alternative imaging modality in patients with known contraindications to CMR or in patients with inadequate images from other noninvasive methods.

CMR is often the preferred imaging modality for cardiac mass evaluation largely due to its superior soft tissue characterization (see Fig. 48.13).[33] Relatively high temporal resolution, multiplanar imaging capabilities, and unrestricted field of view, as well as an absence of ionizing radiation are also advantages. Tissue characterization is achieved with various T1- and T2-weighted imaging sequences, as well as rest perfusion and early and delayed enhancement patterns. T1-weighted imaging with and without fat suppression distinguishes the fat content in the mass, whereas T2-weighted imaging with fat suppression determines water content reflecting edema, a feature usually present in malignant tumors and myxomas. Perfusion of the lesion suggests vascularity and is an important characteristic of tumors often indicating malignancy (see Video 48.19). Early and LGE patterns are described in different tumors and further refine the differential diagnosis. Thrombus must be ruled out in the case of every intracardiac tumor by performing a long TI time LGE sequence (as described earlier). Myocardial tagging allows additional evaluation of tumors by assessing myocardial contraction and demonstrating differentiation between contractile and noncontractile tissue for instance in the case of a true intramyocardial mass. Tagging also exquisitely defines tissue planes and in doing so demonstrates the presence or absence of tumor invasion across the tissues.

The role of nuclear imaging in the assessment of cardiac masses is very important. FDG-PET and octreotide imaging are the usual tracers involved. FDG-PET is a standard imaging tool in oncology for the detection and follow-up of neoplasms by assessing the metabolic activity of glucose (see Fig. 48.13). Myocardial metabolism must be switched to a predominantly fatty acid state as in inflammation and infection imaging described earlier. Primary malignant and metastatic cardiac tumors have higher standardized uptake values compared with primary benign tumors.[34] A primary tumor and/or distant metastasis can also

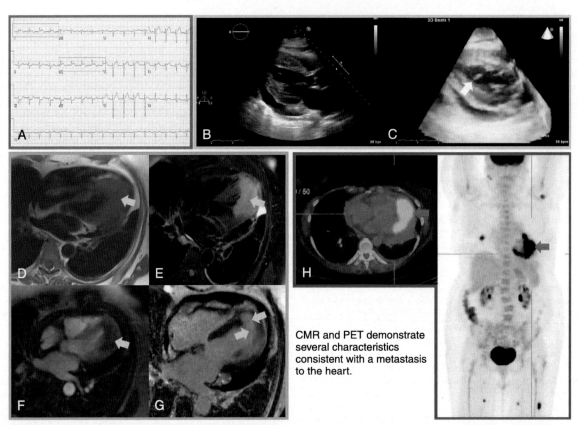

CMR and PET demonstrate several characteristics consistent with a metastasis to the heart.

FIG. 48.13 Cardiac metastasis. A 65-year-old female smoker presented with chest pain and lateral ST elevation on ECG (A). Left heart catheterization revealed nonobstructive coronary disease. A TTE *(orange border)* showed thickening and hypokinesis of the lateral wall and apical segments as well as a mobile echodensity within the LV cavity *(white arrow,* C) and a moderate pericardial effusion (B and C show representative PSLA 2 and 3D TTE images, see Videos 48.17 and 48.18). The patient was referred for a CMR *(gray border),* which demonstrated findings consistent with an infiltrating primary or secondary tumor as indicated by the *green arrows* (isointense on T1 [D], hyperintense on T2 with fat suppression suggesting edema/inflammation [E], abnormal perfusion [F, see Video 48.19] and heterogeneous uptake of gadolinium on myocardial delayed enhancement [G]). Cardiac PET/CT *(purple border)* was subsequently performed according to a sarcoid protocol (previously described), which showed FDG avidity in the lateral wall and apex *(red arrows,* H). The whole body FDG PET revealed FDG avidity in the right lung *(orange arrow,* H), left axilla, right parotid gland and left femur as well as the heart. Biopsy of the lung lesion revealed adenosquamous carcinoma of the lung. *CMR,* Cardiac magnetic resonance imaging; *FDG,* F[18]-fluorodeoxyglucose; *LV,* left ventricle; *PET/CT,* positron emission tomography/computed tomography; *PSLA,* parasternal long-axis view; *TTE,* transthoracic echocardiogram.

be identified with FDG-PET imaging. A weakness of this technique is that normal metabolic activity may obscure small lesions and brown fat may also appear positive, for example, lipomatous hypertrophy of the interatrial septum. Octreotide scintigraphy (also known as somatostatin receptor scintigraphy) is used for the detection of carcinoid and neuroendocrine tumors. It is a drug similar to somatostatin and is radiolabeled with indium 111. Of note, nonfunctioning prolactin adenomas are usually positive on ocreotide scintigraphy. Patients with somatostatin receptor–positive neuroendocrine tumors are more likely to respond to octreotide therapy and, like FDG-PET, response to treatment can be monitored with ocreotide scintigraphy.

PERICARDIAL DISEASE

Pericardial disease results in a variety of clinical presentations and may be isolated to the pericardium or associated with a systemic disorder. Acute presentations are usually straight forward, and a combination of the history and physical examination is highly suggestive of the underlying process. However, occasionally more chronic pericardial disease causes a diagnostic dilemma whereby an integrated multimodality imaging approach may provide incremental value. An expert consensus statement on the "Recommendations for Multimodality Cardiovascular Imaging of Patients with Pericardial Disease" was published in 2013, representing the first guideline for the role of imaging in pericardial disease.[35] TTE is the initial imaging method of choice for the evaluation of pericardial diseases. Frequently a further test is required, but there is uncertainty about which is the best next test. As a consequence, patients may get referred for an exhaustive battery of imaging tests with variable yield. Cardiovascular imaging experts are often consulted to ensure that patients do not get inappropriate or unnecessary tests and avoid incomplete or nondiagnostic studies.[36]

Acute pericarditis is a relatively common condition, with the diagnosis usually made based on history, examination, ECG, and laboratory findings. TTE is often requested as a screening tool for an associated pericardial effusion and should be done within 24 hours of presentation. Intrapericardial fibrinous strands indicate an inflammatory etiology or possibly clotted blood. Urgent TTE may also be required to rule out a more sinister cause of ST segment elevation. Although TTE is unreliable for measuring pericardial thickness, TEE has been demonstrated to be reproducible and comparable with CT.[37] Further imaging should be considered when pericarditis is associated with indicators of worse outcome (fever >38°C, subacute course, failure of initial response to standard therapy, or evidence of hemodynamic compromise). The most sensitive subsequent test is CMR.[35] CT or CMR should also be performed when there are therapeutic difficulties or complications following acute pericarditis, such as failure to respond to medical therapy, evolution toward recurrent or chronic pericarditis with possible constrictive features. Pericarditis associated with trauma, neoplastic disorders, aortic dissection, empyema, or acute pancreatitis usually requires additional imaging. CT and CMR clearly visualize the pericardium and identify thickening, whereas inflammation involving the pericardium is demonstrated with CMR (T2-weighted imaging and LGE). Occasionally follow-up CMR is required to monitor improvement or otherwise.

CT is an important adjunct study when localization and quantification of pericardial fluid are important or when the effusion is complex or loculated or clot is present. The attenuation of the pericardial effusion on CT is a very useful parameter, indicating the nature of the accumulated fluid. Low attenuation (<10 HU) usually represents serous or transudative fluid. Measurements close to that of fat (–60 to –80 HU) may represent a chylopericardium. Relatively high attenuation material (>50–60 HU) is more consistent with blood products and likely indicates

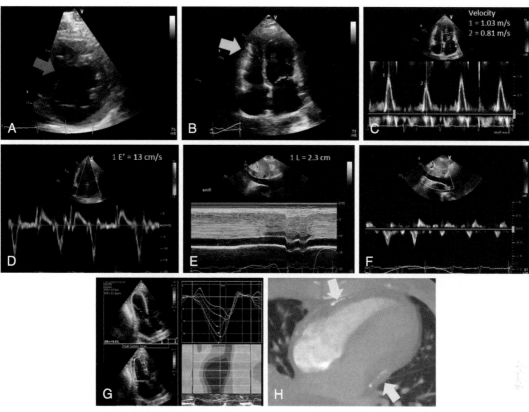

FIG. 48.14 Pericardial constriction (TTE and CT). A 65-year-old male with a history of recurrent pericarditis presented with worsening abdominal distension and ankle swelling. TTE demonstrated a septal bounce (A, PSSA view *[red arrow]*, see Video 48.20), biatrial enlargement with tubular RV (B, A4Ch view *green arrow*, see Video 48.21), respirophasic diastolic filling (C, mitral inflow Doppler), and annulus paradoxus (D, tissue Doppler imaging of the medial annulus). The IVC was dilated (E), and there was increased expiratory diastolic flow reversal in the hepatic veins (F). A normal longitudinal strain pattern is often found in constriction as opposed to reduced values in restrictive cardiomyopathy (G, normal global longitudinal strain −19.6%). A CT scan ordered for a different indication demonstrated pericardial calcification (H, *orange arrows*). *A4Ch,* Apical four-chamber view; *CT,* computed tomography; *IVC,* inferior vena cava; *PSSA,* parasternal short-axis view; *RV,* right ventricle; *TTE,* transthoracic echocardiogram.

a hemopericardium. Exudative effusions as found in purulent pericarditis or malignancy have an attenuation of 10–50 HU. CMR may also allow further characterization of a pericardial effusion. Transudative effusions typically have a low signal intensity on T1-weighted images, whereas hemorrhagic or exudative effusions often have a medium or high signal intensity. Cardiac tamponade is a clinical diagnosis that can be confirmed on TTE. It is also a medical emergency, and referral for CT or CMR is inappropriate because a delay in treatment may be detrimental to the patient. TEE is occasionally performed in postoperative patients who may have poor acoustic windows or a localized pericardial collection resulting in tamponade physiology. CT can be performed to guide therapy in the setting of subacute pericardial tamponade caused by a loculated or complex effusion. It is recommended to perform pericardiocentesis under echocardiographic guidance.

Prior cardiac surgery and idiopathic constrictive pericarditis are now the most common causes of pericardial constriction in the United States and Europe.[38] Tuberculous pericarditis remains the most common in developing countries. Imaging findings are often suggestive but inconclusive, and, as a result, pericardial constriction can be a challenging diagnosis. TTE is performed early in these cases and rules out more obvious causes of dyspnea and symptoms and signs consistent with right heart failure. Although not very sensitive and specific, classical 2D features of constriction include a septal bounce, inferior vena cava (IVC) plethora and myocardial tethering. Transmitral and transtricuspid Doppler findings using simultaneous respirometry, tissue Doppler imaging help to distinguish constriction from restrictive cardiomyopathy. Strain imaging also helps to distinguish; although a reduction in global strain is more pronounced in constriction in the circumferential direction, global strain is profoundly attenuated in the longitudinal direction in restriction.[35] However, echocardiographic findings remain equivocal in a number of cases, which prompts the need for further testing in the form of CT, CMR (Figs. 48.14 and 48.15; Videos 48.20–48.23), or invasive catheterization. As outlined earlier, CT and CMR provide excellent definition

of pericardial thickness (normal <2 mm). A pericardial thickness of 4 mm or greater is suggestive of constriction in the right clinical setting; however, normal pericardial thickness does not exclude the diagnosis.[39] Morphologic features on CT and CMR such as a tubular right ventricle and biatrial enlargement are also suggestive, as well as the presence of a dilated IVC and pleural effusions. Detection of pericardial calcification is excellent with CT but very limited with CMR (see Fig. 48.14). On the other hand, real time imaging with CMR demonstrates the respirophasic septal bounce very well, a feature not evaluated by CT (see Video 48.23). Persistent pericardial inflammation may be noted on CMR. Myocardial tagging sequences on CMR can demonstrate a lack of normal breakage between the tissue planes and indicate adhesions between inflamed visceral and parietal pericardial surfaces. Abrupt cessation of diastolic filling can also be noted on steady-state free precession sequence cine, providing more evidence of a stiff pericardium. A recent study demonstrated that real-time phase-encoding velocimetry (akin to Doppler echocardiography) without ECG gating could demonstrate the characteristic hemodynamic changes of constrictive physiology.[40] Because these findings are not investigated with CT, CMR is often the preferred additional test when echocardiography is nondiagnostic. When the diagnosis remains uncertain after evaluation with multimodality imaging, cardiac catheterization may be indicated. Interventricular dependence is demonstrated with simultaneous catheters in the right and LVs.

Pericardial masses and suspected congenital absence of the pericardium are also indications for CT or CMR. Pericardial masses include tumors, cysts, and diverticulae that are usually picked up on TTE. Imaging with CT or CMR is performed to assess the lesion further. The utility of multimodality imaging for the evaluation of masses is described in section 3. Congenital absence of the pericardium is a rare disorder and may be associated with other congenital anomalies.[41] Patients are usually asymptomatic, and it is most often an incidental finding discovered on chest x-ray, echocardiography, CT, or CMR. Echocardiographic features of this condition are nonspecific and include unusual imaging

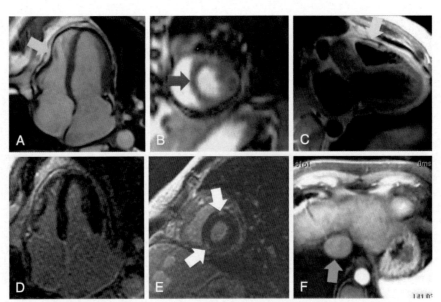

FIG. 48.15 Pericardial constriction (CMR). CMR was performed on the patient described in Fig. 48.14, which confirmed a septal bounce and tubular shape of the RV (A, 4Ch SSFP, *green arrow,* see Video 48.22 and B, short-axis real time, *red arrow,* see Video 48.23). T1-weighted imaging revealed a mild degree of pericardial thickening (4–5 mm, *orange arrows,* C). Patchy pericardial enhancement was noted (D, *white arrow*), and there was late gadolinium enhancement of the RV insertion points, a nonspecific finding (E, *white arrows*). The IVC was also dilated on the CMR (F, *blue arrow*). Collectively, these CMR findings are highly suggestive of pericardial constriction. *4Ch,* four-chamber view; *CMR,* cardiac magnetic resonance imaging; *IVC,* inferior vena cava; *RV,* right ventricle; *SSFP,* steady-state free precession imaging.

windows, the appearance of an enlarged right ventricle, excessive cardiac motion, and abnormal interventricular septal motion. Patients are often referred for CT or CMR on the basis of an enlarged right heart and the concern for an intracardiac shunt. More specific Doppler findings have been reported and include reductions in systolic flow in the superior vena cava and in systolic/diastolic flow ratio in the pulmonary veins.[42] CT and CMR can actually be performed without contrast in order to diagnose congenital absence of the pericardium. However, the need for definitive imaging is questionable in asymptomatic persons (the vast majority) because the diagnosis typically has no clinical consequence.

DISEASES OF THE AORTA

Measurement of the proximal aortic root may be accomplished with TTE, TEE, CT, and CMR. Normal values with reference ranges taking into account age, gender, and body size have been established. The various modalities have near equal standards for assessing aortic root size. Gated CT and MRI are most accurate for the measurement of the proximal aorta, and as a result a lower margin of error is acceptable when monitoring the size of the aortic root, sinotubular junction, and ascending aorta. TTE provides good images of the aortic root, adequate images of the ascending aorta, and aortic arch in most patients and good images of the proximal abdominal aorta. TTE is less helpful for evaluating the descending thoracic aorta. In terms of TEE the close proximity of the esophagus to the thoracic aorta provides high-quality imaging of nearly all aspects of the ascending and descending thoracic aorta. However, a blind spot exists on TEE where a portion of the distal ascending aorta and proximal aortic arch may not be visible due to interposition of the trachea. This may be overcome by deep transgastric views in some cases. Multidetector CT scanners are the preferred technology for aortic imaging. ECG-gated contrast-enhanced CT angiography delivers excellent imaging of the aorta, limiting aortic root artifacts due to cardiac motion. Spatial resolution is second to none. CT angiographic protocols are robust and relatively operator independent. The limiting factors are ionizing radiation and contraindication to iodinated contrast. It is the preferred choice when imaging acute aortic syndromes and is also used for follow-up of aortic pathology. MRI is a useful tool for the evaluation of diseases of the aorta and is used to define aneurysms, aortic wall ulceration, and dissections and to demonstrate areas of wall thickening related to aortitis or intramural hematoma. MRI also provides functional information, including quantification of forward and reverse aortic flow, assessment of aortic wall stiffness and compliance, and aortic valve leaflet morphology

and motion. In patients with severe renal impairment, it is possible to perform an MRA without intravenous contrast. This is achieved by using a 3D navigator segmented steady-state free precession sequence but is particular to a 1.5-T magnet.[43] This technique can be considered in patients with an estimated glomerular filtration rate less than 30 mL/min in whom gadolinium-based contrast is contraindicated.

The term *acute aortic syndrome* describes four different aortic pathologies, including classic aortic dissection, intramural hematoma, penetrating aortic ulcer, and aortic aneurysm rupture (contained or not contained). These conditions are considered under one umbrella term because they require emergency attention due to the risk of rupture and death. Although CT is the overall preferred imaging modality in the case of suspected acute aortic syndrome, each case needs to be considered individually. If a patient is critically ill, it may not be possible to perform a CT, and a bedside TTE and/or TEE are the only options. In the setting of a patient with an iodinated contrast allergy, MRI may be considered. All options must be explored in the presence of severe renal dysfunction with an eGFR less than 30 mL/min, which is usually a contraindication to gadolinium and iodinated contrast agents. Although dialysis patients can receive iodinated contrast agents, local institutional factors such as expertise and availability need to be taken into account. The sensitivity and specificity of CT for the diagnosis of aortic dissection is 100% and 98%, respectively, with high accuracy for the diagnosis of intramural hematoma, penetrating aortic ulcer, and aortic aneurysm rupture. An IRAD (International Registry of Acute Aortic Dissection) publication, including 894 patients, showed that the quickest diagnostic times were achieved when the initial test was CT, whereas the initial use of MRI or catheter-based aortography resulted in significantly longer diagnostic times.[44]

There are a number of conditions that can mimic acute aortic syndrome, for which CT and/or MRI are first line imaging modalities, and include aortitis, atheromatous plaque, prior surgical aorta, artefacts on TEE or CT (gating artifact), and normal structures such as pericardial recess and periaortic fat. Detailed discussion on these conditions is beyond the scope of this chapter.

CONCLUSION

The role of echocardiography in medicine has never been more important, providing crucial information about pathology affecting the heart. In most conditions, echocardiography is also used to monitor stability, improvement, or disimprovement of disease. Multimodality imaging is performed to further evaluate volumes and function, morphology, and anatomy, impact of CAD, characterize tissue, intracardiac masses, pericardial disease, and diseases of the aorta. In many cases, the use of more than one imaging modality is appropriate and complementary to echocardiography. In addition to yielding an abundance of information, echocardiography can guide protocols for other imaging modalities and together definitively characterize the nature and extent of pathology and plan treatment.

Suggested Reading

Fihn, S. D., Gardin, J. M., Abrams, J., et al. (2012). 2012 ACCF/AHA/ACP/AATS/PCNA/SCAI/STS guideline for the diagnosis and management of patients with stable ischemic heart disease: a report of the American College of Cardiology Foundation/American Heart Association Task Force on Practice Guidelines, and the American College of Physicians, American Association for Thoracic Surgery, Preventive Cardiovascular Nurses Association, Society for Cardiovascular Angiography and Interventions, and Society of Thoracic Surgeons. *Circulation, 126*, e354–e471.

Klein, A. L., Abbara, S., Agler, D. A., et al. (2013). American Society of Echocardiography clinical recommendations for multimodality cardiovascular imaging of patients with pericardial disease: endorsed by the Society for Cardiovascular Magnetic Resonance and Society of Cardiovascular Computed Tomography. *Journal of the American Society of Echocardiography, 26*, 965–1012.e1015.

Lang, R. M., Badano, L. P., Mor-Avi, V., et al. (2015). Recommendations for cardiac chamber quantification by echocardiography in adults: an update from the American Society of Echocardiography and the European Association of Cardiovascular Imaging. *Journal of the American Society of Echocardiography, 28*, 1–39.e14.

Nishimura, R. A., Otto, C. M., Bonow, R. O., et al. (2014). 2014 AHA/ACC guideline for the management of patients with valvular heart disease: a report of the American College of Cardiology/American Heart Association Task Force on Practice Guidelines. *Journal of the American College of Cardiology, 63*, e57–e185.

Taylor, A. J., Cerqueira, M., Hodgson, J. M., et al. (2010). ACCF/SCCT/ACR/AHA/ASE/ASNC/NASCI/SCAI/SCMR 2010 appropriate use criteria for cardiac computed tomography. a report of the American College of Cardiology Foundation Appropriate Use Criteria Task Force, the Society of Cardiovascular Computed Tomography, the American College of Radiology, the American Heart Association, the American Society of Echocardiography, the American Society of Nuclear Cardiology, the North American Society for Cardiovascular Imaging, the Society for Cardiovascular Angiography and Interventions, and the Society for Cardiovascular Magnetic Resonance. *Circulation, 122*, e525–e555.

A complete reference list can be found online at ExpertConsult.com.

49 Transesophageal Echocardiography for Cardiac Surgery

Douglas C. Shook

INTRODUCTION

Transesophageal echocardiography (TEE) for intraoperative planning is well established in the armamentarium of surgeons, cardiologists, and anesthesiologists. The use of intraoperative TEE has become the standard of care during cardiac surgery, and the intraoperative echocardiographer (IE), generally an anesthesiologist, has become an integral part of the cardiac surgery care team. This chapter will review the role of the IE and the intraoperative examination.

ROLE OF THE INTRAOPERATIVE ECHOCARDIOGRAPHER

The IE is an integral part of the cardiac surgical team (Box 49.1). The concept of an effective cardiac surgical team needs to emphasized. It is a group of individuals with an expressly agreed common goal who hold themselves mutually accountable for the outcome of the patient, which can depend enormously on how the team functions. Developing a culture of teamwork and effective communication has been shown to reduce mortality in the operative environment.[1] Specifically in cardiac surgery, understanding the complex interactions during a cardiac surgical case likely improves patient safety and effective teamwork.[2,3] The IE needs to develop an understanding of each team member in the cardiac operating room and their individual contribution to the overall success of the procedure at hand. This may be very different from other environments that they are typically used to working in outside the operating room.

The IE should be present during critical components of the operation to optimize their impact on the success of the procedure. The IE is a co-proceduralist, where a successful surgical outcome is dependent on their expert input, based on information obtained from the intraoperative TEE exam, and is communicated to the entire surgical team. As has been reported, information obtained from an intraoperative TEE exam has significant impact on anesthetic patient management, surgical planning, and patient outcomes. The primary objectives of the comprehensive intraoperative exam are to confirm the primary diagnosis and assess for any new pathophysiology, to discuss the exam, including its impact on anesthetic management, and to guide and assess the surgical outcome. The goal is an interdisciplinary plan of action at each stage of the operative procedure (precardiopulmonary bypass [CPB], during CPB, separation from CPB and post-CPB).

BOX 49.1 The Cardiac Surgical Team

Cardiac surgeon
Cardiac anesthesiologist
Intraoperative echocardiographer
Perfusionist
Physician assistants
Nurses
Fellows
Residents
Surgical technicians

IMPACT OF INTRAOPERATIVE TRANSESOPHAGEAL ECHOCARDIOGRAPHY IN CARDIAC SURGERY

Several studies have supported the utilization of TEE in the intraoperative cardiac surgical arena.[4–6] Minhaj et al. reported on 283 consecutive patients undergoing cardiac surgery. There were 106 new TEE findings in 87 patients with half of the new findings involving the mitral valve and a quarter involving the tricuspid valve. The new findings altered surgical management 25% of the time. In addition, information obtained from the intraoperative TEE exam influenced the need for CPB in 3% of patients. In two patients, the TEE exam prompted reinitiating CPB, and in one patient, TEE information cancelled the proposed surgery. Eltzschig et al. reviewed the impact of intraoperative TEE on surgical decisions in 12,566 consecutive patients undergoing cardiac surgery at a single institution. Overall, the intraoperative TEE exam performed before and after CPB influenced the cardiac surgical decision making in more than 9% of all patients studied. TEE had the greatest impact in patients having combined coronary artery bypass grafting (CABG) and a valve procedure (12.3% pre-CBP, 2.2% post-CPB), followed by isolated valve procedures (6.3% pre-CPB, 3.3% post-CPB), and then CAGB alone (5.4% pre-CPB, 1.5% post-CPB). Mishra et al. reported on 5016 consecutive cardiac surgical cases where TEE was utilized during the procedure. Overall, the authors reported that 39% of patients benefited from TEE during the pre-CPB period with similar benefit during the post-CPB exam. TEE guided hemodynamic interventions helped or modified the surgical plan, and identified post-CPB issues, such as the need for bypass graft revision or inadequate valve repair. See Table 49.1 for the most common changes in surgical management and related new intraoperative TEE findings.

Current guidelines by the Society of Cardiovascular Anesthesiologists, the American Society of Anesthesiologists, and the American Society of Echocardiography have further established the role of TEE in cardiac surgery:[7,8]

Cardiac Surgery (for Adult Patients Without Contraindications)

1. TEE should be used in all open heart and thoracic aortic surgical procedures
2. TEE should be considered in patients having coronary artery bypass graft surgery

OBJECTIVES OF THE INTRAOPERATIVE TEE EXAM

The information obtained from a comprehensive intraoperative exam should confirm and refine the preoperative diagnosis (Box 49.2). This is based on studies showing the utility of intraoperative TEE, especially in valve and aortic surgery.[9–14] In addition, intraoperative TEE has been shown to detect new or unsuspected findings as part of the comprehensive pre-CPB exam.[15] The information learned from the pre-CPB exam should be integrated into the anesthetic management of the patient and the surgical plan should be readjusted accordingly. Finally, TEE should assess the results of the surgical intervention to optimize patient outcomes and determine the need to re-initiate CPB if the result of the exam or new findings deem it necessary (Box 49.3).

TABLE 49.1 The Most Common Changes in Surgical Management and New Transesophageal Echocardiography Finding[4–6]

PROCEDURE EITHER ALTERED OR ADDED	NEW FINDINGS ON EXAM
Tricuspid repair or replacement	Tricuspid regurgitation
Mitral repair or replacement	New significant regurgitation Absence of regurgitation Vegetations Leaflet perforation or chordal rupture Annular calcification
Aortic repair or replacement	New significant regurgitation or stenosis Vegetations or abscess Absence of regurgitation Subaortic membrane
Atrial septal defect or patent foramen ovale repair or closure	New or significant defect
Intra-aortic balloon pump insertion	Ventricular failure or ischemia
Ascending aortic aneurysm repair	Aneurysm
Off-pump CABG instead of on-pump	Calcified ascending aorta
VSD closure	New or significant defect
LVAD insertion	Ventricular failure or ischemia
Thrombectomy	Thrombus noted on exam
Case cancelled	Multiple etiologies
Abandon minimally invasive approach	—

CABG, Coronary artery bypass grafting; *LVAD,* left ventricular assist device; *TEE,* transesophageal echocardiography; *VSD,* ventricular septal defect.

BOX 49.2 Objectives of the Intraoperative Transesophageal Echocardiography Exam

Confirm and refine the preoperative assessment
Determine the need for unplanned surgical intervention
Determine cardiac dysfunction that impacts patient management
Cannulation and perfusion strategy
Address surgical procedure-specific issues
Predict complications related to the proposed surgical intervention
Assess surgery specific results after separation from CPB, in addition to a global assessment structure and function

CPB, Cardiopulmonary bypass.

BOX 49.3 Reasons to Re-initiate Cardiopulmonary Bypass[5]

Additional bypass graft or revision
Revision of valve repair or replacement
Additional valve procedure
Ventricular dysfunction
Mass resection or thrombectomy
Dissection or ascending aortic repair
Ventricular septal defect or atrial septal defect
Further de-airing or revision of drug administration

THE INTRAOPERATIVE TRANSESOPHAGEAL ECHOCARDIOGRAPHY EXAM

The best way to examine the role of the IE is to give a detailed example of a patient in the operating room with primary mitral regurgitation for mitral repair. The role of the IE and the steps of the exam can be

TABLE 49.2 The Precardiopulmonary bypass Intraoperative Exam Specific for Mitral Valve Surgery[17]

INTRAOPERATIVE EXAM	EXAMPLES OF FINDINGS
Confirm and refine the preoperative assessment	Confirm and refine the mechanism, location, and severity of mitral regurgitation using 2D/3D imaging and Doppler assessment of the mitral valve
Determine the need for unplanned surgical intervention	Secondary pathophysiology related to severe mitral regurgitation New unexpected findings that should be addressed during the surgical intervention (moderate/severe tricuspid regurgitation)
Determine cardiac dysfunction that impacts patient management	Unexpected ventricular dysfunction Aortic regurgitation Left-sided superior vena cava (impacts coronary sinus retrograde cardioplegia)
Cannulation and perfusion strategy	Finding a significant patent foramen ovale shunt may impact the type of cannulation performed or surgical approach
Address surgical procedure-specific issues	Repair or replace the valve
Predict complications related to the proposed surgical intervention	Postrepair mitral stenosis Systolic anterior motion of the anterior leaflet of mitral valve producing left ventricular outflow tract obstruction Risk of atrial ventricular dissociation due to significant mitral annular calcification debridement Ventricular dysfunction

applied to any surgical procedure where intraoperative echocardiography is utilized.

Ideally, the IE has reviewed all preoperative imaging and already discussed a preliminary assessment of mechanism and function of the mitral valve with the surgeon prior to the patient entering the operating room. This type of collaboration between the surgeon and the IE fosters a relationship that is paramount not only to the current patient's outcome but also to the long-term success of the surgical program.[16] The pre-CPB exam should include confirming and refining the diagnosis, determining the need for unplanned surgical intervention, planning a cannulation and perfusion strategy, addressing surgery-specific issues, and anticipating postrepair complications (Table 49.2).[17]

The initial pre-CPB TEE exam should be comprehensive (see Chapter 4). The information obtained needs to be communicated in a timely manner to other members of the cardiac surgical team as this may impact pre-CPB management of the patient, the cannulation and perfusion strategy, and the need for additional surgical intervention. The focus of the exam then turns to the primary pathology, in this case the mitral valve. The IE should incorporate two-dimensional (2D) and three-dimensional (3D) imaging along with Doppler interrogation of the mitral valve to determine the mechanism, location, and severity of the mitral regurgitation (Fig. 49.1). The IE evaluates all aspects of the mitral apparatus (annulus, leaflets, chordae, papillary muscles, and left ventricle) to determine their individual and collective impact on the mechanism of mitral regurgitation (Figs. 49.2 to 49.7 and Videos 49.1 to 49.5). For successful valve surgery, determining the precise mechanism of valve dysfunction can be the most important aspect of the intraoperative exam (see previous chapters specific to each valve and ventricular pathology).[18] Specific to mitral repair, Shah and Raney recently published a modification of the classic Carpentier description of leaflet motion, which incorporates our greater understanding of leaflet motion pathology since the original publication in 1983 (Table 49.3).[16,19,20]

The results of the intraoperative exam are communicated to the surgical team to discuss the reparability of the valve and to subsequently develop a repair plan. It is essential that the IE knows the surgeon's repair plan based on the TEE exam information provided. Different surgical repair techniques (resecting vs. leaflet sparing), including the choice of annuloplasty ring, impact the success of the surgical procedure and help

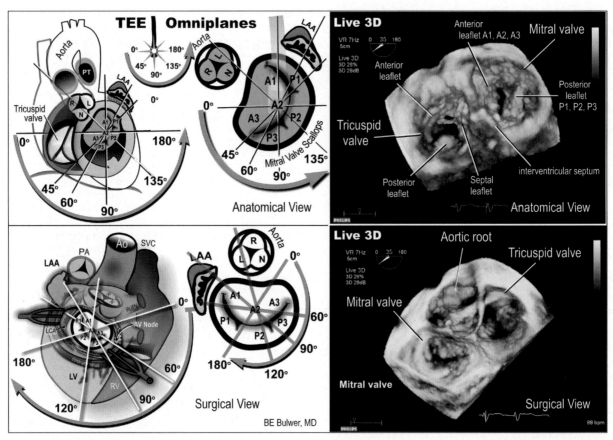

FIG. 49.1 Integration of the cardiac anatomy, two-dimensional imaging planes, and three-dimensional (3D) imaging to determine the mechanism of mitral regurgitation. *Ao,* Aorta; *LAA,* left atrial appendage; *LCA,* left circumflex artery; *LV,* left ventricle; *PA,* pulmonary artery; *RV,* right ventricle; *RUPV,* right upper pulmonary vein; *SVC,* superior vena cava; *TEE,* transesophageal echocardiography. *(Courtesy of Bernard E. Bulwer, MD, FASE.)*

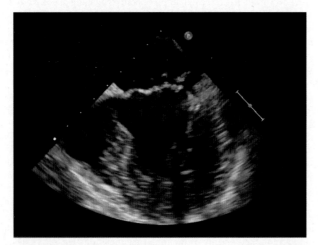

FIG. 49.2 Midesophageal four-chamber view showing a flail posterior leaflet (Carpentier type 2). The anterior leaflet also appears to prolapse above the level of the mitral annulus. See also Video 49.1.

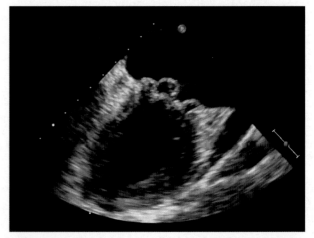

FIG. 49.3 Mid-esophageal commissural view showing a flail posterior leaflet (P2) that appears to have a broad flail width and ruptured chords coming from the posterior-medial papillary muscle. In addition, the P3/A3, A2 body, and A1/P1 leaflets also prolapse above the level of the commissural annulus consistent with bileaflet prolapse. See also Video 49.2.

determine the risk of postrepair dysfunction, such as postrepair left ventricular outflow obstruction (Video 49.6).[18,21]

The dialogue between the echocardiographer and surgeon can have a tremendous impact on success of the surgical intervention. In fact, everyone present in the operating room should be part of the discussion because the information discussed effects every member of the team and their ability to anticipate and optimize the patient's outcome.

The IE's role continues throughout the pre-CPB period as the patient's pathophysiology may change based on altered hemodynamics and cardiac function, which is typical for cardiac surgical patients under general anesthesia. In addition, many institutions utilize epiaortic and epicardial echocardiography for cannulation planning, and as an additional imaging

modality to TEE, especially in patients who have a contraindication to TEE placement.[22–25]

The IE should be present when the surgeon opens the left atrium and begins valve inspection. The surgical findings need to be correlated with imaging findings seen during the pre-CPB exam (Fig. 49.8 and Video 49.7). Every IE develops an expanding mental database that integrates their knowledge of anatomy, imaging, and surgical findings for application to future procedures. This is a critical component of the surgeon-echocardiographer relationship. Each cardiac surgeon has their own individual approach to mitral valve surgery. Therefore, each surgeon incorporates imaging information differently into their planning

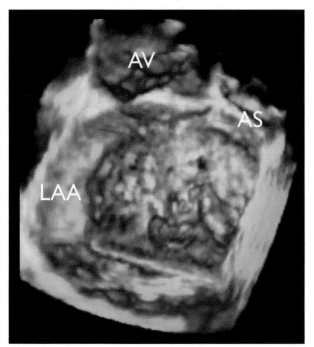

FIG. 49.4 Gated three-dimensional acquisition of the mitral valve with the aortic valve *(AV)* at the top of the image and left atrial appendage *(LAA)* at the left (the surgeon's view of the mitral valve when they open the left atrium). This confirms the P2 flail leaflet with ruptured chords coming from the posterior-medial papillary muscle. In addition, the entire valve (anterior and posterior leaflets) is billowing and prolapsing. This is much easier to see in Fig. 49.5 and Video 49.4. *AS,* Atrial septum.

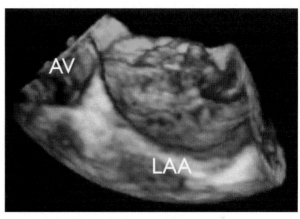

FIG. 49.5 Same gated three-dimensional acquisition from Fig. 49.4; however, the dataset is turned to view the valve at the level of the annulus with the left atrial appendage *(LAA)* in the near field. In this view, it is much easier to see the bileaflet prolapse. *AV,* Atrioventricular.

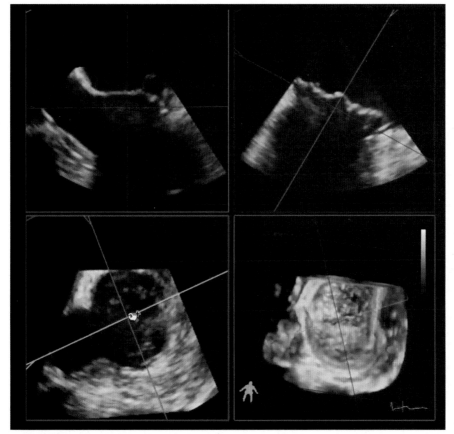

FIG. 49.6 This figure uses multiplanar reconstruction on the same three-dimensional dataset to scan the mitral valve from A1/P1 to A3/P3 in systole (seen in Video 49.5). Using this technique, leaflet lengths and annular dimensions can be accurately measured. In addition, it is much easier to pinpoint areas of valve pathology.

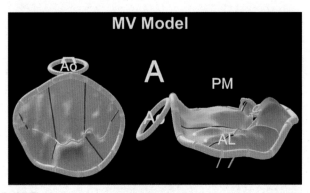

FIG. 49.7 Static systolic models of the mitral valve *(MV)* leaflets and annulus. Note the annulus still has a systolic saddle shape despite the extensive primary valvular disease. *AL,* Anterolateral; *Ao,* aorta; *PM,* posteromedial.

TABLE 49.3 Classification of Mitral Valve Pathology Based on the Intraoperative Echocardiography Exam[16]

TYPE OF LEAFLET MOTION	EXAMPLES
Type 1: Normal leaflet motion	Perforation Leaflet cleft Dilated annulus (without leaflet tethering)
Type 2: Excessive leaflet motion	Flail leaflet Billowing leaflet Bileaflet prolapse with flail segment
Type 3: Restricted leaflet motion	Systolic and diastolic restriction • Rheumatic Symmetric systolic restriction • Dilated cardiomyopathy • Ischemic cardiomyopathy • Dilated annulus with leaflet tethering Asymmetric systolic restriction Focal tethering–segmental ischemic dysfunction
Type 4: Systolic anterior motion of the leaflets	Hypertrophic cardiomyopathy Postrepair SAM Hemodynamic induced SAM • Hypovolemia • Inotropic stimulation • Tachycardia
Type 5: Hybrid conditions	Combination of types 1–4 in the same valve

SAM, Systolic anterior motion.

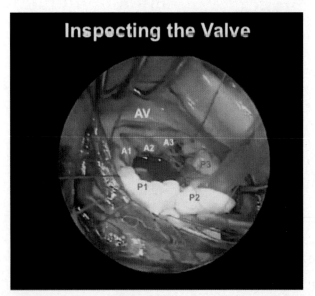

FIG. 49.8 Surgeon's view of the mitral valve. Note the leaflet scallops and location of the aortic valve *(AV)* for orientation. The focus is on the broad-based flail P2 scallop. Note the redundancy of the scallop as seen on intraoperative echo exam. See also Video 49.7. A1, A2, A3, and P1, P2, P3 represent mitral leaflet anatomy as described by Alain Carpentier.

TABLE 49.4 The Postcardiopulmonary Bypass Intraoperative Exam Specific for Mitral Valve Surgery[17]

INTRAOPERATIVE EXAM	EXAMPLES OF FINDINGS
Assess global cardiovascular function (compare to pre-CPB exam)	Ventricular dysfunction Significant tricuspid regurgitation
Diagnose complications and mechanisms specific to the surgical procedure	Residual mitral regurgitation Postrepair mitral stenosis SAM with left ventricular outflow tract obstruction Paravalvular regurgitation (if valve was replaced) Atrioventricular dissociation—rare
Note complications related to cannulation and CPB	Aortic dissection or hematoma Micro-air emboli causing ischemia

CPB, Cardiopulmonary bypass; *SAM,* systolic anterior motion.

process. Part of the IE's responsibility is understanding the surgeon's philosophical repair approach and technique, and how they will integrate the intraoperative exam into their repair process. Likewise, the IE needs to understand the needs of each specific surgeon and tailor their communication to best assist the surgeon in their decision-making process.

Once the patient is on CPB, the IE may still be needed to assess any complications that may arise during the bypass run. Prior to separation from bypass, a detailed explanation of the surgical intervention should to be discussed to assist the IE and the entire surgical team to anticipate post-CPB complications. Specifically, for mitral repair, the discussion must include the repair technique utilized by the surgeon, and the type and size of annuloplasty ring that is placed to support the repair. The IE incorporates this information into their post-CPB assessment, especially if the repair is not optimal, to determine the best way to resolve any issues or complications that may occur. For post-CPB mitral repair, the IE should focus on determining the presence of mitral regurgitation, postrepair stenosis, and left ventricular outflow tract obstruction due to systolic anterior motion of the anterior mitral valve leaflet. By knowing the exact repair performed, the IE can best determine the mechanism for failure, and give guidance for re-repair versus replacement of the valve.

In addition to evaluating the mitral repair, the IE must perform another comprehensive post-CPB TEE exam to assess cardiovascular function, to determine any changes from the pre-CPB exam, and to rule out complications related to CPB, such as aortic dissection from cannulation (Table 49.4). The patient's pathophysiology continually changes throughout the post-CPB period, which requires the IE to assess cardiac structure and function, and to assist the surgical team in the management of the patient until transfer to the intensive care unit. Communication and interdisciplinary decision making is continuous throughout the entire operation with the IE as an integral part of the team assuring the patient the best possible outcome.

IMPACT OF INTRAOPERATIVE TRANSESOPHAGEAL ECHOCARDIOGRAPHY IN NONCARDIAC SURGERY

In addition to utilizing TEE in cardiac surgical patients, there is a role for intraoperative echocardiography in noncardiac surgical patients. Guidelines developed by the Society of Cardiovascular Anesthesiologists, the American Society of Anesthesiologists, and the American Society of Echocardiography have helped define the role of intraoperative TEE in noncardiac surgical patients.[7,8]

Noncardiac Surgery (for Adults Without Contraindications)

• If equipment and expertise is available, TEE should be used when unexplained life-threatening circulatory instability persists despite corrective therapy ("Rescue" TEE).
• TEE (as an intraoperative monitor) may be used when the nature of the planned surgery or the patient's known or suspected cardiovascular pathology might result in severe hemodynamic, pulmonary, or neurologic compromise.

TABLE 49.5 Examples of Patients With Profound Hemodynamic Instability or Cardiac Arrest Where Transesophageal Echocardiography Impacted Care[26,28,29]

TEE FINDING	MANAGEMENT
Normal biventricular function—hypovolemia	Fluid resuscitation
Large PE, RV distension, severe TR	Pulmonary embolectomy
Pericardial tamponade, RV rupture	Surgical RV repair
Left ventricular regional wall motion abnormalities	Management for myocardial infarction
Air in right atrium and ventricle—suspected venous air embolus during neurosurgery	Aspiration from central venous catheter
RV dysfunction—hypotension	Inotropic support
Systolic anterior motion of the mitral valve—hypotension unresponsive to therapy	Changed management from epinephrine to phenylephrine and beta-blockers.

PE, Pulmonary embolism; *RV*, right ventricular; *TR*, tricuspid regurgitation.

BOX 49.4 New Transesophageal Echocardiography Findings in Noncardiac Surgical Patients[15,31,32]

New global or segmental ventricular function abnormalities
Change in ventricular function during the operative procedure
Hypertrophic obstructive cardiomyopathy
Moderate to severe valve stenosis or regurgitation
Left atrial or ventricular thrombus
Significant pericardial or pleural effusion

TABLE 49.6 Impact of Transesophageal Echocardiography in Noncardiac Surgical Patients

INDICATION FOR TEE	PERCENT OF PATIENTS IMPACTED
Cardiac arrest—rescue TEE	80%–90%
Acute, persistent, and life-threatening hemodynamic instability—rescue TEE	60%–70%
Surgical procedures in patients at increased risk for myocardial ischemia or hemodynamic disturbances—TEE as a monitor	20%–50%

TEE, Transesophageal echocardiography.

Not all operative environments can emergently perform a TEE exam when unsuspected life-threatening emergencies occur, such as profound and/or prolonged hypotension or cardiac arrest. If the equipment and personnel are available, there is evidence to support the information provided by intraoperative TEE, which can help to diagnose the underlying pathophysiology, can aide in treatment decisions, and can either suggest or alter surgical intervention.[26–29] The diagnoses typically made with "rescue" TEE include ventricular dysfunction, myocardial ischemia, pulmonary embolism, pericardial effusion, hypovolemia, aortic dissection, and aortic rupture. Just as importantly, these diagnoses also can be ruled out by TEE, so the treating team can focus their care in other directions. One of the benefits of using TEE during operative hemodynamic emergencies and cardiac arrest is that imaging does not disrupt advanced cardiac life support (ACLS) interventions, such as chest compressions. Because of this benefit, TEE not only can help with determining the primary diagnosis but also can monitor the success of ACLS interventions. Examples of how TEE establishes a primary diagnosis and influences decision making in operative patients with significant hemodynamic instability or cardiac arrest can be seen in Table 49.5. When TEE is used, either in rescue situations or during cardiac arrest, it alters or guides surgical intervention 13%–55% of the time.[26,28,29]

Intraoperative TEE has also been shown to effectively monitor cardiac structure and function in appropriately chosen noncardiac operative patients. The greatest impact has been published in neurosurgery, liver transplantation, and orthopedic surgery, and in major vascular, thoracic, and abdominal surgeries. The most common medical interventions based on intraoperative TEE monitoring include fluid boluses, initiating anti-ischemic therapy, and directing vasopressor or inotrope therapy.[30] New TEE findings or other unknown patient pathology was noted in 9%–24% of patients across multiple studies.[15,31,32] Box 49.4 summarizes some of the novel findings noted in the studies. One study noted that TEE directed a change in the surgical procedure approximately 3% of the time in vascular patients.[15]

Overall, the impact of intraoperative TEE in noncardiac surgery is greatest in cases of cardiac arrest, and in patients with profound, unexplained hemodynamic instability. This impact led to the guidelines' recommendation that intraoperative TEE should be used when life-threatening hemodynamic instability persists despite corrective therapy.

When TEE is used as an intraoperative monitor, its impact on guiding therapy and surgical decision making is less well established, but it is greatest in higher risk noncardiac surgeries and in patients with known or suspected cardiovascular pathology that might result in severe hemodynamic, pulmonary, or neurologic compromise (Table 49.6).

The IE is an integral part of the surgical team, and the information the IE provides has a significant impact on anesthetic patient management, surgical planning, and patient outcomes. Intraoperative TEE has become a standard of care for cardiac surgery, and its use in noncardiac surgery is well established. The current guidelines support the utilization of TEE in all open heart and thoracic aortic procedures, and it should be considered in patients having CABG. In noncardiac surgery, rescue TEE should be performed when the equipment and personnel are readily available. Intraoperative TEE as a monitor of cardiovascular function can be a useful adjunct where the planned surgery, or the patient's known or suspected cardiovascular pathology, might result in severe hemodynamic, pulmonary, or neurologic compromise.

Suggested Reading

American Society of Anesthesiologists and Society of Cardiovascular Anesthesiologists Task Force on Transesophageal Echocardiography. (2010). Practice guidelines for perioperative transesophageal echocardiography. An updated report by the American Society of Anesthesiologists and the Society of Cardiovascular Anesthesiologists Task Force on Transesophageal Echocardiography. *Anesthesiology, 112*(5), 1084–1096.

Eltzschig, H. K., Kallmeyer, I. J., Mihaljevic, T., et al. (2003). A practical approach to a comprehensive epicardial and epiaortic echocardiographic examination. *Journal of Cardiothoracic and Vascular Anesthesia, 17*(4), 422–429.

Reeves, S. T., Glas, K. E., Eltzschig, H., et al. (2007). Guidelines for performing a comprehensive epicardial echocardiography examination: recommendations of the American Society of Echocardiography and the Society of Cardiovascular Anesthesiologists. *Journal of the American Society of Echocardiography, 20*(4), 427–437.

Savage, R. M., Aronson, S., & Shernan, S. K. (Eds.). (2011). *Comprehensive textbook of perioperative transesophageal echocardiography* (2nd ed.) (pp. 487–565). Philadelphia: Lippincott Williams & Wilkins.

Shah, P. M., & Raney, A. A. (2011). Echocardiography in mitral regurgitation with relevance to valve surgery. *Journal of the American Society of Echocardiography, 24*(10), 1086–1091.

Wahr, J. A., Prager, R. L., Abernathy, J. H., et al. (2013). Patient safety in the cardiac operating room: human factors and teamwork: a scientific statement from the American Heart Association. *Circulation, 128*(10), 1139–1169.

A complete reference list can be found online at ExpertConsult.com.

Appendix A Reference Tables

TABLE A.1 Normal Values for Two-Dimensional Echocardiographic Parameters of Left Ventricular Size and Function According to Gender

Parameter	MALE Mean ± SD	MALE 2-SD Range	FEMALE Mean ± SD	FEMALE 2-SD Range
LV Internal Dimension				
Diastolic dimension (mm)	50.2 ± 4.1	42.0–58.4	45.0 ± 3.6	37.8–52.2
Systolic dimension (mm)	32.4 ± 3.7	25.0–39.8	28.2 ± 3.3	21.6–34.8
LV Volumes (Biplane)				
LV EDV (mL)	106 ± 22	62–150	76 ± 15	46–106
LV ESV (mL)	41 ± 10	21–61	28 ± 7	14–42
LV Volumes Normalized by BSA				
LV EDV (mL/m²)	54 ± 10	34–74	45 ± 8	29–61
LV ESV (mL/m²)	21 ± 5	11–31	16 ± 4	8–24
LV EF (biplane)	62 ± 5	52–72	64 ± 5	54–74

BSA, Body surface area; *EDV,* end-diastolic volume; *EF,* ejection fraction; *ESV,* end-systolic volume; *LV,* left ventricular; *SD,* standard deviation.
From Lang RM, Badano LP, Mor-Avi V, et al. Recommendations for cardiac chamber quantification by echocardiography in adults: an update from the American Society of Echocardiography and the European Association of Cardiovascular Imaging. *J Am Soc Echocardiogr.* 2015;28(1):1-39.e14.

TABLE A.2 Normal Ranges and Severity Partition Cutoff Values for 2DE-Derived Left Ventricular Ejection Fraction and Left Atrial Volume

	MALE Normal Range	MALE Mildly Abnormal	MALE Moderately Abnormal	MALE Severely Abnormal	FEMALE NORMAL RANGE	FEMALE Mildly Abnormal	FEMALE Moderately Abnormal	FEMALE Severely Abnormal
LV EF (%)	52–72	41–51	30–40	<30	54–74	41–53	30–40	<30
Maximum LA volume/BSA (mL/m²)	16–34	35–41	42–48	>48	16–34	35–41	42–48	>48

BSA, Body surface area; *EF,* ejection fraction; *LA,* left atrial; *LV,* left ventricular.
From Lang RM, Badano LP, Mor-Avi V, et al. Recommendations for cardiac chamber quantification by echocardiography in adults: an update from the American Society of Echocardiography and the European Association of Cardiovascular Imaging. *J Am Soc Echocardiogr.* 2015;28(1):1-39.e14.

TABLE A.3 Normal Ranges for Left Ventricular Mass Indices

	WOMEN	MEN
Linear Method		
LV mass (g)	67–162	88–224
LV mass/BSA (g/m2)	*43–95*	*49–115*
Relative wall thickness (cm)	0.22–0.42	0.24–0.42
Septal thickness (cm)	*0.6–0.9*	*0.6–1.0*
Posterior wall thickness (cm)	*0.6–0.9*	*0.6–1.0*
Two-Dimensional Method		
LV mass (g)	66–150	96–200
LV mass/BSA (g/m2)	*44–88*	*50–102*

Bold italic values, recommended and best validated.
BSA, Body surface area; *LV,* left ventricular.
From Lang RM, Badano LP, Mor-Avi V, et al. Recommendations for cardiac chamber quantification by echocardiography in adults: an update from the American Society of Echocardiography and the European Association of Cardiovascular Imaging. *J Am Soc Echocardiogr.* 2015;28(1):1-39.e14.

TABLE A.4 Expected Findings for Left Ventricular Relaxation, Filling Pressures and 2D and Doppler Findings According to Left Ventricular Diastolic Function

	NORMAL	GRADE I	GRADE II	GRADE III
LV relaxation	Normal	Impaired	Impaired	Impaired
LAP	Normal	Low or normal	Elevated	Elevated
Mitral E/A ratio	≥0.8	≤0.8	>0.8–<2	>2
Average E/e′ ratio	<10	<10	10–14	>14
Peak TR velocity (m/s)	<2.8	<2.8	>2.8	>2.8
LA volume index	Normal	Normal or increased (>34 mL/m²)	Increased	Increased

LA, Left atrial; *LAP,* left atrial pressure; *LV,* left ventricular; *TR,* tricuspid regurgitant.
From Nagueh SF, Smiseth OA, Appleton CP, et al. Recommendations for the evaluation of left ventricular diastolic function by echocardiography: an update from the American Society of Echocardiography and the European Association of Cardiovascular Imaging. *J Am Soc Echocardiogr.* 2016;29(4):277-314.

TABLE A.5 Normal Values for Right Ventricular Chamber Size

PARAMETER	MEAN ± SD	NORMAL RANGE
RV basal diameter (mm)	33 ± 4	25–41
RV mid diameter (mm)	27 ± 4	19–35
RV longitudinal diameter (mm)	71 ± 6	59–83
RVOT PLAX diameter (mm)	25 ± 2.5	20–30
RVOT proximal diameter (mm)	28 ± 3.5	21–35
RVOT distal diameter (mm)	22 ± 2.5	17–27
RV wall thickness (mm)	3 ± 1	1–5
RVOT EDA (cm²)		
Men	17 ± 3.5	10–24
Women	14 ± 3	8–20
RV EDA Indexed to BSA (cm²/m²)		
Men	8.8 ± 1.9	5–12.6
Women	8.0 ± 1.75	4.5–11.5
RV ESA (cm²)		
Men	9 ± 3	3–15
Women	7 ± 2	3–11
RV ESA Indexed to BSA (cm²/m²)		
Men	4.7 ± 1.35	2.0–7.4
Women	4.0 ± 1.2	1.6–6.4
RV EDV Indexed to BSA (mL/m²)		
Men	61 ± 13	35–87
Women	53 ± 10.5	32–74
RV ESV Indexed to BSA (mL/m²)		
Men	27 ± 8.5	10–44
Women	22 ± 7	8–36

BSA, Body surface area; *EDA,* end-diastolic area; *EDV,* end-diastolic volume; *ESA,* end-systolic area; *ESV,* end-systolic volume; *PLAX,* parasternal long-axis view; *RV,* right ventricle; *RVOT,* right ventricular outflow tract; *SD,* standard deviation.
From Lang RM, Badano LP, Mor-Avi V, et al. Recommendations for cardiac chamber quantification by echocardiography in adults: an update from the American Society of Echocardiography and the European Association of Cardiovascular Imaging. *J Am Soc Echocardiogr.* 2015;28(1):1-39.e14.

TABLE A.6 Normal Values for Parameters of Right Ventricular Function

PARAMETER	MEAN ± SD	ABNORMALITY THRESHOLD
TAPSE (mm)	24 ± 3.5	<17
Pulsed Doppler S wave (cm/s)	14.1 ± 2.3	<9.5
Color Doppler S wave (cm/s)	9.7 ± 1.85	<6.0
RV fractional area change (%)	49 ± 7	<35
RV free wall 2D strain (%)[a]	−29 ± 4.5	>−20 (<20 in magnitude with the negative sign)
RV 3D EF (%)	58 ± 6.5	<45
Pulsed Doppler MPI	0.26 ± 0.085	>0.43
Tissue Doppler MPI	0.38 ± 0.08	>0.54
E wave deceleration time (ms)	180 ± 31	<119 or >242
E/A	1.4 ± 0.3	<0.8 or >2.0
e'/a'	1.18 ± 0.33	<0.52
e'	14.0 ± 3.1	<7.8
E/e'	4.0 ± 1.0	>6.0

[a]Limited data; values may vary depending on vendor and software version.
EF, Ejection fraction; *MPI*, myocardial performance (Tei) index; *RV*, right ventricle; *TAPSE*, tricuspid annular plane systolic excursion.
From Lang RM, Badano LP, Mor-Avi V, et al. Recommendations for cardiac chamber quantification by echocardiography in adults: an update from the American Society of Echocardiography and the European Association of Cardiovascular Imaging. *J Am Soc Echocardiogr*. 2015;28(1):1-39.e14.

TABLE A.7 Estimation of Right Atrial Pressure based on Inferior Vena Cava Diameter and Collapse

VARIABLE	NORMAL (0–5 [3] MM HG)	INTERMEDIATE (5–10 [8] MM HG)		HIGH (15 MM HG)
IVC diameter	≤2.1 cm	≤2.1 cm	>2.1 cm	>2.1 cm
Collapse with sniff	>50%	<50%	>50%	<50%
Secondary indices				Restrictive filling by TV inflow Tricuspid E/e' >6 Diastolic flow predominance in hepatic veins (systolic filling <55%)

Ranges are provided for low and intermediate categories, but for simplicity, midrange values of 3 mm Hg for normal and 8 mm Hg for intermediate are suggested. Intermediate (8 mm Hg) RA pressures may be downgraded to normal if no secondary indices of elevated RA pressure are present and upgraded to high if minimal collapse with nasal inhalation (<35%); and secondary indices of elevated RA pressure are present or left at 8 mm Hg if uncertain.
IVC, Inferior vena cava; *RA*, right atrium; *TV*, tricuspid valve.

TABLE A.8 Wilkins Scoring System for Mitral Valvuloplasty

GRADE	LEAFLET MOBILITY	VALVE THICKENING	CALCIFICATION	SUBVALVULAR THICKENING
1	Highly mobile	Minimal thickening	Single area of brightness	Minimal chordal thickening
2	Reduced mobility	Thickened tips	Scattered areas at leaflet margins	Chordal thickening up to ⅓
3	Basal leaflet motion only	Entire leaflet thickened	Brightness extends to mid leaflets	Distal third of chordae thickened
4	Minimal motion	Marked leaflet thickening	Extensive leaflet brightness	Extensive thickening to papillary muscles

A desirable score is 8 or lower.

TABLE A.9 Normal Values for Aortic Size in Adults

Aortic Root	ABSOLUTE VALUES (CM)		INDEXED VALUES (CM/M²)	
	Men	Women	Men	Women
Annulus	2.6 ± 0.3	2.3 ± 0.2	1.3 ± 0.1	1.3 ± 0.1
Sinuses of Valsalva	3.4 ± 0.3	3.0 ± 0.3	1.7 ± 0.2	1.8 ± 0.2
Sinotubular junction	2.9 ± 0.3	2.6 ± 0.3	1.5 ± 0.2	1.5 ± 0.2
Proximal ascending aorta	3.0 ± 0.4	2.7 ± 0.4	1.5 ± 0.2	1.6 ± 0.3

From Lang RM, Badano LP, Mor-Avi V, et al. Recommendations for cardiac chamber quantification by echocardiography in adults: an update from the American Society of Echocardiography and the European Association of Cardiovascular Imaging. *J Am Soc Echocardiogr*. 2015;28(1):1-39.e14.

Tables A.10–A.15 and Figures A.1–A.3 can be found online at ExpertConsult.com.

Appendix B Commonly Utilized Equations in Echocardiography

GENERAL BODY MEASURES

Body Mass Index

$$BMI = \frac{Weight}{Height^2}$$

W weight (kg)
H height (cm)

Body Surface Area (Mosteller Formula)

$$BSA = \frac{\sqrt{W \times H}}{60}$$

W weight (kg)
H height (cm)

ECHOCARDIOGRAPHY

Left and Right Ventricle
Left Ventricular Volume (Teicholz Formula)

$$LVEDV = [7/(2.4 + LVEDD)] \cdot LVEDD^3$$

LVEDV = LV end-diastolic volume (mL)
LVEDD = LV end-diastolic diameter (mm)
LVESD = LV end-systolic diameter (mm)
The same formula is used to calculate the left ventricular end-systolic volume (LVESV), substituting LVESD for LVEDD, and the percent difference is used to calculate the LVEF.
(See Fig. 14.4, in which LVIDd = LVEDD and LVIDs = LVESD)

Left Ventricular Ejection Fraction (Simplified Quinones Equation)

$$LVEF = \frac{LVEDD^2 - LVESD^2}{LVEDD^2} \times 100\% + K$$

LVEDD = LV end-diastolic diameter (mm)
LVESD = LV end-systolic diameter (mm)
K = correction for apical contraction
   +10% if normal
   +5% if hypokinetic
   +0% if akinetic
   −5% if dyskinetic
   −10% if aneurysmal

Left Ventricular Fractional Shortening

$$FS = \frac{LVEDD - LVESD}{LVEDD} \times 100\%$$

LVEDD = LV end-diastolic diameter (mm)
LVESD = LV end-systolic diameter (mm)

Left Ventricular Mass (Linear Method, Cube Formula)

$$LV\,Mass = 0.8\left(1.04(LVEDD + IVSd + PWd)^3 - LVEDD^3\right) + 0.6\,g$$

LVEDD = LV end-diastolic diameter (mm)
LVESD = LV end-systolic diameter (mm)
IVSd = Interventricular septal thickness at end-diastole (mm)
PWd = Posterior wall thickness at end-diastole (mm)

Relative Wall Thickness

$$RWT = \frac{IVSd + PWd}{LVEDD}$$

IVSd = Interventricular septal thickness at end-diastole (mm)
PWd = Posterior wall thickness at end-diastole (mm)
LVEDD = LV end-diastolic diameter (mm)

Myocardial Performance, or Tei Index (Left Ventricular) (Fig. B.1; see also Fig. 14.12)

$$LV\,MPI = \frac{IVCT + IVRT}{LVET} = \frac{MCOT - LVET}{LVET}$$

IVCT = isovolumetric contraction time (ms)
IVRT = isovolumetric relaxation time (ms)
MCOT = mitral valve closure-to-opening time (ms)
LVET = LV ejection time (ms)

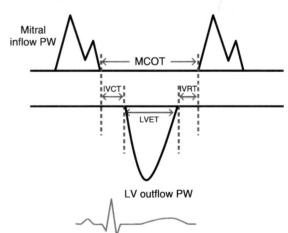

FIG. B.1 Myocardial performance, or Tei index (Left Ventricular).

Myocardial Performance, or Tei Index (Right Ventricular)

$$RV\,MPI = \frac{IVCT - IVRT}{RVET} = \frac{TCOT - RVET}{RVET}$$

$$MPI\,(Tei\,index) = \frac{IVCT + IVRT}{LVET} = \frac{MCOT - LVET}{LVET}$$

483

IVCT = isovolumetric contraction time (ms)
IVRT = isovolumetric relaxation time (ms)
RVET = RV ejection time (ms)
TCOT = tricuspid valve closure-to-opening time (ms)
(Measurements may be performed from pulsed Doppler frames, at similar heart rates, or with a single-tissue Doppler frame. (See Figs. 16.13 and 16.14, as well as Fig. 36.18, in which TCOT = TRT)

Left Ventricular Wall Motion Score Index (for 17 Segment Left Ventricular Model)

$$WMSI = \left(\sum 17 \; segmental \; scores \right) /17$$

Each segment is scored as
1 = normokinetic
2 = hypokinetic
3 = akinetic
4 = dyskinetic

Stroke Volume

$$SV = \pi \left(\frac{LVOT_d}{2} \right)^2 \times VTI_{LVOT}$$

SV = stroke volume (mL)
$LVOT_d$ = LVOT diameter (cm)
VTI_{LVOT} = LVOT velocity time integral (cm)

Cardiac Output

$$CO = SV \cdot HR$$

CO = cardiac output (mL/min) (divide by 1000 for L/m)
SV = stroke volume (mL)
HR = heart rate (beats per min)
Pulmonary-Systemic Flow Ratio Qp/Qs for quantifying intracardiac shunt

$$\frac{Q_P}{Q_S} = \frac{\pi \cdot \left(\frac{RVOT_d}{2} \right)^2 \cdot VTI_{RVOT}}{\pi \cdot \left(\frac{LVOT_d}{2} \right)^2 \cdot VTI_{LVOT}}$$

which by canceling out the same factors in the numerator and denominator, the equation simplifies to

$$= \frac{RVOT_d^2 \cdot VTI_{RVOT}}{LVOT_d^2 \cdot VTI_{LVOT}}$$

Valves, General

Peak pressure gradient, using the modified Bernoulli equation to convert velocity differences to peak instantaneous pressure gradients, is as follows:

$$\Delta P = \left(4V_2^2 - V_1^2 \right)$$

ΔP = peak pressure gradient (mm Hg)
V_2 = velocity distal to stenosis or valve (m/s), e.g., V_{Ao}
V_1 = velocity proximal to stenosis (m/s), e.g., V_{LVOT}

Stroke volume at any annulus can be calculated from PW Doppler recordings and 2D measurements (see Fig. 14.10).

$$SV = CSA \cdot VTI$$

SV = stroke volume (mL)
CSA = cross-sectional area of the annulus
VTI = velocity time integral of flow at annulus by PW Doppler
This is typically used at the LVOT or aortic annulus, and is less frequently at the mitral annulus and pulmonic annulus.

e.g., $LVOT \; SV = CSA_{LVOT} \cdot VTI_{LVOT}$

$$= \pi \left(\frac{LVOT_d}{2} \right)^2 \cdot VTI_{LVOT}$$

$LVOT_d$ = LVOT diameter (cm)
VTI_{LVOT} = LVOT velocity time integral (cm)

Volumetric Methods for Determining Valvular Regurgitation

In normal patients, that is, those with no valvular regurgitation and no shunting, the stroke volume (SV) should be equal through all valve annuli. If one valve is regurgitant, then flow through the affected valve is larger than the other competent valves. The regurgitant volume may then be calculated as the regurgitant valve's SV minus the unaffected valve's SV. For aortic regurgitation (AR), this would be calculated as the LVOT SV – MV (or PV) SV. See AR and mitral regurgitation (MR) below.

Aortic Stenosis

Peak pressure gradient, using the modified Bernoulli equation, is as follows:

$$\Delta P = 4 \left(V_{Ao}^2 - V_{LVOT}^2 \right)$$

ΔP = peak pressure gradient (mm Hg)
V_{Ao} = peak transaortic distal velocity (m/s)
V_{LVOT} = peak LVOT velocity (m/s)

Aortic valve area, using the continuity equation with *either* velocity time integral (VTI) or peak flow velocity (Vmax) data, is calculated as follows:

$$AVA = \pi \left(\frac{LVOT_d}{2} \right)^2 \times \frac{VTI_{LVOT}}{VTI_{Ao}}$$

AVA = aortic valve area (cm²)
$LVOT_d$ = LVOT diameter (cm)
VTI_{LVOT} = LVOT velocity time integral from PW Doppler (cm)
VTI_{Ao} = aortic velocity time integral from CW Doppler (cm)
or

$$AVA = \pi \left(\frac{LVOT_d}{2} \right)^2 \times \frac{V_{LVOT}}{V_{Ao}}$$

AVA = aortic valve area (cm²)
$LVOT_d$ = LVOT diameter (cm)
V_{LVOT} = maximum LVOT velocity from PW Doppler (m/s)
V_{Ao} = maximum aortic velocity from CW Doppler (m/s)
(See Fig. 29.8)

The same formulas yields the effective regurgitant orifice area when used for prosthetic aortic valves.
**Aortic valve areas should be indexed to BSA, particularly for very large or small patients.*

Aortic valve dimensionless index, using *either* velocity time integral (VTI) or peak flow velocity (Vmax) data

$$DI = \frac{VTI_{LVOT}}{VTI_{Ao}}$$

VTI_{LVOT} = LVOT velocity time integral from PW Doppler (cm)
VTI_{Ao} = aortic velocity time integral from CW Doppler (cm)
or

$$DI = \frac{V_{LVOT}}{V_{Ao}}$$

V_{LVOT} = maximum LVOT velocity from PW Doppler (m/s)
V_{Ao} = maximum aortic velocity from CW Doppler (m/s)

Aortic Regurgitation

Effective Regurgitant Orifice Area by proximal isovelocity surface area (PISA) method

$$EROA = \frac{2\pi r^2 \cdot V_A}{V_{max}}$$

EROA = effective regurgitant orifice area (cm^2)
r = PISA radius (cm)
V_A = aliasing velocity (cm/s)
V_{max} = peak AR jet velocity (cm/s)
   (See Fig. 29.14)

Regurgitant Volume by the PISA method

$$RV = EROA \cdot VTI_{AR}$$

RV = regurgitant volume (mL)
EROA = effective regurgitant orifice area (cm^2); see above
VTI_{AR} = AR velocity time integral

Regurgitant Volume by the Continuity Equation (Volumetric Method)

$$RV = LVOT\ SV - MV\ (or\ PV)\ SV$$

RV = regurgitant volume (mL)
LVOT SV = LVOT stroke volume (mL)
MV SV = mitral valve stroke volume, or alternatively
PV SV = pulmonic valve stroke volume

Regurgitant Fraction by the PISA/2D Method

$$RF = \frac{RV}{Transaortic\ SV} \cdot 100\%$$

RF = regurgitant fraction (%)
RV = regurgitant volume (mL); see above
Transaortic SV = transaortic stroke volume (mL),

$$= CSA_{LVOT} \cdot VTI_{LVOT}$$

Mitral Stenosis

Peak pressure gradient, using the modified Bernoulli equation, is as follows:

$$\Delta P = 4\left(V_2^2 - V_1^2\right)$$

ΔP = peak pressure gradient (mm Hg)
V_2 = peak transmitral velocity distal to valve, on LV side (m/s)
V_1 = peak velocity proximal to valve, on LA side (m/s)

Mitral valve area, using *either* the pressure half-time and the deceleration time methods, is as follows:

$$MVA = \frac{220}{PHT}$$

MVA = mitral valve area (cm^2)
PHT = pressure half-time (ms)

$$MVA = \frac{759}{DT}$$

DT = deceleration time (ms)

Mitral valve area, by the PISA method (see Fig. 28.18), is as follows:

$$MVA = \frac{2\pi r^2 \cdot V_A}{V_{max}} \cdot \frac{\alpha}{180}$$

EROA = effective regurgitant orifice area (cm^2)
r = PISA radius (cm)
V_A = aliasing velocity (cm/s)
V_{max} = peak mitral stenosis jet velocity (cm/s)
$\alpha/180$ = correction factor for angle of PISA formation at the MV (typically ~120°)

Mitral Regurgitation

Effective Regurgitant Orifice Area by the PISA method (see Fig. 28.12) is as follows:

$$EROA = \frac{2\pi r^2 \cdot V_A}{V_{max}} \cdot \frac{\alpha}{180}$$

EROA = effective regurgitant orifice area (cm^2)
r = PISA radius (cm)
V_A = aliasing velocity (cm/s)
V_{max} = peak MR jet velocity (cm/s)
$\alpha/180$ = correction factor for angle of PISA formation at the MV (typically ~120°)

Regurgitant Volume by PISA Method

$$RV = EROA \cdot VTI_{MR}$$

RV = regurgitant volume (mL)
EROA = effective regurgitant orifice area (cm^2); see above
VTI_{MR} = MR velocity time integral

Regurgitant Volume by Continuity Equation (Volumetric Method) (see Fig. 28.13)

$$RV = MV\ SV - LVOT\ SV$$

RV = regurgitant volume (mL)
LVOT SV = LVOT stroke volume (mL)
MV SV = mitral valve stroke volume

Regurgitant Fraction by PISA/2D Method

$$RF = \frac{RV}{Transmitral\ SV} \cdot 100\%$$

RF = regurgitant fraction (%)
RV = regurgitant volume (mL), see above
Transmitral SV = transmitral stroke volume (mL)

$$\text{which} = CSA_{MV} \cdot VTI_{MV}$$

CSA_{MV} = cross-sectional area of MV (cm^2)
VTI_{MR} = MR velocity time integral (cm)

Since the mitral annulus is not circular, total LV stroke volume (LV SV) or even pulmonic valve stroke volume (PV SV) is often substituted for transmitral SV, which is valid as long as there is no other regurgitant valve or intracardiac shunt.

Total LV SV = LVOT forward SV + MR RV,
   where LVOT forward SV = $CSA_{LVOT} \cdot VTI_{LVOT}$

and MR RV is as previously calculated.

Alternatively,
Total LV SV can be calculated as

$$LV\ SV = LVEDV - LVESV$$

LVEDV = LV end-diastolic volume,
LVESV = LV end-systolic volume
   (from Simpson's 2D calculations or 3D LV calculations)

Tricuspid Regurgitation

RVSP (for TR)

$$RVSP = 4(TR\ V_{max})^2 + RAP$$

RVSP = right ventricular systolic pressure (mm Hg), which usually = pulmonary artery (PA) end-systolic pressure

TR V_{max} = TR peak velocity (m/s)

RAP = right atrial (RA) pressure, generally estimated as
- 3 (0–5) mm Hg if IVC diameter ≤21 mm and collapses >50%
- 8 (5–10) mm Hg if IVC diameter ≤21 mm and collapses <50%
- 8 (5–10) mm Hg if IVC diameter >21 mm and collapses >50%
- 15 mm Hg if IVC diameter >21 mm and collapses <50%

(See Appendix A, Table A.7 for refinements)

Pulmonic Regurgitation

PA end-diastolic pressure may be estimated as

$$PA\ EDP = 4(PI\ V_{end-diastole})^2 + RAP$$

PA EDP = PA end diastolic pressure (mm Hg)

PI $V_{end\text{-}diastole}$ = velocity of pulmonic insufficiency (PI) flow at end-diastole (m/s)

RAP = RA pressure

(See Fig. 36.5, where PA EDP = dPAP, for an example)

Pulmonary Vascular Resistance

$$PVR = 10\ (TR\ V_{max}/VTI_{RVOT}) + 0.16$$

PVR = Pulmonary vascular resistance (Wood units)

TR V_{max} = TR peak velocity (m/s)

VTI_{RVOT} = right ventricular outflow tract (RVOT) velocity time integral (cm)

*Many of the above-recommended and other methods of calculation for chamber quantification are discussed further in Lang RM, Badano LP, Mor-Avi V, et al. Recommendations for cardiac chamber quantification by echocardiography in adults: an update from the American Society of Echocardiography and the European Association of Cardiovascular Imaging. *J Am Soc Echocardiogr.* 2015;28:1-39.

EXERCISE STRESS TESTING

Maximally predicted heart rate for age (Haskell and Fox formula) is as follows:

$$MPHR = 220 - age$$

MPHR = maximally predicted heart rate for age

Percentage of maximally predicted heart rate for age is as follows:

$$\%\ MPHR = \frac{maximum\ HR\ acheived}{MPHR}$$

Rate-pressure product is as follows:

$$RPP = Max\ HR \times Max\ SBP$$

RPP = rate pressure product

Max HR = maximum heart rate (beats per min)

Max SBP = maximum systolic blood pressure (mm Hg)

Suggested Reading

Baumgartner, H., Hung, J., Bermejo, J., et al. (2009). Echocardiographic assessment of valve stenosis: EAE/ASE recommendations for clinical practice. *Journal of the American Society of Echocardiography, 22,* 1–23.

Grayburn, P. A., Weissman, N. J., & Zamorano, J. L. (2012). Quantitation of mitral regurgitation. *Circulation, 126,* 2005–2015.

Lancellotti, P., Tribouilloy, C., & Hagendorff, A. (2013). Recommendations for the echocardiographic assessment of native valvular regurgitation: an executive summary from the European Association of Cardiovascular Imaging. *European Heart Journal, 14,* 611–644.

Lang, R. M., Badano, L. P., Mor-Avi, V., et al. (2015). Recommendations for cardiac chamber quantification by echocardiography in adults: an update from the American Society of Echocardiography and the European Association of Cardiovascular Imaging. *Journal of the American Society of Echocardiography, 28,* 1–39.

Rudski, L. G., Lai, W. W., Afilalo, J., et al. (2010). Guidelines for the echocardiographic assessment of the right heart in adults: a report from the American Society of Echocardiography endorsed by the European Association of Echocardiography, a registered branch of the European Society of Cardiology, and the Canadian Society of Echocardiography. *Journal of the American Society of Echocardiography, 23,* 685–713.

Index

Note: Page numbers followed by "*f*" indicate figures, "*t*" indicate tables and "*b*" indicate boxes.